D0745844

THE AMERICAN PSYCHIATRIC PRESS

Textbook of Geriatric Neuropsychiatry

SECOND EDITION

The cover depicts T1-weighted coronal magnetic resonance images of the human brain, at the level of the optic chiasm. Reading from left to right, the images depict increasingly severe levels of cortical atrophy and lateral ventricular enlargement, the hallmark changes of brain aging. Yet all three images are selected from a sample of elderly control volunteers living independently in the community, making the point that there is marked variability in the effects of aging on brain structure and behavior.

THE AMERICAN PSYCHIATRIC PRESS

Textbook of Geriatric Neuropsychiatry

SECOND EDITION

EDITED BY

C. Edward Coffey, M.D.
Henry Ford Health System, Detroit, Michgan

Jeffrey L. Cummings, M.D.
UCLA School of Medicine, Los Angeles, California

ASSOCIATE EDITORS

Mark R. Lovell, Ph.D.
Henry Ford Health System, Detroit, Michgan

Godfrey D. Pearlson, M.D.
*Johns Hopkins University School of Medicine,
Baltimore, Maryland*

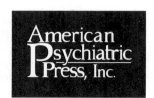

**Washington, DC
London, England**

Manufactured in the United States of America on acid-free paper

Second Edition   03   02   01   00   4   3   2   1

American Psychiatric Press, Inc.
1400 K Street, N.W., Washington, DC   20005
www.appi.org

Library of Congress Cataloging-in-Publication Data
The American Psychiatric Press textbook of geriatric neuropsychiatry /
   edited by C. Edward Coffey, Jeffrey L. Cummings. — 2nd ed.
      p.   cm.
   Includes bibliographical references and index.
   ISBN 0-88048-841-7. — ISBN 0-88048-841-7
   1. Geriatric neuropsychiatry.   2. Clinical neuropsychology.
I. Coffey, C. Edward, 1952–   .   II. Cummings, Jeffrey L., 1948–   .
III. Title: Textbook of geriatric neuropsychiatry.
   [DNLM: 1. Geriatric Psychiatry.   2. Mental Disorders—Aged.
3. Neuropsychology—Aged.   WT 150 A5123 2000 / WT 150 A5123 2000]
RC451.4.A5A516   2000
618.97′689—dc21
DNLM/DLC
for Library of Congress   99-33987
                                                                              CIP

British Library Cataloguing in Publication Data
A CIP record is available from the British Library.

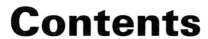

Contents

SECTION I

Introduction to Geriatric Neuropsychiatry

Jeffrey L. Cummings, M.D., and C. Edward Coffey, M.D., Section Editors

SECTION II

Neuropsychiatric Assessment of the Elderly

Mark R. Lovell, Ph.D., Section Editor

SECTION III

Neuropsychiatric Aspects of
Psychiatric Disorders in the Elderly

Godfrey D. Pearlson, M.D., Section Editor

SECTION IV

Neuropsychiatric Aspects of Neurological Disease in the Elderly

Jeffrey L. Cummings, M.D., Section Editor

SECTION V

Principles of Neuropsychiatric Treatment of the Elderly

C. Edward Coffey, M.D., Section Editor

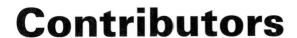

Contributors

Roland M. Atkinson, M.D.
Professor of Psychiatry, School of Medicine, Oregon
Health Sciences University, Portland, Oregon

Karen Blank, M.D.
Associate Clinical Professor of Psychiatry, University of
Connecticut School of Medicine, Farmington,
Connecticut; Senior Research Psychiatrist, Braceland
Center for Mental Health and Aging, The Institute for
Living, Hartford, Connecticut

Daryl E. Bohning, Ph.D.
Associate Professor of Radiology, Director of Advanced
Magnetic Resonance Physics Research, Medical
University of South Carolina, Charleston, South
Carolina

Randall Buzan, M.D.
Assistant Professor of Psychiatry; Director, Outpatient
Services, Department of Psychiatry, University of
Colorado, Denver, Colorado

John J. Campbell III, M.D.
Director of Geriatric Psychiatry and Neuropsychiatry,
Henry Ford Health System, Department of Psychiatry,
Detroit, Michigan

Dawn Cisewski
Indiana University of Pennsylvania, Indiana,
Pennsylvania

Michael R. Clark, M.D., M.P.H.
Assistant Professor and Director, Adolf Meyer Chronic
Pain Treatment Services, Department of Psychiatry and
Behavioral Sciences, Johns Hopkins Medical
Institutions, Baltimore, Maryland

C. Edward Coffey, M.D.
Professor of Psychiatry (Neuropsychiatry) and of
Neurology; Chairman and Kathleen and Earl Ward
Chair, Department of Psychiatry, Henry Ford Health
System, Detroit, Michgan

Paul T. Costa, Jr., Ph.D.
Chief, Laboratory of Personality and Cognition,
Gerontology Research Center, National Institution on
Aging, National Institutes of Health, Baltimore,
Maryland

Jeffrey L. Cummings, M.D.
Augustus S. Rose Professor of Neurology and Professor
of Psychiatry and Biobehavioral Sciences and Director,
UCLA Alzheimer's Disease Center, University of
California, Los Angeles, School of Medicine, Los
Angeles, California

Mark D'Esposito, M.D.
Professor, Neuroscience Institute and Department of
Psychology, University of California, Berkeley, Berkeley,
California

Bruce H. Dobkin, M.D.
Professor of Neurology, Director, Neurologic Rehabilitation and Research Unit, University of California, Los Angeles, School of Medicine, Reed Neurologic Research Center, Los Angeles, California

Steven L. Dubovsky, M.D.
Professor of Psychiatry and Medicine, University of Colorado; Chairman, Department of Psychiatry, University of Colorado, Denver, Colorado

James D. Duffy, M.B., Ch.B.
Director of Consultative Psychiatry, Hartford Hospital; Medical Director, Huntington's Disease Program and Associate Professor of Psychiatry, Connecticut School of Medicine, Farmington, Connecticut

Julie A. Fields
Research Associate, Center for Neuropsychology and Cognitive Neuroscience, Department of Neurology, University of Kansas Medical Center, Kansas City, Kansas

Robert B. Fields, Ph.D.
Assistant Professor of Psychiatry (Psychology), Division of Neuropsychiatry, Medical College of Pennsylvania, Allegheny Campus, Oakdale, Pennsylvania

Mark S. George, M.D.
Professor of Psychiatry, Radiology, and Neurology; Director of the Functional Neuroimaging Division (Psychiatry) and the Brain Stimulation Laboratory, Psychiatry Department, Medical University of South Carolina; Director of Psychiatric Neuroimaging, Ralph H. Johnson Veterans Administration Hospital, Charleston, South Carolina

Andrew Greenshields
Medical student, Medical University of South Carolina, Charleston, South Carolina

Andrew Gustavson, M.D.
Harbor-UCLA Medical Center, Torrance, California

Eleanore Hobbs, M.D.
Department of Psychiatry, University of Connecticut School of Medicine, Farmington, Connecticut

Carolyn C. Hoch, Ph.D.
Assistant Professor of Psychiatry, Department of Psychiatry, University of Pittsburgh, School of Medicine, Western Psychiatric Institute and Clinic, Pittsburgh, Pennsylvania

Daniel P. Holschneider, M.D.
Assistant Professor, Department of Psychiatry and the Behavioral Sciences, and Department of Neurology, University of Southern California, School of Medicine, Los Angeles, California

George R. Jackson, M.D., Ph.D.
Assistant Professor of Neurology, Department of Neurology, University of California, Los Angeles School of Medicine, Los Angeles, California

Ira R. Katz, M.D.
Professor, Department of Psychiatry, University of Pennsylvania, Philadelphia, Pennsylvania

Charles H. Kellner, M.D.
Professor of Psychiatry and Neurology, Director, ECT Program, Medical University of South Carolina, Charleston, South Carolina

William C. Koller, M.D., Ph.D.
Professor of Neurology, Department of Neurology, University of Miami School of Medicine, Miami, Florida

Anthony E. Lang, M.D., F.R.C.P.
Associate Professor of Neurology, Department of Neurology, University of Toronto, and Director, Movement Disorders Clinic, The Toronto Hospital, Toronto, Ontario, Canada

Andrew F. Leuchter, M.D.
Professor of Psychiatry, Director, Quantitative Electroencephalography (QEEG) Laboratory, UCLA Neuropsychiatric Institute and Hospital; Director, Division of Adult Psychiatry and Biobehavioral Sciences, UCLA School of Medicine, Los Angeles, California

Jeffrey P. Lorberbaum, M.D.
Anxiety and Imaging Research Fellow, Psychiatry Department, Medical University of South Carolina, Charleston, South Carolina

Mark R. Lovell, Ph.D.
Director, Division of Neuropsychology, Henry Ford Health System, Detroit, Michigan

Constantine G. Lyketsos, M.D., M.H.S.
Director of the Neuropsychiatry Service, Associate Professor, Department of Psychiatry, Johns Hopkins Hospital, Baltimore, Maryland

Roberta Malmgren, Ph.D.
Adjunct Assistant Professor, Department of Epidemiology, School of Public Health, University of California, Los Angeles, California

Kathleen A. McConnell
Medical student, Medical University of South Carolina, Charleston, South Carolina

Robert R. McCrae, Ph.D.
Research Psychologist, Gerontology Research Center, National Institution on Aging, National Institutes of Health, Baltimore, Maryland

Susan M. McCurry, Ph.D.
Research Assistant Professor, Departments of Psychosocial and Community Health and Psychiatry and Behavioral Sciences, University of Washington, Seattle, Washington

Mario F. Mendez, M.D., Ph.D.
Associate Professor of Neurology, University of California, Los Angeles, School of Medicine, and Chief, Neurobehavior Unit, Psychiatry Service, West Los Angeles Veterans Affairs Medical Center, Los Angeles, California

Bruce L. Miller, M.D.
Professor of Neurology, Department of Neurology, University of California at San Francisco, San Francisco, California

Jacobo Mintzer, M.D.
Professor of Psychiatry and Director of Geriatric Services, Psychiatry Department, Medical University of South Carolina, Charleston, South Carolina

Peter D. Nowell, M.D.
Assistant Professor of Psychiatry, Dartmouth Medical School, Sleep Medicine, Dartmouth-Hitchcock Medical Center, Lebanon, New Hampshire

Godfrey D. Pearlson, M.D.
Professor of Psychiatry and Behavioral Science, and Director, Division of Psychiatric Neuro-Imaging, Johns Hopkins University School of Medicine, Baltimore, Maryland

Pietro Pietrini, M.D., Ph.D.
Professor, Institute of Medical Biochemistry, Department of Human and Environmental Sciences, University of Pisa, Pisa, Italy

Kenneth Podell, Ph.D.
Senior Staff, Division of Neuropsychology, Henry Ford Health System, Detroit, Michigan

Richard E. Powers, M.D.
Associate Professor of Pathology, University of Alabama (Birmingham), and Director, Bureau of Geriatric Psychiatry, Alabama Department of Mental Health and Mental Retardation, Birmingham, Alabama

Stanley I. Rapoport, M.D.
Chief, Section on Brain Physiology and Metabolism, National Institute on Aging, National Institutes of Health, Bethesda, Maryland

Graham Ratcliff, D.Phil.
Adjunct Assistant Professor of Psychiatry and Neurology, University of Pittsburgh, and Director of Neurobehavior Program, HEALTHSOUTH Harmarville Rehabilitation Hospital, Pittsburgh, Pennsylvania

William E. Reichman, M.D.
Associate Professor of Psychiatry, University of Medicine and Dentistry of New Jersey, Robert Wood Johnson Medical School, Piscataway, New Jersey

Charles F. Reynolds III, M.D.
Professor of Psychiatry, Neurology, and Neuroscience, and Director, Sleep and Chronobiology Center, Western Psychiatric Institute and Clinic, University of Pittsburgh, Pittsburgh, Pennsylvania

Robert G. Robinson, M.D.
Professor and Chairman, Department of Psychiatry, University of Iowa College of Medicine, Iowa City, Iowa

Barry W. Rovner, M.D.
Professor, Department of Psychiatry, Jefferson Medical College, Philadelphia, Pennsylvania

Carl Salzman, M.D.
Professor of Psychiatry, Harvard Medical School, and Director of Education, and Director of Psychopharmacology, Massachusetts Mental Health Center, Boston, Massachusetts

Judith Saxton, Ph.D.
Assistant Professor of Psychiatry, University of Pittsburgh, Pittsburgh, Pennsylvania

Douglas W. Scharre, M.D.
Assistant Professor of Clinical Neurology and Psychiatry, Ohio State University, Columbus, Ohio

Javaid I. Sheikh, M.D.
Associate Professor, Department of Psychiatry and Behavioral Sciences, Stanford University School of Medicine, Stanford, California; Chief of Psychiatry, VA Palo Alto Health Care System, Palo Alto, California

J. Edward Spar, M.D.
Professor, Department of Psychiatry and Biobehavioral Sciences, UCLA School of Medicine; Director, Division of Geriatric Psychiatry, UCLA Neuropsychiatric Institute and Hospital, Center for Health Sciences, Los Angeles, California

Sergio E. Starkstein, M.D., Ph.D.
Director, Department of Behavioral Neurology, Raúl Carrea Institute of Neurological Research, Buenos Aires, Argentina

David L. Sultzer, M.D.
Associate Clinical Professor, Department of Psychiatry and Biobehavioral Sciences, UCLA School of Medicine, and Director, Gero/Neuropsychiatry Division, Veterans Administration Greater Los Angeles Healthcare System, Los Angeles, California

Trey Sunderland, M.D.
Chief, Geriatric Psychiatry Branch, National Institute of Mental Health, Bethesda, Maryland

Linda Teri, Ph.D.
Professor, Departments of Psychosocial and Community Health and Psychiatry and Behavioral Sciences, University of Washington, Seattle, Washington

Alexander I. Tröster, Ph.D.
Associate Professor of Neurology, Director, Center for Neuropsychology and Cognitive Neuroscience, Department of Neurology, University of Kansas Medical Center, Kansas City, Kansas

Larry E. Tune, M.D.
Professor, Department of Psychiatry and Behavioral Sciences, Emory University School of Medicine, Atlanta, Georgia

Peter J. Whitehouse, M.D., Ph.D.
Professor of Neurology, Psychiatry, Neuroscience, Psychology, Nursing, Organizational Behavior, and Biomedical Ethics, Case Western Reserve University/University Alzheimer Center, Cleveland, Ohio

Kirk C. Wilhelmsen, M.D., Ph.D.
Associate Professor of Neurology in Residence, Gallo Clinic and Research Center at the University of California, San Francisco, California

George S. Zubenko, M.D., Ph.D.
Professor, Department of Psychiatry, School of Medicine, University of Pittsburgh; Professor, Department of Biological Sciences, Mellon College of Science, Carnegie-Mellon University, Pittsburgh, Pennsylvania

Foreword

The publication of this second edition of *The American Psychiatric Press Textbook of Geriatric Neuropsychiatry* provides an opportunity to reflect on the many advances that have transformed the field since the first edition.

First, increasingly, the term *geriatric* is no longer associated with the feebled or impaired. With improvements in lifestyle and health care, the outer boundary of middle age has now been moved to age 64. Furthermore, the fastest growing sector of the American population is that of those over 80 years of age. Most of the elderly report living satisfying lives, engaged with family, hobbies, religion, and travel. Thus, the importance of geriatric neuropsychiatry must grow commensurate with these demographic changes and should focus increasingly on preventive strategies that maintain healthy brains in the elderly.

Second, the molecular mechanisms responsible for neuronal damage and degeneration that underlie many of the age-related disorders of the brain—stroke, Alzheimer's disease, Parkinson's disease, amyotrophic lateral sclerosis—have been worked out in considerable detail in recent years. For example, five risk genes for Alzheimer's disease have been identified, thereby illuminating the final common pathway leading to senile plaques and selective neuronal vulnerability in this disorder. Through recombinant DNA technology, the human Alzheimer genes have been inserted in the mouse genome, thereby creating mice who develop the neuropathology of Alzheimer's disease. These advances provide molecular targets for the design of drugs that will not simply palliate the disease but will actually prevent it.

A common theme emerging from these studies is the role of reactive oxygen species in causing cumulative damage to neuronal membrane, proteins, and, most importantly, the DNA. The "new agers" obsession with antioxidants now has a scientific basis as aspirin and vitamin E appear to have protective effects in Alzheimer's and Huntington's disease. The cumulative damage to DNA by reactive oxygen species triggers a form of cell suicide known as apoptosis. In the periphery, apoptosis eliminates cells with DNA damage that are likely to become cancerous; however, in the nondividing neurons, it appears to account for neuronal elimination in neurodegenerative disorders. In the future, pharmacologic blockade of neuronal cell suicide may prevent or delay the onset of these neurodegenerative disorders, but the impact of these drugs on carcinogenesis will present a challenge.

Third, remarkable advances in imaging technology now permit noninvasive studies of human brain structure, chemistry, and function with increasingly higher resolution. With advances made in cognitive neuroscience, mental tasks are devised that challenge the systems affected by disorders such as schizophrenia and obsessive-compulsive disorder much like the stress test is used in cardiology. These new, more refined "windows" into the brain are providing opportunities for better understanding the pathophysiology of age-related brain impairments and ways of testing new treatments and rehabilitation techniques.

Finally, the armamentarium of therapeutic agents to treat effectively neuropsychiatric disorders of late life has grown substantially and will continue to expand. The new drugs are generally much more specific in their actions and thus have fewer noxious side effects to which the elderly are particularly vulnerable. The molecular sites of action of most are well characterized so that clinicians now have, for example, antidepressants that act at six different molecular targets alone or in combination.

It is the mind, the product of the brain, that defines our humanity, and it is the loss of mind that most terrifies the elderly. This textbook provides a remarkably comprehensive approach to the identification, diagnosis, and treatment of the broad range of neuropsychiatric conditions that affect the elderly. Given the pace of discovery and the rich knowledge displayed in this textbook, we and our patients can look forward with greater confidence to successful aging.

Joseph T. Coyle, M.D.

Preface

Geriatric neuropsychiatry is an emerging clinical subspecialty that is devoted to the diagnosis and treatment of psychiatric or behavior disorders in aging patients with disturbances of brain structure or function. Such disturbances are particularly common in older individuals, and the continued expansion of the elderly segment of our population has recently resulted in considerable interest in the study of neuropsychiatric illness associated with brain aging.

The first edition of *The American Psychiatric Press Textbook of Geriatric Neuropsychiatry* was published in 1994. Its popularity exceeded even our mothers' expectations. Its publication also generated a number of cards, letters, emails, faxes, and phone calls from readers with appreciation for our efforts as well as suggestions for how future editions of the textbook could be improved. The 6-year interval since the first edition of the textbook has also witnessed a continued aging of the population (by almost exactly 6 years!), as well as the continued explosion in neuroscience research and in our understanding of human behavior.

The second edition of the *Textbook of Geriatric Neuropsychiatry* takes to heart the advice of our previous readers and advisors, embraces the "graying" of our population, and incorporates the very latest in neuroscience research in an updated text designed for clinicians interested in brain-behavior relations. This edition bridges the fields of geriatric neurology and geriatric psychiatry, and emphasizes the relationships that exist between neuropsychiatric illness and aging of the nervous system. The book is intended for healthcare professionals—psychiatrists, neurologists, psychologists, geriatricians, and other clinicians—who desire to understand and manage disturbed behavior in the elderly through a comprehensive approach based upon a thorough knowledge of contemporary neuroscience. This textbook endeavors to establish a link between the neurobiology of idiopathic psychiatric illness and the neurobiology of neurologic disorders that cause disturbed behavior in the elderly and in so doing stimulate consideration of fundamental brain-behavior relationships.

A number of changes have been incorporated in the second edition of the *Textbook of Geriatric Neuropsychiatry*. The text has been expanded by 28%, from 32 to 41 chapters. In addition to the 9 new chapters, all previous chapters have been extensively revised and updated with the latest in published research.

The textbook is organized into five sections, each of which is edited by one or more of the book's editors or associate editors. The section editors have assembled an outstanding collection of world-renowned neuropsychiatrists and neuroscientists who in turn have produced chapters that impart clinically relevant information within the context of the very latest in neuroscience research.

Section I, "Introduction to Geriatric Neuropsychiatry," begins with an overview of the emerging clinical specialty of geriatric neuropsychiatry, followed by chapters on the demography of aging and the neurobiology of brain aging. The final chapter in this section provides an integrative model linking neurobiology with behavior and thus sets the stage for the subsequent sections in the book.

Section II, "Neuropsychiatric Assessment of the Elderly," comprises three practical chapters on clinical and neuropsychological examination of the elderly, a chapter on memory changes in senescence, and four chapters on the role of advanced brain imaging technologies (updated chapters on magnetic resonance imaging [MRI], positron-emission tomography, and computerized topographic electroencephalography, as well as a new chapter on functional MRI and resonance spectroscopy) in the evaluation of the aging patient. This section accomplishes the essential and fundamental task of defining the acceptable limits of "normal" aging as assessed at the bedside and in the neuroscience laboratory.

Sections III and IV provide the clinical core of the book and focus on the neuropsychiatric aspects of psychiatric and neurologic disorders, respectively, in the elderly. Section III, "Neuropsychiatric Aspects of Psychiatric Disorders in the Elderly," includes three new chapters that examine personality disorders in geriatric neuropsychiatry, neuropsychiatric aspects of aging in the mentally retarded population, and aggression in geriatric neuropsychiatry. Section IV, "Neuropsychiatric Aspects of Neurological Disease in the Elderly," includes a new chapter on neurobehavioral syndromes. The comprehensive chapters in these sections highlight the influence of the aging nervous system on the pathophysiology, neuropsychiatric manifestations, clinical course, and prognosis of neurologic and psychiatric illness in the elderly.

Section V, "Principles of Neuropsychiatric Treatment of the Elderly," emphasizes the special considerations that are essential for safe and effective treatment of neuropsychiatric disorders in the elderly. This section features up-to-date chapters on interactions between aging and neuropharmacotherapy, electroconvulsive therapy, psychosocial and family therapies, and extended care. Four new chapters have been added on genetic interventions, behavioral and cognitive rehabilitation, ethical issues, and medico-legal and forensic issues. The discussions and recommendations for treatment are anchored as much as possible in a firm foundation of clinical science research. The new chapters in this section acknowledge the increasingly complex ethical, social, and forensic issues arising in the health care of the elderly.

▍ Acknowledgments

We thank the associate editors, Mark R. Lovell, Ph.D., and Godfrey D. Pearlson, M.D., for the amazing effort they devoted to the textbook. They join us in thanking each of the chapter authors for their contributions—such quality work requires thought, time, and energy, all of which must be redirected from other pressing demands. Pam Harley, Martin Lynds, Anne Barnes, Claire Reinburg, and Carol Nadelson, M.D., of American Psychiatric Press, Inc., provided much guidance and were always available to assist with the many issues that invariably arise with a project of this scale. We are grateful that all of these collaborators—the associate editors, chapter authors, and APPI—shared our vision and made this textbook a priority.

We also acknowledge with special appreciation Tom Royer M.D. and the Henry Ford Medical Group, as well as the Board of Trustees of Henry Ford Behavioral Health, all of whom understand and value the importance of science in the enterprise of clinical medicine. Further, we acknowledge the federal (AG 16529) and state of California research support of Dr. Cummings, as well as the generous support of Mrs. Katherine Kagan and the Sidell-Kagan Foundation. We thank Kathy Bernardin and Janice May for their administrative assistance. Finally, this project was ultimately made possible by the understanding, patience, and support of our families.

C. Edward Coffey, M.D.
Jeffrey L. Cummings, M.D.

SECTION I

Introduction to Geriatric Neuropsychiatry

Jeffrey L. Cummings, M.D., and

C. Edward Coffey, M.D., Section Editors

CHAPTER 1
Geriatric Neuropsychiatry

CHAPTER 2
Epidemiology of Aging

CHAPTER 3
Neurobiology of Aging

CHAPTER 4
Neurobiological Basis of Behavior

1

Geriatric Neuropsychiatry

Jeffrey L. Cummings, M.D.

C. Edward Coffey, M.D.

Grow old along with me!
The best is yet to be,
The last of life, for which the first was made.

Robert Browning
Rabbi Ben Ezra

Neuropsychiatry is the discipline devoted to understanding the neurobiological basis of human behavior. Neuropsychiatry has patient care, research, and educational dimensions emphasizing, respectively, the application, enhancement, and dissemination of neuropsychiatric information. The growth of neuropsychiatry has been stimulated by advances in neuroscience, neuroimaging, neuropsychopharmacology, geriatrics, and psychiatry. *Geriatric neuropsychiatry* represents the application of neuropsychiatry to older individuals. Geriatric neuropsychiatry is an integrative activity bridging the fields of psychiatry, neurology, neuroscience, and geriatrics. The emergence of geriatric neuropsychiatry is a response to the increasing size of the elderly population and the high prevalence of brain diseases and behavioral disorders among them. The practice of geriatric neuropsychiatry reflects commitment to the principle that improved understanding of brain-behavior relationships can lead to a higher quality of life for older individuals through minimization of excess disability,

Supported by National Institute on Aging Alzheimer's Disease Center Grant AG10123, an Alzheimer's Disease Research Center of California grant, and the Sidell-Kagan Foundation (to J. L. C.), and by the Mental Illness Research Association, Detroit, MI (to C. E. C.).

early recognition of diseases, and improved therapeutic interventions in behavioral disturbances.

The *Textbook of Geriatric Neuropsychiatry* is the first volume devoted exclusively to the discipline of geriatric neuropsychiatry. It is intended to serve as a guide to the practice and further development of this area of research and care. In this introductory chapter, we review the major issues in geriatric neuropsychiatry. Our purpose is to provide a neurobiological perspective on behavioral disturbances in elderly individuals, to create a context for the remaining chapters of this book, and to define and describe geriatric neuropsychiatry. In this chapter, we also review important aspects of training and research in geriatric neuropsychiatry.

▌ Geriatric Neuropsychiatry as a Discipline

Geriatric Neuropsychiatry

Most subspecialization or growth of an area of specific knowledge results from concentration on a small part of a parent discipline. With the explosion of information relevant to behavioral alterations in the elderly, however, the emergence of geriatric neuropsychiatry arises from a different imperative. Geriatric neuropsychiatry is an integrative specialty that draws from a diversity of fields (psychiatry, neuropsychiatry, neurology, neuroscience, neuroimaging, neuropsychopharmacology, neuropsychology, gerontology, molecular biology, genetics, epidemiology, and psychodynamics) with the intent of improving the care of elderly individuals with behavioral disorders and to stimulate research in this critical area (Figure 1–1).

The practice of geriatric neuropsychiatry depends on distinguishing normal age-related changes from those of disease and disordered brain function. Slowing of cognition, diminished access to specific bits of memory (e.g., names), and reduced cognitive flexibility may occur in the course of normal aging (Van Gorp and Mahler 1990) (see Chapters 7 and 8 in this volume). These changes must be differentiated from the effects of dementia, depression, and systemic illness. Geriatric neuropsychiatry provides expertise in this area.

Neuropsychiatry and Geriatric Neuropsychiatry

Neuropsychiatry is an old discipline that has been resurrected to assume a prominent place in contemporary psychiatry. There is no consensus definition of *neuropsychiatry.*

Psychiatry	→ Geriatric psychiatry
Psychiatry	→ Neuropsychiatry
Neurology	→ Geriatric neurology
Neurology	→ Behavioral neurology
Medicine	→ Geriatrics
Psychology	→ Neuropsychology
Psychology	→ Geriatric psychology
Pharmacology	→ Neuropsychopharmacology
Radiology	→ Neuroimaging
Basic science	→ Neuroscience
Sociology	→ Gerontology

FIGURE 1–1. Geriatric neuropsychiatry is an integrative discipline importing information from a number of specialties relevant to behavioral alterations in elderly individuals.

Lishman (1992) suggested that it is that aspect of psychiatry that seeks to advance understanding of behavioral problems through increased knowledge of brain structure and function. Yudofsky and Hales (1989a, 1989b) defined *neuropsychiatry* as the discipline concerned with the assessment and treatment of patients with psychiatric illnesses or symptoms associated with brain abnormalities. Trimble (1993) emphasized that neuropsychiatry attempts to understand the effects of central nervous system structural or functional change on behavior, recognizing the essentially dynamic and individualistic nature of behavioral dispositions.

Neuropsychiatry is an umbrella discipline under which geriatric neuropsychiatry is subsumed. Geriatric neuropsychiatry, however, integrates information from geriatrics, gerontology, and aging research not specifically relevant to all areas of the broader discipline of neuropsychiatry.

Geriatric Neuropsychiatry and Geriatric Psychiatry

Geriatric neuropsychiatry has a wide interface with geriatric psychiatry and can be regarded as an integration of geriatric psychiatry and neuropsychiatry. Both geriatric psychiatry and geriatric neuropsychiatry are concerned with care, education, and research related to behavioral changes in elderly individuals. The principal difference between the two is one of emphasis. Geriatric neuropsychiatry emphasizes its relationship to the neurosciences, the application of pharmacological treatments, and the assessment and management of psychiatric aspects of neurological diseases in elderly patients. Geriatric neuropsychiatry is committed to the proposition that the cure of neuropsychiatric disorders of elderly patients, improved management of behavioral disturbances, and amelioration of adverse age-related changes in brain function are linked to advances in neuroscience, as well as to progress in psychology, sociology, and related disciplines. While accepting the incontestable importance of social, cultural, and psychological aspects of aging and diseases of the elderly population, geriatric neuropsychiatry emphasizes importing and developing neuroscience information with the goal of better understanding and treatment of disorders of the elderly.

Geriatric Neuropsychiatry and Behavioral Neurology

No definitional boundaries exist between neuropsychiatry and behavioral neurology or between geriatric neuropsychiatry and behavioral neurology. Traditionally, behavioral neurology has been devoted to the study of "deficit disorders" such as aphasia, amnesia, agnosia, and apraxia, whereas neuropsychiatry has been concerned with the diagnosis and management of syndromes with "productive symptoms" such as hallucinations, delusions, and mood changes. In addition, behavioral neurologists usually have been trained in neurology, whereas neuropsychiatrists usually have had a background in psychiatry. Neither neurology nor psychiatry, however, completely prepares a clinician for the broad range of behavioral disorders associated with acquired and idiopathic brain dysfunction. Both disciplines produce behavioral neuroscientists who use similar concepts to relate abnormal behavior to brain dysfunction. Furthermore, individual patients often manifest both deficit and productive disorders, making it imperative that clinicians have knowledge of both neuropsychiatry and behavioral neurology. This knowledge is particularly important in geriatric neuropsychiatry where the prevalence of acquired brain disease as a cause of altered behavior is high.

A corollary of the absence of boundaries between behavioral neurology and neuropsychiatry is the transcendence of traditional restrictive definitions of individual diseases as "neurological" or "psychiatric." Alzheimer's disease and Parkinson's disease are examples of disorders traditionally considered as "neurological," whereas depression and obsessive-compulsive disorder have been thought of as "psychiatric." Neither of these assumptions proves to be true from the perspective of geriatric neuropsychiatry. Alzheimer's disease and Parkinson's disease both have major behavioral manifestations, whereas depression and obsessive-compulsive disorder are increasingly well understood as brain disorders. It is ever more evident that designating disorders as "neurological" or "psychiatric"—although convenient for some administrative purposes—is arbitrary and may be misleading. These designations are clinically unhelpful and may hinder the evolution of a behavioral neuroscience commensurate with optimum patient care.

Geriatric Neuropsychiatry: Clinical Training

There is a marked lack of availability of individuals with expertise in geriatric neuropsychiatry and a dearth of training programs to provide experience in this area. This reflects the widespread lack of training in clinical care and research regarding both behavioral neuroscience and the care of elderly patients (Cummings et al. 1998). Few United States neurology residencies provide formal research training (Griggs et al. 1987), and only a small number of psychiatric faculty members have postgraduate research training (Burke et al. 1986). Geriatric psychiatry and geriatric medicine are decidedly understaffed (Rowe 1987; Small et al. 1988). Development of a cadre of individuals with expertise in the assessment and management of geriatric neuropsychiatric abnormalities is an essential response to the expanding elderly population. Currently available training programs are inadequate to meet the growing need.

Converging Information in Geriatric Neuropsychiatry

The two principal dimensions in geriatric neuropsychiatry are the psychiatric manifestations of neurological disorders and the neurobiological basis of psychiatric illnesses. One exciting aspect of contemporary neuropsychiatry is the convergence of conclusions emanating from these two avenues of research (Table 1–1). For example, Robinson and Starkstein (1990) have demonstrated that depression is most common among stroke patients when the cerebrovascular lesion involves the anterior structures of the left hemisphere, whereas studies of idiopathic depression have found evidence of reduced frontal lobe volume (Coffey et al. 1993) and metabolism (Baxter et al. 1985, 1989). Thus, both avenues of investigation lead to similar anatomical implications. Neuropathological investiga-

TABLE 1–1. Convergent results of investigations of the psychiatric complications of neurological disorders and the neurobiological basis of psychiatric illness

Neuropsychiatric abnormality	Neurological disorder	Psychiatric illness
Depression	Poststroke depression after left frontal stroke	Reduced metabolism in the frontal lobes in idiopathic depression with PET; reduced frontal lobe volume in depression with MRI
Psychosis	Increased prevalence in temporal lobe disorders	Histological changes in the temporal lobes in schizophrenia
Obsessive-compulsive disorder (OCD)	Increased prevalence of OCD in diseases affecting frontal-subcortical circuits originating in orbitofrontal cortex	Increased glucose metabolism in orbitofrontal cortex in idiopathic OCD
Anxiety	Occurs with lesions of the temporal cortex	Increased blood flow in the temporal lobes during episodes of anxiety

Note.   PET = positron-emission tomography; MRI = magnetic resonance imaging.

tions in schizophrenia have revealed abnormalities in the cellular architectonics in the temporal lobe (Altshuler et al. 1987), and studies of neurological disease with psychosis demonstrated that the temporal lobe is a common site of pathological changes (Cummings 1992b). Again, studies of psychiatric and neurological disorders with similar symptoms suggest shared pathophysiologies.

In studies of idiopathic obsessive-compulsive disorders, Baxter et al. (1987) found increased metabolism in the orbitofrontal cortex, and Cummings (1993) observed that obsessions and compulsions occur in neurological disease when there is involvement of structures participating in the frontal-subcortical circuit originating in orbitofrontal cortical regions. Preliminary studies with positron-emission tomography (PET) have suggested altered regional metabolic activity in anxiety disorders (Reiman et al. 1989; Wu et al. 1991), and anxiety symptoms have been associated with structural lesions of related cortical areas in neurological diseases (Drubach and Kelly 1989). The convergence of information from the neurological and psychiatric approaches to neuropsychiatry has many implications. When clinical neuropsychiatric symptoms are similar, even in seemingly different disorders, there may be involvement of the same underlying neuroanatomical structures and common pathobiological mechanisms. These observations also support the use of the same therapeutic agents in patients with diverse underlying diseases but similar neuropsychiatric symptoms.

These convergent data in neuropsychiatric research justify the working assumption of geriatric neuropsychiatry that the relationship between brain dysfunction and behavioral disturbances is rule governed, that the axioms relating structure and function are discoverable, and

that the rules will apply regardless of the etiology of the underlying disorder (Cummings 1999).

Aging, the Brain, and Geriatric Neuropsychiatry

The brain undergoes various neurochemical, structural, and neurophysiological alterations in the course of normal aging (Creasey and Rapoport 1985; see also Chapters 3, 9, and 10 in this volume). Grossly, there is a small decrease in brain weight in the course of normal aging with widening of cerebral cortical sulci and enlargement of the lateral ventricles.

Microscopically, neuronal loss occurs in specific cortical and subcortical structures (Brody 1982; Terry et al. 1987). In addition, lipofuscin, granulovacuolar changes, neuritic plaques, and neurofibrillary tangles also accumulate in the course of aging, and there is a progressive shrinkage of the dendritic domain of some cortical and subcortical neurons (Brody 1982).

Neurochemical changes also accompany aging. Decreased activity of catecholamine synthesizing enzymes and increased activity of monoamine oxidase (an enzyme involved in catecholamine catabolism) have been documented (Bowen and Davison 1982; Van Gorp and Mahler 1990). These biochemical changes may underlie the psychomotor retardation of elderly individuals, as well as the mild parkinsonian habitus associated with aging, and they may contribute to the occurrence of depression in elderly people (Veith and Raskind 1988). Neurochemical alterations may also have a role in the age-associated memory impairment observed in elderly individuals (see Chapter 8 in this volume).

The underlying mechanisms of aging remain mysterious, but strides are being made in understanding some of the processes that contribute to age-related changes in function. Oxidative metabolism catalyzed by oxygen free radicals damages enzymes, and this in turn leads to a reduced synthetic ability and compromise of the aged organism's ability to respond to changing biological contingencies (Stadtman 1992). Trophic factors may be responsible for maintaining cellular connectivity, and changes in tropism with aging may contribute to some age-related brain alterations (Creasey and Rapoport 1985). Finally, some cells have genetically determined life-spans, whereas other cell populations manifest few, if any, changes in the course of aging (Finch 1990). Deciphering the molecular mechanisms responsible for programmed aging is critical to a comprehensive understanding of the neurobiology of aging.

The brain is continuously changing from its fetal developmental period through senescence. The changes associated with aging are not global, and they affect specific cellular populations, structures, and transmitters more than they do others. The temporal sequence of aging varies among different structures. The neurobiological changes of aging, as well as the differential involvement of functional systems, may influence the types of neuropsychiatric disorders to which elderly people are vulnerable.

Aging, Brain Diseases, and Geriatric Neuropsychiatry

The emergence and growth of geriatric neuropsychiatry are driven by four circumstances: 1) the growth of the size of the elderly population, 2) the increased prevalence of brain diseases among the elderly, 3) a high frequency of psychiatric disorders among elderly people, and 4) the recognition that behavioral disturbances often are manifestations of brain dysfunction.

Demography of Aging

People over age 65 composed only 4% of the United States population in 1900; this population will increase to 13% by the year 2000 and to 22% by 2030 (Department of Health and Human Services 1990; see also Chapter 2 in this volume). The growth of the old-old population is proceeding at a disproportionately rapid pace. Those over age 80 numbered 6 million in 1985 and comprised 22% of the elderly population; by 2005, 31% of elderly Americans will be over

age 80 (Torrey et al. 1987). In 1980, there were approximately 15,000 centenarians in the United States; this number increased to 25,000 by 1986 and is projected to reach 100,000 by the year 2000 (Spencer et al. 1987).

Aging and the diseases of elderly people present a global challenge (Torrey et al. 1987). The world's elderly population is growing at a rate of 2.4% per year, faster than the rest of the population. In 1985, there were 290 million individuals over age 65 in the world; this number will rise to 410 million by the year 2000. Twenty-three countries had 2 million or more elderly individuals in 1985; 50 countries will have this number by 2025. The growth of the world's elderly population will occur disproportionately in the countries least able to provide services; by the year 2025, 69% of the world's elderly people will live in developing countries (Torrey et al. 1987).

Neurological Diseases With Behavioral Manifestations Among the Elderly

The three neurological conditions most responsible for neuropsychiatric morbidity in elderly individuals are 1) Alzheimer's disease and other dementing disorders, 2) Parkinson's disease, and 3) stroke. The prevalence of dementia increases dramatically with age. A demographic study of dementia in Stockholm, Sweden (Fratiglioni et al. 1991), found that 5.7% of individuals 75–79 years old had mental status changes indicative of dementia, and 9.6% of those 80–84 years old had dementia; the proportion rose to 20.4% in those 85–89 years old and to 32% in those over age 90. Evans et al. (1989) found the rate of Alzheimer's disease among the elderly in a United States community to be 3% in those 65–74 years old, 18.7% in those 75–84 years old, and 47.2% in those over age 84. Parkinson's disease also exhibits an age-related prevalence. The reported frequency varies among studies, but a representative investigation (D'Alessandro et al. 1987) revealed a prevalence of 0.8% among people 55–59 years old, 3.8% in those 60–64, 5.7% in those 65–69, 12.4% in those 70–74, 19.5% in those 75–79, and 9.5% in those 80–84 years old. The prevalence of stroke and vascular dementia likewise increases with age. The prevalence of cerebrovascular disease rises from 2.3% in those 55–64 years old to 4.2% in those 65–74, 8.1% in those 75–84, and 10% in those over age 85 (National Center for Health Statistics 1986). The cumulative prevalence of neurological disease among the elderly and the chronic nature of many neurological illnesses make brain diseases a major source of morbidity and mortality among elderly individuals.

Neurological diseases of elderly people are often manifested by alterations in behavior. The dementia syndromes are defined by loss of cognitive abilities, and many patients with dementia also exhibit delusions, depression, anxiety, agitation, and aggressiveness (Cummings and Benson 1992; Cummings et al. 1987; Mega et al. 1997; Merriam et al. 1988; Reisberg et al. 1987; Teri et al. 1988). Dementia occurs in 41% of patients with Parkinson's disease (Mayeux et al. 1992), and 40%–60% of patients with Parkinson's disease have depressive disorders, anxiety, and apathy (Cummings 1992a). With treatment, hallucinations and delusions may emerge. Eighty percent of strokes involve the cerebral hemispheres, where they produce neurobehavioral and neuropsychiatric syndromes such as aphasia, amnesia, visuospatial disturbances, depression, or psychosis (Beckson and Cummings 1991; Robinson and Benson 1981). One-fourth of all patients hospitalized with stroke meet criteria for vascular dementia (Hershey et al. 1987). Thus, behavioral disturbances are the principal clinical manifestations of many brain diseases of elderly people. Recognition and management of geriatric neuropsychiatric disorders is critical in an aging society.

Psychiatric Illness in the Elderly Population

Psychiatric illness is present in 12.3% of the elderly population (Regier et al. 1988; see also Chapter 2 and Section III in this volume). Approximately 5.5% of elderly individuals have anxiety disorders (4.8% phobia, 0.1% panic), 4.9% have severe cognitive impairment, 2.5% have a mood disorder (0.7% major depressive episode; 1.8% dysthymia), 1% manifest alcohol abuse or dependence, 0.8% have obsessive-compulsive disorder, and 0.1% have schizophrenia or a schizophreniform disorder. These figures were derived from a household study (Regier et al. 1988) of individuals in five United States cities using the criteria of DSM-III (American Psychiatric Association 1980). In a similar community survey (Myers et al. 1984), the four most common psychiatric disorders in men over age 65 were severe cognitive impairment, phobia, alcohol abuse and dependence, and dysthymia; in women of the same age, the four most frequent diagnoses were phobia, severe cognitive impairment, dysthymia, and major depressive episode.

Thus, dementia, alcoholism, anxiety, and mood disorders are the most common psychiatric conditions among elderly people. Each of these diseases has an important neurobiological dimension. Dementia is an overt brain disorder produced by Alzheimer's disease, cerebrovascular disease, or other encephalopathic processes (Cummings and Benson 1992). In individuals with alcohol abuse, PET reveals diminished brain glucose metabolism (Volkow et al.

1992), and dysfunction of basal ganglia–limbic circuits is implicated in alcohol craving (Modell et al. 1990). Patients with anxiety disorders have an increased frequency of structural alterations of the right temporal lobe (Fontaine et al. 1990), exhibit regional alterations in metabolism (Reiman et al. 1989; Wu et al. 1991), and evidence functional disturbances involving a variety of neurotransmitter systems (Hoehn-Saric 1982).

Depression occupies a particularly important place in geriatric neuropsychiatry. This disorder is disabling and treatable and may occur for the first time in elderly individuals. If not detected and treated, depression may be fatal; men 65–74 years old have the highest suicide rate of any age group in the United States (Department of Health and Human Services 1990). Imaging studies suggest that depression is associated with alterations in brain structure and function, particularly in elderly people (see Chapter 13 in this volume). Reported structural abnormalities include cortical atrophy (especially of the frontal lobes), ventricular enlargement, and subcortical encephalomalacia (Coffey 1996; Coffey et al. 1993; Duffy and Coffey 1997). These findings may be related to the onset of mental disorders in late life (Coffey 1991), and they are associated with a poor long-term prognosis (Jacoby et al. 1981). Functional imaging studies reveal evidence of altered regional cerebral blood flow and metabolism in depressive disorders. The frontal lobes are most prominently affected (Baxter et al. 1985, 1989; Duffy and Coffey 1997; Sackeim et al. 1990; see also Chapter 13 in this volume). Although relatively few studies have examined elderly subjects, data suggest that functional brain imaging may be useful in distinguishing the neurodegenerative dementias from the dementia of depression. Together, these observations indicate that alterations of brain structure and function may interact with the aging process to facilitate the emergence of affective disorders in late life.

Late-onset psychoses may occur, although they are considerably rarer than late-occurring depression or anxiety (see Chapter 14 in this volume). Investigations of patients with late-onset delusional disorders reveal that about half have an identifiable underlying brain disease (Leuchter and Spar 1985; Miller et al. 1992). Thus, delusions may be the heralding feature of a neurological disease.

Together, these studies indicate that mental disorders are an important aspect of geriatric care, that there is an emerging understanding of the neurobiology of these psychiatric conditions, and that brain abnormalities are associated with many late-onset psychiatric disturbances. Geriatric neuropsychiatry addresses both the neurobiology of idiopathic psychiatric disorders and the psychiatric disturbances associated with neurological conditions.

Cost of Brain Disorders

The annual cost of brain disease has been calculated, and the yearly expense is staggering (National Foundation for Brain Research 1992). The annual cost (direct and indirect total) in billions of dollars for psychiatric illnesses is $136.1; for neurological disease, $103.7; for alcohol abuse, $90.1; and for drug abuse, $71.2. Together, these diseases cost United States society $401.1 billion annually. Fifteen percent of the average annual income of workers in the United States is devoted to brain diseases. Although the costs of diseases of the elderly were not separately calculated, dementia accounted for the largest share (45%) of the costs of all neurological illnesses, and it is obvious that a substantial share of the funds expended on brain disorders concerns diseases of elderly patients.

▍ Aging, Medical Illness, Drugs, and Geriatric Neuropsychiatry

The rise of geriatric neuropsychiatry is fueled in part by the marked rise in medical illness in the elderly population and the increased frequency of associated behavioral disturbances. Medical disorders become increasingly common among elderly people, medications are more frequently administered, and there are changes in drug metabolism with aging (see Chapter 31 in this volume). These alterations create a neurophysiological setting that is conducive to brain dysfunction and behavioral abnormalities (Figure 1–2).

Medical illnesses are common in elderly people, and many of these affect brain function and produce behavioral alterations. Among the 10 most common nonneurological diseases of elderly people are hypertension, ischemic heart disease, diabetes, and arteriosclerosis (Cassel and Brody 1990). These may involve the brain through direct mechanisms such as stroke or through indirect mechanisms including hypoxia and renal failure. Epidemiological studies (Cohen-Cole 1989; Derogatis and Wise 1989) have revealed that approximately 20% of patients with medical illness have significant depressive symptoms and 5%–20% experience major depressive episodes; 10%–15% of patients with medical illness manifest anxiety disorders. The coexistence of medical and psychiatric illness increases the length of stay of hospitalized patients and is associated with a poorer postdischarge prognosis (Mayou et al. 1991; Saravay et al. 1991). Conversely, approximately 50% of elderly patients with psychiatric illness have significant medical illnesses. Nearly 60% of these conditions are undiagnosed before psychiatric admission, and in 10%–20% the behavioral changes are directly attributable to the physical pathology (Koranyi 1982).

The high prevalence of medical illness among elderly people results in an increase in the number of medications ingested (see Chapter 29 in this volume). Elderly people take more prescribed and over-the-counter medications than any other age group. They comprise 12% of the population and take 25%–30% of all prescribed drugs. The average older United States citizen receives 4.5 prescribed medications, and two-thirds also take at least one over-the-counter agent (Beers 1992; Lamy 1985). Forty percent of the elderly individuals who take medications receive prescriptions from more than one physician, and 12% take drugs prescribed for someone else (Lamy 1985). These practices are further complicated by intentional or accidental noncompliance with prescribing instructions. Up to 30% of elderly patients make serious errors in the way they take their medications, and up to 50% default on one or more prescribed agents (Lamy 1985).

Drug metabolism is altered in elderly patients, and the changes may have marked consequences for brain function and the treatment of behavioral abnormalities (see Chapter 34 in this volume). There is an increased sensitivity of receptors for most classes of drugs in the course of aging, making lower levels more effective and "standard" doses more likely to induce toxicity (Avorn and Gurwitz 1990). Changes also occur in drug distribution with aging. There is a relative increase in body fat and decrease in muscle; this produces a greater volume of distribution for fat-soluble drugs (e.g., benzodiazepines) and smaller volume of distribution for drugs absorbed primarily in lean body mass (e.g., lithium). There is reduced liver blood flow and impaired oxidative metabolism by hepatic enzymes in the course of normal aging, leading to reduced hepatic metabolism of many pharmacological agents. Renal function also declines with age; glomerular filtration rate is reduced by approximately one-third in elderly individuals (Avorn and Gurwitz 1990). These changes all tend to increase the risk of toxicity when medications are administered to elderly patients. Adverse drug reactions account for 12%–17% of all hospital admissions of elderly patients, and 21% of all elderly patients experience adverse side effects while in the hospital (Davison 1985; Lamy 1985).

The higher frequency of medical illness in the elderly population and concomitant need for more drug administration place elderly patients at a substantially increased risk of toxic-metabolic neuropsychiatric disturbances. Delirium, dementia, depression, mania, psychosis, and anxiety have all been observed in patients with brain dysfunction secondary to systemic illnesses and drug toxicity (Cummings 1985; Estroff and Gold 1986).

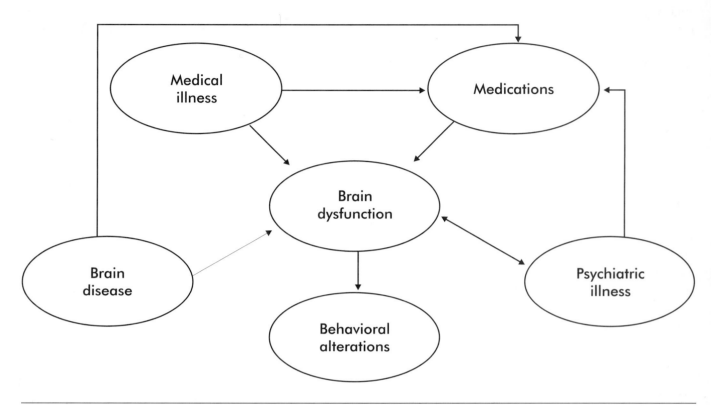

FIGURE 1–2.   Interactions of medical illness, medications, brain disease, and psychiatric disorders to produce brain dysfunction and behavioral changes.

Neuroimaging

The emergence of new diagnostic technologies has accelerated the development of geriatric neuropsychiatry. Among these, neuroimaging has had the greatest impact. Neuroimaging plays an increasingly large role in the diagnosis, differential diagnosis, and treatment monitoring of behavioral disturbances in the elderly. Structural and functional imaging has provided new insights into brain function, the pathophysiology of brain disorders, and the neurobiology of normal aging.

Imaging brain structure, metabolism, and chemical composition are now possible (Mazziotta and Gilman 1992). In addition, specialized techniques allow visualization of arterial and venous blood flow. Images of brain structure are generated by computed tomography (CT) and magnetic resonance imaging (MRI) (see Chapter 4 in this volume). These techniques reveal the brain structure and the ventricular system. Tumors, large strokes, subdural hematomas, large demyelinating lesions, arteriovenous malformations, and hydrocephalus are demonstrated by both techniques. MRI is more sensitive to changes in white matter of the central nervous system and is superior to CT

in revealing evidence of ischemic and inflammatory disease.

MRI has been shown to have a potential role in predicting adverse responses to therapy. Patients with depression who have basal ganglia lesions and increased white matter abnormalities are more likely to exhibit prolonged interictal confusion during electroconvulsive therapy and a higher frequency of antidepressant-induced deliria than are elderly patients with depression who have normal MRI results (Coffey 1996; Figiel et al. 1990). Elderly patients with depression who have enlarged ventricles and cortical atrophy may have a poorer prognosis for recovery than elderly patients with depression but without these structural changes (Jacoby et al. 1981; Nasrallah et al. 1989).

Magnetic resonance spectroscopy is a specialized application of magnetic resonance technology that allows the determination of the concentration of specific chemicals in the brain, and new fast imaging techniques using magnetic resonance can be used to determine cerebral blood flow (see Chapter 11 in this volume). The rapid advances in MRI technology suggest that this tool will be of increasing importance in neuropsychiatry (Prichard and Cummings 1997).

Except for the marked caudate nucleus atrophy associated with Huntington's disease, degenerative brain diseases (e.g., Alzheimer's disease and Parkinson's disease) produce no pathognomonic changes that are detectable on conventional structural imaging. In these disorders, structural imaging techniques such as CT and MRI provide little specific diagnostic information. Moreover, idiopathic neuropsychiatric disorders such as depression, mania, psychosis, and anxiety are not associated with diagnostic structural brain alterations.

Functional brain imaging such as PET and single photon emission computed tomography (SPECT) provides a new approach to these neuropsychiatric disorders. PET may be used to study cerebral glucose metabolism (with radiolabeled glucose), cerebral blood flow (with radiolabeled oxygen), and neurotransmitter function (with radiolabeled receptor ligands and transmitters) (see Chapter 10 in this volume). SPECT is typically used to measure cerebral blood flow but may also be applied to assessment of neurotransmitters and receptors. Degenerative diseases and idiopathic neuropsychiatric illnesses may have distinctive alterations on metabolic imaging studies. For example, Alzheimer's disease typically causes reduced metabolism or perfusion in the temporoparieto-occipital junction region; frontal lobe degenerations cause decreased metabolism or perfusion of the frontal lobes; depression may be associated with diminished frontal lobe metabolism; and obsessive-compulsive disorder has been shown to be associated with increased metabolism of the orbitofrontal cortex (Holcomb et al. 1989).

These investigations demonstrate that reliable relationships exist between behavioral changes and brain metabolism or perfusion. Imaging research is beginning to provide important insights into the pathophysiology of neuropsychiatric disorders.

Advances in Treatment

The value of accurate diagnosis is enhanced when it proceeds in concert with advances in treatment. In this regard, the past decade has seen an unparalleled increase in the availability of medications to treat behavioral disturbances (see Section V in this volume). Antidepressant agents have proliferated and become highly differentiated, with relative selectivity for inhibition of reuptake of norepinephrine or serotonin. A variety of anxiolytics have been discovered, and the clinician can now choose an agent that best fits the patient's needs according to the rapidity of onset, duration of action, and side effects. Conventional neuroleptic agents are rapidly giving way to a new generation of novel antipsychotic drugs that produces fewer acute or chronic

extrapyramidal side effects (Baldessarini and Frankenburg 1991). With the evolution of these agents, patients should experience less risk of dystonia, parkinsonism, or tardive dyskinesia as their psychiatric disorders are controlled. The discovery that anticonvulsants such as carbamazepine and sodium valproate have antimanic benefits has improved the treatment of mania while emphasizing that common neurophysiological processes are shared by some neurological and psychiatric illnesses (Post et al. 1984).

Relevant advances also have been made in the pharmacological treatment of neurological disorders. Most remarkably, vitamin E has been shown to slow the progression of Alzheimer's disease (Sano et al. 1997). This represents a revolutionary treatment advance and the first success in intervening in a degenerative disease. The neuroprotective action of vitamin E implies that the behavioral aspects of Alzheimer's disease such as depression and dementia may also be delayed or ameliorated. In addition, modest symptomatic improvement is observed in patients with Alzheimer's disease treated with cholinesterase inhibitors (Farlow et al. 1992; Rogers et al. 1998), and intensive investigation at the molecular biological level has revealed a systematic cascade of events with individual steps that might be amenable to pharmacological manipulation. Ticlopidine (a potent platelet antiaggregate) has been shown to be more powerful than aspirin in preventing stroke and improving the prognosis for patients with cerebrovascular disease (Gent et al. 1989).

The rapid advances in neuropsychopharmacology provide the clinician with a varied and powerful armamentarium with which to meet the challenges of neuropsychiatric disease in the elderly patient. These developments also require that the clinician be familiar with the pharmacokinetics, side effects, and drug interactions of each of these new agents (see Chapter 34 in this volume). Geriatric neuropsychiatry is the clinical discipline committed to implementation of these advances for the benefit of elderly individuals with behavioral disorders.

Geriatric Neuropsychiatry and Ethical Issues

Ethical issues arise often in geriatric neuropsychiatry (see Chapter 40 in this volume). The main challenges concern the ability of individuals to take responsibility for their own actions and the responsibility of society to preserve the rights of elderly citizens. With regard to driving, for example, at what point are the wishes of the patient to maintain independence and mobility in conflict with the safety of other drivers and pedestrians who might be endangered by the patient? At what point do patients relinquish their right to make decisions regarding disposition of property and money? When do they lose their right to decide when they can no longer live at home? When do they need a surrogate decision maker for questions of life support, treatment of infections, and postmortem autopsy? Who should make decisions for the patients when the patients themselves cannot? Should such decisions be based on family beliefs about what the patient would want, on advanced directives from the patient, or on an assessment of the apparent daily life satisfaction of the individual with dementia (Dresser 1992; Moody 1992; see also Chapter 32 in this volume)? Is euthanasia a viable societal response to severe dementia? These questions do not have categorical answers; they must be answered individually for each patient, taking into account the needs and abilities of the patient, the family context, and other patient-specific contingencies.

Geriatric neuropsychiatric illnesses strike at the self and alter the individual's personal identity; whereas a patient may *have* pneumonia, he or she *is* "demented." How does and how should this change in identity affect decision making for the patient? How can the dignity of the patient be preserved when institutional caregivers know the person only after the onset of disease and are unacquainted with the unique biography of the individual under their care? For the individual with dementia, how can extended care become an extended meaningful life?

The great majority of elderly people, and many of those in institutions, are competent, if physically infirm. How can we best preserve their autonomy, dignity, and quality of life? These ethical dilemmas must be given careful consideration as the elderly population grows, more and more elderly individuals require institutional care, and the resources available to care for them come steadily under more pressure.

An Agenda for Geriatric Neuropsychiatry

Patient Care

The growth of geriatric neuropsychiatry can improve the quality of patient care. Appropriate treatment of neuropsychiatric illness depends on accurate diagnosis, and diagnosis in elderly patients depends on a comprehensive understanding of brain-behavior relationships. In addition, diagnosis increasingly demands familiarity with neuroimaging, electrophysiology, and a variety of laboratory tests, and geriatric neuropsychiatry incorporates data from

these techniques into diagnostic formulations. New medications have been developed and are able to effectively ameliorate many behavioral disturbances and improve the quality of life of elderly patients with brain disorders. Many of these agents have potentially serious side effects, and practitioners in this area must be familiar with the effects, as well as the adverse consequences, of these new agents.

Education

The growth of the elderly population demands greater availability of practitioners of geriatric neuropsychiatry (Benjamin et al. 1995; Cummings and Hegarty 1994; Cummings et al. 1998). This field incorporates information from psychiatry, neurology, geriatrics, and neuroscience. Training opportunities must be developed and expanded.

Research

Geriatric neuropsychiatry is a nascent field (Cummings et al. 1998). Its research agenda must include the application of advanced technologies to diagnosis in the elderly population: the usefulness of PET, SPECT, and magnetic resonance spectroscopy has yet to be defined in detail. Their sensitivity in early disease, specificity in differential diagnosis, and predictive ability for determining prognosis and treatment response have not been established. The correlations between behavior and metabolic and structural brain imaging findings, as well as between behavior and pathological alterations, must be described. Complex behavioral changes such as delusions and mood disorders are unlikely to correspond to single specific lesions, and the shared characteristics of lesions and conditions producing similar syndromes demand investigation. New treatments are continuously emerging and must be integrated into clinical practice to provide the most benefit for elderly patients. The effects, side effects, and drug interactions of these new agents must be discovered. Effective nonpharmacological interventions must also be identified and perfected. Molecular underpinnings of aging must be identified and explored. The appropriate ethical responses of society to severe illness in elderly individuals must be carefully considered. Finally, a means of bridging the gap between neuroscience and human experience must be found. Geriatric neuropsychiatry will succeed to the extent that advances in the neurosciences can be related to the suffering of elderly people and its relief. We hold the conviction that research advances will translate directly into improved care and a higher quality of life for elderly individuals.

References

Altshuler LL, Conrad A, Kovelman JA, et al: Hippocampal pyramidal cell orientation in schizophrenia. Arch Gen Psychiatry 44:1094–1098, 1987

American Psychiatric Association: Diagnostic and Statistical Manual of Mental Disorders, 3rd Edition. Washington, DC, American Psychiatric Association, 1980

Avorn J, Gurwitz J: Demography, epidemiology, and aging, in Geriatric Medicine, 2nd Edition. Edited by Cassel CK, Riesenberg DE, Sorensen LB, et al. New York, Springer-Verlag, 1990, pp 66–77

Baldessarini RJ, Frankenburg FR: Clozapine: a novel antipsychotic agent. N Engl J Med 324:746–754, 1991

Baxter LR Jr, Phelps ME, Mazziotta JC, et al: Cerebral metabolic rates for glucose in mood disorders. Arch Gen Psychiatry 42:441–447, 1985

Baxter LR Jr, Phelps ME, Mazziotta JC, et al: Local cerebral glucose metabolic rates in obsessive-compulsive disorder. Arch Gen Psychiatry 44:211–218, 1987

Baxter LR Jr, Schwartz JM, Phelps ME, et al: Reduction of prefrontal cortex glucose metabolism common to three types of depression. Arch Gen Psychiatry 46:243–250, 1989

Beckson M, Cummings JL: Neuropsychiatric aspects of stroke. Int J Psychiatry Med 21:1–15, 1991

Beers MH: Medication use in the elderly, in Practice of Geriatrics, 2nd Edition. Edited by Calkins E, Ford AB, Katz PR. Philadelphia, PA, WB Saunders, 1992, pp 33–49

Benjamin S, Cummings JL, Duffy JD, et al: Pathways to neuropsychiatry. J Neuropsychiatry Clin Neurosci 7:96–101, 1995

Bowen DM, Davison AN: The biochemistry of the ageing brain, in Neurological Disorders in the Elderly. Edited by Caird FI. London, Wright PSG, 1982, pp 33–43

Brody H: Age changes in the nervous system, in Neurological Disorders in the Elderly. Edited by Caird FI. London, Wright PSG, 1982, pp 17–24

Burke JD Jr, Pincus HA, Pardes H: The clinician-researcher in psychiatry. Am J Psychiatry 143:968–975, 1986

Cassel CK, Brody JA: Demography, epidemiology, and aging, in Geriatric Medicine, 2nd Edition. Edited by Cassel CK, Riesenberg DE, Sorensen LB, et al. New York, Springer-Verlag, 1990, pp 16–27

Coffey CE: Structural brain abnormalities in the depressed elderly, in Brain Imaging in Affective Disorders. Edited by Hauser P. Washington, DC, American Psychiatric Press, 1991, pp 89–111

Coffey CE: Brain morphology in primary mood disorders: implications for ECT. Psychiatric Annals 26:713–716, 1996

Coffey CE, Wilkinson WE, Weiner RD, et al: Quantitative cerebral anatomy in depression: a controlled magnetic resonance imaging study. Arch Gen Psychiatry 50:7–16, 1993

Cohen-Cole SA: Depression and heart disease, in Depression and Co-Existing Disease. Edited by Robinson RG, Rabins PV. New York, Igaku-Shoin, 1989, pp 27–39

Creasey H, Rapoport SI: The aging human brain. Ann Neurol 17:2–10, 1985

Cummings JL: Clinical Neuropsychiatry. New York, Grune & Stratton, 1985

Cummings JL: Depression and Parkinson's disease: a review. Am J Psychiatry 149:443–454, 1992a

Cummings JL: Psychosis in neurologic disease: neurobiology and pathogenesis. Neuropsychiatry Neuropsychol Behav Neurol 5:144–150, 1992b

Cummings JL: Frontal-subcortical circuits and human behavior. Arch Neurol 50:873–880, 1993

Cummings JL: Principles of neuropsychiatry: toward a neuropsychiatric epistemology. Neurocase 5:181–188, 1999

Cummings JL, Benson DF: Dementia: A Clinical Approach, 2nd Edition. Boston, MA, Butterworths, 1992

Cummings JL, Hegarty A: Neurology, psychiatry, and neuropsychiatry. Neurology 44:209–213, 1994

Cummings JL, Miller B, Hill MA, et al: Neuropsychiatric aspects of multi-infarct dementia and dementia of the Alzheimer type. Arch Neurol 44:389–393, 1987

Cummings JL, Coffey CE, Duffy JD, et al: The clinician-scientist in neuropsychiatry: a position statement from the Committee on Research of the American Neuropsychiatric Association. J Neuropsychiatry Clin Neurosci 10:1–9, 1998

D'Alessandro R, Gamberini G, Granieri E, et al: Prevalence of Parkinson's disease in the Republic of San Marino. Neurology 37:1679–1682, 1987

Davison W: Adverse drug reactions in the elderly: general considerations, in The Aging Process: Therapeutic Implications. Edited by Butler RN, Bearn AD. New York, Raven, 1985, pp 101–113

Department of Health and Human Services: Healthy People 2000. Washington, DC, U.S. Government Printing Office, 1990

Derogatis LR, Wise TN: Anxiety and Depressive Disorders in the Medical Patient. Washington, DC, American Psychiatric Press, 1989

Dresser RS: Autonomy revisited: the limits of anticipatory choices, in Dementia and Aging: Ethics, Values, and Policy Choices. Edited by Binstock RH, Post SG, Whitehouse PJ. Baltimore, MD, Johns Hopkins University Press, 1992, pp 71–85

Drubach DA, Kelly MP: Panic disorder associated with a right paralimbic lesion. Neuropsychiatry Neuropsychol Behav Neurol 2:282–289, 1989

Duffy JD, Coffey CE: The neurobiology of depression, in Contemporary Behavioral Neurology. Edited by Trimble MR, Cummings JL. Boston, MA, Butterworth-Heinemann, 1997, pp 275–288

Estroff TW, Gold MS: Medication-induced and toxin-induced psychiatric disorders, in Medical Mimics of Psychiatric Disorders. Edited by Extein I, Gold MS. Washington, DC, American Psychiatric Press, 1986, pp 163–198

Evans DA, Funkenstein H, Albert MS, et al: Prevalence of Alzheimer's disease in a community of older persons: higher than previously reported. JAMA 262:2552–2556, 1989

Farlow M, Gracon SI, Hershey LA, et al: A controlled trial of tacrine in Alzheimer's disease. JAMA 268:2523–2529, 1992

Figiel GS, Coffey CE, Djang WT, et al: Brain magnetic resonance imaging findings in ECT-induced delirium. J Neuropsychiatry Clin Neurosci 2:53–58, 1990

Finch CE: Longevity, Senescence, and the Genome. Chicago, IL, University of Chicago Press, 1990

Fontaine R, Breton G, Dery R, et al: Temporal lobe abnormalities in panic disorder: an MRI study. Biol Psychiatry 27:304–310, 1990

Fratiglioni L, Grut M, Forsell Y, et al: Prevalence of Alzheimer's disease and other dementias in an elderly urban population: relationship with age, sex, and education. Neurology 41:1886–1892, 1991

Gent M, Easton JD, Hachinski VC, et al: The Canadian American Ticlopidine Study (CATS) in thromboembolic stroke. Lancet 2:1215–1220, 1989

Griggs RC, Martin TB, Penn AS, et al: Training clinical neuroscientists. Ann Neurol 21:197–201, 1987

Hershey LA, Modic MT, Greenough PG, et al: Magnetic resonance imaging in vascular dementia. Neurology 37:29–36, 1987

Hoehn-Saric R: Neurotransmitters in anxiety. Arch Gen Psychiatry 39:735–742, 1982

Holcomb HH, Links J, Smith C, et al: Positron emission tomography: measuring the metabolic and neurochemical characteristics of the living human nervous system, in Brain Imaging: Applications in Psychiatry. Edited by Andreasen NC. Washington, DC, American Psychiatric Press, 1989, pp 235–370

Jacoby RJ, Levy R, Bird JM: Computed tomography and the outcome of affective disorder: a follow-up study of elderly patients. Br J Psychiatry 139:288–292, 1981

Koranyi EK: Undiagnosed physical illness in psychiatric patients. Annu Rev Med 33:309–316, 1982

Lamy PP: Patterns of prescribing and drug use, in The Aging Process: Therapeutic Implications. Edited by Butler RN, Bearn AD. New York, Raven, 1985, pp 53–82

Leuchter AF, Spar JE: The late-onset psychoses. J Nerv Ment Dis 173:488–494, 1985

Lishman WA: What is neuropsychiatry? J Neurol Neurosurg Psychiatry 55:983–985, 1992

Mayeux R, Denaro J, Hemenegildo N, et al: A population-based investigation of Parkinson's disease with and without dementia: relationship to age and gender. Arch Neurol 49:492–497, 1992

Mayou R, Hawton K, Feldman E, et al: Psychiatric problems among medical admissions. Int J Psychiatry Med 21:71–84, 1991

Mazziotta JC, Gilman S (eds): Clinical Brain Imaging: Principles and Application. Philadelphia, PA, FA Davis, 1992

Mega MS, Cummings JL, Salloway S, et al: The limbic system: an anatomic phylogenetic and clinical perspective. J Neuropsychiatry Clin Neurosci 9:315–330, 1997

Merriam AE, Aronson MK, Gaston P, et al: The psychiatric symptoms of Alzheimer's disease. J Am Geriatr Soc 36: 7–12, 1988

Miller BL, Lesser IM, Mena I, et al: Regional cerebral blood flow in late-life-onset psychosis. Neuropsychiatry Neuropsychol Behav Neurol 5:132–137, 1992

Modell JG, Mountz JM, Beresford TP: Basal ganglia/limbic striatal and thalamocortical involvement in craving and loss of control in alcoholism. J Neuropsychiatry Clin Neurosci 2:123–144, 1990

Moody HR: A critical view of ethical dilemmas in dementia, in Dementia and Aging: Ethics, Values, and Policy Choices. Edited by Binstock RH, Post SG, Whitehouse PJ. Baltimore, MD, Johns Hopkins University Press, 1992, pp 86–100

Myers JK, Weissman MM, Tischler GL, et al: Six-month prevalence of psychiatric disorders in three communities. Arch Gen Psychiatry 41:959–967, 1984

Nasrallah HA, Coffman JA, Olson SC: Structural brain-imaging findings in affective disorders: an overview. J Neuropsychiatry Clin Neurosci 1:21–26, 1989

National Center for Health Statistics: Statistics on older persons: United States, 1986 (Vital and Health Statistics). Washington, DC, Department of Health and Human Services, 1986

National Foundation for Brain Research: The Cost of Disorders of the Brain. Washington, DC, National Foundation for Brain Research, 1992

Post RM, Uhde TW, Ballenger JC: Efficacy of carbamazepine in affective disorders: implications for underlying physiological and biochemical substrates, in Anticonvulsants in Affective Disorders. Edited by Emrich HM, Okuma T, Muller AA. New York, Elsevier, 1984, pp 93–115

Prichard JW, Cummings JL: The insistent call from functional MRI. Neurology 48:797–800, 1997

Regier DA, Boyd JH, Burke JD Jr, et al: One-month prevalence of mental disorders in the United States. Arch Gen Psychiatry 45:977–986, 1988

Reiman EM, Fusselman MJ, Tox PT, et al: Neuroanatomical correlates of anticipatory anxiety. Science 243:1071–1074, 1989

Reisberg B, Borenstein J, Salob SP, et al: Behavioral symptoms in Alzheimer's disease: phenomenology and treatment. J Clin Psychiatry 48 (suppl):9–15, 1987

Robinson RG, Benson DF: Depression in aphasic patients: frequency, severity, and clinicopathologic correlations. Brain Lang 14:282–291, 1981

Robinson RG, Starkstein SE: Current research in affective disorders following stroke. J Neuropsychiatry Clin Neurosci 2:1–14, 1990

Rogers SL, Farlow MR, Doody RS, et al, and the Donepezil Study Group: A 24-week double-blind, placebo-controlled trial of donepezil in patients with Alzheimer's disease. Neurology 50:136–146, 1998

Rowe J: Report of the Institute of Medicine: academic geriatrics in the year 2000. N Engl J Med 316:1425–1428, 1987

Sackeim HA, Prohovnik II, Moeller JR, et al: Regional cerebral blood flow in mood disorders. Arch Gen Psychiatry 47:60–70, 1990

Sano M, Ernesto C, Thomas RG, et al, for the members of the Alzheimer's Disease Cooperative Study: A controlled trial of selegiline, alpha-tocopherol, or both as treatment for Alzheimer's disease. N Engl J Med 336:1216–1222, 1997

Saravay SM, Steinberg MD, Weinschel B, et al: Psychological comorbidity and length of stay in the general hospital. Am J Psychiatry 148:324–329, 1991

Small GW, Fong K, Beck JC: Training in geriatric psychiatry: will supply meet the demand? Am J Psychiatry 145:476–478, 1988

Spencer G, Goldstein AA, Taeuber CM: America's Centenarians. Washington, DC, U.S. Department of Commerce, Bureau of Statistics, U.S. Government Printing Office, 1987

Stadtman ER: Protein oxidation and aging. Science 257:1220–1224, 1992

Teri L, Larson EB, Reifler BV: Behavioral disturbances in dementia of the Alzheimer's type. J Am Geriatr Soc 36:1–6, 1988

Terry RD, DeTeresa R, Hansen LA: Neocortical cell counts in normal human adult aging. Ann Neurol 21:530–539, 1987

Torrey BB, Kinsella K, Taeuber CM: An Aging World. Washington, DC, U.S. Department of Commerce, Bureau of the Census, U.S. Government Printing Office, 1987

Trimble MR: Neuropsychiatry or behavioral neurology. Neuropsychiatry Neuropsychol Behav Neurol 6:60–69, 1993

Van Gorp W, Mahler M: Subcortical features of normal aging, in Subcortical Dementia. Edited by Cummings JL. New York, Oxford University Press, 1990, pp 231–250

Veith RC, Raskind MA: The neurobiology of aging: does it predispose to depression? Neurobiol Aging 9:101–117, 1988

Volkow ND, Hitzemann R, Wang G-J, et al: Decreased brain metabolism in neurologically intact healthy alcoholics. Am J Psychiatry 149:1016–1022, 1992

Wu JC, Buchsbaum MS, Hershey TG, et al: PET in generalized anxiety disorder. Biol Psychiatry 29:1181–1199, 1991

Yudofsky SC, Hales RE: The reemergence of neuropsychiatry: definition and direction. J Neuropsychiatry Clin Neurosci 1:1–6, 1989a

Yudofsky SC, Hales RE: When patients ask . . . What is neuropsychiatry? J Neuropsychiatry Clin Neurosci 1:362–365, 1989b

Epidemiology of Aging

Roberta Malmgren, Ph.D.

Aging populations present one of the world's major health care challenges. Industrialized countries currently face this challenge; but developing nations, with anticipated increases in the numbers and proportion of their elderly populations, will also soon need to deal with problems of growing geriatric populations (Holden 1996; Steel 1997). Concerns about the elderly population arise from two characteristics of that group: 1) the recent and continuing increases in the population age 65 and older ("65+") and 2) the increasing number and severity of health problems associated with aging. (Unless otherwise noted, "elderly" and "older people" refer to people 65 years old and older.)

Epidemiology characterizes groups rather than individuals. As cultural background and gender play an important role in an individual's health, so, too, do characteristics of an age group, such as the elderly, affect and reflect the well-being of its members. Although the subject of this book is neuropsychiatric disorders, it is important to understand how a range of other factors may affect the neuropsychiatric realm. Therefore, in this chapter my purpose is to define the population at risk, the elderly, and to describe some of the most salient epidemiological characteristics of this population, particularly its physical health. The focus is on the 65+ population in the United States. However, most of the concepts and problems apply to other industri-

alized countries now and presage issues that will affect developing nations in the near future. What, then, are some of the major epidemiological characteristics of the elderly?

Graying of the Population

One of the most remarkable and far-reaching demographic developments of the 20th century has been the "graying" of populations. This phrase often evokes the image of a horrendous set of problems produced by increasing numbers of elderly people. The specific problems—medical, social, financial, and psychological—are not all necessarily new. But what is unique are the great increases in the numbers and proportions of older people.

The graying of the population has three components (Table 2–1). First are the increases in the absolute numbers of people 65 and older. Between 1900 and 1995, the number of elderly people in the United States increased 10-fold, from 3 million to almost 34 million. Second are the increases in the proportion of the population that is elderly. In 1900, the elderly were only 4% of the total United States population; currently they are 13%. Third, the oldest old, those who are 85 or older ("85+"), are growing as a proportion of the 65+ group. In 1995, 3.6 million people in the United States were 85 or older, almost 30 times their num-

TABLE 2–1.   Population 65 and older (65+)—United States, 1900–2050

Population	1900	1950	1995[a]	2010[a]	2030[a]	2050[a]
65+ population (in millions)	3.1	12.3	33.5	39.4	69.4	78.9
(As % of total population)	(4.1%)	(8.1%)	(12.8%)	(13.2%)	(20.0%)	(20.0%)
85+ population (in millions)	0.1	0.6	3.6	5.7	8.5	18.2
(As % of 65+ population)	(4.0%)	(4.7%)	(10.8%)	(14.4%)	(12.2%)	(23.1%)

[a]Middle series projections.
Source.   Adapted from 1900–1990: Hobbs and Damon 1996; 1995–2050: Day 1996.

ber in 1900 and more than double their proportion in the total elderly population.

Table 2–1 shows that the graying of the United States population will continue well into the next century. In the year 2030, there will be close to 70 million elderly people, more than twice as many as there are now. As a proportion of the total population, today one of eight Americans is 65 or older; in 2030, one of five will be. In the next century, the 85+ group will be one of the fastest growing age groups, increasing from 3.6 million in 1995 to 18.2 million in 2050. Currently, 11% of the elderly population is 85+; but in 2050, 23% of the 65+ group will be 85 or older. The major reason for these rapid future increases in the 65+ population is past increases in birth rates: the baby boomers, a large cohort born between 1946 and 1964, will start to turn 65 in 2011, continuing to inflate the numbers of 65+ until 2030 (Day 1996).

Changing Racial Composition

In the coming century, the racial composition of the elderly population will also change (Table 2–2). In 1995, 10% of the United States elderly population was non-white. In 2050, almost one-fifth will be non-white. By 2050, the black elderly population is projected to increase from 8% to 11% of the 65+ group, whereas Hispanic elderly people (who may be of any race) will have quadrupled as a percentage of the United States elderly population. By the middle of the next century, the number of Asian and Pacific Islander elderly will be almost 10 times their current number, an increase from 1.9% to 6.6% of the total 65+ group.

Sex Ratio

Because of increased mortality rates among men, the ratio of men to women decreases strikingly from ages 65–69 (83 men to every 100 women) to ages 90+ (when the ratio is 31 to 100) (Figure 2–1). Many social and medical consequences of aging in developed countries are associated with

the sex ratio imbalance. With increasing age, women are more likely to be unmarried and living alone (Saluter 1996). Both of these characteristics are linked to poverty (Davis et al. 1997; Lewis 1997; Social Security Administration 1996) and other disadvantages, such as increased likelihood of admission to nursing homes (Davis et al. 1997; Hing and Bloom 1990).

Marital Status[1]

Elderly men are more likely to be married, and elderly women are more likely to be widowed. According to the U.S. Bureau of the Census, in 1996 15% of all men 65+ were widowers, whereas 47% of all women 65+ were widows (Saluter and Lugaila 1998). As a corollary of this statistic, 73% of elderly men lived with spouses compared with 40% of elderly women.

Living Arrangements

The percentage of elderly people living alone increases with age and is greater for women than for men. In 1996, 15% of men 65–74 years old lived alone, whereas 31% of women these ages did so; 21% of men 75+ lived alone compared with 53% of women 75+ (Saluter and Lugaila 1998).

Income

The median income of the elderly population decreases with age, is lower for nonmarried people, and is lowest for nonmarried women (Social Security Administration 1998). In terms of median income and total assets, today's elderly people are financially better off than those in the past (Hobbs and Damon 1996; Social Security Administration 1996). Nonetheless, in 1996, 13% of the United States elderly people lived below the poverty level and another 37% would have been below that level had they not had Social Security benefits (Social Security Administration 1998). The risk of poverty is higher for unmarried people, for women, and for black and

---

[1] Statistics for marital status, living arrangements, and income are all based on surveys of noninstitutionalized elderly.

TABLE 2–2.   Racial and ethnic changes in population of people 65 and older (65+)—United States, 1995–2050 (middle series projections)

	1995	2010	2030	2050
All non-whites				
Population (in millions)	3.5	5.0	10.6	14.4
As % of total 65+ population	(10.4%)	(12.7%)	(15.3%)	(18.3%)
Blacks (in millions)	2.7	3.4	6.9	8.6
As % of total 65+ population	(8.1%)	(8.7%)	(10.0%)	(10.9%)
Asians/Pacific Islanders (in millions)	0.6	1.3	3.3	5.2
As % of total 65+ population	(1.9%)	(3.4%)	(4.7%)	(6.6%)
Native Americans[a] (in millions)	0.1	0.2	0.4	0.6
As % of total 65+ population	(0.4%)	(0.6%)	(0.6%)	(0.8%)
Hispanics[b] (in millions)	1.5	2.8	7.8	13.8
As % of total 65+ population	(4.5%)	(7.2%)	(11.2%)	(17.5%)

[a]American Indian, Eskimo, Aleut.
[b]Hispanics may be of any race, including white, so sum of racial/ethnic subgroups exceeds "All non-whites."
Source.   Adapted from Day 1996.

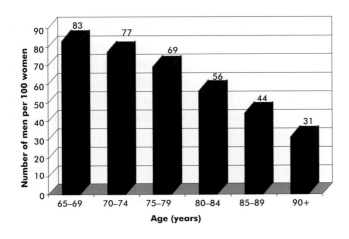

FIGURE 2–1.   Ratio of men to women, by age group—United States, 1995.
Source.   Adapted from Day 1996.

Hispanic elderly people (Hobbs and Damon 1996; Social Security Administration 1998).

Worldwide Aging

The aging of populations is a worldwide phenomenon. In 1995, 371 million people, 6.5% of the world's population, were 65+ (Table 2–3). Their numbers will almost double in 2020, when 9% of the world's population will be 65+. In that year, two-thirds of the world's elderly people will live in developing countries. In the year 2050, one of four people in developed countries, and one of seven in developing countries, will be 65 or older.

Life Expectancy

The single statistic that best summarizes a population's health is life expectancy—the average number of years of life remaining at a certain age. Although life expectancy from birth is the most commonly quoted, life tables generate life expectancy values for all ages of a population. Thus we can compare the longevity of elderly people in different groups or at different times using life expectancy at, for example, age 65 or age 85.

Older Americans have many years of life yet to live. In 1995, a 65-year-old person had a life expectancy of 17.4 years—more than 20% of his or her life still remained (Anderson et al. 1997). In the same year, a 75-year-old person had an expected 11 more years of life, and an 85-year-old could expect to live, on average, 6 more years. Life expectancy for elderly people has, in general, been improving since 1900. At the turn of the century, the life expectancy of a 65-year-old person was 11.9 years and that of an 85-year-old person was 4.0 years (Statistical Bulletin of the Metropolitan Insurance Co 1987). Thus in less than 100 years, life expectancy has increased by about 50% for older Americans.

As is true of virtually all health measures, life expectancy for elderly people varies by race and sex, with elderly women having a definite, but decreasing, survival advantage over men. Table 2–4 lists 1995 life expectancy for older subgroups: a 65-year-old man had a life expectancy of 15.6 years; a 65-year-old woman, 18.9 years. For ages 85+, male-female differences in life expectancy shrank to 1.1 years (5.2 for men versus 6.3 for women). For blacks and whites as well, the gap in life expectancy narrows with age:

TABLE 2–3. World population of people 65 and older, by region: 1995–2050 (medium variant projections)

Region	1995 Number (in millions)	1995 % of total population	2020 Number (in millions)	2020 % of total population	2050 Number (in millions)	2050 % of total population
World	371	6.5	686	8.9	1,416	15.1
More developed regions[a]	158	13.5	225	18.4	287	24.7
Less developed regions[b]	213	4.7	461	7.1	1,129	13.8

[a]North America, Japan, Europe, Australia, New Zealand.
[b]Africa, Latin America/Caribbean, Asia (excludes Japan), Melanesia, Micronesia, and Polynesia.
Source. Adapted from United Nations 1997.

TABLE 2–4. Life expectancy (in years) at ages 65, 75, and 85, by sex and race—United States, 1995

	All races	White	Black
At age 65			
Men	15.6	15.7	13.6
Women	18.9	19.1	17.1
At age 75			
Men	9.7	9.7	8.8
Women	11.9	12.0	11.1
At age 85			
Men	5.2	5.2	5.1
Women	6.3	6.3	6.2

Source. Adapted from Anderson et al. 1997.

in 1995, the life expectancy of a 65-year-old white person was about 2 years greater than that of a black person the same age. However, at age 85, life expectancy of black people was much closer to that of whites: black men and women had life expectancies that were only 0.1 year less than those of their white counterparts. This closing of the gap of racial survival has been reported for many years and reflects a phenomenon known as the "black-white mortality crossover": at very old ages mortality rates for whites exceed those of blacks (Nam 1995).

Mortality Rates

Life expectancy, though a succinct summary of a population's health, tells nothing of the specific components of survival: who dies, what people die from, and how these causes change over time. Mortality data, from which life expectancies are calculated, provide this information. In the United States, 5 of every 100 elderly people die each year (Table 2–5). Mortality rises dramatically with age: in 1995, the death rates were 2.6% for those 65–74 years old,

5.9% for those 75–84 years old, and 15.5% for those 85+. Men are at higher risk of dying than are women; and, up to very old ages, blacks have higher mortality rates than do whites (National Center for Health Statistics 1997a). However, with advancing age, differences in mortality rates lessen between the sexes and between the races; and, as noted previously, at very old ages, mortality rates for blacks of both sexes become lower than those of whites.

High mortality rates in the elderly result in a large turnover of this population in a short time and may result in considerable changes in the characteristics of the 65+ population in a short period. Myers (1990) estimated that 50% of those who were 65+ in 1970 had died by 1980. Thus the elderly population in one decade may be quite different from that in the next in terms of health, lifestyles, and attitudes.

The three leading causes of death in elderly people are heart disease, cancer, and stroke. In 1995, these accounted for two-thirds of all elderly deaths (Anderson et al. 1997). The major fatal cancers in elderly men are lung, prostate, and colon; in elderly women, the major sites are lung, breast, and colon (Yancik 1997). Chronic obstructive pulmonary disease is the fourth leading cause of death, and the combined category of pneumonia/influenza is the fifth. This last cause particularly affects the oldest old: in 1995, the pneumonia/influenza death rate among those 85+ was 18 times that of those 65–74 years old. In 1995, for the first time in the history of vital statistics reports in the United States, Alzheimer's disease (AD) appeared as one of the 10 leading causes of death in the elderly, ranking number eight in the 65+ population (Anderson et al. 1997) (see Chapter 24 in this volume).

In the United States, mortality has been declining for all three older age groups for many years (Figure 2–2). Between 1950 and 1995, mortality rates for people 65–84 years old decreased by more than one-third; for those 85+, the rates declined by approximately one-fourth (National Center for Health Statistics 1997a). Much of this remarkable decline in mortality is a result of improvements in car-

TABLE 2–5. Leading causes of death in the population 65 and older (65+)—United States, 1995

Cause	Death rates per 1,000 people			
	65+	65–74	75–84	85+
All causes	**50.5**	**25.6**	**58.5**	**154.7**
Diseases of the heart	18.4	8.0	20.6	64.8
Malignant neoplasms	11.4	8.7	13.6	18.2
Cerebrovascular diseases	4.1	1.4	4.8	16.4
Chronic obstructive pulmonary diseases	2.6	1.6	3.5	5.3
Pneumonia and influenza	2.2	0.6	2.3	10.4
Diabetes mellitus	1.3	0.9	1.6	2.8
Accidents and adverse effects	0.9	0.4	1.0	2.7
Alzheimer's disease	0.6	0.1	0.7	2.8
Nephritis/nephrosis	0.6	0.2	0.7	2.1
Septicemia	0.5	0.2	0.6	1.7

Source. Adapted from Anderson et al. 1997.

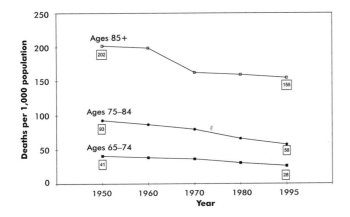

FIGURE 2–2. Death rates in the elderly population, all causes—United States, 1950–1995.
Source. Adapted from National Center for Health Statistics 1997a.

diovascular disease mortality (Bonita and Beaglehole 1996; Centers for Disease Control 1997; Feinleib 1995; Hunink et al. 1997). Between 1950 and 1995, the age-adjusted rates for heart disease for the total United States population dropped by more than 50%; those of stroke, by 70% (National Center for Health Statistics 1997a). These improvements occurred in the elderly population as well: in the past 45 years, death rates from both heart disease and stroke have decreased in all three of the elderly age groups. Unlike cardiovascular mortality, death rates for cancer have been increasing in the elderly (Ries et al. 1998). These long-term increases in cancer mortality have not been enough to offset the effects of improved cardiovascular disease mortality.

In developed countries, virtually all deaths are recorded, so that, of all health status measures, mortality data are the most complete. Cause-specific mortality, however, has a number of limitations, especially for older persons (Havlik and Rosenberg 1992). Diagnostic accuracy of cause of death partly reflects much lower autopsy rates in the elderly (Smith 1997), as well as attending physicians' perceptions of what is normal aging and what is disease. But even with thorough medical assessment of an elderly decedent, determining the underlying cause of death can be difficult because of the presence of multiple, chronic disorders.

AD exemplifies the limitations of mortality data. In a 1976 article on the senile type of AD, Katzman estimated that it was the fourth or fifth leading cause of death in the United States (Katzman 1976), although it was not listed among the 263 leading causes of death listed in United States vital statistics. (Until 1979, there was no specific cause-of-death code for AD.) Katzman's article greatly increased awareness of AD as a major health problem of the elderly population. Also, the International Classification of Diseases (ICD), used to code conditions on death certificates, now has a unique number for AD (U.S. Department of Health and Human Services 1980). Because there is now a specific ICD code for AD and because of increasing physician awareness of this illness, increasingly more deaths are appropriately attributed to this cause. However, even with both improved recognition of AD and assignment of an ICD code for it, current mortality rates still underestimate the public health importance of this disease (Hoyert 1996). Many cases are undiagnosed (Small et al. 1997) or, if diagnosed, AD may not be mentioned on the death certificate (Hoyert 1996).

Risk of Severe Medical Disease

The risk of developing a disease is not the same as the risk of dying from it. Even diseases that are the leading causes of death do not always result in death and so do not give a complete picture of the occurrence of those diseases in a population. The two epidemiological measures most often used to describe the occurrence of disease are incidence and prevalence. Incidence is the number of new cases of a disease or condition arising in a population within a certain period (usually a year). Prevalence is the number of existing cases in a population at a certain point in time (or in a short period). Though incidence is the only valid way to measure risk of developing disease, incidence studies are usually expensive and time-consuming to conduct. Because of this limitation, relatively few community-based incidence studies have been conducted on even the three leading causes of death: heart disease, cancer, and stroke. Fewer still have collected information on any but the youngest of the elderly. Where adequate data exist, they show that the prevalence and incidence of severe diseases increase greatly in elderly people.

Heart Disease

Four-fifths of all heart disease deaths in the United States occur in people 65+ (Anderson et al. 1997). Yet there is remarkably little population-based research on the risk of this population developing heart disease. Rochester, Minnesota, has an excellent medical record linkage system that covers virtually all residents (Leibson et al. 1992). In Rochester, between 1979 and 1982, the average annual incidence of coronary heart disease for people 70+ was 1.7/100 for men and 1.4/100 for women (Elveback et al. 1986). The coronary heart disease rate in men 70+ was almost eight times greater than that observed in 30- to 49-year-old men; the rate in women 70+ was 24 times that of women who were 30–49. As has been shown in other studies, older men have a higher risk of heart disease than do women, but this gender difference narrows with age (Burke et al. 1989; Centers for Disease Control 1992b).

Unlike the clear decline in heart disease mortality over the past three decades, evidence for decreases in risk of developing heart disease (incidence) is very limited. Furthermore, published reports on whether or not there have been changes, and the direction of the changes, are mixed. In Rochester, between 1965–1969 and 1979–1982, the risk of myocardial infarction and sudden unexpected death declined for 50- to 69-year-old men but increased for women (Elveback et al. 1986). For those 70+, rates of these manifestations of heart disease declined only slightly over time

for men (9%) and not at all for women. Croft et al. (1997) calculated changes in age-adjusted hospitalization rates for heart failure in the 65+ population in the United States between 1986 and 1993: heart failure rates increased slightly in this period. The Minnesota Heart Survey found no significant changes in hospitalized myocardial infarction rates in Minneapolis-St. Paul between 1970 and 1985 (Burke et al. 1989). However, for the period 1985–1990, a slight decrease in hospitalization rates for acute myocardial infarction was found (McGovern et al. 1996). Sytkowski et al. (1996) looked at long-term changes in risk of cardiovascular disease in three cohorts of Framingham, Massachusetts, subjects (ages 50–59). The incidence of all cardiovascular diseases decreased by 21% in women and only 6% in men. Most of this decline occurred between 1950 and 1959, with little changes later. For women, the greatest declines occurred in the risk of having a stroke.

With so little change occurring in the risk of developing heart disease, what might be the reason for the large decline in heart disease mortality? A number of authors report improvements in survival of patients with heart disease (Feinleib 1995; Massie and Shah 1997; McGovern et al. 1996; Sytkowski et al. 1996). Thus, intervention efforts appear to be less effective in preventing the onset of heart disease than in reducing its severity (Hunink et al. 1997).

Cancer

The Surveillance and Epidemiology End Results program, a major source of data on cancer incidence in the United States, estimates that 60% of all new cancers in the United States occur in the 65+ population (Yancik 1997) and that people 65+ have a risk of developing cancer that is more than 10 times that of those under 65 (Ries et al. 1998). The leading cancer incidence sites in older women are breast, lung, and colon. In men, they are prostate, lung, and colon (Rosenthal 1998). As is true for cancer mortality, the incidence rates of a number of neoplasms have increased in the 65+ population in the past two decades (Balducci and Lyman 1997). Some of these increased rates may be a result of improved detection methods, for example, prostate-specific antigen screening (Stephenson and Stanford 1997). For other neoplasms, such as lung cancer, these increases are a consequence of lifestyle differences, particularly tobacco use, in older birth cohorts (Levi et al. 1996; Travis et al. 1996). Recently, certain types of cancer appear to be declining in some elderly subgroups: Travis et al. (1996) report decreases in squamous cell carcinoma rates for both black and white men under 75 years of age, as well as declining small cell carcinoma rates for black men under 75.

Stroke

More than heart disease or cancer, stroke is a disease of elderly people. Almost 90% of all stroke deaths occur in the elderly population (Anderson et al. 1997). Stroke is also one of the most disabling conditions to affect elderly people (Kalache and Aboderin 1995; Verbrugge et al. 1989), and its risk increases with age (Sudlow and Warlow 1997). Well-designed studies of stroke incidence indicate that 2%–4% of the 85+ age group have a first-ever stroke each year, and men have a somewhat greater risk of stroke than do women (Malmgren et al. 1987). Some of the best evidence for changes in stroke incidence with time comes from Rochester, Minnesota, where average annual stroke rates were calculated for 5-year periods starting in 1945 (Broderick et al. 1989). Between 1945–1949 and 1975–1979, total age-adjusted stroke rates dropped by 45% in this city (Figure 2–3). However, this decline was followed by a 17% increase in stroke incidence between 1975–1979 and 1980–1984 (Broderick et al. 1989). Over the 40-year period, changes occurred in all age groups, but were most pronounced in the 85+ age group. The most recent data from Rochester, for the years 1985–1989, show that the stroke risk in Rochester has changed little compared with that for the previous 5 years (Brown et al. 1996).

▌ Neuropsychiatric Disorders

Dementia

Progressive loss of cognition and eventual total incapacitation make dementia one of the most dreaded consequences of aging. It is a major cause of functional disability

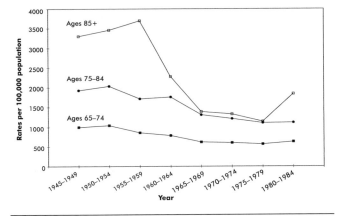

FIGURE 2–3. Average annual stroke incidence in the elderly population—Rochester, Minnesota, 1945–1984. *Source.* Adapted from Broderick et al. 1989.

(Barberger-Gateau and Fabrigoule 1997) and the need for long-term care, including admission to nursing homes (Hing et al. 1989). Dementia is also an enormous burden to family caregivers (Office of Technology Assessment Task Force 1988; Schulz et al. 1995; Small et al. 1997).

If there is an "epidemic" among the elderly population, it is AD and related dementias (see Chapter 24 in this volume). An estimated 4 million people in the United States have AD, with a 6%–8% prevalence in the 65+ group and 30% in those 85+ (Small et al. 1997). Studies have been done in many parts of the world and have produced widely differing estimates of dementia prevalence (Corrada et al. 1995). However, for no other disorder of the elderly are methodological issues of conducting community-based studies so complex or variation in study design so great (Chandra et al. 1994; Jorm 1991; van Duijn 1996). These methodological variations, rather than true differences in frequency of dementia, are a major reason why estimates of prevalence rates of dementia are so disparate.

Another cause of differences in rates of overall prevalence of dementia is the type of dementia identified. The Office of Technology Assessment Task Force (1988) lists more than 80 conditions that cause or simulate dementia (see Chapters 23 and 24 in this volume). In many countries, AD is the most common cause and vascular dementia the second most common (Hebert and Brayne 1995; Small et al. 1997). The exact proportion of dementia attributable to each cause depends in part on the stroke risk in the population of interest: where stroke risk is higher, for example, among blacks (Broderick et al. 1998; Centers for Disease Control 1992a) or among Asian populations (Kalache and Aboderin 1995; Malmgren et al. 1987; van Duijn 1996), the proportion of dementia attributable to vascular causes will be higher. Similarly, secular declines in stroke risk should have an effect on the total risk of dementia, as well as on the type of dementia seen.

Few population-based studies of dementia incidence have been conducted (Keefover 1996; Kokmen et al. 1996). In Rochester, Minnesota, data were collected on all new cases occurring between 1970 and 1974 (Kokmen et al. 1983). The average annual incidence rates of all dementias there were 1.4/1,000 for those 60–69 years old, 6.4/1,000 for those 70–79 years old, and 20.5/1,000 for those 80+. AD was the diagnosis in 38% of new dementia cases in people who were 60–69, 71% of those 70–79, and 82% in those 80+. Some studies suggest a somewhat greater frequency of AD in women (Jorm 1990; Seshadri et al. 1997; Small et al. 1997); however, others find no significant differences by sex (Corrada et al. 1995; Hebert and Brayne 1995; van Duijn 1996).

Only a few studies have looked at secular changes in

the incidence of dementia. In Lundby, Sweden, residents were followed from 1947 until 1972 (Rorsman et al. 1986). No change in the incidence of "age psychosis" was detected. Similarly, in Rochester, Minnesota, incidence rates for dementia were stable between 1960 and 1984, except for a slight increase in the very old (Kokmen et al. 1996).

Other Mental Disorders

Except for dementia, the frequency of most mental disorders does not appear to increase in the elderly population. Though conducted 15 years ago, the Epidemiologic Catchment Area Program still provides one of the largest samples of population-based data on mental illness in elderly Americans (Eaton et al. 1989; Fichter et al. 1996). In the early 1980s, staff from this research program interviewed residents in five cities (Baltimore, Maryland; St. Louis, Missouri; Los Angeles, California; New Haven, Connecticut; and Durham, North Carolina), identifying major types of mental disorders by using a questionnaire based on DSM-III criteria (American Psychiatric Association 1980). The prevalence of all types of mental disorder in elderly people was 12.3%, lower than that for any other age group (Regier et al. 1988) (Table 2–6). By type of disorder, the prevalence was also lower in all categories except severe cognitive impairment: as measured by the Mini-Mental State Exam (Folstein et al. 1975), 5% of the elderly in this sample had severe cognitive impairment. For some of the disorders, differences by sex were found: the prevalence of alcohol abuse was six times greater in elderly men than in elderly women (see Chapter 16 in this volume), whereas the prevalence of affective disorders in women was more than double that in men (see Chapter 13 in this volume). Elderly men had a higher prevalence of severe cognitive impairment than did women at ages 65–74 and a similar rate at ages 75–84, but for those 85+, the prevalence in men was less than half that observed in women (8.2% compared with 19.5%).

The Epidemiologic Catchment Area Program re-interviewed subjects 1 year after the baseline interview to determine the incidence (rate of new cases) in their population (Eaton et al. 1989). The authors found that the onset of major depressive disorder was rare in elderly subjects (except in St. Louis), as was the onset of panic disorders (see Chapters 13 and 15 in this volume). Not surprisingly, the risk of developing severe cognitive impairment increased with age: approximately 5 of every 100 subjects 65+ developed severe cognitive impairment each year. Unlike the prevalence data, the incidence of alcohol abuse increased after age 60: in men 75+ older, the rate was six times as high as that for men 65–74 (see Chapter 16 in this volume). For women, the incidence was twice as high in the 75+ group as in the 65–74 age group.

Reported prevalences of depression among the elderly vary widely (Roberts et al. 1997). Low estimates may be a result, in part, of methodological issues resulting in underascertainment (Garrard et al. 1998; Heithoff 1995; Pearson et al. 1997; Roberts et al. 1997; Slater and Katz 1995). Furthermore, depression is a significant cause of morbidity and mortality in older people (Zisook and Downs 1998). Suicide rates in older white males are currently the highest suicide rate of all age groups: in 1995, the rates for white men were 30/100,000 for those 65–74, 48/100,000 for those 75–84, and 68/100,000 for the 85+ group (National Center for Health Statistics 1997a) (see Chapter 13 in this volume). Since the early 1980s, the suicide rates for white males 85 and older have been rising (McIntosh 1995; National Center for Health Statistics 1997a). An urgent research question is whether or not the incidence and prevalence of depression are also increasing in this high-risk group (Roberts et al. 1997).

▎ Prevalence of Chronic Conditions

In addition to their high risk of fatal illnesses, many older adults suffer from less serious, but nevertheless affecting, chronic disorders. A major source of information about the

---

TABLE 2–6. Epidemiologic Catchment Area Program 1-month prevalence of mental disorders in persons 65 and older (per 100 subjects)

	Anxiety disorders[a]	Severe cognitive impairment	Affective disorders[b]	Alcohol abuse	Schizophrenia	Antisocial personality
Both sexes	5.5	4.9	2.5	0.9	0.1	0.0
Men	3.6	5.1	1.4	1.8	0.1	0.1
Women	6.8	4.7	3.3	0.3	0.1	0.0

[a]Phobia, panic, and obsessive-compulsive disorders.
[b]Manic episode, major depressive episode, and dysthymia.
Source. Adapted from Regier et al. 1988.

prevalence of chronic conditions in the United States is the National Health Interview Survey, a continuing survey of the noninstitutionalized United States population (Havlik et al. 1987). Table 2–7 lists 10 of the most prevalent chronic conditions reported by the 65+ population. Almost 50% of older Americans living in the community report that they have arthritis, a third say that they are deaf or have other hearing impairments, and 8% are blind or visually impaired (not corrected by glasses). Surprisingly, the prevalence of many of these conditions does not increase with age. However, the National Health Interview Survey excludes nursing home residents. In very old subjects, some of the listed conditions are likely to result in institutionalization or death, removing subjects with these conditions from the community-dwelling population. Incontinence, too, is common among the 65+ population: Fultz and Herzog (1996) estimate that 30% of noninstitutionalized older people have urinary incontinence.

Many of the most prevalent conditions in the elderly population are not fatal but still have a major impact on the quality of life. Arthritis has been targeted as a major health problem in the elderly because of its high prevalence and impact (Boult et al. 1996; Callahan et al. 1996; Verbrugge and Patrick 1995). Both visual and hearing problems often lead to significant physical, social, and emotional problems (Crews 1994; Jerger et al. 1995; Maino 1996). Incontinence is associated with an increased risk of depression, social isolation, and institutionalization (Busby-Whitehead and Johnson 1998; Thom et al. 1997).

TABLE 2–7. Percentage of self-reported conditions of noninstitutionalized elderly individuals—United States, 1990–1992

Condition	Age		
	65+	65–74	75+
Arthritis	48	43	55
Hypertension	37	36	37
Hearing impairment	32	26	41
Heart disease	30	26	36
Deformity/orthopedic impairment	22	20	24
Cataract	17	12	23
Chronic sinusitis	15	16	14
Diabetes	10	11	9
Tinnitus	9	9	8
Visual impairment	8	6	11

Source. Adapted from National Center for Health Statistics 1997b.

Comorbidity

Comorbidity, the coexistence of multiple conditions, is common in elderly individuals. The Supplement on Aging, a supplement to the 1984 National Health Interview Survey, focused on the elderly population (Fitti and Kovar 1987). Half of the Supplement's subjects 60+ reported two or more of nine medical conditions, the most frequent combination being arthritis and high blood pressure (Guralnik et al. 1989). Comorbidity complicates diagnosis and management of health problems in elderly patients and is associated with a number of health problems, including functional limitations (Guralnik 1996; Guralnik et al. 1996; Verbrugge et al. 1991) and mortality (Dunn et al. 1992).

Psychiatric disorders also often coexist with organic illnesses of the elderly (Zisook and Downs 1998). For example, depression is frequently reported in AD (Cummings and Mendez 1997) (see Chapter 24 in this volume), stroke (Finch et al. 1992) (see Chapter 27 in this volume), and Parkinson's disease (Tom and Cummings 1998) (see Chapter 26 in this volume). Methodological problems beset the accurate estimation of comorbidity and complicate the determination of whether depression accompanying organic illness is secondary or unrelated to the illness (Tandberg et al. 1997). Moreover, these disorders have clinical features that overlap with those of depression and make assessment difficult (Kramer and Reifler 1992; Tom and Cummings 1998; Zisook and Downs 1998). Whatever the precise risk of depression in AD, stroke, or Parkinson's disease, any such comorbidity in these devastating disorders will add to an already heavy burden of dysfunction. Because depression can often be alleviated in such patients, it is important that they be evaluated for depression (Cummings and Mendez 1997; Tom and Cummings 1998).

Functional Limitations

The well-being of the elderly population is measured primarily in terms of functional abilities. Kane (1990) wrote, "Function is the common language of gerontology" (p. 15). Impairment of physical and psychological function is associated with an enormous number of health problems, including greater risk of specific conditions and injuries, such as fractures, increased probability of institutionalization, and higher mortality (Guralnik et al. 1996, 1997).

If, however, function is the lingua franca of geriatric neuropsychiatric research and practice, it is a language with many dialects: functional ability has many components, and for each there is a multitude of assessment instruments (Guralnik and LaCroix 1992; Guralnik et al. 1996), each with its own set of problems of application and interpretation (Rodgers and Miller 1997; Thomas et al. 1998; Wiener et al. 1990). In population-based surveys, the most common assessments are of activities of daily living (ADLs) and instrumental activities of daily living (IADLs). ADLs reflect basic personal care activities: eating, bathing, dressing, getting in and out of bed or a chair ("transferring"), using the toilet, and mobility. IADLs measure more complex functions of daily living such as preparing meals, using the telephone, managing money, and doing housework.

The Survey of Income and Program Participation, conducted by the U.S. Bureau of the Census, provides estimates of functional limitations for the noninstitutionalized United States population. Figure 2–4 shows the percentage of elderly people who reported difficulties with ADLs. Difficulty in walking was the most prevalent ADL limitation: 14% of the 65+ group and 35% of those 85+ had problems walking. However, only 2% of all elderly in the community and 4% of those 85+ had difficulties with eating activities. The most frequent IADL difficulty was with light housework (Figure 2–5).

Most studies indicate that the prevalence of functional limitations is greater in women than in men (Guralnik et al. 1996; Hobbs and Damon 1996; Manton 1997). This increased prevalence in women appears to be a result primarily of the longer survival of women with disabilities rather than true differences in risk (i.e., incidence) of developing functional limitations (Guralnik et al. 1997; Manton 1997).

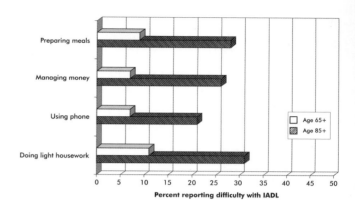

FIGURE 2–5. Instrumental activity of daily living (IADL) difficulties in the elderly noninstitutionalized population, ages 65+ and 85+—United States, 1991.
Source. Adapted from Hobbs and Damon 1996.

Institutionalization

For the elderly population, ultimate dependency is symbolized by admission to nursing homes (see Chapter 37 in this volume). Murtaugh et al. (1997) estimate that 40% of all people reaching age 65 will enter a nursing home at some time in their lives. Nevertheless, at any one time, the proportion of the United States elderly population in nursing homes is not high. According to data from the 1995 National Nursing Home Survey, the percentage of elderly in nursing homes is 4.2% (National Center for Health Statistics 1997a); but the percentage increases from 1% for those 65–74 years old to 5% for those 75–84 years old and to 20% for those 85+. A greater proportion of women are in nursing homes, a difference that becomes especially pronounced at very old ages (Figure 2–6). This disparity by sex is the result of a number of factors including the higher prevalence of disability among women and the fact that, with their greater longevity, women are less likely to have spouses available as caretakers (Chenier 1997). Older whites are more likely to be institutionalized than elderly blacks (Wallace et al. 1998).

Conclusions

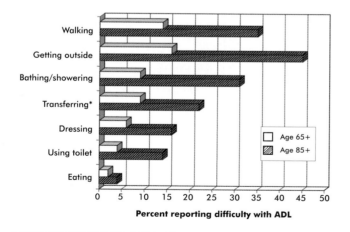

FIGURE 2–4. Activity of daily living (ADL) difficulties in the elderly noninstitutionalized population, ages 65+ and 85+—United States, 1991. *Getting in and out of bed or chair.
Source. Adapted from Hobbs and Damon 1996.

Aging is associated with increased vulnerability to a number of interacting and accumulating disadvantages: physical, functional, social, psychological, and economic. Assessment of all these dimensions is needed to give a complete picture of the health of the elderly individual (Fillenbaum 1990; Turpie et al. 1997). Beyond the specific

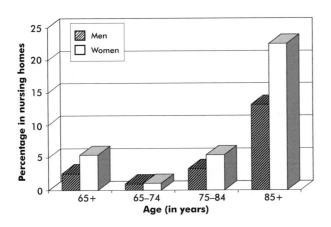

FIGURE 2–6. Percentage of elderly residents in nursing homes, by age and sex—United States, 1995.
Source. Adapted from National Center for Health Statistics 1997a.

impact that each dimension has on the well-being of elderly people, together they create a complex matrix of cause and effect (Fried and Wallace 1992). Furthermore, the health of an elderly person often greatly affects others. In 1991, 4.5 million elderly living in the community needed help with ADLs (Hobbs and Damon 1996). More than one-third of caregivers are themselves over 65 years old (Stone and Kemper 1989). Informal caregivers, often female relatives, are at increased risk for health problems, both physical and psychological (Chenier 1997; Schulz et al. 1995; Wijeratne 1997). In many instances, the caregiver is as appropriate an intervention target as the patient (Chenier 1997) (see Chapter 36 in this volume).

Characterizing and treating health problems of the elderly population is much more complex than doing so in younger groups. The traditional medical model of diseased versus not diseased is often too simplistic to address health issues in older populations, and health professionals need to expand and refocus expectations regarding health and prevention. As an example, elderly patients may have several impairments, with no obvious link to a specific disease. Halting or slowing progression of any one of these impairments may make a critical difference in their quality of life and ability to remain independent.

One of the most overlooked characteristics of the elderly population is its diversity in health. Age "65+" encompasses people whose ages range from 65 to greater than 100. Most research confirms that, with each successive 10 years of age, health worsens. Functional limitations, incidence and prevalence of specific conditions, and mortality all increase enormously. However, people who are extremely old (100+ years) appear to be healthier than those just younger than them (Perls 1995, 1997; Smith 1996,

1997). Also, for every morbidity statistic presented in this chapter, there is a complementary one of health. For example, 75% of the noninstitutionalized elderly population receive no help with ADLs and IADLs (Hing and Bloom 1990); and four-fifths of the 85+ population live in the community, not in nursing homes (National Center for Health Statistics 1997a).

The demographic heterogeneity of elderly Americans explains, in part, the diversity of health. Sex and race are associated with different health risks (Manton 1997). As has been described, women live longer than men, but risks for specific types of morbidity vary between the sexes. The elderly population is also racially diverse. Each of the minority elderly groups in the United States has a different health profile (Bernard et al. 1997; Clinics in Geriatric Medicine 1995; Markides et al. 1996; Mouton 1997; Tanjasiri et al. 1995). With future changes in the racial and ethnic characteristics of the 65+ population, the health needs of American elderly will change as well.

As the 65+ population in the United States is diverse, so are the elderly in other countries, both within those countries and compared with the data presented in this chapter. Although many of the general concepts outlined here will apply to the elderly in other nations, measures of specific morbidity, functional limitations, and institutionalization are not always comparable. Even when standardized methods are used to study the elderly populations of other countries, cultural, social, and economic differences may affect clinical presentation, as well as use of health services.

Much has been written about the compression of morbidity, that is, delaying or preventing the onset of illness and disability so that the amount of active, self-sufficient life in the elderly person increases as a proportion of total life expectancy (Campion 1998; Diehr et al. 1998; Fries 1980, 1996; Katz et al. 1983). There is a great deal of debate regarding whether many measures of health, such as functional ability, are being compressed (Crimmins et al. 1997; Kane et al. 1990). But there is no doubt that, according to mortality and some morbidity measures, the health of the elderly population is improving (Leibson et al. 1992; Manton et al. 1998), or is at least susceptible to improvement (Fried and Guralnik 1997; Fries 1997; Goldberg and Chavin 1997; Vita et al. 1998). Increasingly there are calls to study the vigorous, or successful, elderly (Rowe and Kahn 1997) and to enhance life, as well as to extend it (Lonergan 1991). More than for any other age group, the health of the elderly population is a continuum, and their heterogeneity strongly suggests that much ill-health in the elderly is preventable.

Besides health, other factors are changing that are

likely to have a positive effect on the well-being of older people. For example, in 1991, 8.5% of noninstitutionalized women 65+ had completed at least 4 years of college; this percentage is expected to increase to 22% in the year 2030 (Hobbs and Damon 1996). Because of such changes, women will be more able to make lives outside their immediate families. When they reach advanced ages, these women are likely to be more socially and financially independent than their past cohorts.

In spite of much debate about the health and welfare of our older population in the 21st century, much evidence suggests that this group will be healthier and financially more secure than the elderly of today (Vatter 1998). For geriatric health professionals, a commitment to understanding the unique characteristics of elderly people and the complexity of their health will help ensure that, in the coming century, these improvements will take place.

■ References

American Psychiatric Association: Diagnostic and Statistical Manual of Mental Disorders, 3rd Edition. Washington, DC, American Psychiatric Association, 1980

Anderson RN, Kochanek KD, Murphy SL: Report of final mortality statistics, 1995. Monthly Vital Statistics Report 45(11) (suppl 2), 1997

Balducci L, Lyman GH: Cancer in the elderly: epidemiologic and clinical implications. Clin Geriatr Med 13(1):1–14, 1997

Barberger-Gateau P, Fabrigoule C: Disability and cognitive impairment in the elderly. Disabil Rehabil 19:175–193, 1997

Bernard MA, Lampley-Dallas V, Smith L: Common health problems among minority elders. J Am Diet Assoc 97:771–776, 1997

Bonita R, Beaglehole R: The enigma of the decline in stroke deaths in the United States: the search for an explanation. Stroke 27:370–372, 1996

Boult C, Altmann M, Gilbertson D, et al: Decreasing disability in the 21st century: the future effects of controlling six fatal and nonfatal conditions. Am J Public Health 86:1388–1393, 1996

Broderick J, Brott T, Kothari R, et al: The Greater Cincinnati/Northern Kentucky Stroke Study: preliminary first-ever and total incidence rates of stroke among blacks. Stroke 29:415–421, 1998

Broderick JP, Phillips SJ, Whisnant JP, et al: Incidence rates of stroke in the eighties: the end of the decline in stroke? Stroke 20:577–582, 1989

Brown RD, Whisnant JP, Sicks JD, et al: Stroke incidence, prevalence, and survival: secular trends in Rochester, Minnesota, through 1989. Stroke 27:373–380, 1996

Burke GL, Sprafka JM, Folsom AR, et al: Trends in CHD mortality, morbidity, and risk factor levels from 1960 to 1986: the Minnesota Heart Survey. Int J Epidemiol 18 (suppl 1):S73–S81, 1989

Busby-Whitehead J, Johnson T: Urinary incontinence. Clin Geriatr Med 14:285–295, 1998

Callahan L, Rao J, Boutaugh M: Arthritis and women's health: prevalence, impact, and prevention. Am J Prev Med 12:401–409, 1996

Campion EW: Aging better (editorial). N Engl J Med 338:1064–1066, 1998

Centers for Disease Control: Cerebrovascular disease mortality and Medicare hospitalization: United States, 1980–1990. MMWR Morb Mortal Wkly Rep 41:477–480, 1992a

Centers for Disease Control: Coronary heart disease incidence, by sex: United States, 1971–1987. MMWR Morb Mortal Wkly Rep 41:526–529, 1992b

Centers for Disease Control: Trends in ischemic heart disease deaths—United States, 1990–1994. MMWR Morb Mortal Wkly Rep 46:146–150, 1997

Chandra V, Ganguli M, Ratcliff G, et al: Studies of the epidemiology of dementia: comparisons between developed and developing countries. Aging (Milano) 6:307–321, 1994

Chenier M: Review and analysis of caregiver burden and nursing home placement. Geriatric Nursing 18:121–126, 1997

Clinics in Geriatric Medicine: Ethnogeriatrics (entire issue). Clin Geriatr Med 11(1), 1995

Corrada M, Brookmeyer R, Kawas C: Sources of variability in prevalence rates of Alzheimer's disease. Int J Epidemiol 24:1000–1005, 1995

Crews JE: The demographic, social, and conceptual contexts of aging and vision loss. J Am Optom Assoc 65:63–68, 1994

Crimmins EM, Saito Y, Reynolds SL: Further evidence on recent trends in the prevalence and incidence of disability among older Americans from two sources: the LSOA and the NHIS. J Gerontol B Psychol Sci Soc Sci 52:S59–S71, 1997

Croft JB, Giles WH, Pollard RA, et al: National trends in the initial hospitalization for heart failure. J Am Geriatr Soc 45:270–275, 1997

Cummings JL, Mendez MF: Alzheimer's disease: cognitive and behavioral pharmacotherapy. Conn Med 61:543–552, 1997

Davis M, Moritz D, Neuhaus J, et al: Living arrangements, changes in living arrangements, and survival among community dwelling older adults. Am J Public Health 87:371–377, 1997

Day JC: Population Projections of the United States by Age, Sex, Race, and Hispanic Origin: 1995 to 2050. U.S. Bureau of the Census, Current Population Reports (P-25, No 1130). Washington, DC, U.S. Government Printing Office, 1996

Diehr P, Patrick D, Bild D, et al: Predicting future years of healthy life for older adults. J Clin Epidemiol 51:343–353, 1998

Dunn JE, Rudberg MA, Furner SE, et al: Mortality, disability, and falls in older persons: the role of underlying disease and disability. Am J Public Health 82:395–400, 1992

Eaton WW, Kramer M, Anthony JC, et al: The incidence of specific DIS/DSM-III mental disorders: data from the NIMH Epidemiologic Catchment Area Program. Acta Psychiatr Scand 79:163–178, 1989

Elveback LR, Connolly DC, Melton LJ: Coronary heart disease in residents of Rochester, Minnesota, VII: incidence, 1950 through 1982. Mayo Clin Proc 61:896–900, 1986

Feinleib M: Trends in heart disease in the United States. Am J Med Sci 310 (suppl 1):S8–S14, 1995

Fichter MM, Narrow WE, Roper MT, et al: Prevalence of mental illness in Germany and the United States: comparison of the Upper Bavarian Study and the Epidemiologic Catchment Area Program. J Nerv Ment Dis 184:598–606, 1996

Fillenbaum GG: Assessment of health and functional status: an international comparison, in Improving the Health of Older People: A World View. Edited by Kane R, Evans J, MacFayden D. Oxford, England, Oxford University Press, 1990, pp 69–90

Finch EJ, Ramsay R, Katona CL: Depression and physical illness in the elderly. Clin Geriatr Med 8:275–287, 1992

Fitti JE, Kovar MG: The Supplement on Aging to the 1984 National Health Interview Survey. Vital Health Stat (1) 21:1–115, 1987

Folstein MF, Folstein SE, McHugh PR: Mini-Mental State: a practical method for grading the cognitive state of patients for the clinician. J Psychiatr Res 12:189–198, 1975

Fried L, Guralnik J: Disability in older adults: evidence regarding significance, etiology, and risk. J Am Geriatr Soc 45:92–100, 1997

Fried L, Wallace R: The complexity of chronic illness in the elderly: from clinic to community, in The Epidemiologic Study of the Elderly. Edited by Wallace R, Woolson R. New York, Oxford University Press, 1992, pp 10–19

Fries J: Aging, natural death, and the compression of morbidity. N Engl J Med 303:130–135, 1980

Fries J: Physical activity, the compression of morbidity, and the health of the elderly. J R Soc Med 89:64–68, 1996

Fries J: Can preventive gerontology be on the way? (editorial). Am J Public Health 87:1591–1593, 1997

Fultz NH, Herzog AR: Epidemiology of urinary symptoms in the geriatric population. Urol Clin North Am 23:1–10, 1996

Garrard J, Rolnik S, Nitz N, et al: Clinical detection of depression among community-based elderly people with self-reported symptoms of depression. J Gerontol A Biol Sci Med Sci 53:M92–M101, 1998

Goldberg T, Chavin S: Preventive medicine and screening in older adults. J Am Geriatr Soc 45:344–354, 1997

Guralnik J: Assessing the impact of comorbidity in the older population. Ann Epidemiol 6:376–380, 1996

Guralnik J, LaCroix A: Assessing physical function in older populations, in The Epidemiologic Study of the Elderly. Edited by Wallace R, Woolson R. New York, Oxford University Press, 1992, pp 159–181

Guralnik J, LaCroix A, Everett D, et al: Aging in the eighties: the prevalence of co-morbidity and its association with disability (advance data). Vital Health Stat 170:1–8, 1989

Guralnik J, Fried L, Salive M: Disability as a public health outcome in the aging population. Annu Rev Public Health 17:25–46, 1996

Guralnik J, Leveille S, Hirsch R, et al: The impact of disability in older women. J Am Med Womens Assoc 52:113–120, 1997

Havlik R, Rosenberg H: The quality and application of death records of older persons, in The Epidemiologic Study of the Elderly. Edited by Wallace R, Woolson R. New York, Oxford University Press, 1992, pp 262–280

Havlik R, Liu B, Kovar M, et al: Health statistics on older persons: United States, 1986. Vital Health Stat (3) 25:1–157, 1987

Hebert R, Brayne C: Epidemiology of vascular dementia. Neuroepidemiology 14:240–257, 1995

Heithoff K: Does the ECA underestimate the prevalence of late-life depression? J Am Geriatr Soc 43:2–6, 1995

Hing E, Bloom B: Long-term care for the functionally dependent elderly. Vital Health Stat (13) 104:1–50, 1990

Hing E, Sekscenski E, Strahan G: The National Nursing Home Survey: 1985 summary for the United States. Vital Health Stat (13) 97:1–249, 1989

Hobbs F, Damon B: 65+ in the United States. U.S. Bureau of the Census. Current Population Reports, Special Studies (P23-190). Washington, DC, U.S. Government Printing Office, 1996

Holden C: New populations of old add to poor nations burdens. Science 273:46–48, 1996

Hoyert D: Mortality trends for Alzheimer's disease, 1979–91. Vital Health Stat 20 Data Natl Vital Stat Syst 28, 1996

Hunink M, Goldman L, Tosteson A, et al: The recent decline in mortality from coronary heart disease, 1980–1990. JAMA 277:535–542, 1997

Jerger J, Chmiel R, Wilson N, et al: Hearing impairment in older adults: new concepts. J Am Geriatr Soc 43:928–935, 1995

Jorm AF: The Epidemiology of Alzheimer's Disease and Related Disorders. London, Chapman & Hall, 1990

Jorm AF: Cross-national comparisons of the occurrence of Alzheimer's and vascular dementias. Eur Arch Psychiatry Clin Neurosci 240:218–222, 1991

Kalache A, Aboderin I: Stroke: the global burden. Health Policy Plan 10:1–21, 1995

Kane RL: Introduction, in Improving the Health of Older People: A World View. Edited by Kane R, Evans J, MacFayden D. Oxford, England, Oxford University Press, 1990, pp 15–18

Kane RL, Radosevich DM, Vaupel JW: Compression of morbidity: issues and irrelevancies, in Improving the Health of Older People: A World View. Edited by Kane R, Evans J, MacFayden D. Oxford, England, Oxford University Press, 1990, pp 30–49

Katz S, Branch LG, Branson MH, et al: Active life expectancy. N Engl J Med 309:1218–1224, 1983

Katzman R: The prevalence and malignancy of Alzheimer disease. Arch Neurol 33:217–218, 1976

Keefover R: The clinical epidemiology of Alzheimer's disease. Neurol Clin 14:337–351, 1996

Kokmen E, Chandra V, Schoenberg B: Trends in incidence of dementing illness in Rochester, Minnesota, in three quinquennial periods, 1960–1974. Neurology 38:975–980, 1988

Kokmen E, Beard C, O'Brien P, et al: Epidemiology of dementia in Rochester, Minnesota. Mayo Clin Proc 71:275–282, 1996

Kramer SI, Reifler BV: Depression, dementia, and reversible dementia. Clin Geriatr Med 8:289–297, 1992

Leibson CL, Ballard DJ, Whisnant JP, et al: The compression of morbidity hypothesis: promise and pitfalls of using record-linked data bases to assess secular trends in morbidity and mortality. Milbank Q 70:127–154, 1992

Levi F, La Vecchia C, Lucchini F, et al: Worldwide trends in cancer mortality in the elderly, 1955–1992. Eur J Cancer 32A:652–672, 1996

Lewis M: An economic profile of American older women. J Am Med Womens Assoc 52:107–112, 1997

Lonergan E (ed): Extending Life, Enhancing Life: A National Research Agenda on Aging. Washington, DC, National Academy Press, 1991

Maino J: Visual deficits and mobility: evaluation and management. Clin Geriatr Med 12:803–823, 1996

Malmgren R, Warlow C, Bamford J, et al: Geographical and secular trends in stroke incidence. Lancet 2:1196–1200, 1987

Manton K: Demographic trends for the aging female population. J Am Med Womens Assoc 52:99–105, 1997

Manton K, Stallard E, Corder L: The dynamics of dimensions of age-related disability 1982 to 1994 in the U.S. elderly population. J Gerontol 53A:B59–B70, 1998

Markides K, Stroup-Benham C, Goodwin J, et al: The effect of medical conditions on the functional limitations of Mexican-American elderly. Ann Epidemiol 6:386–391, 1996

Massie B, Shah N: Evolving trends in the epidemiologic factors of heart failure: rationale for preventive strategies and comprehensive disease management. Am Heart J 133:703–712, 1997

McGovern P, Pankow J, Shahar E, et al: Recent trends in acute coronary heart disease: mortality, morbidity, medical care and risk factors. N Engl J Med 334:884–890, 1996

McIntosh J: Suicide prevention in the elderly (age 65–99). Suicide Life Threat Behav 25:180–192, 1995

Mouton C: Special health considerations in African-American elders. Am Fam Physician 55:1243–1253, 1997

Murtaugh C, Kemper P, Spillman B, et al: The amount, distribution, and timing of lifetime nursing home use. Med Care 35:204–218, 1997

Myers G: Demography of aging, in Handbook of Aging and the Social Sciences, 3rd Edition. Edited by Binstock R, George L. San Diego, CA, Academic Press, 1990, pp 19–44

Nam C: Another look at mortality crossovers. Soc Biol 42:133–142, 1995

National Center for Health Statistics: Health, United States, 1996–97 and Injury Chartbook. Hyattsville, MD, National Center for Health Statistics, 1997a

National Center for Health Statistics: Prevalence of selected chronic conditions: United States, 1990–92. Vital and Health Statistics. Hyattsville, MD, U.S. Department of Health and Human Services, 1997b

Office of Technology Assessment Task Force: Confronting Alzheimer's Disease and Other Dementias. Washington, DC, Science Information Resource Center, 1988

Pearson J, Conwell Y, Lyness J: Late-life suicide and depression in the primary care setting. New Dir Ment Health Serv 76:13–38, 1997

Perls T: The oldest old. Sci Am, January 1995, pp 70–75

Perls T: Centenarians prove the compression of morbidity hypothesis, but what about the rest of us who are genetically less fortunate? Med Hypotheses 49:405–407, 1997

Regier DA, Boyd JH, Burke JD, et al: One-month prevalence of mental disorders in the United States. Arch Gen Psychiatry 45:977–986, 1988

Ries L, Kosary C, Hankey B, et al. (eds): SEER Cancer Statistics Review, 1973–1995. Bethesda, MD, National Cancer Institute, 1998

Roberts R, Kaplan G, Shema S, et al: Does growing old increase the risk for depression? Am J Psychiatry 154:1384–1390, 1997

Rodgers W, Miller B: A comparative analysis of ADL questions in surveys of older people. J Gerontol B Psychol Sci Soc Sci 52 (special issue):21–36, 1997

Rorsman B, Hagnell O, Lanke J: Prevalence and incidence of senile and multi-infarct dementia in the Lundby study: a comparison between the time periods 1947–1957 and 1957–1972. Neuropsychobiology 15:122–129, 1986

Rosenthal D: Changing trends. CA Cancer J Clin 48:4–5, 1998

Rowe J, Kahn R: Successful aging. Gerontologist 37:433–440, 1997

Saluter A: Marital status and living arrangements: March 1994. U.S. Bureau of the Census, Current Population Reports (Series P-20, No 484). Washington, DC, U.S. Government Printing Office, 1996

Saluter A, Lugaila T: Marital status and living arrangements: March 1996. U.S. Bureau of the Census, Current Population Reports, Population Characteristics (P20-496). Washington, DC, U.S. Government Printing Office, 1998

Schulz R, O'Brien A, Bookwala J, et al: Psychiatric and physical morbidity effects of dementia caregiving: prevalence, correlates, and causes. Gerontologist 35:771–791, 1995

Seshadri S, Wolf P, Beiser A, et al: Lifetime risk of dementia and Alzheimer's disease: the impact of mortality on risk estimates in the Framingham Study. Neurology 49: 1498–1504, 1997

Slater S, Katz I: Prevalence of depression in the aged: formal calculations versus clinical facts (editorial). J Am Geriatr Soc 43:78–79, 1995

Small G, Rabins P, Barry P, et al: Diagnosis and treatment of Alzheimer disease and related disorders: consensus statement of the American Association for Geriatric Psychiatry, the Alzheimer's Association, and the American Geriatrics Society. JAMA 278:1363–1371, 1997

Smith D: Cancer mortality at very old ages. Cancer 77: 1367–1372, 1996

Smith D: Centenarians: human longevity outliers. Gerontologist 37:200–207, 1997

Social Security Administration: Income of the aged chartbook, 1994. Washington, DC, U.S. Government Printing Office, 1996

Social Security Administration: Income of the population 55 or older, 1996. Washington, DC, U.S. Government Printing Office, 1998

Statistical Bulletin of the Metropolitan Insurance Co: Trends in longevity after age 65. Stat Bull Metrop Insur Co 68:10–17, 1987

Steel K: Research on aging: an agenda for all nations individually and collectively (editorial). JAMA 278:1374–1375, 1997

Stephenson R, Stanford J: Population-based prostate cancer trends in the United States: patterns of change in the era of prostate-specific antigen. World J Urol 15:331–335, 1997

Stone RI, Kemper P: Spouses and children of disabled elders: how large a constituency for long-term care reform? Milbank Q 67:485–506, 1989

Sudlow C, Warlow C: Comparable studies of the incidence of stroke and its pathological types: results from an international collaboration. Stroke 28:491–499, 1997

Sytkowski P, D'Agostino R, Belanger A, et al: Sex and time trends in cardiovascular disease incidence and mortality: the Framingham Heart Study, 1950–1989. Am J Epidemiol 143:338–350, 1996

Tandberg E, Larsen J, Aarsland D, et al: Risk factors for depression in Parkinson disease. Arch Neurol 54:625–630, 1997

Tanjasiri S, Wallace S, Shibata K: Picture imperfect: hidden problems among Asian Pacific Islander elderly. Gerontologist 35:753–760, 1995

Thom D, Haan M, Van Den Eeden S: Medically recognized urinary incontinence and risks of hospitalization, nursing home admission and mortality. Age Ageing 26:367–374, 1997

Thomas V, Rockwood K, McDowell I: Multidimensionality in instrumental and basic activities of daily living. J Clin Epidemiol 51:315–321, 1998

Tom T, Cummings J: Depression in Parkinson's disease: pharmacological characteristics and treatment. Drugs Aging 12:55–74, 1998

Travis W, Lubin J, Ries L, et al: United States lung carcinoma incidences trends. Cancer 77:2464–2470, 1996

Turpie I, Strang D, Darzins P, et al: Health status assessment of the elderly. Pharmacoeconomics 12:533–546, 1997

United Nations: The sex and age distribution of the world populations: the 1996 revision. New York, United Nations, 1997

U.S. Department of Health and Human Services: The International Classification of Diseases, 9th Revision, Clinical Modification (DHHS Publ No 80-1260. Washington, DC, U.S. Government Printing Office, 1980

van Duijn C: Epidemiology of the dementias: recent developments and new approaches. J Neurol Neurosurg Psychiatry 60:478–488, 1996

Vetter R: Boomers enter the golden fifties. Stat Bull Metrop Insur Co 79:2–9, 1998

Verbrugge L, Patrick D: Seven chronic conditions: their impact on U.S. adults' activity levels and use of medical services. Am J Public Health 85:173–182, 1995

Verbrugge L, Lepkowski J, Imanaka Y: Comorbidity and its impact on disability. Milbank Q 67:450–484, 1989

Verbrugge L, Lepkowski J, Konkol L: Levels of disability among U.S. adults with arthritis. J Gerontol Soc Sci 46:S71–S83, 1991

Vita A, Terry R, Hubert H, et al: Aging, health risks, and cumulative disability. N Engl J Med 338:1035–1041, 1998

Wallace S, Levy-Storms L, Kington R, et al: The persistence of race and ethnicity in the use of long-term care. J Gerontol B Psychol Sci Soc Sci 53:S104–S112, 1998

Wiener J, Hanley R, Clark R, et al: Measuring the activities of daily living: comparisons across national surveys. J Gerontol 45:S229–S237, 1990

Wijeratne C: Review: pathways to morbidity in carers of dementia sufferers. Int Psychogeriatr 9:69–79, 1997

Yancik R: Cancer burden in the aged: an epidemiologic and demographic overview. Cancer 80:1273–1283, 1997

Zisook S, Downs N: Diagnosis and treatment of depression in late life. J Clin Psychiatry 59 (suppl 4):80–91, 1998

3

Neurobiology of Aging

Richard E. Powers, M.D.

The human brain undergoes senescent changes governed by a complex mixture of biological, behavioral, and environmental factors. The boundary between normal aging and age-related disease can be difficult to mark. Most causes of age-related neurological degeneration involve a combination of senescent brain changes and physiological alterations outside the central nervous system (CNS).

The human brain reaches full maturity in the second or third decade of life, and senescent alterations usually become apparent after age 40 to the neuropathologist. Each human brain has a unique mixture of age-related alterations that vary in pathology, location, and intensity. The rate of progression ranges from linear to parabolic; however, the aging process is progressive in most instances.

Neuroscientists do not know whether human brain aging follows Gompertz Law, stating that mortality rates increase exponentially with age. Theories attributed to the gerontologist James Fries indicate that the body naturally wears out around age 85 (Comfort 1979). Newer theories suggest that death rates may level off for the oldest old (Barinaga 1992). Biodemographic longevity studies show deceleration of mortality rates after age 80 (Vaupel et al. 1998). The presence of dementia predicts poor 7-year survival after age 85 (Aevarsson et al. 1998).

Most mammalian species undergo neurological aging identifiable with gross, microscopic, molecular biological, and chemical techniques. These alterations may be affected by genetic (Hayflick 1985) and environmental variables (Van Gool et al. 1987), as well as systemic disease outside the CNS. Human brain aging research is fraught with conceptual and technical problems. Methodological problems limit the precision of comparing brain alterations to behavioral changes in nonprimate species whose life cycle is sufficiently short to allow easy study of aging (Baxter and Gallagher 1996).

Theories of Aging

Many theories attempt to explain the age-related degeneration that occurs across mammalian species. Aging theories can be divided into the organ-based, physiological, and genomic hypotheses (Hayflick 1985). Organ-based theories hypothesize that human aging results from incremental loss of organ function driven by the immune system or alterations in neuroendocrine function of the CNS. Physiological theories suggest that toxic levels of cellular waste products accumulate over time resulting from free radical damage, incapacitation of neuroprotective mechanisms, or cross-linkage of vital molecules, for example, collagen, deoxyribonucleic acid (DNA), and vital proteins.

The genomic theories hypothesize aging as the consequence of somatic mutations, multiple genetic errors, or programmed cell death. Life span studies suggest that heritability accounts for less than 35% of variance in human survival duration. Human twin studies show that nonshared environmental factors account for over 65% of variance in survivals (Finch and Tanzi 1997).

A conceptual disagreement exists between theories that human senescent brain alterations result from disuse versus overuse (i.e., the "use it or lose it" theory) and those that attribute aging to cumulative damage (i.e., the "wearing it out" theory) (Davies 1991; Greenamyre 1991; McEwen 1991; Scheff 1991; Swaab 1991). Most experimental aging data come from nonhuman models and provide the basis for this conceptual disagreement. Mammalian aging is most often described in the rodent, in which metabolic rates may influence the rate of aging (Hofman 1983, 1991). A 40% reduction of rodent calorie intake will extend life span by 40%–50%. Diminished feeding of rodents will slow aging and prolong reproductive life span (Swaab 1991). Such dietary restriction may lower oxidative stress by slowing metabolism. Consistent exercise will enhance brain vascularity (Black et al. 1987). The effect of environmental factors on human aging is unknown, although rodent studies demonstrate a positive relationship between environmental stimulation and brain size (Anthony and Zerweck 1979; Van Gool et al. 1987). The effect of chronic physical and emotional stress on aging is unclear, but elevated glucocorticoids are toxic to rodent hippocampal neurons (Sapolsky 1987a, 1987b).

Aging and Genomic Function

The role of genetics in aging is illustrated by life spans that vary from 1 day for mayflies to 150 years for some turtles. The human aging process is accelerated as a consequence of several common, complex genetic disorders, for example, Turner's and Down's syndromes, but accelerated aging is the primary manifestation in several disorders termed progeria, for example, Hutchinson-Gilford and Werner's syndromes (Brown 1990). Progeria is a rare syndrome occurring in 1 per 8 million individuals, and affected patients survive about 12 years from birth. Most victims (80%) die from myocardial infarctions produced by disseminated atherosclerosis. These children retain normal intellect but manifest many age-related physical changes (e.g., cataracts, balding, osteoporosis, neoplasms). Werner's syndrome may represent an autosomal recessive disorder, and recent genetic evidence in Hutchinson-Gilford syndrome implicates a mutated DNA helicase as the gene responsible for defective DNA metabolism producing the accelerated aging (Yu et al. 1996). These rare disorders demonstrate the role of genetic dysfunction in systemic aging.

The role of genetic regulation on human brain aging is less clear, as is the effect of aging on genetic function. Most aging research is conducted in rodents because methodological obstacles limit the study of DNA and RNA obtained from human brain tissues. Messenger RNAs for many proteins are present in low abundance and are difficult to study in all species (Finch and Morgan 1990). Integrity of genomic function depends on accuracy of base-pair sequences, as well as on histone content, three-dimensional conformation, methylation states, and multiple other biochemical variables that affect the accuracy and speed of genetic transcription. Studies in rodents and primates suggest that aging may simultaneously alter DNA base-pair sequence, genetic repair mechanisms, mRNA metabolism, posttranslational modification, protein biochemistry, and axonal transport. Telomere loss may control senescence and might constitute a "mitotic clock" (Ehrenstein 1998; Fossel 1998). The telomere is synthesized by the ribonucleoprotein enzyme telomerase, and this segment of amino acid repeats is located at the ends of each chromosome. Every human chromosome must have telomeres of sufficient length to ensure replicative function. A threshold telomerase activity may be necessary to sustain sufficient telomere length to protect this replicative ability. Telomeric dysregulation may promote several age-related diseases such as cancer or macular degeneration (Bodnar 1998).

Other genetic theories suggest that aging results from multiple genomic errors accumulated over time. Experimental models involving irradiated animals or others exposed to mutagens fail to show accelerated aging (Hayflick 1985). Age-related reactivation of X-linked genes may increase the expression in females of steroid sulfatase and monoamine oxidase A (MOA-A) (Wareham et al. 1987). Age-related demethylation of 5-methyldeoxycitidine can also occur in aging. Aged rodent DNA shows age-dependent change of excision repair and reduction of single-strand break repair (Niedermuller et al. 1985). Nongenomic mitochondrial DNA lacks repair mechanisms. Specific biomarkers for oxidative damage are increased 10-fold in human mitochondrial DNA over nuclear DNA and 15-fold in neuronal DNA from individuals over age 70. Although mitochondrial DNA exhibits high rates of age-related defects, mitochondria DNA damage is not clearly linked to neuronal death (Tomei and Umansky 1998). The quantity of mutated mitochondrial DNA may be small in comparison to the size of available genetic material. Mitochondrial mutations may need to exceed 50%—80% of the mitochondrial genomic pool for clinical expression (Johnson 1999). The significance of cumulative age-related oxidate damage to DNA is unclear (Johnson et al. 1999).

Brain RNA content changes with age. The RNA repertoire is not drastically altered with aging; however, selected RNAs are increased or decreased (Finch and Morgan 1990). For instance, the abundance of pro-opiomelanocortin mRNA decreases by 30% in aging rodents, whereas luteinizing hormone-releasing hormone production remains constant (Finch and Morgan 1990). Total RNA content and poly(A) RNA do not significantly change in aging rodent or primate brain, but selected human RNA, such as tachykinin message in hypothalamus, is increased (Rance and Young 1991). Reductions of nuclear or nucleolar size in neurons of elderly humans suggest diminished gene or RNA activity. Selected human neuronal populations have reductions in nuclear and nucleolar volumes that reflect perikaryal atrophy. Nucleolar shrinkage may result from decreased transcription of ribosomal RNA cistrons and diminished assembly of ribosomes. Neuron populations damaged by neurofibrillary tangles have reduced RNA metabolism as well (Doebler et al. 1987).

Studies in aging rodents show slowing of protein synthesis and axonal transport. Increased amounts of conformationally altered, inactive enzymes accumulate in aging rodents (Finch and Morgan 1990; Ingvar et al. 1985). Some proteins are produced simultaneously by astrocytes and neurons. The interpretation of neuronal protein content is complicated by age- and disease-related increases in the numbers of astrocytes (Frederickson 1992). For example, stability in the number of adrenergic receptors in aging rodents may reflect diminished numbers of neuronal receptors counterbalanced by increased numbers of astrocytes with this molecule. The increased number of astrocytes in aging human brain may obscure similar alterations (Finch and Morgan 1990).

Age-related changes in posttranslational modification of proteins can produce accumulations of advanced glycation end-products in pyramidal neurons. The production of these complex molecules is increased by oxidative stress and inhibited by free radical scavengers or thiol antioxidants (Münch et al. 1996, 1998). This family of glycosylated proteins may contribute to free radical damage, amyloid deposition, and neurofibrillary degeneration (Münch et al. 1997).

Apoptosis

Apoptosis, a word derived from Greek *apo* (away from) and *ptosis* (falling), refers to cell death mediated by intrinsic cellular physiology. Multiple stimuli trigger apoptosis such as

DNA damage, steroid hormones, deficiency of trophic factors, and expression of specific genetic regulators like the Bak gene (Johnson 1999; Obaini et al. 1999). Neuronal apoptosis occurs during normal brain development as well as in pathological states such as ischemia or β-amyloid peptide toxicity (Bredesen 1995). The biochemical mechanisms of neuronal apoptosis are unclear. Initiation factors produce cellular alterations such as nuclear chromatin condensation and DNA fragmentation. Multiple cellular events may induce this cascade including mitochondrial dysfunction (Tatton and Chalmer-Redmon 1998). Apoptotic neurons are difficult to identify, but research suggests that apoptosis may occur in Alzheimer's disease and Parkinson's disease (Bredesen 1995).

Aging and Oxidative Stress

Oxidative stress may contribute to aging and neurodegenerative diseases (Joseph et al. 1998; Mecocci et al. 1993). Oxidative damage is produced by extrametabolic insults, for example, pollution and radiation or intrinsic metabolic sources. Approximately 2%–3% of oxygen consumed by cells results in oxygen-free radicals. Electron transport systems within mitochondrial membrane produce oxygen-derived superoxide (O_{2-}) in response to free radicals as well as multiple other toxic products, for example, hydrogen peroxide (H_2O_2) and hydroxyl radicals (OH). Nitric oxide is another free radical that may contribute to N-methyl-D-aspartate–mediated neurotoxicity from stroke.

Multiple antioxidant defenses remove excess superoxides and H_2O_2 including superoxide dismutase catalase and multiple peroxidases. Glutathione, vitamin E, and ascorbic acid also function as antioxidants.

Healthy aging may require a proper balance of free radical production and detoxification. Oxidative stress may result from increased sensitivity to free radical damage, decreased antioxidant protection, altered calcium homeostasis, or impaired ability to repair damage. Human serum antioxidant levels remain constant over time. Serum antioxidant levels like those of ascorbic acid and β-carotene are positively related to cognitive function in subjects over age 65 (Perrig et al. 1997). Mitochondrial failure and free radical damage are hypothesized causes of both Parkinson's and Alzheimer's diseases as well as amyotrophic lateral sclerosis (Beal 1998; Mizuno et al. 1998), supporting the use of antioxidants to prevent neurological damage.

Normal Versus Abnormal Brain Aging

The neuropathological distinctions between "normal" aging and disease are frequently obscure and confused by conflicting literature. For example, senile plaques, amyloid deposits, and cholinergic deficits were considered disease markers until studies demonstrated similar alterations in brains of some cognitively intact elderly humans (Ball et al. 1997; Berg et al. 1998; Braak and Braak 1997; Crystal et al. 1988; Jellinger 1997; Troncoso et al. 1996) (Table 3–1). Subtle anoxic neuronal injury can be extremely difficult to identify, and considerable ischemic damage may escape detection by standard histopathological methods (Garcia 1992). Clinicopathological correlations can be confused by the lack of diagnostic sophistication and understanding of neurodegenerative disorders by pathologists (Powers et al. 1989). Some neuropathologists propose a continuum from normal aging through pathological aging to disease states (Dickson 1997). These unresolved clinical and pathological distinctions between aging and disease will continue until more sophisticated markers of disease are available (Table 3–1).

Neurons, astrocytes, oligodendrocytes, microglia, and blood vessels are the major cellular constituents of human CNS (Figure 3–1). The neuropil is the woven fabric of the cortex that includes neuronal and astrocytic processes. A normal neuron has a large nucleus, prominent nucleolus, conspicuous dendrites, and straight, thin axons that are difficult to visualize in routine preparations (Figure 3–1). Neuronal atrophy is defined by a decrease in size of the cell body (perikaryon), nucleus, and nucleolus and retraction or loss of dendritic arborization. Neural vulnerability to age-related damage depends on connectivity and neuronal physiology. Senescent changes of glia and vascular tissue

may contribute to neural dysfunction or neurodegenerative disorders as well as to atrophy or death of neurons. Neurons do not replicate in the mature brain; however, plasticity allows them to reorganize synapses and dendritic arborizations. Age-related changes can influence the availability of a specific neurotransmitter by altering production, release, reuptake, and transport. The number and affinity of receptors can either increase or decrease for transmitters depleted by senescent changes. The molecular promoters of neuronal plasticity and reinnervation are altered in aging. Trophic factors, such as nerve growth factor, may play important roles in preventing or slowing the aging process. Each of these brain components changes with senescence; however, none will discriminate normal brain aging from disease. No scientific consensus exists for the definition, causes, or consequences of normal brain aging. Few studies examine these issues in the very old (i.e., those who are over age 85).

In this chapter, I describe important gross, microscopic, neurochemical, and molecular biological alterations of aging human brain. Aging human neurons may enter a complicated cascade of atrophy, hypertrophy, synaptic reorganization, or death. The presence of changes such as cortical atrophy, senile plaques, amyloid deposits, or cholinergic deficits does not always predict neuropsychiatric sequelae. The severity of histopathological alterations, lesion location, and other cumulative brain damage is also important.

Neuronal Alterations in Aging: The Hippocampus as a Model

Normal Intrinsic Hippocampal Connections

The hippocampus is frequently studied because most mammalian species have hippocampi with well-defined neuronal population, consistent morphology, and similar connectivity (Rosene and Van Hoesen 1986). The hippocampus is the center of a series of interconnected structures termed the limbic lobes (Figure 3–2).

The hippocampus is an allocortical structure (i.e., three-layered cortex) and adjacent parahippocampal cortex is neocortex (i.e., six-layered cortex). These structures are usually altered in human aging and damaged in neurodevelopmental as well as neurodegenerative diseases (Braak and Braak 1991; Powers 1999). Brain imaging studies in large numbers of nondemented aged subjects demonstrate hippocampal atrophy in 29% of normal elders with diminished volume correlated to increasing age

TABLE 3–1. Comparison of age- and disease-related alterations usually present in brains of elderly (65 years or older) people

Pathology	Cortical alterations in elderly, cognitively intact subjects	Cortical alterations in subjects with Alzheimer's disease
Atrophy or ventriculomegaly	0–2+	0–3+
Senile plaques	0–2+	3+
Neurofibrillary tangles	0–1+	0–3+
Presence of amyloid	0–2+	0–3+
Dystrophic neurites	0–1+	1+–3+

Note.   0 = none; 1+ = mild; 2+ = moderate; 3+ = severe.

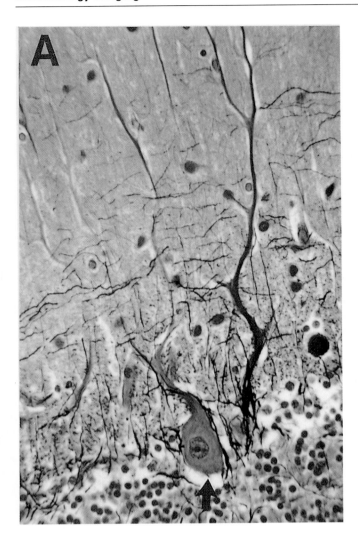

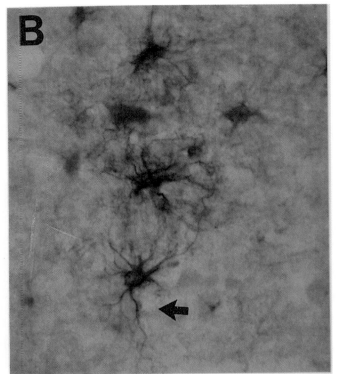

FIGURE 3–1. Normal neurons and reactive astrocytes. *Panel A:* A silver preparation of human cerebellum demonstrating Purkinje cell (*arrow*) with a prominent nucleus and nucleolus. Many straight, thin axons are seen. *Panel B:* An immunocytochemical stain of reactive astrocytes using antibodies to glial fibrillary acidic protein (GFAP). These astrocytes have many long, thin processes and variable amounts of cytoplasm (*arrow*).

(DeLeon et al. 1997) (Figure 3–3).

The hippocampus, entorhinal cortex, and associated parahippocampal cortices span 3.5 cm of the mesial temporal lobe (Figure 3–2). The hippocampal formation is important for short-term memory, and transmission through this allocortical structure proceeds in an orderly fashion (Figure 3–3, *panels A* and *B*). Afferent inputs originate from layer II of entorhinal cortex and synapse on dendrites of granule cells in the molecular layer of the dentate gyrus (Figures 3–3 and 3–4). Transmission proceeds to the CA4-CA3 region via mossy fibers and then to the CA1 subiculum via axons termed the Schaffer collaterals. Information is relayed out to the deeper layers of the entorhinal cortex, that is, layer IV, and to neocortical regions such as the temporal lobe (Figure 3–3, *panel C*). Important basal forebrain cholinergic inputs project to the dentate gyrus (Decker 1987) and synapse on the dendrites of granule cells in the molecular layer (Rosene and Van Hoesen 1986). Noradrenergic and serotonergic fibers project onto neu-

rons in the CA4 through CA1 (Powers et al. 1988; Rosene and Van Hoesen 1986). Adrenergic and serotonergic receptors are present in hippocampus, and rodent studies show that these catecholamines will facilitate or synchronize hippocampal transmission (Rosene and Von Hoesen 1986).

GABAergic[1] and peptidergic neurons are present in CA4 and provide inhibitory transmission. Proper hippocampal function depends on a balance of these excitatory, inhibitory, and neuromodulatory transmitters.

Cellular Hippocampal Alterations With Normal Aging

A range of neuronal alterations occurs in hippocampus of aging human brains. An age-related decline in volume and numbers of hippocampal neurons (Simic et al. 1997), particularly in CA1 and subiculum is confirmed by stereo-

---

[1] GABA, γ-aminobutyric acid.

logical techniques that provide the most accurate assessments (West 1993). Older studies show that the number of granule cell neurons in the dentate gyrus is reduced by 15% when comparing young to old subjects (Dam 1979) (Table 3–2). These small neurons provide a useful model for age-related changes (Figure 3–4). The dendritic tree of granule cells increases in 50- to 70-year-old humans and declines in the very old (those over 90) or those with Alz-

heimer's disease (Flood and Coleman 1988). This proliferation may reflect attempts by intact granule cell neurons to compensate for the senescent loss of neighboring neurons (Flood et al. 1985). Loss of inputs from neurons in entorhinal cortex results in sprouting by axons from other afferent neurons to fill the vacant synapses. Collateral axons develop from cholinergic neurons, intrinsic hippocampal neurons, and neurons of other temporal lobe areas

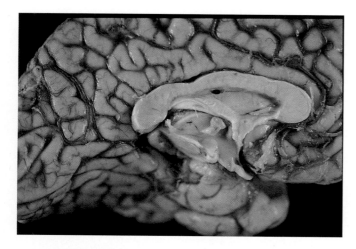

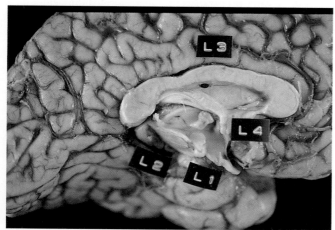

FIGURE 3–2.   The limbic lobe is a system of interconnected structures including temporal lobe (L1 and L2), cingulate gyrus (L3), and basal forebrain (L4). This mid-sagittal section of brain demonstrates corpus callosum and mesial temporal lobe structures visualized after removal of brainstem. Four major components of the limbic system include: 1) amygdala and associated uncinate cortices, 2) hippocampus and parahippocampal cortices, 3) cingulate gyrus, and 4) hypothalamus where the fornix enters the mammillary bodies. The hippocampus courses lateral to the mesial temporal cortex (L1 and L2), spanning approximately 3.5 cm of the temporal lobe and swings around the splenium of the corpus callosum. Entorhinal cortex spreads over the uncinate gyrus at the level of rostral hippocampus (L1) and tapers down to a narrow band of cells in mid-level hippocampus (L2).

FIGURE 3–3.   Gross and microscopic appearance of hippocampus from elderly control subjects and an individual with Alzheimer's disease. A schematic drawing depicts hippocampal neuronal pathways. (See Figure 3–4 for the cytoarchitectonics discussed here.) Coronal hippocampal sections are dissected from the mid-segment of mesial temporal lobe, that is, L2 in Figure 3–2. *Panel A:* Comparison of temporal lobes and hippocampi (*arrows*) from an elderly control subject (*upper*) and a subject with Alzheimer's disease (*lower*). A normal hippocampus and inferior horn of lateral ventricle are seen in the control subject. The subject with Alzheimer's disease has atrophy of the hippocampus, widening of the collateral sulcus, and ventriculomegaly. *Panel B:* A low-magnification photomicrograph of a normal hippocampus stained with cresyl violet. Important anatomical regions include dentate gyrus (d), the cornu ammonis (Ammon's horn [CA_4 through CA_1]), the subiculum (SUB), entorhinal cortex (ERC), parahippocampal cortex (P) aside the collateral sulcus (CS), and fimbria (f). This hippocampus is depicted in *panel C.* The granule cell layer is part of the dentate gyrus. Boundaries between the four fields CA_4 through CA_1 are determined by microscopic examination. *Panel C:* Schematic drawing of hippocampus depicting the complicated neuronal interactions in a typical 65-year-old human. Inputs from ERC neurons synapse on granule cell dendrites in the molecular layer (ML) of the dentate (intact afferents). Axons (mossy fibers) from the granule cells (GCL) synapse on CA_4-CA_3 neurons that project to CAl-subiculum neurons via Schaffer collateral axons. Neurons in CA_1-subiculum complete the loop with axons that synapse on neurons in ERC or temporal cortex. Each granule cell neuron is receiving many types of inputs from intact (IA) and damaged afferents (DA), from temporal cortices (e.g., from neurons in ERC), aminergic inputs from noradrenaline- or serotonin-producing neurons in brainstem (Al), cholinergic inputs from basal forebrain neurons, trophic factors (TF) such as nerve growth factor, and inhibitory inputs (II) such as γ-aminobutyric acid. Age-related decrease or loss of each type of input can affect granule cell firing and synaptic density. The vacant dendritic fields of some damaged granule cells may be partially occupied by dendritic sprouting (S) from adjacent healthy granule cells. Age-related loss of neurons in CA_1 region or subiculum (Sub) will eliminate targets for axons from CA_3 neurons. Loss of neurons in deep layers of ERC will disrupt outflow from CA_1-subicular neurons. Hippocampal neurons and astrocytes (A) also respond to alterations of blood-brain barrier resulting from vascular damage (BV) such as arteriolosclerosis. F = fimbria.

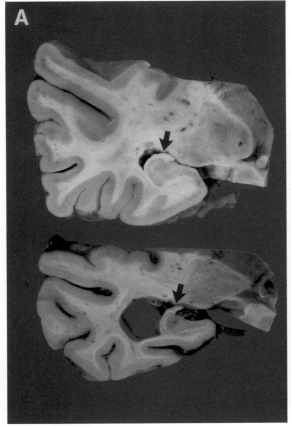

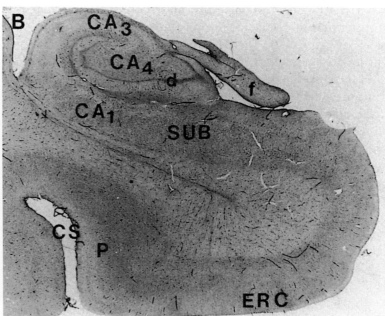

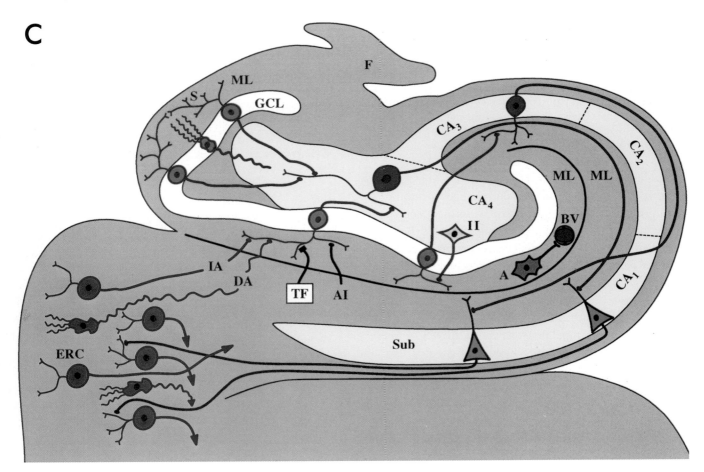

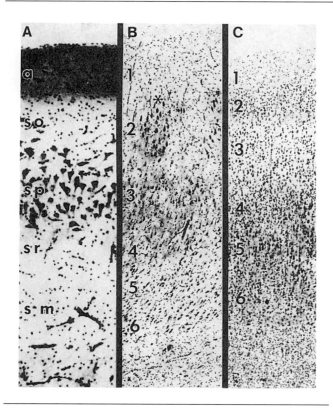

FIGURE 3–4. Three types of cortex seen in human mesial temporal lobe. (See Figure 3–3 for the macroscopic appearance.) *Panel A:* Three-layered cortex from the CA₃ region of hippocampus. This allocortex has an outer layer consisting of the alveus (a) and stratum oriens (so), a middle layer comprised of pyramidal cells (sp), and an inner layer comprised of the stratum radiatum (sr) and stratum moleculare (sm). *Panel B:* The entorhinal cortex, a transition region from three-layered to six-layered cortex. Neurons in layer 2 (*star*) are damaged early in pathological aging and Alzheimer's disease. *Panel C:* Six-layered isocortex in the parahippocampal gyrus.

(Geddes and Cotman 1991). Dendritic extent in the neighboring CA3-CA2 region shows no change with aging (Figure 3–3, *panel C*), although neuronal loss may occur at up to 5.4% per decade from age 50 through 90 years (Ball 1977). Dendritic length of CA1 neurons also remains constant in normal aging but is significantly shortened in Alzheimer's disease (Hanks and Flood 1991). Loss of neurons may provoke gliosis (i.e., increased numbers of astrocytes with more conspicuous amounts of cytoplasm) (Figure 3–1, *panel B*). Hippocampal neurons are sensitive to a range of metabolic insults including hypoxia, hypoglycemia, and excitotoxic damage. For example, the hippocampus contains high densities of corticosteroid receptors. Elevation of adrenal steroids causes dendritic regression in rodents and may damage hippocampal circuits in humans (McEwen 1998). Steroid sensitivity may provide a link between stress and structural brain alterations.

The number of entorhinal cortex neurons remains stable with normal aging. Stereological counts show that a loss of 40%–60% of entorhinal neurons is required to produce mild cognitive impairment as opposed to 90% depletions for severe dementia (Gomez-Isla et al. 1996). (Figures 3–3, *panel A*, and 3–4). Selective injury to one group of neurons in the hippocampal circuit can disconnect the hippocampus and is a mechanism proposed in Alzheimer's disease (Hyman et al. 1984). Cholinergic, serotonergic, and noradrenergic inputs can be lost early as a result of damage to neurons in the basal forebrain (Decker 1987), raphe, or locus ceruleus (Tables 3–2 and 3–3). Intrinsic hippocampal neurons that employ excitatory amino acids can be damaged by neurofibrillary tangles, ischemic injury, or other processes. These processes, disturbing the inherent balance of excitatory and inhibitory transmission, also damage intrinsic inhibitory GABAergic and peptidergic neurons. While the process of neuronal injury and death proceeds, undamaged hippocampal neurons attempt reinnervation and reorganization (Figure 3–3, *panel C*).

Age-related alterations in hippocampus demonstrate the complicated cellular events associated with aging and the severity of cellular damage required to impair function. Hippocampal circuits are important because they are severely damaged in a range of neurodegenerative disorders (e.g., Alzheimer's and Pick's diseases) (Hyman et al. 1984). The resulting damage provides a model for aging of more complex circuits in neocortical regions.

Structural Brain Alterations in Aging

Changes in Gross Anatomy

Normally, adult human brain volume varies by approximately 15% (Haug 1987) for given age groups. The average brain weight of a healthy man at age 65 is 1,360 g and at age 90 is 1,290 g (Dekaban and Sadowsky 1978). The male brain is typically 150 g heavier than the female brain. Gender differences in neuronal counts vary from 0% (Haug 1987; Haug and Eggers 1991) to 16% fewer neurons in female brains (Pakkenberg and Gundersen 1997). Rates of atrophy are similar among the sexes for some structures (Kemper 1984), but not all (Coffey et al. 1998; Cowell et al. 1994; Kaye et al. 1992; also see Chapter 9 in this volume). Brain volume for both sexes is reduced by 0.4% per year after age 60, as determined by radiographic measurements (Akiyama et al. 1997). Autopsy studies show a loss of 2–3 g per year after age 60 with an average lifetime loss of 7%–10% of brain weight (Table 3–2).

The dura mater contains the meningeal artery and

TABLE 3–2. Alterations in the number of neurons in selected brain regions of individuals over age 65

Location of neuronal count	Brain region	Change in neuronal count	Studies
Cortex	Middle frontal gyrus	0–10%	Terry et al. 1987
		28%–40% decrease in large neurons	Coleman and Flood 1987
		0–28% increase in small neurons	
	Calcarine (area 17)	None	Leuba and Kraftsik 1994; Haug and Eggers 1991
Hippocampus	Ammon's horn	19%–43% decrease	Dam 1979; Simic et al. 1997; West et al. 1994
Cerebellum	Purkinje cell layer	10%–40% decrease	Hall et al. 1975
Brainstem	Substantia nigra	35% decrease	McGeer et al. 1977
	Locus ceruleus	0–40% decrease	Mann et al. 1983; Ohm et al. 1997
	Inferior olivary complex	0–20% decrease	Moatamed 1966; Coleman and Flood 1987

TABLE 3–3. Senescent changes of selected cholinergic and catecholaminergic markers usually present in aging human brain

Transmitter	Location of neurons	Senescent change in neuronal numbers	Receptor location	Alterations of receptor densities with aging
Acetylcholine	Nucleus basalis of Meynert	No change or decrease	Neocortex	Decrease in M_1 and M_2
				Decrease in N
	Medial septal region	?	Hippocampus	Decrease in M_1, M_3, and M_4
				Decrease in N
Serotonin	Raphe	?	Neocortex	Decrease in 5-HT$_1$
				Decrease in 5-HT$_2$
Noradrenaline	Locus ceruleus	Decrease	Neocortex	Decrease in α-adrenergic
				Decrease in β-adrenergic
Dopamine	Substantia nigra	Decrease	Basal ganglia	Increase in postsynaptic D_1
				Decrease in postsynaptic D_2
				Decrease in presynaptic D_1
				Decrease in presynaptic D_2

Note. Abbreviations and symbols: ?, definitive data unavailable; 5-HT$_1$, serotonin (5-hydroxytryptamine), subtype 1; 5-HT$_2$, serotonin, subtype 2; D_1, dopamine, subtype 1; D_2, dopamine, subtype 2; M_1, muscarinic, subtype 1; M_2, muscarinic, subtype 2; N, nicotinic.
Source. Adapted from Coleman and Flood 1987; Giacobini 1990; Gottfries 1990; Mendelsohn and Paxinos 1991; Muller et al. 1991; Court et al. 1997; Hubble 1998.

venous sinus systems that include arachnoid granulations. This fibrous covering can thicken and ossify with age. Cortical atrophy expands the arachnoid space, increases the length of bridging veins spanning from the cerebral hemisphere to the sagittal sinus, and may account for the higher rate of subdural hematomas in elderly people (Adams and Duchen 1992; see also Chapter 28 in this volume).

Cerebral cortical volume is reduced in aging based on premortem image analysis estimates (see Chapter 9 in this volume) and autopsy studies. Postmortem brain volume

peaks in the second or third decade and begins a gradual decline that is readily apparent after age 60 (Haug and Eggers 1991). The volume of the frontal lobes decreases approximately 10% with aging, and white matter is reduced 11% when brain volumes from younger subjects (20–40 years) are compared with those of elderly subjects (75–85 years) (Haug and Eggers 1991) (Figure 3–5).

"Atrophy" is defined as widening of sulci and narrowing of gyri (Figures 3–6, 3–7, and 3–8). Frontal (Figure 3–5), parasagittal, and temporal lobe atrophy are present in

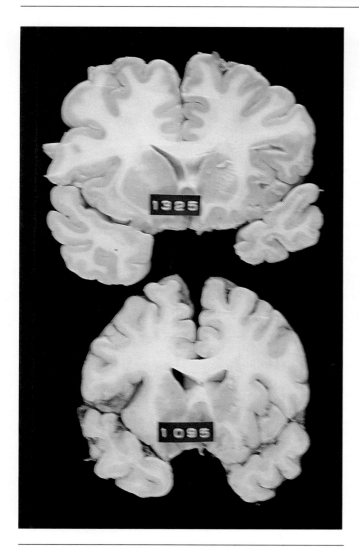

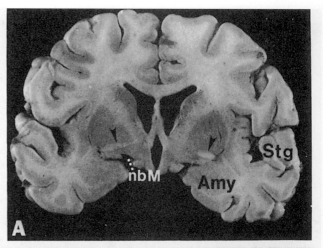

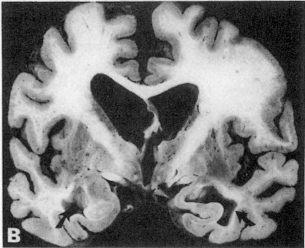

FIGURE 3–5. Normal age-related atrophy. Coronal brain sections of frontal and temporal lobe contrast brain atrophy in an 85-year-old patient with nonspecific age-related atrophy (*bottom*) in a 15-year-old with a brain weight of 1325 g (*top*). Volume loss occurs in frontal, parasagittal, and temporal cortices.

FIGURE 3–6. The coronal sections of normal (*panel A*) and atrophic (*panel B*) brain. *Panel A:* The brain from a 67-year-old control subject with minimal atrophy and normal ventricle size. The anterior commissure is highlighted by *arrowheads,* and the nucleus basalis of Meynert (nbM) is seen immediately beneath the anterior commissure (*arrow*). Normal-appearing amygdala (Amy) and superior temporal gyrus (Stg) are present. The third ventricle is normal in size, and hypothalamic nuclei are located immediately adjacent to the third ventricle. Histological examination of this brain showed occasional senile plaques. *Panel B:* A coronal brain section from a 70-year-old subject with Alzheimer's disease demonstrating atrophy, ventriculomegaly, and dilation of the lateral sulci. The inferior horns of the lateral ventricles (*arrows*) and lateral ventricles are dilated. The hippocampus, entorhinal cortex, and amygdala are reduced in volume. The third ventricle is moderately dilated. Histological examination of this brain showed high densities of senile plaques, neurofibrillary tangles, and neuronal loss (see Figure 3–10).

both aging and Alzheimer's disease (Blessed et al. 1968; Kemper 1984; Tomlinson et al. 1970) (Figure 3–8). Severe cortical atrophy is rare in individuals whose cognition is intact (Table 3–1); however, mild to moderate ventriculomegaly is sometimes present (Blessed et al. 1968; Kemper 1984; Tomlinson et al. 1970) (Figure 3–5). The volumes of basal ganglia and thalamus are reduced by approximately 20% in aging (Haug et al. 1983; Murphy et al. 1992). The volume of the parieto-occipital region is found to be constant (Eggers et al. 1984) when comparing autopsy specimens from young individuals (20–40 years) to subjects over age 75.

Cellular Changes in Aging

The cellular substrate of brain volume reduction is obscure. Atrophy may result from a net loss of neurons,

neuronal perikaryal volume, fibers, and synapses. The number of neurons in human brain ranges from 13.9 billion in both sexes (Haug and Eggers 1991) to 19 billion in females and 23 billion in males (Pakkenberg and

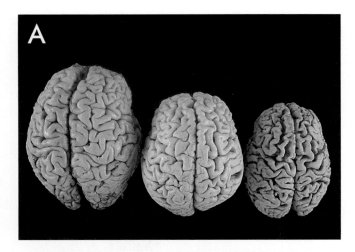

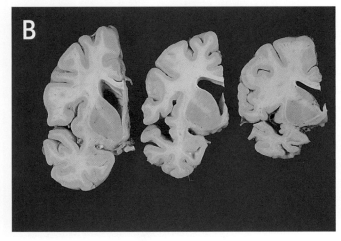

FIGURE 3–7. Disease-related brain atrophy: *Panel A:* Demonstrates the external features from elderly subjects not demented (*left*), moderately demented (*middle*), and severely demented (*right*). The brain volume is reduced, and gyral atrophy becomes more conspicuous. *Panel B:* Coronal sections through each brain demonstrate moderate atrophy seen in a patient with moderate dementia and severe atrophy present in a patient with end-stage Alzheimer's disease. Note the volume reduction of temporal lobes.

diameter and diminished cortical thickness (Table 3–2). This neuronal atrophy begins around age 60 and may be layer specific. For example, neurons in layer 3 of gyrus rectus are shrunken, but those in layer 5 remain constant in subjects over age 65 (Haug et al. 1984). Neuronal atrophy is reported after age 40 in a few cortical regions, such as area 6 (Haug and Eggers 1991). Neuronal shrinkage may explain the net increase in the numbers of small neurons with aging (i.e., shrunken large neurons are counted with small neurons) (Finch 1993). Dendritic changes are common in aging neurons. Dendritic atrophy begins with loss of dendritic spines followed by alterations of horizontal branches and final loss of the dendritic shaft. Quantitative studies using Golgi stains of cortical areas 10 and 18 from aged human brains demonstrate an 11% reduction of dendritic length, but a 50% reduction in numbers of dendrite spines when compared with subjects under age 50 (Jacobs and Driscoll 1997).

Synaptic density declines with aging (Haug and Eggers 1991), and presynaptic terminals are reduced by 20% over age 60 (Masliah et al. 1993). Synaptic proteins associated with dendritic or axonal structural plasticity that control remodeling are reduced with aging (Hatanpaa et al. 1999). Brains showing Alzheimer's disease have substantial synaptic loss, and tangle-bearing neurons contribute to this reduction (Callahan and Coleman 1995; Dickson et al. 1995). Senescent reduction of synaptic numbers varies by brain region. Haug and Eggers (1991) cited stable numbers of synapses in area 6 but diminished (10%) numbers in area 11 (gyrus rectus) of subjects over 65. Synaptic damage may better predict functional loss than neuronal depletion predicts it. Rodents with hippocampal learning deficits and normal numbers of hippocampal neurons (Rapp and Gallagher 1996) demonstrate that clinical deficits may occur from synaptic loss rather than neuronal depletion. The age-related regression of synaptic density predicts synaptic numbers similar to those in demented patients at age 120 (Katzman 1997).

Reduction in the volume of neurons may be offset by a net increase in the number or volume of astrocytes. Studies in aged rodents and humans have demonstrated increased glial fibrillary acidic protein (Figure 3–1), an intermediate filament specific for astrocytes, and increased glial markers (e.g., glutamate synthetase) (Finch and Morgan 1990; Frederickson 1992). However, some authors have described a minimal increase in astrocytic numbers in aging (Haug and Eggers 1991; Haug et al. 1984). A distinct population of astrocytes in the hippocampus, striatum, and periventricular zones of normal age subjects accumulates cytoplasmic inclusions that may result from oxidative stress (Schipper 1996).

Gundersen 1997). Although early studies described generalized senescent neuronal loss (Brody 1955), reports show relatively stable numbers of cortical neurons in many brain regions as compared with those found in younger subjects (Haug and Eggers 1991). Stereological methods demonstrate a 10% reduction in neuronal numbers through age 90 (Morrison and Hof 1997). Hippocampal and subcortical neurons are depleted in subjects over age 65 (Coleman and Flood 1987; Katzman et al. 1988) (Tables 3–2 and 3–3). Some discrepancies may result from methodological problems, such as variations of sampling, and shrinkage artifact. Several authors (Haug 1987; Haug and Eggers 1991; Haug et al. 1984) have demonstrated stable numbers of cortical neurons with age-related reduction of neuronal perikaryal

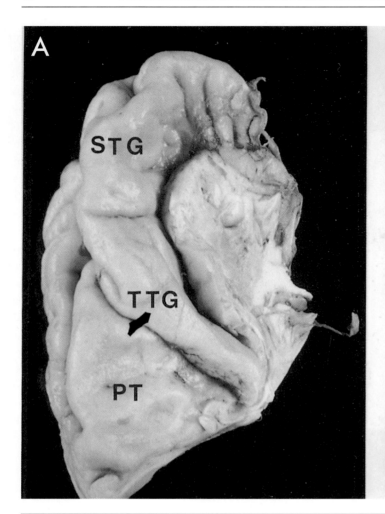
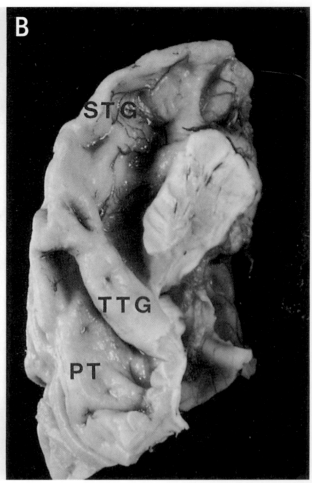

FIGURE 3–8.   Comparison of the supratemporal plane (STP) of an 82-year-old control subject (*panel A*) with that of a patient with Alzheimer's disease (*panel B*). The temporal poles are oriented upward, and the superior surfaces of dissected temporal lobes are shown. The three main components of the supratemporal plane include the superior temporal gyrus (STG), the transverse temporal gyrus (TTG), and the planum temporale (PT); these appear normal in *panel A*. The supratemporal plane from the subject with Alzheimer's disease demonstrates severe atrophy of superior temporal gyrus (auditory association cortex); however, transverse temporal gyrus (primary receptive cortex) is less severely shrunken. Association cortex is preferentially damaged in Alzheimer's disease over primary sensory cortex.

Postmortem morphological studies of aged brains demonstrate variable neuronal loss, relative stability of dendritic length but significant reductions in numbers of dendritic spines and synapses. Neuronal plasticity continues into later life and the loss of spines and synapses may be altered by life-long cognitive stimulation.

Alterations of White Matter With Aging

The integrity of myelin and oligodendrocytes is important to neural transmission, and alterations of white matter occur in aging. Brain imaging changes of white matter pathology are extensively reviewed elsewhere (see Chapter 9 in this volume), and white matter ischemia is described elsewhere in this chapter.

Standard autopsy techniques were used to show an 11% reduction in total white matter volume of elderly subjects (Haug and Eggers 1991). With stereological methods, a 15% age-related reduction in white matter and 17% reduction in total volume of myelinated fibers are estimated, although individual variation is so great that these alterations were not statistically significant (Tang et al. 1997). The estimated total length of myelinated fibers in white matter was 118,000 km in young versus 86,000 km in old subjects. The 27% loss of myelinated fibers may explain diminished white matter volume (Tang et al. 1997). Other postmortem studies demonstrate age-related loss of white matter volume up to 28% (Pakkenberg and Gundersen 1997), with estimates of white matter loss of 2 mL/year over age 60 (Double et al. 1996).

Studies in human occipital cortex from ages 30 through 90 reveal a linear, age-dependent myelin loss in the stripe of Gennari (Lintl and Braak 1983). The optic nerve loses more than 5,600 axons per year (Lintl and Braak 1983) from childhood through senescence. Morphological data on white matter are limited by methodological problems with measuring the volume of myelin or packing densities of axis cylinders in postmortem material.

The confusing clinical and radiographic terminology for white matter alterations includes subcortical hyperintensities, leukoaraiosis (Hachinski et al. 1987), subcortical encephalomalacia, Binswanger's disease, and subcortical arteriosclerotic leukoencephalopathy (Coffey and Figiel 1991; Giaquinto 1988). White matter lucencies are reported in 4%–35% of computed tomography evaluations of elderly individuals and up to 92% of magnetic resonance imaging examinations of elderly control subjects (Awad et al. 1986; Coffey et al. 1992). White matter alterations are also present in Alzheimer's disease (Bennett et al. 1992), depression (Coffey et al. 1993), hypertension, and cardiovascular disease (see Chapter 9 in this volume).

Neuropathological correlates to radiological white matter lesions range from normal myelin to Binswanger's disease (Coffey and Figiel 1991; Gupta et al. 1988; Kirkpatrick and Hayman 1987; Sze et al. 1986). Hypertensive vascular changes (i.e., arteriosclerosis) are frequently noted (Inzitari et al. 1987) in areas of abnormal white matter, as are dilated perivascular spaces and vascular ectasias (Awad et al. 1986; see also Chapter 9 in this volume) (Figure 3–17, *panel A*).

Although the number of brain astrocytes increases with age (Figure 3–1), alterations in the number of oligodendrocytes are not reported. Some oligodendrocytes in aging monkeys demonstrate bulbous inclusions and myelin degeneration (A. Peters 1996). Few studies have examined the composition of myelin and the biological activity of oligodendrocytes in aging human brain. No evidence exists indicating that aging oligodendrocytes develop degenerative changes (as found in neurons) or hypertrophy (as found in astrocytes). The composition of myelin and phospholipids remains relatively constant over time.

Molecular Neuropathology of Aging

Aging neurons undergo a series of histological and molecular biological changes. Lipofuscin, a brown, wear-and-tear pigment, begins to accumulate within neuronal bodies (Figure 3–9, *panel A*). Neuromelanin, a brown pigment common to catecholamine-producing neurons, becomes visible in the brains of adolescent humans and progressively accumulates over years (Graham 1979) (Figure 3–9,

panel B). Neuronal inclusions, such as Hirano bodies, and granulovacular degeneration begin to appear in hippocampal pyramidal neurons (Figure 3–9, *panels C* and *D*). Lewy bodies are seen usually in catecholamine-producing neurons and occasionally in cortical neurons (Figure 3–9, *panel E*). Corpora amylacea, dense spherical inclusions, appear around the ventricles and in the neuropil, where they are numerous in aging and neurodegenerative disorders (Adams and Duchen 1992).

The neuronal cytoskeleton undergoes important, age-related alterations. The cytoskeleton is the delicate meshwork of microtubules, neurofilaments, and other proteins (e.g., microtubule-associated proteins). This matrix, barely visualized with the electron microscope, provides structure to neurons and organizes neuronal transport. The cytoskeleton is a dynamic system constantly cycling through production, transport, and degradation (Peng et al. 1986). Age-related alteration of axonal transport in human neurons is unknown, but slow transport is decreased by 30% in aging rodent brain (Finch and Morgan 1990). The production of antibodies to specific cytoskeletal antigenic sites (i.e., epitopes) allows the identification of molecular constituents within neurons. Immunocytochemical methods show abnormal collections of cytoskeletal constituents in neurons of human neocortex and allocortex in the fifth or sixth decade before developing neurofibrillary tangles (Figure 3–10, *panel A*). For example, phosphorylated neurofilament epitope is normally present in the axon, but not in the neuronal perikarya (Goldman and Yen 1986). Immunocytochemical methods demonstrate accumulation of phosphorylated neurofilament epitope in the body of aging neurons.

Microtubules serve as an intracellular ladder with microtubule-associated proteins as the rungs. Kinesins are specific motor proteins that pull materials, for example, vesicles, down the ladder through the axon (Mandelkow et al. 1995). Hyperphosphorylation of tau is integral to paired helical filaments (Morishima-Kawashima et al. 1995). Tau, a low-molecular-weight, microtubule-associated protein, is present in most forms of age- and disease-related microscopic pathology. Tau gene mutations are implicated in frontotemporal dementia (Tolnoy and Probst 1999).

Cytoskeleton is a major constituent of many age- and disease-related cellular histopathologies. Hirano bodies contain actin (Goldman 1983) (Figure 3–9, *panel C*), granulovacuolar degenerations contain tubulin (Maurer et al. 1990) (Figure 3–9, *panel D*), Lewy bodies contain filaments (Ince et al. 1998) (Figure 3–9, *panel E*), dystrophic neurites contain paired helical filament and tau, and neurofibrillary tangles contain multiple cytoskeletal constituents (Maurer et al. 1990) (Figure 3–10).

Selected groups of neurons are vulnerable to age-related damage, for example, nigrostriatal neurons in Parkinson's disease or corticocortical projections in Alzheimer's disease. Connectivity neurochemistry and cellular physiology can define these populations. Neurons that contain high levels of neurofilaments in the somatodendritic compartment demonstrate more intense damage whereas those with high levels of calcium-binding proteins are less vulnerable (B. M. Morrison et al. 1998). Connectivity and neuronal physiology combine to render specific neuronal populations vulnerable to age-related damage while adjacent neurons remain undamaged.

■ Vascular Alterations in Aging

Vascular pathology produces multiple neuropsychiatric disorders including depression and dementia (see Chapters 13 and 23 in this volume). Population studies indicate that up to one-third of subjects over age 65 have ischemic brain damage that is detectable with brain imaging (Bryan et al. 1997). Four major types of cerebrovascular pathology occur in aging: 1) atherosclerosis, 2) arteriosclerosis, 3) congophilic angiopathy, and 4) hypoperfusion (Table 3–4). Atherosclerosis is damage to the intima of large-caliber vessels, in contrast to arteriosclerosis, which is damage to the media of small-caliber vessels. Congophilic angiopathy is the deposition of amyloid around small vessels in the arachnoid, pia, or brain parenchyma. Hypoperfusion results from hypoxia or poor cardiac function. Cumulative brain damage may occur from a combination of each pathology whose risk varies according to age, gender, ethnicity, and systemic medical conditions.

Appropriate neuronal function depends on the provision of adequate nutrients, like, oxygen and glucose, via cerebral blood flow. Vascular pathology, autoregulatory dysfunction, or cardiac disease can produce focal or diffuse abnormalities of cerebral perfusion. Imaging studies demonstrate a gradual reduction of cerebral blood flow with aging (Choi et al. 1998).

Autoregulation controls the response of cerebral blood vessels based on systemic blood pressure, oxygen tension, CO_2 tension, and cerebral metabolism. Cerebral autoregulation may be affected by age-related diseases such as atherosclerosis, hypertension, and diabetes (Choi et al. 1998).

The brain composes 2% of body weight but receives 17% of cardiac output and requires 20% of the body's oxygen to maintain normal function. The circle of Willis meets the brain's metabolic demand via an extensive anastomotic network that sustains adequate cerebral perfusion despite occlusion of major vessels, for example, the internal carotid artery (Figure 3–11). The tapering of blood vessel diameter in distal branches of major arteries dampens the effect of blood pressure on penetrating vessels. Vessels that branch directly from large-diameter arteries, for example, lenticulostriates of basal ganglia, frequently demonstrate hypertensive damage.

The large cerebral white matter structures such as the centrum semiovale are perfused by long, penetrating vessels that arise at right angles from arteries within the arachnoid space and radiate inward (Figure 3–12). Deep white matter is perfused by branches that originate from vessels located beneath the ventricular surface and radiate outward. The outer vessels are termed centripetal and the inner are termed ventriculofugal. White matter vessels do not arborize, but perpendicular side branches, termed distributing vessels, perfuse adjacent white matter (Pantoni and Garcia 1997). This overlapping system is vulnerable to changes in blood pressure. Subcortical U-fibers are

FIGURE 3–9. Eight hematoxylin and eosin preparations showing microscopic alterations frequently observed in the brains of elderly humans, including lipofuscin (*panel A*), ischemic neuronal injury (*panel B*), Hirano bodies (*panel C*), granulovacuolar degenerations (*panel D*), Lewy bodies (*panel E*), loss of neuromelanin-containing neurons (*panel F*), atherosclerosis (*panel G*), and arteriosclerosis (*panel H*). *Panel A:* Several neurons are shown. Two (*straight arrows*) contain abundant lipofuscin, a light-brown pigment. A normal neuron with abundant Nissl substance is present (*curved arrow*). *Panel B:* Photomicrograph of human hippocampus from a 68-year-old cognitively intact individual who had experienced brief cerebral hypoxia. Normal neurons surround a single shrunken pyramidal neuron in the center of the field with ischemic, eosinophilic degeneration (*arrow*). *Panel C:* Hirano bodies in hippocampal neurons from CA$_1$ region. A Hirano body, the cigar-shaped, eosinophilic rod immediately adjacent to the nucleus, is seen in the center of the field (*arrow*). *Panel D:* Granulovacuolar degenerations in the pyramidal neurons of CA$_3$ region. In the cytoplasm of the neuron in the center of the field, there are multiple, round, clear spaces with a central, slightly basophilic core (*arrow*). *Panel E:* Lewy bodies, circular eosinophilic masses with a thin, peripheral clear space (*arrow*) that displaces the neuromelanin, in the cytoplasm of substantia nigra neurons. Neurons that contain neuromelanin are also present. *Panel F:* Age-related damage of substantia nigra. Two normal-appearing pigmented neurons are shown (*arrows*); however, most neuromelanin is present in rnacrophages or in the neuropil (*arrowheads*). *Panel G:* Atherosclerotic damage in a branch of the posterior cerebral artery. The intima is detached and badly damaged with cholesterol deposition (CD), but the media is intact. *Panel H:* Arteriosclerosis in basal ganglia from a 74-year-old hypertensive individual. A small penetrating blood vessel in the center of the field contains pink, hyalinized material in the media and adventitia.

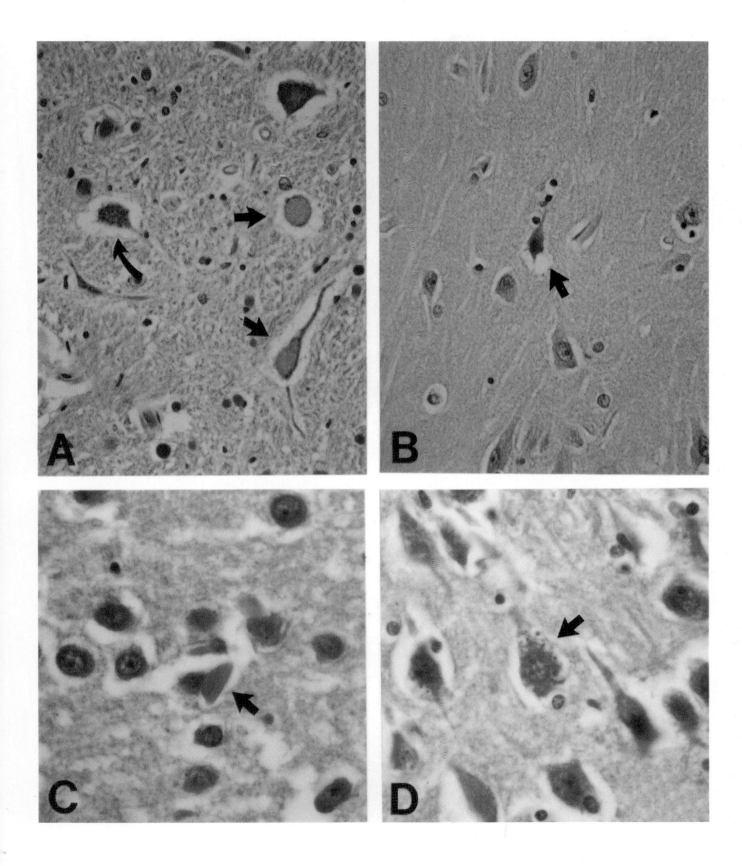

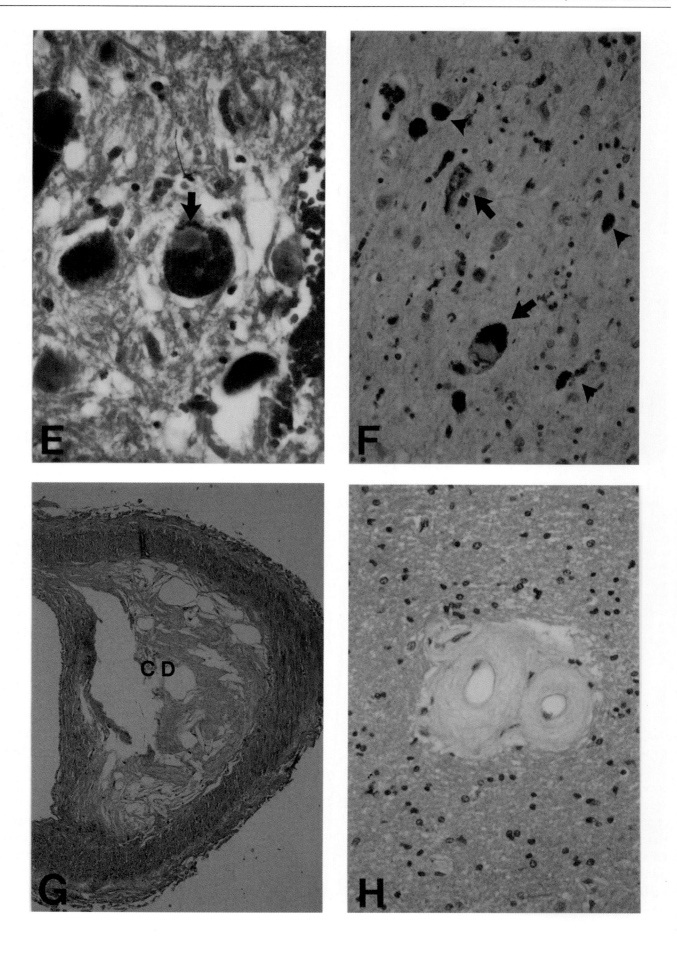

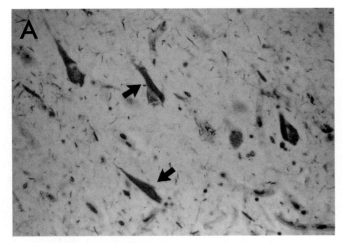

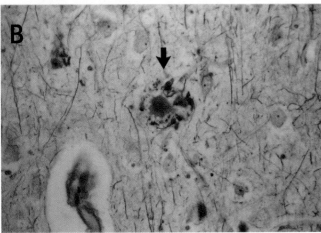

FIGURE 3–10. Photomicrographs showing the appearance of neurofibrillary tangles (*panel A*) and senile plaques (*panel B*) in a 100-year-old subject. *Panel A:* Four hippocampal pyramidal neurons with neurofibrillary tangles (i.e., flame-shaped masses of filamentous material [*arrows*]). Tangles were not present in neocortex. *Panel B:* A silver preparation of neocortex. A senile plaque (*arrow*) contains swollen neurites, an amyloid core, glia, and microglia. Insufficient numbers were present in neocortex to warrant diagnosis of Alzheimer's disease.

perfused by short branches of cortical vessels. The U-fibers are association bands immediately beneath the cortical ribbon, and this distinct perfusion reduces vulnerability to ischemia (Pantoni and Garcia 1997).

Arteries contain three layers: intima, media, and adventitia. The intima includes endothelial lining cells and a connective tissue stroma that prevent thrombosis and control movement of molecules, that is, a blood-brain barrier. Media contains smooth muscle that regulates diameter and accommodates to blood pressure. Adventitia contains a loose connective tissue stroma. Arterioles, capillaries, and veins lack the distinctive muscular media present in arteries.

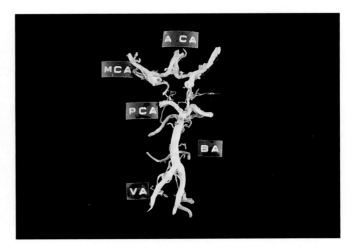

FIGURE 3–11. The circle of Willis as dissected from the base of the brain. The internal carotid artery divides to form the anterior cerebral artery (ACA) and middle cerebral arteries (MCA). Anterior and posterior communicating arteries are not labeled. The vertebral arteries (VA) fuse to form the basilar artery (BA), which then divides to form the posterior cerebral arteries (PCA). This anastomotic network ensures adequate brain perfusion despite occlusion of single major vessels. See Figure 3–13A for in situ appearance.

Atherosclerosis results in damage to the intima of large- or medium-diameter vessels and contributes to most strokes in elderly individuals (Figure 3–13). Atherosclerotic changes are described in vessels of Egyptian mummies, and the frequency or severity of this vascular pathology varies by age, gender, and ethnic background. Atherosclerosis appears as discrete areas of white or yellow discoloration within thickened segments of blood vessel wall. The microscopic appearance includes loss or fibrosis of intima, lipid or cholesterol deposits beneath endothelial cells, narrowing of vessel lumen, and thrombosis on the plaques (Figure 3–9, *panel G*). Hemorrhage within a plaque can occlude the vessel lumen. Systemic atherosclerosis begins in the second decade of life (5%) and accelerates after the third decade. Only 4% of individuals over age 90 avoid atherosclerotic damage (Gorelich 1993). Fatty streaks occur within the aortic walls in the first decade of life followed by fatty streaks in coronary arteries or extracranial carotid vessels in the second. Fibrous plaques appear in vertebral arteries in subjects over age 30 (Moossy 1993) (Table 3–4).

Atherosclerosis has a complex pathogenesis including hyperlipidemia, homocystine deficiency, hypertension, elevated platelet numbers, and a myriad of other factors (Figure 3–13). Intimal damage from atherosclerosis can lead to thrombotic occlusion of vessels or embolization into distal arteries, with resulting cerebral infarction. Extracranial vascular pathology frequently produces cerebral damage. Embolization also results from either atrial fibrillation or

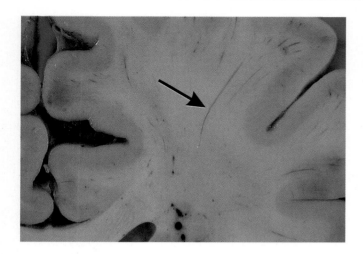

FIGURE 3–12.   White matter vessels. The *thin dark lines* are long, penetrating vessels that pass through the cortical ribbon, traverse into the centrum semiovale, and perfuse a cylinder of white matter adjacent to the vessel (*arrow*). Deeper white matter is perfused by branches originating from beneath the lateral ventricle (*lower left*). White matter structures are sensitive to certain types of anoxic injury, and these vessels sustain hypertensive vascular damage.

myocardial infarction when a mural thrombus forms in either the atrium or the left ventricle (Ott et al. 1997) (Figure 3–14). Liquefactive necrosis and encephalomalacia, that is, discrete loss of brain parenchyma that is apparent to gross inspection, occur weeks or months following brain infarction (Figure 3–15). Abrupt revascularization may convert a pale or ischemic infarct into a red or hemorrhagic infarct (Figure 3–16, *panel A*). Smaller emboli lodge in arterioles where discrete segments of cortical ribbon are infarcted (Figure 3–16, *panel B*). Tiny emboli produce microinfarctions, which are difficult to visualize with imaging and require microscopic examination for identification. Radiographic white matter hyperintensities are also associated with atherosclerosis of internal carotid arteries (Bots et al. 1993).

Hypertension produces a variety of lesions via arteriolosclerosis and damage to medium- and small-caliber arteries and arterioles (Table 3–4). Arteriolosclerosis is damage to the muscular media of small penetrating arteries or arterioles that occurs commonly in small, nonarborizing branches from large-caliber arteries, for example, the lenticulostriate system (Figure 3–17). Vessels with arteriolosclerosis have hyalinization or necrosis of the media that leads to thrombosis or leakage (Figure 3–9, *panel H*). Hypertensive brain lesions include loss of neuropil around small, penetrating arteries, arteriolar sclerosis, lacunar infarcts, and intracerebral hemorrhages. Lacunar infarcts are slitlike lesions measuring 1–10 mm in the cerebral hemisphere (Figure 3–17, *panel C*) and 1–5 mm in the brainstem (Figure 3–17, *panel D*). These punched-out lesions are common in deep nuclei, hemispheric white matter, brainstem, and cerebellar peduncles. Lacunar infarcts are present in up to 49% of autopsy brains, with lesions most commonly found in hemispheric white matter (Figure 3–17) and subcortical nuclei (Dozono et al. 1991). Lacunar infarcts are associated with older age, increased diastolic blood pressure, heavy smoking, internal carotid artery stenosis exceeding 50%, and diabetes mellitus (Longsteth et al. 1998). Hypertensive vascular pathology can also produce extensive damage via intracerebral hemorrhage (Figure 3–18) and associated complications such as bleeding into the ventricles or subarachnoid space. Cumulative hypertensive vascular damage may explain the association of hypertension with impaired psychomotor skills and cognitive loss (Skool et al. 1996; Starr and Whalley 1992).

Congophilic angiopathy is common in patients over age 90. Proteinaceous material is deposited in the media or adventitia of small arachnoidal or cortical arterioles (Table 3–4). Although amyloid angiopathy increases the risk for intracerebral hemorrhage, its effect on cerebral perfusion is unclear. Congophilic deposits probably alter blood-

TABLE 3–4.   **Common causes of vascular brain damage**

Type	Anatomic distribution	Location of lesion	Etiology	Complications
Atherosclerosis	Large-caliber vessels	Intima	Hyperlipidemia Diabetes Hypertension	Stroke
Arteriosclerosis	Penetrating vessels	Media	Hypertension	Lacunes Hemorrhages
Congophilic angiopathy	Arachnoidal and parenchymal vessels	Adventitia	Amyloid production	Unclear
Hypoperfusion	Watershed zone	Cardiovascular dysfunction	Low blood pressure	Pale or red infarcts

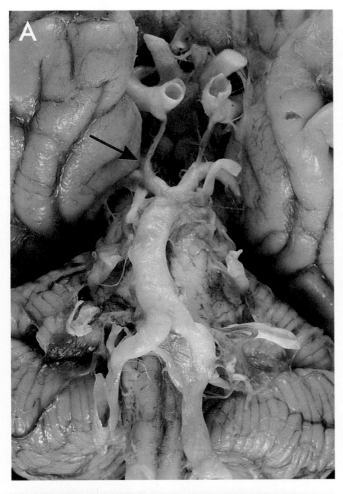

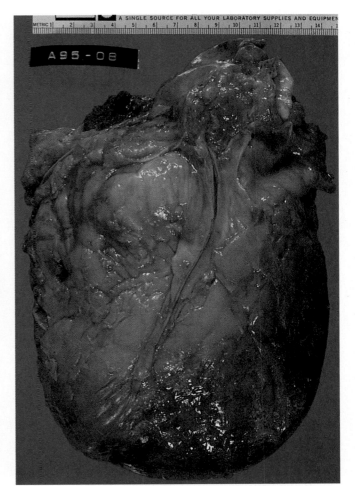

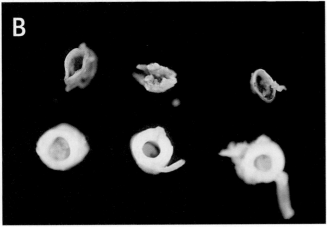

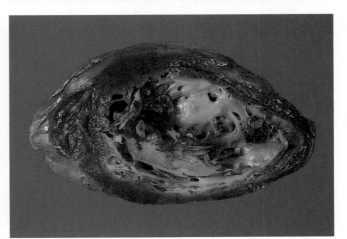

FIGURE 3–13. Atherosclerosis of the circle of Willis. *Panel A:* Typical atherosclerosis in a basilar artery from a 68-year-old subject. Normal basilar artery has a translucent appearance, whereas this atherosclerotic artery has a thickened tortuous wall and an opaque white appearance. Thin posterior communicating arteries connect posterior cerebral to internal carotid arteries. *Panel B:* Cross-sections of normal and atherosclerotic arteries. The *top field* demonstrates normal, paper-thin muscular arteries, whereas the *lower field* contains serial sections through the thickened, narrowed atherosclerotic vessel.

FIGURE 3–14. Cerebrovascular damage from heart disease. Cardiac disease produces arrhythmias and emboli that damage brain. This patient had hypotensive and embolic infarcts caused by atherosclerotic cardiomyopathy (*top*) with a 15% ejection fraction and an apical thrombus in the left ventricle (*bottom*).

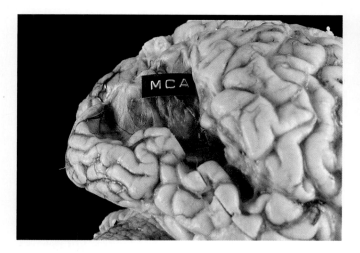

FIGURE 3–15. A stroke in the distribution of the middle cerebral artery (MCA). Encephalomalacia of the inferior parietal, anterior occipital, and superior temporal gyrus regions produces a cavity after a stroke.

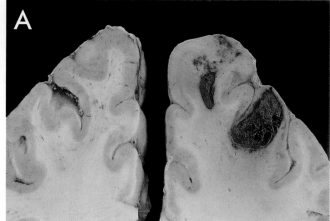

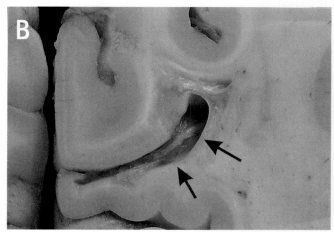

FIGURE 3–16. Reperfusion and embolic infarctions. *Panel A:* Coronal sections of frontal lobe from an individual who sustained hypotensive brain injury after a cardiac arrest (see Figure 3–14). Hemorrhage occurs in necrotic brain tissue located between the superior and middle frontal gyri, a common boundary zone location. Hemorrhagic or red infarcts are produced by reperfusion of infarcted brain parenchyma or lysis of thrombi within occluded blood vessels. *Panel B:* A small infarction in the occipital parietal cortex. A discrete strip of cortical ribbon in the center of the field is absent, but adjacent cortex is intact. This discrete loss of cortical ribbon results from embolic occlusion of small arteries (*arrows*).

brain barrier function in aging (Figure 3–19).

Low perfusion from systemic hypotension can damage brain parenchyma while providing few observable alterations (Table 3–4). Watershed or boundary zones are cortical regions that are located between distal vascular perfusion areas of the cerebral arteries. For example, cortex adjacent to the superior frontal sulcus is vulnerable to hypoperfusion during episodes of systemic hypotension because this region is perfused by distal branches of the anterior and middle cerebral arteries (Figures 3–16, *panel A*, and 3–20). Neuronal vulnerability to anoxia may increase with aging as the brain's capacity to meet energy demands decreases its ability to reinstitute homeostasis and excitability (Roberts 1997). Specific regions such as hippocampus have selective vulnerability to anoxia and excitotoxic damage. Cognitive loss in subjects with poor cardiac pump function (i.e, cardiac arrhythmias), systemic hypotension (Sulkava and Erkinjuntti 1987), and cardiac left ventricular ejection fraction less than 30% (Zuccala et al. 1997) may result from low flow to vulnerable brain regions.

Age-related changes develop in all segments of the cerebrovascular system. Although atherosclerosis and arteriosclerosis are common in large- or medium-diameter vessels, changes also occur in the microvascular system. The density of hippocampal capillary clusters decrease, but the mean diameter of capillaries and arterioles increases in aging (Bell and Ball 1981). Cortical microvasculature studies show intertwining of small arterial branches (Akima 1986), convoluted vessels, and mild perivascular glial proliferation (Ravens 1978). Veins demonstrate fibrous thickening with aging that may slow venous return and increase

edema in white matter. This periventricular veinous collagenosis occurs in 65% of individuals over age 60 and may promote leukoaraiosis, that is, white matter thinning (Moody et al. 1995).

Aging brain is vulnerable to multiple types of vascular damage. Each brain manifests a mixture of embolic, atherosclerotic, hypertensive, or hypotensive damage. This range of pathology explains the difficulty in specifying types or locations of damage that cause vascular dementia.

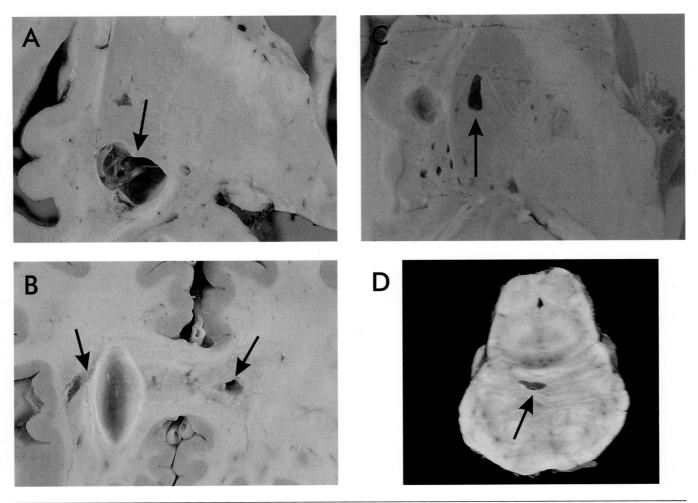

FIGURE 3–17. Hypertensive brain damage. *Panel A:* Demonstrates loss of neuropil around penetrating vessels in basal ganglia (*arrow*). The intact vessel remains within the cavity. *Panel B:* Demonstrates periventricular leukomalacia. Computed tomography scan showed that this patient had extensive white matter thinning. The neuropil about the frontal horn of the lateral ventricle is thin and demonstrates a granular appearance (*arrows*). Extensive atherosclerosis is present in the anterior cerebral arteries bending around the genu of the corpus callosum. *Panel C:* A lacunar infarction present in the putamen. This slitlike lesion is well demarcated (*arrow*). Hemorrhage from such lesions causes intracerebral hematoma (see Figure 3–18). *Panel D:* Lacunar infarct in the pons. This slitlike lesion in the basis pontis can produce nonlateralizing neurological symptoms (*arrow*).

■ Age-Related Changes of the Blood-Brain Barrier

The blood-brain barrier has two major functions: transport of essential materials and protection of brain homeostasis. Although nutrients can reach the brain via spinal fluid, the volume of the blood-brain barrier is 5,000 times greater than the cerebrospinal fluid (CSF)–brain boundary (de la Torre 1997). The blood-brain barrier is located in the brain's microvasculature and consists of tight junctions and fenestration of brain capillary endothelium that use selective pinocytosis to control movement of molecules. Unlike capillaries of non-CNS organs, brain capillary pores do not allow free movement of substances. Carrier-mediated transports in the brain capillaries select specific substances

for entrance into the CNS. This barrier function is mediated by tight junctions between endothelial cells (Giaquinto 1988). The blood-brain barrier is the locus of three essential functions: 1) transport for critical nutrients, hormones, or drugs; 2) export of metabolic waste products; and 3) protection against influx of toxins and osmotically damaging agents (Mooradian 1988).

Histochemical studies of brains from human subjects over age 45 show alterations in the biochemical composition of arterioles, capillaries, and venules (Sobin et al. 1992). Aging of brain microvasculature, described elsewhere in this chapter, may result in minor leakage through the blood-brain barrier. Human serum proteins, such as IgG, IgA, IgM, and α_2-macroglobulin, leak into cortical tissue of elderly subjects and are found in some neurons

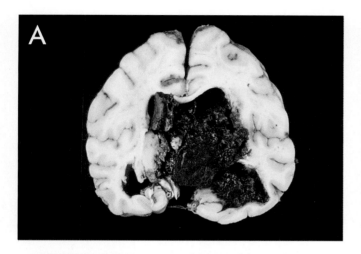

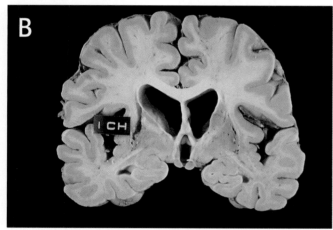

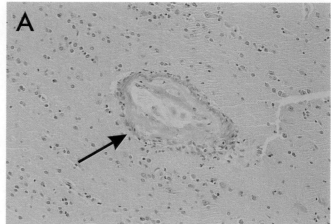

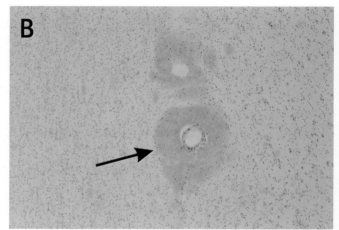

FIGURE 3–18. Hypertensive vascular disease. Coronal sections from different brains that demonstrate acute and long-term consequences of hypertensive damage. *Panel A:* An acute hemorrhage into basal ganglia and thalamus producing cerebral edema and death. *Panel B:* An old healed intracerebral hemorrhage causes a lens-shaped lesion (ICH) in the putamen and internal capsule that produced a spastic hemiparesis. This lesion would also damage ascending catecholaminergic fibers.

FIGURE 3–19. Perivascular amyloid visualized by Congo red and immunoperoxidase stains in the brain of a 91-year-old subject. *Panel A:* The faint-red discoloration of amyloid deposition within adventitia blood vessel stained by Congo red (*arrow*). Polarizing light confirmed the amyloid. *Panel B:* Immunoperoxidase stains of blood vessel, with anti-amyloid antibody demonstrating pale-brown amyloid deposits (*arrow*) around small cortical blood vessels.

(Mooradian 1988). Common systemic diseases in the elderly such as hypertension and diabetes mellitus damage the blood-brain barrier. Hypertension and mild ischemia increase transport of high-molecular-weight proteins through accelerated transendothelial transport and transcytosis. Leakage across blood-brain barriers increases proportionally to severity of ischemia—damage that loosens the tight junctions of endothelium.

Cerebrospinal Fluid and Aging

CSF is clear liquid produced by the choroid plexus within the ventricles and reabsorbed via the arachnoidal granulations located along the sagittal sinus. CSF, produced at 0.3–0.4 mL/min, contains electrolytes, protein, sugar, and

a small number of cells. The rate of CSF production is reduced in aging, and CSF protein content is increased (May et al. 1990). The number or type of inflammatory cells in CSF is unchanged. The physiology of CSF reabsorption is poorly defined, and obstruction of return flow into the arachnoidal granulations may produce normal pressure hydrocephalus. Transmitter metabolic content of CSF changes in aging (Table 3–5).

Pathological Overlap of Aging and Neurodegenerative Diseases

The pathological hallmarks of Alzheimer's disease include senile plaques, neurofibrillary tangles, amyloid deposits,

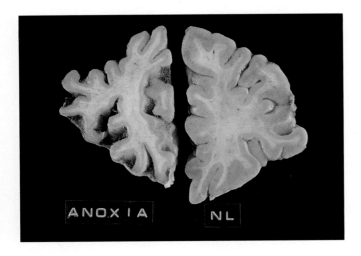

FIGURE 3–20. Diffuse anoxic injury. A normal (nl) frontal lobe (*right*) is contrasted with a coronal section from an individual who suffered prolonged anoxia (*left*). The sulcal gyral pattern remains intact; however, the cortical ribbon is markedly reduced. Microscopic examination revealed severe neuronal loss and gliosis.

TABLE 3–5. Age-related alterations of transmitter metabolites reported in human cerebrospinal fluid

Transmitter system	Marker	Effect with age
Cholinergic	Acetylcholinesterase	Increase
Noradrenergic	MHPG	Increase
Serotonergic	5-HIAA	No change
Dopaminergic	Homovanillic acid	No change
Peptidergic	Somatostatin	No change
	β-Endorphin	No change

Note. MHPG, 3-methoxy-4-hydroxyphenylglycol; 5-HIAA, 5-hydroxyindoleacetic acid.
Sources. Adapted from Giaquinto 1988; Gottfries 1990; Hartikainen et al. 1991.

and neuronal or synaptic loss (Markesbery 1997; McKhann et al. 1984). Senile plaques are abnormal collections of neurites, microglia, and astrocytes that disrupt the normal woven appearance of the neuropil (Figure 3–21). Senile plaques have a range of features and may contain amyloid deposits or cores (Figures 3–10 and 3–21). The appearance of senile plaques ranges from "immature" or diffuse (i.e., amorphous amyloid deposits) to "burned-out" with few remaining neurites (Probst et al. 1987) and amyloid cores. Neuritic plaques contain many dystrophic neurites and glia (Table 3–1). Diffuse plaques are common in normal elders, however the number of neuritic plaques correlates better with cognitive decline (Davia et al. 1999).

Neurofibrillary tangles are masses of abnormal straight and paired helical filaments (Figure 3–10). Neurofibrillary tangles are usually located within neuronal perikarya, although "ghost" tangles are seen in the neuropil. This neuronal pathology occurs first in the entorhinal cortex and later in the hippocampus and amygdala (see Figures 3–2, 3–3, and 3–5). Neurofibrillary tangles probably disrupt neuronal function (Figures 3–10 and 3–21). The nucleolus of tangle-bearing hippocampal neurons is smaller than the nucleolus of normal adjacent neurons, suggesting that neurofibrillary damage reduces metabolic capacity (Jellinger 1997) before neuronal death. Neurons that contain NFTs may survive for 20 years, but genetic function is altered in these damaged cells (Morsch et al. 1999). The density of tangles may correlate with severity of dementia in Alzheimer's disease (Gomez-Isla et al. 1996).

Amyloid deposits include β pleated sheets of fibrillar material composed partially of β protein (A4), the cleavage product of β-amyloid precursor protein, a large transmembrane protein (Mattson and Rydel 1992). Amyloid deposition occurs in aging and Alzheimer's disease (Braak and Braak 1991; Coria et al. 1992; Ikeda et al. 1989; Coria et al. 1992) and is present around blood vessels, in senile plaques, and in the neuropil (Figure 3–18). Autopsy evaluation of brains from cognitively intact elders demonstrates that 75% of specimens contain cerebral amyloid angiopathy (Davis et al. 1999). The role of amyloid in aging and disease is controversial and is the focus of considerable research.

Dystrophic neurites are swollen, tortuous neuronal processes that contain multiple cytoskeletal constituents including tau and paired helical filaments (Figure 3–21). Dystrophic neurites may be axons or dendrites, and these swollen, kinked processes may be degenerative or regenerative. Neurites contain many types of neurotransmitters (Powers et al. 1988; Struble et al. 1987) and are seen in aging, Alzheimer's disease (Braak and Braak 1991; Braak et al. 1986), and other degenerative disorders including diffuse Lewy body disease.

National Institute of Neurological and Communicative Disorders and Stroke (NINCDS) criteria for Alzheimer's disease are consensus values that are based on age-adjusted numbers of senile plaques per square millimeter in the neocortex (Markesbery 1997; McKhann et al. 1984). Senile plaque counts in the hippocampus are not used because the hippocampus is frequently damaged in normal aging. In fact, mesial temporal cortex is damaged in the early stages of Alzheimer's disease (Braak and Braak 1991). The morphological features of aging and disease frequently overlap in this brain region.

Two important contradictions to the consensus crite-

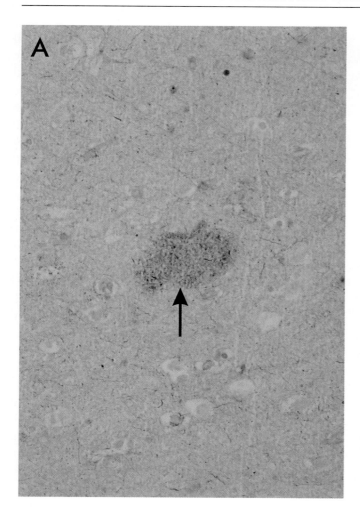
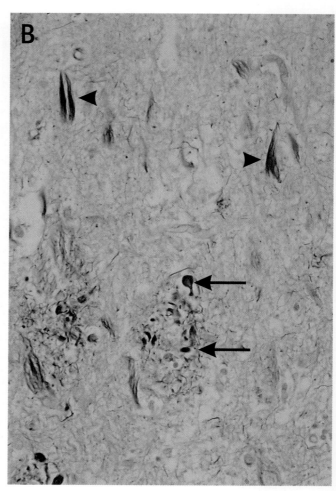

FIGURE 3–21. Immature versus neuritic plaque shown in silver stains of a brain with Alzheimer's disease. *Panel A:* Demonstrates an immature senile plaque with diffuse silver-stained deposits within undisturbed neuropil. Discrete neurites are not present. *Panel B:* Depicts the appearance of a neuritic plaque with dystrophic neurites (*arrows*) and disruption of neuropil. Dystrophic neurites are also present outside the senile plaque. Neurofibrillary tangles are seen in the upper field (*arrow heads*).

ria for Alzheimer's disease include 1) a group of cognitively intact elderly individuals with large numbers of senile plaques in neocortex (Katzman et al. 1988) and 2) a small group of elderly subjects with dementia and morphologically normal brains (Heilig et al. 1985). Some cognitively intact elderly patients can have numerous senile plaques, occasional neurofibrillary tangles (Figure 3–9), and amyloid deposits (Crystal et al. 1988; Katzman et al. 1988; J. L. Price et al. 1991). Longitudinal autopsy studies (see Matsuyama and Nakamura 1978) demonstrated an age-dependent increase in the intensity of Alzheimer's disease pathology. In a retrospective study of neurologically intact patients ages 55–64, Ulrich (1982) demonstrated Alzheimer's disease–type pathology in 25% of brains. Katzman et al. (1988) first described a subpopulation (10%) of cognitively intact elderly individuals who met

NINCDS histopathological criteria for Alzheimer's disease as well as demonstrated cholinergic deficits, an observation reported by multiple other investigators. A longitudinal study of a community of elderly Catholic nuns has provided data on a group of women with limited environmental, intellectual, and neurotoxic variables, for example, diet, alcohol abuse, and daily routine (Berg et al. 1998; Markesbery 1997; Price 1991; Troncoso et al. 1996). Clinicopathological studies of prospectively studied elderly nuns demonstrate Alzheimer's disease pathology in cognitively intact nuns and a higher risk for cognitive loss in nuns with vascular damage. High premorbid intellectual function or professional achievement appears to lessen the risk of dementia, suggesting that cognitive or neuronal reserve, that is, synaptic density, plasticity, etc., may affect onset of dementia

(Snowden 1997; Snowden et al. 1996, 1997).

Neurofibrillary tangles may be a more reliable indicator of brain damage despite a subpopulation of subjects with Alzheimer's disease but without neurofibrillary degeneration (Berg et al. 1998; Terry et al. 1987). No single histopathological, neurochemical, or molecular biological marker always distinguishes normal aging from Alzheimer's disease (Table 3–1); however, some researchers contend that cognitively intact individuals with Alzheimer's disease histopathology would have developed clinical symptoms over time. Other scientists contend that some elderly individuals develop nonprogressive injury (i.e., senile plaques) in selected brain regions. This overlap of pathology between aging and Alzheimer's disease explains the difficulty in creating a premortem marker for Alzheimer's disease (Katzman 1997).

Lewy bodies, spherical neuronal inclusions with an eosinophilic core and clear halo, are comprised of neurofilaments (Goldman et al. 1983) (Figure 3–9). Lewy bodies are present in catecholamine-producing neurons in normal aging (Giaquinto 1988), as well as in diseases such as idiopathic parkinsonism and Lewy body dementia (Figure 3–22). These neuronal inclusions are present in 10 different degenerative diseases and 25% of patients with Alzheimer's disease (Ince et al. 1998). The Lewy body consists of cytoskeletal proteins cross-linked by advanced glycation (Münch et al. 1998) as well as ubiquitin, that is, cell stress–related proteins. Cortical Lewy bodies lack the distinctive halo of their brainstem counterparts and appear as eosinophilic neuronal inclusions best stained with antisera to ubiquitin (Figure 3–23). The frequency, distribution, and natural history of cortical Lewy bodies in normal aging are poorly defined.

The distinction between aging and disease may differ for the young-old, those 65–75, versus the old-old, those over age 90. Neuronal loss and Alzheimer's disease pathology are distinct for each group (Girnnakopoulos et al. 1996), although study populations over age 90 are usually small. Several conclusions are shared by multiple investigators who examined large numbers of aged brains: 1) the number of subjects without senile plaques, neurofibrillary tangles, or amyloid deposits decreases with age; 2) appearance of neurofibrillary tangles can precede amyloid deposition; 3) changes can occur in younger individuals, that is, those age 50–65; and 4) cortical neurofibrillary tangles are more specific for dementia. Prevalence studies based on neuropathological assessment of large numbers of brains predict that 100% of individuals will meet histopathological criteria for Alzheimer's disease at age 100 (Braak and Braak 1997; Davis et al. 1999; Duyckaerts and Haue 1997).

Alterations of Transmitter Systems in Aging

The impact of aging on transmitter systems can be measured at the presynaptic or postsynaptic level. Presynaptic levels of chemical transmitters can be reduced by death or dysfunction of neurons that produce the transmitter, diminished release, and alterations of reuptake. Postsynaptic effects include alteration of postsynaptic receptor density, alterations of the receptor, and changes in signal transduction mechanisms that translate the receptor activation into cellular or membrane events. Signal transmission may be altered at several levels, confusing the interpretation of human data. Although many human brain transmitter markers are altered in aging, in this chapter I focus on systems of most importance to the geriatric neuropsychiatrist (Tables 3–2 and 3–3).

Cholinergic Systems

Acetylcholine innervation is widely present throughout the mammalian CNS (see Chapter 4 in this volume). Most cortical cholinergic fibers originate from neurons in the nucleus basalis of Meynert, a band of large neurons in the basal forebrain that is most conspicuous beneath the anterior commissure (Hedreen et al. 1984; Mesulam and Geula 1988) (Figure 3–6). This band begins anteriorly in the medial septal region and is present posteriorly beneath the basal ganglia. This nucleus has an organized projection to cortex, with medial septal neurons projecting to hippocampus.

A plexus of cholinergic fibers is seen in cortex (Divac 1975; Mesulam et al. 1983), and immunocytochemical methodologies with antisera directed against nicotinic receptors demonstrate postsynaptic densities over neurons in layers 2, 3, and 5 (Schroder et al. 1991) of neocortex. Cholinergic fibers are altered in elderly humans and old primates (Decker 1987), and cholinergic deficits in rodents, primates, and humans are correlated to cognitive impairment (Olton et al. 1991).

No consistent loss of acetylcholine content is found in the brains of cognitively intact elderly humans (Table 3–3). Although acetylcholine transferase, the synthetic enzyme for acetylcholine, is reduced in Alzheimer's disease, the conflicting data in normal aging (Giaquinto 1988; Muller et al. 1991) demonstrate minimal reductions or no change. This minor senescent cholinergic loss may reflect complex alterations in the number and size of neurons in the nucleus basalis of Meynert with aging (Figure 3–6). The diameters of some human forebrain cholinergic neurons increase until age 60. Nucleus basalis of Meynert neurons in elderly humans (over age 60) begin to atrophy, and neuronal loss varies according to region sampled (e.g., 0% in the anterior portion and 65% in posterior subdivisions) (de Lacalle et al. 1991; Finch 1993). A similar sequence of changes is seen in rodent and monkey. The large cholinergic neurons of the nucleus basalis of Meynert are frequently referred to as "magnocellular" and may contain occasional neuro-fibrillary tangles or Lewy bodies in older human subjects. Loss of these magnocellular neurons accounts for cholinergic deficits in Alzheimer's disease (Whitehouse et al. 1981). Aging has a minimal effect on high-affinity choline uptake, the rate-limiting step in the production of acetyl-choline. Levels of acetylcholinesterase are increased in CSF of elderly subjects (Hartikainen et al. 1991; Muller et al. 1991) (Table 3–5).

The density of cholinergic receptors changes with aging (Table 3–3). Release of acetylcholine may be reduced in aging brains because of diminished autoreceptor sensitivity. Alterations occur in both muscarinic and nicotinic receptor systems. Although five types of muscarinic receptors (ml–m5) are distinguished via genetic identification and four via pharmacological techniques (M1–M4), little is known about age-related alterations within either group or their encoding messages (Levey 1996). Aging brain has a 10%–30% reduction of muscarinic receptors in samples of cortex, hippocampus, and striatum and diminished nicotinic receptors in hippocampus. However, in thalamus, density of nicotinic receptors decreases, but density of muscarinic receptors increases (Giacobini 1990, 1991). Nicotinic receptor binding is mildly reduced in neocortex with aging, but significant reductions occur in entorhinal cortex and presubiculum over age 40 (Court et al. 1997). The nicotinic cholinergic receptor family is composed of α and β subunits with seven α and three β subunit genes. In normal elderly subjects, the α_4 nicotinic receptor subunit appears stable, but the α_2 subunit is diminished (Tohgi et al. 1998b). Nicotinic receptors are also reduced in Alzheimer's disease (Nordberg and Winblad 1986).

It is unknown whether the structure of cholinergic receptors is altered in aging or Alzheimer's disease. The ef-fect of human aging on the ratios of receptor subtypes and encoding messages is unknown. Studies in rodents demonstrate age-related decrease in receptor plasticity and diminished neural response to acetylcholine stimulation (Giacobini 1990; Muller et al. 1991).

Although our knowledge of senescent alterations of cholinergic systems is incomplete, a relationship exists between cholinergic deficits and cognitive impairment (Fields et al. 1986). Cholinergic systems are damaged in many neurodegenerative disorders including Alzheimer's disease, progressive supranuclear palsy, parkinsonism with dementia, and other disorders.

Noradrenergic Systems

Noradrenergic systems in human brain include an extensive network of fibers and receptors in neocortex, allocortex, selected diencephalic structures, and brainstem (Fallon and Loughlin 1987). In the human forebrain, noradrenaline is produced by the locus ceruleus, two bands of neurons located immediately beneath the fourth ventricle in the pons that range in number from 11,000 to 25,000 (Ohm et al. 1997) (Figure 3–22). A variable mixture of α- and β-adrenergic receptors is present throughout the cerebral cortices (Mendelsohn and Paxinos 1991; Reznikoff et al. 1986). Conventional counting methodologies demonstrate a progressive loss of noradrenergic neurons throughout the aging human brainstem, commencing between ages 30 and 40 and progressing with a linear relationship to age (Mann et al. 1983, 1984) (Tables 3–2 and 3–3). In the locus ceruleus, 40% of pigmented neurons are lost by age 90, and similar losses are sustained by the A-2 cell groups in the medulla (i.e., the dorsal motor nucleus of the vagus). Stereological estimates suggest smaller age-related loss of pigmented neurons (Ohm et al. 1997) in the locus ceruleus. Occasional neurofibrillary tangles or Lewy bodies are present in these neurons after age 60. Noradrenergic neurites (i.e., abnormal, swollen processes that contain dopamine β hydroxylase) are present in the neuropil and within senile plaques of elderly subjects (Powers et al. 1988), as well as within the pineal gland

FIGURE 3–22. Comparison of midbrain and pons from elderly control subjects and individuals with depigmentation. Regions that produce dopamine and noradrenaline can be distinguished by the brown-black neuromelanin pigment. Serotonin-producing neurons are located in the midline of the brainstem (i.e., raphe [R]) but cannot be distinguished from adjacent structures with either gross or microscopic examination. The ventral tegmental area (V) is present in the midline between the substantia nigrae (SN) and above the interpeduncular fossa (*arrow*). *Panel A:* From an 85-year-old subject, a substantia nigra with some mild loss of pigment. *Panel B:* From a subject with Alzheimer's disease, a substantia nigra with moderate depigmentation. *Panels C and D:* Specimens from a patient with idiopathic parkinsonism with more severe depigmentation on the left than on the right. *Panel E:* The appearance of locus ceruleus in an elderly control subject: a discrete area of brown-black pigment beneath the fourth ventricle (*arrow*). *Panel F:* Depigmentation in locus ceruleus of an aging subject with diffusion of neuromelanin into adjacent neuropil (*arrow*).

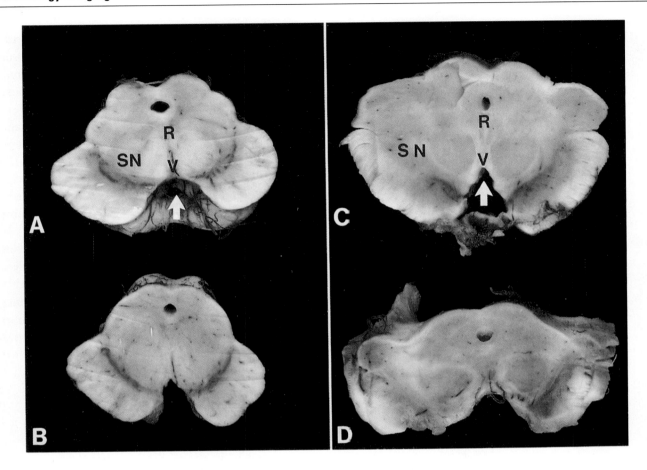

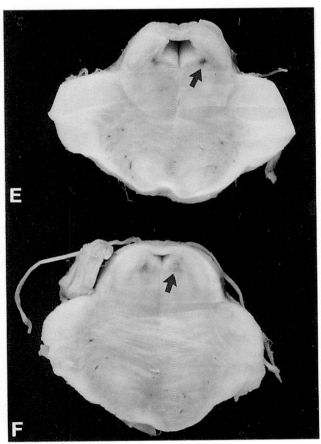

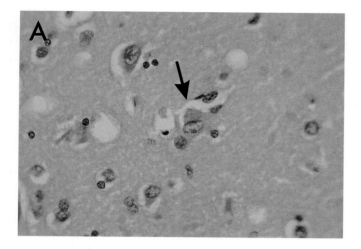

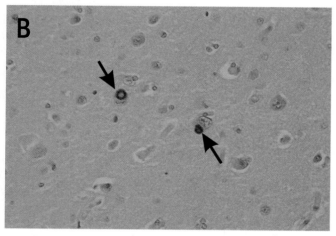

FIGURE 3–23. The appearance of cortical Lewy bodies. *Panel A:* Hematoxylin and eosin–stained preparation through parahippocampal cortex from a patient with diffuse Lewy body disease. The indistinct eosinophilic cytoplasmic inclusion in the neuron in the middle of the field is the Lewy body (*arrow*). *Panel B:* Antibodies to ubiquitin intensely stain two circular Lewy bodies, that is, brown sphere in neurons in center of field (*arrows*).

(Jengeleski et al. 1989). Enzymatic activities are reduced for tyrosine hydroxylase, the rate-limiting enzyme in the production of both dopamine and noradrenaline, as well as dopamine β-hydroxylase, the committed enzyme for the production of noradrenaline. Brain concentrations of methoxyhydroxylphenylglycol may remain constant in aging (Gottfries 1990), but CSF levels are increased (Table 3–5).

Age-related loss of β-adrenergic receptors is region dependent (Table 3–3). Receptor numbers remain constant in the frontal cortex (Kalaria et al. 1989); however, cingulate, precentral, temporal, and occipitotemporal regions demonstrate a linear age-dependent loss (Mendelsohn and Paxinos 1991).

Adrenergic receptors demonstrate a substantial decline in aging human brain (Pascual et al. 1992). Rodent studies also demonstrate age-related loss of adrenergic receptors in all regions except cortex, a phenomenon possibly a result of diminished receptor synthesis (Miller and Zahniser 1988; Scarpace and Abrass 1988). Pharmacological studies in rodent show a progressive age-dependent loss of postsynaptic response to noradrenaline and serotonin (Bickford-Wimer et al. 1988). This cumulative evidence suggests a gradual senescent loss of noradrenergic production and region-dependent loss of adrenergic receptors in human brain.

A relation may exist between the aging of the human catecholaminergic system and neuropsychiatric diseases such as depression (Mann 1991; Procter and Bowen 1987; Veith and Raskind 1988). Poststroke depression may be linked to catecholaminergic function (Robinson et al. 1984, 1987), and depression in Alzheimer's disease may correlate with loss of neurons in the locus ceruleus (Zubenko and Moossy 1988).

Serotonergic Systems

Serotonin is produced by raphe nuclei, clusters of indistinct neurons in the midline of the midbrain and pons (Fallon and Loughlin 1987) (Figure 3–22). Methodological problems limit quantitation of nonpigmented serotonergic neurons in human brainstem. Extensive serotonergic innervation is found in human neocortex, allocortex, and some diencephalic structures. Serotonin content is reduced in selected neocortical and allocortical regions of aging human brain (Gottfries 1990; Morgan and Finch 1987). Concentrations of 5-hydroxyindoleacetic acid, the primary metabolite of serotonin, are not reduced in brain or CSF (Table 3–5). However, imipramine binding, a putative marker for serotonin reuptake, is reduced in aging. Activity of tryptophan hydroxylase, the synthetic enzyme for the production of serotonin, is reduced in the brains of aging rodents.

Multiple subtypes of serotonin (5-hydroxytryptamine [5-HT]) receptors are described using autoradiographic or in situ hybridization methodology (Bloom and Morales 1998; Burnet et al. 1995), and the densities of 5-HT_1 and 5-HT_2 are reduced in brains of elderly humans (Table 3–3). The density of 5-HT_2 is reduced 20%–50%, and 5-HT_1 declines up to 70% (Mendelsohn and Paxinos 1991). Studies of serotonin receptor subtypes are limited; however, the density of 5-HT_{1A} receptors is diminished in aging (Dillon et al. 1991). Depletion of neurons in the raphe nuclei would explain the decreased serotonin content, but not the decreased serotonin receptor density. These limited data on serotonergic systems in human aging suggest a gradual loss of serotonin production and receptor.

Dopaminergic Systems

Dopaminergic systems are altered in aging and in many neurodegenerative disorders, including Alzheimer's disease, idiopathic parkinsonism, and progressive supranuclear palsy (Gibb et al. 1989; Morgan and Finch 1987; Morgan et al. 1987). The brainstem neurons of the mesocortical and nigrostriatal dopaminergic pathways are well defined in human brain (Figure 3–22). Although dopaminergic neurons are present in the human septal and hypothalamic regions (Gaspar et al. 1985), the tubero-infundibular system is poorly defined in humans. A progressive loss of neurons in the substantia nigra occurs in aging and disease (Uchihara et al. 1992). The number of pigmented neurons in the substantia nigra may begin to drop between ages 40 and 50, and substantial loss (35%) is reported after age 65 (Mann et al. 1984; McGeer et al. 1977) (Table 3–2). Nucleolar volume of substantia nigra neurons is reduced after age 65, and neurofibrillary tangles or Lewy bodies begin to appear in small numbers (Mann et al. 1984) (Figures 3–9 and 3–22). Cytochrome *c* oxidase defects indicate an alteration of the respiratory chain function within nigral neurons (Itoh et al. 1996). Relatively few extrapyramidal symptoms are produced by senescent decline because 80% of nigral neurons must be lost to produce the symptoms of parkinsonism.

Age-related loss of neurons in the ventral tegmental area has not been determined (Hirai 1968; Jellinger 1987), but the ventral tegmental area is damaged by Alzheimer's disease (Torack and Morris 1988). Surviving catecholaminergic neurons progressively accumulate neuromelanin (Graham 1979), which displaces perikaryal RNA and reduces nucleolar volume (McGeer et al. 1977). Senescent alterations of dopamine-producing neurons in hypothalamus are unknown. Concentrations of dopamine are reduced in the striatum of individuals over age 65; however, homovanillic acid content, the primary dopamine metabolite, remains constant in tissue and CSF (Gottfries 1990; Hartikainen et al. 1991) (Table 3–5).

Immunocytochemical and receptor autoradiographic studies show an extensive plexus of dopaminergic fibers, terminals, and receptors in frontal, temporal, hippocampal, and parahippocampal cortices as well as basal ganglia (Joyce et al. 1997; Lewis and Akil 1997). Abnormalities of multiple forms of the dopamine receptor are described in schizophrenia (Gjedde et al. 1996; Joyce et al. 1997; Okubo 1997; Sanyal and van Tol 1997). In aging, the density of the D_2 receptor that binds haloperidol in caudate nucleus declines about 1% per year after age 18 (Wong et al. 1997) and 0.6% per year over age 30 for ^{11}C-raclopride binding in putamen (Antonio et al. 1993). The dopamine transporter system also declines in basal ganglia during normal aging (Volkow et al. 1994). D_1 receptor binding declines 6.9% per decade in the caudate and 7.4% per decade in the putamen (Wong et al. 1998). Similar D_1 reductions are also described in the frontal and occipital cortex (Hubble 1998) (see Table 3–3).

Postmortem studies demonstrate diminished expression of mRNA for D_2 receptors in putamen with no alteration of D_1 mRNA levels (Tohgi et al. 1998a), alterations that can result from senescent loss of neurons in the basal ganglia. This decline of striatal dopaminergic activity is associated with loss of fine motor functions and impaired neuropsychological performance, for example, in the Wisconsin Card Sorting (Heaton 1985) or Stroop Color-Word test (Stroop 1935; Volkow et al. 1998).

Alterations of Monoamine Oxidase and Aging

Monoamine oxidase (MAO) activity is significantly altered in the aging human brain. MAO-A, which facilitates the oxidative deamination of noradrenaline, serotonin, and partially dopamine, is not drastically altered in aging. MAO-B, which catalyzes the oxidative deamination of several amines and partially dopamine, increases with age (Fowler et al. 1997; Gottfries 1990). The importance of these age-related alterations is unclear, although increased quantities of this catabolic enzyme may result in depletion of dopamine and other catecholamines. MAO activity is also significantly altered in neurodegenerative disorders such as Alzheimer's disease (Morgan and Finch 1987; Perry et al. 1991; Procter and Bowen 1987).

Alterations of Other Transmitter Systems

A wide array of neuropeptides function as neuromodulators and colocalize with other classical transmitters such as noradrenaline and serotonin. Corticotropin-releasing factor is diminished in aging; however, other more abundant peptides such as somatostatin and neuropeptide Y are not (Giaquinto 1988; Gottfries 1990). Age-related alterations of precursor proteins for substance P and enkephalin suggest a preferential loss of neurons in putamen that produce GABA and substance P (Tohgi et al. 1997). A variety of neuropeptides are present in dystrophic neurites and senile plaques of elderly subjects and include somatostatin, neuropeptide Y, and corticotropin-releasing factor (Struble et al. 1987). CSF contents (Table 3–5) of somatostatin and endorphin are not changed in elderly humans (Hartikainen et al. 1991). Peptide receptors are not adequately characterized in human cortex to assess age-related alterations (Mendelsohn and Paxinos 1991). Studies in aging rodents show no loss of enkephalinergic receptors or diminished receptor affinity (Ueno et al. 1988). Excitatory amino acids are common transmitters in the human brain, and excitotoxic damage is implicated in stroke, anoxic brain damage, and a range of neurodegenerative disorders (Olney et al. 1997; Whetsell 1996). Regional tissue levels of glutamate and aspartate appear altered in aging (Banay-Schwartz 1992). Inhibitory transmitter systems are also altered in aging. GABAergic systems in human hippocampus and cortex are altered with decreased GABA content and diminished GAD activity.

Signal Transduction and Aging

Signal transduction is transmitter dependent and mediated through a variety of cellular mechanisms. Senescent alterations of second-messenger systems are unclear. Phosphoinositide-derived second messengers and protein kinase–derived systems are altered in several neurodegenerative disorders such as Alzheimer's disease and Parkinson's disease. Although second-messenger systems appear stable in postmortem tissue, limited data are available for normal human aging (Pacheco and Jope 1996). Psychiatric disorders such as schizophrenia and depression, as well as subtle alterations of signal transduction systems, can occur in the brains of elderly subjects (Fowler et al. 1992).

Trophic Factors and Aging

Trophic factors are substances produced by neurons or glia that maintain or promote the growth and integrity of cell populations. Receptors exist for trophic factors (Hefti and Mash 1989), and synthesis of these substances can be regulated by specific transmitter systems (Thoenen et al. 1991). The neurotrophins include nerve growth factor, brain-derived neurotrophic factor, neurotrophin-3, and neurotrophin-4 (Fuxe and Agnati 1992). Glial cell line–derived neurotrophic factor (GDNF) is produced from glial cells and affects neurons (Gash et al. 1998).

Nerve growth factor is best characterized by and is comprised of three subunits: α, β, and γ. Biological activity appears to be present in the β subunit. Nerve growth factor receptors are present in the human nucleus basalis of Meynert (Figure 3–6) and in sympathetic neurons (Hefti and Mash 1989; Hefti et al. 1989). This peptide promotes neurite extension and stimulates the activity of tyrosine hydroxylase and dopamine β-hydroxylase (Fuxe and Agnati 1992). Nerve growth factor is essential to the normal development and maintenance of cholinergic neurons. Administration of nerve growth factor to aging rodents will reverse the age-related dendritic spine loss of cortical pyramidal neurons (Mervis et al. 1991).

At the cellular level, nerve growth factor may increase the degradation of superoxide radicals and hydrogen peroxides. Human data suggest an age-related reduction in the synthesis of nerve growth factor (Hefti et al. 1989). Nerve growth factor protects damaged cholinergic forebrain neurons in monkeys, and a similar protective role is postulated for human neurons.

Other peptides such as insulin-like growth factor, platelet-derived growth factor, and fibroblast growth factor affect the production of neurites, development of glia, and regulation of nigrostriatal neurons in nonhuman models. GDNF is one of many new molecules that promote recovery of damaged neurons. GDNF has distinct neuronal receptors and activity on dopaminergic neurons. Infusion of GDNF into rhesus monkey increases dopaminergic neuronal size and neurite extent (Gash et al. 1998). Growth factors such as GDNF can arrest or reverse some of the atrophic changes in aging and are a focus of pharmacological research for neurodegenerative diseases like Alzheimer's or Parkinson's disease.

▋ Neuroendocrinology of Aging

Senescent endocrinological changes of the pancreas, thyroid, and ovary produce significant direct or secondary brain alterations. Multiple other endocrine systems develop important age-related alterations mediated by changes in the hypothalamicopituitary axis (Table 3–6). The human hypothalamus consists of multiple nuclei adjacent to the third ventricle (Figure 3–6). The hypothalamus receives noradrenergic, serotonergic, and cholinergic innervation (Mendelsohn and Paxinos 1991) affecting control of many pituitary-releasing factors. These small clusters of neurons control the pituitary gland via direct neuronal input or via factors released into the hypophysial portal system. The pituitary gland is a small collection of cells in the sella turcica and is divided into an anterior and posterior lobe. The anterior pituitary secretes multiple hormones, that is, growth hormone, thyroid-stimulating hormone, etc., while the posterior pituitary secretes oxytocin and vasopressin. Hypothalamic control of neuroendocrine functions is regulated by catecholaminergic inputs that influence the release of inhibiting factors.

Aging humans undergo a series of senescent sexual and

TABLE 3–6.   **Endocrinology of aging**

System	Primary abnormality	Clinical consequence	Effective therapy
Pituitary gland			
Pituopause	↓ GH ↓ LH ↓ FSH	↑Frailty	Unclear
Thyroid gland			
Thyropause	↓ T_3/T_4	↑TSH Subclinical hypothyroidism	Yes
Male gonad			
Andropause	↓ Testosterone	Unclear	No
Female gonad			
Menopause	↓ Estrogen	Osteoporosis Atherosclerosis Alzheimer's disease	Yes
Adrenal gland			
Adrenopause	↓ DHEA ↓ DHEAS ↓↑ Cortisol	↑Frailty	Unclear
Pancreas			
Pancreopause	↓ Insulin	Diabetes mellitus	Yes

Note. This table demonstrates major endocrinological alterations associated with aging. Values represent consensus opinions from multiple sources. Therapy indicates treatments that are available, effective, and cost efficient. DHEA = dehydroepiandrosterone; DHEAS = dehydroepiandrosterone sulfate; FSH = follicle-stimulating hormone; GH = growth hormone; LH = luteinizing hormone; T_3/T_4 = triiodothyronine/tetraiodothyronine; TSH = thyroid-stimulating hormone.

neuroendocrinological alterations (Rance et al. 1993). Circulating gonadotropins and hypothalamic nuclei manifest age-dependent, gender-specific alterations. Senescent hypothalamic neurons can atrophy, hypertrophy, or remain constant.

The sexually dimorphic nucleus and the preoptic area of the human hypothalamus contain neurons whose density and size are gender specific (Hofman and Swaab 1989). These neurons undergo a series of orderly, predictable changes with age. Sexually dimorphic structures have a sex-dependent pattern of growth and decay (Hofman and Swaab 1989). Males have a 43% reduction and females have a 62% reduction of the volume of the sexually dimorphic nucleus-preoptic area of young (20–30 years) versus old (70–90 years) control subjects. This contrasts with 6% reductions of net brain volume and 20%–25% reductions of basal forebrain structures (Hofman and Swaab 1989). Alterations of these nuclei may reflect the gender-dependent patterns of human sexual aging.

Menopause occurs in most women around age 50 and includes many physiological and psychological alterations. Menopause is caused by disruption of the gonadal-hypothalamic-pituitary cycle through loss of cyclical ovarian estrogen production (Lamberts et al. 1997; Rance 1992). The number of human ova peaks in utero at mid-gestation (7 million) and is 1 million at birth. This number falls to 400,000 at menarche. This gradual ovarian attrition from ages 20 to 50 ends in ovarian follicles unresponsive to gonadotropins. Levels of serum follicle-stimulating hormone and luteinizing hormone rise as levels of serum estrogens fall (Evans and Williams 1992; Hazzard et al. 1990). Estrogen is important because this hormone probably retards atherosclerotic heart disease, osteoporosis, and Alzheimer's disease in women (Grady et al. 1992). The precise neural protective mechanisms of estrogen are unclear, although this hormone may interact with nerve growth factor and may be neuroprotective for hippocampal neurons. Estrogen replacement for postmenopausal women may slightly increase risk for breast or endometrial cancer. Each postmenopausal woman should be considered for estrogen replacement, weighing the modest risk of malignancy or hysterectomy against substantial risk of heart disease, osteoporosis, and dementia (Rowe and Kehn 1998).

The cyclical nature of the menstrual cycle may be partially driven by neurons in the anterior hypothalamus, which receive a variety of catecholaminergic inputs (Wise et al. 1987). Rodent studies have indicated that the release of luteinizing hormone is influenced by noradrenergic, serotonergic, dopaminergic, and peptidergic inputs. In postmenopausal senescent women, some hypothalamic nuclei hypertrophy to include marked increase in the diameter of infundibular neurons expressing estrogen receptors (Rance et al. 1990) and increased tachykinin message in selected hypothalamic nuclei (Rance and Young 1991).

The senescent changes of gonadotropic nuclei that provoke the decline of sexual function in elderly men are undefined. The male sexually dimorphic nucleus also is reduced in size with aging. Testosterone levels fall after age 50, and more than 60% of older men have levels below younger men (Lamberts et al. 1997), thus producing "andropause" (Table 3–6). The number of testicular Leydig cells is reduced in older men. The physiological significance of low testosterone on sexual function, muscle bulk, and mood is unclear. The preventive use of exogenous testosterone by healthy older men is limited by concerns over the hormone's hypertrophic effect on the prostate gland (Rowe and Kahn 1998).

The function of the hypothalamic-pituitary-adrenal axis has been extensively described in elderly patients, producing the concept of "adrenopause" (Lamberts et al. 1997) (Table 3–6). Basal levels of plasma cortisol may increase with age, but the reactivity of the axis as determined by suppression with oral dexamethasone is unchanged (Hazzard et al. 1990; Veith and Raskind 1988). The pattern of cortisol secretion varies significantly in elders, but the secretion of adrenocorticotropic hormone remains relatively stable (Lupien et al. 1996).

A second, important adrenal hormone is dehydroepiandrosterone (DHEA) and its sulfate DHEAS. This steroid is 10 times more abundant than is cortisol, and the age-related decline of DHEA/DHEAS levels is associated with loss of physical and functional ability. These precursor steroids are transformed into active androgens or estrogens in peripheral target tissue. Plasma DHEA levels peak at age 20 and decline with age, resulting in levels at 70% normal around age 60 and 20% at age 85. In older men, lower DHEA levels are associated with higher mortality rates at 2 and 4 years following assessment (Berr et al. 1996). DHEA replacement may benefit elders, but the risk of long-term therapy is unclear. Thus, DHEA supplementation is not recommended for elderly subjects (Rowe and Kahn 1998).

Growth hormone is released from the pituitary gland in pulses that remain constant during aging; however, the pulse amplitude, and hormone secretion are diminished (Table 3–6). The fall in circulating growth hormone causes the liver and other organs to reduce production of insulin-like growth factor 1. Noradrenaline affects the release of growth hormone via control of growth hormone–releasing factor and somatostatin. Growth hormone secretion is increased by adrenergic and dopaminergic receptor activation and inhibited by adrenergic stimulation. The peak of growth hormone secretion occurs in adolescence, followed by a progressive decline over years and a diminished number of growth hormone immunoreactive pituicytes in the glands of elderly subjects (Veith and Raskind 1988). Studies have shown that growth hormone injection in older humans produces a short-term increase of lean body mass (8.8%), skin thickness (7.1%), and bone density, while lowering adipose tissue mass (14.4%) (Rudman et al. 1990); however, these improvements may diminish after 12 months. Growth hormone replacement is expensive (Schoen 1991), and its potential side effects limit the usefulness of this therapeutic modality (Schoen 1991). Functional ability may not improve with growth hormone supplements, and replacement therapy is not recommended for elderly patients (Feller and Rudman 1997; Papadakis et al. 1996; Rowe and Kahn 1998).

Abnormalities of thyroid function are common in elderly patients (Table 3–6). Between 4% and 12% of subjects over age 60 may have chemical hypothyroidism. Individuals over age 60 have a sevenfold increase in the prevalence of hyperthyroidism (Evans and Williams 1992). Fifteen percent of patients over age 60 will have elevated blood levels of thyroid-stimulating hormone, and one-third will develop thyroid failure when followed for 4 years. Some elderly individuals have diminished pituitary responsiveness to thyrotropin-releasing hormone (Evans and Williams 1992), although blunting of thyroid-stimulating hormone response is present with depression (Veith and Raskind 1988).

Glucose intolerance occurs in approximately 40% of individuals over age 65, and almost half are undiagnosed. Diabetes is a significant risk factor for cerebrovascular disease. Diabetic complications such as renal disease, neuropathy, or blindness produce significant neuropsychiatric disability. Insulin production by beta cells of the pancreas falls with aging, and peripheral insulin resistance rises. Preventive measures such as weight control, dietary moderation, and exercise significantly improve glucose control in elders.

▮ Age-Related Alterations of the Special Senses

Aging may affect all five of the special senses. Increased thresholds for touch-pressure, vibration, and cooling are present in aging. Patient deficits of olfaction, sight, and hearing are immensely important to neuropsychiatrists because they affect psychological testing and clinical management of patients.

Taste

Taste is mediated by a chemosensory mechanism located in tongue, cheek margin, soft palate, and other oral structures. Impaired taste perception is common in older patients. More than 250 medications alter taste, and dentures that cover the soft plate diminish taste perception. Taste impairment is classified as ageusia (absence of taste) and hypogeusia (diminished taste sensitivity). Taste thresholds for both detection and recognition are elevated in aging. Detection thresholds in elders are 2.7 times higher for sweets and 11.6 times higher for salts, and such taste alteration may cause elderly people with diabetes to use more sugar and those with hypertension to use more salt (Schiffman 1997). The neuropsychiatric sequelae of diminished taste include weight loss, poor compliance with dietary restrictions, and loss in quality of life.

Olfaction

Aging humans lose multiple olfactory abilities (Kesslak et al. 1988) including the ability to perceive odors, odor discrimination, odor recognition, and olfactory memory (Giaquinto 1988). Alteration of nasal mucosa, cribriform plate stenosis, airway pathology, and other factors contribute to olfactory loss (Doty 1991). Age-related olfactory histopathology, such as neurofibrillary tangles, begins to occur in individuals over age 50 (Doty 1991). Olfaction association areas such as amygdala and uncal cortices are fre-

quently damaged in aging (Braak and Braak 1991; Kemper 1984). Patients with Alzheimer's disease demonstrate olfaction deficits and neuropathology in all components of the olfactory pathway (Hyman et al. 1991; Kesslak et al. 1988; Talamo et al. 1989). The loss of taste and smell can reduce the drive to eat, a problem corrected with simple dietary or behavioral intervention, for example, flavor and odor enhancement of foods (Schiffman 1997).

Vision

Senescent visual loss results from environmental, genetic, metabolic, and vascular etiologies (Evans and Williams 1992; Hazzard et al. 1990). Visual impairment is common in elderly individuals, and frequent causes include opacification of the cornea (cataracts), increased intraocular pressure (glaucoma), retinal damage (diabetic retinopathy), deterioration of the macula (macular degeneration), or disturbance of ocular optics (presbyopia) (Table 3–7) (Abrams et al. 1995). Visual thresholds begin to decline between ages 30 and 40. Approximately 17% of all elders and 36% of individuals over age 80 have opacification of the lens (Giaquinto 1988). Low vision and blindness are common in those over age 85; however, one-half may never seek specialty care, and many can be assisted with simple interventions such as improved home lighting (Evans and Williams 1992). Diabetic retinopathy accounts for 10%–20% of blindness in subjects 65–74 years old and macular degeneration, for 50% of those over age 85 (Evans and Williams 1992; Hazzard et al. 1990) (Table 3–7).

The central visual fields, that is, area 17, include 140

TABLE 3–7. Common causes and treatment of low vision in the elderly

Type	Location of lesion	Etiology	Therapy	Clinical symptoms
Cataract	Lens	Age-related lens degeneration	Lens extraction	Like a blurry film over the eye
Glaucoma	Anterior chamber	Increased intraocular pressure		Progressive insidious loss of peripheral vision
		• Open angle 80%	• Medication	
		• Angle-closure 10%	• Surgery or medication	
Macular degeneration	Retinal area for central vision	Primary retinal degeneration		Patient cannot focus clearly on an object as a result of loss of central vision
		• Wet type 10%	• Laser surgery	
		• Dry type 90%	• None	
Diabetic retinopathy	Multiple foci on retina	Diabetic vascular disease and hemorrhage	• Laser therapy • Prevention	Multifocal, variable loss of vision—described as looking through the top of a salt shaker

Note. This table describes common causes of visual loss encountered during the treatment of elderly patients.

million neurons in adult brain. A minimal number of neurons are lost with aging, and age-related reduction of visual cortical surface area may result from loss of neuropil, for example, in synapses (Leuba and Kraftsik 1994).

Primate studies show that visual information is processed along two pathways involving temporal and parietal cortices. A striate-inferior temporal circuit processes information about form and color distinction (J. H. Morrison et al. 1991). A striate-parietal pathway processes visuo-spatial and motor data. The effect of aging on these interconnected, high-level association cortices is not known; however, these brain regions are damaged in Alzheimer's disease (Hof and Morrison 1990) and other dementias.

Low vision can worsen neuropsychiatric symptoms and complicate management. Recognition of low vision, correction of refractive error, and maximal use of environmental light are important in management of the geriatric population (Table 3–7).

Auditory Functions

Hearing impairment is a chronic condition that affects 30% of individuals over age 65. Auditory impairment worsens with age and affects 60% of individuals ages 71–80 (Davis et al. 1990). High-frequency hearing loss increases with aging and is usually caused by mechanical failure. Causes of hearing loss in elderly people include disorders of the outer, middle, and inner ear. Cerumen impaction is a common problem of the outer ear (Gulya 1992). Hearing loss from damage to the inner ear has four primary causes: 1) sensory presbycusis, 2) neural presbycusis, 3) strial presbycusis, and 4) cochlear conductive presbycusis. Precise epidemiological data are limited because correlative histopathological studies of the auditory apparatus are few, and many conditions have mixed pathology. Most age-related hearing loss is mechanical, and age-related histopathology (e.g., senile plaques or neurofibrillary tangles) is not reported in the peripheral auditory system. Conductive or sensorineural hearing loss can be improved with appropriate hearing amplification. The auditory cortex can be severely damaged in Alzheimer's disease (Esiri et al. 1986), in which a specific pattern of atrophy shows shrinkage of the association cortex (i.e., the superior temporal gyrus [Brodmann's areas 22 and 52]), with sparing of the primary auditory cortex (i.e., the transverse temporal gyrus [Brodmann's areas 41 and 42]) (Figure 3–8).

Subtle auditory impairment may be difficult to detect in the elderly patient who has developed accessory methods such as lip and face reading. Even mild (10 dB) hearing loss can significantly lower quality of life (Bess et al. 1989). Hearing loss can remain undetected by caregivers, and this communication problem can be misinterpreted by caregivers as patient obstinacy. Unrecognized hearing loss can produce neuropsychiatric symptoms that are preventable or reversible such as confusion or irritability.

Aging of the Autonomic and Peripheral Nervous Systems

Autonomic regulation involves a balance between sympathetic and parasympathetic innervation. These two systems include neurons in hypothalamus, brainstem, spinal cord, and peripheral ganglia. Small-diameter myelinated and unmyelinated axons conduct impulses to target organs (McLeod and Tuck 1987). The number and density of peripheral or autonomic myelinated fibers are reduced in aging rodents and humans (Knox et al. 1989).

Aging of the human sympathetic nervous system results in a mixture of clinical alterations. Essential hypertension is an age-related disorder that has both central and peripheral causes (Evans and Williams 1992), and orthostatic hypotension is a common problem in the elderly. Postural hypotension occurs in 20% of selected geriatric patients and complicates the prescription of psychotropic medications (Mader 1989; see also Chapter 29 in this volume). Antihypertensive agents can cause depression in elderly patients. Individuals over age 65 are sensitive to the orthostatic effects of the tricyclic antidepressants. Although senescent changes occur in brainstem and spinal cord (Clark et al. 1984), the age-related alterations of central nuclei that control autonomic function are unknown. A progressive, age-related loss of sympathetic neurons occurs in the intermediolateral column of the spinal cord. These neurons span from T1 to L2 and are involved with vasomotor tone.

Sympathetic control of blood pressure is maintained through a complicated interaction of central, peripheral, and neuroendocrine interactions. The sympathetic nervous system is inhibited in the medullary brainstem and spinal cord through centrally located adrenergic mechanisms. Obesity is associated with increasing plasma norepinephrine levels, and older subjects have higher total body fat. Plasma norepinephrine is elevated in aging; however, the net effect of aging on the peripheral sympathetic tone is unknown (Rowe 1987). Senescent alterations are reported for sympathetic innervation to other organs.

Age-related pathologies (e.g., neurofibrillary tangles, senile plaques, and dystrophic neurites) occur rarely in the human spinal cord and peripheral nervous system, although neurofibrillary tangles are reported in the human superior cervical ganglion (Kawasaki et al. 1987). Aging humans have reduced numbers of neurons in myenteric ganglia (Gomes et al. 1997). Lewy bodies are present in Auerbach's and Meissner's plexuses in elderly subjects, as well as in those with Parkinson's disease (Wakabayashi et al. 1988). Sympathetic innervation of human spleen is not described, but aging rodents have markedly diminished splenic noradrenergic innervation (Madden et al. 1998).

The aging of the human parasympathetic nervous system is poorly understood. A senescent loss of small-diameter peripheral nerve fibers may contribute to parasympathetic dysfunction. Sacral parasympathetic neurons are damaged in parkinsonism (Oyanagi et al. 1990). Many drugs with anticholinergic side effects alter parasympathetic tone (N. L. Peters 1989).

The spinal cord and peripheral nervous system demonstrate subtle age-related changes. The number of anterior horn cells declines with aging, possibly in response to changes in trophic factors such as neurotrophin 3, neurotrophin 4, and insulin-like growth factor 1. The number of swollen axons in spinal cord increases with aging, and amyotrophic lateral sclerosis is a disease of older individuals (Clark et al. 1984). Age-related loss of vibratory, tactile, and thermal response over lower extremities may reflect loss of myelinated axons in the peripheral nervous system (Flanigan et al. 1998).

Aging and the Immune System

The interaction of brain aging and the immune system can be viewed two ways: the effect of aging brain on immune function or the effect of an aging immune system on the brain. Components of the immune system, such as spleen, thymus, and lymph nodes, receive direct noradrenergic innervation and respond to substances (e.g., cortisol) produced by the neuroendocrine system. Selected products of the immune system are CNS-active and may complete the feedback loop to the CNS (Cotman et al. 1987; Madden et al. 1998).

The brain does not have a system of lymphatics or lymphoid tissue like other organs do (e.g., lung or gastrointestinal tract) (Adams and Duchen 1992). Microglia, the immune cells of the brain, are either hematogenous or CNS constituents. Subjects without neurological disease who are over age 60 have increased numbers of activated microglial cells that express the cytokine interleukin-1, and the number of enlarged or phagocytic microglial cells is increased, whereas quiescent cells are unchanged (Mrak et al. 1997; Thomas 1992).

Interleukin-1, a cytokine that mediates acute phase re-

action, innervates key endocrine and autonomic neurons in human hypothalamus that affect many components of the acute phase immune reaction (Breder et al. 1988). Interleukin-2 is centrally active and affects firing of locus ceruleus neurons (Nistic and De Sarro 1991). Interleukin-1 mRNA content is increased in aging brain.

Many systemic diseases of the elderly population, such as arthritis, are immune mediated. The intact blood-brain barrier provides some protection against autoimmunity; however, age- and disease-related changes increase its permeability for selected immunoglobulins. Brain-directed autoantibodies are absent in young subjects, but some older humans produce antibodies that recognize neurons and astrocytes (Gaskin et al. 1987), including cholinergic neurons (Lopez et al. 1991). Astrocytes and microglial cells participate in the immune response of the brain by presenting antigen to T cells (Cotman et al. 1987). Microglia are present in senile plaques (Figures 3–10 and 3–21) and associated with intracellular and extracellular neurofibrillary tangles (Cras et al. 1991). Anti-inflammatory drugs may slow the progression of Alzheimer's disease by altering the brain's immune response to degenerative changes.

Nutritional Deficiencies in Aging

A linear decline of food intake occurs from age 20 to 80. The increased obesity in aging may result from decreased physical activity or metabolic changes. The physiology of age-related anorexia is unclear, but increased circulating cholecystokinin in older subjects may diminish food intake and appetite (Morley 1997). Elderly individuals have significant risks for vitamin deficiencies that produce direct or indirect CNS complications.

Cobalamin or vitamin B_{12} deficiency is common in the elderly, and subnormal serum cobalamin levels are present in approximately 5% of elderly individuals, although estimates range as high as 40% (Stabler et al. 1997). Vitamin B_{12} deficiency is caused by poor nutrition or impaired gastric absorption (Carmel 1997), although this disorder rarely produces pernicious anemia. Low vitamin B_{12} can lead to neurological disorders, and this deficiency can be avoided by supplementing the diet with 1 mg/day (Rowe and Kahn 1998).

Folic acid is available in green leafy vegetables, fruits, and liver, and its deficiency will elevate serum homocysteine. Accelerated atherosclerosis is common in young patients with homocystinuria, and high serum homocysteine is associated with increased risk for stroke, heart disease, and cognitive decline in elders. Low serum folate may worsen cognitive loss in patients with dementia

(Fioravanti et al. 1997). Folate and cobalamin are essential to DNA synthesis and repair. Folic acid deficiency can be avoided by daily supplementation of 400 µg/day (Rowe and Kahn 1998).

Falls and fractures are serious patient complications to the geriatric neuropsychiatrist. Normal serum calcium levels in elders do not predict normal bone density. Older individuals at risk for osteoporosis should have a simple, cost-effective bone density screening using the dual energy X-ray absorption test. The daily calcium requirement for healthy elders is 1200 mg, but the average diet supplies 200–800 mg/day, requiring a supplement of 500 mg/day. Elders need 700 IU of vitamin D/day to sustain calcium absorption from the intestine (Rowe and Kahn 1998). Additional therapeutic interventions are used for patients with documented osteoporosis.

Neurobiology of Aging in Patients With Chronic Mental Illnesses

The neurobiology of aging in patients with chronic mental illnesses can differ from that of healthy individuals. Assessment of age-related alterations in patients with chronic mental illness is complicated by the effect of chronic neuroleptic usage, nutrition, environment, and health status. Current hypotheses suggest that schizophrenia results from neuronal migrational abnormalities, genetic factors, and environmental influences (Barta et al. 1990; Weinberger 1987). Subtle changes in temporal lobe, frontal cortex, and hippocampus are described in brain imaging and autopsy studies (Powers 1999). Other disorders such as mental retardation, autism, and dyslexia (Galaburda et al. 1985; Hier et al. 1978) can involve abnormalities of neuronal migration in brain regions such as hippocampus and planum temporale (Figure 3–8). The neurobiology of aging in migrationally disordered brain is unknown.

Patients with chronic mental illness have normal aging of organs in cardiovascular, pulmonary, and renal systems. Excessive rates of natural death can result from complications of physical disorders produced by psychosocial factors (Black et al. 1987), such as medical noncompliance, poverty, and unavailability of health care services. Medical illness in patients with serious mental illness is underdiagnosed by one-third of primary care doctors and one-half of psychiatrists (Jeste 1996).

Studies of brains from elderly patients with chronic schizophrenia have demonstrated conflicting data on the numbers of senile plaques, neurofibrillary tangles, and vascular alterations as compared with those of age-matched control subjects (Arnold et al. 1998; Purohit et al. 1998). A meta-analysis of 10 postmortem studies showed that elderly patients with schizophrenia have age-related pathology similar to age-matched control subjects (Baldessarini et al. 1997). Postmortem studies of patients who receive long-term neuroleptic therapy demonstrate no specific pathology, and normal levels of iron are found in basal ganglia. The expression of the cytoskeletal epitopes, that is, microtubule-associated protein 2 and microtubule-associated protein 5, is altered in hippocampal subicular neurons (Arnold et al. 1991) of subjects with schizophrenia and of patients with serious mental illness. Such alterations of cytoskeleton may reflect abnormal development as opposed to abnormal aging.

Animal Models for the Neurobiology of Aging

Animal aging models include sheep, monkey, bear, dog, and others (Brizzee et al. 1978; Cork et al. 1988; Maurer et al. 1990). Brain weights of aging monkeys remain relatively constant over time (Herndon et al. 1998). Dystrophic neurites and senile plaques are described in all animals models, and substantial numbers of neurofibrillary tangles are described in the brains of aging bears and sheep (Cork et al. 1988). Other age-related changes such as granulo-vacuolar degeneration, Hirano bodies, and Lewy bodies are not described (Figures 3–9 and 3–23). Hypertensive rodents demonstrate some brain alterations (Wyss and Van Groen 1992; Wyss et al. 1992). Monkeys with surgically induced hypertension will manifest cognitive deficits and multiple cortical infarctions. Animal models for Parkinson's disease have significant limitations, and some degenerative diseases, such as frontotemporal dementia, diffuse Lewy body disease, etc., exist only in humans.

Aging primates demonstrate subtle cognitive decline similar to that of elderly humans (D. L. Price et al. 1991). Senescent cognitive deficits in aging rhesus monkeys correlate with alterations in prefrontal cortex and brainstem nuclei that project to neocortex, as well as damage to central myelin (A. Peters et al. 1996). Unlike aging humans, aged monkeys demonstrate neither cortical atrophy nor severe hippocampal damage (Herndon et al. 1998). Minimal synaptic loss is present in the dentate gyrus of monkey hippocampus (Tigges et al. 1996a, 1996b), and neurons in layer II of entorhinal cortex are spared in aging macaques (Gazzaley et al. 1997). Aging monkey brain can develop senile plaques, dystrophic neurites, and congophilic angiopathy closely resembling those of aging humans.

Apolipoprotein E is present in senile plaques of aging orangutans (Gearing et al. 1997). The $A\beta_{40}$ peptide length predominates in aging monkeys as opposed to the $A\beta_{42}$ length in humans with Alzheimer's disease. Very old dogs also develop amyloid deposits in the frontal cortex with early neuritic pathology (Satou et al. 1997). Neurofibrillary tangles are seen in aging bears, sheep, and very old primates with advanced disease (Cork et al. 1998; Nelson and Saper 1995). Individual bear and monkey neurons will atrophy, accumulate abnormal cytoskeletal proteins, and express amyloid precursor protein. Markers for cholinergic, noradrenergic, serotonergic, and peptidergic systems are decreased in brains of aging primates, suggesting that age-related pathology is not species specific but rather reflects the longevity of the animal (D. L. Price et al. 1991).

Healthy Aging

The aging process alters most organ systems in the human body; however, age-related loss of function is frequently overestimated in disease-free organ systems of elderly patients. Cardiovascular alterations, resulting from common diseases in the elderly such as hypertension and atherosclerosis, are immensely important to the geriatric neuropsychiatrist. Age-related loss of cardiovascular function is not dramatic in elders without heart disease (Evans and Williams 1992; Hazzard et al. 1990). Loss of exercise tolerance is partially explained by disuse (Evans and Williams 1992), rather than by atrophy. Age-related effects on systemic organ systems are displayed in Table 3–8, and alterations of pharmacodynamics are discussed elsewhere (see Chapter 34 in this volume). Epidemiological studies show that walking 30 minutes per day, avoiding depression, and maintaining a network of five friends will increase the likelihood of successful aging (Rowe and Kahn 1998; Seeman et al. 1995). Walking 30 minutes per day will decrease yearly hospitalizations for atherosclerotic heart disease by one-third, and elderly patients can regain some exercise capacity through supervised endurance training.

Although frequently overlooked, simple preventive measures remain effective in the elderly. Prevention of psychological and physical health problems can significantly retard the aging processes despite the role of genetics in longevity. Syndrome X refers to a collection of preventable, high-risk physical characteristics that include obesity, glucose intolerance, hypertension, and elevated serum lipids. Syndrome X is common in elders and predicts vascular disease. Pseudodiabetes of aging includes elevated glucose and elevated insulin levels. Weight reduction and exercise, especially for "potbellied" obesity, improve glucose

TABLE 3–8. Age-related alterations of cardiovascular, renal, and pulmonary function in the absence of intrinsic diseases

Function	Alteration
Cardiac	
Heart rate	No significant change
Ejection fraction	No significant change
Physical exercise capacity	Slight decrease
Pulmonary	
Total lung capacity (TLC)	No significant change
Forced vital capacity (FVC)	Decrease
Diffusion capacity (CDco)	Decrease
Physical work capacity ($VO_{2\,max}$)	Decrease
Partial pressure of arterial oxygen (PaO_2)	Decrease
Renal	
Renal mass	Decrease
Renal blood flow	Decrease
Glomerular filtration rate (GFR)	Decrease

Source. Adapted from Evans and Williams 1992; Hazzard et al. 1990.

metabolism and lower morbidity from syndrome X. Injuries, osteoporosis, vitamin or nutritional deficiencies, and some sensory deficits are preventable conditions that increase morbidity and lower functional ability (Table 3–6).

Conclusions

The secret of successful aging is unknown. The distinction between "normal" senescent phenomena and age-related disease remains unclear. Human neuronal aging includes a complex mixture of atrophy, hypertrophy, synaptic reorganization, and cell death. Genetic, environmental, systemic, and immunological factors may influence human brain aging. Smoking, exercise, and body mass in mid to late life predict survival and disability. Elders with good health habits survive longer and compress end-of-life disability into fewer years (Vita et al. 1998). Simple, cost-effective preventive measures for physical and psychological health can slow the aging process and sustain function in elders (Strawbridge et al. 1996).

▊ References

Abrams WB, Beers MH, Berkow R (eds): The Merck Manual of Geriatrics, 2nd Edition. Whitehouse Station, Merck & Co., Inc., 1995

Adams JH, Duchen LW (eds): Greenfield's Neuropathology, 5th Edition. New York, Oxford University Press, 1992

Aevarsson O, Svanborg A, Skoog I: Seven-year survival rate after age 85 years: relation to Alzheimer disease and vascular dementia. Arch Neurol 55:1226–1232, 1998

Akima M, Nonaka H, Kagesama M, et al: A study of the microvasculature of the cerebral cortex. Lab Invest 55:482–489, 1986

Akiyama H, Meyer JS, Mortel KF, et al: Normal human aging: factors contributing to cerebral atrophy. J Neurol Sci 152:39–49, 1997

Anthony A, Zerweck C: Scanning-integrating micro-densitometric analysis of age-related changes in RNA content of cerebrocortical neurons in mice subjected to auditory stimulation. Exp Neurol 65:542–551, 1979

Antonio A, Leenders KL, Reist H, et al: Effect of age on D_2 dopamine receptors in normal human brain measured by positron emission tomography and ^{11}C-raclopride. Arch Neurol 50:474–480, 1993

Arnold SE, Lee VA, Gur RE, et al: Abnormal expression of two microtubule-associated proteins (MAP2 and MAP5) in specific subfields of the hippocampal formation in schizophrenia. Proc Natl Acad Sci U S A 88:10850–10854, 1991

Arnold SE, Trojanowski JQ, Gur RE, et al: Absence of neurodegeneration and neural injury in the cerebral cortex in a sample of elderly patients with schizophrenia. Arch Gen Psychiatry 55:225–232, 1998

Awad IA, Johnson PC, Spetzler RF, et al: Incidental subcortical lesions identified on magnetic resonance imaging in the elderly, II: postmortem pathological correlations. Stroke 17:1090–1097, 1986

Baldessarini RJ, Hegarty JD, Bird ED, et al: Metaanalysis of postmortem studies of Alzheimer's disease–like neuropathology in schizophrenia. Am J Psychiatry 154:861–863, 1997

Ball MJ: Neuronal loss, neurofibrillary tangles and granulovacuolar degeneration in the hippocampus with ageing and dementia: a quantitative study. Acta Neuropathol (Berl) 37:111–118, 1977

Ball MJ, Braak H, Coleman P, et al: Consensus recommendations for the postmortem diagnosis of Alzheimer's disease. Neurobiol Aging 18(S4):S1–S2, 1997

Banay-Schwartz M, Lajtha A, Palkovits M, et al: Regional distribution of glutamate and aspartate in adult and old human brain. Brain Res 594:343–346, 1992

Barinaga M: Mortality: overturning received wisdom. Science 258:398–399, 1992

Barta PE, Pearlson GD, Powers RE, et al: Auditory hallucinations and smaller superior temporal gyral volume in schizophrenia. Am J Psychiatry 147:1457–1462, 1990

Baxter MG, Gallagher M: Neurobiological substrates of behavioral decline: models and data analytic strategies for individual differences in aging. Neurobiol Aging 17(3):491–495, 1996

Beal MF: Excitotoxicity and nitric oxide in Parkinson's disease pathogenesis. Ann Neurol 44(1):S110–S114, 1998

Bell MA, Ball MJ: Morphometric comparison of hippocampal microvasculature in ageing and demented people: diameters and densities. Acta Neuropathol 53:299–318, 1981

Bennett DA, Gilley DW, Wilson RS, et al: Clinical correlates of high signal lesions on magnetic resonance imaging in Alzheimer's disease. J Neurol 239:186–190, 1992

Berg L, McKeel W, Miller JP, et al: Clinicopathologic studies in cognitively healthy aging and Alzheimer disease. Arch Neurol 35:326–335, 1998

Berr C, Lafont S, Debuire B, et al: Relationships of dehydroepiandrosterone sulfate I the elder with functional, psychological, and mental status, and short-term mortality: a French community-based study. Proc Natl Acad Sci U S A 93:13410–13415, 1996

Bess FH, Lichtenstein MJ, Logan SA: Hearing impairment as a determinant of function in the elderly. J Am Geriatr Soc 37:123–128, 1989

Bickford-Wimer PC, Granholm A-CH, Gerhardt GA: Cerebellar noradrenergic systems in aging: studies in situ and in oculo grafts. Neurobiol Aging 9:591–599, 1988

Black DW, Winokur G, Nasrallah A: Is death from natural causes still excessive in psychiatric patients? a follow-up of 1593 patients with major affective disorder. J Nerv Ment Dis 175:674–680, 1987

Blessed G, Tomlinson BE, Roth M: The association between quantitative measures of dementia and of senile change in the cerebral grey matter of elderly subjects. Br J Psychiatry 114:797–811, 1968

Bloom FE, Morales M: The central 5-HT$_3$ receptor in CNS disorders. Neurochem Res 23:653–659, 1998

Bodnar AG, Ouelette M, Frolkis M, et al: Extension of life span by introduction of telomerase into normal human cells. Science 279:349–352, 1998

Bots ML, Van Swieten JC, Breteler MMB, et al: Cerebral white matter lesions and atherosclerosis in the Rotterdam study. Lancet 341:1232–1237, 1993

Braak H, Braak E: Neuropathological staging of Alzheimer's-related changes. Acta Neuropathol (Berl) 82:239–259, 1991

Braak H, Braak E: Frequency of stages of Alzheimer-related lesions in different age categories. Neurobiol Aging 18(4):351–357, 1997

Braak H, Braak E, Grundke-Iqbal I, et al: Occurrence of neuropil threads in the senile human brain and in Alzheimer's disease: a third location of paired helical filaments outside of neurofibrillary tangles and neuritic plaques. Neurosci Lett 65:351–355, 1986

Breder CD, Dinarello CA, Saper CB: Interleukin-1 immunoreactive innervation of the human hypothalamus. Science 240:321–324, 1988

Bredesen DE: Neural apoptosis. Ann Neurol 38:839–851, 1995

Brizzee KR, Ordy JM, Hofer H, et al: Animal models for the study of senile brain disease and aging changes in the brain, in Alzheimer's Disease: Senile Dementia and Related Disorders. Edited by Katzman R, Terry RD, Bick KL. New York, Raven, 1978, pp 515–553

Brody H: Organization of the cerebral cortex, III: a study of ageing in the cerebral cortex. J Comp Neurol 102:511–556, 1955

Brown WT: Genetic diseases of premature aging as models of senescence. Annual Review of Gerontology and Geriatrics 10:23–42, 1990

Bryan RN, Wells SW, Miller TJ, et al: Infarctlike lesions in the brain: prevalence and anatomic characteristics at MR imaging of the elderly—data from the cardiovascular health study 1. Radiology 202:47–54, 1997

Burnet PWJ, Eastwood SL, Lacey EK, et al: The distribution of 5-HT$_{1A}$ and 5-HT$_{2A}$ receptor mRNA in human brain. Brain Res 676:157–168, 1995

Callahan LM, Coleman PD: Neurons bearing neurofibrillary tangles are responsible for selected synaptic deficits in Alzheimer's disease. Neurobiol Aging 16(3):311–314, 1995.

Carmel R: Cobalamin, the stomach, and aging. Am J Clin Nutr 66:750–759, 1997

Choi JY, Morris JC, Hsu CY: Aging and cerebrovascular disease. Neurologic Clinics of North America 16(3) 687–710, 1998

Clark AW, Parhad IM, Griffin JW, et al: Neurofilamentous axonal swellings as a normal finding in the spinal anterior horn of man and other primates. J Neuropathol Exp Neurol 43:253–262, 1984

Coffey CE, Figiel GS: Neuropsychiatric significance of subcortical encephalomalacia, in Psychopathology and the Brain. Edited by Carroll BJ, Barrett JE. New York, Raven, 1991, pp 243–264

Coffey CE, Wilkinson WE, Parashos IA, et al: Quantitative cerebral anatomy of the aging human brain: a cross-sectional study using magnetic resonance imaging. Neurology 42:527–536, 1992

Coffey CE, Wilkinson WE, Weiner RD, et al: Quantitative cerebral anatomy in depression: a controlled magnetic resonance imaging study. Arch Gen Psychiatry 50:7–16, 1993

Coffey CE, Lucke JF, Saxton JA: Sex differences in brain aging: a quantitative magnetic resonance imaging study. Arch Neurol 55:169–179, 1998

Coleman PD, Flood DG: Neuron numbers and dendritic extent in normal aging and Alzheimer's disease. Neurobiol Aging 8:521–545, 1987

Comfort A: The Biology of Senescence, 3rd Edition. New York, Elsevier, 1979

Coria F, Moreno A, Torres A, et al: Distribution of Alzheimer's disease amyloid protein precursor in normal human and rat nervous system. Neuropathol Appl Neurobiol 18:27–35, 1992

Cork LC, Powers RE, Selkoe DJ, et al: Neurofibrillary tangles and senile plaques in aged bears. J Neuropathol Exp Neurol 47:629–641, 1988

Cotman CW, Brinton RE, Galaburda A, et al (eds): The Neuro-Immune-Endocrine Connection. New York, Raven, 1987

Court JA, Lloyd S, Johnson M, et al: Nicotinic and muscarinic cholinergic receptor binding in the human hippocampal formation during development and aging. Brain Res Dev Brain Res 101(1–2):93–105, 1997

Cowell PE, Turetsky BI, Gur RC, et al: Sex differences in aging of the human frontal and temporal lobes. J Neurosci 14(8):4748–4756, 1994

Cras P, Kawai M, Siedlak S, et al: Microglia are associated with the extracellular neurofibrillary tangles of Alzheimer disease. Brain Res 558:312–314, 1991

Crystal H, Dickson D, Fuld P, et al: Clinicopathologic studies in dementia: nondemented subjects with pathologically confirmed Alzheimer's disease. Neurology 38:1682–1687, 1988

Dam AM: The density of neurons in the human hippocampus. Neuropathol Appl Neurobiol 5:249–264, 1979

Davies I: Comments on review by Swaab: brain aging and Alzheimer's disease: "wear and tear" versus "use it or lose it." Neurobiol Aging 12:328–330, 1991

Davis AC, Ostri B, Parving A: Longitudinal study of hearing. Acta Otolaryngol (Stockh) 476 (suppl):12–22, 1990

Davis DG, Schmitt FA, Wekstein DR, et al: Alzheimer neuropathologic alterations in aged cognitively normal subjects. J Neuropathol Exp Neurol 58(4):376–388, 1999

Decker MW: The effects of aging on hippocampal and cortical projections of the forebrain cholinergic system. Brain Res Brain Rs Rev 12:423–438, 1987

Dekaban AS, Sadowsky BS: Changes in brain weights during the span of human life: relation of brain weights to body height and weight. Ann Neurol 4:345–357, 1978

de la Torre JC: Cerebromicrovascular pathology in Alzheimer's disease compared to normal aging. Gerontology 43:26–43, 1997

de Lacalle S, Iraizoz I, Ma Gonzalo L: Differential changes in cell size and number in topographic subdivisions of human basal nucleus in normal aging. Neuroscience 43:445–456, 1991

DeLeon MJ, George AE, Golomb J, et al: Frequency of hippocampal formation atrophy in normal aging and Alzheimer's disease. Neurobiol Aging 18:1–11, 1997

Dickson DW, Crystal HA, Bevona C, et al: Correlations of synaptic and pathological markers with cognition of the elderly. Neurobiol Aging 16(3):285–304, 1995

Dickson DW: Neuropathological diagnosis of Alzheimers disease: a perspective from longitudinal clinicopathological studies. Neurobiol Aging 18(54):521–526, 1998

Dillon KA, Gross-Isseroff R, Israeli M, et al: Autoradiographic analysis of serotonin 5-HT$_{1A}$ receptor binding in human brain postmortem: effects of age and alcohol. Brain Res 554:56–63, 1991

Divac I: Magnocellular nuclei of the basal forebrain project to neocortex, brainstem, and olfactory bulb: review of some functional correlates. Brain Res 93:385–398, 1975

Doebler JA, Markesbery WR, Anthony A, et al: Neuronal RNA in relation to neuronal loss and neurofibrillary pathology in the hippocampus in Alzheimer's disease. J Neuropathol Exp Neurol 46:28–39, 1987

Doty RL: Olfactory capacities in aging and Alzheimer's disease: psychophysical and anatomic considerations. Ann N Y Acad Sci 640:20–27, 1991

Double KL, Halliday GM, Kril JJ, et al: Topography of brain atrophy during normal aging and Alzheimer's disease. Neurobiol Aging 17:513–521, 1996

Dozono K, Ishii N, Nishihara Y, et al: An autopsy study of the incidence of lacunes in relation to age, hypertension, arteriosclerosis. Stroke 22:993–996, 1991

Duyckaerts C, Hauw JJ: Prevalence, incidence and duration of Braak's stages in the general population: can we know? Neurobiol Aging 18(4):362–369, 1997

Eggers R, Haug H, Fischer D: Preliminary report on macroscopic age changes in the human prosencephalon: a stereologic investigation. J Hirnforsch 25:129–139, 1984

Ehrenstein D: Immortality gene discovered. Science 279:177, 1998

Esiri MM, Pearson RCA, Powell TPS: The cortex of the primary auditory area in Alzheimer's disease. Brain Res 366:385–387, 1986

Evans JG, Williams TF (eds): Oxford Textbook of Geriatric Medicine. New York, Oxford University Press, 1992

Fallon JH, Loughlin SE: Monoamine innervation of cerebral cortex and a theory of the role of monoamines in cerebral cortex and basal ganglia, in Cortex, Vol 1. Edited by Jones EG, Peters A. New York, Plenum, 1987, pp 41–127

Feller AX, Rudman IW: Growth hormone and function in the elderly persons (letter). Ann Intern Med 126:7, 1997

Fields SD, MacKenzie CR, Charlson ME, et al: Reversibility of cognitive impairment in medical inpatients. Arch Intern Med 146:1593–1596, 1986

Finch CE: Neuron atrophy during aging: programmed or sporadic? Trends Neurosci 16:104–110, 1993

Finch CE, Morgan DG: RNA and protein metabolism in the aging brain. Annu Rev Neurosci 13:75–88, 1990

Finch CE, Tanzi RE: Genetics of aging. Science 278:17, 1997

Fioravanti M, Ferrario E, Massaia M: Low folate levels in the cognitive decline of elderly patients and the efficacy of folate as a treatment for improving memory deficits. Archives of Gerontology and Geriatrics 26:1–13, 1997

Flanigan KM, Lauria G, Griffin JW, et al: Age-related biology and diseases of muscle and nerve. The Neurology of Aging 16(3):659–668, 1998

Flood DG, Coleman PD: Neuron numbers and sizes in aging brain: comparisons of human, monkey, and rodent data. Neurobiol Aging 9:453–463, 1988

Flood DG, Buell SJ, Defiore CH, et al: Age-related dendritic growth in dentate gyrus of human brain is followed by regression in the "oldest old." Brain Res 345:366–368, 1985

Fossel M: Telomerase and the aging cell: implications for human health. JAMA 279(21):1732–1735, 1998

Fowler CJ, Cowburn RF, O'Neill CO: Brain signal transduction disturbances in neurodegenerative disorders. Cell Signal 4:1–9, 1992

Fowler JS, Volkow ND, Wang GJ: Age-related increases in brain monoamine oxidase B in living healthy human subjects. Neurobiol Aging 18(4):431–435, 1997

Frederickson RCA: Astroglia in Alzheimer's disease. Neurobiol Aging 13:239–253, 1992

Fuxe K, Agnati LF: Neurotrophic factors and central dopamine neurons. Neuroscience Facts 3:81, 1992

Galaburda AM, Sherman GF, Rosen GD, et al: Developmental dyslexia: four consecutive patients with cortical anomalies. Ann Neurol 18:222–233, 1985

Garcia JH: The evolution of brain infarcts: a review. J Neuropathol Exp Neurol 51:387–393, 1992

Gash DM, Zhang Z, Gerhardt G: Neuroprotective and neurorestorative properties of GDNF. Ann Neurol 44(1): S121–S125, 1998

Gaskin F, Kingsley BS, Fu SM: Autoantibodies to neurofibrillary tangles and brain tissue in Alzheimer's disease and aging, in Molecular Neuropathology of Aging. Edited by Davies P, Finch CE. Cold Spring Harbor, NY, Cold Spring Harbor Laboratory, 1987, pp 321–336

Gaspar P, Berger B, Alvarez C, et al: Catecholaminergic innervation of the septal area in man: immunocytochemical study using TH and DBH antibodies. J Comp Neurol 241:12–33, 1985

Gazzaley AH, Thakker MM, Hof PR, et al: Preserved number of entorhinal cortex layer II neurons in aged macaque monkeys. Neurobiol Aging 18(5):549–553, 1997

Gearing M, Tigges J, Mori H, et al: β-Amyloid (Aβ) deposition in the brains of aged orangutans. Neurobiol Aging 18(2):139–146, 1997

Geddes JW, Cotman CW: Plasticity in Alzheimer's disease: too much or not enough? Neurobiol Aging 12:330–333, 1991

Giacobini E: Cholinergic receptors in human brain: effects of aging and Alzheimer disease. J Neurosci Res 27:548–560, 1990

Giacobini E: Nicotinic cholinergic receptors in human brain: effects of aging and Alzheimer. Adv Exp Med Biol 296:303–315, 1991

Giaquinto S: Aging and the Nervous System. New York, Wiley, 1988

Gibb WRG, Mountjoy CQ, Mann DMA, et al: The substantia nigra and ventral tegmental area in Alzheimer's disease and Down's syndrome. J Neurol Neurosurg Psychiatry 52:193–200, 1989

Girnnakopoulos P, Hof PR, Dovari E, et al: Distinct patterns of neuronal loss and Alzheimer's disease lesion distribution in elderly individuals older than 90 years. J Neuropathol Exp Neurol 55:1210–1220, 1996

Gjedde A, Jakob R, Wong DF: In schizophrenia, some dopamine D_2-like receptors are still elevated (letter). Psychiatry Res 67:159–162, 1996

Goldman JE: The association of actin with Hirano bodies. J Neuropathol Exp Neurol 42:146–152, 1983

Goldman JE, Yen S-H: Cytoskeletal protein abnormalities in neurodegenerative diseases. Ann Neurol 19:209–223, 1986

Goldman JE, Yen S-H, Chiu F-C, et al: Lewy bodies of Parkinson's disease contain neurofilament antigens. Science 221:1082–1084, 1983

Gomes OA, de Souza RR, Liberti EA: A preliminary investigation of the effects of aging on the nerve cell number in the myenteric ganglia of the human colon. Gerontology 43:210–217, 1997

Gomez-Isla T, Price JL, McKeel DW Jr, et al: Profound loss of layer II entorhinal cortex neurons occurs in very mild Alzheimer's disease. J Neurosci 16(14):4491–4500, 1996

Gorelich P: Distribution of atherosclerotic vascular lesions: effects of age, race, and sex. Stroke 24(12):I16–I–21, 1993

Gottfries CG: Neurochemical aspects on aging and diseases with cognitive impairment. J Neurosci Res 27:541–547, 1990

Grady D, Rubin S, Petitti DB, et al: Hormone therapy to prevent disease and prolong life in postmenopausal women. Ann Intern Med 117:1016–1037, 1992

Graham DG: On the origin and significance of neuromelanin. Arch Pathol Lab Med 103:359–362, 1979

Greenamyre JT: Neuronal bioenergetic defects excitotoxicity and Alzheimer's disease: use it or lose it. Neurobiol Aging 12:334–336, 1991

Gulya AJ: Disorders of hearing, in Oxford Textbook of Geriatric Medicine. Edited by Evans JG, Williams TF. New York, Oxford University Press, 1992, pp 580–585

Gupta SR, Naheedy MH, Young JC, et al: Periventricular white matter changes and dementia: clinical, neuropsychological, radiological, and pathological correlation. Arch Neurol 45:637–641, 1988

Hachinski VC, Potter P, Merskey H: Leuko-araiosis. Arch Neurol 44:21–23, 1987

Hall TC, Miller AKH, Corsellis JAN: Variations in human Purkinje cell population according to age and sex. Neuropathol Appl Neurobiol 1:267–292, 1975

Hanks SD, Flood DG: Region-specific stability of dendritic extent in normal human aging and regression in Alzheimer's disease, I: CA1 of hippocampus. Brain Res 540:63–82, 1991

Haroutunian V, Perl DP, Purohit DP, et al: Regional distribution of neuritic plaques in the nondemented elderly and subjects with very mild Alzheimer disease. Arch Neurol 55:1185–1191, 1998

Hartikainen P, Soininen H, Reinikainen KJ, et al: Neurotransmitter markers in the cerebrospinal fluid of normal subjects: effects of aging and other confounding factors. Journal of Neural Transmission: General Section 84:103–117, 1991

Hatanp K, Isaacs KR, Shirao T, et al: Loss of proteins regulating synaptic plasticity in normal aging of the human brain and in Alzheimer's disease. J Neuropathol Exp Neurol 58:637–643, 1999

Haug H: Brain sizes, surfaces, and neuronal sizes of the cortex cerebri: a stereological investigation of man and his variability and a comparison with some mammals (primates, whales, marsupials, insectivores, and one elephant). American Journal of Anatomy 180:126–142, 1987

Haug H, Eggers R: Morphometry of the human cortex cerebri and corpus striatum during aging. Neurobiol Aging 12:336–338, 1991

Haug H, Barmwater U, Eggers R, et al: Anatomical changes in aging brain: morphometric analysis of the human prosencephalon, in Brain Aging: Neuropathology and Neuropharmacology. Edited by Cerves-Navarro J, Sarkander HI. New York, Raven, 1983, pp 1–11

Haug H, Kühl S, Mecke E, et al: The significance of morphometric procedures in the investigation of age changes in cytoarchitectonic structures of human brain. J Hirnforsch 25:353–374, 1984

Hayflick L: Theories of biological aging. Exp Gerontol 20:145–159, 1985

Hazzard WR, Andres R, Bierman EL, et al (eds): Principles of Geriatric Medicine and Gerontology, 2nd Edition. New York, McGraw-Hill, 1990

Heaton RK: Wisconsin Card Sorting Test. Odessa, FL, Psychological Assessment Resources, 1985

Hedreen JC, Struble RG, Whitehouse PJ, et al: Topography of the magnocellular basal forebrain system in human brain. J Neuropathol Exp Neurol 43:1–21, 1984

Hefti F, Mash DC: Localization of nerve growth factor receptors in the normal human brain and in Alzheimer's disease. Neurobiol Aging 10:75–87, 1989

Hefti F, Hartikka J, Knusel B: Function of neurotropic factors in the adult and aging brain and their possible use in the treatment of neurodegenerative diseases. Neurobiol Aging 10:515–533, 1989

Heilig CW, Knopman DS, Mastri AR, et al: Dementia without Alzheimer pathology. Neurology 35:762–765, 1985

Herndon JG, Tigges J, Klumpp SA, et al: Brain weight does not decrease with age in adult rhesus monkeys. Neurobiol Aging 19(3):267–272, 1998

Hier DB, LeMay M, Rosenberg PB, et al: Developmental dyslexia: evidence for a subgroup with a reversal of cerebral asymmetry. Arch Neurol 35:90–92, 1978

Hirai S: Histochemical study on the regressive degeneration of the senile brain, with special reference to the aging of the substantia nigra. Advances in Neurological Science (Tokyo) 12:845–849, 1968

Hof PR, Morrison JH: Quantitative analysis of a vulnerable subset of pyramidal neurons in Alzheimer's disease, II: primary and secondary visual cortex. J Comp Neurol 301:55–64, 1990

Hofman MA: Energy metabolism, brain size and longevity in mammals. Q Rev Biol 58:495–512, 1983

Hofman MA: From here to eternity: brain aging in an evolutionary perspective. Neurobiol Aging 12:338–340, 1991

Hofman MA, Swaab DF: The sexually dimorphic nucleus of the preoptic area in the human brain: a comparative morphometric study. J Anat 164:55–72, 1989

Hubble JP: Aging and the basal ganglia. Neurol Clin 16(3):649–657, 1998

Hyman BT, Van Hoesen GW, Damasio AR, et al: Alzheimer's disease: cell-specific pathology isolates the hippocampal formation. Science 225:1168–1170, 1984

Hyman BT, Arriagada PV, Van Hoesen GW: Pathologic changes in the olfactory system in aging and Alzheimer's disease. Ann N Y Acad Sci 640:14–19, 1991

Ikeda SI, Allsop D, Glenner GG: Morphology and distribution of plaque and related deposits in the brains of Alzheimer's disease and control cases: an immunohistochemical study using amyloid-protein antibody. Lab Invest 60:113–122, 1989

Ince PG, Perry EK, Morris CM: Dementia with Lewy bodies. A distinct non-Alzheimer dementia syndrome? Brain Pathol 8:299–324, 1998

Ingvar MC, Maeder P, Sokoloff L, et al: Effects of ageing on local rates of cerebral protein synthesis in Sprague-Dawley rats. Brain 108:155–170, 1985

Inzitari D, Diaz F, Fox A, et al: Vascular risk factors and leuko-araiosis. Arch Neurol 44:42–47, 1987

Itoh K, Weis S, Mehraein P, et al: Cytochrome c oxidase defects of the human substantia nigra in normal aging. Neurobiol Aging 17(6):843–848, 1996

Jacobs B, Driscoll L, Schall M: Life-span dendritic and spine changes in areas 10 and 18 of human cortex: a quantitative golgi study. J Comp Neurol 386:661–680, 1997

Jellinger KA: Quantitative changes in some subcortical nuclei in aging, Alzheimer's disease and Parkinson's disease. Neurobiol Aging 8:556–561, 1987

Jellinger KA: Neuropathological staging of Alzheimer'related lesions: The challenge of establishing relations to age. Neurobiol Aging 18(4):369–375, 1997

Jengeleski CA, Powers RE, O'Connor DT, et al: Noradrenergic innervation of human pineal gland: abnormalities in aging and Alzheimer's disease. Brain Res 481:378–382, 1989

Jeste DV: Medical comorbidity in schizophrenia. Schizophr Bull 22:413–430, 1996

Johnson BF, Sinclair DA, Guarente L: Molecular biology of aging. Cell Press 96:291–302, 1999

Joseph JA, Denisova N, Fisher D, et al: Age-related neuerodegeneration and oxidative stress. The Neurology of Aging 16(3):747–755, 1998

Joyce JN, Goldsmith SG, Gurevich EV: Limbic circuits and monoamine receptors dissecting the effects of antipsychotics from disease processes. J Psychiatr Res 31:197–217, 1997

Kalaria RN, Andorn AC, Tabaton M, et al: Adrenergic receptors in aging and Alzheimer's disease: increased receptors in prefrontal cortex and hippocampus. J Neurochem 53:1772–1781, 1989

Katzman R: The aging brain: limitation in our knowledge and future approaches (editorial). Arch Neurol 54:1201–1205, 1997

Katzman R, Terry R, DeTeresa R, et al: Clinical, pathological, and neurochemical changes in dementia: a subgroup with preserved mental status and numerous neocortical plaques. Ann Neurol 23:138–144, 1988

Kawasaki H, Murayama SA, Tomonaga M, et al: Neurofibrillary tangles in human upper cervical ganglia: morphological study with immunohistochemistry and electron microscopy. Acta Neuropathol 75:156–159, 1987

Kaye JA, DeCarli C, Luxenberg JS, et al: The significance of age-related enlargement of the cerebral ventricles in healthy men and women measured by quantitative computed x-ray tomography. J Am Geriatr Soc 40:225–231, 1992

Kemper T: Neuroanatomical and neuropathological changes in normal aging and dementia, in Clinical Neurology of Aging. Edited by Albert ML. New York, Oxford University Press, 1984, pp 9–52

Kesslak JP, Cotman CW, Chui HC, et al: Olfactory tests as possible probes for detecting and monitoring Alzheimer's disease. Neurobiol Aging 9:399–403, 1988

Kirkpatrick JB, Hayman LA: White-matter lesions in MR imaging of clinically healthy brains of elderly subjects: possible pathologic basis. Radiology 162:509–511, 1987

Knox CA, Kokmen E, Dyck PJ: Morphometric alteration of rat myelinated fibers with aging. J Neuropathol Exp Neurol 48:119–139, 1989

Lamberts SWJ, van den Beld AW, van der Lely A-J: The endocrinology of aging. Science 278:419–424, 1997

Leuba G, Kraftsik R: Changes in volume, surface estimate, three-dimensional shape and total number of neurons of the human primary visual cortex from midgestation until old age. Anat Embryol (Berl) 190:351–366, 1994

Levey A: Muscarinic acetylcholine receptor expression in memory circuits: implications for treatment of Alzheimer's disease. Proc Natl Acad Sci U S A 93:13541–13546, 1996

Lewis DA, Akil M: Cortical dopamine in schizophrenia: strategies for postmortem studies. J Psychiatr Res 31(2):175–195, 1997

Lintl P, Braak H: Loss of intracortical myelinated fibers: a distinctive age-related alteration in the human striate area. Acta Neuropathol (Berl) 61:178–182, 1983

Longstreth WT, Bernick C, Manolio TA, et al: Lacunar infarcts defined by magnetic resonance imaging of 3660 elderly people: the cardiovascular health study. Arch Neurol 55:1217–1225, 1998

Lopez OL, Rabin BS, Huff FJ: Serum auto-antibodies in Alzheimer's disease. Acta Neurol Scand 84:441–444, 1991

Lupien S, Lecours AR, Schwartz G, et al: Longitudinal study of basal cortisol levels in healthy elderly subjects: evidence for subgroups. Neurobiol Aging 17(1):95–105, 1996

Madden KS, Thyagarajan S, Felten DL: Alterations in sympathetic noradrenergic innervation in lymphoid organs with age. Ann N Y Acad Sci 840:262–268, 1998

Mader SL: Aging and postural hypotension: an update. J Am Geriatr Soc 37:129–137, 1989

Mandelkow E, Song YH, Schweers O, et al: On the structure of microtubules, tau, and paired helical filaments. Neurobiol Aging 16(3):347–354, 1995

Mann DMA: Is the pattern of nerve cell loss in aging and Alzheimer's disease a real, or only an apparent, selectivity? Neurobiol Aging 12:340–343, 1991

Mann DMA, Yates PO, Hawkes J: The pathology of the human locus ceruleus. Clin Neuropathol 2:1–7, 1983

Mann DMA, Yates PO, Marcyniuk B: Monoaminergic neurotransmitter systems in presenile Alzheimer's disease and in senile dementia of Alzheimer type. Clin Neuropathol 3:199–205, 1984

Markesbery, WR: Neuropathological criteria for the diagnosis of Alzheimer's disease. Neurobiol Aging 18(S4):S13–S19, 1997

Masliah E, Mallory M, Hansen L, et al: Quantitative synaptic alterations in the human neocortex during normal aging. Neurology 43:192–197, 1993

Matsuyama H, Nakamura S: Senile changes in the brain in the Japanese: incidence of Alzheimer's neurofibrillary change and senile plaques, in Alzheimer's Disease: Senile Dementia and Related Disorders. Edited by Katzman R, Terry RD, Bick KL. New York, Raven, 1978, pp 287–297

Mattson MP, Rydel RE: Amyloid precursor protein and Alzheimer's disease: the peptide plot thickens. Neurobiol Aging 13:617–621, 1992

Maurer K, Riederer P, Beckmann J(eds): Alzheimer's Disease: Epidemiology, Neuropathology, Neurochemistry, and Clinics. New York, Springer-Verlag, 1990

May C, Kaye JA, Atack JR, et al: Cerebrospinal fluid production is reduced in healthy aging. Neurology 40:500–503, 1990

McEwen BS: When is stimulation too much of a good thing? Neurobiol Aging 12:346–348, 1991

McEwen BS: Stress, adaptation, and disease: allostasis and allostatic load. Ann N Y Acad Sci 840:33–44, 1998

McGeer PL, McGeer EG, Suzuki JS: Aging and extrapyramidal function. Arch Neurol 34:33–35, 1977

McKhann G, Drachman D, Folstein M, et al: Clinical diagnosis of Alzheimer's disease: report of the NINCDS-ADRDA work group under the auspices of Department of Health and Human Services Task Force on Alzheimer's Disease. Neurology (NY) 34:939–944, 1984

McLeod JG, Tuck RR: Disorders of the autonomic nervous system, I: pathophysiology and clinical features. Ann Neurol 21:419–430, 1987

Mecocci P, MacGarvey U, Kaufman AE: Oxidative damage to mitochondrial DNA shows marked age-dependent increases in human brain. Ann Neurol 34:609–616, 1993

Mendelsohn FAO, Paxinos G (eds): Receptors in the Human Nervous System. San Diego, CA, Academic Press, 1991

Mervis RF, Pope D, Lewis R, et al: Exogenous nerve growth factor reverses age-related structural changes in neocortical neurons in the aging rat: a quantitative Golgi study. Ann N Y Acad Sci 640:95–103, 1991

Mesulam M-M, Geula C: Nucleus basalis (ch 4) and cortical cholinergic innervation in the human brain: observations based on the distribution of acetylcholinesterase and choline acetyltransferase. J Comp Neurol 275:216–240, 1988

Mesulam M-M, Mufson EJ, Levey AI, et al: Cholinergic innervation of cortex by the basal forebrain: cytochemistry and cortical connections of the septal area, diagonal band nuclei, nucleus basalis (substantia innominata), and hypothalamus in the rhesus monkey. J Comp Neurol 214:170–197, 1983

Miller JA, Zahniser NR: Quantitative autoradiographic analysis of pindolol binding in Fischer 344 rat brain: changes in adrenergic receptor density with aging. Neurobiol Aging 9:267–272, 1988

Mizuno Y, Yoshino H, Ikebe S, et al: Mitochondrial dysfunction in Parkinson's disease. Ann Neurol 44(1):S99–S109, 1998

Moatamed F: Cell frequencies in human inferior olivary nuclear complex. J Comp Neurol 128:109–115, 1966

Moody DM, Brown WR, Challa VR, et al: Periventricular venous collagenosis: association with leukoaraiosis. Radiology 194:469–476, 1995

Moody D, Brown WR, Challa VR, et al: Cerebral microvascular alterations in aging, leukoaraiosis, and Alzheimer's disease. Ann N Y Acad Sci 826:103–116, 1997

Mooradian AD: Effect of aging on the blood-brain barrier. Neurobiol Aging 9:31–39, 1988

Moossy J: Pathology of cerebral atherosclerosis: influence of age, race, and gender. Stroke 24 (suppl I):I22–I23, 1993

Morgan DG, Finch CE: Neurotransmitter receptors in Alzheimer's disease and nonpathological aging, in Molecular Neuropathology of Aging. Edited by Davies P, Finch CE. Cold Spring Harbor, NY, Cold Spring Harbor Laboratory, 1987, pp 21–35

Morgan DG, Marcusson JO, Nyberg P, et al: Divergent changes in D-1 and D-2 dopamine binding sites in human brain during aging. Neurobiol Aging 8:195–201, 1987

Morishima-Kawashima M, Hasegawa M, Takio K, et al: Hyperphosphorylation of tau in PHF. Neurobiol Aging 16(3):365–380, 1995

Morley JE: Anorexia of aging: physiologic and pathologic. Am J Clin Nutr 66:760–773, 1997

Morrison BM, Hof PR, Morrison JH: Determinants of neuronal vulnerability in neurodegenerative diseases. Ann Neurol 44(1):S32–S44, 1998

Morrison JH, Hof PR: Life and death of neurons in the aging brain. Science 278:412–419, 1997

Morrison JH, Hof PR, Bouras C: An anatomic substrate for visual disconnection in Alzheimer's disease. Ann N Y Acad Sci 640:36–43, 1991

Morsch R, Simon W, Coleman PD: Neurons may live for decades with neurofibrillary tangles. J Neuropathol Exp Neurol 58(2):188–197, 1999

Mrak RE, Griffin WST, Graham DI: Aging-associated changes in human brain. J Neuropathol Exp Neurol 56(12): 1269–1275, 1997

Muller WE, Stoll L, Schubert T, et al: Central cholinergic functioning and aging. Acta Psychiatr Scand 366 (suppl):34–39, 1991

Münch G, Thome J, Foley P, et al: Advanced glycation endproducts in ageing and Alzheimer's disease. Brain Research Reviews 23:134–143, 1997

Münch G, Gerlach M, Sian J, et al: Advanced glycation end products in neurodegeneration: more than early markers of oxidative stress? Ann Neurol 44 (suppl 1):S85–S88, 1998

Murphy DGM, DeCarli C, Schapiro MG, et al: Age-related differences in volumes of subcortical nuclei, brain matter, and cerebrospinal fluid in healthy men as measured with magnetic resonance imaging. Arch Neurol 49:839–845, 1992

Nelson PT, Saper CB: Ultrastructure of neurofibrillary tangles in the cerebral cortex of sheep. Neurobiol Aging 16(3): 315–323, 1995

Niedermuller H, Hofecker G, Skalicky M: Changes of DNA repair mechanisms during the aging of the rat. Mech Ageing Dev 29:221–238, 1985

Nistic G, De Sarro G: Is interleukin 2 a neuromodulator in the brain? Trends Neurosci 14:146–150, 1991

Nordberg A, Winblad B: Reduced number of [^{3}H]nicotine and [^{3}H]acetylcholine binding sites in the frontal cortex of Alzheimer brains. Neurosci Lett 72:115–119, 1986

Obonai T, Mizuguchi M, Takashima S: Developmental and aging changes of Bak expression in the human brain. Brain Res 783:167–170, 1998

Ohm TG, Busch C, Bohl J: Unbiased estimation of neuronal numbers in the human nucleus coeruleus during aging. Neurobiol Aging 18(4):393–399, 1997

Okubo Y, Suhara T, Suzuki K: Decreased prefrontal dopamine D$_1$ receptors in schizophrenia revealed by PET (letter). Nature December 4, 1996, pp 34–36

Olney JW, Wozniak DF, Farber NB: Excitotoxic neurodegeneration in Alzheimer's disease: new hypothesis and new therapeutic strategies. Arch Neurol 54:1234–1240, 1997

Olton D, Markowska A, Voytko ML, et al: Basal forebrain cholinergic system: a functional analysis. Adv Exp Med Biol 295:353–371, 1991

Ott A, Breteler MMB, deBruyne MC, et al: Atrial fibrillation and dementia in a population-based study: The Rotterdam Study. Stroke 28(2):316–321, 1997

Oyanagi K, Wakabayashi K, Ohama E, et al: Lewy bodies in the lower sacral parasympathetic neurons of a patient with Parkinson's disease. Acta Neuropathol (Berl) 80:558–559, 1990

Pacheco MA, Jope RS: Phosphoinositide signaling in human brain. Prog Neurobiol 50:255–273, 1996

Pakkenberg B, Gundersen JG: Neocortical neuron number in humans: effect of sex and age. J Comp Neurol 384(2): 379–482, 1997

Pantoni L, Garcia JH: Cognitive impairment and cellular/vascular changes in the cerebral white matter. Ann N Y Acad Sci 826:92–101, 1997

Papadakis MA, Grady D, Black D, et al: Growth hormone replacement in healthy older men improves body composition but not functional ability. Ann Intern Med 124: 708–716, 1996

Pascual J, del Arco C, Gonzàlez AM, et al: Quantitative light microscopic autoradiographic localization of adrenoceptors in the human brain. Brain Res 585:116–127, 1992

Peng I, Binder LI, Black MM: Biochemical and immunological analyses of cytoskeletal domains of neurons. J Cell Biol 102:252–262, 1986

Perrig WJ, Perrig P, St. Helin HB: The relation between antioxidants and memory performance in the old and very old. J Am Geriatr Soc 45:718–724, 1997

Perry EK, McKeith I, Thompson P, et al: Topography, extent, and clinical relevance of neurochemical deficits in dementia of Lewy body type, Parkinson's disease, and Alzheimer's disease. Ann N Y Acad Sci 640:197–202, 1991

Peters A: Age-related changes in oligodendrocytes in monkey cerebral cortex. J Comp Neurol 371:153–163, 1996

Peters A, Rosene DL, Moss MB, et al: Neurobiological bases of age-related cognitive decline in the rhesus monkey. J Neuropathol Exp Neurol 55(8):861–874, 1996

Peters NL: Snipping the thread of life: antimuscarinic side effects of medications in the elderly. Arch Intern Med 149:2414–2420, 1989

Powers RE, Struble RG, Casanova MF, et al: Innervation of human hippocampus by noradrenergic systems: normal anatomy and structural abnormalities in aging and in Alzheimer's disease. Neuroscience 25:401–417, 1988

Powers RE, Powell SK, Schlough CN, et al: Autopsy services for dementia patients. Gerontologist 29:120–123, 1989

Powers R: The neuropathology of Schizophrenia. J Neuropathol Exp Neurol 58(7):679–690, 1999

Price DL, Martin LJ, Sisodia SS, et al: Aged non-human primates: an animal model of age-associated neurodegenerative disease. Brain Pathol 1:287–296, 1991

Price JL, Davis PB, Morris JC, et al: The distribution of tangles, plaques and related immunohistochemical markers in healthy aging and Alzheimer's disease. Neurobiol Aging 12:295–312, 1991

Probst A, Brunnschweiler H, Lautenschlager C, et al: A special type of senile plaque, possibly an initial stage. Acta Neuropathol (Berl) 74:133–141, 1987

Procter AW, Bowen DM: Aging, the cerebral neocortex, and psychiatric disorder, in Molecular Neuropathology of Aging. Edited by Davies P, Finch CE. Cold Spring Harbor, NY, Cold Spring Harbor Laboratory, 1987, pp 3–21

Purohit DP, Perl DP, Haroutunian V, et al: Alzheimer's disease and related neurodegenerative diseases in elderly patients with schizophrenia. Arch Gen Psychiatry 55:205–211, 1998

Rance NE: Hormonal influences on morphology and neuropeptide gene expression in the infundibular nucleus of post-menopausal women. Prog Brain Res 93:221–236, 1992

Rance NE, Young WS III: Hypertrophy and increased gene expression of neurons containing neurokinin-B and substance-P messenger ribonucleic acids in the hypothalami of postmenopausal women. Endocrinology 128:2239–2247, 1991

Rance NE, McMullen NT, Smialek JE, et al: Postmenopausal hypertrophy of neurons expressing the estrogen receptor gene in the human hypothalamus. J Clin Endocrinol Metab 71:79–85, 1990

Rance NE, Uswandi SV, McMullen NT: Neuronal hypertrophy in the hypothalamus of older men. Neurobiol Aging 14:337–342, 1993

Rapp PR, Gallagher M: Preserved neuron number in the hippocampus of aged rats with spatial learning deficits. Neurobiology (Bp) 93:9926–9930, 1996

Ravens JR: Vascular changes in the human senile brain. Adv Neurol 20:487–501, 1978

Reznikoff GA, Manaker S, Rhodes CH, et al: Localization and quantification of beta-adrenergic receptors in human brain. Neurology 36:1067–1073, 1986

Roberts EL, Ching-Ping C, Rosenthal M: Age-related changes in brain metabolism and vulnerability to anoxia. Advances in Experimental Medicine and Biology 411:83–89, 1997

Robinson RG, Kubos KL, Starr LBN, et al: Mood disorders in stroke patients: importance of location of lesion. Brain 107 (pt 1):81–93, 1984

Robinson RG, Bolduc PL, Price TR: Two-year longitudinal study of poststroke disorders: diagnosis and outcome at one and two years. Stroke 18:837–843, 1987

Rosene DL, Van Hoesen GW: The hippocampal formation of the primate brain: a review of some comparative aspects of cytoarchitecture and connections, in Cerebral Cortex, Vol 6. Edited by Jones EG, Peters A. New York, Plenum, 1986, pp 345–456

Rowe JW: Plasma norepinephrine as an index of sympathetic activity in aging man, in Molecular Neuropathology of Aging. Edited by Davies P, Finch CE. Cold Spring Harbor, NY, Cold Spring Harbor Laboratory, 1987, pp 137–143

Rowe JW, Kahn RL: Successful Aging. New York, Pantheon Books, 1998

Rudman D, Feller AG, Nagraj HS, et al: Effects of human growth hormone in men over 60 years old. N Engl J Med 323:1–6, 1990

Sanyal S, van Tol HHM: Review the role of dopamine D_4 receptors in schizophrenia and antipsychotic action. J Psychiatr Res 31(2):219–232, 1997

Sapolsky RM: Glucocorticoids and hippocampal damage. Trends Neurosci 10:346–349, 1987a

Sapolsky RM: Protecting the injured hippocampus by attenuating glucocorticoid secretion, in Molecular Neuropathology of Aging. Edited by Davies P, Finch CE. Cold Spring Harbor, NY, Cold Spring Harbor Laboratory, 1987b, pp 191–201

Satou T, Cummings BJ, Head E, et al: The progression of β-amyloid deposition in the frontal cortex of the aged canine. Brain Res 774:35–43, 1997

Scarpace PJ, Abrass IB: Alpha- and beta-adrenergic receptor function in the brain during senescence. Neurobiol Aging 9:53–58, 1988

Scheff SW: Use or abuse. Neurobiol Aging 12:349–351, 1991

Schiffman SS: Taste and smell losses in normal aging and disease. JAMA 278:1357–1362, 1997

Schipper H: Astrocytes, brain aging and neurodegeneration. Neurobiol Aging 17:467–480, 1996

Schoen EJ: Growth hormone in youth and old age (the old and new déjà vu) (letter). J Am Geriatr Soc 39:839, 1991

Schroder H, Giacobini E, Struble RG, et al: Cellular distribution and expression of cortical acetylcholine receptors in aging and Alzheimer's disease. Ann N Y Acad Sci 640:189–192, 1991

Seeman TE, Berkman LF, Charpentier PA, et al: Behavioral and psychosocial predictors of physical performance: MacArthur studies of successful aging. J Gerontol A Biol Sci Med Sci 50(4):177–183, 1995

Simic G, Kostovic I, Winblad B, et al: Volume and number of neurons of the human hippocampal formation in normal aging and Alzheimer's disease. J Comp Neurobiol 379(4):482–494, 1997

Snowdon DA: Aging and Alzheimer's disease: lessons from the nun study. Gerontologist 37(2):150–156, 1997

Snowdon DA, Kemper SJ, Mortimer JA, et al: Linguistic ability in early life and cognitive function and Alzheimer's disease in late life. JAMA 275(7):528–532, 1996

Snowdon, DA, Greiner LH, Mortimer JA, et al: Brain infarction and the clinical expression of Alzheimer's disease: the nun study. JAMA 277(10):813–817, 1997

Sobin SS, Bernick S, Ballard KW: Histochemical characterization of the aging microvasculature in the human and other mammalian and non-mammalian vertebrates by the periodic acid-Schiff reaction. Mech Ageing Dev 63:183–192, 1992

Stabler P, Lindenbaum J, Allen RH: Vitamin B-12 deficiency in the elderly: current dilemmas. Am J Clin Nutr 66:741–749, 1997

Starr JM, Whalley LJ: Senile hypertension and cognitive impairment: an overview. J Hypertens 10 (suppl 2):S31–S42, 1992

Strawbridge WJ, Cohen RD, Shema SJ, et al: Successful aging: predictors and associated activities. Am J Epidemiol 144(2):135–141, 1996

Stroop JR: Studies of Interference of serial verbal reaction. J Exp Psychol 18:643–662 , 1935

Struble RG, Powers RE, Casanova MF, et al: Neuropeptidergic systems in plaques of Alzheimer's disease. J Neuropathol Exp Neurol 46:567–584, 1987

Sulkava R, Erkinjuntti T: Vascular dementia due to cardiac arrhythmias and systemic hypotension. Acta Neurol Scand 76:123–128, 1987

Swaab DF: Brain aging and Alzheimer's disease, "wear and tear" versus "use it or lose it." Neurobiol Aging 12:317–324, 1991

Sze G, De Armond SJ, Brant-Zawadzki M, et al: Foci of MRI signal (pseudo lesions) anterior to the frontal horns: histologic correlations of a normal finding. AJNR Am J Neuroradiol 7:381–387, 1986

Talamo BR, Rudel RA, Kosik KS, et al: Pathological changes in olfactory neurons in patients with Alzheimer's disease. Nature 337:736–739, 1989

Tang Y, Nyengaard JR, Pakkenberg B: Age-induced white matter changes in the human brain: a stereological investigation. Neurobiol Aging 18:609–615, 1997

Tatton WG, Chalmer-Redmon RME: Mitochondria in neurodegenerative apoptosis: an opportunity for therapy? Ann Neurol 44 (suppl 1):S134–S141, 1998

Terry RD, Hansen LA, DeTeresa R, et al: Senile dementia of the Alzheimer type without neocortical neurofibrillary tangles. J Neuropathol Exp Neurol 46:262–268, 1987

Thoenen H, Zafra F, Hengerer B, et al: The synthesis of nerve growth factor and brain-derived neurotrophic factor in hippocampal and cortical neurons is regulated by specific transmitter systems. Ann N Y Acad Sci 640:86–90, 1991

Thomas WE: Brain macrophages: evaluation of microglia and their functions. Brain Res Brain Res Rev 17:61–74, 1992

Tigges J, Herndon JG, Rosene DI: Mild age-related changes in the dentate gyrus of adult rhesus monkeys. Acta Anat (Basel) 157:39–48, 1996a

Tigges J, Herndon JG, Rosene DI: Preservation into old age of synaptic number and size in the supragranular layer of the dentate gyrus in rhesus monkeys. Acta Anat (Basel) 157:63–72, 1996b

Tohgi H, Utsugisawa K, Yoshimura M, et al: Reduction in the ratio of β-preprotachykinin to preproenkephalin messenger RNA expression in postmortem human putamen during aging and in patients with status lacunaris: implications for the susceptibility to Parkinsonism. Brain Res 768:86–90, 1997

Tohgi H, Utsugisawa K, Yoshimura M, et al: Age-related changes in D_1 and D_2 receptor mRNA expression in postmortem human putamen with and without multiple small infarcts. Neurosci Lett 243:37–40, 1998a

Tohgi H, Utsugisawa K, Yoshirmura M, et al: Alterations with aging and ischemia in nicotinic acetylcholine receptor subunits α_4 and β_2 messenger RNA expression in porsmortem human putamen: implications for susceptibility to parkinsonism. Brain Res 791:186–190, 1998b

Tolnay M, Probst A: Review: tau protein pathology in Alzheimer's disease and related disorders. Neuropathol Appl Neurobiol 25:171–187, 1999 @reference = Tomei LD, Umansky SR: Aging and apoptosis control. Neurologic Clinics of North America 16(3):735–745, 1998

Tomlinson BE, Blessed G, Roth M: Observations on the brains of demented old people. J Neurol Sci 11:205–242, 1970

Torack RM, Morris JC: The association of ventral tegmental area histopathology with adult dementia. Arch Neurol 45:497–501, 1988

Troncoso JC, Martin LJ, dal Forno G, et al: Neuropathology in controls and demented subjects from the Baltimore Longitudinal Study of Aging. Neurobiol Aging 17(3):365–371, 1996

Uchihara T, Kondo H, Kosaka K, et al: Selective loss of nigral neurons in Alzheimer's disease: a morphometric study. Acta Neuropathol (Berl) 83:271–276, 1992

Ueno E, Liu DD, Ho IK, et al: Opiate receptor characteristics in brains from young, mature and aged mice. Neurobiol Aging 9:279–283, 1988

Ulrich J: Senile plaques and neurofibrillary tangles of the Alzheimer type in nondemented individuals at presenile age. Gerontology 28:86–90, 1982

Van Gool WA, Pronker HF, Mirmiran M, et al: Effect of housing in an enriched environment on the size of the cerebral cortex in young and old rats. Exp Neurol 96:225–232, 1987

Vaupel JW, Carey JR, Christensen K, et al: Biodemographic trajectories of longevity. Science 280:855–860, 1998

Veith RC, Raskind MA: The neurobiology of aging: does it predispose to depression? Neurobiol Aging 9:101–117, 1988

Vita AJ, Terry RB, Hubert HB, et la: Aging, health risks, and cumulative disability. N Engl J Med 338:1035–1041, 1998

Volkow ND, Fowler JS, Wang GJ, et al: Decreased dopamine transporters with age in healthy subjects. Ann Neurol 36:237–239, 1994

Volkow ND, Gur RC, Wang GJ, et al: Association between decline in brain dopamine activity with age and cognitive and motor impairment in healthy individuals. Am J Psychiatry 155:344–349, 1998

Wakabayashi K, Takahashi H, Takeda S, et al: Parkinson's disease: the presence of Lewy bodies in Auerbach's and Meissner's plexuses. Acta Neuropathol (Berl) 76:217–221, 1988

Wang Y, Chan GLY, Holden JE, et al: Age-dependent decline of dopamine D1 receptors in human brain: a PET study. Synapse 30:56–61, 1998

Wareham KA, Lyon MF, Glenister PH, et al: Age-related reactivation of an X-linked gene. Nature 327:725–727, 1987

Weinberger DR: Implications of normal brain development for the pathogenesis of schizophrenia. Arch Gen Psychiatry 44:660–669, 1987

West MJ: New stereological methods for counting neurons. Neurobiol Aging 14:275–285, 1993

West MJ, Coleman PD, Flood DG: Differences in the pattern of hippocampal neuronal loss in normal ageing and Alzheimer's disease. Lancet 344:769–772, 1994

Whetsell WO: Current concepts of excitotoxicity. J Neuropathol Exp Neurol 55(1):1–13, 1996

Whitehouse PJ, Price DL, Clark AW, et al: Alzheimer disease: evidence for selective loss of cholinergic neurons in the nucleus basalis. Ann Neurol 10:122–126, 1981

Wise PM, Cohen IR, Weiland NG: Hypothalamic monoamine function during aging: its role in the onset of reproductive infertility, in Molecular Neuropathology of Aging. Edited by Davies P, Finch CE. Cold Spring Harbor, NY, Cold Spring Harbor Laboratory, 1987, pp 159–164

Wong DF, Young D, Wilson PD, et al: Quantification of neuroreceptors in the living human brain, III: D_2-like dopamine receptors: theory, validation, and changes during normal aging. J Cereb Blood Flow Metab 17:316–330, 1997

Wyss JM, Van Groen T: Early breakdown of dendritic bundles in the retrosplenial granular cortex of hypertensive rats: prevention by antihypertensive therapy. Cereb Cortex 2:468–476, 1992

Wyss JM, Fisk G, Van Groen T: Impaired learning and memory in mature spontaneously hypertensive rats. Brain Res 592:135–140, 1992

Yu CE, Ishima J, Fu YH, et al: Positional cloning of the Werner's syndrome gene. Science 272(12):258–262, 1996

Zubenko GS, Moossy J: Major depression in primary dementia: clinical and neuropathologic correlates. Arch Neurol 45:1182–1186, 1988

Zuccala G, Cattel C, Manes-Gravina E, et al: Left ventricular dysfunction: a clue to cognitive impairment in older patients with heart failure. J Neurol Neurosurg Psychiatry 63:509–512, 1997

4

Neurobiological Basis of Behavior

Jeffrey L. Cummings, M.D.

C. Edward Coffey, M.D.

All behavior and experience are mediated by the brain. No behavior, thought, or emotion lacks a corresponding cerebral event, and abnormalities of human behavior are frequently a reflection of abnormal brain structure and are accompanied by aberrant brain function. This premise does not deny the influence of learning, life events, education, or the sociocultural dimension of human existence; these factors create the context of human behavior and exert powerful biological, developmental, and situational influences. In all cases, however, psychological and sociocultural effects are mediated through brain function. Thus, a comprehensive approach to human behavior demands an understanding of the neurological basis of human cognition, emotion, and psychopathology.

A life-span perspective adds another dimension to understanding behavior: brain function alters dramatically from uterine life through infancy, childhood, adolescence, adulthood, and old age. Physiological functions vary more widely in elderly people than in young people, tolerance of injury and potential for recovery are diminished in elderly patients, and the types of behaviors associated with brain dysfunction often differ depending on the age of the patient.

In this chapter, we provide a review of the neuroanatomical and neurochemical basis of human behavior. First, we present a synoptic model of behavioral neuroanatomy as a framework for the remaining discussion. The model divides the nervous system into three behaviorally relevant zones: an inner zone surrounding the ventricular system, a middle zone encompassing the basal ganglia and limbic system, and an outer zone comprised primarily of the neocortex. We present the anatomy of each zone and describe the behavioral consequences of injury to each. Next, we describe two distributed systems; these cross the three zones to allow information to enter the brain (thalamocortical system) and allow impulses mediating action to exit the brain (frontal-subcortical circuits). We also present neuropsychiatric syndromes associated with abnormalities of these systems. Finally, we integrate the biochemical basis of behavior with this anatomical approach.

A Model of Behavioral Neuroanatomy

Paul Yakovlev developed a comprehensive model of the nervous system in terms relevant to behavior (Yakovlev 1948, 1968; Yakovlev and Lecours 1967). He adopted an evolutionary perspective and noted that the brain consists of three general regions: a median zone surrounding the ventricular system, containing the hypothalamus and related structures; a paramedian-limbic zone consisting primarily of limbic system structures, basal ganglia, and parts of the thalamus; and a supralimbic zone containing the neocortex.

In this chapter, we present the Yakovlev approach—updated with information from more recent anatomical studies (Benarroch 1997; Mesulam 1985)—as a foundation for understanding brain-behavior relationships (Figure 4–1). The *median zone* is immediately adjacent to the central canal, is poorly myelinated, and has neurons with short axons that synapse on nearby cells, as well as on cells with longer axons that project to more distant nuclei. The median zone contains the hypothalamus, medial thalamus, and periventricular gray matter of the brainstem as well as functionally related areas of the amygdala and insular cortex. The system mediates energy metabolism, homeostasis, peristalsis, respiration, and circulation. The median zone contains the reticular activating system and the nonspecific thalamocortical projections that maintain consciousness and arousal in the awake state and participate in sleep mechanisms. No lateral specialization is evident in the median zone. This system is fully functional at birth and is responsible for the early survival of the infant.

The *paramedian-limbic zone* has neurons that are more well myelinated than the median zone, and neurons here are grouped in nuclear structures that are connected in series. Many of the thalamic nuclei, the basal ganglia, cingulate gyrus, insula, orbitofrontal region, hippocampus, and parahippocampal gyri are included in this zone. The paramedian-limbic zone includes the structures composing the limbic system (Papez 1937). Structures of this zone mediate the experiential aspects of emotional states. They also mediate posture and the outward expression of emotion in vocalization, gestures, and facial affective display. There is little lateral specialization of the paramedian structures. Phylogenetically, this level of brain development is present in reptiles (MacLean 1990). The paramedian-limbic zone is partially functional at birth, and

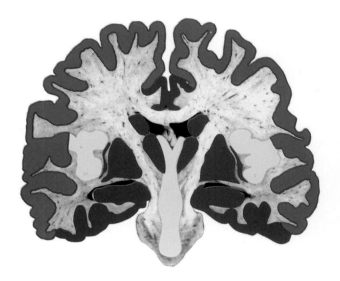

FIGURE 4–1.   Updated version of Yakovlev's model of the nervous system demonstrating the median zone (*yellow*), paramedian-limbic zone (*green*), and supralimbic zone (*red*) *Source.*   Modified with permission from Yakovlev PI, Lecours A-R: "The Myelogenetic Cycles of Regional Maturation of the Brain," in *Regional Development of the Brain in Early Life.* Edited by Minkowski A. Oxford, England, Blackwell Scientific, 1967, pp. 3–65.

its emerging integrity becomes evident in smiling and crawling. Disorders of motivation, mood, and emotion are associated with paramedian-limbic dysfunction, and this zone is the anatomic site of structures involved in many neuropsychiatric disorders. Parkinson's disease with its depression, apathy, akinesia, masked face, hypophonic voice, and marked postural changes is an example of a common disease of elderly people affecting the paramedian-limbic zone.

The *supralimbic zone* is outermost in the brain and includes the neocortex and the lateral thalamic nuclei. The neurons of this zone have long, well-myelinated axons that project via white matter tracts to more distant targets. The supralimbic neocortex contains the neurons mediating higher cortical (association) functions, as well as the pyramidal neurons projecting to limbs, lips, and tongue. It mediates highly skilled, fine motor movements evident in human speech and hand control. Ontogenetically, this zone first finds expression in the pincer grasp and articulate speech. Phylogenetically, the supralimbic zone first appears in mammals and is most well developed in humans (MacLean 1990). The supralimbic zone is expressed in human cultural achievements including art, manufacture, speech, and writing. The supralimbic zone exhibits lateral specialization with marked differences between the functions of the neocortex within the two hemispheres.

The supralimbic zone is vulnerable to some of the most common neurological disorders associated with aging, including stroke and Alzheimer's disease. For example, the expansion of the neocortex has been at the expense of a secure vasculature. The enlarged association areas have created border zone areas between the territories of the major intracranial blood vessels that are at risk of stroke because of limited interconnections and poor collateral flow; reduced cerebral perfusion with carotid artery disease or cardiopulmonary arrest regularly results in border zone infarctions at the margins between these vascular territories. In addition, penetrating branches form arterial end zones that have no collateral supply as they project through the white matter to the borders of the ventricles. This vascular anatomy creates an area of vulnerability to ischemia at the margins of the lateral ventricles. Periventricular brain injury has been associated with depression (Coffey et al. 1988), vascular dementia, and Binswanger's disease. Along with the hippocampus, the supralimbic zone is the major site of pathological changes in Alzheimer's disease. Focal lesions of the neocortex result in restricted neurobehavioral deficits such as aphasia, apraxia, and agnosia.

This model of behavioral neuroanatomy provides an ontogenetic life-span perspective showing the emerging function of these structures in early life and their disease-related vulnerability in later life. The model reflects an evolutionary perspective of the brain emphasizing its development through time and its increasing complexity in response to evolutionary pressures. From a clinical point of view, most neuropsychological deficit syndromes such as disorders of language and praxis are associated with dysfunction of the supralimbic neocortex, whereas disorders of mood, psychosis, and personality alterations are more likely to occur with abnormalities in the paramedian-limbic system. The median zone is responsible for more basic life-sustaining functions, and disturbances there are reflected in disorders of consciousness and abnormalities of metabolism, respiration, and circulation. Thus the patterns of neuropsychiatric disturbance occurring with brain disorders are highly organized events that reflect the history, structure, and function of the nervous system.

▮ Neocortex (Supralimbic Zone)

Histological Organization of the Cortex and Behavior

Brodmann originally described 46 cortical areas with distinctive histological characteristics, and Brodmann's maps have remained the classic guide to the histological organization of the cerebral mantle. Within Brodmann's areas, three types of cortex relevant to understanding behavior have been identified: a three-layered allocortex, a six-layered neocortex, and an intermediate paralimbic cortex. The limbic system cortex such as the hippocampus has a three-layered allocortical structure, whereas the sensory, motor, and association cortices of the hemispheres have a six-layered organization (Kelly 1991). In the neocortex, layer I is outermost and consists primarily of axons connecting local cortical areas; layers II and III have a predominance of small pyramidal cells and serve to connect one region of cortex with another; layer IV has mostly nonpyramidal cells, receives most of the cortical input from the thalamus, and is greatly expanded in primary sensory cortex; layer V is most prominent in motor cortex and has large pyramidal cells that have long axons descending to subcortical structures, brainstem, and spinal cord; and layer VI is adjacent to the hemispheric white matter and contains pyramidal cells, many of which project to thalamus (Kelly 1991) (Figure 4–2). Layers II and IV have the greatest cell density and the smallest cells; conversely, layers III and V have the lowest density and the largest cells. Cell size correlates with the extent of dendritic ramification, implying that cells of the layers III and V projecting to other cortical regions have the largest dendritic domains (Schade and Groeningen 1961).

Functional Organization of the Neocortex

The *neocortex* is highly differentiated into primary motor and sensory areas and unimodal and heteromodal association regions (Mesulam 1985) (Table 4–1). Figure 4–3 shows the anatomical distribution of the different cortical types in the cerebral hemispheres. Association cortex occupies 84% of the human neocortex, whereas primary motor and sensory areas account for only 16%; this indicates the marked importance of association cortex in human brain function (Rapoport 1990). The neocortex is organized in a mosaic of cortical columns, and local circuit neurons (confined to the cortex) compose approximately 25% of the cellular population (Rapoport 1990). Cortical regions receive and send information via white matter tracts.

Primary motor cortex occupies the motor strip in the posterior frontal lobe and serves as the origin of the pyramidal motor system (Figure 4–1). Lesions of the motor cortex produce contralateral weakness, particularly of the leg flexors and arm extensors, hyperreflexia, and an extensor plantar response. *Primary somatosensory cortex* is located in the postcentral gyrus in the anterior parietal lobe, *primary auditory cortex* occupies Heschl's gyrus in the superior tem-

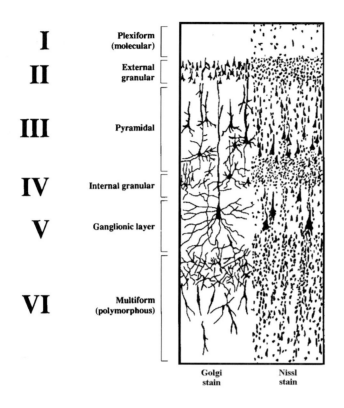

I — Plexiform (molecular)
II — External granular
III — Pyramidal
IV — Internal granular
V — Ganglionic layer
VI — Multiform (polymorphous)

Golgi stain   Nissl stain

FIGURE 4–2. Histological structure of six-layered neocortex.
Source. Reprinted with permission from Carpenter MB: *Core Text of Neuroanatomy*, 4th Edition. Baltimore, MD, Williams & Wilkins, 1991, p. 391. Copyright 1991 Williams & Wilkins.

poral lobe anterior to Wernicke's area, and *primary visual cortex* is situated in the calcarine region of the occipital lobe (Figure 4–4). Lesions of these regions typically result in contralateral hemisensory deficits (the auditory system is an exception).

Unimodal association areas mediate the second level of information processing in the cerebral cortex after the primary sensory cortex. Unimodal somatosensory cortex is located in the superior parietal lobule, unimodal auditory cortex is situated in Wernicke's region in the left hemisphere and the equivalent area of the posterior superior temporal cortex of the right hemisphere, and unimodal visual cortex occupies peristriate, midtemporal, and inferotemporal cortical regions (Figure 4–5). Lesions of these regions produce deficits confined to a single sensory modality; the syndromes associated with dysfunction of these regions reflect the higher level of information processing. Wernicke's area lesions produce fluent aphasia; lesions of right-sided auditory unimodal cortex produce sensory aprosodia (i.e., the inability to comprehend speech inflection and melody); and lesions of the unimodal visual association cortex produce visual agnosias (e.g., visual object agnosia, prosopagnosia, and environmental agnosia) (Kirshner 1986).

The highest level of information processing in the cerebral hemispheres occurs in the *heteromodal association cortices*. It is also primarily in these regions that sensory information from primary sensory and unimodal association cortex is integrated with limbic and paralimbic input

TABLE 4–1. Structure and function of different types of cerebral cortex

Cortex	Layer number	Brain regions	Relevant behaviors
Neocortex			
Primary cortex			
Koniocortex	6	Primary sensory cortex (parietal)	Vision, hearing, somatic sensation
Macropyramidal	6	Primary motor cortex (motor cortex)	Movement
Unimodal association cortex	6	Secondary association (parietal, temporal, occipital cortex)	Modality-specific processing of vision, hearing, and somatic sensation
Heteromodal association cortex	6	Multimodal association (inferior parietal lobule, prefrontal cortex)	Higher-order association
Allocortex			
Archicortex	3	Hippocampus	Memory
Paleocortex	3	Piriform cortex	Olfaction
Paralimbic (mesocortex)	4, 5	Orbitofrontal cortex, insula, temporal pole, parahippocampal gyrus, cingulate gyrus	Emotional behavior

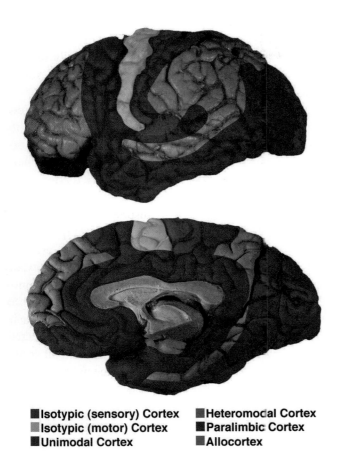

■ **Isotypic (sensory) Cortex** ■ **Heteromodal Cortex**
■ **Isotypic (motor) Cortex** ■ **Paralimbic Cortex**
■ **Unimodal Cortex** ■ **Allocortex**

FIGURE 4–3. Distribution of different histological types of cortex in the human cerebrum. The hippocampal allocortex is shown in *white*, paralimbic cortex in *green*, unimodal association cortex in *yellow*, multimodal association cortex in *red*, and primary motor and sensory cortex in *blue*.
Source. Image courtesy of M. Mega and the UCLA Laboratory of Neuroimaging.

(Mesulam 1985). Two heteromodal association regions are recognized in the human brain: the inferior parietal lobule and the prefrontal cortex (Figure 4–6). Dysfunction of these areas produces complex behavioral deficits that transcend single modalities. Lesions of the left inferior parietal lobule produce the angular gyrus syndrome with alexia, agraphia, acalculia, right–left disorientation, finger agnosia, anomia, and constructional disturbances (Benson et al. 1982). Right-sided inferior parietal lesions produce visuospatial deficits affecting constructions, spatial attention, and body-environment orientation. Prefrontal cortical dysfunction produces deficits in motor programming, memory retrieval, abstraction, and judgment (Stuss and Benson 1986). Posterior heteromodal association cortex dysfunction observed with inferior parietal lobe lesions reflects abnormalities of the highest level of processing of incoming sensory information; anterior heteromodal associ-

ation cortex dysfunction in conjunction with prefrontal disturbances produces deficits in active organizational or executive behaviors.

Thus a behavioral neuroanatomy can be discerned in the organization of the cerebral cortex. Information processing proceeds through progressively more complicated levels of analysis and integration and is then translated into action through a series of executive processes (using anterior heteromodal cortex and supplementary and primary motor cortex). Each cortical region carries on specific types of information processing activities, and regional injury or dysfunction produces a signature syndrome. From a clinical perspective, neurobehavioral and neuropsychological abnormalities such as aphasia, aprosodia, and agnosia are products of dysfunction of neocortical association cortex or connecting pathways. Although each region has unique functions, each also contributes to more complex integrative processes required for human experience and behavior.

White Matter Connections

White matter of the brain consists of myelinated axons of neurons and contains three types of fibers: 1) projection fibers that connect the cortex with the basal ganglia,

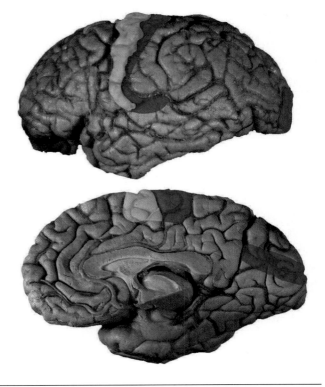

FIGURE 4–4. Primary motor (*red*) and sensory (*blue*) cortex. *Source.* Image courtesy of M. Mega and the UCLA Laboratory of Neuroimaging.

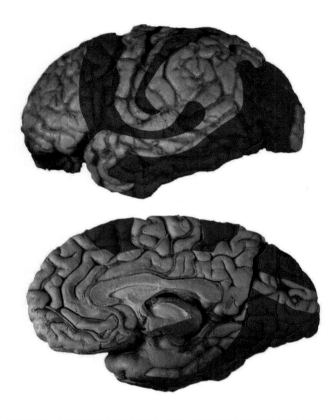

FIGURE 4–5.   Unimodal association cortex (*yellow*).
Source.   Image courtesy of M. Mega and the UCLA Laboratory of Neuroimaging.

thalamus, brainstem, and spinal cord; 2) association fibers that interconnect cortical regions of the same hemisphere; and 3) commissural fibers that connect the two hemispheres with each other (Carpenter and Sutin 1983). The principal *projection tracts* include the efferent corticostriatal projections; corticothalamic connections; corticobulbar, corticopontine, and corticospinal fibers; and the afferent thalamocortical radiations. There are also short and long *association fibers*. The short association or "U" fibers connect adjacent sulci; the long association fibers form large tracts connecting more distant regions within each hemisphere (Figure 4–7). The main long association tracts are the uncinate gyrus connecting the orbitofrontal region with the anterior temporal cortex, the arcuate fasciculus projecting between the temporal lobe and the superior and middle frontal gyri, the superior longitudinal fasciculus reaching between parieto-occipital and frontal cortices, the inferior longitudinal fasciculus connecting the parieto-occipital region with the temporal lobe, and the cingulum containing fibers connecting frontal and parietal regions with the hippocampus. The *commissural fibers* are situated in the massive corpus callosum interconnecting all lobes of one hemisphere with areas of the contralateral

hemisphere and in the more diminutive anterior commissure interconnecting the olfactory regions and the middle and inferior temporal gyri of the hemispheres (Figure 4–8).

Intact cerebral function depends on the integrity of the axons of the white matter, as well as on the activity of the neurons of the gray matter. White matter diseases with diffuse or multifocal demyelination produce memory abnormalities, dementia, depression, mania, delusions, and personality alterations. Focal lesions of white matter tracts produce a number of *disconnection syndromes* that arise when critical neuronal areas are uncoupled by an intervening lesion (Geschwind 1965; Kirshner 1986). Table 4–2 summarizes the principal disconnection syndromes.

Disruption of *commissural fibers* by stroke, surgery, or trauma disconnects the left and right hemispheres, and several commissural or callosal syndromes are recognized clinically. With an anterior callosal lesion, the right hemisphere controlling the left hand becomes disconnected from the left hemisphere; thus the left hand no longer has access to the verbal and motor skills of the left hemisphere, and callosal apraxia, left-hand tactile anomia, and left-hand agraphia result. When the splenium of the corpus callosum is damaged in association with injury to the left occipital

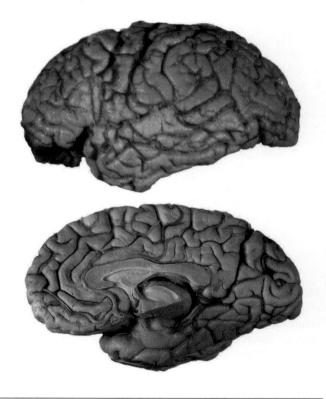

FIGURE 4–6.   Heteromodal association cortex (*red*).
Source.   Image courtesy of M. Mega and the UCLA Laboratory of Neuroimaging.

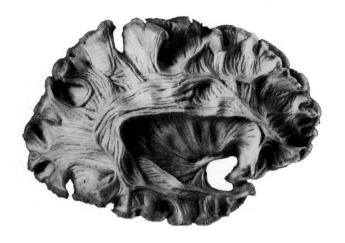

FIGURE 4–7. Brain dissection shows short cortico-cortical connections and intrahemispheric connections.
Source. Image courtesy of M. Mega and the UCLA Laboratory of Neuroimaging.

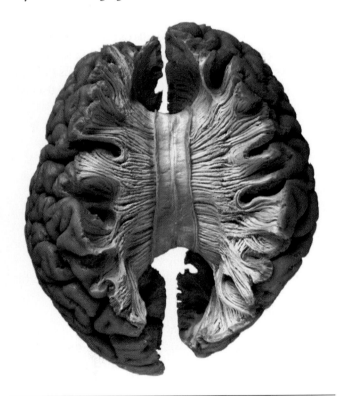

FIGURE 4–8. Commissural fibers of the hemispheres including the corpus callosum (*blue*) and the anterior commissure (*red*).
Source. Image courtesy of M. Mega and the UCLA Laboratory of Neuroimaging.

cortex (usually from a left posterior cerebral artery occlusion), the visual information available to the right hemisphere cannot be transferred to the left for semantic decoding, and alexia without agraphia ensues.

Disconnection syndromes also occur with lesions of association fiber tracts. Interruption of the arcuate fasciculus is responsible for conduction aphasia and parietal apraxia. Lesions of the right inferior longitudinal fasciculus produce prosopagnosia and environmental agnosia, whereas bilateral inferior longitudinal fasciculus damage causes visual object agnosia. Hemisensory deficits and homonymous hemianopsia result from lesions affecting the thalamocortical projections, and hemimotor syndromes occur with lesions of the descending corticospinal projections. The locked-in syndrome occurs with bilateral lesions of descending corticobulbar and corticospinal projection tracts at the pontine level.

The complex histological organization of the cerebral cortex, with its different cytoarchitectonic areas subsuming different processing tasks (as described above), is reflected in the complex connectivity of the cerebral white matter. White matter tracts connect specialized cortical regions, and neuropsychological syndromes may reflect focal cortical injury or disconnection of the cortical regions through injury to the white matter connections. Disconnection syndromes occur with lesions of commissural, long association, or projection fibers. Discrete neurobehavioral syndromes have been identified and occur primarily when lesions of callosal or association fibers disconnect unimodal association areas (e.g., interruption of visual processing in the agnosias or motor activities in the apraxias).

Hemispheric Specialization, Laterality, and Dominance

Anatomic asymmetries.   The two cerebral hemispheres, although grossly symmetrical, differ in some aspects of development, structure, and biochemical composition. Differences between the right and left hemispheres have been shown in both the upper surface of the temporal lobes and the inferolateral surface of the frontal lobe. The temporal lobe area corresponding to Wernicke's area (in 65% of cases) and the frontal region corresponding to Broca's area are both larger than the corresponding right-brain regions (in 83% of cases) (Falzi et al. 1982; Galaburda et al. 1978). The superior temporal surface is longer and the total area is approximately one-third larger in the left hemisphere. The sylvian fissure is longer and more horizontal on the left, whereas it is curved upward on the right (Galaburda et al. 1978). Cytoarchitectonic differences correspond to these morphological asymmetries: there is a larger region corresponding to Wernicke's area on the left compared to that on the right.

TABLE 4–2.   Fiber tracts and related disconnection syndromes of the cerebral hemispheres

Fiber type	Tract	Symptoms
Commissural	Corpus callosum	Left-hand tactile anomia, left-hand agraphia, left-hand apraxia, inability to match hand postures or tactile stimuli of the two hands, reduced constructional skills in the right hand
	Splenium	Alexia without agraphia (this syndrome occurs when there is a left occipital injury and right homonymous hemianopsia in addition to the splenial lesion)
Association	Arcuate fasciculus	Conduction aphasia
	Arcuate fasciculus	Parietal apraxia
	Inferior longitudinal fasciculus (right)	Prosopagnosia, environmental agnosia
	Inferior longitudinal fasciculus (bilateral)	Visual object agnosia
Projection	Corticospinal tract	Locked-in syndrome

Other gross asymmetries of the human brain include a wider and longer left occipital lobe, wider right frontal lobe, larger left occipital horn of the lateral ventricular system, and a tendency for the left descending pyramidal tract to decussate before the right in the medulla (Galaburda et al. 1978). Asymmetries of neurotransmitter concentrations also have been identified. Cortical choline acetyltransferase activity is greater in the left than in the right temporal lobe (Amaducci et al. 1981).

Cerebral asymmetries do not occur in the brains of nonprimates but are present in gorillas, chimpanzees, and orangutans, as well as in humans (LeMay 1976). Studies of endocasts of fossil skulls reveal that brain asymmetries similar to those of modern humans were evident in the brains of Neanderthal people 40,000 years ago and may have been present as early as 400,000 years ago in Peking man (Galaburda et al. 1978).

Investigations of asymmetries between the two hemispheres have identified differences at the gross morphological level, in the cytoarchitectonic structure of the hemispheres, in the shape of the brain, in the shape of specific aspects of the ventricular system, and in the concentrations of neurotransmitters. The magnitude of these differences is relatively small and does not correspond to the marked differences in hemispheric function. The means by which the dramatic differences in function of the two hemispheres are achieved remain enigmatic. The advantage of hemispheric specialization and lateralized development of functional capacities is that the capacity of the human brain is nearly doubled (Levy 1977). The principal disadvantage is that reduced redundancy exaggerates the effects of lateralized cerebral injury; in humans, a unilateral lesion often has devastating behavioral consequences because of the limited compensatory capability of the contralateral hemisphere.

Asymmetric cognitive function of the hemispheres.   Hemispheric specialization refers to the differential functions of the two hemispheres. Nearly all human behavior has contributions from both hemispheres, and complex behavior requires the integrated action of both halves of the brain. Almost no skills are completely unique to one hemisphere. Nevertheless, the two hemispheres differ substantially in their potential for many skills and are differentially engaged in most tasks. Numerous attempts have been made to identify antinomies of function that characterize the right and left hemispheres (i.e., verbal versus nonverbal, propositional versus appositional, and holistic versus analytic); none of these have been entirely successful, and it is unlikely that the brain is organized along such polar dimensions. A more accurate approach is to acknowledge that the two hemispheres perform different but not necessarily correlated or complementary roles. Table 4–3 lists capacities mediated to a significantly different extent by the two hemispheres.

Language is the best known example of a lateralized function. The right hemisphere mediates the prosodic apects of verbal expression; the left brain mediates propositional speech. The left hemisphere is specialized for symbol usage including words (spoken, written, heard, and read), mathematical symbols, symbolic gesture, and verbal memory. The left brain is language dominant in nearly all right-handed individuals and in most left-handed people. The lateralization of language functions is not complete, and rudimentary language skills are present in the right brain.

Praxis refers to the ability to execute learned movements on command. This ability is mediated by the left hemisphere, and most instances of apraxia occur in pa-

TABLE 4–3. Abilities mediated primarily by the right or left hemisphere and corresponding clinical deficits resulting from lateralized lesions

Hemispheric function	Correlated clinical deficit
Left hemisphere	
Language	Aphasia
Execution	Nonfluent aphasia
Comprehension	Comprehension defect
Reading	Alexia
Writing	Agraphia
Verbal memory	Verbal amnesia
Verbal fluency (word list generation)	Reduced verbal fluency
Mathematical abilities	Anarithmetia
Praxis	Apraxia
Musical rhythm (execution)	Impaired rhythm in singing
Contralateral spatial attention	Right-sided neglect
Contralateral motor function	Right hemiparesis
Contralateral sensory function	Right hemisensory loss
Contralateral visual field perception	Right homonymous hemianopia
Right hemisphere	
Speech prosody	Aprosodia
Executive	Executive aprosodia
Receptive	Receptive aprosodia
Nonverbal memory	Nonverbal amnesia
Design fluency (novel figure generation)	Reduced design fluency
Elementary visuospatial skills	
Depth perception	Reduced depth perception
Angle discrimination	Reduced angle discrimination
Complex visuospatial skills	
Familiar face recognition	Prosopagnosia
Familiar place recognition	Environmental agnosia
Unfamiliar face discrimination	Impaired facial discrimination
Visuomotor abilities	
Constructional ability	Constructional disturbance
Dressing (body-garment orientation)	Dressing disturbance
Musical melody (perception and execution)	Amusia
Contralateral spatial attention	Left-sided neglect
Contralateral motor function	Left hemiparesis
Contralateral sensory function	Left hemisensory loss
Contralateral visual field perception	Left homonymous hemianopia
Miscellaneous	
Familiar voice recognition	Phonagnosia

tients with left-sided brain injury.

The right hemisphere is dominant for *visuospatial functions*, but the left hemisphere has considerable visuospatial ability and left-hemisphere injuries frequently produce at least minor visuospatial deficits. The most marked and enduring visuospatial abnormalities occur with lesions of the posterior right hemisphere. Elementary visuoperceptual skills (e.g., judging line orientation and depth perception), complex visual discrimination and recognition abilities (e.g., discriminating between two unfamiliar faces or recognizing familiar faces), and visuomotor skills (e.g., drawing, copying, and dressing) are mediated primarily by the right hemisphere (Kimura and Durnford 1974).

Components of *music* appear to be differentially processed in the hemispheres. At least in nonprofessionals, the left hemisphere appears to be involved primarily in the mediation of rhythm, whereas the right brain mediates the perception and execution of melody (Gordon 1983).

Cortically mediated processes are well lateralized, and neurobehavioral phenomena such as aphasia, alexia, agraphia, amusia, abnormalities of visual discrimination and recognition, and altered affective expression occur with local damage to the left or right hemisphere. The cortex is comprised of regionally specialized modules that can be rendered dysfunctional by local cortical injury or by disconnection from other regions by white matter lesions.

Limbic System (Paramedian Zone)

Limbic system structures comprise a critical neuroanatomic substrate for the mediation of mood, emotion, and motivation. Limbic dysfunction contributes to a variety of neuropsychiatric syndromes including psychosis, depression, mania, personality alterations, and obsessive-compulsive disorder.

"Limbic" means "border" or "hem" and was first used in an anatomical context by Broca, the French anatomist, to describe the structures that lie beneath the neocortex and that surround the brainstem (Isaacson 1974). In 1937, Papez authored the landmark article, titled "A Proposed Mechanism of Emotion," in which he hypothesized that these structures surrounding the upper brainstem formed a functional system mediating human emotion. Since then, research and clinical observations have largely confirmed the idea that limbic structures are involved in the mediation of behaviors and experiences that share the common feature of having an emotional component.

As currently conceived, the limbic system includes the hippocampus, olfactory cortex, caudal orbitofrontal cortex, insula, temporal pole, parahippocampal gyrus, cingulate cortex, amygdala, septal nuclei, hypothalamus, and selected thalamic nuclei (Carpenter 1991; Mesulam 1985) (Figure 4–9). The limbic system is poised between the hypothalamus with its neuroendocrine control systems of the internal milieu and the neocortex mediating action on the external environment.

The principal known function of the hippocampus is the mediation of new learning and recent memory. Localized injury to hippocampus produces an amnestic disorder with deficient storage of new information. This syndrome has been described with hippocampal damage secondary to stroke, anoxia, trauma, early Alzheimer's disease, and herpes encephalitis.

Paralimbic cortex includes the orbitofrontal area, insula, temporal pole, parahippocampal gyrus, and cingulate gyrus. Paralimbic cortex is represented in brain regions critical to emotional control, social judgment, civility, and motivated behavior. Lesions of the orbitofrontal cortex produce marked personality changes with disinhibition, impulsiveness, loss of tact, and coarsened behavior. Cingulate dysfunction results in marked apathy with disinterest and loss of motivation (Cummings 1993).

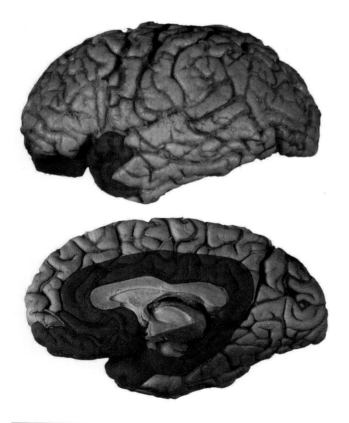

FIGURE 4–9. Paralimbic cortex.
Source. Image courtesy of M. Mega and the UCLA Laboratory of Neuroimaging.

Portions of the basal ganglia are included in the limbic system. The head of the caudate nucleus consists of ventromedial and dorsolateral portions. The ventromedial section has major limbic system connections and receives projections from the hippocampus, amygdala, cingulate cortex, and the orbitofrontal cortex. The dorsolateral portion, in contrast, receives projections from the lateral prefrontal cortex and has little limbic input (Nauta 1986). The globus pallidus is divided similarly into dorsal-nonlimbic portions and ventral-limbic portions. As predicted by these anatomic observations, basal ganglia diseases are commonly accompanied by emotional dysfunction and psychopathology.

Various clinical neuropsychiatric disorders are associated with limbic system dysfunction (Cummings 1985; Doane 1986) (Table 4–4). The limbic system serves no single unifying function, and the only common feature shared by limbic system disorders is that they have an emotional dimension. Limbic system lesions produce emotional disturbances and rarely cause intellectual deficits. (An exception is the amnesia produced by hippocampal system lesions.)

Psychosis, mood disorders, obsessive-compulsive behavior, personality alterations, and disturbances of sexual behavior have all been linked to limbic system dysfunction. *Psychosis* occurs with lesions of the temporal lobes and subcortical limbic system structures. The schizophrenia-like disorder of epilepsy occurs almost exclusively in patients with seizure foci in the temporolimbic cortex (Perez et al. 1985). Stroke, tumors, herpes encephalitis, and Alzheimer's disease are other disorders that affect the temporal cortex and produce psychotic features in the elderly. At the subcortical limbic level, Huntington's disease, idiopathic basal ganglia calcification, and lacunar state are examples of conditions with pathology of the limbic system and increased frequencies of psychosis.

Mood disorders also have been related to limbic system dysfunction (Duffy and Coffey 1997). Depression occurs with basal ganglia dysfunction in stroke, movement disorders, and idiopathic depressive disorders (Baxter et al. 1985; Cummings 1992; Starkstein et al. 1987, 1988a). Manic behavior has been associated with disorders affecting the caudate nuclei, thalamus, and basotemporal areas (Bogousslavsky et al. 1988; Cummings and Mendez 1984; Folstein 1989; Starkstein et al. 1988b).

Investigation of idiopathic *obsessive-compulsive behavior* has revealed increased metabolism in the orbitofrontal cortex (Baxter et al. 1987). Focal lesions and neurological disorders producing obsessive-compulsive behavior frequently involve the caudate nucleus or globus pallidus (Cummings and Cunningham 1992).

TABLE 4–4.   Neuropsychiatric disorders with evidence of limbic system dysfunction

Neuropsychiatric disorder	Anatomical structure implicated	Diseases affecting structure
Amnesia	Hippocampus, hypothalamus	Stroke, anoxia, trauma, tumors, herpes encephalitis
Psychosis	Temporal cortex	Epilepsy, stroke, tumors, herpes encephalitis, Alzheimer's disease
	Striatum	Huntington's disease, idiopathic basal ganglia calcification, lacunar state, schizophrenia
Depression	Striatum	Stroke, Huntington's disease, Parkinson's disease, idiopathic basal ganglia calcification, idiopathic depression
Mania	Striatum	Huntington's disease, idiopathic basal ganglia calcification
	Thalamus	Stroke
	Temporal cortex	Stroke, trauma
OCD	Orbitofrontal cortex	Idiopathic OCD
	Striatum	Huntington's disease, Sydenham's chorea, PEPD, manganese intoxication, carbon monoxide intoxication
Personality alterations	Orbitofrontal cortex	Trauma, tumors, degenerative disorders
	Temporal cortex	Epilepsy
	Amygdala	Herpes encephalitis, trauma
	Striatum	Huntington's disease
Anxiety	Temporal cortex	Idiopathic anxiety
	Striatum	Parkinson's disease
Hyposexuality	Temporal cortex	Epilepsy (interictal)
	Hypothalamus	Trauma (surgical)
Hypersexuality	Orbitofrontal cortex	Tumors, trauma
	Temporal cortex	Epilepsy (ictal)
	Amygdala	Herpes encephalitis, trauma
	Septal nuclei	Trauma
Paraphilias	Hypothalamus	Tumors, trauma, encephalitis
Addictions	Septal nuclei, hypothalamus	Idiopathic addictive behavior

Note.   OCD = obsessive-compulsive disorder; PEPD = postencephalitic Parkinson's disease.

A variety of *personality alterations* have been correlated with limbic system lesions. Orbitofrontal or orbitofrontal-subcortical circuit lesions produce disinhibited, impulsive, and tactless behavior; temporolimbic epilepsy has been associated with a rigid, viscous demeanor with hypergraphia, circumstantiality, hyposexuality, and hyperreligiosity (Brandt et al. 1985); and bilateral amygdala lesions produce behavioral placidity as part of the Klüver-Bucy syndrome (Lilly et al. 1983).

Idiopathic *anxiety* is associated with increased temporal and decreased basal ganglia glucose metabolism (Wu et al. 1991). Anxiety has been associated with temporal lobe and basal ganglia disorders including Parkinson's disease and Alzheimer's disease (Reisberg et al. 1989; Stein et al. 1990).

Apathy is recognized increasingly as a common behavioral change in patients with brain disorders. Reduced motivation, interest, engagement, affection, and activity contribute a syndrome of diminished involvement (Marin 1990). The syndrome varies in severity from mild loss of interest and reduced involvement in previous affairs to an akinetic mute state with markedly reduced movement, speech, and intellectual content. The syndrome most commonly results from lesions of the anterior cingulate cortex or related structures of the cingulate-subcortical circuit including nucleus accumbens, globus pallidus, and thalamus (Cummings 1993).

Disorders of sexual function also may reflect limbic system disturbances. Diminished libido has been associated with hypothalamic injury and with the interictal state of patients with temporal lobe seizure foci. Hypersexuality has been observed in patients with orbitofrontal injury or trauma to the septal region and as an ictal manifestation in the course of temporal lobe seizures (Gorman and Cummings 1992). Paraphiliac behavior including pedophilia, transvestism, sadomasochistic behavior, and exhibitionism has been observed in patients with temporal lobe injury and epilepsy, basal ganglia disorders, and brain tumors involving limbic structures (Cummings 1985; Miller et al. 1986). Opiate and cocaine *addictions* appear to be mediated in part by receptors located in limbic brain regions (Gawin 1991).

Thus neocortical disorders and white matter lesions tend to produce deficit disorders of language, praxis, and gnosis. Limbic system disorders have little associated intellectual impairment and produce diverse "productive" disorders of emotional function with the new appearance of positive neuropsychiatric symptoms.

Limbic System Asymmetries and Lateralized Neuropsychiatric Syndromes

Anatomic and biochemical asymmetries of the limbic system. Asymmetries of subcortical structures are less marked than are asymmetries of cortical regions, but the left globus pallidus, right medial geniculate nucleus of the thalamus, and left lateral posterior nucleus of the thalamus have been found to be larger than the corresponding nuclei of the contralateral hemisphere (Eidelberg and Galaburda 1982; Kooistra and Heilman 1988). Asymmetries of neurotransmitter concentrations in limbic system structures have been identified. The content of dopamine and choline acetyltransferase (a marker of cholinergic function) is increased in the left globus pallidus compared with their content in the right (Glick et al. 1982); norepinephrine concentrations are greater in the left pulvinar and in the right somatosensory nuclei of the thalamus (Oke et al. 1978); and choline acetyltransferase activity is greater in the left than in the right temporal lobe (Amaducci et al. 1981). Transmitter asymmetries may underlie the differential occurrence of mood disorders and anxiety with lesions of the left and right hemispheres.

Lateralized neuropsychiatric syndromes. Some aspects of emotional function are lateralized, with greater representation in one hemisphere than in the other (Coffey 1987). Emotional functions include the perception of emotional stimuli in the environment (e.g., apprehending facial expression, comprehending voice inflection, and inter-

preting postural adjustments), the expression of emotion (e.g., facial affective display and inflection of voice), and the subjective experience of emotion. Emotional perception and expression appear to be mediated primarily by the right hemisphere. For example, the right hemisphere is superior to the left in discriminating among unfamiliar faces, recognizing familiar faces, and interpreting facial emotional expression (Borod et al. 1986). The right brain also is better able to recognize familiar voices than is the left (Van Lancker et al. 1989) and to comprehend the emotional inflection of spoken language (Tucker et al. 1977). Emotion is more intensely expressed on the left side of the face, suggesting that the right brain has more efficient access to cerebral mechanisms required for affective expression (Moscovitch and Olds 1982). Finally, the right hemisphere also shows evidence of electroencephalographic activation when processing emotional stimuli (Davidson 1992), and emotional information may serve to activate the right hemisphere (Bryden and Ley 1984).

Experiential aspects of emotion are more difficult to study, and the underlying neurobiology is less securely established. Information has been derived from depth electrode investigations, from emotional changes reported in association with epileptic seizures, from temporary hemispheric inactivation with intracarotid amobarbital injections (Wada test), and from lesion studies. Stimulating depth electrodes located in and around the amygdala produces the sense of déjà vu, anxiety, visceral sensations, hallucinations (Halgren et al. 1978), and occasionally intense fear or anger (Girgis 1981), irrespective of which hemisphere is stimulated. Fear is the most common affect experienced in the course of spontaneous epileptic seizures. Some studies have found a predominance of right-sided foci (Hermann et al. 1992), but fear is also observed in patients with left-sided lesions, suggesting that this experience is not consistently lateralized (Strauss et al. 1982). Depression is the second most common ictal affect and occurs with both left- and right-sided foci (Williams 1956). A small number of patients have positive emotional experiences as ictal manifestations, and laughter as an ictal behavior may be more common with left- than with right-sided seizure foci (Sackeim et al. 1982), although a consensus is lacking regarding interpretation of this observation (Coffey 1987). Taken together, these data suggest that many experiential aspects of emotion are mediated by nonlateralized limbic system structures.

An important source of information regarding the laterality of emotional processing is the Wada test. In this technique, amobarbital is injected into the carotid artery of patients with epilepsy before temporal lobectomy to establish which side of the brain is dominant for language function. The carotid is the principal arterial supply for the ipsilateral hemisphere, and transient hemispheric inactivation follows the injection. Approximately 50% of patients undergoing this procedure evidence a marked change in emotion soon after the amobarbital perfusion. When the left hemisphere is inactivated, a depressive or catastrophic reaction occurs; when the right hemisphere is involved, patients manifest euphoria or an indifference reaction (Loring et al. 1992).

Studies of emotional changes in patients with unilateral lesions lead to conclusions similar to those suggested by the Wada test. Patients with left-hemisphere lesions have more catastrophic reactions and are more anxious and depressed; patients with right-hemisphere lesions evidence more indifference and tend to joke about, minimize, or deny their disability (Gainotti 1972). Investigation of stroke patients have found a higher prevalence of severe depression among those with left frontal lobe lesions, whereas patients with right-brain lesions exhibited more undue cheerfulness or, occasionally, frank mania (Robinson and Starkstein 1990; see also Chapter 23 in this volume). Van Lancker (1991) observed that many functions of the right hemisphere subserve determination of the personal relevance of environmental stimuli, and Weintraub and Mesulam (1983) reported that children who sustained right-brain injury characteristically had interpersonal difficulties, shyness, and impaired prosody and gesture. An impaired ability to comprehend personally relevant information or to execute interpersonal cues appropriately may lead to difficulties in establishing interpersonal relationships and to subsequent social isolation. In elderly individuals, right-hemisphere dysfunction may contribute to the disengagement and interpersonal abnormalities evident in many patients with right-brain strokes and dementia syndromes.

Another avenue for investigating the hemisphericity of emotion is to search for evidence of lateral brain dysfunction in idiopathic psychiatric disorders. A number of neuropsychological studies have suggested preferential right-hemisphere dysfunction during depressed mood states that normalizes during euthymia, and a few patients have been reported to exhibit frank neurological deficits referable to the right hemisphere that were present only during the depressed period (for a review, see Coffey 1987). Electrophysiological studies have demonstrated electroencephalographic changes referable to the right hemisphere during episodes of depression (Davidson 1992), but studies of regional cerebral blood flow and metabolism have produced conflicting findings, with dysfunction in either or both hemispheres accompanying depression (Baxter et al. 1985; Delvenne et al. 1990; Dolan et al. 1992; Drevets et al. 1992; George et al. 1996; Sackeim et al. 1990).

In other psychiatric disorders, several lines of evidence point toward dysfunction of left temporal lobe structures in schizophrenia, but this hypothesis is controversial (Gruzelier 1983; Sedvall 1992; Suddath et al. 1989). Even more tentative are data suggesting greater left-hemisphere dysfunction in violent individuals and more right-brain involvement in patients with conversion hysteria and alexithymia (Flor-Henry 1983; Nachson 1983; Stern 1983; TenHouten et al. 1986). Most idiopathic disorders have not been found to be strongly linked to a single hemisphere. Table 4–5 summarizes the neuropsychiatric syndromes associated with lateralized brain dysfunction.

Reticular Formation (Median Zone)

The median zone contains the reticular formation including the ascending reticular activating system, the vaso-

TABLE 4–5. Neuropsychiatric disorders associated with lateralized brain dysfunction

Neuropsychiatric disorder	Predominant laterality of an associated lesion
Disorders of personal relevance	
Prosopagnosia (inability to recognize familiar faces)	Right
Environmental agnosia (inability to recognize familiar places)	Right
Phonagnosia (inability to recognize familiar voices)	Right
Affective dysprosody (inability to inflect one's voice or to comprehend emotional inflection)	Right
Mood disorders	
Depression (major)	Left
Catastrophic reaction	Left
Mania	Right
Euphoria, undue cheerfulness	Right
Indifference	Right
Possible hemispheric relationships to other psychiatric disorders	
Schizophrenia	Left
Violent behavior	Left
Obsessive-compulsive behavior	Left
Conversion hysteria	Right
Alexithymia	Right

pressor and respiratory mechanisms, and the central components of the sympathetic and parasympathetic nervous systems (Carpenter 1991). The reticular formation is a dense network of neurons with short and long axons that form nuclei in the periventricular gray areas surrounding the cerebral aqueduct in the midbrain, is adjacent to the floor of the fourth ventricle in the pons, and extends into the medulla. The ascending reticular activating system projects to the intralaminar nuclei of the thalamus, and these in turn project to the cerebral cortex. The intralaminar nuclei project primarily to layer I of the cortex, the layer comprised of parallel fibers whose stimulation results in local cortical activation (Figure 4–10).

The thalamic reticular nucleus is a unique structure that forms a thin shell around the anterior aspects of the thalamus and governs cortical arousal. It receives projections from the cerebral cortex, dorsal intralaminar nucleus, and dorsal specific sensory nuclei. It has no projections to the cerebral cortex but projects back to the dorsal thalamic nuclei. It is positioned to serve as a gate, modifying and censoring information projected from thalamus to cortex, and its principal effect is to inhibit cortical activity (Carpenter and Sutin 1983; Plum and Posner 1980).

Increased input from the brainstem reticular activating system reduces the tonic inhibition of the reticular nucleus and activates the cortex by disinhibiting the cortical projections of other thalamic nuclei (Plum and Posner 1980). The ascending reticular activating system is responsible for the maintenance of consciousness, and disturbances of the system result in impaired arousal varying from drowsiness to obtundation, stupor, and coma.

Nuclei of the reticular formation also are involved in control of heart rate, blood pressure, and respiratory rhythms (Carpenter 1991). Dysfunction of these nuclei results in alterations in blood pressure, cardiac arrhythmias, and respiratory irregularities. The hypothalamus is contained in the median zone, and abnormalities of basic life functions (e.g., appetite, libido, and sleep) may occur in individuals who sustain hypothalamic injury. The hypothalamus influences endocrine function via its connections with the pituitary gland, and endocrine abnormalities are produced by hypothalamic lesions.

Connections Between the Cerebral Cortex and Subcortical Structures

Information enters the nervous system one principal way, and there is one principal exit pathway by which humans act on their environment. The entry pathway is via thalamocortical afferents that receive sensory information from peripheral sensory receptors and convey the data to the cortex. The principal exit pathway is via the descending corticospinal tracts, particularly the pyramidal system. Thus the flow of information is from the thalamus to the primary sensory cortex, unimodal association cortex, and then heteromodal association cortex. From there, the long association fibers connect the posterior heteromodal cortex to the anterior (frontal lobe) heteromodal cortex that in turn connects to the subcortical nuclei. After processing through frontal-subcortical circuits, executive commands flow to the primary motor cortex and then to bulbar and spinal effector mechanisms. The thalamocortical afferents and frontal-subcortical efferents are distributed systems that include portions of both the paramedian (limbic) and supralimbic (neocortical) zones. Activation of brain structures is not limited to the sequence described above; there is simultaneous activation of many brain regions, as well as feedback mechanisms from ongoing activity.

Thalamic-Cortical Relationships

The thalamus plays several crucial roles in human brain function. Specific thalamic nuclei receive input from a relatively restricted number of sources and project to layers III and IV of the cortex.

The specific nuclei include sensory nuclei that process all incoming sensory information except olfaction (ventral posterior, medial geniculate, and lateral geniculate); nuclei

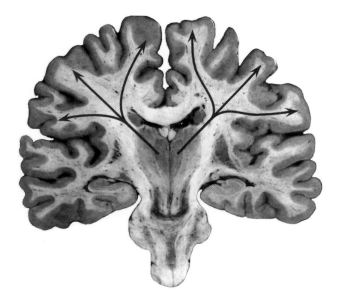

FIGURE 4–10.   Cortical projections from the thalamus.
Source.   Image courtesy of M. Mega and the UCLA Laboratory of Neuroimaging.

that participate in the motor pathways (ventral anterior and ventral lateral); association nuclei that have major connections with frontal (dorsomedial nuclei) or temporoparietal (lateral nuclei) association cortex; and nuclei that are included in the limbic circuits (anterior and medial nuclei) (Carpenter and Sutin 1983; Nauta and Feirtag 1986). Table 4–6 presents a functional classification of thalamic nuclei with their principal afferents and efferents.

A number of distinctive behavioral disorders have been associated with dysfunction of the associative and sensory thalamic nuclei. Disorders of the associative dorsal medial nuclei produce amnesia and a "frontal lobe"–type syndrome (Cummings 1993; Stuss et al. 1988). Apathy also is common after dorsal medial nuclear injury. Lesions of the specific thalamic sensory nuclei cause deficits in primary sensation. Ventral posterior nuclear lesions disrupt all sensory abilities of the contralateral limbs, trunk, and face. In some cases, spontaneous disabling pain of the affected side occurs (Dejerine-Roussy syndrome) (Adams and Victor 1981). Lesions of the lateral geniculate bodies produce a contralateral visual field defect. Mania has been observed in several patients with right-sided thalamic lesions involving the paramedian thalamic nuclei (Bogousslavsky et al. 1988; Cummings and Mendez 1984; Starkstein et al. 1988b).

Frontal-Subcortical Circuits

The frontal lobe is the origin of executive processes that guide action. The output from the frontal lobe is through subcortical circuits that eventually reach motor pathways. Five circuits connecting the frontal lobes and subcortical structures are currently recognized: a motor circuit originating in the supplementary motor area, an oculomotor circuit with origins in the frontal eye fields, and three circuits originating in prefrontal cortex (dorsolateral prefrontal cortex, lateral orbital cortex, and anterior cingulate cortex) (Alexander and Crutcher 1990; Alexander et al. 1986, 1990). The prototypic structure of all circuits is an origin in the frontal lobes, projection to striatal

TABLE 4–6. Function and anatomic relationships of the thalamic nuclei

Nuclei	Input	Output	Function
Limbic nuclei			
Anterior	Mammillary body	Cingulate	Emotional function
Motor nuclei			
Ventroanterior	Globus pallidus	Frontal cortex	Motor function
Ventrolateral	Cerebellum	Frontal cortex	Motor function
Sensory nuclei			
Ventral posterolateral	Sensory tracts from body	Parietal sensory cortex	Touch, temperature vibration, position
Ventral posteromedial	Sensory tracts from face	Parietal sensory cortex	Touch, temperature vibration, position
Lateral geniculate	Optic tracts	Occipital cortex	Vision
Medial geniculate	Inferior colliculi	Temporal cortex	Hearing
Association nuclei			
Dorsomedial	Globus pallidus, amygdala, temporal and frontal cortex	Prefrontal cortex	Intellectual and emotional function
Lateral[a]	Sensory thalamic nucleus, parietal and temporal cortex	Temporoparietal cortex	Intellectual function
Nonspecific nuclei			
Midline	Hypothalamus	Amygdala, cingulate hypothalamus	Visceral function
Intralaminar	Reticular formation, precentral and premotor cortex	Striatum, cortex	Activation
Reticular	Thalamic nucleus and cortex	Dorsal thalamic nuclei	Samples, gates, and focuses thalamocortical output

structures (caudate, putamen, or nucleus accumbens), connections from striatum to globus pallidus and substantia nigra, projections from these two structures to specific thalamic nuclei, and a final link back to the frontal lobe (Figure 4–11).

The *motor circuit* originates from neurons in the supplementary motor area, premotor cortex, motor cortex, and somatosensory cortex (Alexander and Crutcher 1990; Alexander et al. 1986). Throughout the circuit, the discrete somatotopic organization of movement-related neurons is maintained. Distinct types of motor disturbances are associated with lesions at different sites in the motor circuit. Motor initiation abnormalities (akinesia) are associated with supplementary motor area lesions; parkinsonism and dystonia are observed with putaminal dysfunction; and choreiform movements occur with caudate and subthalamic nucleus damage.

The *oculomotor circuit* originates in the frontal eye fields, as well as in the prefrontal and posterior parietal cortex. Acute lesions of the cortical eye fields produce ipsilateral eye deviation, whereas more chronic lesions produce ipsilateral gaze impersistence. Lesions in other areas of the circuit produce supranuclear gaze palsies such as those seen in Parkinson's disease, progressive supranuclear palsy, and Huntington's disease.

Three distinct frontal lobe neurobehavioral syndromes are recognized, and each corresponds to a region of origin of one of the three prefrontal-subcortical circuits. Dysfunction of any of the member structures of the circuits results in similar circuit-specific behavioral complexes, and these frontal-subcortical circuits compose major anatomic axes governing behavior (Cummings 1993). The *dorsolateral prefrontal circuit* originates in the convexity of the frontal lobe and projects primarily to the dorsolateral head of the caudate nucleus (Alexander and Crutcher 1990; Alexander et al. 1986) (Figure 4–12). This caudate region connects to globus pallidus and substantia nigra, and pallidal and nigral neurons of the circuit project to the medial dorsal thalamic nuclei that in turn project back to the dorsolateral prefrontal region. The dorsolateral prefrontal syndrome is characterized primarily by executive function deficits. Abnormalities include developing poor strategies for solving visuospatial problems or learning new information and reduced ability to shift sets. Such behavioral changes are observed in patients with dorsolateral

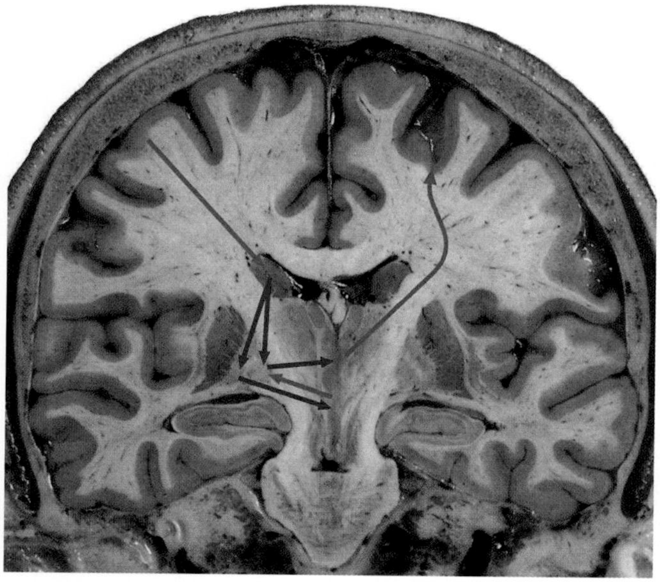

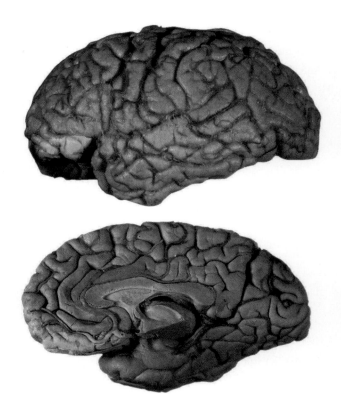

FIGURE 4–11. Organization of the prefrontal-subcortical circuits. The prefrontal cortical regions (dorsolateral prefrontal, orbitofrontal, and anterior cingulate) project to specific striatal regions that in turn project to globus pallidus and substantia nigra. These structures project to thalamic nuclei that connect to frontal lobe, completing the circuit.
Source. Image courtesy of M. Mega and the UCLA Laboratory of Neuroimaging.

FIGURE 4–12. Prefrontal cortical origins of the dorsolateral, anterior cingulate, and orbital circuits.
Source. Image courtesy of M. Mega and the UCLA Laboratory of Neuroimaging.

prefrontal lesions, as well as in those with caudate, globus pallidus, and thalamic dysfunction.

The *orbitofrontal circuit* contains primarily limbic system structures. It begins in the inferolateral prefrontal cortex and projects to the ventromedial caudate nucleus (Alexander and Crutcher 1990; Alexander et al. 1986) (Figure 4–12). This caudate region projects to the pallidum and substantia nigra. Pallidum and nigra connect to medial portions of the ventral anterior and medial dorsal thalamic nuclei that project back to the orbitofrontal cortex. Disorders involving cortical or subcortical structures of the orbitofrontal circuit feature marked changes in personality, including a tendency to be more outspoken, more irritable, and more tactless and to worry less and have an elevated mood.

The *anterior cingulate circuit* begins in the cortex of the anterior cingulate gyrus (Brodmann area 24) and projects to the ventral striatum (also known as the *limbic striatum*), which includes the nucleus accumbens and the ventromedial portions of the caudate and putamen (Alexander and Crutcher 1990; Alexander et al. 1986) (Figure

4–12). The most dramatic cases of anterior cingulate injury exhibit akinetic mutism. The patients are profoundly apathetic: they typically have their eyes open, do not speak spontaneously, answer questions in monosyllables if at all, and are profoundly indifferent. Apathy also has been associated with lesions of nucleus accumbens, globus pallidus, and thalamus, the principal subcortical members of the anterior cingulate circuit. Table 4–7 summarizes the behaviorally relevant frontal-subcortical circuits including the anatomical structures involved, the behavioral disturbances observed with circuit dysfunction, and the common diseases affecting each circuit.

Frontal-subcortical circuits are involved in several neuropsychiatric disorders. In addition to personality alterations (e.g., apathy and disinhibition), mood changes and obsessive-compulsive behaviors are associated with focal brain lesions affecting these circuits. Depression occurs with lesions of the dorsolateral prefrontal cortex and the head of the caudate nucleus, particularly when the left hemisphere is affected (Robinson et al. 1984; Starkstein et al. 1987, 1988a; see also Chapters 13 and 27 in this volume).

TABLE 4–7.   **Behavioral abnormalities associated with frontal-subcortical circuit disorders**

Disease	Personality change	Mania	Depression	Obsessive-compulsive disorder	Neuropsychological impairment
Prefrontal cortical disorders					
Lateral prefrontal syndrome	No	No	Yes	No	Yes
Orbitofrontal syndrome	Yes	Yes	No	Yes	No
Medial frontal syndrome	Yes	Yes	No	No	No
Caudate disorders					
Parkinson's disease	Yes	No	Yes	No	Yes
Progressive supranuclear palsy	Yes	No	Yes	Yes	Yes
Huntington's disease	Yes	Yes	Yes	Yes	Yes
Sydenham's chorea	Yes	No	No	Yes	No
Wilson's disease	Yes	Yes	Yes	No	Yes
Neuroacanthocytosis	Yes	Yes	Yes	Yes	Yes
Fahr's disease	UD	Yes	Yes	No	Yes
Infarction	Yes	No	Yes	Yes	Yes
Globus pallidus disorders					
Postencephalitic Parkinson's disease	Yes	Yes	Yes	Yes	Yes
Manganese toxicity	Yes	UD	UD	Yes	Yes
Carbon monoxide toxicity	Yes	No	No	Yes	Yes
Infarction	Yes	UD	UD	No	Yes
Thalamic disorders					
Infarction	Yes	Yes	No	No	Yes
Degeneration	Yes	UD	UD	UD	Yes

Note.   UD = undetermined.

Positron-emission tomography in patients with idiopathic unipolar depression reveals diminished glucose metabolism in the prefrontal cortex and the caudate nuclei, suggesting that dysfunction of frontal-subcortical circuits may be a shared substrate for both idiopathic and acquired mood disorders (Baxter et al. 1985). Lesions producing secondary mania also involve nuclei and connections of frontal-subcortical circuits. Mania has been observed with lesions of the medial orbitofrontal cortex, diseases of the caudate nuclei such as Huntington's disease, and injury to the right thalamus (Bogousslavsky et al. 1988; Cummings and Mendez 1984; Folstein 1989; Starkstein et al. 1988b).

Both acquired and idiopathic obsessive-compulsive disorders have been related to dysfunction of frontal-subcortical circuits. Obsessive-compulsive behavior has been observed in patients with caudate dysfunction in Huntington's disease and after Sydenham's chorea (Cummings and Cunningham 1992; Swedo et al. 1989), as well as with globus pallidus lesions in postencephalitic Parkinson's disease, progressive supranuclear palsy, manganese-induced parkinsonism, and after anoxic injury (Laplane et al. 1989; Mena et al. 1967; Schilder 1938). Idiopathic obsessive-compulsive disorder has been associated with increased glucose metabolism in the left orbitofrontal frontal gyrus and caudate nuclei (Baxter et al. 1987) and with increased blood flow in the medial frontal area (Machlin et al. 1991).

Frontal-subcortical circuits are affected in patients who have diseases of the basal ganglia. The high frequency of neuropsychological alterations, the increased prevalence of personality and mood disturbances, the occurrence of obsessive-compulsive disorder, and the similarity between behaviors of patients with basal ganglia diseases and patients with frontal lobe injury are attributable to dysfunction of multiple frontal-subcortical circuits in basal ganglia disorders.

▎ Neurochemistry and Behavior

The anatomical organization of the brain is complemented by an equally complex neurochemical organization. Many behavioral disorders reflect biochemical dysfunction, and the most effective interventions available are neurochemical in nature. Neurobehavioral deficits stemming from focal cortical lesions (e.g., aphasia and apraxia) have limited available remediable neurochemical treatments; neuropsychiatric disorders associated with limbic system dysfunction are frequently modifiable through neurochemical interventions.

There are two types of cerebral transmitters: 1) projection or extrinsic transmitters that originate in subcortical and brainstem nuclei and project to brain targets and 2) local or intrinsic transmitters that originate in neurons of the brain and project locally to adjacent or nearby cells. Projection transmitters or their synthetic enzymes must be transported within neurons for long distances from subcortical nuclei to distant regions and are vulnerable to disruption by stroke, tumors, and other processes. Transmitters are highly conserved from an evolutionary point of view, and many function locally in some neuronal systems and function as projection transmitters in others. The classic neurotransmitters have served neuronal communication for 600 million years of evolution (Rapoport 1990). Table 4–8 summarizes the origins and destinations of the extrinsic transmitters. The effects of neurotransmitters are mediated by receptors to which the transmitter binds after it has been released into the synaptic cleft. Receptors may be located on the presynaptic or postsynaptic terminal. Presynaptic receptors (autoreceptors) regulate neurotransmitter synthesis or release. Postsynaptic receptors mediate the effects of the neurotransmitter on the postsynaptic cell. Heteroreceptors (receptors for neurotransmitters other than those produced by the neuron) also regulate synaptic activity. Binding of a neurotransmitter to a receptor results either in opening of an ion channel (ionotropic receptors) or initiation of second messenger cascades via guanosine triphosphate-binding (G) proteins (metabotropic receptors). The neurotransmitter is removed from the synapse (either before or after binding to a receptor) either by enzymatic degradation or by active reuptake into the presynaptic terminal by a high-affinity transporter protein. Behavioral effects can rarely be assigned to alterations in a single transmitter, but some aberrant behaviors are associated with changes that affect predominantly one type of transmitter. Table 4–9 presents the principal transmitter-behavior relationships currently identified.

There are two main *cholinergic projections* from subcortical sites to the brain. The first originates in the reticular formation and projects via the dorsal tegmental pathway to the thalamus. This pathway is the essential component of the ascending reticular activating system (Nieuwenhuys 1985). The second cholinergic projection begins in the cells of the nucleus basalis in the basal forebrain and projects to the hippocampus, hypothalamus, amygdala, and diffusely to the neocortex (Figure 4–13). The afferents to nucleus basalis are primarily from cortical and subcortical limbic system structures establishing the nucleus basalis as a relay between the limbic system afferents and efferents to the neocortex (Mesulam and Mufson 1984).

TABLE 4–8. Origins and destinations of the major extrinsic transmitter projections

Neurotransmitter	Origin	Destination
Acetylcholine		
Reticular system	Reticular formation	Thalamus
Basal forebrain system	Nucleus basalis and nucleus of diagonal band of Broca	Neocortex, hippocampus, hypothalamus, and amygdala
Dopamine		
Nigrostriatal system	Substantia nigra	Putamen and caudate nucleus
Mesolimbic system	Ventral tegmental area	Nucleus accumbens, septal nucleus, and amygdala
Mesocortical system	Ventral tegmental area	Medial temporal and frontal lobes and anterior cingulate cortex
Noradrenaline		
Dorsal pathway	Locus ceruleus	Thalamus, amygdala, basal forebrain, hippocampus, and neocortex
Ventral pathway	Locus ceruleus	Hypothalamus and midbrain reticular formation
Serotonin	Raphe nuclei	Entire nervous system
Histamine	Posterior hypothalamus	Entire nervous system
GABA	Zona incerta	Neocortex, basal ganglia, and brainstem
	Caudate and putamen	Globus pallidus and substantia nigra
	Globus pallidus and substantia nigra	Thalamus
Glutamate	Neocortex	Caudate, putamen, thalamus, and nucleus accumbens
	Subthalamic nucleus	Globus pallidus
	Thalamus	Neocortex
	Hippocampus, subiculum	Septal region
	Entorhinal cortex	Hippocampus

Note. GABA = γ-aminobutyric acid.

Cholinergic function is mediated by either nicotinic (ionotropic) or muscarinic (metabotropic) receptors. Both receptor types are present in the brain, but the latter appear to be of special interest to neuropsychiatry. The muscarinic receptors are classified pharmacologically as M_1 (located postsynaptic) or M_2 (located presynaptic) and have different distributions throughout the brain. Cholinergic systems mediate a wide range of behaviors. Disruption of central cholinergic function (e.g., through the administration of cholinergic receptor-blocking agents such as scopolamine) produces amnesia (Bartus et al. 1982), and intoxication with anticholinergic compounds produces delirium and delusions. Alzheimer's disease is one major disorder associated with cholinergic deficiency. This disease produces atrophy of the nucleus basalis with consequent reduction in the synthesis of choline acetyltransferase, the enzyme that synthesizes acetylcholine; loss of synthetic activity leads to interruption of cortical cholinergic function (Katzman and Thal 1989). Increasing evidence indicates that some of the neuropsychiatric disturbances of Alzheimer's dis-

ease—hallucinations, apathy, disinhibition, purposeless behavior—are produced by the cholinergic deficit (Cummings and Kaufer 1996). Cholinergic hyperactivity has been posited to play a role in the genesis of depression (Dilsaver and Coffman 1989), and in some species cholinergic stimulation of limbic system structures produces aggression (Valzelli 1981).

There are three main *dopaminergic projections* from the brainstem to the cerebral hemispheres: 1) a nigrostriatal projection arising from the compact portion of the substantia nigra and projecting to the putamen and caudate, 2) a mesolimbic projection originating in the ventral tegmental area and projecting to limbic system structures, and 3) a mesocortical system beginning in the ventral tegmental area and projecting to frontal and temporal areas (Nieuwenhuys 1985) (Figure 4–14). Targets of the mesolimbic dopaminergic projection include the nucleus accumbens, septal nucleus, and amygdala. The mesocortical projections terminate primarily in the medial frontal lobe, medial temporal lobe, and the anterior cingulate

TABLE 4–9. Behavioral alterations associated with transmitter disturbances

Neurotransmitter	Reduced function	Increased function
Acetylcholine	Memory impairment, delirium, and delusions	Depression, aggression
Dopamine		
Motor function	Parkinsonism	Chorea, tics
Behavior	Dementia and depression	Psychosis, anxiety, confusion, elation, obsessive-compulsive behavior, and paraphilias
Noradrenaline	Depression, dementia, and reduced attention	Anxiety

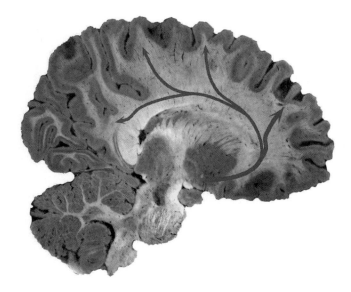

FIGURE 4–13. Cholinergic projections from the nucleus basalis.
Source. Image courtesy of M. Mega and the UCLA Laboratory of Neuroimaging.

region. Less robust projections are distributed to the neocortex.

Dopaminergic function is mediated by metabotropic receptors that can be classified pharmacologically as D_1 (stimulate cAMP) or D_2 (inhibit cAMP). These receptors have different distributions throughout the brain. The D_2 receptors are blocked by the neuroleptics, and it is possible that subtypes of the D_2 receptor differentially mediate the motor and mental effects of dopaminergic drugs.

Dopamine plays a key role in motoric functions and behavior. Dopamine deficiency or blockade leads to parkinsonism; dopamine excess produces chorea, dyskinesia, or tics. Behaviorally, dopamine deficiency causes at least mild cognitive impairment and may contribute to the depression that commonly accompanies Parkinson's disease and other parkinsonian syndromes. Dopamine excess leads to psychosis, elation or hypomania, and confusion. Dopamine hyperactivity may contribute to the pathophysiology

of schizophrenia, obsessive-compulsive behavior, anxiety, and some paraphiliac behaviors (Cummings 1985, 1991).

The locus coeruleus and adjacent nuclei comprise the origin of the *noradrenergic projection system.* A dorsal noradrenergic bundle courses in the dorsal brainstem to the septum, thalamus, amygdala, basal forebrain, hippocampus, and neocortex (Nieuwenhuys 1985) (Figure 4–15). A ventral noradrenergic bundle projects to the hypothalamus and midbrain reticular formation. Adrenergic function is mediated by metabotropic receptors that can be classified pharmacologically as α (inhibit cAMP) or β (stimulate cAMP) receptors. α-Adrenergic receptors can be further subtyped as α_1 or α_2; the former are located postsynaptically and the latter presynaptically and postsynaptically. These receptors have different distributions throughout the brain. Effective treatment for depression is associated with decreased numbers (downregulation) of

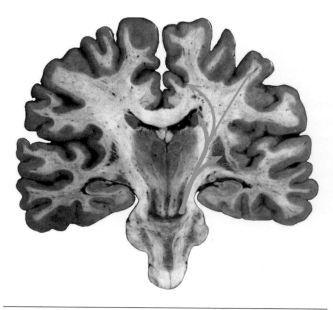

FIGURE 4–14. Nigrostriatal and nigrocortical dopaminergic projections.
Source. Image courtesy of M. Mega and the UCLA Laboratory of Neuroimaging.

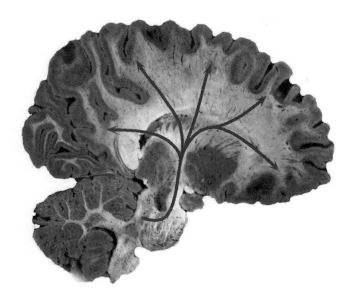

FIGURE 4–15. Noradrenergic projections from the locus coeruleus.
Source. Image courtesy of M. Mega and the UCLA Laboratory of Neuroimaging.

β-adrenergic receptors. Noradrenergic hypofunction has been linked to depression, dementia, and diminished alertness and concentration (Agid et al. 1987). Increased noradrenergic activity has been linked to anxiety (Lechin et al. 1989).

Serotonergic neurons are located almost exclusively in the median and paramedian raphe nuclei of the medulla, pons, and midbrain (Figure 4–16). The projection system of these serotonergic neurons is a complex, highly branched, fiber system that embraces virtually the entire central nervous system (Nieuwenhuys 1985). Serotonergic function is mediated by multiple metabotropic receptors (5-HT$_1$, 5-HT$_2$, 5-HT$_4$) and to a lesser extent by ionotropic receptors (5-HT$_3$). These receptors have different distributions throughout the brain. Serotonin deficiency has been hypothesized to play a major role in suicide, depression, and aggression (Agid et al. 1987), and serotonin hyperactivity can play a role in obsessive-compulsive behavior and anxiety (Lechin et al. 1989; Zohar et al. 1987).

γ-Aminobutyric acid (GABA) is an inhibitory neurotransmitter present in both projection systems and local neuronal circuits. The principal GABA projection system begins in the zona incerta and projects bilaterally to the entire neocortex, basal ganglia, and brainstem (Lin et al. 1990). In subcortical regions, one projection system originates in the caudate and putamen and projects to the globus pallidus and substantia nigra, and another begins in the globus pallidus and substantia nigra with projections to the

thalamus (Alexander and Crutcher 1990; Nieuwenhuys 1985). Local circuit neurons using GABA are found in the raphe nuclei, reticular nucleus of the thalamus, and basal ganglia. Local circuit neurons of the cerebral cortex also use GABA as their principal neurotransmitter (Rapoport 1990). GABA function is mediated by ionotropic (GABA$_A$) and metabotropic (GABA$_B$) receptors, the former being of special interest to neuropsychiatry because they contain the binding sites for alcohol, anticonvulsants, and benzodiazepines. These receptors have different distributions throughout the brain. GABA concentrations are decreased in the basal ganglia of patients with Huntington's disease, and the GABA deficiency may contribute to the dementia, mood disorder, obsessive-compulsive disorder, and psychosis occurring with increased frequency in this condition (Morris 1991).

Glutamate is an excitatory neurotransmitter that is used in the massive projection from the neocortex to the ipsilateral caudate, putamen, and nucleus accumbens. Glutamate is the principal neurotransmitter of projections from cortex to thalamus, from thalamus to cortex, and from one region of cortex to another. Glutamatergic neurons also project from subthalamic nucleus to globus pallidus. Glutamate functions in several hippocampus-related projections, including the perforant pathway projecting from entorhinal cortex to hippocampus and the pathways originating in hippocampus and adjacent subiculum and projecting to the septal region (Alexander and Crutcher 1990; Nieuwenhuys 1985). Glutamatergic function is mediated by ionotropic and metabotropic receptors, with subtypes

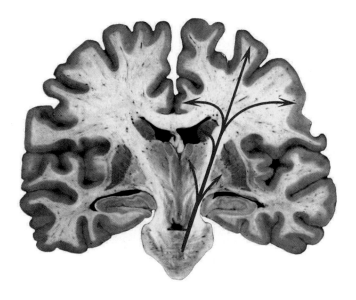

FIGURE 4–16. Serotonergic projections (*blue*).
Source. Image courtesy of M. Mega and the UCLA Laboratory of Neuroimaging.

of the former (e.g., *N*-methyl-D-aspartate receptor) having been implicated in learning, excitotoxicity, and the psychotomimetic effects of phencyclidine. These receptors have different distributions throughout the brain. Glutamate release is inhibited by several drugs recently introduced into clinical practice. These include lamotrigine (anticonvulsant) and riluzole (amyotrophic lateral sclerosis). The behavioral consequences of alterations in glutamate function are unknown.

Several other transmitters occur in behaviorally relevant areas, but their role in human behavior remains to be determined. *Histaminergic* neurons are situated in the posterior hypothalamus and project diffusely to most brain structures including the neocortex, amygdala, septum, caudate, and putamen (Nieuwenhuys 1985). *Glycine* is an inhibitory transmitter that may function in local circuit neurons in the substantia nigra, caudate, and putamen. *Substance P* is present in the projection from caudate and putamen to the substantia nigra, and *enkephalin*-containing neurons project from caudate and putamen to the globus pallidus (Alexander and Crutcher 1990; Nieuwenhuys 1985). *Vasoactive intestinal peptide* neurons are intrinsic to the cortex and participate in local neuronal circuits (Nieuwenhuys 1985).

Summary

The brain consists of a median zone mediating arousal and basic life-sustaining functions, such as respiration, digestion, circulation, and neuroendocrine function; a paramedian-limbic zone mediating extrapyramidal function and many aspects of emotional experience; and a supralimbic-neocortical zone mediating instrumental cognitive functions such as language and praxis (Table 4–10). Injury of the supralimbic-neocortical zone is associated with neurobehavioral deficit syndromes such as aphasia and apraxia; dysfunction of the paramedian-limbic zone correlates with neuropsychiatric disorders including mood disorders, psychoses, anxiety, and obsessive-compulsive disorder. Within each zone, behavioral deficits can be related to dysfunction of specific neurotransmitters. This approach provides a comprehensive framework for understanding brain-behavior relationships.

References

Adams RD, Victor M: Principles of Neurology, 2nd Edition. New York, McGraw-Hill, 1981

Agid Y, Ruberg M, Dubois B, et al: Anatomoclinical and biochemical concepts of subcortical dementia, in Cognitive Neurochemistry. Edited by Stahl SM, Iversen SD, Goodman EC. New York, Oxford University Press, 1987, pp 248–271

Alexander GE, Crutcher MD: Functional architecture of basal ganglia circuits: neural substrates of parallel processing. Trends Neurosci 13:266–271, 1990

Alexander GE, DeLong MR, Strick PL: Parallel organization of functionally segregated circuits linking basal ganglia and cortex. Annu Rev Neurosci 9:357–381, 1986

Alexander GE, Crutcher MD, DeLong MR: Basal ganglia-thalamocortical circuits: parallel substrates for motor, oculomotor, "prefrontal" and "limbic" functions. Prog Brain Res 85:119–146, 1990

Amaducci L, Sorbi S, Albanese A, et al: Choline acetyltransferase (ChAT) activity differs in right and left human temporal lobes. Neurology 31:799–805, 1981

TABLE 4–10. Summary of the anatomy, functions, and syndromes of the median, paramedian-limbic, and supralimbic-neocortical zones of the brain

Zone	Myelination	Neuronal connectivity/anatomy	Ontogeny	Function	Behavioral syndromes
Median	Poor	Feltwork; reticular	Functional at birth	Arousal	Disturbances of arousal, neuro-endocrine control, respiration, and circulation
Paramedian-limbic	Intermediate	Series; limbic system and basal ganglia	Functional within first few months	Emotion and extra-pyramidal function	Neuropsychiatric disorders; movement disorders
Supralimbic-neocortical	Complete	Parallel; neocortex	Functional in adulthood	Sensory cortex, motor cortex, and association cortex	Neurobehavioral disorders

Bartus RT, Dean RL III, Beer B, et al: The cholinergic hypothesis of geriatric memory dysfunction. Science 217:408–417, 1982

Baxter LR Jr, Phelps ME, Mazziotta JC, et al: Cerebral metabolic rates for glucose in mood disorders. Arch Gen Psychiatry 42:441–447, 1985

Baxter LR Jr, Phelps ME, Mazziotta JC, et al: Local cerebral glucose metabolic rates in obsessive-compulsive disorder. Arch Gen Psychiatry 44:211–218, 1987

Benarroch EE: Central Autonomic Network: Functional Organization and Clinical Correlations. Armonk, NY, Futura, 1997

Benson DF, Cummings JL, Tsai SY: Angular gyrus syndrome simulating Alzheimer disease. Arch Neurol 39:616–620, 1982

Bogousslavsky J, Ferrazzini M, Regli F, et al: Manic delirium and frontal-like syndrome with paramedian infarction of the right thalamus. J Neurol Neurosurg Psychiatry 51:116–119, 1988

Borod JC, Koff E, Lorch MP, et al: The expression and perception of facial emotion in brain-damaged patients. Neuropsychologia 24:169–180, 1986

Brandt J, Seidman LJ, Kohl D: Personality characteristics of epileptic patients: a controlled study of generalized and temporal lobe cases. J Clin Exp Neuropsychol 7:25–38, 1985

Bryden MP, Ley RC: Right-left hemispheric involvement in the perception and expression of emotion in normal humans, in Neuropsychology of Human Emotion. Edited by Heilman KM, Satz P. New York, Guilford, 1984, pp 6–44

Carpenter MB: Core Text of Neuroanatomy, 4th Edition. Baltimore, MD, Williams & Wilkins, 1991

Carpenter MB, Sutin J: Human Neuroanatomy, 8th Edition. Baltimore, MD, Williams & Wilkins, 1983

Coffey CE: Cerebral laterality and emotion: the neurology of depression. Compr Psychiatry 28:197–219, 1987

Coffey CE, Figiel GS, Djang WT, et al: Leukoencephalopathy in elderly depressed patients referred for ECT. Biol Psychiatry 24:143–161, 1988

Cummings JL: Clinical Neuropsychiatry. New York, Grune & Stratton, 1985

Cummings JL: Behavioral complications of drug treatment of Parkinson's disease. J Am Geriatr Soc 39:708–716, 1991

Cummings JL: Depression and Parkinson's disease: a review. Am J Psychiatry 149:443–454, 1992

Cummings JL: Frontal-subcortical circuits and human behavior. Arch Neurol 50:873–880, 1993

Cummings JL, Cunningham K: Obsessive-compulsive disorder in Huntington's disease. Biol Psychiatry 31:263–270, 1992

Cummings JL, Kaufer DI: Neuropsychiatric aspects of Alzheimer's disease: the cholinergic hypothesis revisited. Neurology 47:876–883, 1996

Cummings JL, Mendez MF: Secondary mania with focal cerebrovascular lesions. Am J Psychiatry 141:1084–1087, 1984

Davidson RJ: Anterior cerebral asymmetry and the nature of emotion. Brain Cogn 20:125–151, 1992

Delvenne V, Delecluse F, Hubain Ph P, et al: Regional cerebral blood flow in patients with affective disorders. Br J Psychiatry 157:359–365, 1990

Dilsaver SC, Coffman JA: Cholinergic hypothesis of depression: a reappraisal. J Clin Psychopharmacol 9:173–179, 1989

Doane BK: Clinical psychiatry and the physiodynamics of the limbic system, in The Limbic System: Functional Organization and Clinical Disorders. Edited by Doane BK, Livingston KE. New York, Raven, 1986, pp 285–315

Dolan RJ, Bench CJ, Brown RG, et al: Regional cerebral blood flow abnormalities in depressed patients with cognitive impairment. J Neurol Neurosurg Psychiatry 55:768–773, 1992

Drevets WC, Videen TO, Price JL, et al: A functional anatomical study of unipolar depression. J Neurosci 12:3628–3641, 1992

Duffy JD, Coffey CE: The neurobiology of depression, in Contemporary Behavioral Neurology. Edited by Trimble MR, Cummings JL. Boston, MA, Butterworth-Heinemann, 1997, pp 275–288

Eidelberg D, Galaburda AM: Symmetry and asymmetry in the posterior thalamus. Arch Neurol 39:325–332, 1982

Falzi G, Perrone P, Vignolog LA: Right-left asymmetry in anterior speech region. Arch Neurol 39:239–240, 1982

Flor-Henry P: Cerebral Basis of Psychopathology. Boston, MA, John Wright-PSG, 1983

Folstein SE: Huntington's Disease. A Disorder of Families. Baltimore, MD, Johns Hopkins University Press, 1989

Gainotti G: Emotional behavior and hemispheric side of lesion. Cortex 8:41–55, 1972

Galaburda AM, LeMay M, Kemper TL, et al: Right-left asymmetries in the brain. Science 199:852–856, 1978

Gawin FH: Cocaine addiction: psychology and neurophysiology. Science 251:1580–1586, 1991

George MS, Ketter TA, Kimbrell TA, et al: What functional imaging has revealed about the brain basis of mood and emotion. Advances in Biological Psychiatry 2:63–113, 1996

Geschwind N: Disconnection syndromes in animals and man. Brain 88:237–294, 585–644, 1965

Girgis M: Neural Substrates of Limbic Epilepsy. St. Louis, MO, Warren H. Green, 1981

Glick SD, Ross DA, Hough LB: Lateral asymmetry of neurotransmitters in human brain. Brain Res 234:53–63, 1982

Gordon HW: Music and the right hemisphere, in Functions of the Right Cerebral Hemisphere. Edited by Young AW. New York, Academic Press, 1983, pp 65–87

Gorman DG, Cummings JL: Hypersexuality following septal injury. Arch Neurol 49:308–310, 1992

Gruzelier JH: A critical assessment and integration of lateral asymmetries in schizophrenia, in Hemisyndromes: Psychobiology, Neurology, and Psychiatry. Edited by Myslobodsky MS. New York, Academic Press, 1983, pp 265–326

Halgren E, Walter RD, Cherlow DG, et al: Mental phenomena evoked by electrical stimulation of the human hippocampal formation and amygdala. Brain 101:83–117, 1978

Hermann BP, Wyler AR, Blumer D, et al: Ictal fear: lateralizing significance and implications for understanding the neurobiology of pathological fear states. Neuropsychiatry Neuropsychol Behav Neurol 5:205–210, 1992

Isaacson RL: The Limbic System. New York, Plenum, 1974

Katzman R, Thal L: Neurochemistry of Alzheimer's disease, in Basic Neurochemistry, 4th Edition. Edited by Siegel GJ, Agranoff BW, Albers RW, et al. New York, Raven, 1989, pp 827–838

Kelly JP: The neural basis of perception and movement, in Principles of Neural Science, 3rd Edition. Edited by Kandel ER, Schwartz JH, Jessell TM. New York, Elsevier, 1991, pp 283–295

Kimura D, Durnford M: Normal studies on the function of the right hemisphere in vision, in Hemisphere Function in the Human Brain. Edited by Dimond SJ, Beaumont JG. London, Elek Science, 1974, pp 25–47

Kirshner HS: Behavioral Neurology. A Practical Approach. New York, Churchill Livingstone, 1986

Kooistra CA, Heilman KM: Motor dominance and lateral asymmetry of the globus pallidus. Neurology 38:388–390, 1988

Laplane D, Levasseur M, Pillon B, et al: Obsessive-compulsive and other behavioral changes with bilateral basal ganglia lesions. Brain 112:699–725, 1989

Lechin F, van der Dijs B, Amat J, et al: Central neuronal pathways involved in anxiety behavior: experimental findings, in Neurochemistry and Clinical Disorders: Circuitry of Some Psychiatric and Psychosomatic Syndromes. Edited by Lechin F, van der Dijs B. Boca Raton, FL, CRC Press, 1989, pp 49–64

LeMay M: Morphological cerebral asymmetries of modern man, fossil man, and nonhuman primate. Ann N Y Acad Sci 280:349–366, 1976

Levy J: The mammalian brain and the adaptive advantage of cerebral asymmetry. Ann N Y Acad Sci 299:264–272, 1977

Lilly R, Cummings JL, Benson DF, et al: The human Klüver-Bucy syndrome. Neurology 33:1141–1145, 1983

Lin C-S, Nicolelis MAL, Schneider JS, et al: A major direct GABAergic pathway from zona incerta to neocortex. Science 248:1553–1556, 1990

Loring DW, Meador KJ, Lee GP, et al: Amobarbital effects and lateralized brain function. New York, Springer-Verlag, 1992

Machlin SR, Harris GJ, Pearlson GD, et al: Elevated medial-frontal cerebral blood flow in obsessive-compulsive patients: a SPECT study. Am J Psychiatry 148:1240–1242, 1991

MacLean PD: The Triune Brain in Evolution. New York, Plenum, 1990

Marin RS: Differential diagnosis and classification of apathy. Am J Psychiatry 147:22–30, 1990

Mena I, Marin O, Fuenzalida S, et al: Chronic manganese poisoning. Neurology 17:128–136, 1967

Mesulam M-M: Patterns of behavioral neuroanatomy: association areas, the limbic system, and hemispheric specialization, in Principles of Behavioral Neurology. Edited by Mesulam M-M. Philadelphia, PA, FA Davis, 1985, pp 1–70

Mesulam M-M, Mufson EJ: Neural inputs into the nucleus basalis of the substantia innominata (Ch4) in the rhesus monkey. Brain 107:253–274, 1984

Miller BL, Cummings JL, McIntyre H, et al: Hypersexuality or altered sexual preference following brain injury. J Neurol Neurosurg Psychiatry 49:867–873, 1986

Morris M: Psychiatric aspects of Huntington's disease, in Huntington's Disease. Edited by Harper PS. Philadelphia, PA, WB Saunders, 1991, pp 81–126

Moscovitch M, Olds J: Asymmetries in spontaneous facial expressions and their possible relation to hemispheric specialization. Neuropsychologia 20:71–81, 1982

Nachson I: Hemisphere dysfunction in psychopathy and behavior disorders, in Hemisyndromes: Psychobiology, Neurology, and Psychiatry. Edited by Myslobodsky MS. New York, Academic Press, 1983, pp 389–414

Nauta WJH: Circuitous connections linking cerebral cortex, limbic system, and corpus striatum, in The Limbic System: Functional Organization and Clinical Disorders. Edited by Doane BK, Livingston KE. New York, Raven, 1986, pp 43–54

Nauta WJH, Feirtag M: Fundamental Neuroanatomy. New York, WH Freeman, 1986

Nieuwenhuys R: Chemoarchitecture of the Brain. New York, Springer-Verlag, 1985

Oke A, Keller R, Mefford I, et al: Lateralization of norepinephrine in human thalamus. Science 200: 1411–1413, 1978

Papez JW: A proposed mechanism of emotion. Archives of Neurology and Psychiatry 38:725–743, 1937

Perez MM, Trimble MR, Murray NMF, et al: Epileptic psychosis: an evaluation of PSE profiles. Br J Psychiatry 146: 155–163, 1985

Plum F, Posner JB: The Diagnosis of Stupor and Coma. Philadelphia, PA, FA Davis, 1980

Rapoport SI: Integrated phylogeny of the primate brain, with special reference to humans and their diseases. Brain Res Rev 15:267–294, 1990

Reisberg B, Franssen E, Sclan SG, et al: Stage specific incidence of potentially remediable behavioral symptoms in aging and Alzheimer's disease. Bulletin of Clinical Neurosciences 54:95–112, 1989

Robinson RG, Starkstein SE: Current research in affective disorders following stroke. J Neuropsychiatry Clin Neurosci 2:1–14, 1990

Robinson RG, Kubos KL, Starr LB, et al: Mood disorders in stroke patients: importance of location of lesion. Brain 107:81–93, 1984

Sackeim HA, Greenburg MS, Weiman AL, et al: Hemispheric asymmetry in the expression of positive and negative emotions. Arch Neurol 39:210–218, 1982

Sackeim HA, Prohovnik I, Moeller JR, et al: Regional cerebral blood flow in mood disorders. Arch Gen Psychiatry 47:60–70, 1990

Schade JP, Groeningen VV: Structural organization of the human cerebral cortex. Acta Anat (Basel) 47:79–111, 1961

Schilder P: The organic background of obsessions and compulsions. Am J Psychiatry 94:1397–1416, 1938

Sedvall G: The current status of PET scanning with respect to schizophrenia. Neuropsychopharmacology 7:41–54, 1992

Starkstein SE, Robinson RG, Price TR: Comparison of cortical and subcortical lesions in the production of post-stroke mood disorders. Brain 110:1045–1059, 1987

Starkstein SE, Robinson RG, Berthier ML, et al: Differential mood changes following basal ganglia vs thalamic lesions. Arch Neurol 45:725–730, 1988a

Starkstein SE, Boston JD, Robinson RG: Mechanisms of mania after brain injury: twelve case reports and review of the literature. J Nerv Ment Dis 176:87–100, 1988b

Stein MB, Heuser IJ, Juncos JL, et al: Anxiety disorders in patients with Parkinson's disease. Am J Psychiatry 147:217–220, 1990

Stern DB: Psychogenic somatic symptoms on the left side: review and interpretation, in Hemisyndromes: Psychobiology, Neurology, and Psychiatry. Edited by Myslobodsky MS. New York, Academic Press, 1983, pp 415–445

Strauss E, Risser A, Jones MW: Fear responses in patients with epilepsy. Arch Neurol 39:626–630, 1982

Stuss DT, Benson DF: The Frontal Lobes. New York, Raven, 1986

Stuss DT, Guberman A, Nelson R, et al: The neuropsychology of paramedian thalamic infarction. Brain Cogn 8:348–378, 1988

Suddath RC, Casanova MF, Goldberg TE, et al: Temporal lobe pathology in schizophrenia: a quantitative magnetic resonance imaging study. Am J Psychiatry 146:464–472, 1989

Swedo SE, Rapoport JL, Cheslow DL, et al: High prevalence of obsessive-compulsive symptoms in patients with Sydenham's chorea. Am J Psychiatry 146:246–249, 1989

TenHouten WD, Hoppe KD, Bogen JE, et al: Alexithymia: an experimental study of cerebral commissurotomy patients and normal control subjects. Am J Psychiatry 143:312–316, 1986

Tucker DM, Watson RT, Heilman KM: Discrimination and evocation of affectively intoned speech in patients with right parietal disease. Neurology 27:947–950, 1977

Valzelli L: Psychobiology of Aggression and Violence. New York, Raven, 1981

Van Lancker D: Personal relevance and the human right hemisphere. Brain Cogn 17:64–92, 1991

Van Lancker D, Kreiman J, Cummings JL: Voice perception deficits: neuroanatomical correlates of phonagnosia. J Clin Exp Neuropsychol 11:665–674, 1989

Weintraub S, Mesulam M-M: Developmental learning disabilities of the right hemisphere. Arch Neurol 40:463–468, 1983

Williams D: The structure of emotions reflected in epileptic experiences. Brain 79:29–67, 1956

Wu JC, Buchsbaum MS, Hershey TG, et al: PET in generalized anxiety disorder. Biol Psychiatry 29:1181–1199, 1991

Yakovlev PI: Motility, behavior and the brain. J Nerv Ment Dis 107:313–335, 1948

Yakovlev PI: Telencephalon "impar," "semipar," and "totopar." International Journal of Neurology 6:245–265, 1968

Yakovlev PI, Lecours A-R: The myelogenetic cycles of regional maturation of the brain, in Regional Development of the Brain in Early Life. Edited by Minkowski A. Oxford, England, Blackwell Scientific, 1967, pp 3–65

Zohar J, Mueller EA, Insel TR, et al: Serotonergic responsivity in obsessive-compulsive disorder. Arch Gen Psychiatry 44:946–951, 1987

SECTION II

Neuropsychiatric Assessment of the Elderly

Mark R. Lovell, Ph.D., Section Editor

CHAPTER 5

Neuropsychiatric Assessment

CHAPTER 6

Mental Status Examination

CHAPTER 7

Neuropsychological Assessment

CHAPTER 8

Age-Associated Memory Impairment

CHAPTER 9

Anatomic Imaging of the Aging Human Brain:
Computed Tomography and Magnetic Resonance Imaging

CHAPTER 10

Functional Brain Imaging:
Cerebral Blood Flow and Glucose Metabolism in
Healthy Human Aging

CHAPTER 11

Functional Brain Imaging:
Functional Magnetic Resonance Imaging and
Magnetic Resonance Spectroscopy

CHAPTER 12

Quantitative Electroencephalography:
Neurophysiological Alterations in Normal Aging and
Geriatric Neuropsychiatric Disorders

5

Neuropsychiatric Assessment

John J. Campbell III, M.D.

Neuropsychiatry is an ambiguous construct. Its precise definition remains elusive (Cummings and Hegarty 1994; Lishman 1992; Trimble 1993). In practice, however, a neuropsychiatric approach permits a broad conceptualization of a particular clinical problem that transcends a basic neurological or psychiatric paradigm. This is of particular relevance for the geriatric patient, in whom the interplay between biology and psychology is complex and pervasive. A thorough neuropsychiatric examination can reconcile this dichotomy and form the basis for a comprehensive treatment plan. Several outstanding reviews have detailed the areas relevant to a proper assessment (Cummings 1985a; Mueller and Fogel 1997; Ovsiew 1997; Strub and Black 1993; Weintraub and Mesulam 1985).

Mueller and Fogel (1997) have elaborated on the neuropsychiatric gestalt. The approach represents a fundamental departure from traditional psychiatry and neurology in several ways. Collateral confirmation of historical details is emphasized. Neuropsychiatric syndromes often affect recall and insight, thus requiring supplementary history from those who know the patient. The reciprocal influences of psychology and cerebral dysfunction are appreciated. Both processes are, of course, brain related; however, each has its own unique and significant influence on behavior. Localization of signs and symptoms in the brain takes precedence over standard psychiatric diagnoses. Therefore, a more comprehensive and flexible assessment of mental status is undertaken.

The neuropsychiatric assessment is data driven. The collection of the data and their synthesis into a coherent formulation serve to establish neuropsychiatry as a unique clinical discipline. In this chapter, I provide an overview of the neuropsychiatric assessment of the geriatric patient, emphasizing the relationship between functional neuroanatomy and neuropathology. The basic framework of this assessment includes taking a history, doing a mental status examination, performing a physical examination, and making a formulation.

Clinical Interview

The geriatric neuropsychiatry clinical interview has unique aspects. Patients commonly experience hearing impairment, diminished cognitive efficiency, attentional impairments, lack of insight, impaired memory, and dysphasias, all of which challenge the skills of the interviewer. In addition, the caregiver must be an integral source of historical information. Caregivers play an increasingly important role as the patient experiences functional declines and requires increasing assistance. The presence of impaired memory and insight may interfere with the gathering of the history to such an extent that the caregiver provides the essential collateral information.

Further, the ongoing responsibility of taking care of an impaired individual can lead to demoralization, isolation, and depression, which serve to diminish the effectiveness of the caregiver. This can result in a possibly preventable accident, such as falling and fracturing a hip, nursing home placement, or even elder abuse. Thus, inquiring as to how the caregivers are dealing with their own stresses is part of the geriatric neuropsychiatric assessment.

The neuropsychiatric history explores two interrelated realms of human existence—the development of a central nervous system and the development of a person. As such, our exploration begins before conception, with the *genetic history of the parents*, through gestation and birth, up to the day of the examination. The clinical interview below has been organized along a time line in order to address issues of psychological development along with the typical starting points for important behavioral and neurological considerations, such as occurrence of depression or onset of Parkinson's disease, for example. It emphasizes that the patients are products of their past experiences regardless of the presenting complaint. The completed history will establish a qualitative functional baseline, along with an appreciation of inherited and acquired influences on development, their impact, and the role of biological and psychological attempts at compensation (see Table 5–1).

Gestation and Birth

The central nervous system develops in an orderly sequence notable for the germination, migration, and differentiation of neurons and glia throughout gestation. During this period, cerebral and somatic development are vulnerable to numerous perturbations from many causes. Maternal drug use, infection, and injury can negatively influence the developmental process. Labor and delivery impose additional stresses on the neonatal brain. Fetal distress from maternal hemorrhage, circulatory impairment, and cranial trauma can result in hypoxic injury, cerebral contusions, and intracerebral hemorrhage, all of which may negatively affect neurodevelopment.

The *gestational and birth history* is not generally accessible with geriatric patients. Ideally, higher functioning pa-

tients or caregivers can provide this information. When not available, several clues in the history and physical examination may raise the index of suspicion. Early hemispheric damage often leads to subtle contralateral hemiatrophy. Careful observation of the face or comparison of the hands can reveal somatic asymmetry and developmental anomaly. For example, manifestations of fetal alcohol syndrome include facial changes with epicanthal eye folds, poorly formed concha, small teeth with faulty enamel, and microcephaly with mental retardation (Streissguth and Landesman-Dwyer 1980). Delays in the timely *achievement of developmental milestones* are another possible sign of inherited or acquired dysfunction. Scholastic difficulties with speech, language, and arithmetic may reflect left hemispheric anomaly. In addition, Rourke (1989) has described a syndrome of social impairment and dysprosodia localized to the right hemisphere.

Ovsiew (1997) listed several additional signs that may suggest developmental abnormality. These include an abnormal head circumference, fine "electric" hair, more than one hair whorl, abnormal epicanthic folds of the eyes, abnormal interorbital distance, low-set or malformed ears, high palate, and furrowed tongue. Peripheral signs include curved fifth finger, single palmar crease, wide gap between first and second toes, partial fusion of the toes, and third toe longer than second toe.

Handedness is a variable that may reflect anomalous cerebral development. Geschwind and Galaburda (1985) have proposed a model of handedness based on intra-

TABLE 5–1.   Elements of the clinical interview

Gestational and birth history

Achievement of developmental milestones

Handedness

Genetic history of the parents and siblings

School history: academic and disciplinary

History of violence or criminal behavior

History of head injury

Psychiatric history

Substance abuse history

Behavioral and cognitive baseline

Occupational history

Medical and surgical history

Medication regimen

Review of systems

Survey of the vegetative functions

Assessment of activities of daily living

History of recent changes in behavior and cognition

uterine influences on development. They describe a continuum of handedness ranging from strongly right-handed to ambidextrous to strongly left-handed and suggest that the degree of left-handedness reflects compensation for negative intrauterine influences on left hemisphere development.

Childhood

The challenges of childhood include refining social and scholastic skills. School represents an intellectual and behavioral laboratory where deficits may be revealed, and the *school history* requires thorough probing. It is important to obtain information about any remedial classes or a history of being held back. Often, formal testing was done and a report may be available. This is a more recent development in United States education, however, and such information may not be obtainable for elderly persons.

A *history of disciplinary troubles* may reflect the presence of attention-deficit/hyperactivity or disruptive behavior disorders. Asking patients to describe their behavior in the classroom is a helpful probe, if recall is sufficient. Signs of inattention in the classroom include making careless mistakes, failing to finish schoolwork, easy distractibility, and forgetfulness in daily activities. Signs of hyperactivity and impulsivity include fidgeting, frequently leaving the seat, intrusiveness, and running about excessively. Attention-deficit/hyperactivity disorder is believed to continue into adulthood in some cases (Wender 1981; Zametkin et al. 1990). The presentation in adults is somewhat different and includes difficulty being organized, low frustration tolerance, impulsivity, restlessness, and mood swings (Woods 1986). It is not known whether residual attention-deficit/hyperactivity disorder extends into senescence.

Behavioral patterns are typically established in childhood. A repetitive pattern of aggression to people and animals, destruction of property, deceitfulness or theft, and serious violations of social norms is evidence for a conduct disorder (American Psychiatric Association 1994). Conduct disorder may represent the presence of developmental anomaly (Nachson 1991). One must inquire about any *history of violence or criminal behavior* beginning in childhood and adolescence. Violent behaviors can also appear as sequelae to numerous central nervous system disorders (Elliott 1992).

Many neurological disorders that may be relevant later in life occur during childhood, including Gilles de la Tourette's syndrome, epilepsy, meningitides, and closed head injury. These conditions are often associated with cognitive and behavioral sequelae that may persist into senescence. Older individuals may have contacted many neurological diseases now considered to be rare, such as poliomyelitis, dementia paralytica, or encephalitis lethargica.

Adolescence

During adolescence, individuals develop a social identity and begin to form strong attachments outside the family. They may also join the workforce. Maladaptive patterns of behavior established during childhood can continue into adolescence. Adolescents also begin to experiment with drugs, occasionally resulting in substance abuse and dependence. Risk-taking behaviors, such as reckless driving, are not uncommon. Injury is a common cause of morbidity in adolescence. A *history of head injury* should be elicited. Many head injuries do not result in gross cerebral trauma. Asking patients if their ability to think was affected by an injury can often elicit evidence of subtle cerebral pathology. Lishman reported that the degree of anterograde and retrograde amnesia after a head injury is a predictor of postinjury cognitive sequelae (Lishman 1987). The history should define the window of amnesia preceding and subsequent to the injury.

A thorough review of *past psychiatric history* is an essential part of the neuropsychiatric history. Numerous psychiatric illnesses have their onset during adolescence, including anxiety, mood, and thought disorders. Psychiatric illness can reflect neurobiological anomaly and certainly affects psychological development. Schizophrenia is believed to result from structural abnormality in the brain. One line of evidence supports an abnormal migration of hippocampal neurons during gestation (Roberts 1990). Other investigations have focused on prefrontal and temporal heteromodal association cortex pathology rendering an individual vulnerable to hallucinations and psychosis (Shenton et al. 1992; Weinberger 1988). Mood disorders are associated with diminished metabolism in prefrontal and subcortical regions (Ketter et al. 1996; Mayberg et al. 1997).

The *substance abuse history* must be thoroughly explored. Substance abuse can lead to acquired neurological insult and chronic symptoms. Intoxication with alcohol or other substances increases the risk for accidents and head injury. Alcohol and prescription drug abuse in the elderly are often missed by clinicians. Use of cocaine can precipitate stroke (Levine et al. 1990). The use of the designer drug 1-methyl-4-phenyl-1,2,3,6-tetrahydropyridine (MPTP) led to an acute parkinsonian syndrome (Tetrud et al. 1989). Lysergic acid diethylamide (LSD) use is occasionally associated with recurrent visual hallucinatory experiences, known as hallucinogen persisting perception disorder (American Psychiatric Association 1994). Sharing hypodermic needles exposes individuals to numerous infectious agents, including human immunodeficiency virus, which can cross the blood-brain barrier and affect cognition (Gibbs et al. 1990; Tross and Hirsch 1988) while also predisposing the user to opportunistic central nervous system infections.

Adulthood

Adulthood heralds the establishment of a stable *pattern of behavior and cognitive performance*, representing an important baseline. Elderly individuals typically present for neuropsychiatric evaluation after a decline from these prior levels of functioning, so this baseline must be clearly identified in the history. Patients establish an *occupational history* during adulthood that should be explored for continuity, stability, and possible exposure to toxic substances.

The persistence of maladaptive behaviors from adolescence into adulthood introduces an element of chronicity that may have relevance for the neuropsychiatric evaluation. Chronic use of alcohol is thought to result in an alcoholic dementia (Charness et al. 1989; Lishman 1990). Malnutrition associated with heavy alcohol use can precipitate thiamine deficiency and the Wernicke-Korsakoff syndrome (Greenberg and Diamond 1986). A pattern of poorly managed aggression and violence can lead to traumatic brain injury, creating a downward spiral of further maladaptive behaviors and cognitive impairment.

Neurological problems that have particular relevance to the neuropsychiatric evaluation, and typically arise before the age of 65, include brain tumors, Huntington's disease, inflammatory disorders such as lupus erythematosus, and multiple sclerosis. Health habits such as nicotine dependence that place an individual at risk for cerebrovascular disease, along with the onset of medical conditions such as hypertension, diabetes mellitus, and hypercholesterolemia, are also noted during adulthood.

Senescence

The elderly person presenting for neuropsychiatric evaluation has a wealth of life experiences that contribute to current functioning. Erikson et al. (1994) described the primary challenge of this life epoch as consolidating these experiences into a cohesive sense of integrity. The alternative is a feeling of despair that goals have not been accomplished, dreams have not been realized, and that time is running out. Neuropsychiatric disorders represent a significant threat to this sense of integrity. Important neurological conditions that arise in senescence, in addition to

those previously listed, include Parkinson's disease and the various cortical degenerative disorders such as Alzheimer's disease, frontotemporal dementias, dementia with Lewy bodies, normal pressure hydrocephalus, and subdural hematoma.

Elderly persons are far more likely to have chronic medical problems and to be prescribed multiple medications. The history should include a *comprehensive medical and surgical history*, along with a thorough *review of systems*, to screen for any current medical conditions such as urinary tract infections, endocrine disorders, acute neurological deficits, cardiac symptoms, or respiratory conditions that may precipitate an acute confusional state. The presence of bowel or bladder incontinence should be determined. Elderly patients often report somatic and cognitive symptoms in the context of major depressive disorder. The review of systems should include a *survey of the vegetative functions* affected by mood disorder including sleep, appetite, libido. At times, an alteration in the vegetative functions may be the only way to differentiate between a primary psychiatric diagnosis such as depression and a neuropsychiatric syndrome such as acquired apathy. Individuals with depression would have sleep and appetite changes, whereas patients with apathy syndromes, also known as pseudodepression, will eat when presented with food and do not experience significant sleep disruption. Recent changes in a patient's *medication regimen* can precipitate a confusional state or ataxia and should be documented. Any medication capable of crossing the blood-brain barrier has the potential to cause myriad central nervous system side effects in the elderly.

Many elderly patients are functioning well with a "preclinical" dementia but lose their functional reserve and appear to have frank dementia or a depressive disorder in the context of acute medical conditions. The aging brain, with a limited cortical reserve and an often tenuous blood supply, is quite vulnerable to acute dysfunction from systemic illness and is more susceptible to cognitive and behavioral toxicity of many commonly prescribed medications. Recovery from these confusional states is often slow to proceed. The "acute dementia" or "acute depression" will slowly resolve upon adequate treatment of the underlying condition.

The clinical interview of the geriatric patient should also include an *assessment of activities of daily living* to explore functional status. These activities include cooking, dressing, performing household chores, shopping, driving, maintaining personal hygiene, and paying bills. Several instruments have been developed to assess functional status in the elderly (Applegate et al. 1990). They provide the clinician with useful measures to document and monitor a person's level of independence. The degree of autonomy and effectiveness at functioning in one's environment is a crucial historical domain that must be thoroughly assessed.

Historical information, particularly a *history of recent changes in behavior and cognition*, must be organized in order to direct the focus of the mental status and physical examinations. The various neural systems in the brain are associated with rather discrete behavioral and cognitive functions. The signs of neuropsychiatric illness reflect dysfunction in these neuronal networks. The neuropsychiatric examination must, therefore, have localizing value. Through an understanding of functional neuroanatomy and neuropathology, the neuropsychiatrist will be able to clarify problems identified in the history and expand upon them through strategic use of bedside testing to arrive at a more complete understanding of the clinical problem.

Major Neuropsychiatric Syndromes of the Elderly

Elderly patients frequently present for neuropsychiatric evaluation with chief complaints of forgetfulness, personality change, or mental status change. The differential diagnosis for these symptoms includes virtually all medical conditions prevalent in the elderly. Careful neuropsychiatric evaluation can assist the clinician by discriminating between a depressive disorder, a confusional state, a benign condition of age-related cognitive decline, or intellectual impairment caused by more significant cerebral or somatic dysfunction. Major neuropsychiatric syndromes affecting cognition will typically involve, in addition to memory, other cognitive domains, as well as the executive, motor, and limbic systems. These syndromes are described below to assist in the focus of the clinical interview and to begin to structure the approach to the mental status examination.

Clinical Characteristics of Age-Related Cognitive Changes

Cognitive decline is not an inevitable consequence of aging. However, numerous studies have demonstrated intellectual impairment of mild to moderate severity in a significant proportion of elderly individuals not diagnosed with a dementia (Ebly et al. 1995; Peterson et al. 1992; Rapp and Amaral 1992). The cognitive domain that is primarily affected appears to be memory and, in particular, acquisition or learning (Petersen et al. 1992). Elderly individuals appear to acquire less information but retain the ability to store and recall the learned material.

The issue of when aging ends and disease begins re-

mains to be resolved. A longitudinal study of healthy, independent seniors with an isolated, mild memory impairment showed that approximately 10%–15% of these individuals experienced progression to clinically diagnosable dementia of the Alzheimer type each year (Petersen et al. 1997). Age-associated memory impairment is discussed in greater detail elsewhere in this text.

Clinical Characteristics of Prefrontal Systems Dysfunction

Prefrontal systems dysfunction is recognized as a condition that can cause gross disruption of behavior while sparing basic motor, sensory, and cognitive functions. The metacognitive functions subserved by prefrontal systems are essential for adaptive functioning in one's environment. Despite their vital role in human behavior, the so-called executive cognitive functions are not routinely tested in common cognitive screening instruments such as the Mini-Mental State Exam (Folstein et al. 1975) or the Short Portable Mental Status Questionnaire (Pfeiffer 1975). However, an understanding of their contributions to adaptive behavior, together with an appreciation of the cardinal signs of prefrontal dysfunction, can lead to a proper diagnosis and treatment plan. Signs of prefrontal systems dysfunction range from the dramatic personality changes associated with orbitofrontal and mesial frontal dysfunction to a perplexing inability to function well in the presence of only mild motor, sensory, or cognitive impairment, as is often seen with dysfunction of the dorsolateral convexity network (Table 5–2).

Dorsal convexity dysexecutive syndrome. The high-level cognitive functions mediated by the dorsolateral prefrontal lobe and its connections include cognitive flexibility, temporal ordering of recent events, planning ahead, regulating actions based on environmental stimuli, and learning from experience (Goldman-Rakic 1993). Patients exhibiting dysfunction in these cognitive domains are concrete and perseverative and show impairment in reasoning and flexibility. The examiner should probe the ability to pay bills on time, organize daily activi-

TABLE 5–2. **Regional prefrontal syndromes**

Region	Cardinal signs
Orbitofrontal system	Behavioral disinhibition
	Environmental dependency
Dorsolateral convexity system	Cognitive disorganization
Mesial frontal system	Apathy syndrome

ties, such as going to the bank or market, keep a tidy house, or cook balanced meals. The "tea and toast" diet frequently results from loss of the organizational capacity to purchase diverse groceries in response to dwindling home supplies and to plan and prepare a meal consisting of several items. In addition, such patients are characterized by a paucity of spontaneous behavior. They often appear apathetic and may become irritable during mental status testing when fatigue easily ensues.

Orbitofrontal disinhibition syndrome. The orbitofrontal cortex has discrete connections with paralimbic cortex and thus plays a role in the elaboration and integration of limbic drives. This area receives highly processed information concerning the individual's experience of an environmental stimulus and the anticipated consequences of various behavioral responses to it (Malloy and Duffy 1992). This process allows a person to maintain consistent behavior in keeping with his or her self-concept. Patients with orbitofrontal damage often exhibit poor impulse control, explosive aggressive outbursts, inappropriate verbal lewdness, jocularity, and a lack of interpersonal sensitivity. The fatuous behaviors observed with orbitofrontal system dysfunction are known as moria or witzelsucht. The stimulus-bound behaviors noted with this syndrome are commonly noted in nursing homes, where residents frequently wander and happen upon numerous stimuli. A doorknob will be turned and a room entered. A sleeve hanging from a drawer is an invitation to disrobe and put on the newly discovered clothes. A shower stall is an open invitation for a shower. These patients often become agitated and aggressive when interfered with. The diagnosis of the orbitofrontal disinhibition syndrome is primarily clinical. Such gross disruption of behavior often leads to a misdiagnosis of mania. Careful review of the history will not, however, demonstrate insomnia, pressured speech, religiosity, or grandiose delusions.

Mesial frontal apathetic syndrome. Mesial frontal pathology affects the functional balance between the cingulum and supplementary motor area. Disruption of this network leads to a dysmotivational syndrome ranging from apathy to akinetic mutism (Duffy and Campbell 1994). These patients often appear depressed, yet they lack the dysphoria, negative cognitions, and neurovegetative signs of a major depression. The diagnosis of a mesial frontal apathy syndrome is entirely clinical. One patient, after a gunshot wound to the frontal lobes, lapsed into a state of inertia when left alone. When questioned, he related an awareness of a personality change. He denied boredom and described it as a "loss of motivation" in that he entertained numerous ideas for activities, but felt no impetus to act on them. His facial expression was one of casual indifference, and he would often respond with simple gestures instead of speaking. Caregivers for patients with apathy syndromes are commonly frustrated with what they incorrectly perceive as willful indifference to the home environment.

Clinical Characteristics of Generalized Cortical Systems Disorders

The neurodegenerative disorders that compose the classic dementias typically affect the cerebral cortex in regional patterns. Alzheimer's disease appears to preferentially affect heteromodal association cortex and the limbic system (Hyman et al. 1984; Pearson et al. 1985). Mesencephalic projection nuclei including dopaminergic, cholinergic, serotonergic, and noradrenergic systems are variably involved (Jellinger 1987). Common clinical findings include amnesia, aphasia, apraxia, agnosia, and visuospatial impairment. The degree of involvement of these cognitive domains is quite variable between patients. Dementia with Lewy bodies may represent a clinicopathological variant of Alzheimer's disease. Patients present with a mixed picture of cortical and subcortical pathology, characterized by global cognitive impairment along with fluctuating attention, visual hallucinations, and spontaneous motor features of parkinsonism (McKeith et al. 1996). Frontotemporal dementias involve limbic and paralimbic degeneration in the prefrontal and temporal regions. Clinical signs of frontotemporal dementia include gross disruption of social comportment with an eventual transition to an apathetic state (Chang Chui 1989).

Clinical Characteristics of Focal Cortical Dementia Syndromes

Focal degeneration syndromes can present in a slowly progressive manner and are regularly noted. Their etiology is not well understood, but autopsy findings in some cases reveal hallmarks of generalized cortical dementias, including senile plaques, neurofibrillary tangles, Pick's bodies, and Lewy bodies (Benson and Zaras 1991; Brun 1987; Hof et al. 1989; Morris et al. 1984). Thus, these syndromes may represent uncommon presentations of more common disorders. Caselli (1995) identified four general syndromes, including progressive frontal lobe syndromes, progressive aphasias, progressive perceptual motor syndromes, and progressive bitemporal syndromes. The progressive frontal lobe syndromes are described above.

Progressive aphasias. The progressive aphasias described in the literature include fluent and nonfluent types, as well as anomic and mixed types. Fluent aphasia, also known as Wernicke's aphasia, receptive aphasia, and posterior aphasia, is characterized by effortless, yet incomprehensible speech, together with difficulty comprehending the speech of others. This aphasia is most commonly caused by damage to unimodal association cortex in area 22 of the left hemisphere (A. R. Damasio 1992). This area is located in the superior temporal gyrus in the posterior regions adjacent to the supramarginal gyrus.

Nonfluent aphasia is also known as Broca's aphasia, expressive aphasia, and anterior aphasia. This aphasia is notable for effortful, agrammatic or telegraphic speech in which the patient has great difficulty using words such as "if," "and," "or," "but," "to," "from," and so on. Anterior aphasia results from damage to the inferior left frontal gyrus in the left hemisphere. Deficits in anomic aphasias are limited to word finding and naming. Anomic aphasia can result from damage to numerous sites in the left hemisphere. The mixed aphasia syndrome appears to involve numerous aspects of language function and is associated with degeneration in the left temporal and perisylvian regions. Other commonly noted aphasia syndromes such as global aphasia, conduction aphasia, transcortical aphasias, and pure word deafness are typically vascular in origin and are not commonly the product of progressive cortical degeneration (H. Damasio 1989).

Progressive perceptual-motor syndromes. The progressive perceptual-motor syndromes are divided into visual syndromes and motor syndromes. The progressive visual syndromes involve occipitoparietal and occipitotemporal networks and include progressive asimultanagnosia, Balint's syndrome, and visual agnosia.

Focal pathology in the occipitoparietal system bilaterally affects higher order processing of visual information into a coherent whole. Consequently, asimultanagnosia describes the inability to adequately appreciate important aspects of a visual scene, a problem known as visual disorientation. Patients can describe certain details but cannot integrate the entirety of the information (A. R. Damasio 1985). Balint's syndrome consists of asimultanagnosia along with optic apraxia, an impairment of voluntary gaze, and optic ataxia, an inability to point accurately at a target under visual guidance (Balint 1909). Bilateral dysfunction in the occipitotemporal system results in visual agnosia, an inability to name visualized objects. Prosopagnosia is a particular type of visual agnosia with a circumscribed deficit of facial recognition (A. R. Damasio et al. 1982).

Two progressive motor syndromes have been described that involve the parietofrontal junction (Caselli 1995). The syndromes are not specifically named. The first

consists of hemispasticity, hemiparesis, and hemisensory impairment in the form of astereognosis or agraphesthesia, and myoclonus. The second motor syndrome is defined by a mixed apraxia, or disorder of higher order motor integration, consisting of limb apraxia, gestural apraxia, dressing apraxia, constructional apraxia, and writing apraxia. Limb apraxia is characterized by difficulty executing simple motor tasks such as combing the hair or brushing the teeth. Gestural apraxia is a form of limb apraxia in which the patient has great difficulty imitating symbolic movements. Dressing apraxia is the inability to dress despite absence of significant sensorimotor disturbance. Constructional and writing apraxias involve impaired ability to draw or write.

Progressive bitemporal syndromes. The progressive bitemporal syndromes include progressive amnesia, progressive prosopagnosia, and Klüver-Bucy syndrome. The Klüver-Bucy syndrome results from bilateral destruction of the amygdalae and is characterized by hyperorality, emotional placidity, hypersexuality, compulsive exploration of the environment, known as hypermetamorphosis, and psychic blindness (Klüver and Bucy 1939; Lilly et al. 1983).

Clinical Characteristics of Subcortical Systems Disorders

Basal ganglia dysfunction. The basal ganglia have a significant functional relationship with specific regions of frontal cortex. Alexander and Crutcher (1990) identified five independent neural loops uniting striatum, globus pallidus, dorsomedial thalamus, and frontal cortex. The physical integrity of these loops appears to be critical to optimal functioning of the behaviors unique to each circuit. The supplementary motor area participates in a circuit responsible for the integration of motor function. Similarly, a loop involving the frontal eye fields subserves oculomotor function. The dorsolateral prefrontal, lateral orbitofrontal, and anterior cingulate areas participate in discrete circuits subserving cognitive organization, social comportment, and motivation, respectively (Duffy and Campbell 1994). These circuits have particular relevance to neuropsychiatry because of their essential roles in adaptive behavior. The cardinal signs of basal ganglia pathology represent suboptimal participation of the striatum in these networks, resulting in cognitive impairment, motor dysfunction, and mood disorders.

The motor signs of basal ganglia dysfunction may be readily apparent during the clinical interview. The classic triad of movement disorder includes tremor, rigidity, and akinesia. It is helpful to observe the gait when the patient first arrives. A shuffling gait may represent an early clue. Other signs include a bland expression with infrequent blinking, difficulty sitting down with ease, and a paucity of movement. "Striatal hand" may be evident and is characterized by an ulnar deviation with flexion of the fingers at the metacarpal phalangeal joints. A "pill rolling" tremor of 4–7 Hz involving the thumb and forefinger is frequently noted. When these signs are noted, the examiner should probe further for progressive symptoms of stiffness, loss of agility, involuntary movements, or difficulty walking. Chorea may be observed with other striatal disorders such as Huntington's disease. Patients often attempt to mask these involuntary movements by quickly stroking their hair or adjusting an article of clothing.

Controversy exists over the presence of cognitive impairment associated with basal ganglia pathology (McHugh 1989). Carefully conducted studies have, however, identified the presence of a pattern of deficits that appears to reflect derangement of the frontal-subcortical contribution to cognition (Brown and Marsden 1990). Albert et al. (1974) and McHugh and Folstein (1975) have described a "subcortical dementia" consisting of mental torpor, cognitive dilapidation, apathy, and depression, without impairment of learning, speech and language, or other "cortical" functions such as praxis or mathematical calculating. The ability to retrieve stored material is often impaired (Brown and Marsden 1990). Patients will require prompts to produce historical information such as the names of recent presidents. The number of prompts required to recall material is a good indicator of the degree of the retrieval deficit. Other signs of subcortical dementia notable during the mental status examination include impersistence and slowed completion of tasks. Pathological conditions that involve the basal ganglia include Parkinson's disease, Huntington's disease, état lacunaire, tumors, progressive supranuclear palsy, multisystem atrophy, Wilson's disease, and corticobasal degeneration.

Vascular dementias are a heterogeneous group resulting from cerebral infarctions of any etiology. Wallin and Blennow (1994) organized the vascular dementias into multi-infarct, strategic-infarct, and subcortical white matter subtypes. They found a reliable clinicopathological correlation between subcortical white matter dementia and a subcortical dementia pattern. The clinical presentation of multi-infarct- and strategic-infarct-related dementias varies widely in accordance with extent of involvement and lesion location. The concept of vascular dementia is currently being reexamined with the hope of refining clinicopathological relationships (Erkinjuntti and Hachinski 1993).

Mental Status Examination

The mental status examination is an assessment of brain function. A proper assessment should enable the examiner to estimate a patient's cognitive capacities in terms of domains of relative strength and impairment. Several general cognitive screening instruments are commonly used by clinicians to investigate intellectual impairment. These include the Mini-Mental State Exam (Folstein et al. 1975), Cognitive Capacities Screening Examination (Jacobs et al. 1977), and the Short Portable Mental Status Questionnaire (Pfeiffer 1975). Screening instruments developed to assess dementing processes include the Dementia Rating Scale (Mattis 1973), Blessed Dementia Scale (Blessed et al. 1968), and the Alzheimer Disease Assessment Battery (Devenny et al. 1992). The Executive Interview (Royall et al. 1992) and Frontal-Subcortical Assessment Battery (Rothlind and Brandt 1993) have been developed to more specifically assess frontal systems dysfunction.

Malloy et al. (1997) have reviewed the merits of these instruments as cognitive screens. However, the geriatric patient presenting for neuropsychiatric evaluation requires a flexible and comprehensive cognitive assessment not permitted by these standard instruments. No single instrument surveys the commonly assessed cognitive and metacognitive domains adequately. The principal drawbacks include substantial false-negative rates, indicating a lack of sensitivity for mild dementia, and inadequate evaluation of right hemisphere and frontal systems function (Nelson et al. 1986).

The clinical assessment of cognition is an area of significant neglect. In a recent survey of neuropsychiatric clinicians, only 57% of respondents reported the use of formal assessment of cognitive status (Coffey et al. 1994). Many respondents routinely requested formal neuropsychological testing as their primary means for assessing cognition. This approach is neither clinically nor economically acceptable. Bedside mental status testing has been demonstrated to be a reasonable clinical indicator of cognitive impairment as a result of cerebral dysfunction of many etiologies (Malloy et al. 1997).

Neuropsychological (NP) assessment should be considered as an adjunct in the geriatric neuropsychiatric assessment. Formal NP testing is an expensive and time-consuming process that can be very helpful for certain indications. When not indicated, however, NP testing frequently does not provide any additional information to assist in treatment planning. Proper indications include the establishment of a quantitative cognitive baseline to track over time, clarification of confusing or variable findings at the bedside, more thorough assessment of specific cognitive domains, or addressing a question of malingering or conversion disorder. It is helpful to compare closely the bedside cognitive findings with those of the NP testing. NP findings should concur with the findings of the bedside assessment. A common cause of discrepancy is suboptimal bedside technique or misinterpretation of the bedside findings. In these situations, the neuropsychologist can assist the bedside examiner by reviewing the technique or recommending other more reliable tests to add to the bedside armamentarium.

Cognitive Assessment

A thorough approach to bedside cognitive testing is provided elsewhere in this text. Throughout the administration of the cognitive tasks, the examiner should consider the performance in terms of quality, localizing value, and functional status. The popular cognitive screening instruments provide numerical scores as a reflection of cognitive capacity. However, cognitive performance falls on a qualitative continuum. All results must be considered in terms of an expected level of performance. Simply relying on a numerical descriptor may result in a false-negative assessment for many patients, particularly those with significant cognitive strengths, who are left with ample reserve despite cognitive decline.

Furthermore, the diagnosis of most dementing disorders is primarily clinical. No laboratory assays exist to confidently differentiate Alzheimer's disease from most other dementias, and brain biopsy is not part of a general workup of progressive cognitive dysfunction. Neuropsychiatric syndromes in the elderly typically involve either widespread pathology or more focal lesions. The pattern of deficits can thus differentiate between a generalized process such as Alzheimer's disease and a focal process such as a left parietal lobe infarction. Organizing the cognitive examination to assess regional functions can assist with this process.

The findings of the neuropsychiatric evaluation should fit with the person's functional status in his or her usual setting and help to explain and understand current difficulties. In some instances, the findings may conflict with the history. A common scenario is finding a patient who appears to be cognitively intact, but who reports an obvious decline in ability to function effectively at home. This is likely the result of a so-called dysexecutive syndrome. The structure of the office provides an artificially optimal environment for cognitive assessment. Patients having executive dysfunction will benefit from this external structure and may appear much less impaired on mental

status testing unless frontal systems are carefully assessed. In addition, the tasks that make up the mental status examination are rather arbitrary and do not necessarily assess the neural networks relied upon for daily living, which have evolved over millions of years without being shaped by the environmental stressor of mental status testing.

Neurobehavioral Assessment

Formal assessment of mental status includes a review of pertinent domains of psychiatric functioning including mood and affect, anxiety, compulsive and repetitive behaviors, personality changes, thought process and content, and perceptions. Upon completion of the clinical interview, the examiner will have acquired numerous clues to guide more thorough exploration of these areas.

Assessment of Mood and Affect

Depressive symptoms are more commonly encountered in the elderly than in individuals under 65 years of age. Despite this, major depressive disorder, as defined by DSM-IV (American Psychiatric Association 1994), has a lower prevalence among the elderly. In addition, common neuropsychiatric disorders such stroke (Robinson and Price 1982) and Parkinson's disease (Starkstein et al. 1990) are associated with a higher incidence of depressive illness. Bipolar disorder is occasionally encountered after stroke and traumatic brain injury (Robinson et al. 1988).

Affect is the outwardly directed manifestation of mood and serves as a nonverbal communication of one's emotional state. In neurologically intact individuals, affect remains congruent with the mood state. Neuropsychiatric disorders can disconnect affect from mood and thus disrupt a person's ability to effectively and accurately communicate their prevailing mood. Right hemisphere pathology can produce an expressive dysprosodia through which facial expression, gesticulation, and speech inflection become limited. Such persons often appear depressed despite denying feelings of dysphoria (Ross 1985). Frontal systems dysfunction resulting in apathy syndromes and Parkinson's disease are also associated with limited affective expression of internal mood states. Pseudobulbar palsy presents with excessive displays of affect in response to minimal emotional stimuli and results from bilateral damage to corticobulbar tracts, generally in the setting of cerebrovascular disease.

Assessment of Anxiety

Anxiety is often evoked during the neuropsychiatric evaluation and can affect a person's ability to concentrate and perform optimally on cognitive examination. The examiner should promptly identify signs of anxiety and make efforts to moderate the patient's distress. Gentle reassurances are usually all that are required for the patient to continue with the examination. The examiner should also inquire about the presence of any specific or recurrent worries that the patient experiences. Anxiety disorders are among the most common psychiatric syndromes in the elderly. Blazer et al. (1991) reported a 6-month prevalence of 19.7% for any anxiety disorder in the elderly.

Assessment of Compulsions and Repetitive Behavior

Obsessive-compulsive symptoms are occasionally sequelae of neuropsychiatric illness. Positron-emission tomographic studies of symptomatic individuals have shown disturbances in orbitofrontal-basal ganglia networks (Baxter et al. 1988). Disorders affecting the basal ganglia can be associated with symptoms of obsessive-compulsive disorder, including intrusive thoughts, repetition, preoccupation with cleanliness, and ruminations (Tomer et al. 1993).

Assessment of Personality Changes

Personality changes detailed above are commonly encountered in the setting of frontal systems dysfunction. Affected individuals often lack awareness of any change in social comportment. The inquiry into pertinent personality changes should therefore include the caregiver's perceptions of change. Ott et al. (1996) found that right hemisphere pathology is associated with a reduction in insight.

Assessment of Thought

Disordered thinking is a common symptom in the elderly. Both thought process and thought content are vulnerable to derangement by numerous neuropsychiatric conditions (Cummings 1985b). The influence of primary psychiatric diagnoses such as mania and schizophrenia on thought process is well known. However, frontal systems dysfunction can mimic these presentations by disrupting the ability to screen out irrelevant stimuli and maintain a given behavioral set. Consequently, stimulus-bound individuals may reveal tangential thinking or flight of ideas. Patients with apathy syndromes may appear to have a poverty of thoughts. Their paucity of speech precludes confident assessment of the thought process. Damage to the posterior language areas can present as rambling, incoherent speech, which may be misdiagnosed as thought derailment.

Disorders of thought content are known to arise late in life. Monosymptomatic or content-specific delusions, in particular, have been reported as sequelae of a number of generalized and focal neurological conditions affecting the brain (Malloy and Richardson 1994). The delusional themes include the duplication of person (Capgras's syndrome) or place (reduplicative paramnesia), sexual themes of infidelity (Othello syndrome) or love (de Clerambault syndrome), or physical changes such as being infested with parasites (Ekbom's syndrome) or being dead (Cotard's syndrome). Lesions affecting the heteromodal association cortex of the right hemisphere appear to be especially likely to result in the occurrence of monosymptomatic delusions (Cutting 1991).

Assessment of Perceptions

Disordered perception in the elderly typically presents as illusions or hallucinations. Illusions are a misperception of a sensory stimulus, such as mistaking a shoe for a cat, and are often experienced by cognitively impaired individuals with diminished vision or hearing, especially at night. These problems are readily treated with correction of the visual problem, use of a hearing aid, or improved lighting. Hallucinations, the experience of a sensory perception in the absence of a stimulus, may indicate the presence of encephalopathy and can occur with any sensory modality.

Sensorimotor Examination

Sensorimotor impairments significantly affect functional status in the elderly and require thorough assessment. The major neuropsychiatric syndromes described above are often associated with sensorimotor findings. Careful identification of sensorimotor impairments is necessary to provide remedial interventions. Elderly individuals with gait impairment are at increased risk for falls, which may be prevented by some form of ambulatory assistance such as a cane or walker, by avoiding doses of medication known to cause ataxia, or by optimizing treatment of the underlying cause, such as Parkinson's disease. In addition, in situations where the cognitive examination reveals a focal pattern of deficits, sensorimotor signs can further refine the bedside localization of cerebral pathology. For an outstanding review of the neurological examination, the reader is referred to Haerer (1992). The examination discussed below is limited to information that is more directly applicable to the neuropsychiatric assessment.

Observation

A great deal of information can be gleaned from the patient through simple observation. The gait can be scrutinized as the patient walks to the examiner's office. The posture may reveal the simian stance of Parkinson's disease or spinal abnormalities such as kyphosis, lordosis, or scoliosis brought on by osteoporosis. Diminished arm swing may be a sign of Parkinson's disease. Frontal systems disease is often associated with a gait apraxia in which the patient's feet appear to stick to the floor like magnets. Circumduction of one leg may be caused by spasticity resulting from an upper motor neuron lesion. Ataxia is frequently noted as a side effect of many psychotropic medications with anticholinergic or antidopaminergic properties. Walking heel-to-toe can elicit dystonic posturing of a hand and arm, suggesting contralateral hemispheric injury. Impaired tandem gait can also be a result of peripheral sensory loss, pain, or focal weakness.

Observation of the face during the neuropsychiatric examination may reveal a Horner's syndrome resulting from ipsilateral carotid atherosclerosis. The full Horner's syndrome includes unilateral ptosis, meiosis, and anhidrosis. A flattened nasolabial fold can indicate a facial plegia from a contralateral lesion such as a stroke. A masked, bland facies with diminished blinking is a common sequela of Parkinson's disease. Exophthalmos may be a sign of hyperthyroidism.

Failure to shave or apply cosmetics to the left side of the face is often seen with left hemineglect as a result of a right hemisphere lesion.

Vision and Hearing

Vision and hearing should be assessed. Elderly patients may not be fully aware of a gradual decline in these sensory modalities and often present with significant impairment. Providing elderly patients with proper eyeglasses and hearing aids can immediately improve functional status and diminish risk of accidents. Ocular and ear diseases are also associated with increased risk for modality-specific release hallucinations (Hammeke et al. 1983; White 1980). Anterior visual pathology can lead to the Charles Bonnet syndrome, characterized by well-formed visual hallucinations (Berrios and Brook 1984). Diminished ability to discriminate others' speech may exacerbate a tendency toward paranoia in susceptible individuals (Cooper and Curry 1976).

Oculomotion

Examining eye movement provides a wealth of information with localizing value. Patients who cannot track the examiner's moving finger without also moving their head may be stimulus bound from frontal systems disease. A unilateral lesion of the frontal eye fields will lead to an ipsilateral gaze preference. The pupils will not cross the midline with voluntary gaze to the contralateral hemispace. Difficulty with voluntary saccades can be an early sign of Huntington's disease in susceptible individuals (Grafton et al. 1990). Internuclear ophthalmoplegia reflects brainstem pathology, commonly a result of multiple sclerosis. Damage to the right medial longitudinal fasciculus will cause failure of the left eye to cross the midline to the right, while the right eye will track normally but exhibit monocular nystagmus. Inability to track a downward moving finger below the midline may be a sign of progressive supranuclear palsy. Lid lag with downward gaze may be a sign of hypothyroidism.

Examination of the visual fields by confrontation can help to localize temporal, parietal, and occipital lesions from damage to the optic radiations. Visual information from the superior quadrants is carried by the inferior aspect of the optic radiations, known as Meyer loop. Temporal lobe lesions will produce a contralateral superior quadrantanopia. Inferior parietal lesions can cause a contralateral inferior quadrantanopia. Patients with left hemineglect caused by a right hemisphere lesion may appear to have a complete contralateral hemianopia. However, visual fields testing in this situation is very difficult because of the strong tendency to neglect left-sided stimuli.

Extrapyramidal Motor Examination

Diseases of the basal ganglia are commonly encountered in geriatric neuropsychiatric practice. The clinical assessment of extrapyramidal motor function is an essential element of proper diagnosis and treatment. The typical gait and tremor of a patient with Parkinson's disease has been described above. In addition to the shuffling quality of the gait, festination is noted, whereby the patient will tend to increase speed and fall forward. Patients cannot turn around easily and tend to turn slowly by shuffling in place. Extrapyramidal muscular rigidity is present throughout the entire range of motion of the neck, trunk, and extremities. A jerky yielding of resistance known as cogwheeling is often noted when examining nuchal, truncal, or limb flexor tone. Repeated rapid opening and closing of the hands will demonstrate a gradual reduction in speed and amplitude. Diffuse increases in tone are noted with lacunar states, but are not associated with cogwheeling unless a parkinsonian tremor is also present.

An additional sign of upper motor neuron and extrapyramidal pathology is gegenhalten, a direct resistance to passive changes in position and posture. Patients who actively move their limb with the examiner despite requests to remain passive demonstrate mitgehen, a finding often noted with frontal systems dysfunction. The pronator drift test can often elicit subtle changes in motor tone as a result of hemispheric dysfunction. A slow pronation of the contralateral wrist with slight flexion of the elbow and fingers along with downward and lateral drift of the hand is noted. After the pronator drift test, the patient can be examined for propulsion and retropulsion by giving the patient a sudden push in either direction. Patients with Parkinson's disease cannot rapidly execute counteractive muscle groups and will stumble in the direction of the push.

Reflexes

Examination of muscle stretch reflexes, and in particular, the biceps, triceps, brachioradialis, patellar, and Achilles reflexes, not only assesses the integrity of the sensory and motor systems, but also has localizing value. Focal lesions involving upper motor neurons originating in the precentral gyrus or their axonal tracts coursing caudally through the internal capsule to form the corticospinal tract can cause a contralateral increase in reflex response. The presence of a Babinski sign, dorsiflexion and fanning of the toes in response to stimulating the sole of the foot, is an additional important lateralizing sign of corticospinal pathology. Geriatric patients with dementia are often variably cooperative with neuropsychiatric testing. However, the reflexes can be reliably tested despite a lack of complete cooperation by the patient.

The value of frontal release signs in neuropsychiatry tends to be overstated. The integrity of the frontal systems is reflected by the quality of the person's behavior over time. A clinical history of behavioral change as noted above, along with impaired performance on bedside tests of frontal functions, is sufficient to offer a diagnosis of executive impairment. The absence of snout, glabellar, and palmomental reflexes in this situation would not exclude the diagnosis. Further, the presence of these reflexes in the absence of behavioral changes or impairment with frontal tests does not suggest the presence of frontal systems dysfunction.

Formulation: Localizing the Findings

An important aspect of the biological domain of the formulation is to place the findings in the brain. The diagnostic necessity for this is discussed earlier in the context of wide-spread impairments in the cortical dementias. However, patterns of deficits are commonly noted. These patterns often reflect regional impairments caused by localized pathology such as a stroke or a tumor. The data from the clinical interview, mental status examination, and sensorimotor examination can be organized in a regional fashion. Table 5–3 is intended to assist the reader with neuropsychiatric localization. The table illustrates the relationship between the three areas of inquiry and can serve as a rough guideline for the cardinal signs and symptoms of regional cerebral dysfunction.

Summary

The neuropsychiatric formulation is the synthesis of the collected data into a cohesive clinical picture. The data are best organized in terms of the biopsychosocial model (Engel 1980). Biological deficits always have some psychological response. Furthermore, the patient's support persons will have a response of their own to the patient, which influences the effectiveness of the patient's attempts at adaptation. A case example follows.

An elderly woman presented to the neuropsychiatry clinic with the complaint of progressive memory impairment. She noted a significant decrease in her ability to manage the household. Her husband had taken up many chores formerly done by the patient. She believed that the need for assistance meant that she was "a failure" and that she was "a burden on her husband." He tended to downplay the patient's memory problem and believed she was being "lazy." Her sleep and appetite were diminished, and she experienced less interest in pleasurable activities. She had a history of poorly controlled hypertension.

Mental status testing demonstrated difficulty with alternating motor sequences as described by Luria (1980), mirroring the examiner's movements on a go/no-go task, and perseveration when copying an alternating design. She also had diminished storage and retrieval of new verbal information and required prompting to complete a chronological list of recent presidents. The sensorimotor examination revealed a mild bilateral increase in muscular tone and reflexes, greater on the right side. Computed tomography of the brain showed mild to moderate generalized cortical atrophy along with several lacunar infarcts in the basal ganglia bilaterally.

Without going into further clinical detail, *biologically*, the patient had acquired a syndrome of impaired cognition and depressed mood. Her cognitive and neuroimaging findings suggested frontotemporal systems dysfunction of a possibly mixed cortical degenerative and subcortical vascular pattern, exacerbated by the depressive syndrome.

TABLE 5–3.   **Localizing neuropsychiatric findings**

Region	History	Mental status	Sensorimotor
Frontal	Disorganization Disinhibition	High-level attention deficit Luria motor sequences deficit Go/no-go task deficit Decrease in verbal fluency Perseveration Losses of set Confabulation Witzelsucht	Gait apraxia Mitgehen Ipsilateral gaze preference Primitive reflexes
	Apathy	Dilapidation	Hypokinesis
Subcortical	Motor impairment Social withdrawal Cognitive impairment	Dilapidation Mental torpor Retrieval deficit	Hypokinesis Masked facies Simian stance Festinating gait Adventitious movement Muscular rigidity Cogwheeling Gegenhalten Downward gaze palsy

Right hemisphere	Confusional state
	Delusions
	Spatial disorientation
	Neglect
	Denial of deficit
	Dressing difficulties
	Left-sided motor impairment
		Dysprosodia
		Visuoconstructive deficit
		Spatial analysis deficit
		Left hemineglect
		Visual memory deficit
		Dressing apraxia
			Left hypertonus
			Left Babinski sign
			Left astereognosis
			Left dysgraphesthesia
			Double simultaneous
			  extinction
			Posturing of left hand/arm
			  with tandem gait
			Left pronator drift
			Left quadrantanopia

Left hemisphere	Right-sided motor impairment Language impairment Math impairment	Ideomotor apraxia Dysphasia Dyslexia Dyscalculia Dysgraphia Right/left disorientation Finger agnosia	Right hypertonus Right Babinski sign Right astereognosis Right dysgraphesthesia Posturing of right hand/arm with tandem gait Right pronator drift Right quadrantanopia
Bitemporal	Placidity Hyperorality Hypersexuality	Amnesia Agnosia Visual: right Auditory: left Anomia Prosopagnosia	Superior quadrantanopia
Biparietal	Spatial disorientation	Asimultanagnosia	Inferior quadrantanopia Ocular apraxia Optic ataxia

Psychologically, she equated being an effective household manager with being a good person. The executive deficits threatened her fragile sense of self-esteem. She also experienced a significant threat from the diminished autonomy associated with her deficits and the need to rely on her seemingly unempathic husband. Her husband appeared to deny the possibility of a progressive dementing syndrome, which may have protected him from acknowledging the potential loss of his partner through dementia. *Socially*, her husband struggled with assisting her, which compounded her dysphoria by making her feel like a burden. Her depressive syndrome made her anergic and even less able to meet the demands of household management.

Once a case is summarized in this fashion, the treatment plan can be constructed to address the depression, dementia, issues with the partner, the partner's issues with the patient's deteriorating condition, and the couple's suboptimal communication.

Conclusions

Geriatric neuropsychiatry provides clinicians with a comprehensive approach for understanding and helping elderly persons with cerebral dysfunction of any etiology. The progressive increase in longevity of the United States population means that an increasing proportion of the populace will be at risk for acquiring a neuropsychiatric syndrome. The ability to diagnose these varied conditions in their early stages and institute aggressive therapeutic and remedial measures will prolong the independent functioning of our patients, improve the quality of their lives, and diminish the significant expense of caring for elderly persons unable to function autonomously. Recent advances in understanding the brain function in healthy and pathological states will provide us with opportunities to offer more effective treatments in the future. However, the time-honored skills of inquiry, listening, and physical examination will remain the cornerstone of the practice of our specialty.

References

Albert ML, Feldman RG, Willis AL: The "subcortical dementia" of progressive supranuclear palsy. J Neurol Neurosurg Psychiatry 37:121–130, 1974

Alexander GE, Crutcher MD: Functional architecture of basal ganglia circuits: neural substrates of parallel processing. Trends Neurosci 13:266–271, 1990

American Psychiatric Association: Diagnostic and Statistical Manual of Mental Disorders, 4th Edition. Washington, DC, American Psychiatric Association, 1994

Applegate WB, Blass JD, Williams TF: Instruments for the functional assessment of older patients. N Engl J Med 322:1207–1214, 1990

Balint R: Seelenahmung des "schauens," optische ataxie, raumliche storung der autmerksamkeit. Monatsschr Psychiat Neurol 25:51–81, 1909

Baxter LR Jr, Schwartz JM, Mazziotta JC, et al: Local cerebral glucose metabolic rates in non-depressed patients with obsessive-compulsive disorder. Am J Psychiatry 145:1560–1563, 1988

Benson DF, Zaras BW: Progressive aphasia. A case with postmortem correlation. Neuropsychiatry Neuropsychol Behav Neurol 4:215–223, 1991

Berrios GE, Brook P: Visual hallucinations and sensory delusions in the elderly. Br J Psychiatry 144:662–684, 1984

Blazer D, George LK, Hughes D: The epidemiology of anxiety disorders: an age comparison, in Anxiety in the Elderly. Edited by Salzman C, Lebowitz BD. New York, Springer, 1991, pp 17–30

Blessed G, Tomlinson BE, Roth M: The association between quantitative measures of dementia and of senile change in the cerebral grey matter of elderly subjects. Br J Psychiatry 114:797–810, 1968

Brown RG, Marsden CD: Cognitive function in Parkinson's disease: from description to theory. Trends Neurosci 13:21–28, 1990

Brun A: Frontal lobe degeneration of the non-Alzheimer type, I: neuropathology. Archives of Gerontology and Geriatrics 6:193–208, 1987

Caselli RJ: Focal and asymmetric cortical degeneration syndromes. The Neurologist 1:1–19, 1995

Chang Chui H: Dementia: a review emphasizing clinicopathologic correlation and brain-behavior relationships. Arch Neurol 46:806–814, 1989

Charness ME, Simon RP, Greenberg DA: Ethanol and the nervous system. N Engl J Med 321:442–453, 1989

Coffey CE, Cummings JL, Duffy JD, et al: Assessment of treatment outcomes in neuropsychiatry: a report from the Committee on Research of the American Neuropsychiatric Association. J Neuropsychiatry Clin Neurosci 7:287–289, 1994

Cooper AF, Curry AR: The pathology of deafness in the paranoid and affective psychoses of later life. J Psychosom Res 20:97–105, 1976

Cummings JL (ed): The neuropsychiatric interview and mental status examination, in Clinical Neuropsychiatry. Orlando, FL, Grune & Stratton, 1985a, pp 5–16

Cummings JL (ed): Secondary psychoses, delusions, and schizophrenia, in Clinical Neuropsychiatry. Orlando, FL, Grune & Stratton, 1985b, pp 163–182

Cummings JL, Hegarty A: Neurology, psychiatry, and neuropsychiatry. Neurology 44:209–213, 1994

Cutting J: Delusional misidentification and the role of the right hemisphere in the appreciation of identity. Br J Psychiatry 14 (suppl):70–75, 1991

Damasio AR: Disorders of complex visual processing: agnosias, achromatopsia, Balint's syndrome, and related difficulties of orientation and construction, in Principles of Behavioral Neurology. Edited by Mesulam M-M. Philadelphia, PA, FA Davis, 1985, pp 259–288

Damasio AR: Aphasia. N Engl J Med 326:531–539, 1992

Damasio AR, Damasio H, Van Hoesen GW: Prosopagnosia: anatomic basis and behavioral mechanisms. Neurol 32: 331–341, 1982

Damasio H: Neuroimaging contributions to the understanding of aphasia, in Handbook of Neuropsychology, Vol 2. Edited by Boller F, Grafman J. Amsterdam, Elsevier, 1989, pp 3–46

Devenny DA, Hill AL, Patxot O, et al: The Alzheimer's Disease Assessment Scale: useful for both early detection and staging of dementia of the Alzheimer type. Alzheimer Dis Assoc Disord 6:89–102, 1992

Duffy JD, Campbell JJ: The regional prefrontal syndromes: a theoretical and clinical overview. J Neuropsychiatry Clin Neurosci 6:379–387, 1994

Ebly EM, Hogan DB, Parhad IM: Cognitive impairment in the non-demented elderly. Arch Neurol 52:612–619, 1995

Elliott FA: Violence. The neurologic contribution: an overview. Arch Neurol 49:595–603, 1992

Engel GL: The clinical application of the biopsychosocial model. Am J Psychiatry 137:535–544, 1980

Erikson EH, Erikson JM, Kivnich HG: Vital Involvement in Old Age. New York, WW Norton, 1994

Erkinjuntti T, Hachinski VC: Rethinking vascular dementia. Cerebrovasc Dis 3:3–23, 1993

Folstein MF, Folstein SE, McHugh PR: Mini-Mental State: a practical method for grading the cognitive state of patients for the clinician. J Psychiatr Res 12:189–198, 1975

Geschwind N, Galaburda AM: Cerebral lateralization: biological mechanisms, associations, and pathology. Arch Neurol 42:428–459, 521–552, 634–654, 1985

Gibbs A, Andrewes DG, Szmukler G, et al: Early HIV-related neuropsychological impairment: relationship to stage of viral infection. J Clin Exp Neuropsychol 12:766–780, 1990

Goldman-Rakic PS: Specification of higher cortical functions. J Head Trauma Rehabil 8:15–23, 1993

Grafton ST, Mazziota JC, Pahl JJ, et al: A comparison of neurological, metabolic, structural, and genetic evaluations in persons at risk for Huntington's disease. Ann Neurol 28: 614–621, 1990

Greenberg DA, Diamond I: Wernicke-Korsakoff syndrome, in Alcohol and the Brain: Chronic Effects. Edited by Tarter RE, Van Thiel DH. New York, Plenum, 1986, pp 295–314

Haerer AF (ed): DeJong's The Neurologic Examination, 5th Edition. Philadelphia, PA, JB Lippincott, 1992

Hammeke TA, McQuillen MP, Cohen BA: Musical hallucinations associated with acquired deafness. J Neurol Neurosurg Psychiatry 46:570–572, 1983

Hof PR, Bouras C, Constantinidis J, et al: Balint's syndrome in Alzheimer's disease: specific disruption of the occipito-parietal visual pathway. Brain Res 49:368–375, 1989

Hyman BT, Van Hoesen GW, Damasio AR, et al: Alzheimer's disease: cell-specific pathology isolates the hippocampal formation. Science 225:1168–1170, 1984

Jacobs JW, Bernard MR, Delgado A, et al: Screening for organic mental syndromes in the medically ill. Ann Intern Med 86:40–47, 1977

Jellinger K: Neuropathological substrates of Alzheimer's disease and Parkinson's disease. J Neural Transm 24 (suppl):109–129, 1987

Ketter TA, George MS, Kimbrell TA, et al: Functional brain imaging, limbic function, and affective disorders. The Neuroscientist 2:55–65, 1996

Klüver H, Bucy PC: Preliminary analysis of functions of the temporal lobes in monkeys. Archives of Neurology and Psychiatry 42:979–1000, 1939

Levine SR, Brust JCM, Futrell N, et al: Cerebrovascular complications of the use of the "crack" form of alkaloidal cocaine. N Engl J Med 323:699–704, 1990

Lilly R, Cummings JL, Benson DF, et al: The human Klüver-Bucy syndrome. Neurol 33:1141–1145, 1983

Lishman WA (ed): Head injury, in Organic Psychiatry: The Psychological Consequences of Cerebral Disorder, 2nd Edition. Oxford, England, Blackwell Scientific, 1987, pp 137–181

Lishman WA: Alcohol and the brain. Br J Psychiatry 156: 635–644, 1990

Lishman WA: What is neuropsychiatry? J Neurol Neurosurg Psychiatry 55:983–985, 1992

Luria AR: Higher Cortical Function in Man. New York, Basic Books, 1980

Malloy PF, Duffy JD: The frontal lobes in neuropsychiatric disorders, in Handbook of Neuropsychology, Vol 8. Edited by Boller F, Spinnler H. New York, Elsevier, 1992, pp 203–232

Malloy PF, Richardson ED: The frontal lobes and content specific delusions. J Neuropsychiatry Clin Neurosci 6: 455–466, 1994

Malloy PF, Cummings JL, Coffey CE, et al: Cognitive screening instruments in neuropsychiatry: a report of the Committee on Research of the American Neuropsychiatric Association. J Neuropsychiatry Clin Neurosci 9:189–197, 1997

Mattis S: Dementia Rating Scale Professional Manual. Odessa, FL, Psychological Assessment Resources, 1973

Mayberg HS, Brannan SK, Mahurin RK, et al: Cingulate function in depression: a potential predictor of treatment response. Neuroreport 8:1057–1061, 1997

McHugh PR: The neuropsychiatry of basal ganglia disorders: a triadic syndrome and its explanation. Neuropsychiatry Neuropsychol Behav Neurol 2:239–247, 1989

McHugh PR, Folstein MF: Psychiatric syndromes of Huntington's chorea: a clinical and phenomenologic study, in Psychiatric Aspects of Neurologic Disease. Edited by Benson DF, Blumer D. New York, Grune & Stratton, 1975, pp 267–286

McKeith IG, Galasko D, Kosaka K, et al: Consensus guidelines for the clinical and pathologic diagnosis of dementia with Lewy bodies (DLB). Neurology 47:1113–1124, 1996

Morris JC, Cole M, Banker BQ, et al: Hereditary dysphasic dementia and the Pick/Alzheimer spectrum. Ann Neurol 16:455–466, 1984

Mueller J, Fogel BS: Neuropsychiatric evaluation, in Neuropsychiatry. Edited by Fogel BS, Schiffer RB, Rao SM. Baltimore, MD, Williams & Wilkins, 1996, pp 11–28

Nachson I: Neuropsychology of violent behavior: controversial issues and new developments in the study of hemispheric function, in Neuropsychology of Aggression. Edited by Miller JS. Boston, MA, Kluwer Academic, 1991, pp 93–116

Nelson A, Fogel BS, Faust D: Bedside cognitive screening instruments: a critical assessment. J Nerv Ment Dis 174: 73–83, 1986

Ott BR, Noto RB, Fogel BS: Apathy and loss of insight in Alzheimer's disease: a SPECT imaging study. J Neuropsychiatry Clin Neurosci 8:41–46, 1996

Ovsiew F: Bedside neuropsychiatry: eliciting the clinical phenomena of neuropsychiatric illness, in The American Psychiatric Press Textbook of Neuropsychiatry. 3rd Edition. Edited by Yudofsky SC, Hales RE. Washington, DC, American Psychiatric Press, 1997, pp 121–164

Pearson RCA, Esiri MM, Hiorns RW, et al: Anatomical correlate of the distribution of the pathologic changes in the neocortex in Alzheimer's disease. Proc Natl Acad Sci U S A 82:4531–4534, 1985

Petersen RC, Smith G, Kokmen E, et al: Memory function in normal aging. Neurology 42:396–401, 1992

Petersen RC, Smith GE, Waring SC, et al: Aging, memory, and mild cognitive impairment. International Psychogeriatrics 9 (suppl 1):65–69, 1997

Pfeiffer E: A short portable mental status questionnaire for the assessment of organic brain deficit in elderly patients. J Am Geriatr Soc 23:433–441, 1975

Rapp PR, Amaral DG: Individual differences in the cognitive and neurobiological consequences in normal aging. Trends Neurosci 15:340–345, 1992

Roberts GW: Schizophrenia: the cellular biology of a functional psychosis. Trends Neurosci 13:207–211, 1990

Robinson RG, Price TR: Post-stroke depressive disorders: a follow up study of 103 patients. Stroke 13:635–641, 1982

Robinson RG, Boston JD, Starkstein SE, et al: Comparison of mania with depression following brain injury. Am J Psychiatry 145:172–178, 1988

Ross ED: Modulation of affect and nonverbal communication by the right hemisphere, in Principles of Behavioral Neurology. Edited by Mesulam M-M. Philadelphia, PA, FA Davis, 1985, pp 239–257

Rothlind JC, Brandt J: A brief assessment of frontal and subcortical functions in dementia. J Neuropsychiatry Clin Neurosci 5:73–77, 1993

Rourke BP: Nonverbal Learning Disabilities. The Syndrome and the Model. New York, Guilford, 1989

Royall DR, Mahurin RK, Gray KF: Bedside assessment of executive cognitive impairment: the Executive Interview. J Am Geriatr Soc 40:1221–1226, 1992

Shenton ME, Kikinis R, Jolesz FA: Abnormalities of the left temporal lobe and thought disorder in schizophrenia: a quantitative magnetic resonance imaging study. N Engl J Med 327:605–612, 1992

Starkstein SE, Bolduc PL, Mayberg HS, et al: Cognitive impairment and depression in Parkinson's disease: a follow up study. J Neurol Neurosurg Psychiatry 53:597–602, 1990

Streissguth AP, Landesman-Dwyer S: Teratogenic effects of alcohol in humans and laboratory animals. Science 209:353, 1980

Strub RL, Black FW: The Mental Status Examination in Neurology, 3rd Edition. Philadelphia, PA, FA Davis, 1993

Tetrud JW, Langston JW, Garbe PL, et al: Mild parkinsonism in persons exposed to 1-methyl-4-phenyl-1,2,3,6-tetrahydropyridine (MPTP). Neurology 39:1483–1487, 1989

Tomer R, Levin BE, Weiner WJ: Obsessive-compulsive symptoms and motor asymmetries in Parkinson's disease. Neuropsychiatry Neuropsychol Behav Neurol 6:26–30, 1993

Trimble MR: Neuropsychiatry or behavioral neurology. Neuropsychiatry Neuropsychol Behav Neurol 6:60–69, 1993

Tross S, Hirsch DA: Psychological distress and neuropsychological complications of HIV infection and AIDS. Am Psychol 43:929–934, 1988

Wallin A, Blennow K: The clinical diagnosis of vascular dementia. Dementia 5:181–184, 1994

Weinberger DR: Schizophrenia and the frontal lobe. Trends Neurosci 11:367–370, 1988

Weintraub S, Mesulam M-M: Mental state assessment of young and elderly adults in behavioral neurology, in Principles of Behavioral Neurology. Edited by Mesulam M-M. Philadelphia, PA, FA Davis, 1985

Wender PH: Attention deficit disorder ("minimal brain dysfunction") in adults. Arch Gen Psychiatry 38:449–456, 1981

White NJ: Complex visual hallucinations in partial blindness due to eye disease. Br J Psychiatry 136:284–286, 1980

Woods D: The diagnosis and treatment of attention deficit disorder, residual type. Psychiatric Annals 16:23–28, 1986

Zametkin AJ, Nordahl TE, Gross M, et al: Cerebral glucose metabolism in adults with hyperactivity of childhood onset. N Engl J Med 323:1361–1366, 1990

6

Mental Status Examination

David L. Sultzer, M.D.

Mental status examination is a critical part of the neuropsychiatric assessment of older patients. The examination reveals the integrity of cognitive skills, which are those intellectual abilities that facilitate thinking, perception, communication, and problem solving. Several cognitive domains are assessed, including attention, memory, language, visuospatial skills, calculation, and executive skills.

Cognitive evaluation adds an important dimension to neuropsychiatric assessment. The psychiatric examination reveals abnormal experiences, thoughts, interpersonal skills, and behavior. The neurological evaluation focuses primarily on the motor and sensory system. The cognitive mental status examination assesses the integrity of a broad range of brain structures and can reveal the presence of cerebral pathology that contributes to the expression of psychiatric symptoms or intellectual deficits. Although a trichotomy is implied, the psychiatric, cognitive, and neurological examinations overlap considerably. Together they identify a pattern of neuropsychiatric signs that the clinician uses to formulate a differential diagnosis, direct further evaluation, and monitor change over time.

Assessing cognitive skills is particularly important in older patients because the prevalence of delirium, demen-

tia, and psychiatric symptoms related to neurological conditions increases with age. Other goals of mental status assessment in older patients include

1. Distinguishing cognitive changes of normal aging from deficits resulting from dementia;
2. Distinguishing cognitive changes of dementia from those associated with depression or delirium;
3. Promoting early recognition and treatment of dementia because even moderate cognitive decline is often not detected by family members (Ross et al. 1997) or the primary physician (Callahan et al. 1995; Eefsting et al. 1996);
4. Identifying and localizing cerebral pathology that is neurologically silent;
5. Monitoring response to treatment for dementia and other cognitive disorders; and
6. Identifying cognitive strengths in patients with mild overall impairment. Use of preserved cognitive skills can maximize a patient's functional skills.

Mental status assessment is not exclusively reserved for neuropsychologists or other subspecialists. Although complex cases may benefit from referral to a specialist, the basic

Supported in part by National Institute of Mental Health Grant MH56031 and the Department of Veterans Affairs.

examination can be performed efficiently by many practitioners. Thoughtful, focused evaluations can rapidly and accurately reveal the necessary information for diagnosis and treatment.

In this chapter, I review the technique of clinical mental status examination, the regional neuroanatomical pathology associated with cognitive deficits, common syndromes of cognitive impairment, and the use of rating scales for cognitive assessment. Individual neuropsychiatric syndromes in the elderly are described in Sections III and IV of this volume and an overview of the neuroanatomical and neurochemical underpinnings of human cognition and emotion is provided in Chapter 4 this volume. The role of mental status assessment in the diagnosis of dementia has been described in several recent clinical guidelines (American Psychiatric Association 1997; Costa et al. 1996; Small et al. 1997; U.S. Department of Veterans Affairs 1997).

Clinical History

The mental status examination begins with a historical review of symptoms. The patient should be invited to describe current or past difficulties with memory and thinking, such as problems concentrating, forgetting recent events, forgetting where things are located, difficulty finding the right word to say, difficulty understanding what others are saying, getting lost in previously familiar places, or difficulty with routine financial transactions or record keeping. Specific features and time course of the difficulties are diagnostically relevant and point toward those cognitive domains that should be explored in more detail during the examination. A history of head trauma, meningitis, encephalitis, seizure disorder, psychiatric symptoms, neurological symptoms, or substance abuse should be identified.

Because memory or language impairment can interfere with the patient's ability to provide an accurate history, information from a family member or close friend is useful. Family members may feel uncomfortable discussing difficulties with the patient present; if so, a separate interview should be conducted. The patient's age, educational background, cultural background, occupation, and handedness should be noted because these factors affect the interpretation of cognitive performance.

Examination Technique

The length and depth of the mental status evaluation depends on the clinical circumstances and the specific goals

(e.g., screening of elderly persons without obvious neuropsychiatric illness, evaluating suspected dementia, or monitoring response to treatment for a cognitive disorder). All patients with suspected neuropsychiatric illness require at least a brief screen for competence in each cognitive domain. In some cases, the history of symptoms or the results of a screening evaluation point toward a cognitive area that needs to be investigated in detail or warrants formal neuropsychological assessment. Rating scales can be particularly useful for diagnostic screening or for following a patient's symptoms over time.

The examiner develops and tests hypotheses during the course of the examination, beginning with observations of behavior and language during the history taking. Observing how the patient behaves during the assessment and how he or she approaches cognitive challenges is essential. Throughout the examination, the *kind* of errors that occur is as important as the *presence* of errors.

A patient may become anxious or defensive during the evaluation. A brief description of the purpose and content of the examination at the beginning usually helps reduce anxiety. The patient should be reminded that "some of these questions may seem relatively easy and others may be very difficult." The evaluation is not an interrogation; an empathic approach improves the interpersonal quality of the interview and increases the reliability of the assessment. In some circumstances, completing the assessment over several brief meetings is preferable to one long examination.

The principal cognitive functions are listed in Table 6–1. These domains are not hierarchical, but competence in some domains is required for adequate performance in others. Adequate *attention* (arousal and concentration) is required for optimal performance of all other cognitive tasks. A patient who is stuporous or markedly distractible will have difficulty with other tasks. Some *executive skills* require competence in other cognitive areas because integrating several elementary cognitive abilities may be necessary. As a result of these two principles, attention is usually assessed at the beginning of the evaluation, and executive skills are often assessed at the end.

Clinical Mental Status Examination

Attention

Attention is the ability to focus, sustain, and appropriately shift mental activity. Arousal and concentration both contribute to attention. *Arousal*, alertness, and "level of consciousness" are terms that describe the patient's awareness

TABLE 6–1. Cognitive domains assessed in the mental status examination

Attention
    Arousal
    Concentration
Memory
    Learning
    Recall
    Recognition
Language
    Spontaneous output; fluency
    Comprehension
    Repetition
    Naming
Visuospatial skills
Calculation
Praxis
Executive skills
    Drive
    Programming
    Response control
    Synthesis

of stimuli. Level of arousal is evident during the interview and falls along a continuum from fully alert to comatose. Intermediate levels of arousal include lethargy, obtundation, and stupor (Plum and Posner 1982), and these levels are defined by the amount of stimulus required to maintain an awake state. A patient with mild impairment of arousal appears drowsy or may fall asleep during the interview. Marked impairment of arousal can be monitored using the Glasgow Coma Scale (Teasdale and Jennett 1974).

Poor *concentration* is manifest as difficulty focusing on a conversation or task. The patient may be easily distracted by extraneous events in the room, the television, or a sound outdoors. Concentration is further assessed by testing:

1. *Digit span.* The patient is asked to repeat a string of digits that is presented by the examiner at a rate of one digit per second. A string of three digits is initially presented, followed by a string of four digits, then five digits, etc. Repeating a string of at least five digits correctly is considered normal performance.
2. *Reverse digit span.* The examiner presents a string of digits, and the patient is asked to repeat the string in reverse order. Normal aging is associated with a mild decline in the ability to perform reverse digit span, but forward digit span is relatively unaffected by age

(Lezak 1995). Normal elderly can reverse a string of at least three digits.

3. *Serial 7s.* The patient is asked to subtract 7 from 100, and to continue subtracting 7 from the result. Arithmetic skills are a prerequisite for accurate performance, and the patient's educational background and occupation provide clues to the expected level of performance.
4. *Reverse sequences.* The patient is asked to state the days of the week, or the months of the year, in reverse order (e.g., "December, November, October, . . . "). These tasks may be preferable for patients who have limited education or do not routinely work with numbers.
5. *Continuous performance.* The patient is asked to tap the table "each time you hear the letter A." The examiner then presents a string of random letters that contains embedded A's. Letters are presented at a rate of one per second, and the task continues for at least 30 seconds. Errors of omission (not tapping for an A) and errors of commission (tapping for a non-A) are noted. Normally no errors occur.

Arousal is maintained by the reticular activating system. This system originates with cells of the pons and midbrain and projects diffusely to cortical and subcortical regions of the brain via the thalamic projection system. Concentration requires an intact reticular activating system as well as intact cortical (particularly frontal) and limbic structures that focus and modulate attention. Specific disorders of attention are discussed later in this chapter. Patients with impaired arousal or concentration have difficulty with other cognitive tasks because attention is required to stay awake, understand directions, and maintain the mental control required for optimal performance. Thus, all cognitive deficits must be interpreted cautiously when attention is impaired. Diagnoses of dementia or amnesia cannot be reliably made when there is marked disturbance of arousal or concentration.

Memory

Recent studies have helped to clarify the neuropsychology and neurobiology of memory. The synaptic changes and neuroanatomic systems responsible for various aspects of memory function have been defined (Kupfermann 1991; Tranel and Damasio 1995), and neuropsychological constructs of memory processing and memory subtypes have been elaborated (Baddeley 1995). However, although strategies to assess specific aspects of memory function are available (Lezak 1995), such techniques may be complex and require instruments not available in typical clinical settings.

For the purpose of routine clinical assessment, memory can be divided into the ability to learn, retain, and recall information. Learning and recall can be assessed using a *word list test*. A list of words is read aloud to the patient who is asked to immediately recall as many words as possible from the list. The process is repeated, using the same list, three or four times. This strategy assesses the patient's immediate or working memory, which requires intact attention. Immediate recall of more words on subsequent trials indicates that learning is occurring. Later in the mental status examination, the patient is asked to recall the word list. Patients with normal memory recall the majority of the words. The examiner should give the patient category clues for those words that are not recalled spontaneously (e.g., "an article of clothing"), followed by multiple choices for words that are not recalled with category clues (e.g., "Was the word 'hat,' 'belt,' or 'shoes'?"). Poor free recall of the word list and inability to recognize the words with clues indicate that the information has not been learned and retained. Poor free recall but accurate recognition of many of the words when given clues suggests dysfunction of the memory retrieval process and indicates that some learning and retention has occurred. Although a word list containing 3 words may suffice for cognitive screening, a longer list of 8–10 words can demonstrate the learning curve and can provide a more sensitive and specific test of learning and recall. *Orientation* questions to test learning and recall of the date and location also assess memory function.

Learning requires the integrity of limbic structures: the medial temporal lobes, the fornix, the dorsomedial thalamic nuclei, and the mammillary bodies (Squire 1987; Tranel and Damasio 1995). Severe memory impairment is usually a result of bilateral or midline brain dysfunction; unilateral brain pathology (often a medial temporal lobe lesion) can cause mild memory impairment. Preferential impairment of verbal memory occurs with left hemisphere dysfunction, whereas impairment in visuospatial memory often occurs with right hemisphere dysfunction (Signoret 1985). Verbal memory is assessed with the word list test. Visuospatial memory can be assessed by asking the patient to reproduce drawings, either immediately after a brief presentation (working memory) or later in the examination (learning, retention, and recall). Alternatively, visuospatial memory can be assessed by asking the patient to locate objects that were previously hidden in the room while the patient observed. Assessing visuospatial memory is particularly important in patients with significant aphasia who may fail verbal memory tests on the basis of language, not memory, deficits.

Tests of *remote memory* assess the ability to recall information that was learned in the distant past. Accurate remote memory requires the integrity of diffuse cortical systems that are required for storage and recall of data. Patients with limbic dysfunction who are unable to learn new information (as in Korsakoff's syndrome or after head trauma or herpes encephalitis) may be able to recall information that was learned before limbic disturbance. Remote memory is assessed by asking the patient to recall historical data: birthplace, family birthdays, work history, past presidents, or details of important historical events. For reliable assessment, the correct information must have clearly been learned in the past by the patient (and be known by the examiner). Therefore, it is helpful to validate remote memory loss with collateral sources.

Language

Language skills are essential for human communication. Language competence is also required for accurate performance in other cognitive domains because most of the information essential to routine cognition is verbally mediated. Right- or left-*handedness* should be noted in the examination because handedness predicts which hemisphere is dominant for language. Nearly all right-handed individuals and the majority of left-handers are left hemisphere dominant for language. Some left-handers, particularly those with a strong family history of left-handedness, have language function distributed across both hemispheres.

Language assessment explores four principal areas: spontaneous verbal output, comprehension, repetition, and naming. *Spontaneous verbal output* is evaluated during the clinical interview by listening to the linguistic features of the patient's discourse. Dysarthria, a motor disorder of speech, is distinguished from aphasia, a disorder of language. Two categories of aphasia in the patient's spontaneous verbal output are considered. In *fluent aphasia*, language output is generally effortless, with normal or increased number of words per minute, normal melody and inflection (prosody), and normal phrase length. Paraphasias, or intrusions of incorrect words or phonemes, can occur (e.g., "I was *leading* the newspaper"). The information content, or "efficiency" of language, is usually low: long sentences may contain many grammatical connecting words, nonspecific nouns ("thing," "the other one"), and limited meaning ("empty speech"). *Nonfluent aphasia*, in contrast, is characterized by effortful but reduced word output, short phrase length, and dysprosody. Dysarthria is often present and sentences efficiently convey meaning with few words. Grammar and syntax are usually abnormal.

Fluent aphasia occurs with lesions of the posterior left hemisphere, whereas nonfluent aphasia occurs with lesions of the left frontal cortex or underlying white matter.

Comprehension is assessed by asking the patient to

1. *Follow simple commands.* Single-step or multiple-step commands are given, such as "Point to your nose" or "Point to the window, then to the floor, and then to the chair."
2. *Follow commands, using objects.* Several items are placed on the table (e.g., a pen, a key, a paper clip, and a nickel). The patient is asked to follow instructions, such as "Touch the pen, then pick up the paper clip," or "With the key, touch the nickel, then point to the floor."
3. *Answer yes/no questions.* Examples are "Does a rock float on water?" and "Do you put your shoes on before your socks?"

Reading comprehension can be assessed by presenting similar commands and questions to the patient in writing. Reduced hearing in the elderly can contribute to impaired performance with spoken commands. Language comprehension deficits occur with dysfunction of the left posterior temporal or parietotemporal cortex.

Repetition is assessed by asking the patient to repeat sentences of increasing length and linguistic complexity. Abnormal repetition occurs with disruption of perisylvian structures of the left hemisphere.

A disturbance of *naming* may be evident as word-finding difficulty in the course of spontaneous speech. Naming is further assessed by asking the patient to identify objects or parts of the body. Both high-frequency names (elbow, nose, shoe, watch, pen) and low-frequency names (eyebrow, earlobe, sole of the shoe, watch crystal) are tested. Poor naming may result from focal brain lesions (usually the left inferior parietal lobule) or with diffuse hemispheric dysfunction. Other tasks, such as *verbal fluency* (asking the patient to name as many animals as possible in 1 minute), *reading skills*, and *writing ability*, can help identify specific aphasic disorders and can provide additional information on regional brain function (Strub and Black 1993). The syndromes of aphasia are discussed later in this chapter.

Visuospatial Skills

Visuospatial impairment is one of the most sensitive indicators of brain dysfunction. Patients with mild delirium or with posterior brain lesions that are otherwise neurologically silent may have marked visuospatial deficits. In contrast, patients with primary psychiatric illness usually have minimal difficulty with visuospatial tasks.

Visuospatial skills include visually guided attention, perception, use of internal visual images, visuospatial memory, and constructional abilities. The history can reveal important evidence of visuospatial impairment: getting lost in previously familiar environments, difficulty estimating distance, or difficulty orienting objects to complete a task. Visuospatial skills can be clinically assessed by asking the patient to copy drawings provided by the examiner or by asking the patient to spontaneously draw a clockface, a house, or a person. Drawings to be copied should include a simple geometric shape, a design that is not easily verbally described, and a complex drawing with three-dimensional perspective. Examples are shown in Figure 6–1. The patient's drawings may reveal a variety of visuospatial errors: poor use of the space available to draw, hemineglect, unusual drawing strategy (focusing on detail while missing overall layout), overlapping or "closing in" on the stimulus drawing, loss of details, loss of three-dimensionality, or poor spatial relationships among elements of the drawing (reversals, rotations, inaccurate angles). Examples of inaccurate reproduction drawings are shown in Figure 6–2. Asking the patient to draw a clockface and put hands on the clock to indicate a particular time may rapidly reveal a visuoconstructive deficit (Mendez et al. 1992) and may reveal impaired executive skills (Royall et al. 1998). Visual acuity and motor skills are obviously required for accurate drawing. Complete understanding of visuospatial deficits may require formal neuropsychological assessment using standardized tests of block design, object assembly, and line orientation (Lezak 1995).

Visuospatial impairment is more common and usually more severe among patients with a focal brain lesion in the posterior hemisphere (Black and Strub 1976). Patients with right hemisphere lesions more often have visuospatial deficits than those with left hemisphere lesions. Characteristic visuoconstructive deficits that depend on the laterality of brain injury have been identified, although the specificity of these findings is limited (Benson and Barton 1970). Features of the deficits associated with lateralized lesions are shown in Table 6–2. Executive skills, in addition to visuospatial abilities, are apparent in the organizational strategy used by the patient to draw a figure (e.g., Figure 6–2, *panel B*).

Among the elderly, visuospatial disturbance is a sensitive indicator of *delirium* and can occur in any *dementia* syndrome. Patients with *Alzheimer's disease* typically have visuospatial impairment early in the course of illness. Visuospatial impairment may also occur with a *focal brain lesion* resulting from cortical infarction or tumor.

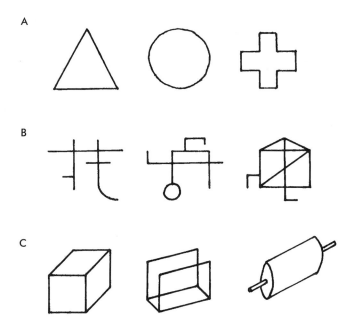

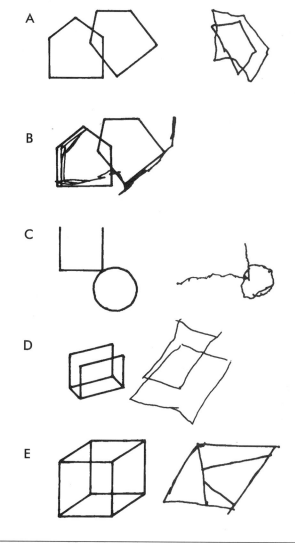

FIGURE 6–1. Examples of designs to be reproduced to assess visuospatial skill. *Panel A:* Simple geometric shapes. *Panel B:* Designs that are not easily verbally described. *Panel C:* Three-dimensional designs.

Calculation

Calculation skill is assessed by asking the patient to perform simple addition and multiplication (e.g., $7 + 6$, 5×7, 8×9) and then more difficult arithmetic (e.g., $18 + 29$, 15×7) without using paper and pencil. Calculation is further assessed by asking the patient to answer arithmetic questions with paper and pencil (e.g., $129 + 87$, 423×18). The ability to perform calculations requires attention, an understanding of mathematic operations (addition, subtraction, multiplication, division), memorized knowledge of simple sums and the "times table," and the visuospatial ability to maintain number alignment. The patient's educational background and premorbid arithmetic skills must be considered in assessing current performance.

Dyscalculia may result from a variety of neurological conditions. Patients with impaired concentration as a result of delirium usually perform poorly, as do patients with diffuse degenerative brain conditions such as Alzheimer's disease. Dyscalculia has been demonstrated in patients with focal involvement of a wide range of brain regions, although it often occurs in association with aphasia and is most common with lesions of the dominant parietal lobe (Luria 1980).

Executive Skills

Executive skills are those mental abilities that facilitate performance of complex cognitive tasks or behaviors. A con-

FIGURE 6–2. Examples of inaccurate reproduction drawings. The design to be reproduced is shown on the left; the patient's reproduction is to the right. *Panel A:* Inaccurate angles and rotation of one of the pentagons; patient with delirium. *Panel B:* Stimulus boundedness; the patient's drawing overlaps the stimulus figure; patient with Alzheimer's disease. *Panel C:* Missing parts of the design and evidence of tremor; patient with Alzheimer's disease. *Panel D:* Missing parts of the design and loss of three-dimensionality; patient with vascular dementia. *Panel E:* Simplified drawing with loss of three-dimensionality; patient after resection of a left occipital astrocytoma.

stellation of skills that extend beyond memory, language, and visuospatial competence is included: planning strategies to accomplish tasks, implementing strategies, adjusting strategies as needed, monitoring performance, recognizing patterns, appreciating time sequence, and formulating abstract ideas (Duffy and Campbell 1994; Tranel et al. 1994). Such skills are critical for routine daily activities. Executive deficits are associated with disruptive

TABLE 6–2. Visuoconstructive deficits characteristic of left-hemisphere versus right-hemisphere brain lesions

Left-hemisphere lesions

    Few lines in drawings

    "Simplified" drawings with few details

    Preserved symmetry of drawings

    Drawing is done slowly

    Drawing skill improves with practice

Right-hemisphere lesions

    Complicated structure and elaborate details

    Extra lines in drawings; extraneous scribbling

    "Piecemeal" approach to drawing

    Particular impairment of three-dimensional drawings

    Left hemineglect

    Drawing is done rapidly

    Drawing skill does not improve with visual cues or

behaviors and self-care limitations among patients with Alzheimer's disease (Chen et al. 1998) and among heterogeneous groups of community-dwelling and institutionalized elderly (Royall et al. 1992).

Executive skills can be divided into four categories: drive, programming, response control, and synthesis (Table 6–3). These categories provide a useful framework for assessing executive function, although there is overlap among the categories. Executive skills can be adequately assessed in the clinic, although an informant's description of the patient's ability to accomplish tasks, negotiate social situations, and respond to environmental contingencies can be particularly revealing (Malloy and Richardson 1994).

Drive includes the initiation of cognitive activity and sustained motivation to perform tasks. Drive is subjectively assessed during the mental status examination. Reduced drive usually has a marked impact on performance in other cognitive domains.

Programming is the ability to recognize patterns and to generate motor programs to perform motor sequences. Two ways that programming skill can be assessed include

1. *Alternating programs.* The examiner provides the patient with an alternating pattern. The patient is asked to copy the pattern and continue the pattern across the page. Examples of inability to generate or maintain a pattern are shown in Figure 6–3.
2. *Hand sequences.* The patient is asked to perform a three-step hand sequence: "slap" (palm down on the table), "fist" (hand in a fist on the table), and "cut" (side of the hand on the table) (Christensen 1975). The examiner demonstrates the sequence, and then the patient attempts to produce the sequence. Normally, a subject will learn to perform the pattern smoothly after about five trials. If there is difficulty, the patient is encouraged to "say the words out loud as you do each step" ("slap," "fist," "cut"). Inability to produce smooth three-step sequences and verbal-manual dissociation (saying "fist," while doing "slap") are noted.

Response control is the ability to plan and efficiently execute a strategy to complete a complex cognitive task. Mental flexibility and a balance between independent thought and use of environmental cues are required for response control. Tasks that assess response control at the bedside include

TABLE 6–3. Categories of executive skills

Category	Executive skills
Drive	Spontaneous initiation of activity
	Motivation
	Sustained performance
Programming	Recognizing patterns
	Recognizing timing sequence
	Fluid output of alternating or rhythmic patterns
Response control	Divided attention
	Inhibition of incorrect responses
	Nonperseverative responses
	Cognitive speed and fluency
	Planning; ordering the steps to accomplish a task
	Mental flexibility: changing strategies, as required
	Use of memory to adjust performance
	Use of feedback to adjust performance
	Freedom from environmental dependence: ability to resist imitation, utilization, or stimulus-bound behavior
Synthesis	Abstraction
	Similarities
	Proverb interpretation
	Monitoring cognitive performance
	Anticipation

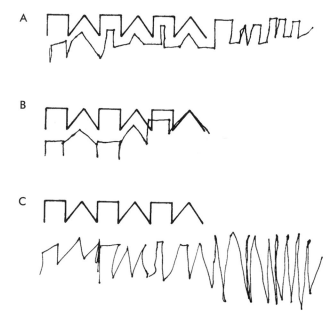

FIGURE 6–3. Alternating patterns. The patient is asked to copy the pattern (shown at the top of each example) and to continue the pattern across the page.   *Panel A:* The patient's drawing initially moves toward the stimulus and the alternating pattern deteriorates as it continues across the page. *Panel B:* The patient's drawing "closes in" on the stimulus and is not continued after the stimulus ends. The patient, with mild dementia and severe bifrontal hypoperfusion on SPECT scan, was able to understand and repeat the instructions. *Panel C:* Marked inability to maintain the alternating pattern.

1. *Divided attention.* The patient is asked to continue the sequence, "1-A, 2-B, 3-C, . . ."
2. *Verbal fluency.* The patient is asked to name as many animals as possible in 1 minute. Alternatively, the patient is asked to name as many words as possible that begin with the letter "F." Initiation, strategy, and perseveration are noted. Normal performance is at least 12 animals or 10 "F" words in 1 minute.
3. *Reciprocal programs and "go/no-go."* The patient is asked to tap the table twice if the examiner taps the table once and to tap once if the examiner taps twice (reciprocal programs). The examiner then randomly taps once or twice and notes the patient's response. When this task is mastered (usually after only a few presentations), the patient is told, "Now I am going to change the rule. If I tap once, you tap twice, but if I tap twice, you should not tap at all" (go/no-go). The patient's ability to respond to the rule change and to resist the impulse to tap is noted.
4. *Multiple loops.* The patient is asked to draw a set of loop figures with the same number of loops as drawn

by the examiner. Perseveration of loop drawing is noted, as shown in Figure 6–4.

5. *Clock drawing strategy.* The patient is asked to draw a clockface. The spontaneous reproduction reveals executive function, as well as visuospatial ability. Planning and organization are observed. Poor spacing of clockface numbers or perseveration can occur (Figure 6–5), as well as incorrect representations on the clockface (Figure 6–6).
6. *Stimulus boundedness.* The patient is asked to draw the hands on a clockface as they would appear when the time is 11:10. The patient may be unable to resist placing the hands on the stimulus numbers (11 and 10) (Figure 6–7). In another task, the examiner writes the word "brown" in large black letters. The patient is asked to name the *color* that the word is written in. The patient may be unable to ignore the *word* "brown." Stimulus boundedness may also appear in a patient's reproduction drawings with overdrawing of the stimulus figure (Figure 6–2, *panel B*).
7. *Imitation behavior.* The examiner rapidly flexes and extends her or his thumb, while pointing to it with the other hand. The patient is asked, "What is this finger called?" Spontaneous movement of the patient's thumb is noted.

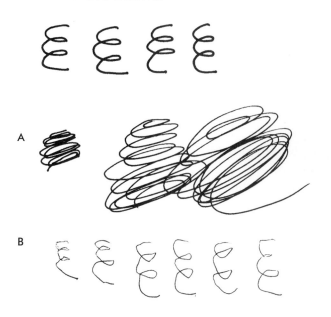

FIGURE 6–4. Multiple loops. The patient is asked to draw loop figures that contain the same number of loops as the examples provided by the examiner (*top*). The patient, who had recently undergone resection of a left frontal astrocytoma, had great difficulty terminating each loop figure drawn with her right hand, which felt "out of control" (*panel A*). She was able to draw the correct number of loops with her left (nondominant) hand (*panel B*).

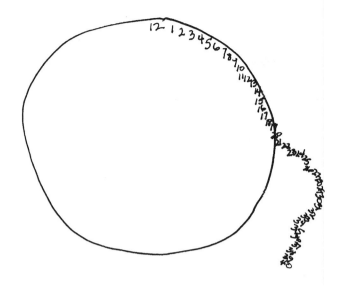

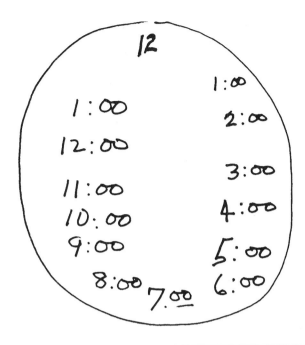

FIGURE 6–5. Poor planning and perseveration on the clockface drawing. The patient, with moderate subcortical dementia and parkinsonism, was asked to put numbers on the clockface in their appropriate places. The spacing between numbers on the patient's drawing is not correct for 12 evenly spaced numbers, and there is perseveration of micrographic number writing up to 40. The patient was able to correctly state that a clock has 12 numbers on it and was able to put all 12 numbers in correct position on a clockface (not shown), when the examiner dictated the numbers to him one by one in random order.

FIGURE 6–6. Intrusion on the clockface drawing. The patient's clockface has a "12" at the top but then includes representations of time in digital format. The intrusion of digital time and the mismatch between time as conventionally written and the true appearance of a clockface reflect the executive deficit. Numbers are also incorrectly located on the clockface and the sequence continues beyond 12:00. The patient has a history of heavy alcohol use and moderate dementia.

Synthesis is the ability to appreciate metaphoric meaning, form an intellectual gestalt, and monitor cognitive performance. These skills are influenced by educational background. Clinical assessment includes evaluation of

1. *Similarities.* The patient is asked to describe how a pair of words are alike. Examples are: rabbit/elephant, bicycle/train, watch/ruler.
2. *Proverbs.* The patient is asked to describe the meaning of a proverb, such as "Don't change horses in the middle of a stream." The patient's appreciation of the abstract meaning is noted.
3. *Monitoring.* The patient's ability to learn from errors and to self-correct while performing cognitive tasks is observed during the examination.

Executive skills require the integrity of diffuse or multifocal neuronal systems. Drive, programming, and response control depend on intact function of discrete circuits that include the frontal cortex, basal ganglia, thalamus, and connecting white matter tracts (Malloy and Richardson 1994; Mega and Cummings 1994). These skills are often impaired with frontal lobe damage (Grafman

1994; Mesulam 1986; Shallice and Burgess 1991; Stuss and Benson 1986; Stuss et al. 1994), although they may occur in patients with focal lesions or degenerative processes distant from the frontal cortex (Cripe 1996; Stuss et al. 1994; Tranel et al. 1994).

Performance on some structured tests of executive skills declines in psychiatrically healthy people after age 60 (Tranel et al. 1994). More extensive impairment of executive skills can result from a variety of conditions: toxic/metabolic disturbance, cerebrovascular disease, head trauma, cerebral neoplasm, cerebral or systemic infection, and degenerative brain diseases such as Alzheimer's disease, frontotemporal dementias, and Parkinson's disease (Duffy and Campbell 1994; Royall and Polk 1998). Older patients with schizophrenia can also exhibit deficits in executive skills (Almeida et al. 1995) (Figure 6–7). Drive, programming, and response control may be particularly impaired in older patients with dysfunction of frontal cortex, as in Pick's disease, frontal lobe degeneration, and some cases of Alzheimer's disease, or with disruption of frontal-subcortical circuits that occurs in basal ganglia disorders such as Parkinson's disease or Huntington's disease. Patients with vascular dementia as a result of cerebrovascular

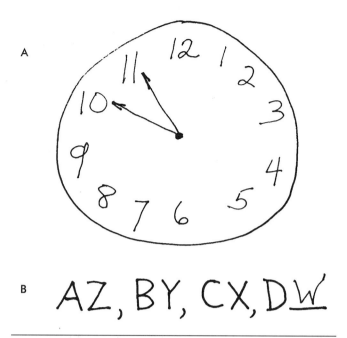

FIGURE 6–7. Stimulus boundedness. The patient is asked to put the hands on the clock as they would appear when the time is 11:10. *Panel A:* The hands are placed on the "11" and the "10," as the patient is unable to resist the stimulus numbers. This example was drawn by a 73-year-old man with schizophrenia, who showed no evidence of memory, language, calculation, or visuospatial deficits. Other executive skills were intact; he was able to correctly identify the letter that follows the "D" in the sequence of letters shown in *panel B*.

disease in subcortical nuclei or white matter tracts that link frontal cortex to other brain regions frequently demonstrate executive deficits (Duffy and Campbell 1994; Ishii et al. 1986).

Other Cognitive Skills

Apraxia. The term "apraxia" is used with variable meaning. Generally, it refers to the inability of a patient with normal elementary motor function to execute the required sequence of skilled movements to complete a complex motor task (Luria 1980). In "dressing apraxia," for example, the coordinated sequence of movements required to put on clothes is disrupted: the steps are out of order or coordinated simultaneous movements do not occur. This type of apraxia (*ideational apraxia*) usually reflects right parietal or bilateral diffuse brain dysfunction.

In *ideomotor apraxia*, the patient is unable to pantomime a motor task on command that can be performed spontaneously (Geschwind 1975). Ideomotor apraxia is revealed by asking the patient to briefly pantomime a motor act that involves muscle groups of the face, trunk, or limbs.

Examples include, "Show me how you blow out a match, . . . suck through a straw, . . . hold a baseball bat, . . . wave good-bye, . . . brush your teeth." Ideomotor apraxia is an inability to smoothly perform the movement altogether or the substitution of a part of the body for the imitated object (e.g., substituting a finger for the toothbrush). Ideomotor apraxia reflects left hemisphere dysfunction or lesion of the anterior corpus callosum.

Agnosia. Patients with agnosia have intact primary sensation and normal perception but lack the ability to recognize or associate meaning to the sensory perception. In *visual agnosia*, the patient can "see" the outline, color, and lighting of an object but is unable to recognize what the object is or what it is used for (Benson and Greenberg 1969). Visual agnosia occurs with bilateral lesions of visual association cortex. Patients with *prosopagnosia* have normal visual perception and do not have visual agnosia, except for impaired recognition of familiar faces. In *environmental agnosia*, the patient can describe details of a familiar environment, but the scene lacks any sense of familiarity (Landis et al. 1986). In *astereognosis*, the patient with normal somatosensory perception is unable to recognize an object by tactile exploration with eyes closed (Adams et al. 1997). Agnosia in an elderly patient is usually caused by a discrete cortical infarction.

Syndromes of Cognitive Impairment

Disorders of Attention

Abnormal attention is the hallmark of *delirium*, or acute confusional state, which is one of the most common causes of behavioral disturbance among hospitalized elderly (see Chapter 19 in this volume). Poor attention is also an important clinical feature that distinguishes delirium from dementia (see Chapters 23 and 24 in this volume).

Reduced arousal occurs on a spectrum: drowsiness, obtundation, stupor, or coma. These states occur with impairment of the reticular activating system or widespread cortical dysfunction. Conditions that cause reduced arousal in older patients include: brainstem infarction or compression, metabolic disturbances, drug intoxication, bilateral cortical infarction, brain infection, and head trauma. *Increased arousal* with anxiety, hypervigilance, and signs of autonomic activation can occur with drug intoxication (stimulants), drug withdrawal (alcohol, benzodiazepine, opioid, or barbiturate), or metabolic disturbances.

Akinetic mutism and catatonia resemble the syndrome

of reduced arousal. Patients with *akinetic mutism* appear alert and may follow stimuli with their eyes. However, spontaneous movement and speech are rare and tend to occur in brief episodes in response to vigorous stimulation (Benson 1990; Mega and Cummings 1994; Plum and Posner 1982). Akinetic mutism is caused by lesions of the midbrain, bilateral cingulate gyri, or septal area. Patients with *catatonia* can present with a variety of motor signs and alterations of attention, including reduced response to stimuli, mutism, posturing, waxy flexibility, and repetitive stereotypic movements (Taylor 1990). Catatonia may occur in patients with schizophrenia, mood disorders, diffuse neurological illness, or metabolic disorders. Focal brain lesions can also cause catatonia. Lesions of the frontal lobes or subcortical structures are most often implicated.

Unilateral *neglect* is a syndrome of inattention to half the body or half the external space. In sensory neglect, sensory input from one hemispace is neglected or extinguished. Sensory neglect can occur in a single sensory modality (e.g., somatosensory, visual) or can be multimodal. In motor neglect, movement in or toward one hemispace is reduced. Neglect of the left hemispace occurs more frequently than neglect of the right hemispace. The extent of neglect does not depend on the extent of primary sensory or motor impairment. With either sensory or motor neglect, the patient is strikingly unaware of the neglected half-space. Sensory neglect usually occurs with right parietal dysfunction, and motor neglect can occur with frontal lesions, although the neuroanatomic specificity of the sensory versus motor components of neglect syndromes is limited (Mesulam 1985).

Patients with normal arousal but poor *concentration* appear awake and alert, but they are easily distracted and have difficulty focusing on cognitive tasks. Poor concentration can result from dysfunction of the brainstem, midbrain, limbic system, or diffuse cortical systems that modulate and focus mental activity. Poor concentration can occur either with metabolic, toxic, or infectious conditions that affect brain function diffusely or with bilateral cortical lesions, as in head trauma or bilateral infarction. The prefrontal cortex and anterior cingulate appear to play important roles in modulating concentration (Knight 1991; Stuss et al. 1995). Older patients with primary psychiatric disorders such as schizophrenia, mania, major depression, and dissociative states may also have reduced ability to concentrate.

Memory Disorders

Amnesia is the inability to learn new information. Patients with amnesia are often able to recall information that was learned before the onset of the memory disorder. *Anterograde amnesia* is the inability to learn during the time that begins with cerebral insult and extends forward in time. *Retrograde amnesia* refers to the lack of recall for events that occurred during the period preceding the cerebral insult. Amnesia occurs with bilateral damage to the medial temporal lobes or midline limbic structures. Conditions that cause amnesia in the elderly include dementia, head trauma, posterior cerebral artery occlusion, anoxia, neoplasms involving midline limbic structures, herpes encephalitis, and Korsakoff's syndrome. Many of these conditions cause cognitive deficits in addition to amnesia, although those affecting only medial temporal or midline limbic structures, such as Korsakoff's syndrome, may result in isolated memory impairment. With stable neurological lesions, anterograde amnesia can improve over time and there can be concomitant shrinkage of the period of retrograde amnesia.

Age-associated memory impairment is the term applied to subtle alterations in recent memory that occur with normal aging (see Chapter 8 in this volume). The elderly often describe a subjective sense of poor memory, may require more trials to learn a word list, and may be less efficient in memory retrieval.

Memory impairment along with other cognitive deficits occurs in patients with dementia. Patients with *Alzheimer's disease* have difficulty learning new information (anterograde amnesia) as well as difficulty recalling information that was learned before onset of the dementia. The recall deficit is a result of widespread impairment of diffuse cortical systems that are required for continued storage and recall of memory and may be mild in the early stage of illness. In *frontotemporal dementias* including Pick's disease, memory impairment often occurs after the onset of behavioral changes, whereas in Alzheimer's disease, memory or language impairment is often the first indication of illness. In *subcortical dementias*, such as those associated with Parkinson's disease or Huntington's disease, memory impairment usually occurs early in the course of dementia, as in Alzheimer's disease. However, the memory impairment of subcortical dementia is characterized by improvement in recall when clues are given, spared recognition memory, and relatively spared declarative memory (facts, knowledge) compared with procedural memory (acquisition of motor skills or cognitive strategies) (Huber and Shuttleworth 1990; Tranel and Damasio 1995). The memory impairment of patients with Alzheimer's disease does not markedly improve when clues are given and deficits in declarative memory are greater than deficits in procedural memory (Cummings and Benson 1992).

Aphasia

Syndromes of aphasia are distinguished by the pattern of specific language skills that are impaired: fluency, comprehension, repetition, or naming (Cummings 1985; Goodglass and Kaplan 1983). The principal aphasia syndromes, the specific language skills that are impaired in each syndrome, and the region of the brain involved are shown in Table 6–4. The disorders of language provide relatively sensitive and specific indications of regional brain dysfunction.

Among elderly patients with language impairment and no other cognitive deficits, the aphasia syndromes usually occur as a result of *infarction, hemorrhage,* or *tumor* that affects the brain regions identified in Table 6–4. Occlusion of the left middle cerebral artery causes global aphasia and right hemiparesis, if the occlusion disrupts perfusion of a wide area of the left hemisphere. If the occlusion is more distal, Broca's aphasia, conduction aphasia, or Wernicke's aphasia may occur, depending on the vascular territory that is compromised. Border zone infarctions, resulting from anoxia, hypotension, or carotid stenosis, affect the watershed regions between the vascular territories served by the anterior, middle, and posterior cerebral arteries and produce transcortical motor or transcortical sensory aphasia.

Elderly patients with dementia often have aphasia along with other cognitive deficits. The involvement of language skills depends on the distribution of brain lesions that cause the dementia. In *Alzheimer's disease,* a characteristic pattern of language disturbance occurs. Very early in the illness, word-finding difficulty and mild anomia are usually present. Subsequently, "empty speech" (language output that contains little information), mild comprehension deficit, and reduced fluency (e.g., measured as number of animals named per minute) occur. Paraphasias may be apparent in spontaneous speech. Elements of transcortical sensory aphasia occur during the course of Alzheimer's disease, reflecting the concentration of neuropathological changes of Alzheimer's disease in the inferior parietal lobe.

In *vascular dementia,* speech abnormalities are more common than in Alzheimer's disease (Sultzer et al. 1993). Language disturbance also occurs. The characteristics of language impairment depend on the brain regions affected by cerebrovascular disease. In general, patients with vascular dementia are more likely to have nonfluent aphasia than are patients with Alzheimer's disease and less likely to have naming impairments (Cummings and Mahler 1991). Marked impairment of language does not occur in patients with dementia associated with *subcortical extrapyramidal disorders* (Huber and Shuttleworth 1990).

TABLE 6–4.   Principal syndromes of aphasia

Aphasia syndrome	Language skills				Regional brain dysfunction[a]
	Fluency	Comprehension	Repetition	Naming	
Broca's	Nonfluent	Intact	Impaired	Impaired	Left frontal operculum, left insular cortex, and adjacent white matter
Transcortical motor	Nonfluent	Intact	Intact	Impaired	Left supplementary motor area
Global	Nonfluent	Impaired	Impaired	Impaired	Wide area of left hemisphere convexity
Wernicke's	Fluent	Impaired	Impaired	Impaired	Posterior, superior left temporal lobe; left inferior parietal lobe may also be involved
Transcortical sensory	Fluent	Impaired	Intact	Impaired	Left inferior parietal lobule
Conduction	Fluent	Intact	Impaired	Impaired	Left arcuate fasciculus (usually in the left parietal operculum) or left insula and adjacent white matter
Anomic	Fluent	Intact	Intact	Impaired	Left angular gyrus or left posterior middle temporal gyrus

[a]In patients with left hemisphere dominance for language.

Frontal Lobe Disorders

The frontal lobe disorders are particularly important in neuropsychiatric evaluation of the elderly because the brain lesions that are responsible are often not detected by the traditional neurological examination and the psychiatric symptoms that occur do not usually fit the characteristic pattern of common psychiatric disorders. Patients with frontal lobe disorders often present with unusual combinations of cognitive, psychiatric, and behavioral symptoms. Neuropsychiatric symptoms that occur in each of the three principal frontal lobe syndromes and those symptoms that are not well localized to specific frontal subregions are shown in Table 6–5 (Malloy and Richardson 1994; Mega and Cummings 1994; Salloway 1994; Stuss and Benson 1986). Symptoms may occur with a lesion in specific regions of the frontal cortex or in linked cortical or subcortical structures. Lesions in subcortical nuclei or white matter tracts may have marked effects on frontal function (Sultzer et al. 1995a). The relationship between anatomy and symptomatology is incomplete: patients with extensive frontal dysfunction may not manifest the full spectrum of "frontal" symptoms, and these symptoms may occur following lesions outside the frontal circuits.

The *medial frontal syndrome* is primarily a disturbance of motivation and includes a range of symptoms from mild disinterest to akinetic mutism (Stuss and Benson 1986). Aspontaneity, blunted affect, and reduced spontaneous movement may occur. The syndrome occurs with lesions of the anterior cingulate gyrus, ventral striatum, medial dorsal thalamus, or tracts that connect these structures. More severe symptoms usually occur with bilateral lesions. Conditions that cause the medial frontal syndrome in the elderly include anterior cerebral artery occlusion, thalamic infarction, hydrocephalus, and tumors of the diencephalon or third ventricle.

Lesions of the *dorsolateral frontal convexity* produce a syndrome of disorganized cognitive performance (Fuster 1997; Malloy and Richardson 1994). Executive dysfunction often appears on the mental status examination, including perseveration (e.g., extra loops on the multiple loops, intrusion of a prior response in a new task), impaired motor programming, stimulus-bound behavior, difficulty with alternating programs or changing mental set, or reduced verbal or design fluency. Dorsolateral frontal convexity insults include head trauma, frontal infarction, frontal lobe tumor, and degenerative dementias, particularly those that preferentially affect frontal structures. Lesion of the dorsolateral caudate nucleus may produce a similar pattern of executive deficits.

The *orbitofrontal syndrome* occurs with lesions of the inferior aspect of the frontal lobe. This region of the frontal lobe is intimately associated with the limbic system, and dysfunction often appears as a striking change of personality (Duffy and Campbell 1994). Disinhibition and aggression are common, and patients may show a marked inability to conform behavior to social customs (Salloway 1994). Mood is often expansive or irritable, affect is labile, and impulsive outbursts of jocularity can occur. When lesions are confined to the orbitofrontal cortex, there may be no formal neurological deficits or other cognitive deficits. Orbitofrontal damage occurs with head trauma, inferior

TABLE 6–5. **Neuropsychiatric symptoms that occur with lesions of the frontal lobe or related subcortical structures**

Site of lesion	Symptoms
Medial frontal	Low motivation
	Blunted affect
	Motor retardation
	Reduced verbal output
	Grasp reflex
Dorsolateral frontal convexity	Poor selective attention
	Deficits in working memory
	Perseveration
	Excessive stimulus dependence
	Impaired motor programming
	Motor impersistence
	Reduced verbal or design fluency
Orbitofrontal	Disinhibition
	Failure to appreciate social customs
	Childlike jocularity
	Labile affect
	Expansive mood
	Irritability
	Lack of empathy
Heterogeneous frontal cortical regions	Apathy
	Impulsivity
	Poor directed attention
	Poor sustained attention
	Difficulty with temporal sequencing
	Inability to change rules

frontal meningiomas, rupture of anterior cerebral artery aneurysms, and frontal dementias.

Screening for Cognitive Impairment

My focus in this chapter is on comprehensive cognitive assessment, but some clinical settings may not be ideally structured to complete a thorough evaluation. Detection rate for dementia in some care settings is low (Callahan et al. 1995; Eefsting et al. 1996). Screening can improve case detection and is most important when the prevalence of cases in the clinic population is high.

Efficient screening can be accomplished by asking questions related to cognitive decline in the patient's history or by very brief mental status testing. A complaint of cognitive difficulty may emerge spontaneously or the clinician can ask if the patient has difficulty learning new information, handling complex tasks, finding his or her way, or using words correctly. Functional abilities can be rapidly assessed using tools such as the Functional Activities Questionnaire (Pfeffer et al. 1982), which has good discriminant ability (Costa et al. 1996). Brief tests such as the Blessed Orientation-Memory-Concentration Test (Katzman et al. 1983) can quickly measure a patient's overall cognitive abilities and are described in the next section of this chapter. Screening techniques will not reveal all cases with cognitive impairment, particularly when deficits are mild, and do not substitute for a complete assessment, but they can facilitate recognition of cases that might otherwise be missed. When screening reveals possible impairment, the patient should undergo more thorough diagnostic assessment to determine the extent and etiology of cognitive deficits.

Rating Scales for Cognitive Assessment

Rating scales can be used to screen for cognitive impairment, provide a framework for more thorough clinical assessment, or quantify the results of a mental status examination. Measurement of cognitive deficits allows the clinician to identify changes over time or to determine the response to treatment. Structured assessment also facilitates reliable communication among clinicians.

Many different rating scales are available, and reviews of their use have been published (Camicioli and Wild 1997; Kluger and Ferris 1991; Raskin and Niederehe 1988; Siu 1991; Weiner et al. 1996). Rating scales differ in the time required for administration and the spectrum of symptoms assessed (cognition, functional skills, psychiatric symptoms, behavior disturbance). Some scales are screening instruments; others are more comprehensive. Some scales provide subscores for individual cognitive domains, whereas others generate only an overall score. Each rating scale accomplishes a different clinical goal:

1. *Blessed Orientation-Memory-Concentration Test*, a six-item screening instrument that assesses concentration and memory (Katzman et al. 1983). Sensitivity, specificity, and diagnostic value of this brief instrument are acceptable and comparable to those of longer instruments (Stuss et al. 1996).
2. *Short Test of Mental Status*, a brief screening instrument (Kokmen et al. 1987). The eight items assess attention, orientation, memory, calculation, and visuoconstructive skill. Sensitivity has been shown to be acceptable.
3. *Mini-Mental State Examination (MMSE)*, a 30-item instrument that is widely used to screen for cognitive impairment and to assess the severity of impairment (Folstein et al. 1975). The examination takes about 10 minutes and provides a reliable overall cognitive score. Sensitivity for mild impairment is limited (Tombaugh and McIntyre 1992), and older individuals with low "normal" scores are at high risk for developing dementia over subsequent years (Braekhus et al. 1995). Age and educational level must be considered in interpreting the MMSE score (Crum et al. 1993).
4. *Neurobehavioral Cognitive Status Examination*, which assesses attention, memory, calculation, visuoconstructive skills, language, and abstraction. A subscore for each of these cognitive domains is generated (Kiernan et al. 1987). The examination requires specific testing materials and takes about 20 minutes to complete with an impaired patient.
5. *Mattis Dementia Rating Scale*, which assesses a wider range of cognitive skills, including executive abilities (Mattis 1976). The instrument requires about 30–45 minutes to complete with an impaired patient. It provides an overall cognitive score, with a maximum of 144 points.
6. *Neurobehavioral Rating Scale*, a 28-item instrument that measures psychiatric and behavioral disturbances, in addition to cognitive impairment (Levin et al. 1987). The evaluation takes about 40 minutes to complete. The instrument provides six factor scores that measure the cognitive and noncognitive symptoms (Sultzer et al. 1992); reliability and validity are acceptable (Sultzer et al. 1995b).

7. *Global Deterioration Scale*, a seven-point scale that measures the overall severity of dementia (Reisberg et al. 1988). Cognitive deficits, psychiatric symptoms, and functional impairment are all considered by the clinician in assigning the global severity score.

8. *Executive Interview*, a brief measure of executive skills (Royall et al. 1992). Measures of executive skills may help to clarify diagnosis (Royall and Polk 1998) and suggest risk for impairment in activities of daily living or behavioral disturbance (Chen et al. 1998).

Functional Assessment

The ability to accomplish functional activities at home is important information that complements the assessment of cognitive skills in the mental status examination. Reduced functional skills can be a sensitive indicator of dementia (Barberger-Gateau et al. 1992; Costa et al. 1996). Functional assessment also reveals the impact of medical problems and cognitive deficits on living skills and indicates the need for assistance with activities, which are both of prime importance to the patient and family.

At least a brief review of functional skills should be included in the assessment of each geriatric patient, and whether the patient currently drives a car should be noted. Two groups of activities are considered in functional assessment: physical activities of daily living (ADLs) and instrumental activities of daily living (IADLs) (Lawton and Brody 1969). Physical ADLs include the basic skills required for self-maintenance: dressing, bathing, toileting, transferring, and feeding. IADLs include more complex skills required for independent living: shopping, cooking, housekeeping, laundry, using the telephone, using transportation, managing money, and managing medications. An observer determines whether the patient is independently able to perform each of these activities. Rating scales such as the IADL Scale (Lawton 1988) or the Functional Activities Questionnaire (Pfeffer et al. 1982) can be used to improve the reliability of functional assessment or to screen for cognitive disorders.

Summary

The mental status examination is a fundamental part of the neuropsychiatric assessment of older patients. The examination focuses on cognitive abilities, which include perception, "thinking," intellect, and problem-solving skills. Several cognitive domains are explored: attention, memory, language, visuospatial skills, calculation, praxis, and executive skills. The extent of cognitive assessment depends on the particular clinical circumstances and the goals of the evaluation; at least a screening evaluation is recommended for all geriatric patients. Rating scales can be used to help screen for cognitive impairment or to quantify the extent of impairment in patients with known deficits.

The pattern of deficits is used to identify syndromes of cognitive impairment, such as delirium, other disorders of attention, dementia, aphasia, amnesia, and frontal lobe disorders. The results of the mental status examination can also reveal the contribution of regional brain dysfunction to the expression of psychiatric symptoms in older patients.

References

Adams RD, Victor M, Ropper AH: Principles of Neurology, 6th Edition. New York, McGraw-Hill, 1997

Almeida OP, Howard RJ, Levy R, et al: Cognitive features of psychotic states arising in late life (late paraphrenia). Psychol Med 25:685–698, 1995

American Psychiatric Association: Practice guidelines for the treatment of patients with Alzheimer's disease and other dementias of late life. Am J Psychiatry 154 (suppl):1–39, 1997

Baddeley AD: The psychology of memory, in Handbook of Memory Disorders. Edited by Baddeley AD, Wilson BA, Watts FN. New York, Wiley, 1995, pp 3–25

Barberger-Gateau P, Commenges D, Gagnon M, et al: Instrumental activities of daily living as a screening tool for cognitive impairment and dementia in elderly community dwellers. J Am Geriatr Soc 40:1129–1134, 1992

Benson DF: Psychomotor retardation. Neuropsychiatry Neuropsychol Behav Neurol 3:36–47, 1990

Benson DF, Barton MI: Disturbances in constructional ability. Cortex 6:19–46, 1970

Benson DF, Greenberg JP: Visual form agnosia. Arch Neurol 20:82–89, 1969

Black FW, Strub RL: Constructional apraxia in patients with discrete missile wounds of the brain. Cortex 12:212–220, 1976

Braekhus A, Laake K, Engedal K: A low, "normal" score on the Mini-Mental State Examination predicts development of dementia after three years. J Am Geriatr Soc 43:656–661, 1995

Callahan CM, Hendrie HC, Tierney WM: Documentation and evaluation of cognitive impairment in elderly primary care patients. Ann Intern Med 122:422–429, 1995

Camicioli R, Wild K: Assessment of the elderly with dementia, in Handbook of Neurologic Rating Scales. Edited by Herndon RM. New York, Demos Vermande, 1997, pp 125–160

Chen ST, Sultzer DL, Hinkin CH, et al: Executive dysfunction in Alzheimer's disease: association with neuropsychiatric symptoms and functional impairment. J Neuropsychiatry Clin Neurosci 10:426–432, 1998

Christensen A-L: Luria's Neuropsychological Investigation: Text. New York, Spectrum, 1975

Costa PTJ, Williams TF, Somerfield M, et al: Recognition and initial assessment of Alzheimer's disease and related dementias. Clinical Practice Guideline No. 19. Rockville, MD, U.S. Department of Health and Human Services, Public Health Service, Agency for Health Care Policy and Research, 1996

Cripe LI: The ecological validity of executive function testing, in Ecological Validity of Neuropsychological Testing. Edited by Sbordone RJ, Long CJ. Delray Beach, FL, GR Press/St. Lucie Press, 1996, pp 171–202

Crum RM, Anthony JC, Bassett SS, et al: Population-based norms for the Mini-Mental State Examination by age and educational level. JAMA 269:2386–2391, 1993

Cummings JL: Disorders of verbal output: mutism, aphasia, and psychotic speech, in Clinical Neuropsychiatry. New York, Grune & Stratton, 1985, pp 17–35

Cummings JL, Benson DF: Subcortical dementias in the extrapyramidal disorders, in Dementia: A Clinical Approach, 2nd Edition. Boston, MA, Butterworth-Heinemann, 1992, pp 95–152

Cummings JL, Mahler ME: Cerebrovascular dementia, in Neurobehavioral Aspects of Cerebrovascular Disease. Edited by Bornstein RA, Brown GG. New York, Oxford University Press, 1991, pp 131–149

Duffy JD, Campbell JJ: The regional prefrontal syndromes: a theoretical and clinical overview. J Neuropsychiatry Clin Neurosci 6:379–387, 1994

Eefsting JA, Boersma F, Van Den Brink W, et al: Differences in prevalence of dementia based on community survey and general practitioner recognition. Psychol Med 26: 1223–1230, 1996

Folstein MF, Folstein SE, McHugh PR: Mini-Mental State: a practical method for grading the cognitive state of patients for the clinician. J Psychiatr Res 12:189–198, 1975

Fuster JM: The Prefrontal Cortex: Anatomy, Physiology, and Neuropsychology of the Frontal Lobe, 3rd Edition. Philadelphia, PA, Lippincott-Raven, 1997

Geschwind N: The apraxias: neural mechanisms of disorders of learned movement. American Scientist 63:188–195, 1975

Goodglass H, Kaplan E: Major aphasic syndromes and illustrations of test patterns, in The Assessment of Aphasia and Related Disorders, 2nd Edition. Philadelphia, PA, Lea & Febiger, 1983, pp 74–100

Grafman J: Alternative frameworks for the conceptualization of prefrontal lobe functions, in Handbook of Neuropsychology, Vol 9. Edited by Boller F, Grafman J. New York, Elsevier, 1994, pp 187–201

Huber SJ, Shuttleworth EC: Neuropsychological assessment of subcortical dementia, in Subcortical Dementia. Edited by Cummings JL. New York, Oxford University Press, 1990, pp 71–86

Ishii N, Nishihara Y, Imamura T: Why do frontal lobe symptoms predominate in vascular dementia with lacunes? Neurology 36:340–345, 1986

Katzman R, Brown T, Fuld P, et al: Validation of a short orientation-memory-concentration test of cognitive impairment. Am J Psychiatry 140:734–739, 1983

Kiernan RJ, Mueller J, Langston JW, et al: The Neurobehavioral Cognitive Status Examination: a brief but differentiated approach to cognitive assessment. Ann Intern Med 107:481–485, 1987

Kluger A, Ferris SH: Scales for the assessment of Alzheimer's disease. Psychiatr Clin North Am 14:309–326, 1991

Knight RT: Evoked potential studies of attention capacity in human frontal lobe lesions, in Frontal Lobe Function and Dysfunction. Edited by Levin HS, Eisenberg HM, Benton AL. New York, Oxford University Press, 1991, pp 139–153

Kokmen E, Naessens JM, Offort KP: A short test of mental status: description and preliminary results. Mayo Clin Proc 62:281–288, 1987

Kupfermann I: Learning and memory, in Principles of Neural Science, 3rd Edition. Edited by Kandel ER, Schwartz JH, Jessell TM. New York, Elsevier, 1991, pp 997–1008

Landis T, Cummings JL, Benson DF, et al: Loss of topographic familiarity: an environmental agnosia. Arch Neurol 43:132–136, 1986

Lawton MP: Scales to measure competence in everyday activities. Psychopharmacol Bull 24:609–614, 1988

Lawton MP, Brody EM: Assessment of older people: self-maintaining and instrumental activities of daily living. Gerontologist 9:179–186, 1969

Levin HS, High WM, Goethe KE, et al: The Neurobehavioral Rating Scale: assessment of the behavioral sequelae of head injury by the clinician. J Neurol Neurosurg Psychiatry 50: 183–193, 1987

Lezak MD: Neuropsychological Assessment, 3rd Edition. New York, Oxford University Press, 1995

Luria AR: Higher Cortical Functions in Man, 2nd Edition. New York, Basic Books, 1980

Malloy PF, Richardson ED: Assessment of frontal lobe functions. J Neuropsychiatry Clin Neurosci 6:399–410, 1994

Mattis S: Mental status examination for organic mental syndrome in the elderly patient, in Geriatric Psychiatry. Edited by Bellak R, Karasu TE. New York, Grune & Stratton, 1976, pp 77–121

Mega MS, Cummings JL: Frontal-subcortical circuits and neuropsychiatric disorders. J Neuropsychiatry Clin Neurosci 6:358–370, 1994

Mendez MF, Ala T, Underwood KL: Development of scoring criteria for the clock drawing task in Alzheimer's disease. J Am Geriatr Soc 40:1095–1099, 1992

Mesulam M-M: Attention, confusional states, and neglect, in Principles of Behavioral Neurology. Edited by Mesulam M-M. Philadelphia, PA, FA Davis, 1985, pp 125–168

Mesulam M-M: Frontal cortex and behavior (editorial). Ann Neurol 19:320–325, 1986

Pfeffer RI, Kurosaki TT, Harrah CH: Measurement of functional activities in older adults in the community. J Gerontol (A) 37:323–329, 1982

Plum F, Posner JB: The Diagnosis of Stupor and Coma, 3rd Edition. Philadelphia, PA, FA Davis, 1982

Raskin A, Niederehe G (eds): Assessment in diagnosis and treatment of geropsychiatric patients. Psychopharmacol Bull 24:501–810, 1988

Reisberg B, Ferris SH, de Leon MJ, et al: Global deterioration scale. Psychopharmacol Bull 24:661–663, 1988

Ross GW, Abbott RD, Petrovitch H, et al: Frequency and characteristics of silent dementia among elderly Japanese-American men. JAMA 277:800–805, 1997

Royall DR, Polk M: Dementias that present with and without posterior cortical features: an important clinical distinction. J Am Geriatr Soc 46:98–105, 1998

Royall DR, Mahurin RK, Gray KF: Bedside assessment of executive cognitive impairment: the executive interview. J Am Geriatr Soc 40:1221–1226, 1992

Royall DR, Cordes JA, Polk M: CLOX: an executive clock drawing task. J Neurol Neurosurg Psychiatry 64:588–594, 1998

Salloway SP: Diagnosis and treatment of patients with "frontal lobe" syndromes. J Neuropsychiatry Clin Neurosci 6:388–398, 1994

Shallice T, Burgess P: Higher-order cognitive impairments and frontal lobe lesions in man, in Frontal Lobe Function and Dysfunction. Edited by Levin HS, Eisenberg HM, Benton AL. New York, Oxford University Press, 1991, pp 125–138

Signoret J-L: Memory and amnesias, in Principles of Behavioral Neurology. Edited by Mesulam M-M. Philadelphia, PA, FA Davis, 1985, pp 169–192

Siu AL: Screening for dementia and investigating its causes. Ann Intern Med 115:122–132, 1991

Small GW, Rabins PV, Barry PP, et al: Diagnosis and treatment of Alzheimer disease and related disorders. Consensus statement of the American Association for Geriatric Psychiatry, the Alzheimer's Association, and the American Geriatrics Society. JAMA 278:1363–1371, 1997

Squire LR: Memory and Brain. New York, Oxford University Press, 1987

Strub RL, Black FW: The Mental Status Examination in Neurology, 3rd Edition. Philadelphia, PA, FA Davis, 1993

Stuss DT, Benson DF: The Frontal Lobes. New York, Raven, 1986

Stuss DT, Eskes GA, Foster JK: Experimental neuropsychological studies of frontal lobe functions, in Handbook of Neuropsychology, Vol 9. Edited by Boller F, Grafman J. New York, Elsevier, 1994, pp 149–185

Stuss DT, Shallice T, Alexander MP, et al: A multidisciplinary approach to anterior attentional functions. Ann N Y Acad Sci 769:191–211, 1995

Stuss DT, Meiran N, Guzman A, et al: Do long tests yield a more accurate diagnosis of dementia than short tests? Arch Neurol 53:1033–1039, 1996

Sultzer DL, Levin HS, Mahler ME, et al: Assessment of cognitive, psychiatric, and behavioral disturbances in patients with dementia: the Neurobehavioral Rating Scale. J Am Geriatr Soc 40:549–555, 1992

Sultzer DL, Levin HS, Mahler ME, et al: A comparison of psychiatric symptoms in vascular dementia and Alzheimer's disease. Am J Psychiatry 150:1806–1812, 1993

Sultzer DL, Mahler ME, Cummings JL, et al: Cortical abnormalities associated with subcortical lesions in vascular dementia: clinical and PET findings. Arch Neurol 52:773–780, 1995a

Sultzer DL, Berisford MA, Gunay I: The Neurobehavioral Rating Scale: reliability in patients with dementia. J Psychiatr Res 29:185–191, 1995b

Taylor MA: Catatonia; a review of a behavioral neurologic syndrome. Neuropsychiatry Neuropsychol Behav Neurol 3:48–72, 1990

Teasdale G, Jennett B: Assessment of coma and impaired consciousness; a practical scale. Lancet 2:81–84, 1974

Tombaugh TN, McIntyre NJ: The Mini-Mental State Examination: a comprehensive review. J Am Geriatr Soc 40:922–935, 1992

Tranel D, Damasio AR: Neurobiological foundations of human memory, in Handbook of Memory Disorders. Edited by Baddeley AD, Wilson BA, Watts FN. New York, Wiley, 1995, pp 27–50

Tranel D, Anderson SW, Benton A: Development of the concept of 'executive function' and its relationship to the frontal lobes, in Handbook of Neuropsychology, Vol 9. Edited by Boller F, Grafman J. New York, Elsevier, 1994, pp 125–148

U.S. Department of Veterans Affairs, University HealthSystem Consortium: Dementia Identification and Assessment: Guidelines for Primary Care Practitioners. Oak Brook, IL, University HealthSystem Consortium, 1997

Weiner MF, Koss E, Wild KV, et al: Measures of psychiatric symptoms in Alzheimer patients: a review. Alzheimer Dis Assoc Disord 10:20–30, 1996

Neuropsychological Assessment

Kenneth Podell, Ph.D.

Mark R. Lovell, Ph.D.

The neuropsychological evaluation of older adults has become increasingly important over the past decade and is often a standard component of the neuropsychiatric evaluation. Neuropsychological assessment can be considered a more in-depth extension and quantification of the mental status examination (see Chapter 6 in this volume) and, as such, is focused on the psychometric assessment of cognitive processes. A thorough neuropsychological evaluation can add much to the clinical diagnostic process and can complement information gathered through electrophysiological, neuroanatomical, and functional neuroimaging technologies (see Chapters 9–11 in this volume).

In this chapter, we review the applications of neuropsychological assessment to geriatric patients and discuss relevant issues regarding the establishment of appropriate normative databases for this population. The selection and use of neuropsychological tests, the interpretation of test results, and the use of these results in the treatment planning process are specifically discussed. We also discuss the use of traditional fixed neuropsychological test batteries and contrast them with more flexible approaches to the assessment of elderly patients.

Goals of the Geriatric Neuropsychological Evaluation

Neuropsychological test results are used in various ways depending on the training of the neuropsychologist, the setting, the referral question, and the treatment program. However, despite differing approaches to assessment, the three primary goals of neuropsychological assessment are generally the same: 1) to establish an individual's cognitive and behavioral strengths and weaknesses, 2) to interpret findings from a diagnostic viewpoint (e.g., differential diagnosis such as depression versus dementia or age-appropriate cognitive decline versus dementia), and 3) to extrapolate treatment and rehabilitation recommendations from the neuropsychological assessment findings (La Rue 1992). In addition to providing specific information that may be useful in differential diagnosis and the localization of brain dysfunction, the neuropsychological evaluation is relatively unique among neurodiagnostic techniques in its ability to document the functional capabilities of geriatric patients. This aspect of neuropsychological assessment has become increasingly important as a greater number of individuals are living well into their eighth decade or beyond. Clinicians are routinely faced with decisions regarding their patients' ability to live alone, operate an automobile, make competent decisions about health care, and manage their financial affairs.

Methodological Issues in Geriatric Neuropsychology

The aging process is accompanied by subtle declines in specific domains of cognitive functioning (Albert 1981; Kaszniak 1987; Wilson et al. 1997), with motor speed, speed of cognitive processing, and mental flexibility most affected (La Rue 1992). This decline is a function of the synergistic effects of the "normal aging process" in combination with the multitude of medical and psychosocial variables that affect the cognition of elderly individuals. The concept of "normal aging," particularly as it pertains to memory decline in older adults, is an extremely important issue and is discussed more thoroughly in Chapter 8 in this volume. However, a brief discussion of how this issue has affected the clinical neuropsychological evaluation of the geriatric patient is germane to the current chapter.

The clinical neuropsychological evaluation is highly dependent on appropriate comparison groups that allow the cognitive dysfunction related to pathological processes to be separated from the decline secondary to the normal aging process. The normative sample provides the basis for this comparison of individual patient performance to established standards for a given age group and is an important prerequisite to the assessment process. However, to date, the usefulness of neuropsychological testing with older adults has been limited by a relative dearth of normative data. The development of valid normative data for geriatric patients continues to be a major challenge for geriatric neuropsychology, particularly with regard to the psychometric assessment of patients over the age of 75 years. This is particularly pertinent for urban geriatric patients, in which case demographic characteristics have a significant impact on normative values. The evidence is starting to show that age, education, literacy, and ethnicity affect performance in various cognitive domains differentially. This issue is starting to be addressed with normative

data being collected on urban- and rural-dwelling patients of varying ethnic origins, educational backgrounds, and literacy levels (Hohl et al. 1999; Lichtenberg et al. 1998; Manly et al. 1999; Marcopulos et al. 1997; Strick et al. 1998).

Substantial limitations still exist in age-based normative data, with limited heterogeneity of education and health variables among normative samples (La Rue 1992) as well as poor reliability, validity, and normative data relevant to "old-old" patient groups (i.e., those 75 or older) (Kaszniak 1989). This lack of an adequate normative base has at times fostered a reliance on norms obtained on younger subject groups—a practice that can lead to an overdiagnosis of pathological cognitive impairment in geriatric patients.

In the absence of age-appropriate and current normative data, some clinicians have tended to rely on data that were collected many years earlier and from samples of geriatric subjects who may have differed significantly from the individual patient whose performance is being evaluated. Given generational differences in the availability of medical treatment, education, nutrition, and a host of other factors that can influence performance on neuropsychological tests, it is risky to compare the test performance of an elderly patient in the 1990s to normative data gathered during the 1970s or before. This cohort effect (Schaie and Schaie 1977) limits the usefulness of previously established normative data to current samples of patients.

One additional problem with using age-appropriate normative data in a geriatric population is making sure that the normative data, even if they have large sample sizes with appropriate age and education ranges, have adequate psychometric properties. This becomes extremely problematic on more difficult tests of memory and executive control, which are particularly important cognitive domains in assessing geriatric populations. For example, normative data are available for performance on the Wisconsin Card Sorting Test (WCST) extending through the eighth decade (Heaton et al. 1993). The WCST, a difficult test even for younger, more educated individuals, is extremely difficult for older, less educated patients. Because of this, the potential for a significant floor effect is very real. Even some seasoned neuropsychologists tend to ignore this problem. It has very real implications in terms of test interpretation and translation to "real world" activities or ecological validity. We believe that not only does one need to ensure adequate norming in terms of demographic variables, but that the test must accurately reflect the range of abilities in the age group and must also have appropriate psychometric properties (e.g., minimizing ceiling or floor effects).

In neuropsychology, because we often do not have predisease or baseline data on patients, we tend to use level of education (among other variables) as a marker of premorbid cognitive abilities. We use this to compare current performance to determine if there has been a meaningful decline. However, level of education for geriatric patients most likely does not have the same meaning as the educational level of someone in their 30s, for example. It has been our experience that level of education, unless very high or very low, may not have the same predictive abilities as we assume with a younger population. Therefore, in our clinic, to help predict life-long cognitive abilities, we also rely upon measures considered highly resilient to any type of central nervous system dysfunction. One such measure is single-word reading recognition and vocabulary skills (Bayles et al. 1985).

Yet another methodological issue that has affected the neuropsychological evaluation of elderly patients has been differing definitions of what constitutes the expected cognitive pattern of "normal aging." For example, some researchers have distinguished between *usual aging*, in which the effects of the aging process are influenced by extrinsic factors such as nutrition and psychosocial factors, and *successful aging*, in which these factors play a neutral or positive role (Rowe and Kahn 1987). Still others have studied unusually healthy groups of geriatric subjects, documenting cognitive functioning in patients who are uncharacteristically free of the medical problems that often afflict the elderly (MacInnes et al. 1983). Obviously, the comparison of a patient's performance to norms gathered from these disparate samples could lead to markedly different conclusions regarding pathological cognitive decline in a given patient. Comparison of the typical elderly patient with norms derived from a sample of unusually healthy individuals may result in an overdiagnosis of pathological cognitive dysfunction (Albert 1981).

Despite past limitations in the development of normative data on cognitive functioning in geriatric patients, there has been significant improvement in the development of neuropsychological tests that provide geriatric norms. For example, the Wechsler Memory Scale—Revised (WMS-R) (Wechsler 1987) and the Wechsler Adult Intelligence Scale—Revised (WAIS-R) (Wechsler 1981), two of the most popular tests used by neuropsychologists, have supporting normative data through age 74. Even more recently, these norms have been augmented by data specific to the old-old population that provide information on normal subjects into their ninth decade (Ivnik et al. 1992). And now with the introduction of WAIS-III and WMS-III (Wechsler 1997a, 1997b), normative data on the same tests have been collected on updated samples through

the eighth decade. Along similar lines, demographic corrections have been developed for the Halstead-Reitan Neuropsychological Battery (HRNB) (Heaton et al. 1991), and the normative data for the Hopkins Verbal Learning Test has been updated (Benedict et al. 1998), whereas others have renormed existing tests (Hohl et al. 1999; Lichtenberg et al. 1998; Manly et al. 1999). Relatively new cognitive screening instruments have also included older-age normative data that permit appropriate global mental status examinations in the elderly (Osato et al. 1989).

Medication side effects on cognitive abilities is another factor that is sometimes underappreciated and not taken into account both in terms of neuropsychological assessment and treatment. Commonly prescribed medications, such as cimetidine, can produce alterations in cognition. Similarly, the use of anticholinergic and antidopaminergic medications must be taken into consideration because of their known deleterious effects on memory (Drachman and Leavitt 1974) and executive control skills, respectively (see Fuster 1989).

Finally, a distinction between age-appropriate cognitive abilities, as defined by performance relative to normative data, and functional abilities needed for the individual's given situation must be clearly defined and addressed in a neuropsychological evaluation. What may be age-appropriate cognitive functioning (e.g., for an 85-year-old individual), may not be sufficient for the level of independent functioning required in the individual's living situation. For example, the same individual may be cognitively intact enough relative to age-appropriate normative data to return to live in an assistive living apartment building where she or he has some increased supervision, but may not be cognitively intact enough to live alone and be independently responsible for instrumental activities of daily living and medical management.

Neuropsychological Evaluation Process

The neuropsychological assessment is a complex process requiring the integration of knowledge from several different areas of medicine (including neurology, psychiatry, neurobiology), clinical psychology and aging, psychometrics, and, of course, neuropsychology and aging (Kaszniak 1989). The evaluation typically consists of a clinical interview, test selection, scoring and interpretation of test results (e.g., functional level, brain systems involved, and possible etiologies), diagnosis, and treatment and rehabilitation recommendations.

The primary goal of the clinical interview should be to develop hypotheses regarding the patient's overall cognitive status, current problems and symptoms, and his or her capacity to engage in further neuropsychological evaluation. In addition, the clinical interview provides an opportunity for the examiner to develop rapport with the patient, explain the nature of the evaluation, and answer any of the patient's questions, which may help to alleviate initial anxiety.

Sometimes the elderly patient is not capable of giving a precise and thorough history. Thus, in our clinic we request that a significant other accompany the patient. After obtaining permission from the patient, we routinely interview the significant other or a relative to verify and/or obtain appropriate history. The significant other is asked to complete the Geriatric Evaluation by Relative's Rating Instrument (GERRI; Schwartz 1983). A questionnaire rating the patient's functional abilities in the realms of cognition, mood, and social abilities. A thorough interview should yield relevant demographic background information (e.g., age, education, occupational history, and handedness), a review of medical and psychiatric history (including past and present medication use), substance use or abuse, familial (both medical and psychiatric) and developmental information, current living situation, and support network. We also do a complete review of sensory and motor systems; homeostasis; and changes in cognition and affect, emphasizing recent changes in language, memory, thinking, and affect; any recent stressors (e.g., death of a spouse or loss of driving license); information pertaining to activity level and hobbies; motivation; and the patient's understanding of why he or she was referred for neuropsychological evaluation.

Through the clinical interview and direct interaction with the patient, the neuropsychologist gathers important qualitative information regarding cognitive functioning. This includes a general sense of the patient's orientation, attentional capacity, motivation, awareness of impairment, willingness to engage in neuropsychological testing, and social appropriateness. Integrity of gross language and motor function, memory capacity, and stamina should also be assessed. The older patient may have limitations that affect his or her performance during the neuropsychological evaluation, including reduced vision and hearing and the effects of overmedication (Goreczny and Nussbaum 1994; Russell 1984). As a result of these factors, the questions may need to be repeated and presented louder and at a slower rate.

Similarly, the method of test administration must sometimes be altered to conform to the patient's sensorial limitations. For example, a subject with poor hearing but intact vision may have to read a word list presented on cue cards rather than listen to the list presented auditorily. This clearly violates standard administration. However, it allows for a "qualitative" analysis and can yield useful information for an experienced neuropsychologist. In addition, the patient should be encouraged to continue working on tasks even after specified time limits have been reached. This testing-the-limits approach can help to establish the patient's capacity to perform a cognitive task when motor abnormalities (e.g., as in Parkinson's disease) and sensory deficits might limit her or his ability to complete the testing within specified time boundaries.

The administration of neuropsychological tests usually begins directly after the clinical interview. Selection of tests should be based on the following five factors: 1) the referral question, 2) level of functioning of the patient as ascertained during the clinical interview, 3) hypotheses regarding the differential diagnosis, 4) physical limitations of the patient, and 5) the need to document cognitive deficiencies and relative strengths. The latter point has relevance to the patient's ability to function in everyday life.

The selection of tests may differ based on individual patient needs. For example, older patients with severe cognitive or medical disturbances may lack the stamina or attentional capacity to undergo an intensive neuropsychological evaluation. For these patients, the selection of tests that tap specific domains of cognitive functioning in combination with the use of a more broad-based screening instrument may be the most useful approach. In contrast, a patient with relatively preserved cognitive abilities and without serious medical complications may be engaged in a more thorough cognitive assessment involving the in-depth assessment of multiple domains of neuropsychological functioning (Russell 1984). Regardless of the estimated level of cognitive functioning or the hypothesized nature of the cognitive impairment, we recommend the use of a brief cognitive screen as part of the interview process with the older patient. This permits not only an initial assessment of the patient's general cognitive capacity, but also provides direction for the selection of instruments to be used in the neuropsychological evaluation. The use of cognitive screening instruments within the more general context of the neuropsychological evaluation also promotes the comparison of test results across different testing sessions, even when the patient has deteriorated to a degree that precludes a more comprehensive evaluation (for a discussion of representative screening instruments and rating scales, see Chapter 6 in this volume).

Although brief screening instruments are extremely useful in detecting (i.e., diagnosing) the presence dementia

(Stuss et al. 1996), they do not provide information regarding functional abilities, placement and competency issues, or recommendations. These limitations should be considered when interpreting results based solely upon a brief screening instrument.

Various demographic variables can influence performance scores on brief screening instruments. For example, advanced age and lower education can produce an overestimate of cognitive impairments on the Mini-Mental State Exam (Malloy et al. 1997; Naugle and Kawczak 1989). Some have taken the step of renorming some of the existing screening tests to take age and education into account (e.g., Dementia Rating Scale; Lucas et al. 1998) to obtain better sensitivity (van Gorp et al. 1999). Others continue to develop new, highly focused, very brief screening instruments for memory loss in dementia (e.g., Memory Impairment Screen; Buschke et al. 1999). Moreover, others have found that brief screening instruments can be somewhat insensitive to mild forms of dementia (particularly the memory component), thus increasing Type II errors (false negatives) (Benedict and Brandt 1992; Pfeffer et al. 1981). Other screening instruments, such as the Neurobehavioral Cognitive Status Examination, or Cognistat (Kiernan et al. 1987), offer better delineation of the patient's cognitive deficits, but may not offer good discrimination for dementia type (van Gorp et al. 1999). Depending on the history and referral question, the use of a brief cognitive screening instrument to solely determine the need for further testing may cause an inaccurate assessment in either direction.

Approaches to the Neuropsychological Evaluation of Geriatric Patients

As a discipline, clinical neuropsychology is generally concerned with the study of brain-behavior relationships. However, clinical approaches to the assessment of these relationships vary widely (Kane 1991). Currently well-accepted strategies for neuropsychological assessment include the use of fixed batteries of neuropsychological tests, flexible evaluation strategies, and use of a combination of both of these approaches. It appears now, with the need to better define cognitive and behavioral deficits and changes associated with different dementia types, that appropriately choosing tests to suit the individual assessment may be the most productive method (Benton 1985; Costa 1983). In this section, we review the application of these different approaches with adults 65 years old or older (see Lezak 1995 and Russell 1998 for more detailed

discussions on using fixed versus flexible battery approaches).

Fixed Test Battery Approaches

In a fixed battery approach, the same test instruments or tests are administered to every patient in a standard manner regardless of the patient's presenting illness or referral question (Kane 1991; Kaszniak 1989). The two most popular neuropsychological batteries are currently the HRNB and the Luria-Nebraska Neuropsychological Battery (see Incagnoli et al. 1986; Lezak 1995). Advantages of the fixed battery approach to neuropsychological assessment include that it provides a comprehensive assessment of multiple cognitive domains and, because of its standardized format, that the test data can be incorporated into databases for clinical and scientific analysis. Disadvantages of the fixed battery approach include time and labor intensiveness and a lack of flexibility in different clinical situations.

Use of fixed test batteries with geriatric patients. A large literature exists on the psychometric properties of fixed batteries such as the HRNB (Anthony et al. 1980; Heaton and Pendleton 1981; Kane 1991; Parsons 1986; Reitan 1976; Reitan and Davison 1974; Reitan and Wolfson 1985) and the Luria-Nebraska Neuropsychological Battery (Golden and Maruish 1986; Golden et al. 1980; Kane 1991; Purisch and Sbordone 1986). However, relatively little empirical research exists regarding the psychometric properties of flexible or fixed battery approaches with the elderly population (Kaszniak 1989).

Halstead-Reitan Neuropsychological Battery. The HRNB represents one of the most popular battery approaches to neuropsychological assessment (Table 7–1). This battery measures cognitive functioning across a number of cognitive domains but is often too difficult for elderly individuals with more than mild cognitive impairment. Despite its widespread use in nongeriatric patients, the use of this battery with the elderly (as well as with younger patients) has been criticized (Fastenau and Adams 1996). Several studies have established age and education as important moderator variables for several of the battery's subtests (Heaton et al. 1986, 1991). Older or more poorly educated subjects were misclassified on the HRNB Impairment Index (a summary score based on seven different measures) as having brain damage more often than two other matched groups. Finally, the sample sizes for individual groups were not given in the published normative data, and evidence suggests that some of the normative groups had very few subjects in them (Fastenau and Adams 1996)

TABLE 7–1. Halstead-Reitan Neuropsychological Battery with measures of general intellect and memory

Halstead-Reitan Battery
    Tactual performance test
    Total time[a]
    Localization[a]
    Memory[a]
    Finger oscillation test (dominant hand)[a]
    Category test[a]
    Seashore rhythm test[a]
    Speech sounds perception test[a]
    Aphasia screening test
    Sensory-perceptual examination
    Strength of grip test
    Tactile form recognition test

General intelligence
    Wechsler Adult Intelligence Scale–Revised

Memory
    Wechsler Memory Scale–Revised

[a]These scores make up the Impairment Index.
Source.   Adapted from Heaton et al. 1991.

and that use of a regression model produced a higher rate of missed diagnoses (Fastenau 1998).

The principal concerns with reliance on the HRNB in assessment of older adults are 1) the HRNB may overestimate brain impairment in otherwise nonneurologically impaired older adults; 2) the amount of time and effort required to complete the HRNB may be inappropriate for elderly patients who are prone to fatigue easily; 3) the HRNB may not adequately assess both the strengths and weaknesses of the elder patient because it uses subtests that measure primarily fluid abilities (i.e., novel problem-solving, reasoning, and spatial processes) known to decline with normal aging; and 4) the HRNB potentially has poor psychometric properties, especially for older groups. For these reasons, some have argued against the use of the HRNB with the elderly (La Rue 1992).

Despite these concerns, some subtests from the HRNB are useful and included in neuropsychological evaluations. Subtests that can provide useful clinical information during an assessment include the Trail Making test (parts A and B) as a measure of cognitive flexibility and attention, the aphasia screening test as a gross measure of language, and the finger oscillation test as a measure of bilateral fine motor speed. Additionally, efforts have been made

to develop HRNB age and education corrections for older adults (see Heaton et al. 1991), and a short form of the HRNB has been developed (Storrie and Doerr 1980).[1]

Luria-Nebraska Neuropsychological Battery. The Luria-Nebraska Neuropsychological Battery yields a number of empirically derived summary scores (Table 7–2). This battery requires less time to administer than the HRNB (which takes 2–3 hours), thus minimizing any fatigue effect in elderly patients. However, some have argued that specific administration and scoring parameters of the Luria-Nebraska Neuropsychological Battery places the geriatric patient at an undue disadvantage, as well as potentially increasing the chance of misdiagnosis (Lezak 1995).

Flexible Approach to Neuropsychological Assessment

In using a flexible approach to neuropsychological testing, individual tests are chosen based upon the patient's presenting illness or referral question (Goodglass 1986; Kane 1991; Kaszniak 1989; Lezak 1995; Schear 1984). Primary advantages of the flexible approach to neuropsychological evaluation include a potentially shorter administration time, economical favorability, and adaptability to differing patient situations and needs. Some (Goodglass 1986; Russell 1984) have argued that the flexible approach permits better specification of the deficits within a given cognitive domain as well as their underlying neural systems rather than simply documenting the presence or absence of brain damage. Others use the flexible approach because it permits easy evaluation of qualitative features such as the patient's use of problem-solving strategies (Kaplan 1983). Finally, the flexible approach can be modified easily and therefore is adaptable to a wide variety of clinical situations (Kane 1991).

Disadvantages of the flexible approach include the need for greater clinical experience; a lack of standardization of administration rules for some tests, as well as the tests administered; a potential lack of comprehensiveness; and limitations in establishing systematic databases (Kane 1991; Tarter and Edwards 1986). Also, examiners who use the flexible battery approach may require more extensive clinical training and experience because the interpretation of test results involves qualitative results as well as quantitative data. An understanding of developmental normal aging, age-related cognitive decline, neuropsychological principles, neuropathological conditions in the elderly, and other issues pertinent to differential diagnosis are

---

[1] Some of these tests have published normative data, independent of the HRNB normative data (Heaton et al. 1991).

TABLE 7–2. Luria-Nebraska Neuropsychological Battery

Clinical scales

Scale 1 (Motor functions)
Scale 2 (Rhythm)
Scale 3 (Tactile functions)
Scale 4 (Visual functions)
Scale 5 (Receptive speech)
Scale 6 (Expressive speech)
Scale 7 (Writing)
Scale 8 (Reading)
Scale 9 (Arithmetic)
Scale 10 (Memory)
Scale 11 (Intellectual functions)
Scale 12 (Intermediate memory)

Summary scales

S1 (Pathognomonic)
S2 (Left hemisphere)
S3 (Right hemisphere)
S4 (Profile elevation)
S5 (Impairment)

Localization scales

L1 (Left frontal)
L2 (Left sensorimotor)
L3 (Left parietal-occipital)
L4 (Left temporal)
L5 (Right frontal)
L6 (Right sensorimotor)
L7 (Right parietal-occipital)
L8 (Right temporal)

Source. Adpated from Incagnoli et al. 1986.

particularly important when using the flexible neuropsychological assessment approach with elderly patients.

The flexible approach does not lend itself well to empirical investigation because of the individualized nature of the tasks and the difficulty comparing results across institutions or centers. However, this individualized approach to neuropsychological assessment remains popular with many neuropsychologists because of its adaptability, flexibility, clinical usefulness of qualitative information, efficiency with severely impaired patients, and applicability with patients who are vulnerable to fatigue, distress, or sensory limitations (Kane 1991; La Rue 1992). For these reasons, the flexible neuropsychological evaluation appears to be a useful, and possibly the best, approach for the clinical assessment of older adults (Benton 1985; Costa 1983).

Recently, test batteries and screening instruments have been designed specifically to address cognitive decline in the elderly patient, as well as test batteries or screens used for differential diagnosis of dementia type (Morris et al. 1989; see Lezak 1995 for a more detailed dis-

cussion). The distinction between a screening test for dementia and an extended mental status examination can be somewhat arbitrary. See Table 7–3 for a listing of a few tests used as screening instruments for dementia.

Individual Tests of Cognitive Functioning

Even when a flexible approach to neuropsychological assessment is adopted, a broad range of cognitive processes should be evaluated. The major domains of cognitive functioning that should be assessed include attention and concentration, general intelligence, conceptual processes and executive functioning, memory and learning, visuospatial skills, language, fine motor speed, coordination, strength, and emotional status (see Albert and Moss 1988; Russell 1984). In addition, we like to include the assessment of functional abilities in terms of completing activities of daily living, or ADLs, and to obtain ratings by relatives or significant others. We find that by including these last two areas to our comprehensive geriatric neuropsychological assessment, we are better able to address issues of competency, improve our ecological validity, better address ability to live alone, and obtain a more accurate picture of the individual's current functioning. Table 7–3 lists individual neuropsychological tests that are commonly used in evaluating the major domains of cognitive functioning in older adults. (A complete review of these cognitive domains and the instruments that measure them is beyond the scope of this chapter; for excellent reviews on this topic, see Albert and Moss 1988; La Rue 1992; LaRue and Swanda 1997; Lezak 1995.)

Assessment of Attentional Processes

After the informal assessment of the patient's basic level of arousal, alertness, and orientation, the patient's attentional capacity should be evaluated. Assessment of attention is necessary because attention is a prerequisite for successful performance in other cognitive domains (Albert 1981). If the patient appears to fatigue in the course of testing, it may be necessary to reassess attention to determine the effect of exhaustion on test performance.

Attention is not a unitary phenomenon; it is a multifactorial and complex cognitive activity. Attentional processes can be impaired in patients with delirium and with dementing disorders, but may also be significantly impaired in the geriatric patient with depression and in patients with focal brain lesions. For the purposes of the clini-

TABLE 7–3. Cognitive domains and representative neuropsychological tests

Attention
Digit Span (Wechsler Adult Intelligence Scale–Revised [WAIS-R; Wechsler 1981], Wechsler Memory Scale–Revised [WMS-R; Wechsler 1987])
Visual Memory Span (WMS-R)
Cancellation tests (number, letter, or figure)
Continuous Performance Test (Rosvold and Mirsky 1956; Loong 1988)
Stroop Test (Golden 1978)
Trail Making Test (see Reitan and Wolfson 1985)

Memory
WMS-R
California Verbal Learning Test (Delis et al. 1987)
Rey-Osterrieth Complex Figure Test (memory) (Osterrieth 1944)
Hopkins Verbal Learning Test (Brandt 1991)
Rey Auditory-Verbal Learning Test (Rey 1964)

Intelligence
WAIS-R

Executive functions
Category Test (see Reitan and Wolfson 1985)
Wisconsin Card Sorting Test (Berg 1948; Heaton 1981)
Tower of London (Shallice 1982)
Trail Making Test
Tinkertoy Test (Lezak 1983)
Porteus Maze Test (Porteus 1965)
Stroop Test
Executive Control Battery (Goldberg et al. 1996)

Language
Boston Diagnostic Aphasia Examination (Goodglass and Kaplan 1972)
Multilingual Aphasia Examination (Benton and Hamsher 1978)
Reitan-Indiana Aphasia Screening Test (see Reitan and Wolfson 1985)
Wepman Auditory Discrimination Test (Wepman and Jones 1961)

Visuospatial and visuomotor processes
Facial Recognition Test (see Benton et al. 1983)
Judgment of Line Orientation (see Benton et al. 1983)
Visual Form Discrimination Test (see Benton et al. 1983)
Benton Visual Retention Test (Benton 1974)
Rey-Osterrieth Complex Figure (copy) (Osterrieth 1944)

Motor processes
Finger Oscillation Test (see Reitan and Wolfson 1985)
Grooved Pegboard Test (Matthews and Kløve 1964)
Purdue Pegboard Test (Purdue Research Foundation 1948)
Strength of Grip Test (see Reitan and Wolfson 1985)

cal evaluation of the geriatric patient, it is useful to evaluate both verbal and nonverbal aspects of attention, as these components of attention can be variably impaired depending on the etiology of the cognitive dysfunction.

Auditory attentional processes are most readily assessed by the use of span procedures. The WMS-R and WMS-III have span procedures that are both auditorily and visually based. A verbally based procedure, called Digit Span, asks the patient to repeat auditorily presented strings of numbers in increasing length in both forward and backward order. The nonverbal, spatially analogous version, called Visual Span, requires the patient to repeat the tapping order of progressively longer sequences of colored boxes printed on a card, after watching the test administrator do so. The patient's ability to perform this task in both forward and backward order is evaluated. Letter and number cancellation tasks (Talland and Schwab 1964) can be used to assess visual attentional processes and require the patient to cross off designated stimuli on a sheet of paper within a short period of time. Visual cancellation tests are particularly useful in patients with hearing loss but are contraindicated in patients with decreased visual acuity.

Divided attention (i.e., the ability to ignore extraneous information, while focusing on specific stimuli) can be assessed by the Stroop Test (Golden 1978; Stroop 1935). This test first involves the presentation of a 100-item list of words, which the patient reads aloud. Next, the patient is required to name the colors of a series of Xs. Finally, the patient is presented with a list of words that are printed in a different color ink than the word implies and is asked to name the color of the ink, ignoring the word. For example, the word *Red* is presented in green ink and the patient must suppress the tendency to read the word rather than name the color. This test is considered to be a measure of executive functioning, as well as divided attention. Patents with frontal lobe lesions (Holst and Villki 1988) or mild to moderate dementia (Fisher et al. 1990) have demonstrated the Stroop effect (i.e., slowing on the interference trials). However, one particular problem about using this test in the elderly population is color discrimination. Occasionally, the elderly subject is not capable of adequately discriminating between the different colors used in the Stroop Test. A simple way of determining this is to randomly select some of the color Xs and ask the subject to name the color. If they can do this correctly, they are capable of completing the test. Similarly, the elderly subject's visual acuity may not be adequate, and this can be tested by asking the subject to read some of the words from the first trial.

Once the patient's ability to focus and sustain attention has been evaluated, the patient's level of cognitive functioning in other domains can be evaluated. If the patient's ability to attend is judged to be severely impaired, further neuropsychological assessment beyond a brief cognitive screen may not be useful.

Assessment of Intellectual Processes

Intellectual processes are differentially affected by the aging process and by dementing disorders. Overlearned crystallized intellectual functions (Cattell 1963) such as fund of general information and vocabulary development are often preserved, whereas the ability to use abstract reasoning and cognitive flexibility (fluid intelligence) usually declines both with normal aging and with disease-associated processes. The WAIS-R and WAIS-III are the most commonly used tests of general intelligence but either may take more than 2 hours to administer to an elderly patient, making it impractical in many cases. When the complete administration of the WAIS-R or WAIS-III is not possible because of limitations in the patient's stamina or severity of cognitive impairment, the administration of selected subtests can be useful. In particular, the Vocabulary and Information subtests are relatively good indicators of the patient's premorbid level of functioning. The ability to think abstractly is most commonly assessed through the use of the Similarities subtest of the WAIS-R, the Comprehension subtest provides a sample of the patient's judgment when placed in hypothetical situations, and Block Design measures visuoconstructive abilities. The Wechsler Abbreviated Scale of Intelligence (Psychological Corporation 1999) is a two or four subtest version of the WAIS-III with normative data extending into the eighth decade.

Memory

The evaluation of memory represents an extremely critical component of the neuropsychological assessment of the geriatric patient and can yield important diagnostic information. The patient's performance can help discriminate the effects of brain impairment from normal aging and can also help differentiate between psychiatric disorders (e.g., depression) and dementia etiology. For example, one dissociation of memory performance includes the difference between impaired free recall and recognition of recent information versus impaired free recall but relatively preserved recognition of recent information. Impaired free recall and recognition performance may be classified as a "pure amnesia" with concomitant dysfunction of encoding and storage. This type of memory loss is typically associated with medial-temporal lobe damage, particularly to the hippocampus, and is characteristic of Alzheimer's disease.

Impaired free recall with relatively preserved recognition performance suggests a retrieval deficit consistent with dysfunction of the frontal-subcortical circuitry and characteristic of subcortical dementias (Cummings 1992; Delis et al. 1991). However, some evidence shows that, when controlled for dementia severity, there may not be any difference in memory performance between Alzheimer's and multi-infarct dementia (La Rue 1989).

Both verbal and visuospatial memory should be assessed and may have relevance for the localization of brain dysfunction to either the left or right hemisphere, respectively. Verbal memory processes are most often assessed through the use of word lists that are presented a specified number of times or through the presentation of "stories" that the patient is asked to recall at some later time (i.e., immediately after presentation and after a 20-minute delay). The Rey Auditory-Verbal Learning Test (Rey 1964) and the California Verbal Learning Test (Delis et al. 1987) are commonly used list-learning tasks, although these tests are challenging because of the length of the lists (15 and 16 words, respectively) and the five required repetitions of the lists. These tests may be too difficult for geriatric patients who have more than a mild level of dementia or who have reduced stamina. The Hopkins Verbal Learning Test (HVLT) (Benedict et al. 1998; Brandt 1991) and California Verbal Learning Test—Dementia Version (Libon et al. 1996) may be preferable because they use shorter word lists and, in the case of HVLT, less number of repetitions. The most common story recall tasks used to evaluate verbal memory are taken from the WMS-R or WMS-III.

Evaluation of the patient's ability to learn and remember abstract spatial information is also an important component of the neuropsychological assessment process, and disruption of spatial memory relative to other test results may suggest right hemisphere dysfunction. Testing most often involves the reproduction and subsequent recall of abstract designs such as are provided by the Visual Reproduction subtest of the WMS-R or WMS-III, the Rey-Osterrieth Complex Figure Test (which is prone to floor effects in the elderly), and the Brief Visuospatial Memory Test—Revised (Benedict 1997). The Brief Visuospatial Memory Test—Revised is unique among published visuospatial memory tests in that it has multiple trials. This allows one to study the subject's visuospatial learning and thus can be compared to the subject's learning curve on a verbal word list–learning test.

In the evaluation of spatial memory, it is particularly important to dissociate the patient's ability to reproduce the designs (constructional disturbance) from memory, per se. One way of conveniently accomplishing this is by asking the patient to copy the design before the memory component of the evaluation is completed, such as in the administration of the Rey-Osterrieth Complex Figure Test. Figure 7–1 provides an example of severe constructional disturbance in a 77-year-old patient with suspected Alzheimer's disease. In addition, other assessment procedures such as the Benton Visual Retention Test (Benton 1992) allow separation of constructional disturbance from impairment of spatial memory by providing normative data for both the reproduction (i.e., copy) and retention of figural information, separately. Finally, nonverbal memory can be assessed by using a recognition paradigm. Here the subject is exposed to a series of geometric stimuli. This is followed by a long series of geometric designs. Most are new (e.g., not part of the initial stimuli shown to the subject previously), but some repeat (e.g., the designs shown initially). The subject is asked to say "yes" if the stimulus looks familiar and "no" if it does not. This type of paradigm has absolutely no graphomotor component, but it also has no free recall component (Paolo et al. 1998).

Remote memory, also referred to as *tertiary memory*, refers to the recall of events that occurred during the early years of one's life (La Rue 1992). Interestingly, older adults typically report the ability to recall events from remote memory (e.g., names of grade school teachers), while complaining of anterograde memory loss for recent events (e.g., what they had for lunch that day). Traditional measures of remote memory include the Famous Faces Test or Famous Events Test (see Lezak 1995), which assess the individual's ability to recall famous faces or events during different decades of the 20th century.

As found with measures of new learning (e.g., word list learning), performance on tests of remote memory can differentiate between cortical (e.g., Alzheimer's disease) and subcortical (e.g., Huntington's disease) dementias. The former tends to show the typical temporal gradient in recall of past events (better recall the older the event), whereas the latter tends to be equally impaired across decades. A similar explanation of poor consolidation versus retrieval, respectively, has been proposed (see Salmon and Bondi 1997). The assessment of remote memory is difficult because the examiner is usually uncertain about the amount of initial exposure or the subsequent rehearsal of this information the subject had with the stimuli (Craik 1977). In other words, what may appear as remote memory failure in a given patient may actually be a lack of exposure to the event in question or even possibly an anterograde amnesia that developed at an earlier time. Research documents significant age differences in a comparison of remote memory (public events) between young, middle-aged, and older adults (Howes and Katz 1988). Specifically, the elderly group demonstrated significantly poorer performance in recall of remote events during the time periods when both groups had lived. However, the elderly demonstrated consistent recall across the five decades.

The issue of whether older subjects demonstrate consistent recall across decades remains a controversial issue (Squire 1974; Warrington and Sanders 1971). Overall, remote memory appears to be affected by age, but this finding should continue to be interpreted with caution because methodological differences remain across studies (La Rue 1992).

In summary, assessment of memory in the geriatric patient should be thorough, encompassing aspects of learning, retention, and recognition as well as remote memory. This is important because it aids in differential diagnosis and also because various components of memory deferentially decline with age (see Lezak 1995).

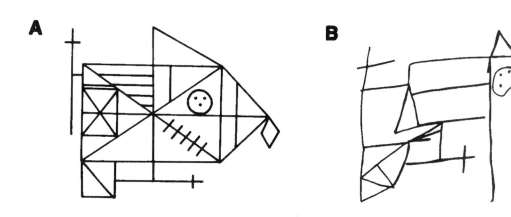

FIGURE 7–1.   Rey-Osterrieth Complex Figure Test (*panel A*) and reproduction of this figure by a 77-year-old man with suspected Alzheimer's disease (*panel B*). The patient's copy of the figure demonstrates severe impairment of visuoconstructional processes often associated with parietal lobe damage.

Executive Functioning

Along with memory, executive control skills show significant decline with normal aging (Libon et al. 1994; see La Rue 1992). In fact, some have postulated that the cognitive changes in normal aging are most pronounced in executive control functioning (Mittenberg et al. 1989). This may be due to greater cortical (Terry et al. 1987) and neurotransmitter (Carlsson 1981; Goldman-Rakic and Brown 1981) loss in the frontal lobe, as well as a greater decline in metabolic activity (Shaw et al. 1984; Smith 1984). This indicates that age-appropriate normative data on measures of executive control are highly relevant to an older population. It also suggests that just simply "renorming" an existing test of executive control may be somewhat problematic. Renorming the test for older patients who are known to decline on that measure increases the chance of that test's having poor psychometric properties for the older population. For example, the WCST is the typical "gold standard" for assessing executive control skills. However, it is particularly prone to floor effects in older populations and thus loses its clinical utility.

Executive control functioning is a constellation of multicompartmental cognitive skills that encompasses mental planning and organization, novel problem solving (e.g., cognitive flexibility), set development and shifting, and error monitoring. These components can be assessed individually or in combination. The WCST is used to assess cognitive flexibility (e.g., novel problem solving) and set shifting. However, as mentioned previously, it may have poor clinical utility in older patients. Tests such as Trail Making can be used to assess sequencing and visual search skills, although these skills also decline sharply with advancing age. Planning can be assessed through a qualitative analysis of how the patient approaches tasks such as the Block Design subtest of the WAIS-R or WAIS-III or the Rey-Osterrieth Complex Figure (Meyers and Meyers 1995; Osterrieth 1944) (Figure 7–1). Planning also may be evaluated formally using the Tinkertoy Test (Lezak 1983), which requires the patient to build a design using a 50-piece Tinkertoy set. The test has shown good construct validity as a measure of executive control functioning (Mahurin et al. 1993) and sensitivity to detecting dementia (Koss et al. 1998) and dementia type (Mendez and Ashla-Mendez 1991).

Two additional measures of executive control functioning that are showing promising results in the clinical assessment of elderly patients are the Executive Control Battery (ECB) (Goldberg et al. 1996) and Cognitive Bias Test (CBT). ECB was designed to quantify the qualitative features of executive dyscontrol as developed by A. R. Luria

and E. Goldberg. The ECB consists of four relatively simple subtests: Competing Programs, Manual Postures, Graphical Sequences, and Motor Programming. The subtests are quick and easy to administer and can be given individually. The battery measures perseveration, field dependency, impulsivity, and sequencing errors. The battery, or portions of it, is sensitive to prefrontal lesions (Podell et al. 1992a, 1992b; Zimmerman et al. 1994), the decline in executive control associated with advanced normal aging (Libon et al. 1994), and the differential effects of Alzheimer's versus cerebrovascular dementia on graphomotor perseverations (Lamar et al. 1997). See Figure 7–2 for examples of graphomotor perseverations elicited on the Graphical Sequences subtest of ECB.

The CBT is an innovative computerized test that assess the subject's response preference along a continuum of context-dependent/independent responding. For example, after being presented with a stimulus, does the subject use it as a context for which to make a subsequent judgment (context dependent)? Or does the subject make all choices independent of any context (i.e., context independent)? CBT performance is sensitive to prefrontal functions with laterality and sexual dimorphic effects (Goldberg et al. 1994; Podell et al. 1995). Research in an elderly population has shown this test's sensitivity to the disease progression in Alzheimer's disease (Goldberg et al. 1997).

Visuospatial and Visuoconstructive Processes

Just as it is important to separate disorders of visual memory from difficulties secondary to impairment of constructional processes, it is also necessary to separate disorders of visuospatial analysis from those of visuoconstructive processes. This dissociation can have localizing value, aid in differential diagnosis, and address functional abilities. The separation of these different, but related, neuropsychological processes can be most effectively accomplished by comparing the results of constructional tasks such as Block Design from the WAIS-R or WAIS-III to performance on motor-free spatial tasks such as the Visual Form Discrimination Test, Judgment of Line Orientation, and Facial Recognition tests developed by Benton and his colleagues (Benton et al. 1983). The Rey-Osterrieth Complex Figure Test, used in combination with these motor-free tasks, can be useful in separating visuospatial from visuoconstructive deficits. Poor performance in copying the figure, with better performance on motor-free tests, suggests a constructional rather than visuospatial disorder. We find a clock-drawing test (command and copy trials) useful in distinguishing between visuospatial, constructional, and

Hyperkinetic Perseverations - The elementary motor act cannot be terminated.

Item:	cross	circle	square	cross
Response:				

Perseveration of Elements - The substitution, or addition, of a previously occurring element, or part of an element, into the current response.

Item:	cross	cross	circle	square
Response:				

Perseveration of Features - No specific component of the element is perseverated. Instead a general characteristic, or feature, of the element intrudes upon the present response.

Item:	triangle	cross	square	cross
Response:				

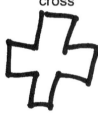

FIGURE 7–2. Types of graphomotor perseverations from the Graphical Sequences subtest of the Executive Control Battery.

executive control (planning) components. This test is relatively quick and easy to administer and has been extensively studied in dementia (Freedman et al. 1994).

One caveat we would like to add addresses the issue of primary vision and assessment of visuospatial and constructional abilities. The examiner must be aware of, and sensitive to, the patient's primary visual acuity (e.g., effects from glaucoma, cataracts, and macular degeneration). We recommend a cursory visual acuity check (e.g., using a Snellen eye chart) for all geriatric patients undergoing any neuropsychological testing using visual stimuli. One must consider the utility of administering these tasks, or the need for using enlarged stimuli, if the patient's primary visual acuity is poor.

Speech and Language

Clinical evaluation of speech and language processes is also a necessary component in the neuropsychological evaluation of geriatric patients. Language processes in the elderly can be affected by the normal aging process (Albert and Moss 1988), depression (Speedie et al. 1990), and dementia (Hill et al. 1989), and a thorough evaluation of language can help differentiate these disorders clinically. In particular, disorders of object naming (tested by presenting the patient with pictures of common objects) have been found to be associated with dementing illness (Albert 1981; Hill et al. 1989) and, to a lesser degree, with cognitive impairment secondary to depression (Speedie et al. 1990).

Other aspects of language should also be assessed during the neuropsychological evaluation, including comprehension and verbal fluency, as well as reading and writing. Verbal fluency can be easily assessed via the Animal Naming subtest of the Boston Diagnostic Aphasia Examination (Goodglass and Kaplan 1972) or the Controlled Oral Word Association Test (Benton and Hamsher 1978). Both types of verbal fluency tests provide the patient with 1 minute to produce as many words that fall under the category of "animals" or that begin with a specific letter. The total number of words generated by the patient in 1 minute represents a total verbal fluency score and is compared to age-appropriate normative data. Comparison between the two fluency tasks can distinguish between a primary deficit in lexical-semantic accessing versus an impairment in executive control functioning. For example, impaired performance on novel fluency (e.g., a specific letter) but intact semantic fluency is an indication of executive dyscontrol (e.g., poor novel generation). The converse, intact fluency for a novel cue but impaired animal naming, is indicative of impaired lexical-semantic accessing skills. The Aphasia Screening Test (Halstead and Wepman 1959) from the HRNB is also useful and provides a brief assessment of multiple aspects of language, as well as allowing an evaluation of basic reading, writing, and calculation abilities.

Motor Processes and Psychomotor Speed

Although motor speed and coordination decrease with normal aging, impairment of motor processes can also signal underlying neuropathological process. Decreased motor strength or speed can suggest a lateralized brain lesion, such as a stroke, tumor, or metastases, or may occur as part of a dementing disorder. In addition, a disruption in the ability to produce complex motor acts (e.g., dressing and eating) may represent an apraxia and may point to dysfunction of specific brain systems. Finally, evidence indicates that tests of impairments in fine and complex motor skills are almost as sensitive as other cognitive measures in differentiating between healthy normal and the mild, early stages of dementia (Kluger et al. 1997).

Motor speed is most commonly evaluated through the use of the Finger Oscillation Test (Finger Tapping) from the HRNB, the Grooved Pegboard Test (Matthews and Kløve 1964), or Purdue Pegboard Test (Purdue Research Foundation 1948). In general, better performance is expected of the dominant (usually right) hand relative to the nondominant hand, and the reversal of this pattern can help to localize a brain lesion to the contralateral hemisphere. The cautions concerning the use of age-appropriate norms are particularly germane to a discussion of the evaluation of motor processes. Comparison of an elderly patient's performance on a motor task to that of a younger normative group will result in spurious and misleading information. Finally, the examiner must be attuned to the contribution of peripheral factors upon motor performance. Peripheral, or non–central nervous system, diseases such as gout, arthritis, or peripheral neuropathies all effect motor performance and, if not taken into consideration, can lead to erroneous and incorrect interpretations.

Daily Functional Abilities

Direct assessment of functional abilities (i.e., instrumental activities of daily living, or IADLs) has become increasingly more important in neuropsychological test batteries. Therefore, some clinicians now advocate the assessment of functional capacity by using instruments specifically designed for this purpose (La Rue and Swanda 1997). Additionally, such instruments play an important role in determining level of legal competency, which has become an increasingly more frequent referral question in neuropsychological assessments of older adults (Grisso 1994).

Functional abilities can be assessed through individual or collateral interviews or questionnaires (e.g., the Instrumental Activities of Daily Living Scale [Lawton and Brody 1969] and the Blessed Dementia Rating Scale [Blessed et al. 1968]) or by direct evaluation of the patient. However, evidence indicates that individual or collateral reports do not correlate well with actual performance (see Grisso 1994). Having a subject actually perform the given tasks or the requisite skills needed for the task is a more accurate and valid assessment of his or her functional abilities.

In our clinic, we have recently incorporated the direct assessment of functional abilities as part of our standard geriatric assessment. Specifically, we have used the Independent Living Scales (ILS) (Loeb 1996). Through a series of verbal responses and actual task completion (e.g., writing a check or using a telephone), the ILS assesses several different areas—Memory/Orientation, Managing Money, Managing Home and Transportation, Health and Safety, and Social Adjustment—vital to independent functioning and competency. The instrument is well normed and has been extensively validated on several different populations. In fact, unpublished data from our clinic (Baird et al. 1999) has shown a strong correlation ($r = .73$) between performance on the ILS and level of dementia as assessed on the Dementia Rating Scale.

Use of Neuropsychological Testing in Differential Diagnosis

As highlighted throughout this chapter, geriatric patients are at risk for a number of neuropathological disorders that affect cognitive functioning, which are often difficult to distinguish clinically. Although the neuropsychological evaluation can often be helpful in the differential diagnosis of neurological disorders, it must be emphasized that the results of neuropsychological testing should not be interpreted "in a vacuum," but should be integrated with other diagnostic information gathered within the broader context of the neuropsychiatric evaluation. This should involve a thorough medical, social, and psychiatric history; mental status examination; the application of appropriate neuroimaging technologies; and appropriate laboratory studies. With these guidelines in mind, we briefly review the use of neuropsychological testing in the differential diagnostic process. For a more detailed review, see La Rue 1992.

Dementia

Dementing disorders are not a homogeneous group of conditions; they vary greatly with regard to etiology, neurological substrate, disease course, and treatment (see Chapters 19, 20, and 24 in this volume). Therefore, it is not surprising that different types of dementia are associated with different neuropsychological profiles (Table 7–4).

One of the more recent developments in the differential diagnosis of dementia is a new classification of individuals who do not conform to a formal diagnosis of dementia (i.e., impairment in multiple cognitive domains) but have a circumscribed memory impairment greater than what can be expected for their age and background. This classification has been termed *mild cognitive impairment* or MCI (Flicker et al. 1991; Petersen et al. 1999). MCI is considered a transitional period between normal aging and the

development of dementia (usually the Alzheimer's variant). However, there is debate whether all individuals diagnosed with MCI develop dementia.

The neuropsychological profile of Alzheimer's disease is most often characterized by impairment of memory, executive control, visuospatial processes, intellectual processes, complex motor skills, and language, although impairment in all of these areas may not be present in every patient, particularly early in the disease. Memory impairment is usually the first sign of the disorder, although detailed neuropsychological evaluation may reveal subtle deficits in other areas (e.g., executive functioning). Dysnomia, decreased verbal fluency, and poor semantic processing are also common, even early in the disease process. The memory impairment is characterized by a relatively spared span of apprehension (as measured by the Digit Span procedure) but marked impairment in the retention of newly learned material. Intrusive errors (i.e., the inclusion of extraneous items, usually semantically related) are common both on list learning (Delis et al. 1991) and story recall tasks.

Early in Alzheimer's disease, often subtle impairment of mental flexibility and executive functioning may be viewed by the patient (and by his or her family) as being part of the normal aging process. Visuospatial impairment may be evident in the patient's drawings and may range from mild distortions of designs to a complete inability to repro-

TABLE 7–4. Profiles of neuropsychological dysfunction in elderly patients

Syndrome	Neuropsychological profile
Alzheimer's disease	Impaired recent memory, intrusive errors on list-learning tasks, poor performance on memory recognition and retention measures, impaired naming and other signs of aphasia, visuospatial processing deficits, general intellectual decline, apraxia, and agnosia (in advanced illness)
Frontotemporal dementias	Executive functioning deficits (perseveration, impaired planning, stimulus boundedness, impaired synthesis, impaired mental flexibility), reduced fluency (verbal and nonverbal), impaired insight, marked personality change early in illness characterized by apathy and inertia, impaired selective attention, and relatively preserved memory
Vascular dementia	"Patchy" pattern of deficits depending on location of infarcts, general intellectual decline over time, stepwise decline in cognitive functioning over time, and lateralized cognitive deficits depending on site of infarct or infarcts
Subcortical dementias	Psychomotor slowing, prominent memory impairment, speech or motor-system difficulties, impaired concept formation and mental flexibility, impaired insight, and depression
Dementia with Lewy bodies	Progressive insidious cognitive decline; pronounced fluctuations in attention and arousal; recurrent, well-formed, and detailed visual hallucinations; motor features consistent with parkinsonism; and usually neuroleptic sensitivity
Dementia syndrome of depression	Mildly impaired naming, impaired attentional processes, and immediate memory but intact depression retention of new material, normal primacy effects on memory tasks, normal learning curve on list-learning tasks, normal retrieval and recognition of material, and intact visuospatial processing

duce even simple two-dimensional copies. At later stages in the disease, more severe impairment of intellectual processes is observed, and agnosia and apraxia are often seen. Severe visuospatial impairment may take the form of an inability to tell time on an analogue clock or by spatial disorientation. This problem can become so severe that the patient is unable to find his or her room consistently. Personality and affective changes are common, especially in the later stages. Sundowning is often associated with Alzheimer's disease in the mid to late stages of the disease.

The label *frontotemporal dementia* is used to describe a number of disorders (such as Pick's disease, progressive subcortical gliosis, and dementia of the frontal lobe type) that primarily affect the prefrontal and temporal regions of the brain. Frontotemporal dementia is most often characterized by marked insidious personality change and impairment of executive functioning affecting all aspects of cognition (Cummings 1992; Moss et al. 1992). Although memory impairments can be present, they are usually associated with a preponderance of an executive control impairment (e.g., poor retrieval).

Unlike dementia of the Alzheimer type, the first signs of frontotemporal dementia are usually neuropsychiatric rather than cognitive in nature. Personality changes can be characterized by two distinct behavioral syndromes: apathy and behavioral inertia in the dorsolateral syndrome or hypomanic-like, puerile, sometimes irritable disinhibition in the orbitofrontal variant (Fuster 1989). Executive functioning impairment takes the form of perseveration, abulia or lack of initiation, stimulus boundedness (or field dependency), impaired synthesis and planning, and poor error monitoring. In contrast to those with the dementia of Alzheimer's disease, patients with frontotemporal dementia often have preserved visuospatial abilities and relatively better preserved memory functions (Neary and Snowden 1991). Although basic motor processes are usually intact, executive processes that involve a significant motor component are typically impaired. Language comprehension and expression are often preserved, but echolalia and a progressive expressive aphasia can develop. The neuropsychiatric and cognitive difficulties seen in frontotemporal dementia can become so severe as to limit the patient's ability to complete a comprehensive evaluation. Short bedside procedures are often useful and should be part of the mental status examination (see Chapter 6 in this volume).

Vascular dementia refers to a group of dementing disorders of a cerebrovascular nature consisting of an abrupt onset with a stepwise decline over time. Vascular dementia is characterized by "patchy" performance on neuropsychological measures with islands of preserved and impaired performance, depending on the site of the infarct(s) or ischemia. As the disease progresses, a stepwise decline in cognitive functioning is typically observed and can be documented through serial neuropsychological evaluations. Left hemisphere lesions often result in language and verbal memory impairment, whereas right hemisphere lesions result in greater impairment of visuospatial processes and visual memory. Small infarcts that do not affect motor or speech areas may go unnoticed by the patient or family but can be documented through neuroimaging and neuropsychological evaluation.

The subcortical dementias are a group of disorders that are characterized by primary dysfunction in subcortical brain areas. Unlike dementing conditions that primarily affect cortical areas, leading to aphasia, apraxia, agnosia, and anomia, subcortical dementia features motor dysfunction, speech impairment, memory dysfunction, characterized primarily by deficits in retrieval (Delis et al. 1991), executive disorders, and disturbances in mood and personality (Cummings 1985). Subcortical dementia occurs with extrapyramidal syndromes such as Parkinson's disease, Wilson's disease, progressive supranuclear palsy, multisystems atrophy, and Huntington's disease. Although there is often a general decline in intellectual processes over time, this decline is usually much less severe than in other dementing disorders. Performance on neuropsychological testing in Parkinson's disease varies across patients, but deficits are often found on tests that require psychomotor speed, visuospatial processing, executive functioning, and memory (Pirozzolo et al. 1982). In addition, performance may be impaired on tests that measure concept formation and problem solving in new situations (Matthews and Haaland 1979), category fluency, and mental flexibility (Beatty et al. 1989).

Patients with Huntington's disease often exhibit executive functioning impairment that involves difficulty with mental flexibility and abstraction but with relatively preserved "overlearned" verbal skills (i.e., on the Information and Vocabulary subtests on the WAIS-R). Memory impairment also commonly occurs with Huntington's disease and is characterized by impairment in the acquisition and retrieval of new information, as well as by impaired remote memory later in the disease process (Albert et al. 1981). In contrast with patients with Alzheimer's disease, who are characterized by dysnomia, patients with Huntington's disease can exhibit normal performance on confrontation naming tests (Butters et al. 1978).

Dementia with Lewy bodies (DLB) is a progressive, degenerative dementia that is often overlooked when making a differential diagnosis of dementia type, but one that has important implications for appropriate treatment (McKeith et al. 1996; for a review, see Hansen and Galasko

1992). As many as 15%–25% of patients undergoing autopsy may have Lewy bodies present in the brainstem and cerebral cortex. The core cognitive features include progressive, insidious cognitive decline with pronounced fluctuations in attention and arousal; recurrent, typically well-formed and detailed visual hallucinations; and motor features consistent with parkinsonism. Memory deficits may not be evident in the early stages, but impairments in executive control and visuospatial and visuomotor skills are mostly likely early prominent features. Other supportive features include syncope, repeated falls, hallucinations in various modalities, and fixed delusional system(s). Patients with DLB are usually neuroleptic sensitive, which in fact is considered a core feature in diagnosis. This is very important in terms of psychiatric treatment. Elderly patients who present with recent onset of a fixed delusional system with visual hallucinations should be considered for a diagnosis of DLB, and the use of a neuroleptic should be carefully considered (see McKeith et al. 1996).

Depression-Related Cognitive Dysfunction

It is estimated that from 10% to 20% of patients with depression have significant cognitive impairment (Reynolds and Hoch 1988). In addition, depression frequently accompanies neurological disorders such as Alzheimer's disease (Kaszniak 1987), stroke (Robinson and Price 1982), and extrapyramidal diseases such as Parkinson's and Huntington's (Cummings 1985). The labels *pseudodementia* (Kiloh 1961), *dementia syndrome of depression* (Folstein and McHugh 1978), *depression-induced organic mental disorder* (McAllister 1983), and *depression-related cognitive dysfunction* (Stoudemire et al. 1989) have been used to describe the reversible cognitive impairment in elderly patients with depression. Since Kiloh's initial characterization of pseudodementia (1961), numerous articles have described the clinical features of cognitive impairment secondary to depression and its differentiation from progressive and irreversible conditions such as Alzheimer's disease (Bulbena and Berrios 1986; Cummings 1989; Jeste et al. 1990; Kaszniak 1987; see Christensen et al. 1997 and Veiel 1997 for reviews). Although the concept of depression-related cognitive impairment is well accepted and has had value in identifying potentially treatable forms of dementia, the term *pseudodementia* has come under criticism (Arie 1983; Lamberty and Bieliuskas 1993; Reifler 1982; Shraberg 1978, 1980). These criticisms have stemmed primarily from the implication that cognitive dysfunction secondary to depression does not represent a "real" or "organic" phenomenon. Additional criticisms have been based on the

lack of diagnostic specificity of the term and from the lack of utility of the concept in predicting response to treatment.

Understanding of the complexity of cognitive dysfunction in elderly patients with depression has increased substantially over the last decade, and an increasing number of systematic studies have been designed to assist in the separation of the potentially reversible (and treatable) dementia of depression from irreversible and often progressive conditions such as Alzheimer's disease and vascular dementia. Although currently no universally accepted neuropsychological template exists for the differentiation of depression-related cognitive dysfunction from cognitive impairment secondary to specific brain disease, research has suggested that neuropsychological test results may be useful in this regard. For example, several studies have pointed to the usefulness of confrontation naming tests, such as the Boston Naming Test (Kaplan et al. 1983), in the differential diagnostic process (Caine 1981; Hill et al. 1989; Petrick and Mittenberg 1992), although this finding has not been found by all researchers (Speedie et al. 1990). Further complicating the issue is research suggesting that depression might represent an early marker for later developing progressive dementia (Kral and Emery 1989; Nussbaum et al. 1991; Reding et al. 1985). Others have recommended that detailed historical information and behavioral features, along with qualitative aspects of neuropsychological performance, are helpful in making a differential diagnosis (Kaszniak and Christenson 1994).

Christenson et al. (1997) recently performed a meta-analysis of studies looking at the cognitive effects of depression. Two types of studies were analyzed: patients with depression versus psychiatrically healthy control subjects and patients with depression versus patients with Alzheimer's disease. Essentially, patients with depression show impaired performance across all cognitive domains with very little intact cognitive skills. One of the greatest effect size was in executive control skills. However, relative to psychiatrically healthy control subjects, patients with depression were mostly impaired on speeded tasks and vigilance tasks. No difference in the effect size was found when comparing free recall to recognition memory, semantic processing, or using verbal versus nonverbal material. Patients with depression were equivalent to those with Alzheimer's disease on recall compared with recognition and verbal compared with nonverbal processing and were significantly better in all other cognitive domains. The notion that the difference between depression and dementia (especially that of the Alzheimer's type) is a result of effortful (including speeded tasks) versus noneffortful tasks received some support in the meta-analysis. Thus, patients with depression being impaired only on effortful (and speeded) tasks, but patients with dementia being impaired on both effortful and noneffortful tasks (Hartlage et al. 1993), may have important use in the differential diagnosis between depression and dementia. But not all noneffortful tasks discriminated well. Also, the notion that recognition versus recall distinguished depression from dementia was not supported by the meta-analysis. The possibility that speed of processing or attentional components might distinguish depression from dementia was proposed by the authors. This was also supported by another meta-analysis that compared younger patients with depression to psychiatrically healthy control subjects (Veiel 1997). The issue of cognitive dysfunction in elderly patients with depression is a complicated one that deserves further study.

Ecological Validity of Neuropsychological Tests

Because neuropsychologists are increasingly asked to render decisions about functional capacity and competency of the elderly patient, ecological validity of standard neuropsychological tests is a central and important issue. Indeed, the utility of neuropsychological assessment lies not only in its ability to aid in the diagnostic process, but also in its capacity to provide information regarding the patient's ability to function in his or her natural environment. Neuropsychological test performance and outcome measures have only a moderate relationship (Acker 1990; Chelune and Moehle 1986), but have a greater predictive accuracy for functional skills demanding complex information processing, such as writing a check, than for basic functional capacity, such as performance of a personal hygiene skill (Baird et al. 1999; Goldstein et al. 1992; Loeb 1996; McCue et al. 1990; Rogers et al. 1994).

Even with the good predictive validity neuropsychological tests have for general functional abilities, little direct evidence indicates that neuropsychological test results can predict specific functional abilities such as driving or appropriate residential placement (see Blaustein et al. 1988; Kaszniak and Nussbaum 1990). Unfortunately, relatively few empirical data exist to support the predictive validity of neuropsychological test performance on these functional domains in older patients. The development of new neuropsychological tasks that more closely parallel ADLs is much needed (Zappala et al. 1989). Currently, decisions are more often based on estimates of the patient's performance on more traditional neuropsychological measures that have no direct corollary "in real life." In particu-

lar, decisions regarding the patient's ability to drive are often based on performance on visuospatial, attentional, memory, and executive functioning tasks, as these processes are generally thought to be requisite to the safe operation of an automobile. The development of ecologically valid neuropsychological tests to more directly assess the patient's ability to perform real-life activities requires continued attention and represents one of the biggest challenges for the field of geriatric neuropsychology. To this end, we see the direct assessment of functional abilities (such as the Independent Living Scale) as one method for trying to fill this void. We find that we are better able to address the issues of functional capacity and level of competency by using standardized neuropsychological tests in conjunction with the direct assessment of functional abilities. Although not a perfect solution, this certainly is a step in the right direction.

Conclusions and Future Directions

In this chapter, we have reviewed several important issues related to the neuropsychological assessment of older patients. First, the use of a flexible, individualized approach to neuropsychological assessment with older patients is advocated because it typically requires less time than standard fixed batteries, is cost-effective, and is patient driven, thus providing the opportunity to address specific cognitive deficits. Second, despite recent developments in geriatric neuropsychology, a continued need exists for empirical-clinical investigation of the utility of different evaluation approaches to the assessment of older adults. Third, age-appropriate normative data for individuals over the age of 74 are still inadequate. Although progress has been made in this area, a need for normative data for individuals in this age group remains. Fourth, the use of neuropsychological testing in the differential diagnosis of dementing illnesses, particularly subcortical versus cortical dementia and depression versus dementia, remains an important area deserving of continued attention. Fifth, the ecological validity of neuropsychological assessment is a relatively new area of concern that deserves sophisticated empirical investigation. Cognitive tests that predict the functional capacity of older patients are just being developed and incorporated into the formal neuropsychological test battery. They have the potential of adding valuable information in addressing a wide range of referral questions. Finally, continued specialized training of the clinical neuropsychologist in the assessment and treatment of older patients is needed.

References

Acker MB: A review of the ecological validity of neuropsychological tests, in The Neuropsychology of Everyday Life. Edited by Tupper DE, Cicerone KD. Boston, MA, Kluwer Academic, 1990, pp 19–55

Albert MS: Geriatric neuropsychology. J Consult Clin Psychol 49:835–850, 1981

Albert MS, Moss MB: Geriatric Neuropsychology. New York, Guilford, 1988

Albert MS, Butters N, Brandt J: Development of remote memory loss in patients with Huntington's disease. Journal of Clinical Neuropsychology 3:1–12, 1981

Anthony WZ, Heaton RK, Lehman RAW: An attempt to cross-validate two actuarial systems for neuropsychological test interpretation. J Consult Clin Psychol 48:317–326, 1980

Arie T: Pseudodementia. BMJ 286:1301–1302, 1983

Baird AD, Podell K, Lovell MR: Predicting functional status in older adults (abstract). Archives of Clinical Neuropsychology 14:44–45, 1999

Bayles KA, Tomoeda CK, Boone DR: A view of age-related changes in language function. Developmental Neuropsychology 1:231–264, 1985

Beatty W, Staton RD, Weir WS, et al: Cognitive disturbances in Parkinson's disease. J Geriatr Psychiatry Neurol 2:22–23, 1989

Benedict RHB: Brief Visuospatial Memory Test—Revised. Odessa, FL, Psychological Assessment Resources, 1997

Benedict RHB, Brandt J: Limitations of The Mini-Mental State Examination for the detection of amnesia. J Geriatr Psychiatry Neurol 5:233–237, 1992

Benedict RHB, Schretlen D, Groninger L, Brandt J: Hopkins Verbal Learning Test—Revised: Normative data and analysis of inter-form and test-retest reliability. Clinical Neuropsychologist 12:43–55, 1998

Benton AL: The Revised Visual Retention Test, 4th Edition. New York, Psychological Corporation, 1974

Benton AL: Some problems associated with neuropsychological assessment. Bulletin of Clinical Neurosciences 50:11–15, 1985

Benton AL: The Benton Visual Retention Test, 5th Edition. San Antonio, TX, Psychological Corporation, 1992

Benton AL, Hamsher K: Multilingual Aphasia Examination. Iowa City, IA, University of Iowa Press, 1978

Benton AL, Hamsher K, Varney N, et al: Contributions to Neuropsychological Assessment: A Clinical Manual. New York, Oxford University Press, 1983

Berg GE: A simple objective test for measuring flexibility in thinking. J Gen Psychol 39:15–22, 1948

Blaustein MJL, Filipp CL, Dungan C, et al: Driving in patients with dementia. J Am Geriatr Soc 36:1087–1091, 1988

Blessed G, Tomlinson BE, Roth M: The association between quantitative measures of dementia and senile change in the cerebral gray matter of elderly subjects. Br J Psychiatry 114:797–811, 1968

Brandt J: The Hopkins verbal learning test: development of a new memory test with six equivalent forms. Clinical Neuropsychologist 5:125–142, 1991

Bulbena A, Berrios GE: Pseudodementia: facts and figures. Br J Psychiatry 148:87–94, 1986

Buschke H, Kuslansky G, Katz M, et al: Screening for dementia with the Memory Impairment Screen. Neurology 52: 231–238, 1999

Butters N, Sax D, Montgomery K, et al: Comparison of the neuropsychological deficits associated with early and advanced Huntington's disease. Arch Neurol 35:585–589, 1978

Caine ED: Pseudodementia: current concepts and future directions. Arch Gen Psychiatry 38:1359–1364, 1981

Carlsson A: Aging and brain neurotransmitters, in Strategies for the Development of an Effective Treatment for Senile Dementia. Edited by Crook T, Gershon S. New Canaan, CT, Mark Powley Associates, 1981, pp 93–104

Cattell RB: Theory of fluid and crystallized intelligence: a critical experiment. Journal of Educational Psychology 54: 1–22, 1963

Chelune GJ, Moehle KA: Neuropsychological assessment and everyday functioning, in The Neuropsychology Handbook: Behavioral and Clinical Perspectives. Edited by Wedding AM, Horton J, Webster J. New York, Springer, 1986, pp 489–525

Christensen H, Griffiths K, MacKinnon A: A quantitative review of cognitive deficits in depression and Alzheimer's-type dementia. J Int Neuropsychol Soc 3:631–651, 1997

Costa L: Clinical neuropsychology: a discipline in evolution. J Clin Neuropsychol 5:1–11, 1983

Craik FIM: Age differences in human memory, in Handbook of the Psychology of Aging. Edited by Birren JE, Schaie KW. New York, Van Nostrand Reinhold, 1977, pp 384–420

Cummings JL: Clinical Neuropsychiatry. Orlando, FL, Grune & Stratton, 1985

Cummings JL: Dementia and depression: an evolving enigma. J Neuropsychiatry Clin Neurosci 1:236–242, 1989

Cummings JL: Neuropsychiatric aspects of Alzheimer's disease and other dementing illnesses, in The American Psychiatric Press Textbook of Neuropsychiatry, 2nd Edition. Edited by Yudofsky SC, Hales RE. Washington, DC, American Psychiatric Press, 1992, pp 605–620

Delis D, Kramer JH, Kaplan E, et al: The California Verbal Learning Test—Adult Version. San Antonio, TX, Psychological Corporation, 1987

Delis DC, Massman PJ, Butters N, et al: Profiles of demented and amnesic patients on the California Verbal Learning Test: implications for the assessment of memory disorders. Psychological Assessment 3:19–26, 1991

Drachman DA, Leavitt J: Human memory and the cholinergic system. A relationship to aging? Arch Neurol 30:113–121, 1974

Fastenau PS: Validity of regression-based norms: An empirical test of the comprehensive norms with older adults. J Clin Exp Neuropsychol 20:906–916, 1998

Fastenau PS, Adams KM: Heaton, Grant and Matthews' Comprehensive Norms: an overzealous attempt. J Clin Exp Neuropsychol 18:444–448, 1996

Fisher LM, Freed DM, Corkin S: Stroop-Color Word Test performance in patients with Alzheimer's disease. J Clin Exp Neuropsychol 12:745–758, 1990

Flicker C, Feris SH, Reisberg B: Mild cognitive impairment in the elderly: Predictors of dementia. Neurology 41:1006–1009, 1991

Folstein MF, McHugh PR: Dementia syndrome of depression, in Alzheimer's Disease: Senile Dementia and Related Disorders. Edited by Katzman R, Terry RD, Bick KL. New York, Raven, 1978, pp 281–289

Freedman M, Leach L, Kaplan E, et al: Clock Drawing: A Neuropsychological Analysis. New York, Oxford University Press, 1994

Fuster JM: The Prefrontal Cortex: Anatomy, Physiology, and Neuropsychology of the Frontal Lobe, 2nd Edition. New York, Raven, 1989

Goldberg E, Podell K, Harner R, et al: Cognitive bias, functional cortical geometry, and the frontal lobes: laterality, sex and handedness. J Cogn Neurosci 6:276–296, 1994

Goldberg E, Podell K, Bilder R, Jaeger J: The Executive Control Battery. Stockholm, PsychologiFöerlaget AB, 1996

Goldberg E, Kluger A, Malts L, et al: Assessment of early frontal-lobe dysfunction in dementia. Paper presented at the Eighth Congress of the International Psychogeriatric Association. Jerusalem, Israel, August 17–23, 1997

Golden CJ: The Stroop Color and Word Test: A Manual for Clinical and Experimental Use. Chicago, IL, Stoelting, 1978

Golden CJ, Maruish M: The Luria-Nebraska Neuropsychological Battery, in Neuropsychological Test Batteries. Edited by Incagnoli T, Goldstein G, Golden CJ. New York, Plenum, 1986, pp 193–227

Golden CJ, Hammeke TA, Purisch AD: The Luria-Nebraska Neuropsychological Battery Manual. Los Angeles, CA, Western Psychological Services, 1980

Goldman-Rakic PS, Brown RM: Regional changes of monamines in cerebral cortex and subcortical structures of aging rhesus monkeys. Neuroscience 6:177–187, 1981

Goldstein G, McCue M, Roger J, et al: Diagnostic differences in memory test based predictions of functional capacity in the elderly. Neuropsychological Rehabilitation 2:307–317, 1992

Goodglass H: The flexible battery, in Neuropsychological Assessment. Edited by Incagnoli T, Goldstein G, Golden CJ. New York, Plenum, 1986, pp 121–131

Goodglass H, Kaplan E: Assessment of Aphasia and Related Disorders. Philadelphia, PA, Lea & Febiger, 1972

Goreczny AJ, Nussbaum PD: Behavioral medicine with military veterans, in Progress in Behavior Modification. Edited by Hersen M, Eisler RM, Miller PM. Sycamore, IL, Sycamore Publishing Company, 1994, pp 99–119

Grisso T: Clinical assessment for legal competence of older adults, in Neuropsychological Assessment of Dementia and Depression in Older Adults: A Clinician's Guide. Edited by Storandt M, VandenBos GR. Washington, DC, American Psychological Association, 1994, pp 119–140

Halstead WC, Wepman JM: The Halstead-Wepman aphasia screening test. Journal of Speech and Hearing Disorders 14:9–15, 1959

Hansen LA, Galasko D: Lewy body disease. Current Opinion in Neurology and Neurosurgery 5:889–894, 1992

Hartlage S, Alloy LB, Vazquez C, Dykman B. Automatic and effortful processing in depression. Psychol Bull 113:247–278, 1993

Heaton RK: The Wisconsin Card Sorting Test Manual. Odessa, FL, Psychological Assessment Resources, 1981

Heaton RK, Pendleton MG: Use of neuropsychological tests to predict adult patient's everyday functioning. J Consult Clin Psychol 49:807–821, 1981

Heaton RK, Grant I, Matthews CG: Differences in neuropsychological test performance associated with age, education, and sex, in Neuropsychological Assessment of Neuropsychiatric Disorders. Edited by Grant I, Adams KM. New York, Oxford University Press, 1986, pp 100–120

Heaton RK, Grant I, Matthews CG: Comprehensive Norms for an Expanded Halstead-Reitan Battery. Odessa, FL, Psychological Assessment Resources, 1991

Heaton RK, Chelune GJ, Talley JL, et al: The Wisconsin Card Sorting Test Manual Revised and Expanded. Odessa, FL, Psychological Assessment Resources, 1993

Hill C, Stoudemire A, Morris R, et al: Dysnomia in the differential diagnosis of major depression, depression-related cognitive dysfunction, and dementia. J Neuropsychiatry Clin Neurosci 4:64–69, 1989

Hohl U, Grundman M, Salmon DP, et al: Mini-Mental State Examination and Mattis Dementia Rating Scale performance differs in Hispanic and Non-Hispanic Alzheimer's disease patients. J Int Neuropsychol Soc 4:301–307, 1999

Holst P, Vilkki J: Effects of frontomedial lesions on performance on the Stroop Test and word fluency tasks (abstract). J Clin Exp Neuropsychol 10:79, 1988

Howes JL, Katz AN: Assessing remote memory with an improved public events questionnaire. Psychol Aging 3:142–150, 1988

Incagnoli T, Goldstein G, Golden CJ (eds): Neuropsychological Test Batteries. New York, Plenum, 1986

Ivnik RV, Malec JF, Smith GE, et al: Mayo's older American study. Clinical Neuropsychologist 6:1–30, 1992

Jeste DV, Gierz M, Harris MJ: Pseudodementia: myths and realities. Psychiatric Annals 20:71–79, 1990

Kane R: Standardized and flexible batteries in neuropsychology: an assessment update. Neuropsychol Rev 2:281–339, 1991

Kaplan E: Process and achievement revisited, in Towards a Holistic Developmental Psychology. Edited by Wapner S, Kaplan B. Hillsdale, NJ, Lawrence Erlbaum Associates, 1983, pp 143–156

Kaplan EF, Goodglass H, Weintraub S: The Boston Naming Test. Philadelphia, PA, Lea & Febiger, 1983

Kaszniak AW: Neuropsychological consultation to geriatricians: issues in the assessment of memory complaints. Clinical Neuropsychologist 1:35–46, 1987

Kaszniak AW: Psychological assessment of the aging individual, in Handbook of the Psychology of Aging. Edited by Birren JE, Schaie KW. San Diego, CA, Academic Press, 1989, pp 427–445

Kaszniak AW, Christenson GD: Differential diagnosis of dementia and depression, in Neuropsychological Assessment of Dementia and Depression. Edited by Storandt M, VandenBos GR. Washington, DC, American Psychological Press, 1994, pp 81–118

Kaszniak AW, Nussbaum PD: Driving in older patients with dementia and depression. Paper presented at the annual meeting of the American Psychological Association, Boston, MA, August 1990

Kiernan RJ, Mueller J, Langston JM, Van Dyke C: The Neurobehavioral Cognitive Status Examination: a brief differentiated approach to cognitive assessment. Ann Intern Med 107:481–485, 1987

Kiloh LG: Pseudo-dementia. Acta Psychiatr Scand 37:336–351, 1961

Kluger A, Gianutsos JG, Golomb J, et al: Motor/psychomotor dysfunction in normal aging, mild cognitive decline, and early Alzheimer's disease: diagnostic and differential diagnostic features. Int Psychogeriatr 9 (suppl 1):307–316, 1997

Koss E, Patterson MB, Mack JL, et al: Reliability and validity of The Tinkertoy Test in evaluating individuals with Alzheimer's disease. Clinical Neuropsychologist 12:325–329, 1998

Kral VA, Emery OB: Long-term follow-up of depressive pseudo-dementia of the aged. Can J Psychiatry 34:445–446, 1989

La Rue A: Patterns of performance on the Fuld Object Memory Evaluation in elderly inpatients. J Clin Exp Neuropsychol 11:409–422, 1989

La Rue A: Aging and Neuropsychological Assessment. New York, Plenum, 1992

La Rue A, Swanda R: Neuropsychological assessment, in Handbook of Neuropsychology and Aging. Edited by Nussbaum PD. New York, Plenum, 1997, pp 360–384

Lamberty CJ, Bieliuskas LA: Distinguishing between depression and dementia in the elderly: a review of neuropsychological findings. Archives of Clinical Neuropsychology 8:149–170, 1993

Lawton MP, Brody EM: Assessment of older people: self-maintaining and instrumental activities of daily living. Gerontologist 9:179–186, 1969

Lemar M, Podell K, Giovannetti T, et al: Perseverative behavior in Alzheimer's disease and subcortical ischaemic vascular dementia. Neuropsychology 11: 523–534, 1997

Lezak M: Neuropsychological Assessment, 3rd Edition. New York, Oxford University Press, 1995

Libon DJ, Glosser G, Malamut BL, et al: Age, executive functions, and visuo-spatial functioning in healthy older adults. Neuropsychology 8:38–43, 1994

Libon DJ, Mattson RE, Glosser G, et al: A nine-word dementia version of The California Verbal Learning Test. Clinical Neuropsychologist 10:237–244, 1996

Lichtenberg PA, Ross TP, Youngblade L, et al: Normative studies research project test battery: detection of dementia in African American and European American elderly patients. Clinical Neuropsychologist 12:146–154, 1998

Loeb PA: The Independent Living Scales. San Antonio, TX, Psychological Corporation, 1996

Loong WK: The Continuing Performance Test. San Luis Obispo, CA, Wang Neuropsychological Laboratory, 1988

Lucas JA, Ivnik RJ, Smith GE, et al: Normative data for the Mattis Dementia Rating Scale. J Clin Exp Neuropsychol 20:536–547, 1998

MacInnes WD, Gillen RW, Golden CJ, et al: Aging and performance on the Luria-Nebraska Neuropsychological Battery. Int J Neurosci 19:179–190, 1983

Mahurin RK, Flanagan AM, Royall DR: Neuropsychological measures of executive function in frail elderly patients. Arch Clin Neuropsychology 7:356, 1993

Malloy PF, Cummings JL, Coffey CE, et al: Cognitive screening instruments in neuropsychiatry: a report of The Committee on Research of The American Neuropsychiatric Association. J Neuropsychiatry Clin Neurosci 9:189–197, 1997

Manly JJ, Jacobs DM, Sano M, et al: Effect of literacy on neuropsychological test performance in nondemented, education-matched elders. J Int Neuropsychol Soc 5: 191–202, 1999

Marcopulos BA, McLain CA, Giuliano AJ: Cognitive impairment or inadequate norms? A study of healthy, rural, older adults with limited education. Clinical Neuropsychologist 11:111–131, 1997

Matthews CG, Haaland KY: The effect of symptom duration on cognitive and motor performance in parkinsonism. Neurology 29:951–956, 1979

Matthews CG, Kløve H: Instruction Manual for the Adult Neuropsychological Text Battery. Madison, WI, University of Wisconsin Medical School Press, 1964

Mattis S. Dementia Rating Scale (DRS). Odessa, FL, Psychological Assessment Resources, 1988

McAllister TW: Overview: pseudodementia. Am J Psychiatry 140:528–533, 1983

McCue M, Rogers J, Goldstein G: Relationships between neuropsychological and functional assessment in elderly neuropsychiatric patients. Rehabilitation Psychology 35: 91–95, 1990

McKeith IG, Galasko D, Kosaka K, et al: Consensus guidelines for the clinical and pathologic diagnosis of dementia with Lewy bodies (DLB): report of the consortium on DLB international workshop. Neurology 47:1113–1124, 1996

Mendez MF, Ashla-Mendez M: Difference between multiinfarct dementia and Alzheimer's disease on unstructured neuropsychological tasks. J Clin Exp Neuropsychol 13: 923–932, 1991

Meyers JE, Meyers KR: Rey Complex Figure Test and Recognition Trial. Odessa, FL, Psychological Assessment Resources, 1995

Mittenberg W, Seidenberg M, O'Leary DS, DiGiulio DV: Changes in cerebral functioning associated with normal aging. J Clin Exp Neuropsychol 11:918–932, 1989

Morris JC, Heyman A, Mohs RC, et al: The Consortium to Establish a Registry for Alzheimer's Disease (CERAD); Part I: clinical and neuropsychological assessment of Alzheimer's disease. Neurology 39:1159–1165, 1989

Moss MB, Albert MS, Kemper TL: Neuropsychology of frontal lobe dementia, in Clinical Syndromes in Adult Neuropsychology: The Practitioner's Handbook. Edited by White RF. Amsterdam, Elsevier, 1992, pp 287–304

Naugle RI, Kawczak BA: Limitations of The Mini-Mental State Examination. Cleve Clin J Med 56:281, 1989

Neary D, Snowden JS: Dementia of the frontal lobe type, in Frontal Lobe Function and Dysfunction. Edited by Levin HS, Eisenberg HM, Benton AL. New York, Oxford University Press, 1991, pp 304–317

Nussbaum PD, Kaszniak AW, Allender J, et al: Cognitive deterioration in elderly depressed: a follow-up study. Paper presented at the annual meeting of the International Neuropsychological Society, San Antonio, TX, February 1991

Osato S, La Rue A, Yang J: Screening for cognitive deficits in older psychiatric patients. Paper presented at the annual meeting of the Gerontological Society of America, Minneapolis, MN, November 1989

Osterrieth PA: Le test de copie d'une figure complexe. Archives de Psychologie 30:306–356, 1944

Paolo AM, Troster AI, Ryan JJ: Continuous Visual Memory Test performance in healthy persons 60 to 94 years old. Archives of Clinical Neuropsychology 13:333–338, 1998

Parsons OA: Overview of the Halstead-Reitan Battery, in Clinical Applications of Neuropsychological Test Batteries. Edited by Incagnoli T, Goldstein G, Golden C. New York, Plenum, 1986, pp 155–189

Petersen RC, Smith GE, Waring SC, et al: Mild cognitive impairment: Clinical Characterization and outcome. Arch Neurology 56:303–308, 1999

Petrick JD, Mittenberg W: The course of naming dysfunction in dementia and depressive pseudodementia. Paper presented at annual meeting of the National Academy of Neuropsychology, Pittsburgh, PA, November 1992

Pfeffer RI, Kurosaki TT, Harrah CH, et al: A survey diagnostic tool for senile dementia. Am J Epidemiol 114:515–527, 1981

Pirozzolo FJ, Hansch EC, Mortimer JA: Dementia in Parkinson's disease: a neuropsychological analysis. Brain Cogn 1: 71–83, 1982

Podell K, Zimmerman M, Rebeta JJ, et al: Assessing frontal lobe dysfunction. Poster presented at the 145th Annual Meeting of the American Psychiatric Association, Washington, DC, May 2–7, 1992a

Podell K, Zimmerman M, Sovastion M, et al: The utility of the Graphical Sequence Test in assessing executive control deficits. Paper presented at The International Neuropsychological Society Annual Meeting, San Diego, CA, 1992b

Podell K, Lovell M, Zimmerman M, Goldberg E: The Cognitive Bias Task and lateralized frontal lobe functions in males. J Neuropsychiatry Clin Neurosci 7:491–501, 1995

Porteus SD: Porteus Maze Test: Fifty Year's Application. Palo Alto, CA, Pacific Books, 1965

Purdue Research Foundation: Examiners Manual for the Purdue Pegboard. Chicago, IL, Science Research Associates, 1948

Purisch AD, Sbordone RJ: The Luria-Nebraska Neuropsychological Battery, in Advances in Clinical Neuropsychology. Edited by Goldstein G, Tarter RE. New York, Plenum, 1986, pp 291–316

Reding M, Haycox J, Blass J: Depression in patients referred to a dementia clinic. Arch Neurol 42:894–896, 1985

Reifler BV: Arguments for abandoning the term pseudodementia. J Am Geriatr Soc 30:665–668, 1982

Reitan RM: Neurological and physiological bases of psychopathology. Annu Rev Psychol 27:189–216, 1976

Reitan RM, Davison LA: Clinical Neuropsychology: Current Status and Applications. New York, Winston-Wiley, 1974

Reitan RM, Wolfson D: The Halstead-Reitan Neuropsychological Test Battery. Tempe, AZ, Neuropsychology Press, 1985

Rey A: L'Examen Clinique En Psychologie. Paris, Press Universitaires de France, 1964

Reynolds CF, Hoch CC: Differential diagnosis of depressive pseudodementia and primary degenerative dementia. Psychiatric Annals 17:743–749, 1988

Robinson RG, Price TR: Poststroke depressive disorders: a follow-up study of 103 patients. Stroke 13:635–641, 1982

Rogers JC, Holm MB, Goldstein G, et al: Stability and change in functional assessment of patients with geropsychiatric disorders. Am J Occup Ther 48:914–918, 1994

Rosvold HE, Mirsky AF: A continuous performance test of brain damage. Journal of Consulting Psychology 20: 343–350, 1956

Rowe JW, Kahn RL: Human aging: usual and unusual. Science 237:143–149, 1987

Russell EW: Theory and development of pattern analysis methods related to the Halstead-Reitan battery, in Clinical Neuropsychology: A Multidisciplinary Approach. Edited by Logue PE, Schear JM. Springfield, IL, Charles C Thomas, 1984, pp 50–62

Russell EW: In defense of the Halstead Reitan Battery: a critique of Lezak's review. Arch Clin Neuropsychol 13:365–382, 1998

Salmon DP, Bondi MW: The neuropsychology of Alzheimer's disease, in The Handbook of Neuropsychology and Aging. Edited by Nussbaum PD. New York, Plenum, 1997, pp 141–158

Schaie KW, Schaie J: Clinical assessment in aging, in Handbook of the Psychology of Aging. Edited by Birren J, Schaie KW. New York, Van Nostrand Reinhold, 1977, pp 692–723

Schear JM: Neuropsychological assessment of the elderly in clinical practice, in Clinical Neuropsychology: A Multidisciplinary Approach. Edited by Logue PE, Schear JM. Springfield, IL, Charles C Thomas, 1984, pp 199–236

Schwartz GE: Development and validation of the Geriatric Evaluation by Relative's Rating Instrument (GERRI). Psychol Rep 53:479–488, 1983

Shallice T: Specific impairment of planning. Philos Trans R Soc Lond B Biol Sci 298:199–209, 1982

Shaw TG, Mortel KF, Meyer JS, et al: Cerebral blood flow changes in benign aging and cerebrovascular disease. Neurology 34:855–862, 1984

Shraberg D: The myth of pseudodementia: depression and the aging brain. Am J Psychiatry 135:601–603, 1978

Shraberg D: Questioning the concept of pseudodementia. Am J Psychiatry 137:260–261, 1980

Smith CB: Aging and changes in cerebral energy metabolism. Trends Neurosci 7:203–208, 1984

Speedie L, Rabins P, Pearlson G, et al: Confrontation naming deficit in dementia and depression. J Neuropsychiatry Clin Neurosci 2:59–63, 1990

Squire LR: Remote memory as affected by aging. Neuropsychologia 12:429–435, 1974

Storrie MC, Doerr HO: Characterization of Alzheimer's type dementia utilizing an abbreviated Halstead-Reitan Battery. Clinical Neuropsychology 2:78–82, 1980

Stoudemire A, Hill C, Gulley LR, et al: Neuropsychological and biomedical assessment of depression-dementia syndromes. J Neuropsychiatry Clin Neurosci 1:347–361, 1989

Strick L, Pittman J, Jacobs DM, et al: Normative data for a brief neuropsychological battery administered to English- and Spanish-speaking community-dwelling elders. J Int Neuropsychol Soc 4:311–318, 1998

Stroop JR: Studies of interference in serial verbal reactions. Journal of Experimental Psychology 18:643–662, 1935

Stuss DT, Meiran N, Guzman A, et al: Do long tests yield a more accurate diagnosis of dementia than short tests? Arch Neurology 53:1033–1039, 1996

Talland GA, Schwab RS: Performance with multiple sets in Parkinson's disease. Neuropsychologia 2:45–53, 1964

Tarter RE, Edwards KL: Neuropsychological batteries, in Clinical Application of Neuropsychological Test Batteries. Edited by Incagnoli T, Goldstein G, Golden CJ. New York, Plenum, 1986, pp 135–152

Terry RD, DeTeresa R, Hansen LA: Neocortical cell counts in normal human adult aging. Ann Neurol 21:530–539, 1987

Van Gorp WG, Marcotte TD, Sultzer D, et al: Screening for dementia: Comparison of three commonly used instruments. J Clin Exp Neuropsychol 21:29–38, 1999

Veiel HOF: A preliminary profile of neuropsychological deficits associated with major depression. J Clin Exp Neuropsychol 19:587–603, 1997

Warrington EK, Sanders HI: The fate of old memories. Q J Exp Psychol 23:432–442, 1971

Wechsler D: Wechsler Adult Intelligence Scale—Revised Manual. New York, Psychological Corporation, 1981

Wechsler D: Wechsler Memory Scale—Revised Manual. New York, Psychological Corporation, 1987

Wechsler D: Wechsler Adult Intelligence Scale—III. San Antonio, TX, Psychological Corporation, 1997a

Wechsler D: Wechsler Memory Scale—III. San Antonio, TX, Psychological Corporation, 1997b

Wechsler Abbreviated Scale of Intelligence. San Antonio, TX, The Psychological Corporation, 1999

Wilson RS, Bennett DA, Swartzendruber A: Age-related change in cognitive function, in Handbook of Neuropsychology and Aging. Edited by Nussbaum PD. New York, Plenum, 1997, pp 7–14

Zappala G, Martini E, Crook T, et al: Ecological memory assessment in normal aging: a preliminary report on an Italian population. Clin Geriatr Med 5:583–594, 1989

Zimmerman M, Poppen B, Podell K, Goldberg E: Lateralized frontal lobe dysfunction in males: the Wisconsin Card Sorting Test vs. The Graphical Sequences Test. Poster presented at The International Neuropsychological Society Annual Meeting, Cincinnati, OH, 1994

8

Age-Associated Memory Impairment

Graham Ratcliff, D.Phil.

Judith Saxton, Ph.D.

In this chapter, we review the memory changes associated with aging, paying particular attention to the phenomenon of age-associated memory impairment (AAMI). We begin the chapter with a brief overview of what is known about memory loss in older adults and a discussion of some current theoretical interpretations of these data. We then turn to the specific, well-defined phenomenon of AAMI, reviewing and critiquing proposed diagnostic criteria for this condition, exploring its clinical significance, and considering alternate constructs. We make the points that age-related memory changes can be conceptualized in a number of different ways and that different constructs, associated with different sets of diagnostic criteria, are appropriate for different purposes. We consider the prime distinguishing feature of currently available constructs to be the comparison group (young adults or the elderly individual's age peers) with reference to which memory is compared, approaches that we see as relevant to the study of normal aging and pathological aging, respectively.

We then undertake a brief review of the characteristics

of individuals who exhibit age-related memory changes and explore some possible biological bases for these conditions. Finally, we discuss some principles and practical considerations relating to clinical memory assessment in elderly individuals and describe some of the tests available for this purpose.

Background

Solid, converging evidence exists from a variety of sources that some otherwise healthy, normally aging individuals experience a deterioration in memory as they grow older (Kaszniak et al. 1986; Poon 1985). The literature of experimental psychology suggests that this decline typically affects secondary memory, also known as *long-term* or *recent memory*, more than it affects primary (*short-term* or *immediate*) memory or tertiary (*remote*) memory (Schacter et al. 1991). Age effects also sometimes appear in working memory (Baddeley 1986), tasks that require the individual not only to hold information in mind for a short time, but also to perform some mental operation on that information or perform another task simultaneously (Bromley 1958; Craik 1977; Dobbs and Rule 1989; Salthouse et al. 1989).

The net main effect of these changes is to reduce the ability to encode new information into memory, hold it over time, and recall it after an interval. Although the processes involved in remembering, particularly encoding and retrieval, become less effective as we grow older, the content of our memories—our knowledge base—can continue to increase (Perlmutter et al. 1987). Older people may, therefore, perform nearly as well as young people on tests such as digit span (in which information need only be held temporarily in a short-term memory store) or on tests assessing general knowledge or vocabulary (which assess well-learned factual or semantic knowledge rather than memory for specific events). Older people are likely to perform less well on tests such as backward digit span or delayed recall of recently presented material exceeding their immediate memory spans.

Psychometric evidence confirms that the decline of memory with increasing age is of substantial proportions. Performance on standard tests of secondary memory declines with age such that the norms for people 70–74 years old on the Wechsler Memory Scales (WMS-R [Wechsler 1987]; WMS-III [Wechsler 1997b]) call for scores up to 50% lower than those expected of young adults, and further declines are seen in individuals age 75 and older (Ivnik et al. 1992b). Age seems to have a more deleterious effect on the subtests involving memory for nonverbal material than on memory for verbal material, recall is more affected than recognition memory, recollection of detail declines more than recall of the general theme in memory for narrative, and the decline on verbal list learning is greater than that for narrative recall (Wechsler 1997b).

In the clinical literature, the phenomenon of "benign senescent forgetfulness" (Kral 1958) has been recognized for more than 30 years. The disorder was described as being the forgetting of details of events without loss of awareness of the events themselves. Remote memories were more affected than recent memories and people who had this disorder were aware of their problem and attempted to compensate for it. Kral et al. (1964) thought that this relatively mild and inconsistent memory impairment was nonprogressive and originally attributed it to normal aging (Kral 1962). They distinguished it in these respects from the "malignant" forgetfulness of the organic amnestic syndrome and dementia.

However, although this general picture is easily discerned and consistent from several viewpoints, the details are less clear and more controversial. In one view, for example, age-related changes in memory are secondary to other

cognitive changes. Thus, reduced speed of information processing with increasing age has been held to play a major role in the memory changes associated with aging and accounts for a substantial proportion of age-related variance in memory tasks (e.g., Luszcz et al. 1997; Salthouse 1996). Similarly, Craik (1990, 1991; Craik and Jacoby, 1996) has argued that the degree of age-related impairment on memory tasks depends on the degree to which the task demands more active, less routine, and more internally organized processing on the part of the subject rather than on the type of memory involved. Older subjects have more difficulty with, or are less inclined to use, this kind of processing and perform less well on tasks that require it.

Other studies have highlighted the relationship between age-related memory changes and the executive functions subserved by the frontal lobes. The frontal lobes may be particularly vulnerable to aging both structurally (Coffey et al. 1992) and functionally. Frontal lobe functions have been reported to be impaired in individuals with AAMI (Hallikainen et al. 1995), and some organizational aspects of memory test performance in the elderly resemble that of younger individuals with frontal lobe lesions (Stuss et al. 1996). Age-related changes in source memory, which has been related to frontal lobe function, have also been reported (Degl'Innocenti and Backman 1996), and performance on tests of executive function explains a significant amount of age-related variance in memory test scores (Troyer et al. 1994).

Certainly, some of the factors that affect the degree of age-related decline on memory test performance affect performance on other cognitive tasks in a similar way. For example, the differential difficulty of verbal and visuospatial memory tests for elderly patients is mirrored in differential rates of decline on the verbal and performance subtests of the Wechsler Adult Intelligence Scales (WAIS-R [Wechsler 1981]; WAIS-III [Wechsler 1997a]), and it may be that the decline in visuospatial memory can be more usefully regarded as a facet of impaired visuospatial ability rather than as a problem primarily of memory (Koss et al. 1991). Similarly, the changes in working memory may be regarded primarily as information-processing deficits rather than as memory impairments, per se, and the age effect seems to appear only when certain kinds of processing are required (Salthouse et al. 1991).

In this view, memory can be regarded as just one aspect of cognition, an emergent property of the human information processing system, which, like other aspects of cognition, is affected by changes in the efficiency of that system. For a further review of these and other resource theories, see A. D. Smith (1996). The implication is that we may learn more about age-related changes in cognition if we do not think of them as changes in memory, perception, attention, and so on, but instead attempt to analyze the memory, perceptual, and attentional tests we use to identify the information-processing requirements involved. Nevertheless, the important end-product for the clinician is that memory, as assessed by clinical memory tests, declines with age in well-established ways.

Just as the magnitude of the age-related decline in memory and the nature of the underlying cognitive processes affected are less well established than the fact of a decline in memory performance, so the defining characteristics, epidemiology, and clinical significance of benign senescent forgetfulness have not been well delineated although the existence of the disorder is recognized. Kral (1958) described some of the characteristics of his subjects' forgetfulness, but he did not define operational criteria for diagnosing the disorder and he did not objectively quantify the impairment. Although he initially regarded the disorder as a part of normal aging (Kral 1962), his subjects were nursing home residents and patients in a psychiatric hospital. More than half of them exhibited neurological signs suggesting lesions in the brain, as did nearly half of his unimpaired subjects. His subjects were thus certainly not drawn from a "normal" population, and Kral himself subsequently speculated (Kral et al. 1964) that benign and malignant forgetfulness might differ only in degree and both might be reflections of a single underlying pathological process. Of course, this would not necessarily make them "abnormal" if the "usually aging" individual who exhibits the range of physiological and even pathological changes typically associated with aging (D. B. Caine et al. 1991), rather than the optimally healthy "successfully aging" individual (Rowe and Kahn 1987), is accepted as the norm.

Constructs of Age-Related Memory Decline

Definitions

Before discussing the specific construct of AAMI (Crook et al. 1986a) in detail, we need to define some of the terms used in this chapter. Our purpose in doing so is emphatically not to introduce yet more terms into the literature; we only wish to simplify communication for the purposes of this review. Many of the apparent disagreements about age-related memory changes are attributable to the inconsistent use of terms. To this end, *age-associated memory impairment* (AAMI) is used in this chapter strictly as defined by Crook et al. (1986a) and designates only phenomena

meeting all the National Institute of Mental Health (NIMH) work group's diagnostic criteria. We also at times refer separately to the NIMH "psychometric criteria for AAMI." By these we mean the conditions set out in criteria c, d, and e, which define memory impairment but not the population eligible for diagnosis (see next section). We also make a general distinction between "age-appropriate forgetfulness," implying a decline in memory from young adult levels (of which AAMI is a specific example), and "age-inappropriate forgetfulness," implying memory impairment in comparison with age peers. The distinction between age-appropriate and age-inappropriate forgetfulness was recognized by Blackford and La Rue (1989) in their definitions of *age-consistent memory impairment* (ACMI) and *late-life forgetfulness* (LLF), the terms apparently being chosen for their similarity to those designating the similar constructs of AAMI and benign senescent forgetfulness, respectively; but we use their terms only to refer to phenomena meeting their specific diagnostic criteria. Finally, we use the general phrase *age-related memory decline* as an all-embracing, vaguely defined term to refer to any and all changes in memory allegedly associated with aging.

Diagnostic Criteria for Age-Associated Memory Impairment

The construct of AAMI was introduced by an NIMH work group (Crook et al. 1986a). It was the group's declared intention to facilitate communication and stimulate research into late-life memory loss, particularly its treatment, by introducing research diagnostic criteria, with the expectation that the criteria would be modified as research in the area developed. Modifications have indeed been suggested (Blackford and La Rue 1989; Larrabee and McEntee 1995, 1996; Rosen 1990; G. Smith et al. 1991), but have not yet been universally agreed on. The NIMH work group made a great contribution by providing a focus for discussion and emphasizing the importance of a detailed operational definition of the construct with which they were dealing. Their original criteria for AAMI are summarized as follows:

a. Age 50 years or over;
b. Complaint of memory loss affecting everyday functioning with gradual onset;
c. Memory test performance at least 1 SD below the mean established for young adults on a standardized test of secondary memory with adequate normative data;
d. Adequate intellectual function as determined by a scaled score of at least 9 on the Vocabulary subtest of

the Wechsler Adult Intelligence Scale (WAIS) (Wechsler 1955);

e. Absence of dementia as determined by a score of 24 or higher on the Mini-Mental State Exam (MMSE) (Folstein et al. 1975); and

f. Exclusion criteria including absence of a number of medical conditions, depression, risk factors for stroke, history of repeated minor or single major head injury, drug or alcohol abuse, or recent use of psychotropic medications that might affect cognitive function together with, in many cases, guidelines for determining whether these conditions were present.

Also, it should be noted that this definition of *age-associated memory impairment* differs from Kral's concept of *benign senescent forgetfulness* (Kral 1958) in several important respects. First, these criteria are attempting to capture a different phenomenon than that described by Kral, and the comparison group is different in the two cases. The AAMI criteria define *impairment* with respect to healthy young adult levels, not to those of the older individual's age peers as was implied in the description of benign senescent forgetfulness. Thus, it would logically be possible for all older individuals to meet criteria for AAMI, by exhibiting poorer memory than young adults, without exhibiting benign senescent forgetfulness in the sense of poorer memory than would be expected of a psychiatrically healthy older individual. Conversely, except for those who failed the AAMI exclusion criteria (including at least 53% of Kral's original group), cases of benign senescent forgetfulness would generally meet criteria for AAMI unless the clinical evidence of forgetfulness was not substantiated by poor performance on standardized memory tests. In practice, this is probably relatively infrequent if the judgment is based on a reasonably thorough clinical evaluation and not just a subjective report of memory impairment. With these provisos, *benign senescent forgetfulness* can be regarded as a subset of *age-associated memory impairment*, but the terms are not equivalent.

Second, the term *age-associated memory impairment* is "non-specific with regard to etiology and does not necessarily imply that the disorder is non-progressive" (Crook et al. 1986a, pp. 269–270). Thus, patients whose memory impairment is subsequently shown to be the earliest stage of a dementing illness are not necessarily excluded from the category of AAMI, and it is sensible to ask how often AAMI is, in fact, a dementia prodrome. This also implies that AAMI is not necessarily to be regarded as nonpathological, although the lengthy and detailed exclusion criteria clearly indicate that Crook and his colleagues had an optimally healthy cohort in mind when they defined it.

Utility of the Construct of Age-Associated Memory Impairment

The construct of AAMI can be criticized on several grounds. First, is the phenomenon it attempts to identify—decline from presumed young adult levels rather than an age-inappropriate impairment of memory relative to older individuals' age peers—the appropriate one to define? Second, if so, do the proposed criteria actually capture it clearly? Third, is the term *age-associated memory impairment* appropriate, and should it be regarded as a diagnosis? Finally, although the specification of diagnostic criteria has undoubtedly helped clarify some issues, is a focus on classification and diagnosis the best way of investigating and describing the changes in memory associated with aging?

When we rate the memory of elderly people, should we compare their memory with the presumably better memory of young adults as Crook et al. (1986a) suggested, or should we compare older adults with each other to identify a subgroup with poorer memory more in the spirit of Kral's benign senescent forgetfulness? Both approaches are feasible and have their merits, but both have practical and theoretical disadvantages. Only the former approach can tell us whether the memories of older people are, in fact, worse than the memories of younger people. However, it is difficult to be sure that the memory of a given older individual has changed over time without reference to test scores obtained from that individual in youth. Cross-sectional studies comparing older individuals' data with normative data collected from young people suffer from the obvious risk of cohort effects, as well as the more general problems involved in referencing performance to published norms based on populations whose demographics are incompletely specified or frankly different. Conversely, only the latter approach can tell us whether an individual has an abnormally poor memory given his or her age, but normative data on cognitive test performance in the old-old has, until recently, been virtually nonexistent, although some progress is being made in this regard. A number of studies from the Mayo Clinic, for example, are useful in the psychometric assessment of the elderly (Ivnik et al. 1992a, 1992b, 1992c), and the most recent version of the Wechsler Memory Scale (WMS-III) (Wechsler 1997b) includes norms for individuals up to 89 years old.

As is often the case, the answer depends on what question one is interested in. Arguing for the "decline from young adult" model, Crook and Ferris (1992) pointed out that elderly people typically complain that their memories are worse than they used to be, not that their memories are worse than those of their age peers, and that the decline is sufficiently common and sufficiently severe to justify therapeutic trials, whether it is normal or not. These researchers compared the situation to other conditions, such as presbyopia, which are "defined by reference to normative standards for young adults and . . . so common among the elderly as to be considered 'normal.' Nevertheless, few clinicians would compare the vision of an 80-year-old with norms established for other people of the same age and prescribe corrective lenses only to those whose visual performance falls outside those norms" (Crook and Ferris 1992, p. 714). If the primary purpose is to select subjects for trials of treatments for a potentially normal age-related decline in memory, the NIMH concept of AAMI is appropriate and the strict exclusion of other possible causes of memory impairment is necessary.

Alternative Approaches to Age-Related Memory Decline

On the other hand, if one is interested in defining a disease state, identifying a dementia prodrome, or performing clinical evaluation of the mass of elderly individuals who are referred for neuropsychological assessment, the "impaired relative to age peers" approach may be more appropriate or, at least, provide a useful additional conceptual framework. Several different ways of defining an age-inappropriate memory impairment have been proposed, and, where the evidence is available, these do seem to identify abnormal memory functioning, although whether the condition is benign has not been conclusively established. In this vein, Larrabee et al. (1986) identified individuals with "senescent forgetfulness" on the basis of memory test performance significantly worse than performance in other cognitive domains and significantly below an age-residualized mean (i.e., they conceptualized it as an age-atypical deficit specific to memory without necessarily implying change from a higher level earlier in life). Senescent forgetfulness defined in this way did not seem simply to be one end of a continuum of memory function because memory test performance in their sample was bimodally distributed, raising the possibility of some causative disease process. Larrabee and Crook (1989) also identified a subgroup of AAMI subjects whose performance on more ecologically valid, everyday memory tests was impaired relative to an age-residualized mean. In both studies, the prevalence of age-inappropriate memory impairment actually increased with increasing age, suggesting that the pathological process involved, if any, is age related. Larrabee and Crook (1989) also pointed out that their age-residualized, cross-sectional data suggest that this form of memory impairment is not evenly distributed across the adult age

range (i.e., those individuals who are shown to be abnormally forgetful after age 65 are not all likely to have been abnormally forgetful earlier in life).

Clinical Significance of Age-Inappropriate Forgetfulness

The value of the construct of an age-inappropriate, selective impairment of memory lies chiefly in its clinical significance, particularly whether it is a correlate of disease and whether it is truly benign or heralds an impending dementia. The evidence on this point is, as yet, inconclusive, although the topic clearly deserves further investigation. Larrabee et al. (1986), for example, failed to find any progression of memory deficit in their subjects with age-inappropriate "senescent forgetfulness" at 1-year follow-up, whereas Katzman et al. (1989) reported that 37% of the "functioning individuals with memory impairment [who] might well have been considered to have benign senescent forgetfulness" in their sample of elderly volunteers had dementia at 5-year follow-up and Parnetti et al. (1996) concluded that some subjects with AAMI may have early Alzheimer's disease. Further, O'Brien et al. (1992) reported an intermediate rate of progression to dementia of 8.8% in a group of 68 patients with benign senescent forgetfulness followed for an average of 3 years. However, these researchers based the diagnosis of forgetfulness entirely on subjective report, specifically excluding subjects who showed objective evidence of memory impairment on psychological tests. This is a different construct from the senescent forgetfulness of Larrabee et al. (1986), which was objectively demonstrable, and highlights the importance of the use of comparable terms in diagnostic criteria.

Another important aspect of the concept of age-inappropriate forgetfulness advanced here and by Larrabee et al. (1986) is that memory should be selectively impaired, or at least disproportionately affected, in comparison with other cognitive functions. This is another difference from the NIMH concept of AAMI, in which the memory impairment could be associated with age-related decline in other cognitive functions, provided that these were not sufficient to justify the diagnosis of dementia and did not substantially affect vocabulary test performance. The disproportionately severe impairment of memory in comparison with other cognitive functions may also distinguish the concept of age-inappropriate forgetfulness advanced here in principle, although possibly not in practice, from other concepts of "mild cognitive impairment not amounting to dementia" (World Health Organization 1978) or "questionable dementia" as used in the Clinical Dementia Rating Scale (Hughes et al. 1982) in which the preservation of nonmnemonic cognitive functions is either not required or only implied. More recently, Petersen and colleagues have proposed broad criteria aimed at identifying individuals with mild cognitive impairment (MCI) who are thought to be at risk for developing dementia (Petersen et al. 1996, 1999). These criteria are broadly similar to age-inappropriate memory decline in that the individual is required to exhibit a significantly abnormal memory performance compared with age-matched peers with relatively normal general cognitive functioning. Although there is still considerable uncertainty regarding the diagnostic criteria for MCI, it had been reported that individuals with MCI progress to Alzheimer's disease at a rate of 12% per year (Petersen et al. 1999) and that those with focal memory impairment, and carrying the APOE-epsilon 4 allele, have increased risk of developing Alzheimer's disease (Petersen et al. 1996). These conversion rates suggest that not all individuals meeting MCI criteria progress to Alzheimer's disease. Indeed, some individuals appear to remain in a plateau for many years, and some may never progress to dementia (Miceli et al. 1996). On the whole, studies using these kinds of classifications seem to find rather higher rates of progression to dementia than those attempting to isolate senescent forgetfulness, although the line of demarcation is not well defined (Dawe et al. 1992). It is not certain for example, to what extent the baseline impairment in Katzman et al.'s subjects (1989) was specific to memory. Although Reisberg et al. (1986) found that the extent to which subjects deteriorated was dependent on initial degree of impairment (i.e., the more impaired subjects tended to show more deterioration), this was based on a global assignment of "magnitude of cognitive decline" rather than on an assessment of memory performance in comparison to other cognitive functions.

The essential difference between the two principal concepts of age-related memory decline discussed so far has been the standard against which memory is compared—the young or the healthy elderly. A third approach is to look for qualitative rather than quantitative differences between the memory of healthy older individuals and the other groups of interest. Generally, the memory of individuals with dementia is much worse than that of healthy elderly people, but not qualitatively different (Huppert 1994). However, Grober and colleagues (Grober and Buschke 1986; Grober et al. 1988) have suggested that a failure to benefit to the normal extent from semantic cuing may distinguish the memory impairment of dementia and this, rather than absolute score, may also be a way of identifying age-inappropriate memory impairment in individuals without dementia.

The significance of abnormal rates of forgetting (Cullum et al. 1990), the severity of memory impairment compared to other cognitive functions (Cullum et al. 1995), overall pattern of neuropsychological test performance (Hänninen et al. 1995), and slow rates of learning (Petersen et al. 1992) have also been emphasized. Although such studies of qualitative aspects of memory in aging are important, we do not believe that they should be incorporated into the diagnostic criteria. The memory of individuals with AAMI may be qualitatively different from the memory of young adults, as well as quantitatively worse; however, the construct of AAMI is not defined by that difference.

To summarize, there are two distinct concepts of age-related memory decline, and both are useful. The concept of a potentially normal age-related decline from young adult levels envisaged by the NIMH criteria for AAMI is appropriate for studies of normal aging and memory. On the other hand, the phenomenon of selective, age-inappropriate forgetfulness in elderly people does appear to exist (Larrabee et al. 1986), and this concept is likely to be more useful in clinical evaluations and research looking for the antecedents of dementia (Barker et al. 1995; Blackford and La Rue 1989; O'Brien and Levy 1992; G. Smith et al. 1991).

Applicability of the Original Diagnostic Criteria for Age-Associated Memory Impairment

Several criticisms of the NIMH criteria for AAMI (Bamford and Caine 1988; Barker et al. 1995; Blackford and La Rue 1989; O'Brien and Levy 1992; Rosen 1990; G. Smith et al. 1991) were reviewed in detail in the first edition of this volume. As Larrabee and McEntee (1995) have pointed out, many of these criticisms referred to psychometric problems that have psychometric solutions, and these issues have become less contentious in the last 5 years. Nevertheless, the issue of precise diagnosis is so important that we review these criticisms briefly here. The reader is referred to the earlier version of this chapter (Ratcliff and Saxton [1994]) and to Larrabee (1996) and Larrabee and McEntee (1995) for further discussion.

First, the criticism of memory test performance 1 SD below the mean for young adults does not make adequate provisions for individuals whose memory functioning as a young adult was substantially above or below average. The former could experience significant deterioration in memory without meeting criteria for AAMI, whereas the latter would meet criteria on reaching age 50 without necessarily experiencing any decline in memory. Similarly, the inclusion criteria of a vocabulary score of at least 9 renders around half of normal adults over the age of 70 ineligible for the diagnosis, and no a priori reason seems to exist to suppose that individuals whose level of intellectual functioning is in the lower half of the average range should not experience age-related declines in memory.

Several authors have suggested ways of overcoming these problems by adjusting memory test scores for presumed level of intellectual function using vocabulary or education as an index and comparing the memory of older individuals with that of young people of an equivalent intellectual level (Goodman and Zarit 1994; Larrabee 1996; Larrabee and McEntee 1995; Ratcliff and Saxton 1994; Rosen 1990). Generally, the effect of these modifications has been to identify a group that seems to reflect the intended construct of AAMI more effectively than the original criteria.

Other criticisms involve the connotation of the term "impairment" in this context (G. Smith et al. 1991), the exclusion of individuals with medical conditions that may be normative in the elderly (Malec et al. 1993; Ratcliff and Saxton 1994), and the use of an MMSE score of 24 as a cutoff for dementia (Ratcliff and Saxton 1994).

A final main criticism of the original NIMH criteria involves the requirement for complaints of memory loss affecting everyday life with gradual onset and without sudden worsening in recent months, and this deserves discussion in more detail. Subjective report of memory impairment has been associated with depressed mood (Kahn et al. 1975; Popkin et al. 1982), neuroticism (Poitrenaud et al. 1989), age stereotypes of failing memory to which the complainant subscribes (Scogin et al. 1985; Zarit et al. 1981), and self-reported health status and number of functional limitations (Cutler and Grams 1988), as well as actual memory impairment (Zelinski et al. 1980).

The frequency with which older individuals "complain" of memory problems is probably also crucially dependent on how the question is asked. Only about half of Cutler and Grams's 14,564 subjects (1988) reported trouble remembering things "frequently" or "sometimes" as opposed to "rarely" or "never," whereas Sunderland et al. (1986) reported a "universal belief" among their elderly subjects that their memories failed them more frequently "now" than "when age 30." Sunderland and colleagues did find evidence of age-related memory impairment on objective tests in their group, but the frequency of reported memory failures was related to performance on only a few of the memory tests, and very few subjects regarded memory failures in everyday life as "even a minor handicap." Sunderland et al. (1986) also reported only moderate agreement between different subjective methods of memory assessment, and their questionnaire (although carefully designed and based on one that had been used effectively with younger individuals with memory impairment resulting from head injury and with their families [Sunderland et al. 1983]) showed low test-retest reliability. Even though studies involving clinical samples show more relationship between complaint and performance than do community-based studies, and progress is being made in the design and selection of appropriate instruments (Zelinski and Gilewski 1988), these observations cast serious doubt on the validity of current methods of subjective memory assessment and imply that subjective complaints of memory impairment should not be uncritically accepted at face value. Nevertheless, they may have a place in the diagnostic criteria for age-related memory decline.

Larrabee and McEntee (1995) point out that the requirement of both subjective complaint and objective deficit may exclude, on the one hand, those individuals who have always functioned at the low end of the normal range throughout adulthood but had noticed no recent decline in memory; whereas, on the other hand, individuals who report memory impairment secondary to psychological factors will not meet the objective-memory test criterion. Neither group constitutes having age-related memory decline. In support of this argument, Larrabee and McEntee quote the data of Koivisto et al. (1995), who found in a large epidemiological study that 76.3% of their sample reported subjective memory impairment and 78.4% were impaired on objective tests, but only 53.8% met both criteria. This appropriate self-exclusion of relatively low-functioning individuals whose memories have not declined probably occurs on a less formal basis in clinical practice, as it is the perception of memory loss rather than poor memory test performance that usually brings patients to the clinic.

It should also be noted that laboratory memory tests may not themselves be good predictors of real-life memory function. Thus, the failure to find correlations between subjective report of memory impairment and poor performance on standard memory tests may be attributable to the fact that laboratory memory test performance does not reflect the everyday memory abilities that are accurately reported by the subjects. In at least one study (Larrabee et al. 1991), good correlations were obtained between performance on a battery of computerized memory tests ingeniously designed to simulate everyday memory functions (Crook et al. 1986b) and responses to a subjective memory questionnaire with good psychometric properties (Crook and Larrabee 1990). Unlike many previous authors, Crook and Larrabee did not find that subjective memory complaint was related to depressed mood. Nevertheless, in spite of this result, subjective reports of memory impairment are currently so difficult to interpret that they should be treated with extreme caution.

Differential Sensitivity of Memory Tests

Even if general diagnostic criteria are agreed upon, the differential sensitivity of different memory tests to aging indicates that the particular test used will determine the size of the population defined. G. Smith et al. (1991) found that at least twice as many of their two groups of elderly subjects met NIMH psychometric criteria for AAMI when a less verbal memory test—Visual Reproduction from the Wechsler Memory Scale (Wechsler 1945) or WMS-R, rather than Logical Memory from the same tests—was used as the index of memory impairment. Even when two verbal tests with a different format (Logical Memory and the Rey Auditory Verbal Learning Test [RAVLT] [Rey 1964]) were compared (Lezak 1983), the proportion of cases identified varied by a factor of more than 4 (20%–96% in one group and 11%–58% in the other). Similar results were reported by Raffaele et al. (1992) with classification rates varying from 22.7% for immediate Logical Memory to 53% for delayed Visual Reproduction. The general tendency is for more subjects to be classified as "impaired" by visuospatial tests than by verbal tests, by delayed recall than by immediate recall, and, at least within the verbal domain, by list learning tasks than by narrative recall. The difference in sensitivity appears to be attributable partly to the modality involved, but also to the psychometric properties (e.g., ceiling effects) of the tests themselves (Raffaele et al. 1992).

Blackford and La Rue (1989) addressed the issue of differential sensitivity of memory tests by requiring that the test battery include at least four memory tests and recommended a number of instruments from which the clinician may select. They defined three levels of impairment on the basis of such a battery: AAMI (performance at least 1 SD below the mean established for young adults on one or more tests); ACMI (performance within + 1 SD of the mean established for age on 75% or more of the tests administered); or LLF (performance between 1 and 2 SD below the mean established for age on 50% or more of the tests administered). Although this reduces the problem of differential sensitivity, it does not eliminate it, as studies using, for example, the four secondary memory tests from the WMS-R would still be expected to yield different rates of LLF than would those including a list learning task like the RAVLT.

A possible compromise is to use a composite score based on the weighted averages of scores on a group of individual tests (rather than looking at the percentage of tests

on which performance falls below a certain level). The General Memory Index and Delayed Recall Index derived from the WMS-R are based on such weighted averages of four tests, including both verbal and nonverbal material, and a composite score based on these tests is considerably more sensitive than each of the component tests individually (G. Smith et al. 1991). Though it may be premature to specify the particular tests that should be used in assessing age-related memory decline as G. Smith et al. (1991) suggested, the WMS-R meets some of the requirements and has the advantages that it is widely used and that normative data for the older old are becoming available.

Age-Associated Memory Impairment as a Diagnostic Entity

It was not the stated intention of the NIMH work group to imply that AAMI was a disease or that it was necessarily abnormal or that it had a known and defined pathological basis for which a diagnostic laboratory test might, in principle, be developed. Instead, as stated above, they proposed to introduce a "diagnostic term" (Crook et al. 1986a) and associated diagnostic criteria to facilitate communication and promote research, particularly into pharmacological treatment for the condition they defined. Nevertheless, a number of subsequent authors have objected to the term on the grounds that it does imply a clinical diagnosis, which in turn implies a disease, although the phenomenon it denotes does not merit such a status (Bamford and Caine 1988; O'Brien and Levy 1992; Rosen 1990). Perhaps because of these kinds of criticism, future diagnostic systems are likely to modify the construct (Caine 1992), distinguishing between age-appropriate and age-inappropriate impairments on the one hand and between those associated with and independent of other systemic or central nervous system disease on the other.

Even if AAMI (or LLF or any other form of age-related memory decline) does constitute a diagnostic entity, one can ask whether the construct is appropriately named and whether it is likely to be useful. Just as the term *benign senescent forgetfulness* can be criticized because it is not clear that the implication of nonprogression is necessarily justified, so the term *age-associated memory impairment* has been criticized because *impairment* connotes abnormality, which is not a necessary part of the AAMI construct (G. Smith et al. 1991). *Decline* or *loss*, which connote deterioration from a previously higher level but not abnormality, might be better. Ironically, the more descriptive and less evaluative term *forgetfulness* has been used in two contexts (*benign senescent forgetfulness* and *late-life forgetfulness*) in which abnormality is implicitly or explicitly involved.

Possible Biological Bases of Age-Related Memory Decline

A number of neuroanatomical and neurochemical changes are known or suspected to occur with aging, and some of these might plausibly be related to deterioration in memory. Modest age-related decreases are known to occur in the size of the mammillary bodies (Raz et al. 1992) and temporal lobe structures (Coffey et al. 1992). Both these brain areas are known to be involved in memory. Hippocampal volume has been reported to be correlated with memory test performance in psychiatrically normal elderly subjects (Golomb et al. 1994) and to be reduced in patients with amnesia (Press et al. 1989) and in patients with Alzheimer's disease (Kesslak et al. 1991; Seab et al. 1988), although Seab and colleagues did not find that the degree of atrophy was related to severity of memory impairment. The possible relationship to frontal lobe function is discussed above. It is also noted above that the majority of the elderly are not completely healthy, and a wide range of comorbidities probably influence memory and other cognitive functions in the elderly. We have found, for example, that individuals with cardiovascular disease even at subclinical levels (Kuller et al. 1994) performed less well on memory tests and on tests of speed, attention, and working memory than did those free of such disease. Cognitive test performance was also related to relatively rare diseases such as diabetes and emphysema. Poor performance on tests of attention, visuospatial ability, and delayed recall from the WMS-R was also associated with history of bypass surgery.

The presence of the APOE-epsilon 4 allele may help distinguish the small subset of individuals whose memory impairment may represent an early, monosymptomatic stage of Alzheimer's disease (Blesa et al. 1996; Petersen et al. 1995). White matter changes documented by computed tomography or magnetic resonance imaging are a frequent incidental finding in the elderly (Coffey et al. 1992). Whereas some authors have found that these are both more severe and related to severity of cognitive impairment in individuals with dementia, this is certainly not universally agreed to be the case (Kozachuk et al. 1990). Similarly, changes in cholinergic neurotransmitter systems are well documented in Alzheimer's disease and may also be found in normal aging (Morgan 1992). These changes have been suggested as a possible basis for AAMI (Bartus et al. 1982). Crook and Larrabee (1988) have reviewed other potential underpinnings of AAMI and recommended trials of pharmacotherapy on this basis, although this approach has not been generally agreed upon.

These and other potential causes of AAMI deserve further study, but to date we are not aware of a consistent body of empirical evidence that conclusively links age-related memory decline to specific neurochemical or anatomical changes. In the search for such evidence, it will be necessary to bear in mind the distinctions between age-appropriate and age-inappropriate forgetfulness and, consequently, to look for correlates in both successfully and unsuccessfully aging individuals.

Future Research Strategies

The availability of diagnostic criteria for AAMI should not thwart the pursuit of other goals for aging research or other approaches to the study of age-related memory decline. As discussed above, memory can be regarded as an emergent property of the human information-processing system as well as a cognitive domain in which an individual may or may not exhibit impaired functioning. The information-processing system could be affected in a number of different ways, any or all of which could cause the individual to meet criteria for AAMI but have different theoretical, prognostic, and, possibly, therapeutic implications. A different kind of research focused on the processes involved in remembering is required to determine what age-related memory decline is, rather than simply whether it is present in a given individual.

We also need to supplement AAMI-oriented research with studies of aging individuals in which some form of psychometrically defined age-related memory decline is the independent variable and medical conditions, demographics, and subjective report are treated as dependent variables rather than as exclusion criteria. Certainly, it is important to know what proportion of the community-resident elderly exhibits a decline in memory and, for those that do, what the typical causes or, at least, correlates of that decline are. As we have seen, the NIMH exclusion criteria render a large proportion of the population ineligible for the diagnosis of AAMI, and many of these individuals do not exhibit memory impairment in spite of the "threats to memory" (G. Smith et al. 1991) represented by the condition causing their ineligibility. Conversely, it is likely that some of the ineligible individuals who do exhibit memory impairment do so because of age-related changes, rather than because of their medical conditions. It is our impression that, in community samples, rather than patient groups, the adverse effect of medical and psychiatric illness on cognition is minimal, although it may be demonstrable in large group studies. In our sample of community-resident elderly individuals (described above), we evaluated self-reported depressive symptomatology in the previous week using the Center for Epidemiological Studies Depression Scale (CES-D) (Radloff 1977) and assessed memory using the WMS-R. Although a significant correlation was found between depression score and Delayed Recall weighted raw score, this accounted for less than 3% of the variance. Furthermore, individuals with CES-D scores exceeding a conventional cutoff score of 17, raising the possibility of clinically significant depression, were found only slightly more frequently among individuals meeting psychometric criteria for AAMI (11% compared with 7% of individuals not meeting these criteria).

Clinical Memory Assessment in the Elderly

The way in which the clinician investigates the memory of the elderly patient and the thoroughness of the assessment will depend on the purposes and circumstances of the evaluation. It is clear that the assessment must involve some form of objective memory test, rather than relying on subjective report. The minimum requirement for such a test is that it involve the delayed recall of recently presented information and be sufficiently difficult that it is not subject to a marked ceiling effect. The word list learning test used by the Consortium to Establish a Registry of Alzheimer's Disease (CERAD) (Morris et al. 1989) meets these minimal requirements, but the three words from the MMSE (Folstein et al. 1975) do not, as the test is too easy to be sensitive to mild or even moderate memory impairment. Preferably, the test should also involve multitrial learning as well as memory, providing a way of comparing the ability to encode, retain, and recall information (e.g., immediate and delayed recall trials); use both verbal and nonverbal material; and have norms for elderly individuals. A combination of measures is probably required if all these requirements are to be met adequately, and some suggestions were made by Blackford and La Rue (1989). A selection of memory tests was also reviewed by Lezak (1983) and by Spreen and Strauss (1998), and the subject was discussed more extensively in *Clinical Memory Assessment of Older Adults* by Poon (1986).

Although it is not ideal, our usual practice is to base routine memory assessments on the Logical Memory and Visual Reproduction subtests of the WMS-R or WMS-III supplemented by a learning task, typically the RAVLT or the revised version of the Hopkins Verbal Learning Test (Benedict et al. 1998). As noted above, the WMS-R and the WMS-III go some way toward overcoming the problem of differential sensitivity of different tests by providing summary scores based on the weighted averages of subtests involving immediate and delayed recall of verbal and nonverbal material. It is true that the more age-sensitive list-learning type of task is underrepresented in these weighted averages, but this is partially compensated by the fact that the Logical Memory subtest (recall of short passages of prose, similar to news items) weighs heavily and is one of the more ecologically valid memory tests in common clinical use (Sunderland et al. 1983). If prediction of everyday memory function is crucial, however, it would be more appropriate to use the Rivermead Behavioral Memory Test (Wilson et al. 1985) or a research instrument of the kind described by Crook et al. (1986b). The WMS also allows one to compare verbal and nonverbal memory, although the tests are not terribly well matched. Norms for the older old are now available for the WMS-R (Ivnik et al. 1992b) and are included in the manual for its recent successor, the WMS-III (Wechsler 1997b). We do not yet have sufficient experience with the WMS-III to form a definite opinion, but it is likely that similar considerations will apply, although the test, while improved in several respects, is more cumbersome to use and it may be more efficient to extract relevant subtests. If so, we would recommend substituting the RAVLT for the list learning and paired associate subtests of the WMS-III on the grounds of greater sensitivity. The addition of a Working Memory Index may also prove very useful.

Summary scores should be used with caution because information is lost and important discrepancies between individual component scores can be concealed. Nevertheless, summary scores can be convenient and, when one is required, we favor the Delayed Recall weighted raw score over the Immediate Recall weighted raw score because it incorporates a delay and can be expected to be more sensitive to memory impairment in general and age-related memory decline in particular. We prefer the weighted raw scores in some circumstances to the indexes, which can be derived from them, because the former are not age corrected so that an individual's scores can be compared with other individuals of any age.

We also find the Rey-Osterrieth Complex Figure (ROCF) (Osterrieth 1944; Rey 1941) to be extremely useful. It is our practice to administer copy, immediate, and 30-minute delayed recall conditions because the comparison of performance on all three stages provides a wealth of information. For individuals too impaired to complete the original ROCF, we have developed a simplified version and have published norms for healthy elderly and individuals with Alzheimer's disease (Becker et al. 1987; Saxton and Becker, in press).

Finally, we usually use the delayed recall scores rather than a forgetting score calculated by subtracting delayed from immediate recall because we believe that, in most populations, it will be more sensitive to memory impairment without sacrificing specificity to an unacceptable degree. The rationale is as follows: whatever aspect of memory is involved (encoding, retrieval, rate of forgetting, and so on), delayed recall will be affected. It is true that other disorders (e.g., aphasia) may cause low delayed recall scores by impairing the ability to process the information to be remembered. These disorders can then masquerade as memory impairments, a state of affairs that could be avoided by use of an immediate-recall-minus-delayed-recall criterion that would reveal that the information had not been encoded into memory at the outset. However, as the memoranda on the WMS-R and most other standardized memory tests exceed memory span, moderate memory impairments may affect immediate, as well as delayed, recall and therefore would not be fully reflected in an immediate-recall-minus-delayed-recall measure of forgetting. In community-resident populations, the incidence of false negatives of this kind is likely to exceed the incidence of false positives secondary to inability to adequately process the stimulus material. Further, in clinical evaluations one should never consider any test score in isolation, always remembering that any test, however well designed, can be failed for multiple reasons. When false negatives do occur, usually independent evidence of the responsible disorder will be present to help the clinician interpret the results.

The assessment of memory in the elderly, like neuropsychological evaluation in all other circumstances, therefore involves weighing an individual's current memory function against the level that would be expected for that individual on the basis of age, education, and level of intellectual functioning and against his or her functioning in other cognitive domains. As we acquire more data on the natural history of aging and memory and learn more about the significance of age-inappropriate forgetfulness, we will be better able to set the balance and interpret the results.

Summary and Conclusions

To what extent does our research and review of the recent literature enable us to amplify or modify the generalizations with which we began this chapter? First, the recent evidence, spurred by the provision of psychometric criteria for AAMI, confirms that memory test performance is typically poorer in the elderly than in the young. Age affects delayed recall more than it affects immediate recall, and visuospatial material is typically less well recalled than verbal material. Accordingly, estimates of the prevalence of AAMI vary widely depending on which kind of material and what form of test is used. Our view is that the great ma-

jority of elderly people are affected to some degree, but that the decline reaches significant proportions only in a subset, the size of which varies widely depending on the criteria used, and is perceived as a significant problem by only a small minority.

Second, there is sufficient evidence to justify distinguishing age-appropriate and age-inappropriate forms (or levels) of age-related memory decline. The former, of which AAMI is an example, represents a normal age-related phenomenon, whereas the latter, the true descendent of benign senescent forgetfulness, is by definition abnormal and, possibly, pathological. Whether age-inappropriate forgetfulness is progressive, whether it can be distinguished from other concepts of mild cognitive decline by virtue of being specific to memory, and whether it is qualitatively different from normal memory or merely worse is not yet certain. The prevalence of age-inappropriate forgetfulness is also undetermined, but it is certainly less common than the age-appropriate form.

Completely satisfactory diagnostic criteria do not yet exist for AAMI or any other concept of age-related decline in spite of valiant efforts (Blackford and La Rue 1989; Crook et al. 1986a). Improved criteria would take an individual's overall level of intellectual functioning or educational background into account when setting the standard against which to rate memory, distinguish age-appropriate from age-inappropriate decline, make reference to the selectivity of memory impairment, modify the requirement for subjective complaint, and recognize the possibility of a number of comorbidities, rather than impose rigid exclusion criteria. The last might be achieved by assigning a level of probability to the diagnosis much as in the research diagnostic criteria for Alzheimer's disease of the National Institute of Nervous and Communicative Disorders and Stroke and the Alzheimer's Disease and Related Disorders Association (McKhann et al. 1984). Because of the varying sensitivities of different memory tests, it may also be necessary to specify the characteristics of suitable tests, if not actually require that specific, named tests be used.

References

Baddeley AD: Working Memory. Oxford, England, Clarendon Press, 1986

Bamford KA, Caine ED: Does "benign senescent forgetfulness" exist? Clin Geriatr Med 4:897–916, 1988

Barker A, Jones R, Jennison C: A prevalence study of age-associated memory impairment. Br J Psychiatry 167: 642–648, 1995

Bartus RT, Dean RL, Beer B, et al: The cholinergic hypothesis of geriatric memory dysfunction. Science 217:408–417, 1982

Becker JT, Boller F, Saxton J, McGonigle-Gibson K: Normal rates of forgetting of verbal and non-verbal material in Alzheimer's disease. Cortex 72:25–29, 1987

Benedict RH, Schretlen D, Groninger L, Brandt J: Hopkins Verbal Learning Test—Revised: normative data and analysis of inter-form and test-retest reliability. Clinical Neuropsychologist 12(1):43–55, 1998

Blackford RC, La Rue A: Criteria for diagnosing age associated memory impairment: proposed improvements from the field. Developmental Neuropsychology 5:295–306, 1989

Blesa R, Adroer R, Santacruz P, et al: High apolipoprotein E epsilon 4 allele frequency in age-related memory decline. Ann Neurol 39:548–551, 1996

Bromley DB: Some effects of age on short-term learning and memory. J Gerontol 13:398–406, 1958

Caine DB, Eisen A, Meneilly G: Normal aging of the nervous system. Ann Neurol 30:206–207, 1991

Caine ED: Nomenclature and diagnosis of cognitive disorders: a US perspective. Abstract presented at Age Related Cognitive Disorders Conference, Nice, France, June 1992

Coffey CE, Wilkinson WE, Parashos IA, et al: Quantitative cerebral anatomy of the aging human brain: a cross-sectional study using magnetic resonance imaging. Neurology 42:527–536, 1992

Craik FIM: Age differences in human memory, in Handbook of the Psychology of Aging. Edited by Birren JE, Schaie KW. New York, Van Nostrand Reinhold, 1977, pp 384–414

Craik FIM: Changes in memory with normal aging: a functional view, in Alzheimer's Disease (Advances in Neurology Series, Vol 51). Edited by Wurtman RJ, Corkin S, Growdon JH, et al. New York, Raven, 1990, pp 202–205

Craik FIM: Memory functions in normal aging, in Memory Disorders: Research and Clinical Practice. Edited by Yanagihara T, Petersen RC. New York, Marcel Dekker, 1991, pp 347–367

Craik FIM, Jacoby LL: Aging and memory: implications for skilled performance, in Aging and Skilled Performance: Advances in Theory and Applications. Edited by Rogers WA, Fisk AD, Neff W. Mahwah, NJ, Lawrence Erlbaum, 1996, pp 113–137

Crook TH, Ferris SH: Age associated memory impairment (letter). BMJ 304:714, 1992

Crook TH, Larrabee GJ: Age associated memory impairment: diagnostic criteria and treatment strategies. Psychopharmacol Bull 24:509–514, 1988

Crook TH, Larrabee GJ: A self rating scale for evaluating memory in everyday life. Psychol Aging 5:48–57, 1990

Crook TH, Bartus RT, Ferris SH, et al: Age-associated memory impairment: proposed diagnostic criteria and measures of clinical change—report of a National Institute of Mental Health work group. Developmental Neuropsychology 2:261–276, 1986a

Crook TH, Salama M, Gobert J: A computerized test battery for detecting and assessing memory disorders, in Senile Dementias: Early Detection. Edited by Bes A, Cahn J, Hayer S, et al. London, John Libby Eurotext, 1986b, pp 79–85

Cullum CM, Butters N, Troster AI, et al: Normal aging and forgetting rates on the Wechsler Memory Scale–Revised. Archives of Clinical Neuropsychology 5:22–30, 1990

Cullum CM, Filley CM, Kozora E: Episodic memory function in advanced aging and early Alzheimer's Disease. J Int Neuropsychol Soc 1:100–103, 1995

Cutler SJ, Grams AE: Correlates of self-reported everyday memory problems. J Gerontol 43:S82–S90, 1988

Dawe B, Procter A, Philpot M: Concepts of mild memory impairment in the elderly and their relationship to dementia: a review. Int J Geriatr Psychiatry 7:473–479, 1992

Degl'Innocenti A, Backman L: Aging and severe memory: influences of intention to remember and associations with frontal lobe tests. Aging Neuropsychology and Cognition 3:307–319, 1996

Dobbs AR, Rule BG: Adult age differences in working memory. Psychol Aging 4:500–503, 1989

Folstein MF, Folstein SE, McHugh PR: "Mini-Mental State." A practical method of grading the cognitive state of patients for the clinician. J Psychiatr Res 12:189–198, 1975

Golomb J, Kluger A, de Leon MJ, et al: Hippocampal formation size in normal human aging: a correlate of delayed secondary memory performance. Learning and Memory 1:45–54, 1994

Goodman CR, Zarit SH: Effects of education: an assessment of age-associated memory impairment. Am J Geriatr Psychiatry 2:118–123, 1994

Grober E, Buschke H: Genuine memory deficits in dementia. Developmental Neuropsychology 3:13–36, 1986

Grober E, Buschke H, Crystal H, et al: Screening for dementia by memory testing. Neurology 388:900–903, 1988

Hallikainen M, Renikainen KJ, Helkala E-L, et al: Decline of frontal lobe functions in subjects with age-associated memory impairment. Neurology 45 (suppl 4):39P, 1995

Hänninen T, Hallikainen M, Koivisto K, et al: A follow-up study of age-associated memory impairment: neuropsychological predictors of dementia. J Am Geriatr Soc 43(9):1007–1015, 1995

Hughes CP, Berg L, Danziger WL, et al: A new scale for the staging of dementia. Br J Psychiatry 140:566–572, 1982

Huppert FA: Memory function in dementia and normal ageing: dimension or dichotomy, in Dementia and Normal Ageing. Edited by Huppert FA, Brayne C, O'Connor D. Cambridge, England, Cambridge University Press, 1994, pp 291–330

Ivnik RJ, Malec JF, Smith GE, et al: Mayo's older Americans normative studies: WAIS-R norms for ages 56–97. Clinical Neuropsychologist 6:1–30, 1992a

Ivnik RJ, Malec JF, Smith GE, et al: Mayo's older Americans normative studies: WMS-R norms for ages 56–94. Clinical Neuropsychologist 6:49–82, 1992b

Ivnik RJ, Malec JF, Smith GE, et al: Mayo's older Americans normative studies: updated AVLT norms for ages 56–97. Clinical Neuropsychologist 6:83–104, 1992c

Kahn RL, Zaret SH, Hilbert NM, et al: Memory complaint and impairment in the aged. Arch Gen Psychiatry 32:1569–1573, 1975

Kaszniak AW, Poon LW, Riege W: Assessing memory deficits: an information processing approach, in Clinical Memory Assessment of Older Adults. Edited by Poon LW. Washington, DC, American Psychological Association, 1986, pp 168–188

Katzman R, Aronson M, Fuld P, et al: Development of dementing illness in an 80-year-old volunteer cohort. Ann Neurol 25:317–324, 1989

Kesslak JP, Nalcioglu O, Cotman CW: Quantification of magnetic resonance scans for hippocampal and parahippocampal atrophy in Alzheimer's disease. Neurology 41:51–54, 1991

Koivisto K, Reinikainen KJ, Hänninen T, et al: Prevalence of age-associated memory impairment in a randomly selected population from eastern Finland. Neurology 45:741–747, 1995

Koss E, Haxby JV, DeCarli C, et al: Patterns of performance preservation and loss in healthy aging. Developmental Neuropsychology 7:99–113, 1991

Kozachuk WE, DeCarli C, Schapiro MB, et al: White matter hyperintensities in dementia of Alzheimer's type and in healthy subjects without cerebrovascular risk factors. Arch Neurol 47:1306–1310, 1990

Kral VA: Neuropsychiatric observations in an old people's home. J Gerontol 13:169–176, 1958

Kral VA: Senescent forgetfulness: benign and malignant. Journal of the Canadian Medical Association 86:257–260, 1962

Kral VA, Cahn C, Mueller H: Senescent memory impairment and its relation to the general health of the aging individual. J Am Geriatr Soc 12:101–113, 1964

Kuller LM, Borhani NO, Furberg C, et al: Prevalence of subclinical atherosclerosis and cardiovascular disease and association with risk factors in the Cardiovascular Health Study. Am J Epidemiol 139:1164–1179, 1994

Larrabee GJ: Age-associated memory impairment: definition and psychometric characteristics. Aging Neuropsychology and Cognition 3:118–131, 1996

Larrabee GJ, Crook TH: Performance subtypes of everyday memory function. Developmental Neuropsychology 5:267–283, 1989

Larrabee GJ, McEntee WJ: Age associated memory impairment: sorting out the controversies. Neurology 45:611–614, 1995

Larrabee GL, Levin HA, High WM: Senescent forgetfulness: a quantitative study. Developmental Neuropsychology 2:373–385, 1986

Larrabee GJ, West RL, Crook TH: The association of memory complaint with computer-simulated everyday memory performance. J Clin Exp Neuropsychol 13:466–478, 1991

Lezak MD: Neuropsychological Assessment, 2nd Edition. New York, Oxford University Press, 1983

Luszcz MA, Bryan J, Kent P: Predicting episodic memory performance of very old men and women: contributions from age, depression, activity, cognitive ability and speed. Psychol Aging 12:340–351, 1997

Malec JF, Ivnik RJ, Smith GE: Neuropsychology and normal aging: the clinician's perspective, in Neuropsychology of Alzheimer's Disease and Other Dementias. Edited by Parks RW, Zec RF, Wilson RS. New York, Oxford University Press, 1993, pp 81–111

McKhann G, Drachman D, Folstein M, et al: Clinical diagnosis of Alzheimer's disease: a report of the NINCDS-ADRDA work group under the auspices of the Department of Health and Human Services Task Force on Alzheimer's Disease. Neurology 34:939–944, 1984

Miceli G, Colosimo C, Daniele A, et al: Isolated amnesia with slow onset and stable course, without ensuing dementia: MRI and PET data and a six-year neuropsychological follow-up. Dementia 7:104–110, 1996

Morgan DG: Neurochemical changes with aging: predisposition toward age-related mental disorders, in Handbook of Mental Health and Aging, 2nd Edition. Edited by Birren JE, Sloane RB, Cohen GD. New York, Academic Press, 1992, pp 174–199

Morris JC, Heyman A, Mohs RC, et al: The consortium to establish a registry for Alzheimer's disease (CERAD), part I: clinical and neuropsychological assessment of Alzheimer's disease. Neurology 39:1159–1165, 1989

O'Brien JT, Levy R: Age associated memory impairment. BMJ 304:5–6, 1992

O'Brien JT, Beats B, Hill K, et al: Do subjective memory complaints precede dementia? A three-year follow-up of patients with supposed benign senescent forgetfulness. Int J Geriatr Psychiatry 7:481–486, 1992

Osterrieth PA: Le test de copie d'une figure complexe: contribution a l'etude de la perception et de la memoire. Archives de Psychologie 30:206–356, 1944

Parnetti L, Lowenthal DT, Presciutti O, et al: 1H-MRS, MRI-based hippocampal volumetry, and 99mTc-HMPAO-SPECT in normal aging, age-associated memory impairment and probable Alzheimer's Disease. J Am Geriatr Soc 44:133–138, 1996

Perlmutter M, Adams C, Berry J, et al: Aging and memory, in Annual Review of Gerontology and Geriatrics, Vol 8. Edited by Schaie KW, Eisdorfer C. New York, Springer, 1987, pp 57–92

Petersen RC, Smith G, Kokmen E, et al: Memory function in normal aging. Neurology 42:396–401, 1992

Petersen RC, Smith GE, Ivnik RJ, et al: Apolipoprotein E states as a predictor of the development of Alzheimer's disease in memory-impaired individuals. JAMA 274:538, 1995

Petersen RC, Waring SC, Smith GE, et al: Predictive value of APOE genotyping in incipient Alzheimer's disease. Ann N Y Acad Sci 802:58–69, 1996

Petersen RC, Smith GE, Waring SC, et al: Aging, memory, and mild cognitive impairment. Int Psychogeriatr 9 (suppl 1):65–69, 1997

Poitrenaud J, Malbezin M, Guez D: Self-rating and psychometric assessment of age-related changes in memory among young-elderly managers. Developmental Neuropsychology 5:285–294, 1989

Poon LW: Differences in human memory with aging: nature causes and clinical implications, in Handbook of the Psychology of Aging, 2nd Edition. Edited by Birren JE, Schaie KW. New York, Van Nostrand Reinhold, 1985, pp 427–462

Poon LW: Clinical Memory Assessment of Older Adults. Washington, DC, American Psychological Association, 1986

Popkin SJ, Gallagher D, Thompson LW, et al: Memory complaint and performance in normal and depressed older adults. Exp Aging Res 8:141–145, 1982

Press GA, Amaral DG, Squire LR: Hippocampal abnormalities in amnesic patients revealed by high-resolution magnetic resonance imaging. Nature 341:54–57, 1989

Radloff LS: The CES-D Scale: a self-report depression scale for research in the general population. Applied Psychological Measurement 1:385–401, 1977

Raffaele KC, Haxby JV, Schapiro MB: Age-associated memory impairment, in Treatment of Age-Related Cognitive Dysfunction: Pharmacological and Clinical Evaluation. Edited by Racagni G, Medlewicz J. Basel, Switzerland, Karger, 1992, pp 69–79

Ratcliff G, Saxton J: Age-associated memory impairment, in Textbook of Geriatric Neuropsychiatry. Edited by Coffey CE, Cummings JL. Washington, DC, American Psychiatric Press, 1994, pp 145–158

Raz N, Torres IJ, Acker JD: Age-related shrinkage of the mamillary bodies: in vivo MRI evidence. Neuroreport 3:713–716, 1992

Reisberg B, Ferris SH, Franssen E, et al: Age associated memory impairment: the clinical syndrome. Developmental Neuropsychology 2:401–402, 1986

Rey A: L'examen psychologique dans les cas d'encephalopathie traumatique. Archives de Psychologie 28:286–340, 1941

Rey A: L'examen clinique en psychologie [Clinical examinations in psychology]. Paris, Presses Universitaires de France, 1964

Rosen TJ: Age-associated memory impairment: a critique. European Journal of Cognitive Psychology 2:275–287, 1990

Rowe JW, Kahn RL: Human aging: usual and successful. Science 237:143–149, 1987

Salthouse TA: General and specific speed mediation of adult age differences in memory. J Gerontol B Psychol Sci Soc Sci 51:P30–P42, 1996

Salthouse TA, Mitchell RP, Palman R: Memory and age differences in spatial manipulation ability. Psychol Aging 4:480–486, 1989

Salthouse TA, Babcock RL, Shaw RJ: Effects of adult age on structural and operational capacities in working memory. Psychol Aging 118–127, 1991

Saxton J, Becker JT: The Rey-Osterrieth Complex Figure and dementia, in The Handbook of Rey-Osterrieth Complex Figure Usage: Clinical and Research Applications. Edited by Knight JA, Kaplan EF. Odessa FL, Psychological Assessment Resources (in press)

Schacter DL, Kaszniak AW, Kihlstrom JF: Models of memory and the understanding of memory disorders, in Memory Disorders: Research and Clinical Practice. Edited by Yanagihara T, Petersen RC. New York, Marcel Dekker, 1991, pp 111–134

Scogin F, Storandt M, Lott L: Memory skills training, memory complaints and depression in older adults. J Gerontol 40:562–568, 1985

Seab JP, Jagust WJ, Wong ST, et al: Quantitative NMR measurements of hippocampal atrophy in Alzheimer's disease. Magn Reson Med 8:200–208, 1988

Smith AD: Memory, in Handbook of the Psychology of Aging. Edited by Birren JE, Schaie KW. New York, Academic Press, 1996, pp 236–250

Smith G, Ivnik RJ, Petersen RC, et al: Age-associated memory impairment diagnoses: problems of reliability and concerns for terminology. Psychol Aging 6:551–558, 1991

Spreen O, Strauss E: A Compendium of Neuropsychological Tests: Administration, Norms, and Commentary, 2nd Edition. New York, Oxford University Press, 1998

Stuss DT, Craik FI, Sayer L, et al: Comparison of older people and patients with frontal lesions: evidence from word list learning. Psychol Aging 11:387–395, 1996

Sunderland A, Harris JE, Baddeley AD: Do laboratory tests predict everyday memory? A neuropsychological study. Journal of Verbal Learning and Verbal Behavior 22:341–357, 1983

Sunderland A, Watts K, Baddeley AD, et al: Subjective memory assessment and test performance in elderly adults. J Gerontol 41:376–384, 1986

Troyer AK, Graves RE, Cullum CM: Executive functions as a mediator of the relationship between age and episodic memory in healthy aging. Aging Neuropsychology and Cognition 1:45–53, 1994

Wechsler D: A standardized memory scale for clinical use. J Psychol 19:87–95, 1945

Wechsler D: Wechsler Adult Intelligence Scale. New York, Psychological Corporation, 1955

Wechsler D: Wechsler Adult Intelligence Scale—Revised Manual. New York, Psychological Corporation, 1981

Wechsler D: Wechsler Memory Scale—Revised Manual. San Antonio, TX, Psychological Corporation, 1987

Wechsler D: Wechsler Adult Intelligence Scale—Third Edition Manual. San Antonio, Psychological Corporation, 1997a

Wechsler D: Wechsler Memory Scale—Third Edition Manual. San Antonio, Psychological Corporation, 1997b

Wilson B, Cockburn J, Baddeley A: The Rivermead Behavioural Memory Test. Reading, England, Thames Valley Test Company, 1985

World Health Organization: Mental Disorders: Glossary and Guide to Their Classification in Accordance With the Ninth Revision of the International Classification of Diseases. Geneva, World Health Organization, 1978

Zarit SH, Cole KD, Guider RL: Memory training strategies and subjective complaints of memory in the aged. Gerontologist 21:158–164, 1981

Zelinski EM, Gilewski MJ: Assessment of memory complaint by rating scales and questionnaires. Psychopharmacol Bull 24:523–529, 1988

Zelinski EM, Gilewski MJ, Thompson LW: Do laboratory tests relate to self assessment of memory ability in the young and old? in New Directions in Memory and Aging: Proceedings of the George A. Talland Memorial Conference. Edited by Poon LW, Fozard JL, Cermak LS, et al. Hillsdale, NJ, Lawrence Erlbaum, 1980, pp 519–544

9

Anatomic Imaging of the Aging Human Brain

Computed Tomography and Magnetic Resonance Imaging

C. Edward Coffey, M.D.

For most of human history, life expectancy was remarkably stable at about 30–40 years (Cutler 1976, 1979). Within the past 150 years, however, advances in medical science (particularly the successful treatment of infectious diseases) have resulted in a dramatic increase in life span, so that men and women born in 1980 can now expect to live for an average of 70.0 and 77.5 years, respectively (Rowe and Katzman 1992). As such, the elderly segment of our population is growing; the number of persons 65 years old or older increased 8-fold from 1900 (3 million) to 1980 (25 million), and the number of those over age 75 (the so-called old old) has increased 11-fold during that same time period (from 900,000 to 10,000,000) (McFarland 1978).

The continued expansion of the elderly segment of our population and a growing awareness of age-related diseases such as dementia have prompted considerable interest in the study of the aging human brain. Central to this study have been efforts to characterize the spectrum and extent of changes in brain morphology that occur with "normal ag-

ing." Such normative data are essential for an understanding of "pathological" brain aging in elderly people (Creasey and Rapoport 1985; DeCarli et al. 1990; Drayer 1988).

Investigations of age-related changes in brain morphology have used two approaches: autopsy studies and brain imaging techniques. Autopsy studies have found consistent age-related reductions in brain weight and volume (about 2% per decade), cortical volume, and regional cortical neuronal number (Creasey and Rapoport 1985; Katzman and Terry 1992; see also Chapter 3 in this volume). Ventricular dilation has also been reported, and the variance of measurements of ventricular size appears to increase with age. However, neuropathological measures of brain morphology are subject to sources of error such as selection bias, technical and fixation artifacts, and the influences of premorbid illness and cause of death (which may be different for young versus elderly cohorts). Brain imaging techniques avoid many of these problems and provide an opportunity to examine brain morphology in healthy living subjects, with increasing anatomical resolution.

In this chapter, I review imaging studies that have examined the effects of aging on brain anatomy. I begin with a discussion of methodological issues relevant to such investigations and then summarize findings regarding the effects of age on brain ventricular and parenchymal structures. Finally, the potential relationship of these structural brain alterations to age-related changes in cognitive function is also discussed.

Methodological Issues Relevant to the Imaging Assessment of Age-Related Changes in Brain Structure

Study Design

Imaging studies of brain aging can be designed as either cross-sectional or longitudinal investigations. In cross-sectional studies, a single imaging evaluation is performed at roughly the same time on a group of subjects whose ages differ across a range of interest. Such studies allow for relatively rapid, efficient, and economical acquisition of large amounts of data, and it is not surprising therefore that most investigations to date have used a cross-sectional design. However, cross-sectional studies may be influenced by secular effects (i.e., the possibility that brain size exhibits systematic changes over successive birth cohorts in the general population). For example, successive generations may have, on average, larger parenchymal volumes and smaller ventricular volumes. If such trends actually exist in the population at large and if they are not secondary to secular trends associated with correlates of brain morphology such as cranial size or years of education, then an assessment of the true effects of aging on brain size will require longitudinal investigation.

In longitudinal studies, imaging evaluations are repeated on the same group of subjects as they age over time. Such studies are thus free of secular effects, but they are labor intensive and may suffer from significant attrition effects (i.e., subject dropout may result in a sample at the end of the investigation that is markedly different from that at the beginning). Longitudinal studies may also outlive their usefulness (the period effect); for example, an ongoing study of ventricular size that began in the era of pneumoencephalography would not be of great interest in today's world of high-resolution computed tomography (CT) and magnetic resonance (MR) imaging.

The interpretation of both cross-sectional and longitudinal investigations must also consider the possible influences of "survivor effects" and heterogeneity within the elderly population (Creasey and Rapoport 1985). *Survivor effect* refers to the overrepresentation in study samples of relatively healthy subjects (the survivors) because others with preexisting illnesses may have died before study entry. Relative to younger populations, the elderly exhibit greater heterogeneity in a variety of physiological variables that could indirectly influence brain structure. In summary, both cross-sectional and longitudinal study designs have strengths and limitations: the choice of one approach over the other will depend on available resources and the specific aims of the investigation.

Subject Selection

Brain morphology may be affected by variables in the subject sample that are associated with the aging process (e.g., concomitant medical illnesses such as hypertension, diabetes mellitus), as well as by other variables that are relatively independent of it (e.g., gender, body or head size, handedness, education, socioeconomic status, and psychiatric and drug-use history). These variables must be considered and appropriately controlled before conclusions can be reached about the effects of aging, per se, on brain anatomy. It should also be noted that the apparent effects of age on brain structure may vary depending on the age range of the sample studied. In general, aging effects have been less robust in samples with restricted age ranges (Appendixes 9–1, 9–2, and 9–3).

Subject sample.   Selection of an appropriate subject sample is obviously a critically important first step in any investigation of aging effects on brain morphology. A sample of healthy volunteers from the community may differ markedly from a sample of medical or psychiatric *patients* with "normal" scans. Although the latter samples provide a convenient and economical source of readily available imaging data, such samples may include individuals with structural brain changes resulting from causes other than aging (Coffey et al. 1998). In addition, patient samples are generally less representative of the variability in brain morphology that exists within samples of healthy volunteers. As noted above, such heterogeneity is especially great among the elderly, a finding that may be related in part to differences between "usual aging" (i.e., no clinically obvious brain disease) and "successful aging" (i.e., minimal decline in neurobiological function in comparison to that of younger subjects) (Coffey et al. 1998; Rowe and Kahn 1987).

Thus, even within studies that examine healthy community volunteers, considerable variability in brain morphology may exist depending on the relative mix of subjects with usual versus successful aging. Whenever possible, studies should attempt to define the extent to which their subjects fall within these two categories, based in part on thorough medical, neuropsychiatric, and neuropsychological evaluations, as well as on correlative assessments of brain function (e.g., with electroencephalography [EEG], single photon emission computed tomography [SPECT], or positron-emission tomography [PET]). Even these evaluations may fail to identify subjects with various other conditions that may affect brain morphology, including those with preclinical disease or with genetic predispositions to disease. In this chapter, I review those studies that have for the most part examined healthy volunteers from the community.

Sample size is also an important factor in interpreting results—negative findings in studies with relatively small samples may be a result of low power.

Gender and body size. Women are smaller (i.e., shorter and lighter) on average than men are, and, as such, their heads and brains also tend to be smaller (Gould 1981). Even within a single-gender study, however, differences in body or head size among subjects may confound apparent age-related differences. Although there is no generally accepted method of correcting for head or body size, this variable may be taken into account either through subject matching (e.g., on height), statistical analysis (e.g., analysis of covariance), or the use of ratio measures (e.g., using intracranial or total brain size as the denominator) (Appendixes 9–1, 9–2, and 9–3). The latter procedure suffers from two limitations (Coffey et al. 1998). First, the ratio approach implicitly assumes that brain size is perfectly correlated with intracranial size. Although the two variables are highly correlated, the assumption of perfect correlation is in my view untenable. Second, the ratio approach creates outcome variables that are necessarily bounded between zero and one. Such variables may have distributions poorly suited for linear regression analysis. Even after controlling for differences in head size, the literature suggests that gender may interact with the aging process to influence changes in brain structure (see below).

Handedness. Several studies have demonstrated differences in regional brain size or symmetry between right-handed and left-handed (or non–right-handed) individuals (Kertesz et al. 1992; Witelson 1992). Surprisingly, only a few investigations of the aging brain have specified the handedness of their subjects (Appendixes 9–1, 9–2, and 9–3). This variable should be assessed with continuous quantitative measures (Coffey et al. 1992), and its effects on brain structure should be controlled either statistically or through subject inclusion criteria (e.g., limiting the sample to those subjects with definite motoric lateralization).

Education and socioeconomic status. Imaging studies have reported a relationship between brain structure and educational level or socioeconomic class (Andreasen et al. 1990; Coffey et al. 1999; Pearlson et al. 1989b). This relationship may be an indirect one, however, with both of these variables (and perhaps also IQ) serving as markers for body or head size (Pfefferbaum et al. 1990). Studies of brain aging should assess the potential impact of these variables statistically (Coffey et al. 1992, 1999) or attempt to control them through subject matching procedures when appropriate (Pfefferbaum et al. 1990).

Psychiatric and drug-use history. Alterations of brain morphology have been described in patients with a variety of psychiatric disorders, including schizophrenia (Pfefferbaum et al. 1990), affective illness (Coffey 1996; Coffey et al. 1990, 1993), and eating disorders (Laessle et al. 1989). Although some earlier studies failed to specify the psychiatric histories of their subjects, more recent investigations have appropriately excluded patients with such histories (Appendixes 9–1, 9–2, and 9–3). Alcohol and perhaps other drug use may also alter brain structure (Cascella et al. 1991; Lishman 1990; Pfefferbaum et al. 1998), but again studies have varied in the extent to which these factors have been considered (Appendixes 9–1, 9–2, and 9–3). Although more recent investigations of brain aging have generally excluded subjects with substance abuse or dependence, the effects of subclinical drug or alcohol consumption on structural brain aging have not been thoroughly assessed. One major impediment to such efforts has been the inability to obtain reliable and accurate data about the extent of lifetime drug use.

Imaging Technique

Imaging modality. Early imaging modalities provided only indirect visualization of the human brain by imaging either the skull (skull radiography), the cerebral vessels (arteriography), or the cerebrospinal fluid (CSF) spaces (pneumoencephalography). More recent developments in computer technology have now made possible in vivo visualization of brain tissue with imaging techniques such as CT and MR imaging. These techniques differ in their safety, anatomical resolution, and sensitivity to tissue contrast.

X-ray CT images are formed when X rays are passed through the brain from several different directions. Detectors opposite the X-ray source measure the extent to which passage of the X-ray beams has been attenuated by the intervening tissues. Computers relate this information to the density of the various structures (e.g., CSF, bone, gray matter, and white matter) and then construct a series of tomographic images of the brain and cranium.

X-ray CT is a relatively quick and inexpensive imaging modality, but because subjects are exposed to irradiation (about 2 rad), serial studies in healthy individuals may not be possible. The method is also limited by relatively low spatial and anatomic resolution, partial volume effects (inaccurate averaging of tissue attenuation values), and beam-hardening artifact (false elevation of brain CT values adjacent to the skull). This latter problem limits the precision with which boundaries can be determined for structures adjacent to bone, including the temporal lobes, the apical cortex, or the inferior frontal lobes, regions of great interest to neuropsychiatrists.

MR images are formed when the alignment of ions (in medical imaging these are typically protons) in a strong magnetic field is disrupted by a brief radiofrequency pulse. When the pulse is terminated, radiofrequency energy is emitted as the protons become realigned within the magnetic field. Computers relate this emitted radiofrequency energy to various tissue (proton) characteristics, from which a series of planar or three-dimensional images can be constructed. Various imaging sequences may be used to examine different tissue characteristics, resulting in images that are relatively T1- or T2-weighted. In general, T1-weighted images provide greater anatomic resolution, whereas T2-weighted images provide higher contrast and greater sensitivity to pathological tissue changes.

Relative to CT, MR imaging provides more accurate structural information because of clear differentiation of gray matter, white matter, and CSF; the absence of beam-hardening artifact; and the capability to image in multiple planes, thereby providing optimal views of regional cerebral structures with less volume-averaging artifact (see below). Additionally, MR imaging has greater sensitivity to detect pathological tissue, particularly hyperintense foci of the subcortical white matter and gray matter nuclei (subcortical hyperintensity) that occur with increasing frequency in elderly people (Coffey and Figiel 1991). Because MR imaging does not use ionizing radiation, serial studies in healthy subjects are possible.

For these reasons, MR imaging appears to be uniquely suited to the study of age-related changes in brain morphology. It should be noted however, that accurate assessment of brain structure with MR imaging may be affected by a number of technical factors, including choice of acquisition sequence parameters (affecting tissue contrast), slice section thickness (adjacent sections that are too thin may result in overlapping profiles and "cross-talk" artifact), and magnetic field homogeneity (inhomogeneous fields may result in spatial distortion of objects and object pixel nonuniformity) (Jack et al. 1988). Movement artifact may also be induced by pulsation of blood and CSF, especially in the limbic system where structures lie in close proximity to the ventricles and the carotid arteries—such artifact can be lessened with the use of cardiac-gating and flow-compensated pulse sequences (Pfefferbaum et al. 1990). Careful consideration of these methodological issues is needed to ensure precision of measurement with MR imaging. MR imaging is a more expensive and often more lengthy procedure than CT, and some subjects may be unable to cooperate with the long imaging time, especially if they feel confined by the scanner and develop claustrophobia; however, recent advances in imaging technology have resulted in considerable shortening of scanning time with MR imaging. Finally, MR imaging cannot be used in subjects who have a pacemaker or intracranial ferromagnetic objects such as surgical clips. Irrespective of whether CT or MR imaging is employed, the quality of the images collected may be affected by several factors.

Plane of imaging.   The optimal orientation from which to visualize brain anatomy will vary depending on the structure of interest. For example, corpus callosum and medial prefrontal cortex are best seen on midsagittal images, axial images provide a good view of subcortical white matter and gray nuclei (i.e., thalamus and basal ganglia), and coronal sections are required for optimal views of the temporal lobes and limbic structures. With brain CT, the plane of imaging is limited by the patient's position in the scanner: because typically the patient is supine, axial images are produced. With MR imaging, the plane of imaging can be determined simply by programming the magnetic gradients, making possible images in the coronal, axial, and sagittal planes, irrespective of patient positioning within the scanner.

Once the appropriate imaging plane has been selected, the images must be acquired in a standardized orientation so that valid comparisons across subjects are possible. Proper alignment of acquisition plane is especially critical for studies of brain asymmetry because head tilt can result in artifactual right-left differences. External landmarks (e.g., the canthomeatal line) are relatively quick and easy to establish for orientation, but they may not be consistently related to brain structure (Homan et al. 1987). Such problems may be obviated by use of internal landmarks (e.g., the anterior commissure–posterior commissure line), but these can be more technically difficult to establish and thus may add to the length of the scanning procedure.

Slice thickness. Image resolution is affected by section thickness, as each image data point (voxel) in the slice represents an average of slice thickness (millimeters) raised to the third power. Thus the thinner the section, the higher the resolution. However, with thin sections, a greater total scanning time is required to image a given volume, and thin sections are also associated with a reduced signal-to-noise ratio (less tissue is present to produce a signal). Furthermore, slice thickness with MR imaging is limited by certain technical factors including gradient strength, quantity of radiofrequency energy used for excitation, and the phenomenon of cross-talk artifact. This latter problem can be partially obviated by leaving space between adjacent sections (interscan gap), but this method excludes a given portion of tissue from direct assessment, thereby reducing the accuracy of volume measurements (particularly of small or irregular structures). Section interleaving is another method for reducing cross-talk artifact, but this procedure doubles scanning time.

Phantom calibration. Verification of the accuracy of imaging data against a known standard (phantom) should be conducted on a regular basis to ensure stability of the imaging hardware. With MR imaging in particular, image data may be affected by variations in the main magnetic field, the magnetic field gradient systems, and the radiofrequency pulse system.

Head movement artifact. Involuntary head movement by subjects is another source of artifact that can degrade image quality. Head movement is more likely as the length of the scanning time increases, and it may be especially troublesome in certain clinical circumstances. For example, at least some elderly subjects with arthritic conditions may be unable to lie still for more than a few minutes, making comparisons with younger nonarthritic subjects problematic. Head movement may be reduced by physical restraints (e.g., Velcro straps or fitted plastic masks) or the use of sedative medications, but the latter are rarely appropriate for use in nonpatient volunteers.

Methods of Image Analysis

General considerations. The quality of imaging data is affected by several factors related to the methodology of image analysis. First, measurements can be made on a variety of different forms of imaging data including radiographs, overhead projections of radiographs, photographs of the image, or displays of the original digital image data on computer consoles (Jack 1991). Computerized digital data systems afford the greatest flexibility and permit standardization of window settings across images, thereby providing for greater consistency and accuracy of measurement than is possible from films, where window settings are fixed. Second, the interpretation of brain imaging data will be affected by the criteria used to define the structure of interest. For example, the measured size of the frontal lobes on MR imaging will vary depending on whether their posterior boundary has been defined by the optic chiasma, the genu of the corpus callosum, or the central sulcus (Coffey et al. 1992; Kelsoe et al. 1988). Anatomic non-uniformity in these landmarks across subjects will also contribute to variability in regional brain measures. Third, the reliability of the measures of brain anatomy will vary with the skill of the rater—both interrater and intrarater reliabilities should be reported for all raters, using either kappa statistics or intraclass correlation coefficients. Finally, it should be clear from the above that assessment of imaging data requires considerable subjective judgment on the part of the rater. As such, all measurements should be performed by raters who are "blind" to subject data (e.g., age, gender, and diagnostic group) or to study hypotheses that could bias such assessments.

Types of measures. The effects of aging on brain morphology have been assessed with both qualitative and quantitative measures. Qualitative measures consist of various scales to determine the presence and severity of parameters of interest, including, for example, cortical atrophy or ventricular enlargement. Qualitative measures are relatively inexpensive and easy to use, do not require sophisticated technological support, are frequently "clinically relevant," and may show good agreement with more quantitative assessments (Zatz et al. 1982a). Qualitative measures have limited resolution and sensitivity, however, and their accuracy is critically dependent on the skill of the particular rater. For this reason, it is often difficult to compare results from different studies, especially when different rating scales have been used.

Quantitative measures of brain size may be either linear (distance measurement), planimetric (area measurement), or volumetric (multisection planimetric). Linear and planimetric measures are relatively quick and inexpensive and are available to researchers who lack sophisticated computerized image processing capabilities. Such measures also correlate reasonably well with volumetric measures, at least for structures of regular shape. For more complicated structures with irregular shapes, however, volumetric measures are much more accurate, especially when the sections are relatively thin (< 5 mm) and contiguous, and when they span the entire extent of the structure of interest. Volumetric measures are also more sensitive than linear and planimetric methods for detecting subtle group differences (Gado et al. 1983; S. Raz et al. 1987). Finally, volumetric measures are especially important for assessing left-right asymmetries because single-section measures are much more susceptible to the confounding effects of head tilt and patient positioning and because bilateral structures may not be aligned in a perfectly parallel position within the left and right hemispheres. In such situations, the left and right sides of a structure could differ with regard to the particular imaging section on which they appeared larger, in which case left-versus-right comparisons based on a single section clearly would not be representative of any asymmetry in the total volume of that structure.

Among quantitative brain imaging studies, differences exist in the technique used to segment the cranial contents into bone, CSF, white matter, and gray matter compartments. Regions of interest may be outlined manually ("trace" technique) or tissue segmentation can be performed automatically by establishing threshold values of pixel intensity for each tissue compartment. These automated procedures should improve substantially test-retest reliability and the speed with which large volumes of imaging data can be analyzed, but they are less adept at segmenting regions with similar pixel intensity values (e.g., separating amygdala from hippocampus).

Effects of Aging on Brain Structure

Ventricular Size

Brain CT and MR imaging investigations have consistently demonstrated *enlargement of the ventricular system* with age (Appendix 9–1). The reported extent of enlargement has varied, however, depending on the way in which ventricular size has been assessed. General estimates from the literature suggest that, over the first nine decades of life, the ventricular/brain ratio (VBR) may increase nonlinearly from 2% to 17% (Barron et al. 1976; Pearlson et al. 1989a; Schwartz et al. 1985; Stafford et al. 1988), the proportion of ventricular fluid volume to brain volume may increase from 2%–4% to 4%–8% (Stafford et al. 1988), and the proportion of ventricular fluid volume to cranial volume may increase from 1%–2% to 2%–4% (R. C. Gur et al. 1991; Jernigan et al. 1990; Murphy et al. 1992; Pfefferbaum et al. 1986). These age effects appear to be similar for the lateral and third ventricles (Coffey et al. 1992; Murphy et al. 1992; Schwartz et al. 1985). The fourth ventricle is rarely reported separately from the total ventricular system (Appendix 9–1). Shah et al. (1991) and Blatter et al. (1995) found no relation between age and fourth ventricular size.

In a study of 76 healthy adult volunteers from our laboratory, we found that increasing age was associated with significantly larger volumes of the lateral ventricles and the third ventricle (Coffey et al. 1992). After adjusting for gender and intracranial size, both lateral ventricular volume and third ventricular volume were found to increase by approximately 3% per year (Figure 9–1). In a second study focusing on elderly volunteers (*N* = 330) living independently in the community, we found age-specific increases in lateral ventricular volume of approximately 0.95 mL/year and in third ventricular volume of approximately 0.05 mL/year, over ages 65–95 years old (Coffey et al. 1998).

We have also conducted blinded ratings of lateral ventricular enlargement to provide a "clinical context" within which to interpret these volumetric changes (Coffey et al. 1992). We found that the frequency of at least mild lateral ventricular enlargement (Table 9–1) increased significantly with age, in agreement with numerous imaging and postmortem studies (Appendix 9–1). The odds of at least mild lateral ventricular enlargement were 0.10 at age 40 and increased by approximately 7.7% per year to 2.22 at age 80. This ventriculomegaly was typically rated as mild in severity, however; and more than one-half (54%) of our elderly subjects did not meet criteria for lateral ventricular

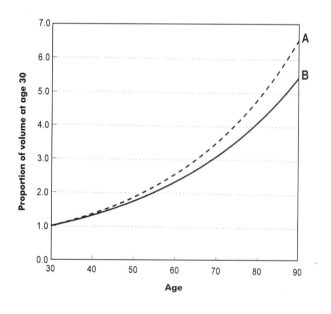

FIGURE 9–1. Increase in brain ventricular volumes with age, relative to volumes at age 30. Linear regression models for $\log_e$ (volume), controlling for the effects of gender and intracranial size, indicated that volume increased exponentially with age for both the lateral ventricles (*line A*) and the third ventricle (*line B*). The rate of volume increase was similar for each region (3.2% per year and 2.8% per year, respectively).

Source. Adapted from Coffey et al. 1992.

enlargement (Table 9–1). These findings are consistent with the increased variation in ventricular size with age that others (Creasey and Rapoport 1985; DeCarli et al. 1990) have observed. Thus, although ventricular volume increases with age, it appears that "clinically rated" ventricular enlargement is not an inevitable consequence of advancing age.

Only a small number of longitudinal studies of age-related ventricular enlargement have been reported (Appendix 9–1). Gado et al. (1983) found a 3.7% increase in the ratio of ventricular volume to cranial volume on CT in 12 elderly subjects followed for 1 year, but no change in linear measures of ventricular size. In a sample of older adults, Shear et al. (1995) reported an average increase in ventricu-

TABLE 9–1.　**Ratings of cortical atrophy, lateral ventricular enlargement, and subcortical hyperintensity**

Rating score	Age (years)					
	30–39	40–49	50–59	60–69	70–79	> 80
Cortical atrophy[a]						
0	6 (60%)	6 (67%)	2 (18%)	3 (18%)	3 (13%)	
1	3 (30%)	2 (22%)	7 (64%)	7 (41%)	6 (25%)	1 (17%)
2 (mild)	1 (10%)	1 (11%)	2 (18%)	7 (41%)	12 (50%)	4 (67%)
3 (moderate)					3 (13%)	1 (17%)
4 (severe)						
Lateral ventricular enlargement						
0	8 (80%)	6 (67%)	5 (46%)	8 (47%)	3 (13%)	
1		2 (22%)	4 (36%)	4 (24%)	7 (29%)	
2 (mild)	2 (20%)	1 (11%)	2 (18%)	2 (12%)	11 (46%)	2 (33%)
3 (moderate)				3 (8%)	3 (13%)	4 (66%)
4 (severe)						
Subcortical hyperintensity[b]						
Deep white matter						
0	8 (80%)	5 (56%)	4 (36%)	7 (44%)	2 (8%)	1 (17%)
1	1 (10%)	3 (33%)	5 (46%)	7 (44%)	15 (63%)	2 (33%)
2	1 (10%)	1 (11%)	1 (9%)	1 (6%)	7 (29%)	1 (17%)
3			1 (9%)	1 (6%)		2 (33%)
Periventricular white matter						
0						
1	10 (100%)	9 (100%)	9 (82%)	15 (94%)	20 (83%)	4 (67%)
2			2 (18%)	1 (6%)	4 (17%)	2 (33%)
3						
Basal ganglia						
0	10 (100%)	8 (89%)	10 (91%)	15 (94%)	20 (83%)	4 (67%)
1 (present)		1 (11%)	1 (9%)	1 (6%)	4 (17%)	2 (33%)
Thalamus						
0	10 (100%)	9 (100%)	10 (91%)	15 (94%)	23 (96%)	5 (83%)
1 (present)			1 (9%)	1 (6%)	1 (4%)	1 (17%)
Pons						
0	10 (100%)	9 (100%)	11 (100%)	10 (63%)	15 (63%)	5 (67%)
1 (present)				6 (37%)	9 (37%)	1 (33%)

[a]See Figure 9–2 for examples of the visual standards used for the ratings of cortical atrophy.
[b]See Figures 9–7 and 9–8 for examples of the visual standards used for the ratings of subcortical hyperintensity.
Source.　Adapted from Coffey et al. 1992.

lar system volume on CT of approximately 0.61 mL/year over an average follow-up period of 2.6 years. Mueller et al. (1998) found a 1.4 mL/year increase in lateral ventricle volume on MR imaging in elderly subjects followed for 3–9 years. In a sample of 28 healthy 21- to 68-year-old men, Pfefferbaum et al. (1998) observed increases in both lateral (approximately 5 mL, or 20%) and third ventricular volumes on MR imaging over a scanning interval of 5 years.

A significant *hemispheric asymmetry* (left greater than right) exists in the volumes of the lateral ventricles (Coffey et al. 1992; Zipursky et al. 1990), but only a few studies have examined whether the right and left lateral ventricles differ with regard to aging effects (Appendix 9–1). Most of these authors have found no differences in aging effects on the two hemispheres (Coffey et al. 1992, 1998; DeCarli et al. 1994; Murphy et al. 1992, 1996; Schwartz et al. 1985), but R. C. Gur et al. (1991) reported that the age-related increase in ratio of ventricular CSF volume to cranial volume was more pronounced in the left hemisphere than in the right, a difference they attributed primarily to elderly men.

Although *gender differences* have been described in the size, symmetry, and function of several brain structures, only a small number of imaging studies have examined the effects of gender on brain aging in nonpatient samples of living humans (see Coffey et al. 1998 for review). Most studies, including recent work from our group, have found no gender effects on the age-related increase in lateral or third ventricular volume (Appendix 9–1). Because age-related ventricular enlargement is presumed to occur as a result of shrinkage of periventricular brain matter, these results are also consistent with other studies that found no effect of gender on the age-related volume loss of structures that form the borders of the lateral ventricles (i.e., the caudate nuclei) (Krishnan et al. 1990; Murphy et al. 1996) or the third ventricle (i.e., the thalamus) (Murphy et al. 1996) (see below). In contrast, Grant et al. (1987) reported that men, but not women, exhibited a significant age-related increase in lateral ventricular volume, although this apparent gender difference was not tested. Likewise, Blatter et al. (1995) observed higher correlations in males than in females between age and lateral ventricle volume (adjusted for intracranial volume [IV]) ($r = .444$ versus $r = .218$, respectively) and between age and third ventricle volume (adjusted for IV) ($r = .634$ versus $r = .406$, respectively), but again these correlations were not statistically compared. Kaye et al. (1992) reported that the precipitous age-related increases in lateral ventricular volume began about a decade earlier in males than in females. Finally, Murphy et al. (1996) found that *females* actually had a greater age-related increase in the ratio of third ventricle volume/IV than did males.

Brain Atrophy

Generalized brain atrophy.   The effects of age on brain size have been assessed with visual estimates (qualitative ratings) of sulcal enlargement, quantitative measurements of CSF spaces, and quantitative measurements of total and regional brain size. Age has been found to be significantly correlated with visual ratings of sulcal enlargement (Coffey et al. 1992; Jacoby et al. 1980; Yoshii et al. 1988) (Appendix 9–1). The only exceptions to these observations are the reports of Laffey et al. (1984) and Wahlund et al. (1990), which limited investigation to elderly subjects.

In our study of 76 healthy adults (Coffey et al. 1992), the odds of a rating of at least mild cortical atrophy were found to increase by approximately 8.9% per year such that, by age 68, subjects had a 50% chance of having acquired cortical atrophy. In spite of this predicted high frequency, the cortical atrophy present in our subjects was typically rated as mild (Figure 9–2). Moderately severe cortical atrophy was uncommon (four [9%] of 46 elderly subjects), and none of our subjects exhibited severe cortical atrophy (Table 9–1). These data suggest that although brain volume declines with age (see below), cortical atrophy (like ventricular enlargement) 1) is not an inevitable correlate of normal aging and 2) when present is typically mild in severity and therefore relatively unlikely to be considered "clinically significant."

Quantitative studies of sulcal CSF spaces have consistently demonstrated increased CSF volume with age (Appendix 9–1), the only exception being two relatively small studies of older adults (Tanna et al. 1991; Wahlund et al. 1990). Estimates of sulcal and cisternal volume range from 1 mL at the second decade of life to 40 mL at the ninth decade (Zatz et al. 1982a). Over the same age span, the proportion of sulcal CSF volume to cranial volume increases from approximately 3% to approximately 10% (R. C. Gur et al. 1991; Jernigan et al. 1990; Murphy et al. 1992), roughly at a rate of 1.0% per decade (Coffey et al. 1998; DeCarli et al. 1994; Pfefferbaum et al. 1994). The age-related increase in sulcal CSF volume may not be linear, however, and appears to be greatest after age 60 (Pfefferbaum et al. 1986; Zatz et al. 1982a). Variability in the measures of sulcal CSF volume also increases substantially with age (Coffey et al. 1998; DeCarli et al. 1994; Pfefferbaum et al. 1986; Zatz et al. 1982a).

Only a small number of *longitudinal studies* of age-related sulcal CSF volume increase have been reported (Appendix 9–1). Gado et al. (1983) found that the ratio of sulcal CSF volume to cranial volume increased by an average of 13% in 12 elderly subjects followed over 1 year.

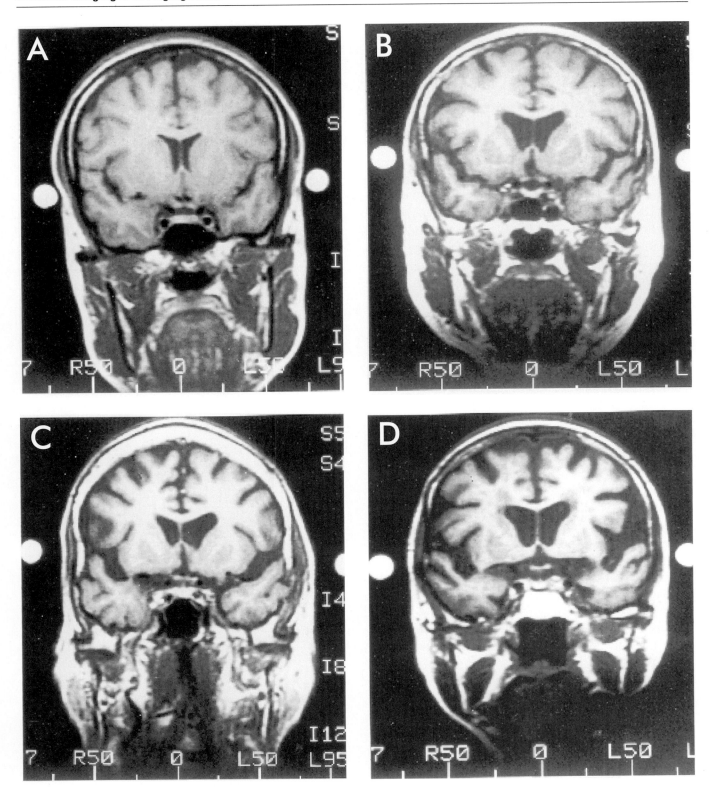

FIGURE 9–2. Visual standards for cortical atrophy score ratings on T1-weighted coronal magnetic resonance images (repetition time = 500 milliseconds, echo time = 20 milliseconds). *Panel A:* Grade 0, 1 = none, borderline. *Panel B:* Grade 2 = mild cortical atrophy. *Panel C:* Grade 3 = moderate cortical atrophy with widening of the interhemispheric fissure. *Panel D:* Grade 4 = severe cortical atrophy, with widening of almost all sulci. This subject also exhibits moderately severe enlargement of the lateral ventricles.
Source. Reprinted with permission from Coffey CE: "Structural Brain Abnormalities in the Depressed Elderly," in *Brain Imaging in Affective Disorders.* Edited by Hauser P. Washington, DC, American Psychiatric Press, 1991, pp. 92–93.

Mueller et al. (1998) found a 1.5 mL/year increase in total CSF volume on MR imaging in elderly subjects followed for 3–9 years. In a sample of 28 healthy 21- to 68-year-old men, Pfefferbaum et al. (1998) observed no significant increase in sulcal CSF volume on MR imaging over a scanning interval of 5 years.

Quantitative investigations that directly measure brain size have consistently found reduced total brain volume with age (Appendix 9–2). The only negative study attempted to estimate brain volume from a single brain section (Yoshii et al. 1988). (It should also be noted that these same subjects did exhibit age-related cortical atrophy as determined from ratings of sulcal enlargement.) Over the first nine decades of life, the ratio of cerebral volume to cranial volume appears to decrease from approximately 93% to approximately 82% (Coffey et al. 1992; Jernigan et al. 1990; Tanna et al. 1991), and brain volume may decrease from an average of approximately 1200–1300 mL to approximately 1100–1200 mL (Coffey et al. 1992; R. C. Gur et al. 1991; Murphy et al. 1992). In our study of 76 healthy adult volunteers, we found that increasing age was associated with a significant decrease in total cerebral hemisphere volume of approximately 0.23% per year (Coffey et al. 1992). In a second study focusing on elderly volunteers ($N = 330$) living independently in the community, we found age-specific reductions in total cerebral hemisphere volume of approximately 2.79 mL/year from ages 65 to 95 years (Coffey et al. 1998). Recent data suggest that genetic factors may contribute to individual differences in both brain parenchymal and CSF volume changes in normal aging (Carmelli et al. 1999).

Only a few *longitudinal studies* of global cerebral volume loss with age have been undertaken (Appendix 9–2). Significant reductions have been observed for whole brain volume (Fox et al. 1996; negative findings reported by Gur et al. 1998) and for total gray matter volume (Pfefferbaum et al. 1998).

Only a few studies have compared the effects of aging on the *right and left cerebral hemispheres,* and none of these has found any difference between hemispheres with regard to age-related total hemisphere volume loss (Appendix 9–2).

Recent literature suggests that *gender differences* may exist in the effects of age on cerebral hemisphere volume loss (see Coffey et al. 1998 for review) (Appendix 9–2). In our study of 330 elderly volunteers, we found that from ages 65 to 95 years males (of average IV) had an increase in peripheral CSF volume of approximately 32% compared with less than a 1% increase in females (Coffey et al. 1998) (Figure 9–3). Gur et al. (1991) also found that the ratio of sulcal CSF volume/IV was greater for elderly (55 years and older) subjects and for men. Similarly, Blatter et al. (1995)

found higher correlations between age and "subarachnoid" CSF volume (adjusted for IV) in males ($r = .653$) than in females ($r = .545$), although these correlations were not statistically compared. Other cross-sectional studies that examined peripheral CSF volume have found no gender effects on age-related increases (Murphy et al. 1996; Sullivan et al. 1993; Yue et al. 1997). In the longitudinal study of Mueller et al. (1998), females apparently showed greater age-related increases in total CSF volume than did males (actual data not reported).

In contrast to the gender differences observed with regard to age-related increases in peripheral CSF, we found no gender differences in the age-related decrease in cerebral hemisphere volume. Similar negative findings have been reported (Coffey et al. 1992; R. C. Gur et al. 1991; Raz et al. 1993c, 1997; Murphy et al. 1996; Sullivan et al. 1993; Yoshii et al. 1988). Although Condon et al. (1988) found that men, but not women, exhibited a significant correlation between age and the ratio of total brain volume/IV, these correlations were not statistically compared. Similarly, Blatter et al. (1995) observed higher correlations in males than in females between age and the ratio of total brain volume/IV ($r = -.675$ versus $r = -.539$, respectively), but again these correlations were not statistically compared. Murphy et al. (1996) reported that males had a significantly greater age-related decrease in the ratio of cerebral hemisphere volume/IV than did females.

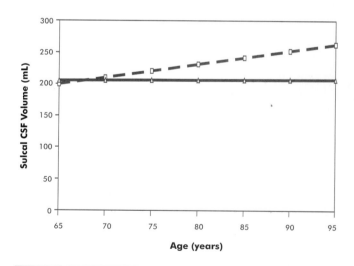

FIGURE 9–3.   Effects of gender on age-specific changes in sulcal cerebrospinal fluid (CSF) volume. Hierarchical regression models for CSF volume, adjusting for the effects of intracranial volume, age, and gender, indicated a significant age-by-gender interaction. Age-specific increases in sulcal CSF volume were significantly greater in men (*dashed line*) than in women (*solid line*) (2.11 mL/year versus 0.06 mL/year, respectively).
Source.   Adapted from Coffey et al. 1998.

Our finding of a significant gender effect on the age-related increase in peripheral CSF volume, in the absence of a gender effect on age-related volume loss of cerebral hemisphere brain matter, is consistent with the observations of R. C. Gur et al. (1991). Taken together, these reports suggest that although peripheral CSF volume may show a greater age-related increase in males than in females (likely as a result of cortical atrophy), such gender differences in cortical atrophy may not be apparent statistically when the size of the cortex is averaged in with a relatively larger structure such as the cerebral hemisphere. We are not aware of any studies that have examined gender effects on age-related tissue loss in the cortex per se.

Regional brain atrophy. Significant age-related reductions have been observed for total *gray matter* volume (Blatter et al. 1995; Guttmann et al. 1998; Lim et al. 1992; Passe et al. 1997; Schwartz et al. 1985) and cortical gray matter volume (Jernigan et al. 1991; Meyer et al. 1994; Pfefferbaum et al. 1994), as well as for specific gray matter structures such as the anterior diencephalon (Jernigan et al. 1991), caudate nucleus (Gunning-Dixon et al. 1998; Hokama et al. 1995; Jernigan et al. 1991; Krishnan et al. 1990; Murphy et al. 1992, 1996; Raz et al. 1993a, 1993c; negative findings reported by Meyer et al. 1994), and putamen or lentiform nucleus (Gunning-Dixon et al. 1998; Hokama et al. 1995; McDonald et al. 1991; Murphy et al. 1992, 1996; Schwartz et al. 1985; negative findings reported by Jernigan et al. 1991; Meyer et al. 1994; Raz et al. 1993a). Conflicting findings have been reported for the thalamus (Murphy et al. 1992, 1996; Schwartz et al. 1985; negative findings reported by Jernigan et al. 1991 and Meyer et al. 1994). The decrease in cerebral gray matter size is likely related in part to age-related neuronal loss or shrinkage or to decreased neuronal interconnectivity (see Chapter 3 in this volume).

Although most studies suggest that total *cerebral white matter* volume does not appear to change significantly with age (Blatter et al. 1995; Jernigan et al. 1991; Lim et al. 1992; Meyer et al. 1994; Passe et al. 1997; Pfefferbaum et al. 1994; Raz et al. 1993b, 1993c, 1997; Schwartz et al. 1985), age effects have been reported for total white matter volume (Guttmann et al. 1998) and for certain regions (e.g., prefrontal) (Raz et al. 1997). Aging is also associated with changes in the tissue characteristics of brain white matter (and some gray matter nuclei), an issue that will be discussed below (see Subcortical Hyperintensity). Studies are consistent in describing age-related size reductions in total and regional corpus callosum (Davatzikos and Resnick 1998; Doraiswamy et al. 1991; Janowsky et al. 1996; Parashos et al. 1995; Salat et al. 1997), an effect that we ob-

serve to be especially prominent in the anterior-most regions (Parashos et al. 1995).

Age-related reductions in brain size have also been described for the frontal lobes ([Cala et al. 1981; Coffey et al. 1992, 1998; Cowell et al. 1994; DeCarli et al. 1994; Jacoby et al. 1980; Murphy et al. 1996; Raz et al. 1997, 1998b]; others observed no age-related changes for the dorsolateral prefrontal cortex [Raz et al. 1993b, 1993c] and the anterior cingulate cortex [Jernigan et al. 1991; Raz et al. 1997]), the temporal lobes (Coffey et al. 1992, 1998; Convit et al. 1995; Cowell et al. 1994; Jack et al. 1992; Murphy et al. 1996; Raz et al. 1997; negative findings reported by DeCarli et al. 1994), the amygdala-hippocampal complex (Coffey et al. 1992; Convit et al. 1995; Doraiswamy et al. 1993; Golomb et al. 1993; Jack et al. 1992, 1997, 1998; Mu et al. 1999; Murphy et al. 1996; O'Brien et al. 1997; Raz et al. 1998b; negative findings reported by Frisoni et al. 1999; Laakso et al. 1998; Raz et al. 1997), and the parietal-occipital lobes (Coffey et al. 1992, 1998; Cowell et al. 1994; Murphy et al. 1996; Raz et al. 1993b, 1993c, 1997, 1998b) (Appendix 9–2).

A relatively small literature has examined posterior fossa structures (Appendix 9–2). Age-related size reductions have been described for the cerebellum (global or regional) (Cala et al. 1981; Deshmukh et al. 1997; Murphy et al. 1996; Oguro et al. 1998; Raz et al. 1998a; negative findings reported by Deshmukh et al. 1997; Escalona et al. 1991; Salat et al. 1997; Shah et al. 1991) and for the midbrain (Doraiswamy et al. 1992; Oguro et al. 1998; Shah et al. 1991), but not for the pons or medulla (Oguro et al. 1998; Salat et al. 1997; Raz et al. 1998a). Oguro et al. (1998) suggested that males demonstrated greater age-related reductions did than females in size of midbrain tegmentum and cerebellar vermis.

In our investigation of 76 adult volunteers (Coffey et al. 1992), we observed that the relative rate of change in cerebral volume with age may differ among individual regions (Figure 9–4). Cerebral hemisphere volume, for example, declined at a rate of about 0.23% per year, a rate that agrees closely with previous postmortem (Davis and Wright 1977; Miller et al. 1980) and imaging studies (Appendix 9–2). In contrast, the rate of volume decrease for the frontal lobes (0.55% per year) was twice as great, indicating that this region may be particularly prone to volume loss associated with aging. This observation is consistent with a small number of imaging studies (Cala et al. 1981; DeCarli et al. 1994; Raz et al. 1997, 1998b) and with previous neuropathological studies demonstrating that the frontal lobes are disproportionately affected by age-related changes such as volume loss, thinning of cortical laminae, widening of superficial sulci, and alterations in neuronal cell populations (Haug 1985; Katzman and Terry 1992).

These data, taken together with findings from our study, may suggest a neuroanatomical substrate for age-related changes in frontal lobe function present in neuropsychological (Mittenberg et al. 1989) (see also Chapter 8 in this volume) and brain metabolic imaging (Alavi 1989; Warren et al. 1985) (see also Chapter 10 in this volume) studies of aging humans. The rates of volume loss for the temporal lobes (0.28% per year) and the amygdala-hippocampal complex (0.30% per year) were similar to those for the cerebral hemispheres.

Only a few *longitudinal studies* of regional cerebral volume loss with age have been undertaken (Appendixes 9–1 and 9–2). Significant reductions have been observed in frontal region (Shear et al. 1995; negative findings reported by R. E. Gur et al. 1998 and Mueller et al. 1998), prefrontal gray matter (Pfefferbaum et al. 1998), temporal lobe (Gur et al. 1998; Kaye et al. 1997; negative findings reported by Mueller et al. 1998), hippocampus (Jack et al. 1998, Mueller et al. 1998), and parietal-occipital region (Fox et al. 1996; Mueller et al. 1998; Pfefferbaum et al.

1998; Shear et al. 1995). Kaye et al. (1997) performed annual brain MR imaging in 30 healthy elderly subjects over an average follow-up of 42 months. Volume loss in the temporal lobes (about 1.27% per year) predicted eventual development of dementia, whereas volume loss in the hippocampus (about 2% per year) or parahippocampus (about 2.5% per year) did not.

Although *hemispheric asymmetries* exist in the size of many brain regions (Bear et al. 1986; Chui and Damasio 1980; Kertesz et al. 1992; LeMay and Kido 1978; Suddath et al. 1989; Weinberger et al. 1982; Weis et al. 1989), only a few studies have examined the interactions between aging and right versus left hemisphere volume loss (Appendix 9–2). No right-left hemispheric differences have been reported for the effects of aging on total gray matter (Schwartz et al. 1985) or total gray matter plus white matter (Schwartz et al. 1985), although Murphy et al. (1992) found that older men (> 60 years old) exhibited a right-greater-than-left asymmetry in lenticular nucleus volume, whereas young men showed the reverse asymmetry. Negative findings have been described by the majority of studies examining the frontal lobes (Coffey et al. 1992, 1998; DeCarli et al. 1994; Raz et al. 1997), although two studies have reported interesting interactions with gender. Cowell et al. (1994) found that the right-greater-than-left asymmetry of frontal lobe volume was larger in females greater than 40 years old than in younger females, a difference that was not seen in males. Murphy et al. (1996) found that age-related volume loss of the frontal lobes was greater in the right hemisphere for males, whereas in females the volume loss was greater in the left hemisphere. No hemispheric differences have been described in the effects of age on the temporal lobes (Coffey et al. 1992, 1998; Cowell et al. 1994; Murphy et al. 1996; Raz et al. 1997), the hippocampus (Coffey et al. 1992; Jack et al. 1997), or the amygdala (Coffey et al. 1992; Jack et al. 1997), although Jack et al. (1997) did observe a left-greater-than-right asymmetry in the age-related volume loss of the parahippocampal gyrus.

Gender differences may exist in the effects of aging on regional brain tissue loss (Appendix 9–2). In our recent study of 330 elderly volunteers (Coffey et al. 1998), we found that the age-associated increase in lateral fissure CSF volume, a marker of frontotemporal (and to a lesser extent, parietal) atrophy, was greater in men than in women. For example, from ages 65 to 95 years, men (of average IV) had an increase in lateral fissure volume of approximately 80%, whereas women had an increase of only approximately 37% (Figure 9–5). Cowell et al. (1994) and Murphy et al. (1996) found that males exhibited greater age-related decreases in the ratio of temporal lobe volume/IV than did females. Similarly, Golomb et al. (1993) found that

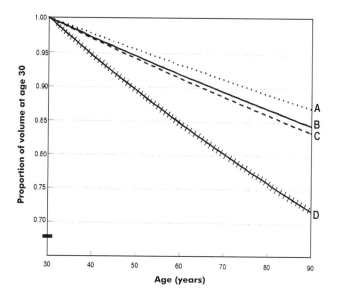

FIGURE 9–4. Decrease in regional cerebral volumes with age, relative to regional volumes at age 30. Linear regression models for $\log_e$ (volume), controlling for the effects of gender and intracranial size, indicated that volume decreased exponentially with age in the cerebral hemispheres (*line A*), the temporal lobes (*line B*), the amygdala-hippocampal complex (*line C*), and the frontal lobes (*line D*). It is apparent that the rate of change in brain volume with age was substantially greater for the frontal lobes (0.55% per year) than for the other regions (range of 0.23% to 0.30% per year). For example, relative to the cerebral hemispheres, frontal lobe volume decreased at a rate of 0.32% per year ($P < .004$).
Source. Adapted from Coffey et al. 1992.

age-related hippocampal atrophy was more common in males than in females, and Raz et al. (1997) observed greater age-related inferior temporal volume loss in males than in females. In contrast, Murphy et al. (1996) actually observed greater temporal lobe atrophy in females than in males. Despite differences in which gender is more affected, these published results suggest that gender may affect the age-related volume loss of the temporal lobe region. These findings may provide a neuroanatomic substrate for the gender differences in age-related verbal memory impairment (see Chapter 8 in this volume).

The literature is also conflicting with regard to the effects of gender on age-related changes in frontal lobe size (Appendix 9–2). Cowell et al. (1994) and Murphy et al. (1996) have both observed greater age-related frontal lobe volume loss in males than in females. In contrast, others have found no interactions between aging and gender effects (Coffey et al. 1992, 1998; Cowell et al. 1994; Raz et al. 1993c, 1997; Sullivan et al. 1993). These discrepant results may reflect differences among studies in samples and brain measurement techniques (e.g., quantitative versus qualitative measures, area measures from a single slice versus volume measures from multiple slices).

With regard to more posterior brain regions, we recently found that the age-related decrease in parietal-occipital region area was greater for males than it was for females. For example, from ages 65 to 95 years, men (of average IA) lost approximately 15% of their parietal-occipital lobe area, whereas women lost only 4% (Coffey et al. 1998) (Figure 9–6). Using a somewhat different definition of this brain region, Cowell et al. (1994) did not find any gender effect on the age-related decrease in the ratio of the posterior cerebral hemisphere volume/IV. Murphy et al. (1996) likewise found no gender differences in the age-related decrease in parieto-occipital region volume/IV, although they actually observed worse atrophy in females for the ratio of parietal lobe volume/IV. Similarly, Raz et al. (1993c) reported that females exhibited greater age-related volume loss in the visual cortex than did males. These widely divergent findings indicate a need for additional research (Appendix 9–2).

Our data also indicate that the rates of age-related changes in regional cerebral volume are greater for ventricular regions (about 3% per year) than for the parenchymal regions described above (0.23%–0.55% per year). This finding suggests that ventricular enlargement

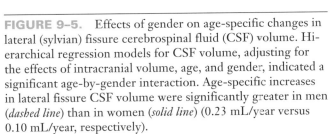

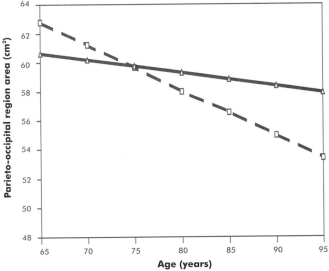

FIGURE 9–5. Effects of gender on age-specific changes in lateral (sylvian) fissure cerebrospinal fluid (CSF) volume. Hierarchical regression models for CSF volume, adjusting for the effects of intracranial volume, age, and gender, indicated a significant age-by-gender interaction. Age-specific increases in lateral fissure CSF volume were significantly greater in men (*dashed line*) than in women (*solid line*) (0.23 mL/year versus 0.10 mL/year, respectively).
Source. Adapted from Coffey et al. 1998.

FIGURE 9–6. Effects of gender on age-specific changes in parieto-occipital region area. Hierarchical regression models for cerebrospinal fluid (CSF) volume, adjusting for the effects of intracranial volume, age, and gender, indicated a significant age-by-gender interaction. Age-specific decreases in parieto-occipital region area were significantly greater in men (*dashed line*) than in women (*solid line*) (–0.31 mL/year versus –0.09 mL/year, respectively).
Source. Adapted from Coffey et al. 1998.

may provide a more sensitive index of brain aging than does cortical atrophy. It has been assumed that age-related ventricular enlargement occurs by ex vacuo expansion that results from shrinkage of periventricular structures. Current work is under way in our laboratory to examine whether age-related changes in the size of these structures (e.g., caudate and thalamic nuclei) are indeed related to the increase in ventricular volume that accompanies aging.

With regard to aging effects on the *shape* of brain structure, Magnotta and colleagues (1999) observed that age was associated with more sharply and steeply curved cortical gyri, as well as with sulci that were flatter and less curved.

In summary, aging is associated with global changes in brain structure, including decreased brain volume and increased CSF volume. In addition, differential effects of aging are observed for specific brain regions and structures. Some structures (e.g., association cortices such as prefrontal) are highly vulnerable to age-related volume loss, whereas others (e.g., medial temporal region) show moderate vulnerability, and still others (e.g., occipital cortex, pons) exhibit only mild sensitivity to aging. Raz (in press) has made the interesting suggestion that this pattern of differential vulnerability follows a rule of "last (phylogenetically and ontogenetically) in—first out." That is, those structures that evolved in more modern species and that matured late in the course of human development appear to suffer greater effects of aging than do the more ancient and mature structures. These late-evolving and maturing structures are also the ones that complete myelination relatively late in the development of the organism. The pathophysiology of these age-related volume changes is unknown, although a variety of mechanisms have been suggested including age-related changes in neurotransmitter concentration or function, excitotoxicity, subclinical inflammation, stress-induced glucocorticoid neurotoxicity, and cumulative effects of systemic illnesses such as hypertension (see Chapter 3 in this volume).

Studies are consistent in demonstrating increased variability in brain anatomic measures with aging—some subjects show marked atrophic changes, whereas others show very little change. Factors that may account for at least some of this variation include general medical health as well as alcohol and other recreational drugs. Recently, we found that education level may also explain some of the individual variation in brain aging (Coffey et al. 1999). In a sample of 320 elderly individuals living independently in the community, years of formal education was significantly associated with peripheral (sulcal) CSF volume, a marker of cortical atrophy. Each year of education was associated with an increase in peripheral CSF of 1.77 mL. Our finding of a greater age-specific increase in peripheral CSF volume

in *normal* elderly persons is consistent with the "reserve" hypothesis that such individuals are afforded greater protection from any clinical manifestations of cortical atrophy. These findings are also consistent with the few imaging studies of Alzheimer's disease demonstrating greater regional brain atrophy and hypoperfusion in those patients with more education. These latter studies suggest that education exerts its "protective" effect, not by reducing the brain changes associated with disease or aging, but by enabling more educated individuals to resist the influence of deteriorating brain structure by maintaining better cognitive and behavioral functioning. The mechanism by which education may be related to preserved cognitive functioning in the setting of cortical atrophy is unknown but may be suggested by our observation of a lack of association between education and age-specific ventricular enlargement. This observation suggests that education is not associated with relatively greater age-related atrophy of those striatal structures (e.g., caudate nucleus) that form the lateral walls of the lateral ventricles. Preserved striatal structure may imply preserved integrity of frontosubcortical circuits critical to executive cognitive functioning, which in turn would afford the individual a greater cognitive "buffer" against any clinical manifestations of brain aging or cortical atrophy.

Neuropsychological Correlates of Age-Related Changes in Brain Structure

Aging may be characterized cognitively by generalized slowing of cognitive function and by decreased working memory (see Chapter 8 in this volume). Despite a relatively large literature on the relationship between cognitive functioning and brain structure in patients with dementia, only a few studies have examined such relationships in nonpatient samples of aging healthy adult volunteers, and results have been conflicting (Appendices 9–1 through 9–4).

Neuropsychological Correlates of Age-Related Changes in Global Brain Structure

With regard to global brain changes, six of nine studies examining *ventricular size* found no relation with a variety of measures of cognitive function (Jacoby et al. 1980; Kaye et al. 1992; Matsubayashi et al. 1992; Pearlson et al. 1989a; Sullivan et al. 1993; Wahlund et al. 1990) (Appendix 9–1). Three positive studies have been reported. Earnest et al.

(1979) performed neuropsychological testing (Trail Making Test, the Digit Symbol and Block Design subtests of the Wechsler Adult Intelligence Scale [WAIS] [Wechsler 1955], and the Visual Reproduction subtest of the Wechsler Memory Scale [Wechsler 1945]) in 59 elderly subjects who had been scanned by CT 1 year earlier (Appendixes 9–1 and 9–2). After adjustments for age, the only significant findings were negative correlations between the Digit Symbol Test and linear ($r = -.40$) and planimetric ($r = -.30$) measures of lateral ventricular size. In a sample of elderly subjects, Soininen et al. (1982) found a negative correlation between a composite neuropsychological test score and linear measures of ventricular size and sylvian fissure size on CT, but the effects of age were not controlled. Although Stafford et al. (1988) reported a negative correlation between a discriminant function of ventricular volume on CT and a discriminant function of neuropsychological tests of naming and abstraction, the effects of subject age on this correlation were apparently not partialled out.

Only a few studies have examined relations between global *brain parenchymal* measures and cognitive function (Appendixes 9–1 and 9–2). Jacoby et al. (1980) found no significant correlations (after adjustments for age) between a test of memory and orientation and ratings of cortical atrophy on CT scanning of elderly subjects. In contrast, Carmelli and colleagues (1999) found that within-pair differences in brain volume on MRI were associated with within-pair differences in memory function in 74 elderly male twin pairs. Two MR imaging investigations have observed relations between IQ and total and regional brain volumes in relatively young samples (Andreasen et al. 1993; Willerman et al. 1991). A third MR imaging investigation found no relation between IQ and either total or regional brain volumes in a mixed-age sample, although global cerebral asymmetry (left greater than right) did predict IQ (Raz et al. 1993b).

Neuropsychological Correlates of Age-Related Changes in Regional Brain Structure

Most studies of the neuropsychological correlates of age-related changes in brain structure have focused on memory and the *temporal lobe* (Appendix 9–2). Golomb et al. (1993) found that elderly subjects with hippocampal atrophy performed worse on the recent verbal memory portion of the Guild Memory Scale, but no group differences were observed in immediate verbal memory, digit span, or recall of designs. A subgroup of these subjects was followed for a mean of 3.8 years, at which time those who had declined to a score of 3 on the Global Deterioration Scale

were found to have had smaller hippocampal volumes at baseline (Golomb et al. 1996). In a study of 40 healthy older volunteers, O'Brien et al. (1997) found a relation between the presence of amygdala-hippocampal atrophy on MR imaging and lower scores on the Cambridge Cognitive Examination (CAMCOG), a relation that was entirely a result of lower scores on the memory subscale. Kohler et al. (1998) studied 26 healthy elderly (approximately 71 years old) subjects and observed a trend for a negative association between hippocampal volume and delayed verbal recall on the California Verbal Learning Test, but no association with visual recall (Visual Reproduction Test of the Wechsler Memory Scale–Revised) or scores on the Mattis Dementia Rating Scale. Parahippocampal gyrus volume was not related to any of the three measures. Raz et al. (1998b) observed no relations between hippocampal and parahippocampal volumes on MR imaging and several memory measures in a sample of 95 healthy adults. In a study of 11 healthy elderly subjects, Lupien et al. (1998) found decreased hippocampal volume on MR imaging, as well as deficits in hippocampal-dependent memory function, in those with significant prolonged elevations of serum cortisol. The authors speculated that elevated glucocorticoid levels, which are known to be toxic to hippocampal cells in animals, may likewise cause hippocampal atrophy and dysfunction in elderly humans.

With regard to *other brain structures*, Salat et al. (1997) found a correlation between corpus callosum area and performance on the Visual Reproduction portion of the Wechsler Memory Scale in females but not males. No relations were found in either gender with scores on the Logical Memory portion of this test or with scores on the Block Design subtest of the WAIS. Hokama et al. (1995) found no correlation between IQ and volumes of basal ganglia nuclei in 15 adult male volunteers. In the MR imaging study of Raz et al. (1998b) described above, relations were observed between the volume of the visual processing areas (pericalcarine cortex) and nonverbal working memory and between prefrontal cortex atrophy and increased perseveration.

Recently, a few studies have examined the neuropsychological and brain MR imaging correlates of the apolipoprotein E e4 allele, a risk marker for Alzheimer's disease and vascular dementia (see Chapters 23 and 24 in this volume). H. Schmidt et al. (1996) found that elderly nondemented apoE carriers performed worse than noncarriers on tests of learning and memory, but the groups did not differ on measures of sulcal and ventricular widening, hippocampal and parahippocampal volumes, or extent of subcortical hyperintensity (see below). In contrast, in a study of elderly twins without dementia,

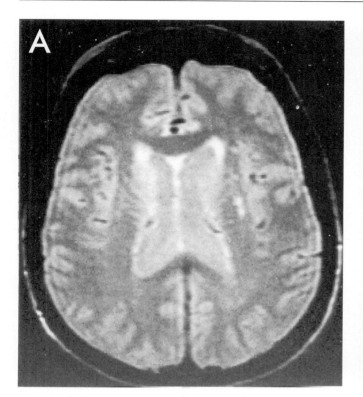

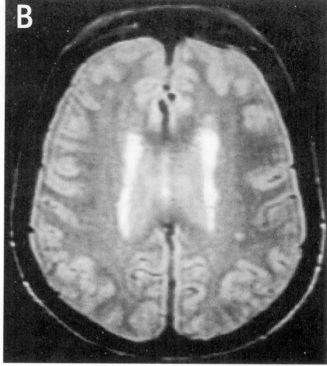

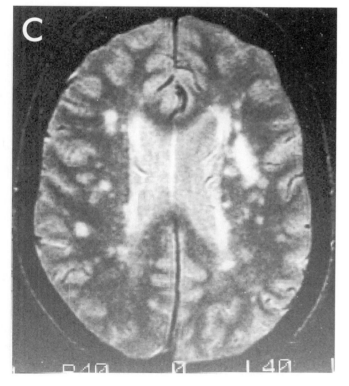

FIGURE 9–7. Visual standards for ratings of hyperintensity in the periventricular white matter on T2-weighted magnetic resonance images (repetition time = 2500 milliseconds; echo time = 80 milliseconds). *Panel A:* Grade 1 = "caps" at anterior tips of frontal horns. *Panel B:* Grade 2 = "halo" along border of lateral ventricles. *Panel C:* Grade 3 = irregular extension of hyperintensity into the deep white matter.
Source. Reprinted with permission from Coffey CE: "Structural Brain Abnormalities in the Depressed Elderly," in *Brain Imaging in Affective Disorders.* Edited by Hauser P. Washington, DC, American Psychiatric Press, 1991, pp. 94–95.

Plassman et al. (1997) found no neuropsychological differences between apoE carriers and noncarriers, although the former had smaller right and left hippocampal volumes.

Subcortical Hyperintensity

Numerous MR imaging studies have demonstrated that aging is associated with an increased prevalence and severity of subcortical hyperintensity (foci of increased signal on T2-weighted images) (see Coffey 1994 for review; Guttmann et al. 1998; Liao et al. 1997; Yue et al. 1997). In our study of healthy adults (Coffey et al. 1992), subcortical hyperintensity was present in the deep white matter in 48 subjects (64.0%), in the periventricular white matter in 9 (12.0%), in the basal ganglia in 9 (12.0%), in the thalamus in 4 (5.3%), and in the pons in 16 (21.3%) (Table 9–1 and Figures 9–7 and 9–8). The odds of subcortical hyperintensity increased by 5% to 9% per year of age, depending on the anatomical region involved (Figure 9–9).

A growing body of neuropathological evidence is defining the pathophysiological significance of subcortical hyperintensity (Coffey and Figiel 1991; Pantonini and Garcia 1997). Periventricular hyperintensities in the form of caps or rims (Figure 9–7, *panel A*) are common in healthy individuals and do not appear to constitute pathology. Histological studies suggest that these periventricular caps

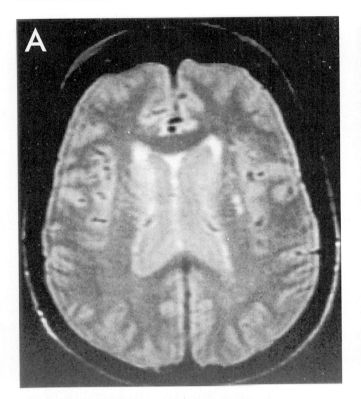

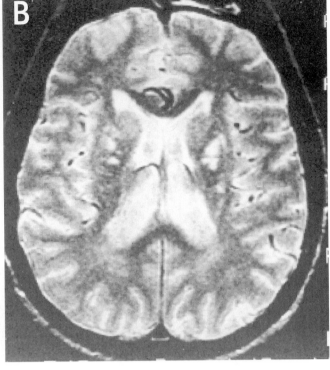

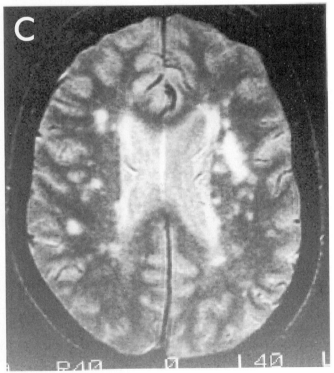

FIGURE 9–8. Visual standards for ratings of hyperintensity in the deep white matter on T2-weighted magnetic resonance images (repetition time = 2500 milliseconds; echo time = 80 milliseconds). *Panel A:* Grade 1 = punctate foci. *Panel B:* Grade 2 = small confluence of foci. *Panel C:* Grade 3 = large confluent areas of signal hyperintensity.

Source. Reprinted with permission from Coffey CE: "Structural Brain Abnormalities in the Depressed Elderly," in *Brain Imaging in Affective Disorders.* Edited by Hauser P. Washington, DC, American Psychiatric Press, 1991, pp. 96–97.

and rims likely reflect increased water content resulting from various factors, including a loose network of axons with low myelin content, a patchy loss of ependyma with astrocytic gliosis ("ependymitis granularis"), and the normal convergence of flow of interstitial fluid within the periventricular region (Sze et al. 1986). For the more severe changes of subcortical hyperintensity, however (Fig-ure 9–7, *panels B* and *C,* and Figure 9–8), a spectrum of histological changes may be present that range from vascular ectasia and dilated perivascular spaces, to edema and demyelination, to frank lacunar infarctions. It has been suggested that these more severe changes are a consequence of chronic brain hypoperfusion stemming from some combination of advancing arteriosclerosis, hypertensive vascular disease, chronic recurrent hypotension, cerebral amyloid angiopathy, the presence of "senile" arteriolar hyaline lesions, age-related thickening of meninges, and impaired autoregulation of cerebral circulation associated with aging. Indeed, evidence on MR imaging of old cerebral "microbleeds" is reported in approximately 6% of neuropsychiatrically normal community volunteers, and is associated with more extensive subcortical hyperintensity (Roob et al. 1999). The prevalence and severity of subcortical hyperintensity are thus increased in the presence of risk factors for vascular disease (Coffey and Figiel 1991; Liao et al. 1997). As conceptualized by Awad et al.

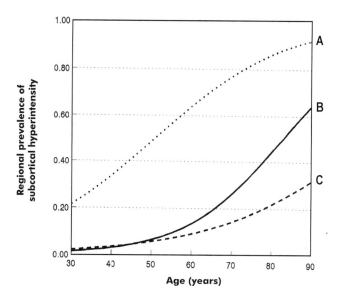

FIGURE 9–9.   Increase in the regional prevalence of subcortical hyperintensity with age. Logistic regression models indicated that the risk of subcortical hyperintensity increased significantly with age in the deep white matter (*line A*) and pons (*line B*), but not in the periventricular white matter or basal ganglia (*line C*). The odds of subcortical hyperintensity increased by approximately 6.3% per year in the deep white matter and by 8.1% per year in the pons. *Source.*   Adapted from Coffey et al. 1992.

(1986), subcortical hyperintensity in otherwise healthy older subjects may reflect "wear and tear" of brain parenchyma that accompanies aging and chronic cerebrovascular disease. Recent data in twins suggest that genetic factors may also contibute to individual differences in volume of subcortical hyperintensity (Carmelli et al. 1999).

Although a growing literature exists with respect to the relation between cognition and changes in subcortical white matter in normal aging (Appendix 9–3), these results are conflicting and the studies are difficult to compare given methodological differences. Most studies find no relation between subcortical hyperintensity and scores on dementia rating scales (Austrom et al. 1990; Harrell et al. 1991; Hendrie et al. 1989; Mirsen et al. 1991; positive findings reported by Steingart et al. 1987 and Matsubayashi et al. 1992). Positive findings have generally been more common among studies using more focal neuropsychological assessment batteries, with measures of frontal lobe function appearing to show the closest relation with subcortical hyperintensity (Austrom et al. 1990; Boone et al. 1992; Carmelli et al. 1999; DeCarli et al. 1995; Rao et al. 1989; Schmidt et al. 1993, 1999; Ylikoski et al. 1993).

In a study from our laboratory (Tupler et al. 1992), we examined the relationship between subcortical hyperintensity on MR imaging and two specific neuropsy-

chological instruments—the Benton Facial Recognition Test (Benton et al. 1983) and the WAIS-R Digit Symbol. The former was chosen because it had yielded the highest level of significance of any test reported to be associated with subcortical hyperintensity; the latter, because it had been reported to be related to subcortical hyperintensity by two independent groups (Appendix 9–3). In addition, both the Benton Facial Recognition Test and the Digit Symbol subtest of the WAIS-R (Wechsler 1981) were favored a priori because subcortical pathology might be expected to disrupt visuospatial perception and visuomotor execution, respectively.

We found that performance on both tests was highly related to age and education, but not to the presence of subcortical hyperintensity. The majority of our subjects had relatively mild findings of subcortical hyperintensity, however, and it thus remains possible that more severe changes might be associated with cognitive dysfunction in otherwise healthy adults (e.g., see Boone et al. 1992; DeCarli et al. 1995; Matsubayashi et al. 1992; Steingart et al. 1987). Indeed, extensive damage to subcortical white matter tracks would disrupt frontal-subcortical circuitry and possibly provide an anatomical substrate for the mental slowing and disturbed executive functioning seen with aging.

In addition, an issue not addressed by our study was whether subcortical hyperintensity might be associated with cognitive changes in patients with various medical, neurological, or psychiatric illnesses (Coffey and Figiel 1991). In this regard, we have previously reported that subcortical hyperintensity is more common in patients with severe depression (Coffey 1991; Coffey et al. 1990, 1993), and correlative studies are currently under way to determine whether the cognitive impairment that frequently afflicts this population might be associated with these brain changes.

Other Brain Imaging Parameters

Intracranial calcification.   Punctate calcification appears as an area of increased density on CT but leaves a signal void on MR imaging. Intracranial calcification may occur in association with many pathological conditions and may also be noted as an incidental finding commonly involving the pineal gland, dura, habenula, petroclinoid ligament, choroid plexus, basal ganglia, and major cerebral vessels (Rhea and DeLuca 1983). Clinical experience and some research suggest that "physiological calcification" of these various structures increases with age (Cohen et al. 1980; Modic et al. 1980), but little systematic information is available in nonclinical elderly samples.

Brain tissue characteristics. Conflicting data exist on whether increasing age is associated with alterations in CT attenuation values (Hounsfield unit) of the subcortical white matter (Cala et al. 1981; Schwartz et al. 1985; Zatz et al. 1982b). However, patchy areas of decreased attenuation in the subcortical white matter do occur with increasing frequency on CT of the elderly (Coffey and Figiel 1991). Such changes likely reflect the effects of hypoperfusion to subcortical structures and are the CT scan equivalent of subcortical hyperintensity on MR imaging (Coffey and Figiel 1991).

Increasing age has also been reported to be associated with regional brain changes in T1 and T2 relaxation time estimates on MR imaging (Appendix 9–4), but such data must be considered preliminary given a number of methodological issues (Drayer 1989).

Magnetic resonance spectroscopy. Magnetic resonance spectroscopy is a noninvasive technique capable of measuring the metabolism and chemical composition of brain tissue (Keshavan et al. 1991). Age-related findings have been reported for magnetic resonance spectroscopy in animals (Herndon et al. 1998; Pettegrew et al. 1990), but this technique has only recently been applied to the systematic study of "normal or usual" aging in humans, with variable findings (Appendix 9–4). Preliminary efforts are under way to explore the role of magnetic resonance spectroscopy in age-related conditions such as dementia and cerebrovascular disease (Dager and Steen 1992; Keshavan et al. 1991; Meyerhoff et al. 1994; Parnetti et al. 1997, see also Chapter 11, this volume).

Brain iron. High-field-strength (1.5 tesla) MR imaging can be used to visualize brain nuclei that are rich in iron. On heavily "T2-weighted" images, brain iron produces reduced signal intensity (the paramagnetic properties of iron accelerate T2 relaxation time) that correlates with the distribution of iron staining in postmortem brains (Coffey et al. 1989; Sachdev 1993). Nuclei of the extrapyramidal system are especially rich in iron, and aging is associated with increased deposition of iron in these regions. Although these age-related changes are maximal during development and early adulthood (Pujol et al. 1992), MR imaging changes consistent with increased iron deposition have been reported in the elderly (Steffens et al. 1996; see also Appendix 9–4).

Magnetic resonance imaging of cerebral blood flow. Because of its sensitivity to flow-related phenomena, MR imaging can be used to image in remarkable detail the extracranial and intracranial vasculature—a form of noninvasive angiography (Caplan et al. 1995;

Ståhlberg et al. 1992). MR imaging may also permit quantitative measurements of blood flow velocity and volume, and possibly of CSF hydrodynamics as well. Measurement of brain perfusion with MR imaging is also possible, permitting noninvasive assessment of brain functional activity comparable to that obtained with PET or SPECT. Such techniques would have obvious applications to the study of normal and abnormal brain aging (see Chapters 10 and 11 in this volume).

Summary

Modern computer-based imaging technologies provide an excellent opportunity to examine in vivo the spectrum and extent of changes in brain morphology that occur with normal aging. Such data are essential for an understanding of pathological brain aging in the elderly. The interpretation of these imaging studies must include careful consideration of a plethora of methodological issues that can obscure, confound, or modify apparent aging effects. Although studies vary in the extent to which such factors have been controlled, general agreement is found in the literature that increasing age is associated with 1) nonlinear increases in lateral and third ventricular volume; 2) increasing sulcal CSF volume; 3) decreasing brain volume, especially of the frontal lobes and of cortical and subcortical gray matter structures; 4) increasing variability in measures of brain size; and 5) increasing frequency and severity of subcortical hyperintensity on MR imaging. The effects of age on the two hemispheres are similar for most structures. Gender differences in the effects of age on brain morphology may exist for some regions or structures (e.g., sulcal CSF volume and possibly the frontotemporal regions), and in most cases such changes are greater in men than they are in women. Further study is needed to characterize in greater detail the effects of "usual versus successful" aging on global and regional brain structure, and the relationship of such age-related changes to cognitive function in aging people.

Research is also needed that identifies strategies to preserve brain function in the face of aging, an issue of increasing interest to the public. As discussed above, we know that the effects of age upon brain structure may be mollified by optimizing general medical health, by minimizing use of alcohol and other recreational drugs, and by avoiding injury to the head (e.g., by wearing bicycle helmets, wearing seat belts, avoiding extreme contact sports). Estrogen replacement therapy may also prove beneficial in maintenance of cognitive functioning in postmenopausal women, and its effects on age-related changes in brain structure should be studied. Finally, we need to understand the value of "brain exercise" as it relates to aging—can we preserve cognitive functioning by maintaining a vigorous intellectual life, much as physical exercise helps preserve muscle functioning in the face of age-related muscle cell loss? I for one certainly hope so, and at any rate, there doesn't seem to be much of a down side to tackling the morning crossword puzzle over a good cup of coffee.

References

Alavi A: The aging brain. J Neuropsychiatry Clin Neurosci 120 (suppl 1):S51–S60, 1989

Andreasen NC, Ehrhardt JC, Swayze VW, et al: Magnetic resonance imaging of the brain in schizophrenia: the pathophysiologic significance of structural abnormalities. Arch Gen Psychiatry 47:35–44, 1990

Andreasen NC, Flaum M, Swayze V, et al: Intelligence and brain structure in normal individuals. Am J Psychiatry 150: 130–134, 1993

Austrom MG, Thompson RF, Hendrie HC, et al: Foci of increased T_2 signal intensity in MR images of healthy elderly subjects: a follow-up study. J Am Geriatr Soc 38: 1133–1138, 1990

Awad IA, Johnson PC, Spetzler RF, et al: Incidental subcortical lesions identified on magnetic resonance imaging in the elderly, II: post mortem correlations. Stroke 17:1090–1097, 1986

Barron SA, Jacobs L, Kinkel WR: Changes in size of normal lateral ventricles during aging determined by computerized tomography. Neurology 26:1011–1013, 1976

Bear D, Schiff D, Saver J, et al: Quantitative analysis of cerebral asymmetries: fronto-occipital correlation, sexual dimorphism and association with handedness. Arch Neurol 43:598–603, 1986

Benton AL, Hamsher KdeS, Varney NR, et al: Contributions to Neuropsychological Assessment: A Clinical Manual. New York, Oxford University Press, 1983

Blatter DD, Bigler ED, Gale SD, et al: Quantitative volumetric analysis of brain MR: normative database spanning 5 decades of life. AJNR Am J Neuroradiol 16:241–251, 1995

Boone KB, Miller BL, Lesser IM, et al: Neuropsychological correlates of white-matter lesions in healthy elderly subjects. Arch Neurol 49:549–554, 1992

Cala LA, Thickbroom GW, Black JL, et al: Brain density and cerebrospinal fluid space size: CT of normal volunteers. AJNR Am J Neuroradiol 2:41–47, 1981

Caplan LR, DeWitt LD, Breen JC: Neuroimaging in patients with cerebrovascular disease, in Neuroimaging. Edited by Greenberg JO. New York, McGraw-Hill, 1995, pp 435–457

Carmelli D, Swan GE, Reed T, et al: Midlife cardiovascular risk factors and brain morphology in identical older male twins. Neurology 52:1119–1124, 1999

Cascella NG, Pearlson G, Wong DF, et al: Effects of substance abuse on ventricular and sulcal measures assessed by computerized tomography. Br J Psychiatry 159:217–221, 1991

Chui C, Damasio AR: Human cerebral asymmetries evaluated by computed tomography. J Neurol Neurosurg Psychiatry 43:873–878, 1980

Coffey CE: Structural brain abnormalities in the depressed elderly, in Brain Imaging in Affective Disorders. Edited by Hauser P. Washington, DC, American Psychiatric Press, 1991, pp 94–95

Coffey CE: Anatomic imaging of the aging human brain, in Textbook of Geriatric Neuropsychiatry. Edited by Coffey CE, Cummings JL. Washington, DC, American Psychiatric Press, 1994, pp 159–194

Coffey CE: Brain morphology in primary mood disorders: implications for ECT. Psychiatric Annals 26:713–716, 1996

Coffey CE, Figiel GS: Neuropsychiatric significance of subcortical encephalomalacia, in Psychopathology and the Brain. Edited by Carroll BJ, Barrett JE. New York, Raven, 1991, pp 243–264

Coffey CE, Alston S, Heinz ER, et al: Brain iron in progressive supranuclear palsy: clinical, magnetic resonance imaging, and neuropathological findings. J Neuropsychiatry Clin Neurosci 1:400–404, 1989

Coffey CE, Figiel GS, Djang WT, et al: Subcortical hyperintensity on magnetic resonance imaging: a comparison of normal and depressed elderly subjects. Am J Psychiatry 147:187–189, 1990

Coffey CE, Wilkinson WE, Parashos IA, et al: Quantitative cerebral anatomy of the aging human brain: a cross-sectional study using magnetic resonance imaging. Neurology 42:527–536, 1992

Coffey CE, Wilkinson WE, Weiner RD, et al: Quantitative cerebral anatomy in depression: a controlled magnetic resonance imaging study. Arch Gen Psychiatry 50:7–16, 1993

Coffey CE, Lucke JF, Saxton JA, et al: Sex differences in brain aging: a quantitative magnetic resonance imaging study. Arch Neurol 55:169–179, 1998

Coffey CE, Saxton JA, Ratcliff G, et al: Relation of education to brain size in normal aging: implications for the reserve hypothesis. Neurology 53:189–196, 1999

Cohen CR, Duchesneau PM, Weinstein MA: Calcification of the basal ganglia as visualized by computed tomography. Neuroradiology 134:97–99, 1980

Condon B, Grant R, Hadley D, et al: Brain and intracranial cavity volumes: in vivo determination by MRI. Acta Neurol Scand 78:387–393, 1988

Convit A, de Leon MJ, Hoptman MJ, et al: Age-related changes in brain: I. Magnetic resonance imaging measures of temporal lobe volumes in normal subjects. Psychiatr Q 66:343–355, 1995

Cowell PE, Turetsky BI, Gur RC, et al: Sex differences in aging of the human frontal and temporal lobes. J Neurosci 14:4748–4755, 1994

Creasey H, Rapoport SI: The aging human brain. Ann Neurol 17:2–10, 1985

Cutler RG: Evolution of longevity in primates. J Hum Evol 5:169–202, 1976

Cutler RG: Evolution of human longevity: a critical overview. Mech Ageing Dev 9:337–754, 1979

Dager SR, Steen RG: Applications of magnetic resonance spectroscopy to the investigation of neuropsychiatric disorders. Neuropsychopharmacology 6:249–266, 1992

Davatzikos C, Resnick SM: Sex differences in anatomic measures of interhemispheric connectivity: correlations with cognition in women but not men. Cereb Cortex 8:635–640, 1998

Davis PJM, Wright EA: A new method for measuring cranial cavity volume and its application to the assessment of cerebral atrophy at autopsy. Neuropathol Appl Neurobiol 3:341–358, 1977

DeCarli C, Kaye JA, Horwitz B, et al: Critical analysis of the use of computer-assisted transverse axial tomography to study human brain in aging and dementia of the Alzheimer type. Neurology 40:872–883, 1990

DeCarli C, Murphy DGM, Gillette JA, et al: Lack of age-related differences in temporal lobe volume of very healthy adults. AJNR Am J Neuroradiol 15:689–696, 1994

DeCarli C, Murphy DG, Tranh M, et al: The effect of white matter hyperintensity on brain structure, congitive performance, and cerebral metabolism of glucose in 51 healthy adults. Neurology 45:2077–2084, 1995

Deshmukh AR, Desmond JE, Sullivan EV, et al: Quantification of cerebellar structures with MRI. Psychiatry Res 75:159–171, 1997

Doraiswamy PM, Figiel GS, Husain MM, et al: Aging of the human corpus callosum: magnetic resonance imaging in normal volunteers. J Neuropsychiatry Clin Neurosci 3:392–397, 1991

Doraiswamy PM, Na C, Husain MM, et al: Morphometric changes of the human midbrain with normal aging: MR and stereologic findings. AJNR Am J Neuroradiol 13:383–386, 1992

Doraiswamy PM, McDonald WM, Patterson L, et al: Interuncal distance as a measure of hippocampal atrophy: normative data on axial MR imaging. AJNR Am J Neuroradiol 14:141–143, 1993

Drayer BP: Imaging of the aging brain, part I: normal findings. Radiology 166:785–796, 1988

Drayer BP: Basal ganglia: significance of signal hypointensity on T2 weighted MR images. Radiology 173:311–312, 1989

Earnest MP, Heaton RK, Wilkinson WE, et al: Cortical atrophy, ventricular enlargement and intellectual impairment in the aged. Neurology 29:1138–1143, 1979

Escalona PR, McDonald WM, Doraiswamy PM, et al: In vivo stereological assessment of human cerebellar volume: effects of gender and age. AJNR Am J Neuroradiol 12:927–929, 1991

Fox NC, Freeborough PA, Rossor MN: Visualisation and quantification of rates of atrophy in Alzheimer's disease. Lancet 348:94–97, 1996

Fox NC, Scahill RI, Crum WR, et al: Correlation between rates of brain atrophy and cognitive decline in AD. Neurology 52:1687–1689, 1999

Frisoni GB, Laakso MP, Beltramello A, et al: Hippocampal and entorhinal cortex atrophy in frontotemporal dementia and Alzheimer's disease. Neurology 52:91–100, 1999

Fukuzako H, Hashiguchi T, Sakamoto Y, et al: Metabolite changes with age measured by proton magnetic resonance spectroscopy in normal subjects. Psychiatry Clin Neurosci 51:261–263, 1997

Gado M, Hughes CP, Danziger W, et al: Aging, dementia, and brain atrophy: a longitudinal computed tomography study. AJNR Am J Neuroradiol 4:699–702, 1983

Golomb J, de Leon MI, Kluger A, et al: Hippocampal atrophy in normal aging: an association with recent memory impairment. Arch Neurol 50:967–973, 1993

Golomb J, Kluger A, de Leon MJ, et al: Hippocampal formation size predicts declining memory performance in normal aging. Neurology 47:810–813, 1996

Gould SJ: The Mismeasure of Man. New York, WW Norton, 1981

Grant R, Condon B, Lawrence A, et al: Human cranial CSF volumes measured by MRI: sex and age influences. Magn Reson Imaging 5:465–468, 1987

Gunning-Dixon FM, Head D, McQuain J, et al: Differential aging of the human striatum: a prospective MR imaging study. AJNR Am J Neuroradiol 19:1501–1507, 1998

Gur RC, Mozley PD, Resnick SM, et al: Gender differences in age effect on brain atrophy measured by magnetic resonance imaging. Proc Natl Acad Sci U S A 88:2845–2849, 1991

Gur RE, Cowell P, Turetsky BI, et al: A follow-up magnetic resonance imaging study of schizophrenia. Arch Gen Psychiatry 55:145–152, 1998

Guttmann CRG, Jolesz FA, Kikinis R, et al: White matter changes with normal aging. Neurology 50:972–978, 1998

Harrell LE, Duvall E, Folks DG, et al: The relationship of high-intensity signals on magnetic resonance images to cognitive and psychiatric state in Alzheimer's disease. Arch Neurol 48:1136–1140, 1991

Haug H: Are neurons of the human cerebral cortex really lost during aging? a morphometric examination, in Senile Dementia of the Alzheimer Type. Edited by Traber J, Gispen WH. Berlin, Springer-Verlag, 1985, pp 150–163

Hendrie HC, Farlow MR, Austrom MG, et al: Foci of increased T_2 signal intensity on brain MR scans of healthy elderly subjects. AJNR Am J Neuroradiol 10:703–707, 1989

Herndon JG, Constantinidis I, Moss MB: Age-related brain changes in rhesus monkeys: a magnetic resonance spectroscopic study. Neuroreport 9:2127–2130, 1998

Hokama H, Shenton ME, Nestor PG, et al: Caudate, putamen, and globus pallidus volume in schizophrenia: a quantitative MRI study. Psychiatry Res 61:209–229, 1995

Homan RW, Herman J, Purdy P: Cerebral localization in international 10-20 system electrode placement. Electroencephalogr Clin Neurophysiol 66:376–382, 1987

Jack CR: Brain and cerebrospinal fluid volume: measurement with MR imaging. Radiology 178:22–24, 1991

Jack CR, Gehring DC, Sharbrough FW, et al: Temporal lobe measurement from MR images: accuracy and left-right asymmetry in normal persons. J Comput Assist Tomogr 12:21–29, 1988

Jack CR, Petersen RC, O'Brien PC, et al: MR-based hippocampal volumetry in the diagnosis of Alzheimer's disease. Neurology 42:183–188, 1992

Jack CR, Petersen RC, Xu YC, et al: Medial temporal atrophy on MRI in normal aging and very mild Alzheimer's disease. Neurology 49:786–794, 1997

Jack CR, Petersen RC, Xu Y, et al: Rate of medial temporal lobe atrophy in typical aging and Alzheimer's disease. Neurology 51:993–999, 1998

Jacoby RJ, Levy R, Dawson JM: Computed tomography in the elderly, I: the normal population. Br J Psychiatry 136:249–255, 1980

Janowsky JS, Kaye JA, Carper RA: Atrophy of the corpus callosum in Alzheimer's disease versus healthy aging. J Am Geriatr Soc 44:798–803, 1996

Jernigan TL, Press GA, Hesselink JR: Methods of measuring brain morphologic features on magnetic resonance images: validation and normal aging. Arch Neurol 47:27–32, 1990

Jernigan TL, Archibald SL, Berhow MT, et al: Cerebral structure on MRI, part I: localization of age-related changes. Biol Psychiatry 29:55–67, 1991

Katzman R, Terry R: Normal aging of the nervous system, in Principles of Geriatric Neurology. Edited by Katzman R, Rowe JW. Philadelphia, PA, FA Davis, 1992, pp 18–58

Kaye JA, DeCarli C, Luxenberg JS, et al: The significance of age-related enlargement of the cerebral ventricles in healthy men and women measured by quantitative computed x-ray tomography. J Am Geriatr Soc 40:225–231, 1992

Kaye JA, Swihart T, Howieson D, et al: Volume loss of the hippocampus and temporal lobes in healthy elderly persons destined to develop dementia. Neurology 48:1297–1304, 1997

Kelsoe JR, Cadet JL, Pickar D, et al: Quantitative neuroanatomy in schizophrenia: a controlled magnetic resonance imaging study. Arch Gen Psychiatry 45:533–541, 1988

Kertesz A, Polk M, Black SE, et al: Anatomical asymmetries and functional laterality. Brain 115:589–605, 1992

Keshavan MS, Kapur S, Pettegrew JW: Magnetic resonance spectroscopy in psychiatry: potential, pitfalls, and promise. Am J Psychiatry 148:976–985, 1991

Kohler S, Black SE, Sinden M, et al: Memory impairments associated with hippocampal versus parahippocampal-gyrus atrophy: an MR volumetry study in Alzheimer's disease. Neuropsychologia 36:901–914, 1998

Krishnan KR, Husain MM, McDonald WM, et al: In vivo stereological assessment of caudate volume in man: effect of normal aging. Life Sci 47:1325–1329, 1990

Laakso MP, Soininen H, Partanen K, et al: MRI of the hippocampus in Alzheimer's disease: sensitivity, specificity, and analysis of the incorrectly classified subjects. Neurobiol Aging 19:23–31, 1998

Laessle RG, Krieg JC, Fichter MM, et al: Cerebral atrophy and vigilance performance in patients with anorexia nervosa and bulimia nervosa. Neuropsychobiology 21:187–191, 1989

Laffey PA, Peyster RG, Nathan R, et al: Computed tomography and aging: results in a normal elderly population. Neuroradiology 26:273–278, 1984

LeMay M, Kido DK: Asymmetries of cerebral hemispheres on computed tomograms. J Comput Assist Tomogr 2:471–476, 1978

Liao D, Cooper L, Cai J, et al: The prevalence and severity of white matter lesions, their relationship with age, ethnicity, gender, and cardiovascular risk factors: the ARIC study. Neuroepidemiology 16:149–162, 1997

Lim KO, Spielman DM: Estimating NAA in cortical gray matter with applications for measuring changes due to aging. Magn Reson Med 37:372–377, 1997

Lim KO, Zipursky RB, Watts MC, et al: Decreased gray matter in normal aging: an in vivo magnetic resonance study. J Gerontol 47:B26–B30, 1992

Lishman WA: Alcohol and the brain. Br J Psychiatry 156:635–644, 1990

Lupien SJ, de Leon M, de Santi S, et al: Cortisol levels during human aging predict hippocampal atrophy and memory deficits. Nature Neuroscience 1:69–73, 1998

Magnotta VA, Andreasen NC, Schultz SK, et al: Quantitative in vivo measurement of gyrification in the human brain: changes associated with aging. Cerebral Cortex 9:151–160, 1999

Matsubayashi K, Shimada K, Kawamoto A, et al: Incidental brain lesions on magnetic resonance imaging and neurobehavioral functions in the apparently healthy elderly. Stroke 23:175–180, 1992

McDonald WM, Husain M, Doraiswamy PM, et al: A magnetic resonance image study of age-related changes in human putamen nuclei. Neuroreport 2:41–44, 1991

McFarland D: The aged in the 21st century: a demographer's view, in Aging into the 21st Century: Middle Ages Today. Edited by Jarvik LF. New York, Gardner, 1978, pp 5–25

Meyer JS, Takashima S, Terayama Y, et al: CT changes associated with normal aging of the human brain. J Neurol Sci 123:200–208, 1994

Meyerhoff DJ, MacKay S, Constans JM, et al: Axonal injury and membrane alterations in Alzheimer's disease suggested by in vivo proton magnetic resonance spectroscopic imaging. Ann Neurol 36:40–47, 1994

Miller AKH, Alston RL, Corsellis JA: Variation with age in the volumes of grey and white matter in the cerebral hemispheres of man: measurements with an image analyzer. Neuropathol Appl Neurobiol 6:119–132, 1980

Mirsen TR, Lee DH, Wong CJ, et al: Clinical correlates of white-matter changes on magnetic resonance imaging scans of the brain. Arch Neurol 48:1015–1021, 1991

Mittenberg W, Seidenberg M, O'Leary DS, et al: Changes in cerebral functioning associated with normal aging. J Clin Exp Neuropsychol 11:918–932, 1989

Modic MT, Weinstein MA, Rothner AD, et al: Calcification of the choroid plexus visualized by computed tomography. Radiology 135:369–372, 1980

Mu Q, Xie J, Wen Z, et al: A quantitative MR study of the hippocampal formation, the amygdala, and the temporal horn of the lateral ventricle in healthy subjects 40 to 90 years old. AJNR 20:207–211, 1999

Mueller EA, Moore, MM, Kerr DCR, et al: Brain volume preserved in healthy elderly through the eleventh decade. Neurology 51:1555–1562, 1998

Murphy DGM, DeCarli C, Schapiro MB, et al: Age-related differences in volumes of subcortical nuclei, brain matter, and cerebrospinal fluid in healthy men as measured with magnetic resonance imaging. Arch Neurol 49:839–845, 1992

Murphy DGM, DeCarli C, McIntosh AR, et al: Sex differences in human brain morphometry and metabolism: an in vivo quantitative magnetic resonance imaging and positron emission tomography study on the effect of aging. Arch Gen Psychiatry 53:585–594, 1996

O'Brien JT, Desmond P, Ames D, et al: Magnetic resonance imaging correlates of memory impairment in the healthy elderly: association with medial temporal lobe atrophy but not white matter lesions. Int J Geriatr Psychiatry 12:369–374, 1997

Oguro H, Okada K, Yamaguchi S, et al: Sex differences in morphology of the brain stem and cerebellum with normal aging. Neuroradiology 40:788–792, 1998

Pantonini L, Garcia JH: Pathogenesis of leukoaraiosis: a review. Stroke 28:652–659, 1997

Parashos IA, Wilkinson WE, Coffey CE: Magnetic resonance imaging of the corpus callosum: predictors of size in normal adults. J Neuropsychiatry Clin Neurosci 7:35–41, 1995

Parnetti L, Tarducci R, Presciutti O, et al: Proton magnetic resonance spectroscopy can differentiate Alzheimer's disease from normal aging. Mech Ageing Dev 97:9–14, 1997

Passe TJ, Rajagopalan P, Tupler LA, et al: Age and sex effects on brain morphology. Prog Neuropsychopharmacol Biol Psychiatry 21:1231–1237, 1997

Pearlson GD, Rabins PV, Kim WS, et al: Structural brain CT changes and cognitive defects in elderly depressives with and without reversible dementia ("pseudodementia"). Psychol Med 19:573–584, 1989a

Pearlson GD, Kim WS, Kubos KL, et al: Ventricle-brain ratio, computed tomographic density, and brain area in 50 schizophrenics. Arch Gen Psychiatry 46:690–697, 1989b

Pettegrew JW, Panchalingam K, Withers G, et al: Changes in brain energy and phospholipid metabolism during development and aging in the Fischer 344 rat. J Neuropathol Exp Neurol 49:237–249, 1990

Pfefferbaum A, Zatz LM, Jernigan TL: Computer-interactive method for quantifying cerebrospinal fluid and tissue in brain CT scans: effects of aging. J Comput Assist Tomogr 10:571–578, 1986

Pfefferbaum A, Lim KO, Rosenbloom M, et al: Brain magnetic resonance imaging: approaches for investigating schizophrenia. Schizophr Bull 16:453–476, 1990

Pfefferbaum A, Sullivan EV, Rosenbloom MJ, et al: Increase in brain cerebrospinal fluid volume is greater in older than in younger alcoholic patients: a replication study and CT/MRI comparison. Psychiatry Res 50:257–274, 1993

Pfefferbaum A, Mathalon DH, Sullivan EV, et al: A quantitative magnetic resonance imaging study of changes in brain morphology from infancy to late adulthood. Arch Neurol 51:874-887, 1994

Pfefferbaum A, Sullivan EV, Rosenbloom MJ, et al: A controlled study of cortical gray matter and ventricular changes in alcoholic men over a 5-year interval. Arch Gen Psychiatry 55:905-912, 1998

Plassman BL, Welsh-Bohmer KA, Bigler ED, et al: Apolipoprotein E e4 allele and hippocampal volume in twins with normal cognition. Neurology 48:985–989, 1997

Pujol J, Junqué C, Vendrell P, et al: Biological significance of iron-related magnetic resonance imaging changes in the brain. Arch Neurol 49:711–717, 1992

Rao SM, Mittenberg W, Bernardin L, et al: Neuropsychological test findings in subjects with leukoaraiosis. Arch Neurol 46:40–44, 1989

Raz N: Aging of the brain and its impact on cognitive performance: integration of structural and functional findings. In Craik FIM, Salthouse TA (eds), Handbook of Aging and Cognition—II. Mahwah NJ, Erlbaum (in press)

Raz N, Torres IJ, Acker JD: Age, gender, and hemispheric differences in human striatum: a quantitative review and new data from in vivo MRI morphometry. Neurobiol Learn Mem 63:133–142, 1993a

Raz N, Torres IJ, Spencer WD, et al: Neuroanatomical correlates of age-sensitive and age-invariant cognitive abilities: an in vivo MRI investigation. Intelligence 17:407-422, 1993b

Raz N, Torres IJ, Spencer WD, et al: Pathoclysis in aging human cerebral cortex: evidence from in vivo MRI morphometry. Psychobiology 21:151-160, 1993c

Raz N, Gunning FM, Head D, et al: Selective aging of the human cerebral cortex observed in vivo: differential vulnerability of the prefrontal gray matter. Cereb Cortex 7: 268–282, 1997

Raz N, Dupuis JH, Briggs SD, et al: Differential effects of age and sex on the cerebellar hemispheres and the vermis: a prospective MR study. AJNR Am J Neuroradiol 19:65–71, 1998a

Raz N, Gunning-Dixon FM, Head D, et al: Neuroanatomical correlates of cognitive aging: evidence from structural magnetic resonance imaging. Neuropsychology 12: 95–114, 1998b

Rey A: L'Examen Clinique En Psychologie. Paris, Press Universitaires de France, 1964

Rhea JT, DeLuca SA: Benign intracranial calcification. Am Fam Physician 27:151–152, 1983

Roob G, Schmidt R, Kapeller P, et al: MRI evidence of past cerebral microbleeds in a healthy elderly population. Neurology 52:991–994, 1999

Rowe JW, Kahn RL: Human aging: usual and successful. Science 237:143–149, 1987

Rowe JW, Katzman R: Principles of geriatrics as applied to neurology, in Principles of Geriatric Neurology. Edited by Katzman R, Rowe JW. Philadelphia, PA, FA Davis, 1992, pp 3–17

Sachdev P: The neuropsychiatry of brain iron. J Neuropsychiatry Clin Neurosci 5:18–29, 1993

Salat D, Ward A, Kaye JA, et al: Sex differences in the corpus callosum with aging. Neurobiol Aging 18:191–197, 1997

Salat DH, Kaye JA, Janowsky JS: Prefrontal gray and white matter volumes in healthy aging and Alzheimer disease. Arch Neurol 56:338–344, 1999

Schmidt R, Fazekas F, Offenbacher H, et al: Neuropsychological correlates of MRI white matter hyperintensities: a study of 150 normal volunteers. Neurology 43:2490–2494, 1993

Schmidt H, Schmidt R, Fazekas F, et al: Apolipoprotein E e4 allele in the normal elderly: neuropsychological and brain MRI correlates. Clin Genet 50:293–299, 1996

Schmidt R, Fazekas F, Kapeller P, et al: MRI white matter hyperintensities: three-year follow-up of the Austrian Stroke Prevention Study. Neurology 53:132–139, 1999

Schwartz M, Creasey H, Grady CL, et al: Computed tomographic analysis of brain morphometrics in 30 healthy men, aged 21 to 81 years. Ann Neurol 17:146–157, 1985

Shah SA, Doraiswamy PM, Husain MM, et al: Assessment of posterior fossa structures with midsagittal MRI: the effects of age. Neurobiol Aging 12:371–374, 1991

Shear PK, Sullivan EV, Mathalon DH, et al: Longitudinal volumetric computed tomographic analysis of regional brain changes in normal aging and Alzheimer's disease. Arch Neurol 52:392–402, 1995

Soher BJ, van Zijl PCM, Duyn JH, et al: Quantitative proton MR spectroscopic imaging of the human brain. Magn Reson Med 35:356–363, 1996

Soininen H, Puranen M, Riekkinen PJ: Computed tomography findings in senile dementia and normal aging. J Neurol Neurosurg Psychiatry 45:50–54, 1982

Stafford JL, Albert MS, Naeser MA, et al: Age-related differences in computed tomographic scan measurements. Arch Neurol 45:409–415, 1988

Ståhlberg F, Ericsson A, Nordell B, et al: MR imaging, flow and motion. Acta Radiol 33:179–200, 1992

Steffens DC, McDonald WM, Tupler LA, et al: Magnetic resonance imaging changes in putamen nuclei iron content and distribution in normal subjects. Psychiatry Res 68:55–61, 1996

Steingart A, Hachinski VC, Lau C, et al: Cognitive and neurologic findings in subjects with diffuse white matter lucencies on computed tomography scan (leuko-araiosis). Arch Neurol 44:32–35, 1987

Suddath RC, Casanova MF, Goldberg TE, et al: Temporal lobe pathology in schizophrenia: a quantitative magnetic resonance imaging study. Am J Psychiatry 146:464–472, 1989

Sullivan EV, Shear PK, Mathalon D, et al: Greater abnormalities of brain cerebrospinal fluid volumes in younger than in older patients with Alzheimer's disease. Arch Neurol 50:359–373, 1993

Sze G, DeArmond SJ, Brant-Zawadzki M, et al: Foci of MRI signal (pseudolesions) anterior to the frontal horns: histologic correlations of a normal finding. AJR Am J Roentgenol 147:331–337, 1986

Tanna NK, Khon MI, Horwich DN, et al: Analysis of brain and cerebral fluid volumes with MR imaging: impact on PET data correction for atrophy. Radiology 178:123–130, 1991

Tupler LA, Coffey CE, Logue PE, et al: Neuropsychological importance of subcortical white matter hyperintensity. Arch Neurol 49:1248–1252, 1992

Wahlund LO, Agartz I, Almqvist O, et al: The brain in healthy aged individuals: MR imaging. Radiology 174:675–679, 1990

Warren LR, Butler RW, Katholi CR, et al: Age differences in cerebral blood flow during rest and during mental activation measurements with and without monetary incentive. J Gerontol 40:53–59, 1985

Wechsler D: A standardized memory scale for clinical use. J Psychol 19:87–95, 1945

Wechsler D: Wechsler Adult Intelligence Scale. New York, Psychological Corporation, 1955

Wechsler D: Wechsler Adult Intelligence Scale—Revised Manual. New York, Psychological Corporation, 1981

Weinberger DR, Luchins DR, Morihisa MD, et al: Asymmetrical volumes of the right and left frontal and occipital regions of the human brain. Ann Neurol 11:97–100, 1982

Weis S, Haug H, Holoubec B, et al: The cerebral dominances: quantitative morphology of the human cerebral cortex. Int J Neurosci 47:165–168, 1989

Willerman L, Schultz R, Rugledge JN, et al: In vivo brain size and intelligence. Intelligence 15:223–228, 1991

Witelson SF: Cognitive neuroanatomy: a new era. Neurology 42:709–713, 1992

Ylikoski R, Ylikoski A, Erkinjuntti T, et al: White matter changes in healthy elderly persons correlate with attention and speed of mental processing. Arch Neurol 50:818–824, 1993

Yoshii F, Barker WW, Chang JY, et al: Sensitivity of cerebral glucose metabolism to age, gender, brain volume, brain atrophy and cerebrovascular risk factors. J Cereb Blood Flow Metab 8:654–661, 1988

Yue NC, Arnold AM, Longstreth WT, et al: Sulcal, ventricular, and white matter changes at MR imaging in the aging brain: data from the cardiovascular health study. Radiology 2:33–39, 1997

Zatz LM, Jernigan TL, Ahumada AJ: Changes in computed cranial tomography with aging: intracranial fluid volume. AJNR Am J Neuroradiol 3:1–11, 1982a

Zatz LM, Jernigan TL, Ahumada AJ: White matter changes in cerebral computed tomography related to aging. J Comput Assist Tomogr 6(1):19–23, 1982b

Zipursky RB, Lim KO, Pfefferbaum A: Volumetric assessment of cerebral asymmetry from CT scans. Psychiatry Res 35:71–89, 1990

APPENDIX 9–1. Imaging studies of human aging and brain cerebrospinal fluid spaces

Study	Subjects	Imaging and measurement technique	Findings
Barron et al. 1976	135 volunteers 9 months to 90 years old Equal gender distribution in all age groups (8 M; 7 F per decade) No history of neurological disease; psychiatric history not reported Handedness not specified	CT Planimetric determination of VBR by single rater (average of three measurements) from Polaroid photograph	Age associated with increased VBR and with increased variability in VBR Interactions with gender or laterality not reported
Earnest et al. 1979	59 volunteer retirees 60–99 years old 11 M; 48 F Living independently and free of neurological disease Handedness not specified	CT Linear and planimetric measures of ventricular size at three different levels, from photographs Linear measurements of four largest sulci No additional data provided Neuropsychological test battery comprised of Trail Making Test, and the Digit Symbol and Block Design subtests of the Wechsler Memory Scale	Subjects 80 years or older ($n = 29$) had larger ratio of ventricular size to intracranial size than did younger subjects ($n = 30$) The sum of the widths of the four sulci was greater in older subjects than in younger subjects Adjusting for age (but not education?), ventricular size correlated only with performance on the Digit Symbol subtest Interactions with gender or laterality not reported
Jacoby et al. 1980	50 healthy elderly volunteers 62–88 years old 10 M; 40 F No history of significant psychiatric or neurological illness Handedness not specified	CT Ratings (small, normal, enlarged) of ventricular size from films by single blinded rater (rater reliability not reported) Planimetric determination of lateral ventricular/skull ratio and Evans' ratio from films by single rater (average of three measurements) with established reliabilities	8 (16%) subjects were rated as having "enlarged" lateral ventricles No correlation between age and lateral ventricular/skull ratio or Evans' ratio Interactions with gender or laterality not reported Adjusting for age, no relation between ventricular size and performance on the Hodkinson test of memory and orientation
Meese et al. 1980	160 healthy volunteers 1–71 years old 10 M and 10 F in each decade No additional data provided	CT Linear measurements of ventricular size and sulcal width from four axial slices (no additional data provided)	Apparent age-related changes in some measures of ventricular size and sulcal width, but these changes not analyzed statistically Interactions with gender or laterality not reported

(continued)

Study	Subjects	Method	Findings
Cala et al. 1981	115 volunteers 15–40 years old 62 M; 53 F No history of migraine, head trauma, or excessive alcohol intake (no additional details provided) All but 8 subjects right-handed	CT ($n = 2$ scanners) Planimetric measurements of ventricular/skull ratio at level of frontal horns (no additional details provided) Axial slices (13 mm thick)	No relationship between age and ventricular/skull ratio Interactions with gender or laterality not reported
Soininen et al. 1982	85 volunteers: 53 from community and 32 from nursing home 75 ± 7 years old 23 M; 62 F No neurological disease (no additional details provided)	CT Linear measurements (from films?) of ventricular and sulcal size Axial slices ($n = 8$–12, 8 mm thick) No additional details provided Composite neuropsychological test score comprised of personal and up-to-date knowledge, orientation, praxis of hand, receptive speech, expressive speech, memory, and general reasoning (arithmetic [Luria], similarities [WAIS], and comprehension [WAIS])	Age correlated with ratios of ventricular width to skull width (frontal horn index and cella media index) Age correlated with mean width of four largest sulci Correlations were found between the composite neuropsychological test score and the size of the lateral and third ventricles, and the left sylvian fissure, but the effects of age and education were not controlled Interactions with gender or laterality not reported
Zatz et al. 1982a	123 volunteers 10–90 years old 49 M; 74 F No history of neurological or major medical disease Handedness not specified	CT Volume measurement derived from computer-assisted pixel segmentation technique (ASI-II program) Axial slices ($n = 9$, 10 mm thick, 10-mm interscan gap)	Age significantly associated with increased ventricular volume (M = F), even after controlling for IV Increased variability of ventricular size with age Age associated with increased sulcal CSF volume, even after controlling for IV
Gado et al. 1983	12 elderly volunteers 64–81 years old 9 M; 3 F No additional clinical data provided	CT Volume measurements derived from computer-assisted pixel segmentation technique (seven axial slices, 8 mm thick) Linear measurements from axial images Number of raters and rater reliabilities not specified	During 1-year follow-up, ratio of ventricular volume to IV increased significantly by an average of 3.7%; no significant changes in linear measures of ventricular size (VBR, third ventricular ratio, frontal horn ratio) During 1-year follow-up, ratio of sulcal volume to IV increased significantly by an average of 13% Interactions with gender or laterality not reported

APPENDIX 9–1. Imaging studies of human aging and brain cerebrospinal fluid spaces *(continued)*

Study	Subjects	Imaging and measurement technique	Findings
Laffey et al. 1984	212 elderly volunteers 65–89 years old 110 M; 102 F No evidence of alcoholism, dementia, or neurological illness	CT Qualitative rating (6-point scale) of ventricular enlargement and sulcal widening from films, by two experienced radiologists with established reliabilities	Age associated with increased ventricular size No association between age and ratings of sulcal widening Interactions with gender or laterality not reported
Schwartz et al. 1985	30 healthy M volunteers 21–81 years old No history of major medical, neurological, or psychiatric illness Handedness not specified	CT Volume measurements derived from computer-assisted pixel segmentation technique (ASI-II program) Axial slices ($n = 7$) starting from the plane of the inferior orbitomeatal line (10 mm thick, 7-mm interscan gap)	Age correlated with areas and volumes of lateral and third ventricles, even after adjusting for height and intracranial area Age correlated with VBR Increased variability of ventricular size with age No laterality effects Age correlated with CSF volume (ventricular plus basal cisterns), even after controlling for IV Increased variability of CSF volume with age
Pfefferbaum et al. 1986	57 healthy volunteers 20–84 years old 27 M; 30 F No additional data provided	CT Volume measurements derived from computer-assisted pixel segmentation technique (modification of Gado et al. 1983) Contiguous axial slices ($n = 5$) starting at the level of the superior roof of the orbits	Age associated with increased ratio of ventricular volume to IV Increased variability in ventricular volume with age Interactions with gender or laterality not reported Age associated with increased ratio of sulcal CSF volume to IV (from single axial slice [8 mm thick] approximately 48 mm from the level of the superior roof of the orbits) Age associated with increased variability of ratio of sulcal CSF volume to IV
Stafford et al. 1988	79 healthy M volunteers 31–87 years old No severe medical or psychiatric illness Handedness not specified	CT CSF volume and CT density measurements derived from computer-assisted pixel segmentation technique (ASI-II program) Axial slices ($n = 3$) at mid-, high-, and supraventricular levels Cognitive test battery comprised of attention (auditory and visual continuous performance), Boston Naming Test, Wechsler Memory Scale (verbal and visuospatial memory), and Gorham Proverb Test	Age associated with increased ratio of ventricular volume to brain volume, with increased ratio of supraventricular CSF volume to brain volume, and with decreased CT density Interactions with laterality not reported Inverse correlation observed between a discriminant function of total CSF volume and a discriminant function of neuropsychological tests of naming and abstraction; no relation with a discriminant function of memory and attention No relation between CT density and any cognitive test measure

Study	Subjects	Method	Findings
Pearlson et al. 1989b	31 healthy elderly volunteers 68.3 ± 1.2 years old 15 M; 16 F No major medical, neurological, or psychiatric illness Handedness not specified	CT Planimetric determination of VBR from films by one of two raters, each with established reliabilities	Age correlated with VBR Interactions with gender or laterality not reported No correlation (n = 14) between VBR and scores on Boston Naming Test or Rey Auditory Verbal Learning Test (Rey 1964)
Kaye et al. 1992	107 healthy volunteers 64 M (21–90 years old); 43 F (23–88 years old) No major medical, neurological, or psychiatric illness Handedness not specified	CT Volume measurements derived from computer-assisted pixel segmentation technique (ASI-II program) Axial slices (10 mm thick, 7-mm interscan gap)	Age associated with increased ventricular volume in both M and F (about 20% per decade); precipitous increases observed beginning in the fifth decade in M and in the sixth decade in F Interactions with laterality not reported Adjusting for age, no relation between ventricular volume and sum of the scores on the WAIS verbal or performance scales
Sullivan et al. 1993	114 healthy volunteers 21–82 years old (51.2 ± 17.7 years) 84 M; 30 F No history of major medical, neurological, or psychiatric illness 90% right-handed	CT Volume measurements derived from computer-assisted pixel segmentation technique (modification of Gado et al. 1983) Axial slices (n = 10, 10 mm thick) Neuropsychological test battery comprised of MMSE, Trail Making Test A and B, WAIS-R subtests—Information, Digit Span, Vocabulary, Digit Symbol, Picture Completion, Block Design, and Object Assembly	Age correlated with total and third ventricular volume, even after adjustments for head size (M = F) No correlation between age-related changes in total or third ventricular volume and age-adjusted performance on any of the 10 neuropsychological tests Age correlated with increased CSF volume in sylvian fissure and in vertex, frontal, and parieto-occipital sulci (M = F) No correlation between age-related changes in sulcal fissure CSF volume and age-adjusted performance on any of the 10 neuropsychological tests
Shear et al. 1995	35 healthy volunteers (included in Sullivan et al. 1993) 67.4 ± 7.4 years old 23 M; 12 F No history of major medical, neurological, or psychiatric illness	CT Longitudinal within-subject follow-up, using blinded volume measurements per technique of Sullivan et al. 1993 High rater reliabilities	Over mean (± SD) follow-up of 2.6 (± 0.96) years, increases were observed in CSF volumes of frontal sulci (0.31 mL/year), sylvian fissure (0.58 mL/year), parieto-occipital sulci (0.05 mL/year), and ventricular system (0.61 mL/year) Interactions with gender not reported

(continued)

APPENDIX 9–1. Imaging studies of human aging and brain cerebrospinal fluid spaces (*continued*)

Study	Subjects	Imaging and measurement technique	Findings
Elwan et al. 1996a	88 healthy "lower middle class" volunteers 40–76 years old (54.8 ± 9.6 years) 57 M; 31 F No major medical, neurological, or psychiatric illness All right-handed	CT Multiple distance measurements (no additional details provided)	Age correlated with maximum width of third ventricle Interactions with gender or laterality not reported
Grant et al. 1987	64 healthy volunteers 18–64 years old 25 M; 39 F No history of neurological disease; psychiatric history not reported Handedness not specified	MR imaging (0.15 tesla) Mathematically derived estimate of ventricular volume and CSF volume from signal intensity measurements made on single sagittal slice (number of raters not specified)	Age associated with increased ventricular volume in M, but not in F; however, this apparent gender difference was not tested statistically Interactions with laterality not reported Age associated with increased total (ventricular plus cisternal) cranial CSF volume (M = F) No control for size of brain or head
Condon et al. 1988	40 volunteers 20–60 years old 20 M; 20 F No additional details provided	MR imaging (0.15 tesla) Volume measurement (two raters) derived from computer-assisted pixel segmentation of contiguous sagittal slices (variable slice thickness and number)	For males but not females, age correlated with ratio of total ventricular volume to IV, total CSF volume to IV, and total sulcal CSF volume to IV
Yoshii et al. 1988	58 healthy volunteers 21–81 years old 29 M; 29 F Neurological and psychiatric histories not reported Handedness not specified	MR imaging (1.0 tesla) Blinded global ratings (4-point scale) of lateral ventricular enlargement from inversion recovery films (axial slices [*n* unspecified], 10 mm thick, 3-mm interscan gap) Numbers of raters and rater reliabilities not specified	Age correlated with ratings of lateral ventricular enlargement (M = F) Interactions with laterality not reported
Jernigan et al. 1990	58 healthy volunteers 8–79 years old 35 M; 23 F No neurological, psychiatric, or medical (e.g., diabetes mellitus and heart disease) illness Handedness not specified	MR imaging (1.5 tesla) Volume estimates (one of two raters) derived from computer-assisted pixel classification of multiple spin-echo axial images (5 mm thick, 2.5-mm interscan gap)	Age associated with increased ratio of ventricular CSF volume to IV Age associated with increased ratio of sulcal CSF volume to IV Interactions with gender or laterality not reported

Study	Subjects	Methods	Results
Wahlund et al. 1990	24 healthy elderly volunteers 75–85 years old (mean = 79 years) 8 M; 16 F No evidence of neurological or psychiatric illness Handedness not specified	MR imaging (0.02 tesla) Visual ratings (5-point scale) of CSF spaces on T2-weighted axial films (slice: 10 mm thick, no gap) by two raters (blind?) with established reliabilities Area measurements of lateral ventricles based on computer-assisted pixel classification technique, from single axial section at level of basal ganglia Neuropsychological test battery comprised of MMSE, WAIS-R subtests (Information, Digit Span, Similarities, Block Design, Object Assembly, Digit Substitution) and Wechsler Memory Scale (Associative Learning, Visual Reproduction)	No correlation between age and visual ratings or area measurements of sulcal CSF or lateral ventricle CSF size No relation between size of sulcal or lateral ventricular CSF and any neuropsychological test measure
Gur et al. 1991	69 healthy volunteers 18–80 years old 34 M; 35 F No neurological or psychiatric illness 66 right-handed; 3 left-handed	MR imaging (1.5 tesla) Volume measurements (any two of four raters) derived from segmentation technique based on two-feature pixel classification of multiple spin-echo axial images (5 mm thick, contiguous)	Older (≥ 55 years) subjects (n = 26) had larger total CSF volume (M > F), larger ratio of ventricular CSF volume to IV (M = F), and larger ratio of sulcal CSF volume to IV (M > F) Effects of age on ratio of ventricular CSF volume to IV were asymmetric (L > R) in M but not in F
Tanna et al. 1991	16 healthy volunteers 52–86 years old 5 M; 11 F No evidence of major medical, neurological, or psychiatric illness Handedness not specified	MR imaging (1.5 tesla) Volume measurements (one of two raters with established reliabilities) derived from segmentation techniques based on two-feature pixel classification of multiple spin-echo axial images (5 mm thick, 2.5-mm interscan gap)	Age correlated with ratio of ventricular CSF volume to total CSF plus total brain volume Trend (nonsignificant) for age to be associated with increasing ratio of sulcal CSF volume to total CSF plus total brain volume Interactions with gender or laterality not reported
Coffey et al. 1992	76 healthy volunteers 36–91 years old 25 M; 51 F No lifetime evidence of neurological or psychiatric illness All right-handed	MR imaging (1.5 tesla) Volume measurements (one of three blinded raters with established reliabilities) using computer-assisted trace methodology of T1-weighted coronal images (n = 30–35, 5 mm thick, contiguous) Blinded clinical ratings (5-point scale) of lateral ventricular enlargement from films (average score of two experienced raters)	Adjusting for IV, age associated with increased volumes of the third (2.8% per year) and lateral (3.2% per year) ventricles (M = F) Age associated with increased odds (7.7% per year) of at least mild lateral ventricular enlargement, from 0.10 at age 40 to 2.22 at age 80 (M = F) No interactions with laterality
Lim et al. 1992	14 healthy M volunteers 8 young (21–25 years old); 6 elderly (68–76 years old) No evidence of significant medical or psychiatric illness Handedness not specified	MR imaging (1.5 tesla) Blinded volume measurements derived from semiautomated pixel segmentation of intermediate and T2-weighted axial imaging (n = 8, 5 mm thick, 2.5-mm interscan gap)	Compared with younger M, older M had higher percentage of CSF volume to IV (8% vs. 20.1%)

(continued)

APPENDIX 9–1. Imaging studies of human aging and brain cerebrospinal fluid spaces (*continued*)

Study	Subjects	Imaging and measurement technique	Findings
Matsubayashi et al. 1992	73 healthy volunteers 59–83 years old 24 M; 49 F No history of major medical, neurological, or psychiatric illness	MR imaging (0.5 tesla) Planimetric determination of VPR No additional details provided Neuropsychological test battery comprised of MMSE, Hasegawa Dementia Scale (Hasegawa 1974), a visuospatial cognitive performance test, and a manual dexterity test	Age correlated with VPR Interactions with gender or laterality not reported Adjusting for age, no relation between VPR and any neuropsychological test measure
Murphy et al. 1992	27 healthy M 19–92 years old No major medical, neurological, or psychiatric illness Handedness not specified	MR imaging (0.5 tesla) Blinded volume measurements derived from semiautomated pixel segmentation of proton density axial images ($n = 36$, 7 mm thick, contiguous) Rater reliabilities established, but number of raters not specified	Compared with younger M (< 60 years old; $n = 10$), older M ($n = 17$) had larger ratio of lateral ventricular volume to IV, larger ratio of third ventricular volume to IV, and larger ratio of peripheral CSF volume (total CSF volume minus ventricular volumes) to IV No interactions with laterality
Raz et al. 1993c	29 healthy volunteers 18–78 years old 17 M; 12 F No major medical, neurological, or psychiatric illness Self-reported right-handers	MR imaging (0.30 tesla) Blinded volume measurements from films using digital planimetry of T1-weighted and proton density sagittal and coronal images Good rater ($n = 2$) reliabilities	Controlling for head size, age associated with increased lateral ventricular volume (M = F) Interactions with laterality not reported
Christiansen et al. 1994	142 healthy volunteers 21–80 years old 78 M; 64 F No major medical or neurological illness	MR imaging (1.5 tesla) Volume measurements using manual tracing of T2-weighted axial images (4 mm thick, 4-mm interscan gap) No additional details provided	Age associated with increased lateral ventricle volume in M (134%) and F (66%), but these apparent gender differences were not statistically compared Interactions with laterality not reported
DeCarli et al. 1994	30 healthy M volunteers 18–92 years old No major medical, neurological, or psychiatric illness 29 right-handed	MR imaging (0.5 tesla) Volume measurements of T1-weighted coronal images (6 mm thick, contiguous) by single rater using computer-assisted pixel segmentation techniques Good rater reliabilities	Age associated with increased volume of sulcal CSF to IV (1.3%/decade), central CSF to IV (0.3%/decade), and third ventricle CSF to IV (0.04%/decade) For all measures, no interactions with laterality

Study	Subjects	Method	Results
Golomb et al. 1994	54 healthy volunteers with MMSE ≥ 28 (overlap with Golomb et al. 1993) 55–87 years old (59.7 ± 7.9 years) 23 M; 31 F. No major medical, neurologic, or psychiatric illness. Handedness not specified	MR imaging (1.5 tesla). Blinded volume measurements of sulcal CSF using computer-assisted trace methodology of T1-weighted coronal images (4 mm thick, 10% gap) by single rater with established reliabilities	Adjusting for head size, age associated with increased sulcal CSF volume
Pfefferbaum et al. 1994	73 healthy M volunteers (included in Pfefferbaum et al. 1993) 21–70 years old (44.1 ± 13.8 years). No major medical, neurological, or psychiatric illness. Left-handers included (n not specified)	MR imaging (1.5 tesla). Blinded volume measurements of T2-weighted axial slices (5 mm thick, 2.5 mm-interscan gap) by four raters using computer-assisted pixel segmentation techniques. Good rater reliabilities	Age associated with increased cortical CSF volume to IV (0.6 mL/year) and with ventricular volume to IV (0.3 mL/year). Interactions with laterality not reported
Blatter et al. 1995	194 healthy volunteers 16–65 years old 89 M; 105 F. No history (by questionnaire) of any neurological or psychiatric illness. 95% right-handed	MR imaging (1.5 tesla). Volume measurements derived from semiautomated pixel segmentation and trace methodologies, of intermediate and T2-weighted axial images (5 mm thick, 2-mm gap). High rater reliabilities (blind)	Adjusting for IV, age associated with increased subarachnoid CSF volume, and lateral and third ventricular volumes, but not with fourth ventricular volume; correlations tended to be higher for M than for F, but these apparent differences were not analyzed. Interactions with laterality not reported
Murphy et al. 1996	69 healthy volunteers 35 M (mean ± SD age = 44 ± 23 years); 34 F (mean ± SD age = 50 ± 21 years). No major medical or psychiatric illness. All right-handed	MR imaging (0.5 and 1.5 tesla). Blinded volume measurements using computer-assisted segmentation and trace methodology of contiguous coronal images (5–6 mm thick). Number of raters not specified	Relative to younger subjects (age 20–35 years), older subjects (60–85 years) had larger ratios of lateral ventricular volume to IV (M = F), third ventricular volume to IV (F > M), and peripheral CSF volume to IV (M = F). No interactions with laterality
Salonen et al. 1997	61 healthy volunteers 30–86 years old 30 M; 31 F. No neurological symptoms or disease; psychiatric history not specified. Handedness not specified	MR imaging (1.0 tesla). Qualitative ratings (5-point scale) of sulcal and lateral ventricular enlargement. Linear measurement of maximum width of third ventricle. T1-weighted axial slices (5 mm thick, 1-mm interscan gap). Number of raters and rater reliabilities not specified	Age associated with increased ratings of sulcal and lateral ventricular enlargement, and with width of third ventricle. Interactions with gender or laterality not reported
Yue et al. 1997	1,488 healthy elderly volunteers from the Cardiovascular Health Study 65–80+ years old. No major medical or neurological illness (psychiatric illness not assessed). Number of M and F not specified. Handedness not specified	MR imaging (0.35 or 1.5 tesla). Blinded ratings of sulcal prominence (10-point scale) and ventricular size (10-point scale) from T1-weighted axial images. Good to excellent rater reliabilities, but number of raters not specified	Age associated with increased sulcal prominence and ventricular enlargement (M = F)

(continued)

APPENDIX 9–1. Imaging studies of human aging and brain cerebrospinal fluid spaces (continued)

Study	Subjects	Imaging and measurement technique	Findings
Coffey et al. 1998	330 elderly volunteers living independently in the community 66–96 years old (74.98 ± 5.09) 129 M; 201 F No lifetime history of neurological or psychiatric illness All right-handed	MR imaging (1.5 tesla, n = 248; 0.35 tesla, n = 82) Blinded volume measurements (one of two raters with established reliabilities) using computer-assisted trace methodology of T1-weighted axial images (5 mm thick, no interscan gap)	Adjusting for IV, age associated with increased peripheral (sulcal) CSF volume, lateral fissure CSF volume, lateral ventricular volume (0.95 mL/year), and third ventricular volume (0.05 mL/year) M showed greater age-related changes than did F for peripheral CSF (2.11 mL/year vs. 0.06 mL/year, respectively) and lateral fissure volumes (0.23 mL/year vs. 0.10 mL/year, respectively) No interactions with laterality
Guttmann et al. 1998	72 healthy volunteers 18–81 years old 22 M; 50 F No history of psychiatric illness, epilepsy, or severe head trauma Handedness not specified	MR imaging (1.5 tesla) Blinded volume measurements using computer-assisted segmentation and trace methodology of contiguous axial images (3 mm thick) Good interrater reliabilities	Age associated with increased ratio of total CSF volume to IV Interactions with gender or laterality not reported
Mueller et al. 1998	46 healthy elderly volunteers 65–74 years old (6 M, 5 F), 75–84 years old (8 M, 7 F), and 85–95 years old (9 M, 11 F) All functionally independent, MMSE ≥ 24, and free of major medical and neurological illness, as well as depression Handedness not specified	MR imaging (1.5 tesla) Volume measurements (nonblind?) using computer-assisted pixel segmentation of contiguous coronal images (4 mm thick) Excellent interrater reliabilities Scanning repeated annually or biannually over 3- to 9-year follow-up	Adjusting for IV, age associated with increased temporal horn volume, but not with total CSF, sulcal CSF, or lateral ventricle volumes Interactions with gender not reported Over the follow-up period, significant increases were seen only in total CSF volume (1.5 mL/year, F > M) and in lateral ventricular volume (1.4 mL/year, M = F)
Pfefferbaum et al. 1998	28 healthy M volunteers (overlap with Pfefferbaum et al. 1994) 21–68 years old (51 ± 13.8 years) No major medical, neurological, or psychiatric illness Left-handers included (n not specified)	MR imaging (1.5 tesla) Blinded volume measurements derived from semiautomated pixel segmentation of intermediate and T2- weighted axial images (n = 17–20, 5 mm thick, 2.5-mm interscan gap) Scanning repeated at 5-year follow-up	Over the follow-up interval, significant increase in volume of lateral (5 mL, or 20%) and third ventricles, but not in cortical sulcal CSF volume

Note. CSF = cerebrospinal fluid; CT = computed tomography; F = female(s); IV = intracranial volume; M = male(s); MMSE = Mini-Mental State Exam; MR = magnetic resonance; VBR = ventricular/brain ratio; VPR = ventricular/parenchymal ratio; WAIS-R = Weschler Adult Intelligence Scale–Revised.

APPENDIX 9–2. Imaging studies of human aging and brain parenchymal atrophy

Study	Subjects	Imaging and measurement technique	Findings
Jacoby et al. 1980	50 healthy elderly volunteers 62–88 years old 10 M; 40 F No history of significant psychiatric or neurological illness Handedness not specified	CT Ratings (4-point scale) of cortical atrophy from films by single blinded rater; five regions rated (frontal, parietal, temporal, insular, and occipital) and scores summed	Age correlated with total cortical atrophy score Interactions with gender or laterality not reported Adjusting for age, no relation between cortical atrophy and performance on the Hodkinson test of memory and orientation
Cala et al. 1981	115 volunteers 15–40 years old 62 M; 53 F No history of migraine, head trauma, or excessive alcohol intake (no additional details provided) All but eight subjects right-handed	CT (n = 2 scanners) Ratings (5-point scale) of cortical atrophy (no additional details provided) Axial slices (13 mm thick)	Age apparently associated with increased frequency of mild (grade 2) atrophy of frontal lobes and cerebellar vermis, but no statistical analysis reported Interactions with gender or laterality not reported
Schwartz et al. 1985	30 healthy M volunteers 21–81 years old No history of major medical, neurological, or psychiatric illness Handedness not specified	CT Volume measurements derived from computer-assisted segmentation technique (ASI-II program) Axial slices (n = 7) starting from the plane of the inferior orbitomeatal line (10 mm thick, 7-mm interscan gap)	Adjusting for IV, age negatively correlated with volume of gray matter and with volume of gray plus white matter, but not with white matter volume Subjects > 60 years old (n = 11) had smaller volumes of thalamus, lenticular nuclei, and total gray matter than younger subjects (n = 19) Effects similar for both hemispheres
Golomb et al. 1993	154 healthy volunteers with MMSE score > 27 55–88 years old (70 ± 8 years) 73 M; 81 F No evidence of active medical, neurological, or psychiatric illness Handedness not specified	CT (n = 51); MR imaging (n = 81); both CT and MR imaging (n = 22) Blinded ratings (4-point scale) of hippocampal atrophy as defined by dilation of transverse choroidal fissure on films, by raters (n = ?) with established reliabilities Neuropsychological test battery comprised of WAIS Digit Span and the Guild Memory Test (Paired Associates, Paragraph Recall, and Design Recall)	Subjects with hippocampal atrophy (rating of 2 or greater in either hemisphere; n = 50) significantly older than those without atrophy More M (41%) than F (25%) with hippocampal atrophy After controlling for age, education, and WAIS vocabulary score, subjects with hippocampal atrophy performed worse on recent verbal memory portion of the Guild Memory Scale; no group differences were observed in digit span or recall of designs

(continued)

APPENDIX 9–2. Imaging studies of human aging and brain parenchymal atrophy (*continued*)

Study	Subjects	Imaging and measurement technique	Findings
Meyer et al. 1994	81 healthy volunteers 27–90 years old 44 M; 37 F No major neurological or psychiatric illness	CT (n = 2 scanners) Blinded measure of tissue density (densitometry) and regional brain volume (trace methodology) from axial slices (8 mm thick)	Age associated with decreased tissue density in cortical gray matter (frontal, temporal, parietal, and occipital) and in white matter (frontal only), but not in subcortical gray matter (caudate, putamen, or thalamus) Age associated with decreased ratios of cortical gray matter volume to IV and subcortical gray matter volume to IV, but not with white matter volume to IV Interactions with gender or laterality not reported
Elwan et al. 1996b	88 healthy "lower middle class" volunteers 40–76 years old (54.8 ± 9.6 years) 57 M; 31 F No major medical, neurological, or psychiatric illness All right-handed	CT Multiple linear measurements (no additional details provided)	No correlation between age and maximal bifrontal distance, bifrontal index, maximal bicaudate distance, maximal septum–caudate distance, or cella media index Interactions with gender or laterality not reported
Condon et al. 1988	40 volunteers 20–60 years old 20 M; 20 F No additional details provided	MR imaging (0.15 tesla) Volume measurement (two raters) derived from computer-assisted pixel segmentation of contiguous sagittal slices (variable slice thickness and number)	For M but not F, age negatively correlated with ratio of total brain volume to IV Interactions with laterality not reported
Yoshii et al. 1988	58 volunteers 21–81 years old 29 M; 29 F Neurological and psychiatric histories not reported Handedness not specified	MR imaging (1.0 tesla) Mathematically derived estimate of brain volume from inversion recovery films, based on planimetric measurement made on single slice (10 mm thick) at level of foramen of Monro Blinded global ratings of cortical atrophy from films (axial slices, [n = ?], 10 mm thick, 3-mm interscan gap) Number of raters and rater reliabilities not specified	No correlation between age and brain volume Age significantly correlated with ratings of cortical atrophy for both M and F

Study	Subjects	Methods	Findings
Jernigan et al. 1990, 1991	58 healthy volunteers 8–79 years old 35 M; 23 F No history of neurological, psychiatric, or medical illness (diabetes mellitus, heart disease) Handedness not specified	MR imaging (1.5 tesla) Volume estimates (one of two raters) derived from computer-assisted pixel classification of multiple spin-echo axial images (5 mm thick, 2.5-mm interscan gap)	Age negatively correlated with ratios of cerebral volume to IV and of gray matter volume to IV Among gray matter structures, age negatively correlated with ratios of cortical gray matter volume to IV, caudate volume to IV, and diencephalon volume to IV; but not with thalamus volume to IV or anterior cingulate volume to IV No correlation between age and ratio of white matter volume to IV Interactions with gender or laterality not reported
Krishnan et al. 1990	39 healthy volunteers 24–79 years old 17 M; 22 F No evidence of major medical, neurological, or psychiatric illness Handedness not specified	MR imaging (1.5 tesla) Stereological measurement (one of two raters) of axial slices (variable number, 5 mm thick, 2.5-mm interscan gap) from intermediate and T2-weighted films	Age negatively correlated with total caudate volume (M = F) Caudate volume was less in subjects older than 50 years (n = 22) No adjustments for cranial size
Doraiswamy et al. 1991	36 healthy volunteers (overlap with subjects of Krishnan et al. 1990) 26–79 years old 16 M; 20 F No evidence of major medical, neurological, or psychiatric illness Handedness not specified	MR imaging (1.5 tesla) Area measurement of T1-weighted midsagittal image using computer-assisted trace methodology Rater reliabilities not reported	Age negatively correlated with corpus callosum area in M but not in F
Escalona et al. 1991	37 healthy volunteers (overlap with subjects of Krishnan et al. 1990) 24–79 years old 16 M; 21 F No evidence of major medical, neurological, or psychiatric illness Handedness not specified	MR imaging (1.5 tesla) Stereological measurement (one of two raters) of axial slices (variable number, 5 mm thick, 2.5-mm interscan gap) from intermediate and T2-weighted films Good rater reliabilities	No association between age and volume of cerebellar hemispheres
Gur et al. 1991	69 healthy volunteers 18–80 years old 34 M; 35 F No neurological or psychiatric illness 66 right-handed; 3 left-handed	MR imaging (1.5 tesla) Volume measurements (any two of four raters) derived from segmentation technique based on two-feature pixel classification of multiple spin-echo axial images (5 mm thick, contiguous)	Older (≥ 55 years) subjects (n = 26) had smaller whole brain volumes than younger subjects (M = F)

(continued)

APPENDIX 9–2. Imaging studies of human aging and brain parenchymal atrophy (*continued*)

Study	Subjects	Imaging and measurement technique	Findings
McDonald et al. 1991	36 healthy volunteers (subjects also included in Krishnan et al. 1990) 24–79 years old 13 M; 23 F No evidence of major medical, neurological, or psychiatric illness	MR imaging (1.5 tesla) Same as Krishnan et al. 1990 (above)	Age negatively correlated with total putamen volume (M = F; left = right), but no adjustments for cranial size
Shah et al. 1991	36 healthy volunteers (overlap with subjects in Krishnan et al. 1990) 26–79 years old 16 M; 20 F No evidence of major medical, neurological, or psychiatric illness	MR imaging (1.5 tesla) Computer-assisted measurements from T1-weighted midsagittal films by single rater with established intrarater reliabilities	Increasing age associated with decreasing midbrain area (M > F?) No age effects on areas of pons, medulla, anterior cerebellar vermis, or fourth ventricle
Tanna et al. 1991	16 healthy volunteers 52–86 years old 5 M; 11 F No evidence of major medical, neurological, or psychiatric illness Handedness not specified	MR imaging (1.5 tesla) Volume measurements (one of two raters with established reliabilities) derived from segmentation techniques based on two-feature pixel classification of multiple spin-echo axial images (5 mm thick, 2.5-mm interscan gap)	Age negatively correlated with ratio of total brain volume to total CSF plus total brain volume Interactions with gender or laterality not reported
Coffey et al. 1992	76 healthy volunteers 36–91 years old 25 M; 51 F No lifetime history of neurological or psychiatric illness All right-handed	MR imaging (1.5 tesla) Volume measurements (one of three blinded raters with established reliabilities) using computer-assisted trace methodology of T1-weighted coronal images (n = 30–35, 5 mm thick, contiguous) Blinded clinical ratings (5-point scale) of "cortical atrophy" (average score of two raters)	Age associated with decreased total volumes of the cerebral hemispheres (0.23% per year), the frontal lobes (0.55% per year), the temporal lobes (0.28% per year), and the amygdala-hippocampal complex (0.30% per year); all effects similar for M and F, and for both hemispheres Increasing age associated with increasing odds (8.9% per year) of "cortical atrophy," from 0.08 at age 40 to 2.82 at age 80
Doraiswamy et al. 1992	75 healthy volunteers (overlap with subjects in Krishnan et al. 1990) 21–82 years old (52.5 ± 18 years) 34 M; 41 F No neurological or psychiatric illness	MR imaging (1.5 tesla) Blinded measurements of midbrain size on T2-weighted axial films (no additional details provided)	Age negatively correlated with midbrain volume and anteroposterior diameter, but not with red nucleus size Effects similar for both M and F

Study	Subjects	Methods	Findings
Jack et al. 1992	22 healthy elderly volunteers 76.3 ± 11.3 years old 10 M; 12 F No major medical or neurological illness; no depression Handedness not specified	MR imaging (1.5 tesla) Volume estimates (single rater) derived from computer-assisted pixel classification of T1-weighted coronal images (4 mm thick, contiguous) Intrarater reliabilities not reported	Age associated with decreased ratio of hippocampal volume to IV and of anterior temporal lobe volume to IV Interactions with gender or laterality not reported
Lim et al. 1992	14 healthy M volunteers 8 young (21–25 years old) and 6 elderly (68–76 years old) No evidence of significant medical or psychiatric illness Handedness not specified	MR imaging (1.5 tesla) Blinded volume measurements derived from semiautomated pixel segmentation of intermediate and T2-weighted axial images ($n = 8$, 5 mm thick, 2.5-mm interscan gap)	Compared to young M, elderly M had lower ratio of gray matter volume to IV (49.7% vs. 38.7%) No group difference in ratio of white matter volume to IV (47.2% vs. 41.2%) Interactions with laterality not reported
Murphy et al. 1992	27 healthy M volunteers 19–92 years old No major medical, neurological, or psychiatric illness Handedness not specified	MR imaging (0.5 tesla) Blinded volume measurements using computer-assisted trace methodology of proton density axial images ($n = 36$, 7 mm thick, contiguous) Manual tracing of subcortical nuclei from enhanced images Rater reliabilities were established, but number of raters not reported	Older M (> 60, $n = 17$) had smaller ratios of total, left, and right hemisphere volume to IV than did younger M Older M had smaller ratios of total caudate volume to IV and of total lenticular nuclei volume to IV than did younger M; no difference in ratio of total thalamus volume to IV Reductions in caudate and lenticular volumes also found when the volumes were normalized to total brain volume, suggesting a differential effect of aging on these structures Older M exhibited a R > L asymmetry in lenticular volumes; the reverse was true in younger M
Doraiswamy et al. 1993	Same as Doraiswamy et al. 1992	MR imaging (1.5 tesla) Blinded linear measurements of interuncal distance on T1-weighted axial image (no additional details provided)	Age associated with larger interuncal distance (NB: this measure was not correlated with amygdala volume in a follow-up study [Early et al. 1993]) Interactions with gender or laterality not reported

(continued)

APPENDIX 9–2. Imaging studies of human aging and brain parenchymal atrophy *(continued)*

Study	Subjects	Imaging and measurement technique	Findings
Raz et al. 1993a, 1993b, 1993c	29 healthy volunteers 18–78 years old (43.8 ± 21.5 years) 17 M; 12 F No history of medical, neurological, or psychiatric illness All right-handed	MR imaging (0.3 tesla) Volume measurements using computer-assisted trace methodology of digitized images from the films, by two blinded raters with high reliabilities T1-weighted axial slices ($n = 9$, 4.2 mm thick, 6.0-mm interscan gap) T2-weighted coronal slices ($n = 17$–21, 6.6 mm thick, 8.6-mm interscan gap) Measures of "fluid" (Cattell Culture-Fair Intelligence Test) and crystallized (Extended Vocabulary) intelligence	After controlling for head size, age associated with decreased volumes of caudate and visual cortex (F > M) No association between age and volumes of dorsolateral prefrontal cortex, anterior cingulate gyrus, prefrontal white matter, hippocampal formation, postcentral gyrus, inferior parietal lobule, or parietal white matter Both measures of intelligence were associated with L > R asymmetry in cerebral hemisphere volume, but not with any other measure of brain size
Christiansen et al. 1994	142 healthy volunteers 21–80 years old 78 M; 64 F No major medical or neurological illness	MR imaging (1.5 tesla) Area and volume measurements using computer-assisted trace methodology of T2-weighted axial slices ($n = 15$, 4 mm thick, 4-mm interscan gap) Number of raters, their "blindness," and their reliabilities not specified	Age associated with decreased volume of cerebral hemispheres Interactions with gender or laterality not reported
Cowell et al. 1994	130 healthy volunteers (overlap with subjects in Gur et al. 1991) 18–80 years old 70 M; 60 F No major medical, neurological, or psychiatric illness All right-handed	MR imaging (1.5 tesla) Volume measurements using a combination of computer-assisted trace methodology and pixel segmentation of three-dimensional images reconstructed from T2-weighted axial images (5 mm thick, contiguous) Good rater reliabilities, but "blindness" not specified	Ratio of *frontal lobe* to IV was smaller in M > 40 years old than in younger M; no such group difference in F In contrast, the R > L asymmetry of frontal lobe to IV was larger in older F than younger F; no such group difference in M Ratio of *temporal lobe* to IV was also smaller in M > 40 years old than in younger M; no such group difference in F; no interactions with laterality Ratio of the *remaining brain volume* to IV was smaller in older than in younger subjects for both sexes; no interactions with laterality

Study	Subjects	Methods	Results
DeCarli et al. 1994	30 healthy M volunteers 19–92 years old No major medical, neurological, or psychiatric illness 29 right-handed	MR imaging (0.5 tesla) Volume measurements using computer-assisted trace methodology of T1-weighted coronal images (6 mm thick, contiguous) through temporal lobe, by single (blind?) rater	Age associated with decreased ratio of frontal lobe volume to IV but not with temporal lobe volume to IV No interactions with laterality
Golomb et al. 1994	54 healthy volunteers (overlap with Golomb et al. 1993) 55–87 years old (59.7 ± 7.9 years) 23 M; 31 F No major medical, neurological, or psychiatric illness Handedness not specified	MR imaging (1.5 tesla) Blinded volume measurements using computer-assisted trace methodology of T1-weighted coronal images (4 mm thick, 10% gap) by single rater with established reliabilities Composite scores of primary (WAIS Digit Span) and secondary memory with immediate and delayed recall (Guild Memory Test, list recall, facial recognition)	Adjusting for head size, age associated with decreased volumes of hippocampal formation and of superior temporal gyrus After adjusting for age, gender, WAIS vocabulary, and subarachnoid CSF volume, hippocampal volume was associated with delayed recall but not with initial recall or digit span Volume of superior temporal gyrus was unrelated to any memory measure
Pfefferbaum et al. 1994	73 healthy M volunteers (included in Pfefferbaum et al. 1993) 21–70 years old (44.1 ± 13.8 years) No major medical, neurological, or psychiatric illness Left-handers included (n not specified)	MR imaging (1.5 tesla) Blinded volume measurements derived from semiautomated pixel segmentation of intermediate and T2-weighted axial images ($n = 17$–20, 5 mm thick, 2.5-mm interscan gap)	Adjusting for head size, age associated with decreased cortical gray matter volume (0.7 mL/year), but not with cortical white matter volume Interactions with laterality not reported
Soininen et al. 1994	32 healthy volunteers from the community, all with MMSE scores > 25 16 with AAMI (67.7 ± 7 years; 4 M, 12 F) 16 control subjects (70.2 ± 4.7 years; 6 M, 10 F) without AAMI All but 1 right-handed	MR imaging (1.5 tesla) Blinded volume measurements using computer-assisted trace methodology of T1-weighted coronal images (1 mm thick, contiguous) through temporal lobe, by single rater with established reliabilities Neuropsychological measures of verbal memory (Buschke-Fuld Selective Reminding Test) and visual memory (Benton Visual Retention Test, Heaton Visual Retention Test)	No group differences in hippocampal volumes, although control subjects (but not AAMI subjects) exhibited significant R > L asymmetry No group differences in amygdala volume or asymmetry No correlation between verbal memory and any volume measurement Visual memory (BVRT) correlated with 1) right hippocampal volume and with degree of R > L asymmetry in total sample only, and 2) with left hippocampal volume and right amygdala volume in AAMI subjects Visual memory (Heaton) correlated with volumes of right and left amygdala in total sample and in AAMI subjects

(continued)

APPENDIX 9–2. Imaging studies of human aging and brain parenchymal atrophy *(continued)*

Study	Subjects	Imaging and measurement technique	Findings
Blatter et al. 1995	194 healthy volunteers 16–65 years old 89 M; 105 F No history (by questionnaire) of any neurological or psychiatric illness 95% right-handed	MR imaging (1.5 tesla) Volume measurements derived from semiautomated pixel segmentation and trace methodologies of intermediate and T2-weighted axial images (5 mm thick, 2-mm gap) High rater reliabilities (blinded status?)	Adjusting for head size, age associated with decreased total brain volume and gray matter volume, but not white matter volume Correlations tended to be higher for M than for F, but these apparent differences were not analyzed. However, only F showed significant age-related reductions in gray matter.
Convit et al. 1995	37 healthy adult volunteers 27 older (14 M, 13 F; 69.2 ± 8.3 years old) 10 younger (5 M, 5 F; 26.1 ± 4.1 years old) No evidence of stroke or major medical or psychiatric illness	MR imaging (1.5 tesla) Blinded volume measurements by single rater (reliabilities?) using computer-assisted trace methods of T1-weighted coronal images (4 mm thick, 10% gap)	Interactions with laterality not reported Controlling for gender and head size, age associated with volume loss in lateral temporal lobe (especially fusiform gyrus) and medial temporal lobe (especially hippocampus and parahippocampus)
Hokama et al. 1995	15 healthy M community volunteers 20–55 years old No lifetime history of major medical, neurological, or psychiatric illness All right-handed	MR imaging (1.5 tesla) Volume measurements of basal ganglia using semiautomated computer assisted trace methodology from T1-weighted coronal and axial sections (1.5 mm thick, contiguous) by raters with established reliabilities	Age associated with decreased volumes of caudate and putamen, but not of globus pallidus No correlation between basal ganglia volumes and IQ as estimated by WAIS-R Information subscale
Parashos et al. 1995	80 healthy volunteers (overlap with subjects in Coffey et al. 1992) 30–91 years old 28 M; 52 F No lifetime history of neurological or psychiatric illness All right-handed	MR imaging (1.5 tesla) Blinded area measurements using computer-assisted trace methodology of T1-weighted midsagittal image (5 mm thick), made by single rater with established rater reliabilities	Adjusting for IV, increasing age associated with smaller total and regional callosal areas, especially of anterior regions (M = F)
Fox et al. 1996	11 adult volunteers with no evidence of memory impairment on testing 5 M, 6 F; 51.3 ± 5.9 years old No additional details provided	MR imaging (1.5 tesla) Volume measurements using computer-assisted pixel segmentation of T1-weighted coronal images (1.5 mm thick, contiguous) Scanning repeated at 12.8 ± 4.3 months and volume differences determined from subtraction images	Over the follow-up period, brain volume decreased by 0.05% (0.03 mL)

Reference	Subjects	Methods	Results
Golomb et al. 1996	44 healthy volunteers (from Golomb et al. 1994) 68.5 ± 7.7 years old 16 M; 28 F No major medical, neurological, or psychiatric illness Handedness not specified	MR imaging (1.5 tesla) Blinded volume measurements using computer-assisted trace methodology of T1-weighted coronal images (4 mm thick, contiguous) Guild Memory Test (Paired Associates, Paragraph Recall, and Design Recall) administered at baseline and at mean of 3.8 years later	After adjusting for age, gender, and years of education, change in paragraph recall scores over the follow-up interval were significantly inversely related to baseline hippocampal volume (adjusted for intracranial volume), but not to baseline superior temporal gyrus size or subarachnoid CSF volume Baseline hippocampal volume (adjusted for intracranial volume) was significantly smaller in the 14 subjects who declined to a score of 3 (mild cognitive impairment) on the Global Deterioration Scale
Janowsky et al. 1996	60 healthy elderly volunteers 66–94 years old (mean 78.2) 15 M; 45 F No major medical, neurological, or psychiatric illness Handedness not specified	MR imaging (1.5 tesla) Area measurement of corpus callosum derived from computer-assisted trace methodology Number of raters and their "blindness" not specified	Age associated with decreased total callosal area, anterior callosal area, and middle callosal area Interactions with gender not reported
Murphy et al. 1996	69 healthy volunteers 35 M (44 ± 23 years old); 34 F (50 ± 21 years old) No major medical or psychiatric illness All right-handed	MR imaging (0.5 and 1.5 tesla) Blinded volume measurements using computer-assisted segmentation and trace methodology of contiguous coronal images (5–6 mm thick) Number of raters not specified	Relative to "young" subjects (age 20–35 years), "old" subjects (60–85 years) had smaller brain matter volume ratios of cerebellum to IV (M = F), cerebrum to IV (M > F), frontal lobe to IV (M > F), temporal lobe to IV (M > F), parietal lobe to IV (F > M), parieto-occipital lobe to IV (M = F), parahippocampal gyrus to IV (M = F), amygdala to IV (M = F), hippocampus to IV (F > M), thalamus to IV (M = F), lenticular nucleus to IV (M = F), and caudate to IV (M = F) For the frontal lobe, the right side decreased more than the left with age in M, but in F the left side decreased more than the right; for all other regions, there were no interactions with laterality
Deshmukh et al. 1997	10 healthy M volunteers 50.1 ± 13.8 years old No evidence of major medical, neurological, or psychiatric illness 9 right-handed; 1 left-handed	MR imaging (1.5 tesla) Volume measures using semiautomated computer-assisted trace methodology from three-dimensional T1-weighted sagittal sections, realigned in the axial plane, by raters with established reliabilities	Age associated with decreased volume of cerebellar lobules VI–VII

(continued)

APPENDIX 9–2. Imaging studies of human aging and brain parenchymal atrophy (*continued*)

Study	Subjects	Imaging and measurement technique	Findings
Jack et al. 1997	126 healthy elderly volunteers 51–89 years old (79.15 ± 6.73 years) 44 M; 82 F No active neurological or psychiatric illness Handedness not specified	MR imaging (1.5 tesla) Blinded volume measurements using computer-assisted trace methodology of T1-weighted three-dimensional volumetric images (1.6 mm thick, contiguous, $n = 124$) by single rater with established reliabilities	Age associated with decreased volume ratio of hippocampus to IV (45.63 mL/year), amygdala to IV (20.75 mL/year), and parahippocampal gyrus to IV (46.65 mL/year); effects similar for M and F Effects were similar for the 2 hemispheres except for the parahippocampal gyrus (L > R)
Kaye et al. 1997	30 healthy elderly volunteers from the community, with MMSE ≥ 24 All ≥ 84 years old; 14 M, 16 F No evidence of major medical, neurological, or psychiatric illness	MR imaging (1.5 tesla) Blinded volume measurements using computer-assisted trace methodology of T1-weighted coronal images (4 mm thick, contiguous) by raters with established reliabilities Scanning repeated annually over a mean of 42 months	12 subjects developed cognitive decline (MMSE < 24) during follow-up (predementia group) Ratio of temporal lobe volume/IV declined at a faster rate in the predementia group (about 1.27%/year) than in the others (0%/year) No group differences in rate of decrease in hippocampal/IV (about 2%/year) or parahippocampal volume/IV (about 2.5%/year)
O'Brien et al. 1997	40 healthy community volunteers 55–96 years old 20 M, 20 F No evidence of major medical or neurological illness, nor of depression or drug abuse	MR imaging (0.3 tesla) Ratings of amygdala-hippocampal atrophy from T1-weighted coronal images (5.1 mm thick, 0.5-mm gap) by two raters with established reliabilities, blind to cognitive scores	Age associated with presence of amygdala-hippocampal atrophy Controlling for the effects of age and education, amygdala-hippocampal atrophy was associated with lower scores on CAMCOG, a relation entirely the result of lower scores on the memory subscale

N. Raz et al. 1997	148 healthy volunteers 18–77 years old 66 M (47.39 ± 8.07 years old); 82 F (45.72 ± 16.48 years old) No major medical, neurological, or psychiatric illness All right-handed	MR imaging (1.5 tesla) Blinded volume measurements (digital planimetry) from scans of T1-weighted reformatted coronal images (1.3 mm thick, contiguous) Good rater reliabilities among eight raters	Adjusted for height, age significantly related to smaller volumes of whole brain (M = F), prefrontal gray matter (M = F), inferior temporal cortex (M > F), fusiform gyrus (M = F), hippocampal formation (M = F), primary somatosensory cortex (M = F), superior parietal cortex (M = F), prefrontal white matter (M = F), and superior parietal white matter (M = F) No age effects were found for anterior cingulate cortex, parahippocampal cortex, primary motor cortex, inferior parietal cortex, visual cortex, and precentral, postcentral, or inferior parietal white matter No interactions with laterality
Salat et al. 1997	76 healthy elderly volunteers 65–95 years old (mean 77.7 years) 31 M; 45 F No major medical or neurological illness, and no depression All right-handed, except 1 left-handed F	MR imaging (1.5 tesla) Area measurements (one of three raters with established reliabilities) of corpus callosum, pons, and cerebellum using trace methodology of T1-weighted midsagittal image Neuropsychological test battery comprised of Wechsler Memory Scale and Block Design subtest of WAIS	Age associated with decreased total, anterior, and middle callosum areas in F but not in M No relation of age to pons or cerebellum areas No relation between any brain measure and verbal memory or visual construction Nonverbal memory correlated with callosum area in F
Coffey et al. 1998	330 elderly volunteers living independently in the community 66–96 years old (74.98 ± 5.09) 129 M; 201 F No history of neurological or psychiatric illness All right-handed	MR imaging (1.5 tesla, n = 248; 0.35 tesla, n = 82) Blinded volume measurements (one of two raters with established reliabilities) using computer-assisted trace methodology of T1-weighted axial images (5 mm thick, no interscan gap)	Adjusting for IV, age associated with decreased cerebral hemisphere volume (2.79 mL/year) (M = F), frontal region area (0.13 mL/year) (M = F), temporal-parietal region area (0.13 mL/year) (M = F), and parietal-occipital region (M > F, 0.31 vs. 0.09 mL/year, respectively) All effects similar in both hemispheres
Davatzikos and Resnik 1998	114 healthy volunteers 56–85 years old 68 M (70.9 ± 7.6 years), 46 F (69.4 ± 8.0 years old) All right-handed No additional details provided	MR imaging (1.5 tesla) Quantitative morphometry of the corpus callosum using computer-assisted trace methodology of T1-weighted midsagittal image (1.5 mm thick); morphometry was quantitated using a template and deformation function No additional details provided	Age associated with decreased total and regional callosal size (M = F), with exception of anterior and posterior extremes

(continued)

APPENDIX 9–2. Imaging studies of human aging and brain parenchymal atrophy *(continued)*

Study	Subjects	Imaging and measurement technique	Findings
Gunning-Dixon et al. 1998	Same as Raz et al. 1997	MR imaging (1.5 tesla) Blinded volume measurements (digital planimetry) from scans of T1-weighted reformatted coronal images (1.3 mm thick, contiguous)	Age associated with decreased caudate volume (L > R in M, R > L in F), decreased putamen volume (R > L, M = F), and decreased globus pallidus volume (M only, R = L)
Gur et al. 1998	17 healthy volunteers (overlap with subjects in Gur et al. 1991 and Cowell et al. 1994) 31.9 ± 8.9 years old 13 M; 4 F	MR imaging (1.5 tesla) Volume measurements using a combination of computer-assisted trace methodology and pixel segmentation of three-dimensional images reconstructed from T2-weighted axial images (5 mm thick, contiguous) Good rater reliabilities, but "blindness" not specified	No significant change over follow-up period in whole brain, CSF, or frontal lobe volumes Significant volume loss was observed for L (7.5%) and R (7.2%) temporal lobes
Guttmann et al. 1998	72 healthy volunteers 18–81 years old 22 M; 50 F No history of psychiatric illness, epilepsy, or severe head trauma Handedness not specified	MR imaging (1.5 tesla) Blinded volume measurements using computer-assisted segmentation and trace methodology of contiguous axial images (3 mm thick) Good interrater reliabilities Scanning repeated an average of 32 months later	Age associated with decreased ratio of total white matter volume to IV and decreased total gray matter volume to IV Interactions with gender or laterality not reported
Jack et al. 1998	24 elderly volunteers 70–89 years old (81.04 ± 3.78 years) 8 M; 16 F No active neurological or psychiatric illness Handedness not specified	MR imaging (1.5 tesla) Blinded volume measurements using computer-assisted trace methodology of T1-weighted three-dimensional volumetric images (1.6 mm thick, contiguous, n = 124) by single rater with established reliabilities	Over a 12-month interval, mean hippocampal volume decreased by 1.55%, and mean temporal horn volume increased by 6.15% (M = F, L = R)
Kohler et al. 1998	26 healthy elderly community volunteers 70.8 ± 6.3 years old 12 M; 14 F No history of neurological or psychiatric impairment, and no dementia or age-associated memory impairment on neuropsychological testing	MR imaging (1.5 tesla) Blinded volume measurements (one of two raters, reliabilities ?) using computer-assisted trace or stereological methods, from T1-weighted coronal images (1.3 mm thick, contiguous) Mattis Dementia Rating Scale and neuropsychological testing of verbal recall (California Verbal Learning Test) and visual recall (Visual Reproduction Test of WMS-R)	Controlling for age, gender, education, and head size, a trend was found for a negative association between hippocampal volume and delayed verbal recall (CVLT) No relations observed between para-hippocampal volume and any memory measure

Study	Subjects	Methods	Findings
Laakso et al. 1998	42 cognitively normal healthy elderly community volunteers 64–79 (72 ± 4) years old 19 M; 23 F	MR imaging (1.5 tesla) Volume measures using computer-assisted trace methods from T1-weighted coronal images (2 mm thick, contiguous) by a single blinded rater with established reliabilities	No relation between age and hippocampal size
Mueller et al. 1998	46 healthy elderly volunteers 65–74 years old (6 M, 5 F), 75–84 years old (8 M, 7 F), and 85–95 years old (9 M, 11 F) All functionally independent, MMSE ≥ 24, and free of major medical and neurological illness, as well as depression Handedness not specified	MR imaging (1.5 tesla) Volume measurements (nonblind?) using computer-assisted pixel segmentation of contiguous coronal images (4 mm thick) Excellent interrater reliabilities Scanning repeated annually or biannually over 3- to 9-year follow-up	Adjusting for IV, age associated with decreased volumes of total brain, cerebral hemispheres, frontal lobes, temporal lobes, basilar–subcortical region, hippocampus, and hippocampal gyrus Interactions with gender not reported Over the follow-up period, significant volume decreases were seen in hippocampus (0.02 mL/year), parahippocampal gyrus (in youngest age group only, 0.05 mL/year), parieto-occipital region (in middle and oldest age groups, 3 mL/year), and basilar region (in middle group only, 0.5 mL/year); no volume decreases were seen in cerebral hemispheres, frontal lobes, or temporal lobes.
Oguro et al. 1998	152 healthy adults 81 M, 71 F Age range 40s–70s No evidence of neurological disease	MR imaging (0.2 tesla) Linear and area measurements using computer-assisted trace methodology from T1-weighted midsagittal image (7 mm thick) and T2-weighted axial images (no details), by raters ($n = ?$) with established reliabilities	Age associated with decreased linear measures of midbrain tegmentum (M only), midbrain pretectum (M and F), and base of pons (M only), but not with pontine tegmentum or fourth ventricle Age associated with decreased area of cerebellar vermis (M only), but not of pons Age associated with decreased ratio of cerebrum to IA (M and F) at level of third ventricle and at level of body of lateral ventricles Interactions with laterality not reported
Pfefferbaum et al. 1998	28 healthy M volunteers (overlap with Pfefferbaum et al. 1994) 21–68 years old (51 ± 13.8 years) No major medical, neurological, or psychiatric illness Left-handers included (n not specified)	MR imaging (1.5 tesla) Blinded volume measurements derived from semiautomated pixel segmentation of intermediate and T2-weighted axial images ($n = 17–20$, 5 mm thick, 2.5-mm interscan gap) Scanning repeated at 5-year follow-up	Over the follow-up interval, significant decrease in total gray matter volume and in regional gray matter volume (prefrontal gray 2 mL, or 7%; posterior parieto-occipital gray 1 mL, or 3.5%); no change in frontal, anterior superior temporal, posterior superior temporal, or anterior parietal region gray matter volume Interactions with laterality not reported

(continued)

APPENDIX 9–2. Imaging studies of human aging and brain parenchymal atrophy *(continued)*

Study	Subjects	Imaging and measurement technique	Findings
Raz et al. 1998a	146 healthy volunteers (overlap with N. Raz et al. 1997) 18–77 years old 64 M (48 ± 18 years); 82 F (46 ± 17 years) No evidence of major medical, neurological, or psychiatric illness All right-handed	MR imaging (1.5 tesla) Blinded volume measurements (digital planimetry) from scans of T1-weighted reformatted coronal and sagittal images (0.8 mm thick, 1.5 mm thick) Good rater reliabilities	Age associated with volume loss in cerebellar hemispheres (2%/decade) vermis, vermian lobules VI and VII (4%/decade), and posterior vermis (lobules VIII–X; 2%/decade), but not in anterior vermis (lobules I–V) or pons
Raz et al. 1998b	95 healthy volunteers (selected from N. Raz et al. 1997) 18–77 (44.02 ± 16.35) years old 41 M (42.98 ± 17.24 years); 54 F (44.82 ± 15.76 years) No major medical, neurological, or psychiatric illness All right-handed	MR imaging (1.5 tesla) Blinded volume measurements (digital planimetry) from scans of T1-weighted reformatted coronal images (1.3 mm thick, contiguous) Good rater reliabilities among eight raters Neuropsychological test measures of executive functions and of verbal and nonverbal working memory, explicit memory, and priming	Age associated with decreased test scores and with decreased volumes of dorsolateral prefrontal cortex, orbitofrontal cortex, pericalcarine cortex, fusiform gyrus, and hippocampal formation Using path analysis, atrophy of prefrontal cortex was related to an index of perseveration (from Wisconsin Carol Sort Test) and atrophy of visual processing areas to nonverbal working memory; volume of limbic structures was unrelated to any cognitive measure
Hokama et al 1995	15 healthy M community volunteers 20–55 years old No lifetime history of major medical, neurologic or psychiatric illness All right-handed	MR imaging (1.5 tesla) Volume measurements of basal ganglia using semiautomated computer-assisted trace methodology from T1-weighted coronal and axial sections (1.5 mm thick, contiguous) by raters with established reliabilities	Age associated with decreased volumes of caudate and putamen, but not of globus pallidus No correlation between basal ganglia volumes and IQ as estimated by WAIS-R Information subscale
Carmelli et al. 1999	148 elderly male monozygotic twins (74 twin pairs) 72.7 ± 2.1 years old Medical history remarkable for hypertension (37%), coronary artery disease (25%), diabetes (13%), and cerebrovascular disease (5%)	MR imaging (1.5 tesla) Volumetric measures using computer-assisted pixel segmentation of T2-weighted axial images (5mm, contiguous) by single blinded rater with established reliability Principal component analysis used to derive a "memory" factor (from California Verbal Learning Test) and a "speed" factor (from Digit Symbol subtest of WAIS-R, Stroop Color Test, and Trail Making Test)	Within-pair differences in brain volume were associated with within-pair differences in lower memory scores, but not with "speed" scores Relations between CSF and cognitive tests not reported

Study	Sample	Imaging method	Findings
Coffey et al. 1999	330 elderly volunteers living independently in the community (overlap with Coffey et al. 1998) 66–96 (74.98 ± 5.09) years old 129 M; 201 F No history of neurologic or psychiatric illness All right-handed	MR imaging (1.5 tesla, n = 248; 0.35 tesla, n = 82) Blinded volume measurements (one of two raters with established reliabilities) using computer-assisted trace methodology of T1-weighted axial images (5 mm thick, contiguous)	Education was associated with age-specific increase in sulcal CSF volume, but not with decreases in total or regional brain volumes or with increased volumes of lateral or third ventricles
Fox et al. 1999	15 healthy older adult volunteers 55.3 ± 14.0 years old Sex and handedness not specified MMSE = 29.5 ± 0.7	MR imaging (1.5 tesla) Volumetric measures using computer-assisted pixel segmentation of coronal images (1.5 mm thick, contiguous) by raters (n not specified) with established reliabilities MR imaging repeated an average (± SD) of 1.7 ± 1.2 years later (minimum interval = 5 months)	Over the follow up interval, brain volume decreased by mean (± SD) of 0.4% (± 0.7%) per year
Frisoni et al. 1999	30 healthy elderly volunteers 53–86 (68 ± 5) years old 10 M; 20 F No evidence of neurologic disease or cognitive deficits	MR imaging (1.5 tesla) Volumetric measures using computer assisted trace methodology of T1-weighted coronal images (2 mm thick, contiguous) by rater with established reliability	No relation between age and volumes of hippocampus or entorhinal cortex
Magnotta et al. 1999	148 healthy volunteers 18–82 (28 ± 9.8) years old No evidence of active psychiatric, neurologic, or general medical disorders	MR imaging (1.5 tesla) Volumetric measures using computer assisted pixel segmentation of T1-, intermediate, and T2-weighted coronal images (1.5 mm thick), by raters with established reliabilities	Age associated with changes in shape of gyri (more sharply and steeply curved) and sulci (more flattened and less curved) (M = F), as well as with decreased cortical thickness (M > F)
Mu et al. 1999	619 healthy adult volunteers 40–90 years old 313 M; 306 F No evidence of cardiovascular, neurologic, or neuropsychologic disease	MR imaging (1.5 tesla) Volumetric measures using computer assisted trace methodology of T1-weighted coronal images (2 mm thick, contiguous) by 5 blinded raters (average used)	Age correlated with decreased ratios of hippocampal formation volume/IV and amygdala volume/IV, and with increased ratio of temporal horn volume/IV
Salat et al. 1999	28 healthy elderly community volunteers (overlap with Kaye et al. 1997) Young group: 65–76 years old; 7M, 7F Old group: 84–95 years old; 7M, 7F No significant medical disease or stroke, and MMSE ≥ 25	MR imaging (1.5 tesla) Volumetric measures using computer assisted trace methodology of T1- and T2-weighted coronal sections (4 mm thick, contiguous) from prefrontal region (8 slices per subject) by single rater with established reliabilities	Old group had smaller volumes of total prefrontal region and of prefrontal white matter, but no group differences in volume of prefrontal gray matter

Note. AAMI = age-associated memory impairment; BVRT = Benton Visual Retention Test; CAMCOG = Cambridge Cognitive Examination; CSF = cerebrospinal fluid; CT = computed tomography; CVLT = California Verbal Learning Test; F = female(s); IV = intracranial volume; L – left; M – male(s); MMSE – Mini-Mental State Exam; MR – magnetic resonance; R – right; WAIS = Weschler Adult Intelligence Scale; WMS-R = Weschler Memory Scale–Revised.

APPENDIX 9–3. Neuropsychological correlates of subcortical encephalomalacia

Study	Subjects	Imaging and measurement technique	Findings
Steingart et al. 1987	105 elderly volunteers 59–91 years old 56 M; 49 F No evidence of dementia or stroke	CT Determination of presence of "leukoaraiosis" by single blinded rater	Subjects with leukoaraiosis ($n = 9$) had lower scores on the Extended Scale for Dementia than did subjects without the finding ($n = 96$), even after controlling for age, gender, education, and presence of infarct
Skoog et al. 1996	134 volunteers without dementia Mean age = 85 years 45 M; 89 F	CT Severity rating (0–3) of white matter attenuation by two blinded radiologists with good agreement (kappa = 0.75%) Neuropsychological examination by blinded psychologist comprised of MMSE, Synonym Test, Figure Classification Test, Block Design Test, Identical forms, Thurstone Picture Memory Test, Digit Span, Clock Test, Coin Test, MIR Memory Test, Prose Recall Test, and Ten-Word Memory Test	Subjects with white matter lesions ($n = 46$) scored lower on MMSE and on tests of verbal ability (Synonyms), spatial ability (Block Design, Clock Test), perceptual speed (Identical Forms), secondary memory (Thurstone Picture Memory), and basic arithmetic (Coin Test)
Brant-Zawadzki et al. 1985	14 elderly volunteers 59–81 years old 6 M; 8 F No medical conditions "associated with cognitive loss"	MR imaging (0.35 tesla) Standardized severity ratings (5-point scale) of white matter hyperintensity made by two raters (interrater agreement not given) from intermediate and T2-weighted scans	No statistical analysis of neuropsychological test data (10 tests) conducted One of the 10 subjects with a hyperintensity rating of 1 or less scored in the "demented range" on the WMS (Russell revision) and WAIS-R Block Design One of the 4 subjects with a hyperintensity rating of 2 or greater had impaired performance on WAIS-R Picture Arrangement
Hendrie et al. 1989	27 elderly volunteers 63–86 years old 10 M; 17 F No evidence of medical or neurological illness	MR imaging (1.5 tesla) Standardized rating by two blinded raters of severity (4-point scale) of white matter hyperintensity from T2-weighted films Cognitive test battery comprised of MMSE, CAMCOG, and WAIS Digit Symbol	No differences (statistical analysis not described) between the 4 severity categories of white matter hyperintensity with regard to scores on the three cognitive measures

Study	Subjects	Methods	Results
Hunt et al. 1989	46 elderly volunteers Mean ± SD age = 78.2 ± 4.6 years old 17 M; 29 F No evidence of major medical illness	MR imaging (1.5 tesla) Single blinded rater determined number (4-point scale) and size (3-point scale) of white matter hyperintensity changes from intermediate and T2-weighted scans Severity score derived from multiplying number by size, summed across five brain regions Neuropsychological test battery from which were derived composite scores for 5 cognitive "domains"—verbal ability (WAIS-R Information, Boston Naming-Revised, Word List Generation Task, and Token Test), spatial ability (WAIS-R Block Design, Rey-Osterreith Complex Figure, and Hooper Visual Organization Test), memory (Wechsler Memory Scale [logical and visual] and Rey-Osterrieth Complex Figure), attention and concentration (MMSE, Blessed Dementia Scale, Jacobs Dementia Scale, and Digit Span), and executive functioning (Luria and Christensen tasks)	When controlling for age, no relation between total severity of white matter hyperintensity and composite neuropsychological performance in any of the five "domains" No apparent difference in neuropsychological performance between subjects with more or less than the median number of white matter lesions (statistical analysis not reported)
Rao et al. 1989	50 healthy middle-aged volunteers 25–60 years old 11 M; 39 F No evidence of major medical, neurological, or psychiatric illness	MR imaging (1.5 tesla) Presence of leukoaraiosis on intermediate and T2-weighted scans (no description of rating methodology provided) Neuropsychological test battery comprised of measures of verbal intelligence (from 6 subtests of the WAIS-R), recent memory (Buschke Verbal Selective Reminding Test, 7/24 Spatial Recall Test, Story Recall Test), remote memory (President's Test), rate of forgetting (Brown-Peterson Interference Test), abstract/conceptual reasoning (Wisconsin Card Sorting Test, Booklet Category Test, Standard Raven Progressive Matrices, Stroop Color/Word Interference Test, and Hooper Visual Organization Test), attention/concentration (WAIS-R Digit Span, Sternberg High Speed Scanning Test, and the Paced Auditory Serial Addition Test), language (Boston Naming Test, Controlled Oral Word Association Test, and Category Word Generation Test), visuospatial skills (Benton Line Orientation, Benton Facial Recognition, and Benton Visual Form Discrimination), and upper extremity motor function (Wisconsin Motor Battery)	Relative to subjects without leukoaraiosis ($n = 40$), subjects with the finding ($n = 10$) performed significantly worse on 3 of the 45 neuropsychological tests (t-tests): Benton Facial Recognition Test, Brown-Peterson Interference Test (18-second delay), and the President's Test
Austrom et al. 1990	27 elderly volunteers 63–86 years old 10 M; 17 F No significant medical or neurological illness	MR imaging (1.5 tesla) Consensus ratings of white matter hyperintensity (4-point scale) from T2-weighted axial slices by two raters with established reliabilities	Subjects without white matter hyperintensity at baseline ($n = 11$) showed a significant improvement on the WAIS Digit Symbol test, whereas subjects with white matter hyperintensity tended to have lower scores at follow-up Neither group showed significant changes in MMSE or CAMCOG scores

(continued)

APPENDIX 9–3. Neuropsychological correlates of subcortical encephalomalacia (*continued*)

Study	Subjects	Imaging and measurement technique	Findings
Harrell et al. 1991	25 healthy elderly volunteers Mean ± SD age = 65.6 ± 6.9 years old Gender not reported No history of significant medical, neurological, or psychiatric illness	MR imaging (0.5 or 1.5 tesla) Standardized severity ratings (6-point scale) of white matter hyperintensity by single blinded rater from T1- and T2-weighted scans	No correlation between severity of either periventricular or deep white matter hyperintensity and scores on MMSE or Mattis Dementia Rating Scale
Mirsen et al. 1991	39 elderly volunteers 73.2 ±5.8 years old 20 M; 19 F 3 subjects with infarcts; an indeterminate number with no evaluation (medical, neurological, or psychiatric), apart from cognitive testing, which was normal	MR imaging (1.5 tesla) Blinded determination by two raters of presence of periventricular hyperintensity and severity (5-point scale) of leukoaraiosis on T1- and T2-weighted films (interrater agreement ranged from 56% to 88%)	No correlations between presence of either periventricular hyperintensity or leukoaraiosis and performance on the Extended Scale for Dementia
R. Schmidt et al. 1991	32 healthy volunteers 22–49 years old 25 M; 7 F Most receiving medication for hypertension, but otherwise no evidence of major medical, neurological, or psychiatric illness	MR imaging (1.5 tesla) Blinded determination of white matter lesions from intermediate and T2-weighted films (no description of rating methodology provided) Neuropsychological test battery comprised of a computerized test of vigilance and reaction time, a test of visual attention (d2 test), and a test of learning and memory (Lern und Gedächtnistest)	No differences between subjects with (*n* = 12) and without (*n* = 20) white matter lesions on any of the neuropsychological tests
Almkvist et al. 1992	23 healthy elderly volunteers All > 75 years 9 M; 14 F No major medical, neurological, or psychiatric illness	MR imaging (0.02 tesla) Computer-assisted volumetric measurements of subcortical hyperintensity by single blinded rater (no intrarater reliabilities reported) Neuropsychological test battery comprised of MMSE, 6 subtests from WAIS-R (Information, Digit Span, Similarities, Block Design, Object Assembly, and Digit Symbol), Wechsler Memory Scale (Associative Learning and Visual Reproduction), Corsi Block Tapping Test, Digit Span Test, Simple Reaction Time Test, Finger Tapping Test, Boston Naming Test, FAS Word Fluency Test, Maze Test (from WISC), Map Orientation Test, Line Bisection Test, and the Tactile Identification of Objects Test	No relationship between total or regional volumes of subcortical hyperintensity and performance on any of the 24 neuro-psychological tests

Study	Subjects	Methods	Results
Boone et al. 1992	100 healthy volunteers 45–83 years old 36 M; 64 F No major medical, neurological, or psychiatric illness	MR imaging (1.5 tesla) Computer-assisted area measurements of subcortical hyperintensity from T2-weighted axial sections by single rater (additional rater information not reported) Neuropsychological test battery comprised of measures of frontal lobe functioning (Wisconsin Cart Sorting Test, Stroop 3, Auditory Consonant Trigrams), general intelligence (WAIS-R), memory (Wechsler Memory Scale-R logical and visual reproduction subtests), attention and information processing speed (WAIS-R Digit Span and Digit Symbol subtests, Stroop 1 and 2), language (Verbal Fluency), and visuospatial skills (Rey-Osterrieth Complex Figure)	Subjects ($n = 6$) with lesion areas greater than 10 cm^2 performed less well on measures of frontal lobe ability (Auditory Consonant Trigrams, Wisconsin Card Sorting Test [Heaton 1985], and Stroop Test), attention (Digit Span), and speed of information processing (Digit Symbol, Stroop Test)
Matsubayashi et al. 1992	73 healthy elderly volunteers 59–83 years old 24 M; 49 F No history of major medical, neurological, or psychiatric illness	MR imaging (0.5 tesla) Standardized severity ratings (4-point scale) of periventricular hyperintensity by single blinded rater (intrarater agreement not reported) Neuropsychological test battery comprised of MMSE, Hasegawa Dementia Scale (Hasegawa 1974), a visuospatial cognitive performance test, and a test of manual dexterity	Subjects with periventricular hyperintensity ratings of 3 or greater ($n = 19$) performed worse on all neuropsychological test measures even after controlling for age effects
Tupler et al. 1992	66 healthy volunteers (overlap with subjects in Coffey et al. 1992) 45–89 years old 24 M; 42 F No evidence of lifetime neurological or psychiatric illness	MR imaging (1.5 tesla) Consensus ratings (4-point scale) of severity of white matter hyperintensity from axial scans by two blinded raters with established reliabilities Two neuropsychological tests were selected a priori: the Benton Facial Recognition Test and the Digit Symbol	After adjustments for age and education, neither test was associated with severity of subcortical hyperintensity
Levine et al. 1993	127 healthy nonelderly volunteers 50 M (35.2 ± 11.8 years old); 77 F (43.3 ± 8.4 years old) No history of significant medical, neurological, or psychiatric illness	MR imaging (0.5 tesla) Presence of subcortical hyperintensity determined by three "experienced neuroradiologists" from intermediate and T2-weighted axial scans (no additional data provided) Neuropsychological test battery comprised of measures of general intellectual functioning (WAIS-R), frontal lobe functioning (Wisconsin Card Sorting Test), attention (Digit Span Task, binaural dichotic listening task), and visuospatial functioning (Benton Line Orientation, Benton Facial Recognition)	Among subjects with subcortical hyperintensity (5 M, 7 F), M exhibited impaired attention on a dichotic listening task, relative to subjects without subcortical hyperintensity

(continued)

APPENDIX 9–3. Neuropsychological correlates of subcortical encephalomalacia *(continued)*

Study	Subjects	Imaging and measurement technique	Findings
R. Schmidt et al. 1993	150 healthy elderly volunteers 44–82 years old (mean = 59.9) 82 M; 68 F No severe medical, neurological, or psychiatric illness	MR imaging (1.5 tesla) Area of SH as assessed by three blinded raters using trace methodology on proton-density axial images (5 mm thick) Neuropsychological test battery assessing verbal intelligence (Mehrfachwahl-wortschatetest), mood (Janke and Debus), learning capacity and intermediate memory (Lern und Gedächtnistest), conceptual reasoning (Wisconsin Card Sorting Test), attention and speed (multiple tests), and visuopractical skills (Purdue Pegboard Test)	Presence of SH associated with Purdue Pegboard Test (complex reaction time, number of errors on the complex reaction time task, the assembly procedure) and form B of the Trail Making Test No relation between the total SH area and any test score
Ylikoski et al. 1993	120 volunteers living in the community 55–85 years old 54 M; 66 F No evidence of neurological illness	MR imaging (0.02 tesla) Blinded severity ratings (4-point scale) of SH from T2-weighted axial and coronal images (10 mm thick, no gaps) by single blinded rater (no reliabilities given) Neuropsychological test battery assessing memory (Fuld Object-Memory Evaluation, WMS-R), verbal intelligence (Information and Similarities subtests of WAIS), construction (Block Design of WAIS), language (Token Test, Boston Naming Test), and speed and attention (Trail Making Test A, Stroop Test)	Controlling for the effects of age, both presence and severity of SH correlated with scores on Trail Making A and Stroop Test (correlations were similar for both hemispheres)
DeCarli et al. 1995	51 healthy community volunteers 19–91 years old 26 M; 25 F No evidence of chronic medical illness, psychiatric illness, or head trauma	MR imaging (0.5 tesla) Computer-assisted volumetric measurements of SH by blinded raters (*n* = ?) with established reliabilities Neuropsychological test battery comprised of WAIS, Wechsler Memory Scale, and frontal lobe tests (Porteus Maze Test, FAS Word List Generation, Trail Making Test A and B, and WAIS Digit Symbol Test)	Controlling for the effects of age and education, SH volume was significantly associated with WAIS IQ, immediate and delayed visual memory, and Trails A and B times
O'Brien et al. 1997	39 healthy community volunteers 55–96 years old No evidence of major medical or neurological illness, or of depression or drug abuse	MR imaging (0.3 tesla) Ratings of SH (0–3) by two raters with established reliabilities, blind to cognitive scores	Age associated with presence of SH Controlling for the effects of age and education, there was no relation between SH and scores on CAMCOG

Study	Sample	Methods	Findings
Carmelli et al. 1999	148 elderly male monozygotic twins (74 twin pairs) 72.7 ± 2.1 years old Medical history remarkable for hypertension (37%), coronary artery disease (25%), diabetes (13%), and cerebrovascular disease (5%)	MR imaging (1.5 tesla) Volumetric measures using computer-assisted pixel segmentation of T2-weigthted axial images (5 mm, contiguous) by single blinded rater with established reliability Principal component analysis used to derive a "memory" factor (from California Verbal Learning Test) and a "speed" factor (from Digit Symbol subtest of WAIS-R, Stroop Color Test, and Trail Making Test)	Within-pair differences in volume of subcortical hyperintensity was associated with within pair differences in lower memory and speed scores
Schmidt et al. 1999	273 elderly community volunteers 60 ± 6.1 years old 131 M, 142 F No evidence of neuropsychiatric disease	MR imaging (1.5 tesla) Consensus global ratings of SH (0–3 scale) by three blinded raters with established reliabilities Neuropsychological test battery comprised of Baumler's Lern-und Gedächtnistest (learning and memory), Wisconsin Card Sort Test, Trail Making Test B, Digit Span (WAIS-R), Alters-Konzentrations-Test, and Purdue Pegboard Test	Over the 3-year follow-up interval, SH progressed in 49 subjects (17.9%), with minor progression in 27 (9.9%) and marked progression in 22 (8.1%) Neuropsychological test performance improved on the Wisconsin Card Sort Test but declined on the Trail Making Test No relation between SH lesion progression and changes on neuropsychological test performance

Note.　Abbreviations: CAMCOG = Cambridge Cognitive Examination; CT = computed tomography; F = female(s); M = male(s); MMSE = Mini-Mental State Exam; MR = magnetic resonance; SH = subcortical hyperintensity; WAIS-R = Wechsler Adult Intelligence Scale–Revised; WMH = white matter hyperintensities; WMS-R = Wechsler Memory Scale–Revised.

APPENDIX 9–4. Imaging studies of human aging and other brain changes

Study	Subjects	Imaging and measurement technique	Findings
T1 and T2 relaxometry			
N. Raz et al. 1990	26 healthy volunteers 18–76 years old (45.8 ± 21.8 years) 15 M; 11 F No history of neurological or psychiatric illness All right-handed	MR imaging (0.3 tesla) T1 relaxometry calculated from multiple images derived from a single coronal slice (6.6 mm thick, 2-mm gap) through anterotemporal lobe Number of raters and their reliabilities not reported	Age correlated positively with T1 in white matter and hippocampus and negatively with ratio of T1 gray matter to T1 white matter Scores on a test of "fluid" intelligence (the Cattell Culture-Fair Test) were associated with shorter white matter T1 (but not gray matter T1) and with higher gray matter to white matter T1 ratio Scores on a test of "crystallized" intelligence (Extended Vocabulary) were associated with shorter gray matter T1
Agartz et al. 1991	79 healthy volunteers 19–85 years old 36 M; 43 F No evidence of major medical illness	MR imaging (0.02 tesla) Multiple T1- and T2–weighted images obtained on single axial slice at level of basal ganglia T1 and T2 relaxation times calculated for regions of interest within right and left frontal white matter, caudate, thalamus, and occipital white matter	T1 relaxation times showed a "cradle-shaped" relation to age, with minimal values at ages 40–45 years; no interactions with gender or laterality No relation between age and T2 relaxation times
Breger et al. 1991	151 healthy volunteers 10–90 years old No evidence of major medical or neurological illness	MR imaging (1.5 tesla) Multiple T1- and T2–weighted images obtained on single slice (level not specified) T1 and T2 relaxation times calculated for regions of interest within right and left anterior white matter, posterior white matter, anterior gray matter, and basal ganglia	Age correlated with T1 relaxation times in white matter and caudate Age correlated with T2 relaxation times in white matter and thalamus No interactions with gender
Laakso et al. 1996	34 volunteers 18 old (74 ± 2 years old); 8 M, 10 F 16 young (26 ± 7 years old); 9 M, 7 F No evidence of neurological illness	MR imaging (1.5 tesla) T2 relaxometry calculated from multiple images derived from four oblique coronal slices (8 mm thick, 2-mm gap) through anterotemporal lobe Number of raters and their reliabilities not specified	Age correlated with T2 relaxation times in temporal and parietal white matter, but not in hippocampus

Study	Method	Subjects	Findings
Salonen et al. 1997	MR imaging (1.0 tesla) T2 relaxometry calculated from axial slices (5 mm thick, 1-mm gap) through the frontal horns Number of raters and rater reliabilities not specified	61 healthy volunteers 30–86 years old 30 M; 31 F No neurological symptoms or disease; psychiatric history not specified Handedness not specified	Age correlated with T2 relaxation times in white matter, but not in caudate, putamen, or thalamus T2 relaxation times were greater in F than in M after age 60
Spectroscopy			
Christiansen et al. 1993	MR imaging (1.5 tesla) MR spectroscopy (stimulated echoes, or STEAM) of volumes of interest (2 mL) from right basal ganglia and frontal, temporal, and occipital hemispheres	16 healthy volunteers 8 young (20–30 years), 8 old (60–80 years) No neurological, cardiovascular, or diabetic diseases, and no medications	Young (but not old) group had higher concentrations of NAA in occipital region than in the other three areas. No regional variations found in either group for concentrations of Cr, PCr, or Cho Young (but not old) group had higher NAA/Cho ratio in occipital region relative to other regions No group differences in T1 or T2 relaxation times for the three metabolites
Charles et al. 1994	MR imaging (1.5 tesla) MR spectroscopy (STEAM) of voxel (27 mL) at level of basal ganglia	34 healthy volunteers 21–75 years old (47 ± 17 years) 15 M, 19 F No evidence from examination of "significant medical or psychiatric condition"	Old (> 59 years old) group had lower Cho, Cr, and NAA in voxel containing cortical and subcortical gray matter. No group differences within white matter or noncortical gray matter voxels Interactions with gender not reported
Meyerhoff et al. 1994	MR imaging (2.0 tesla) MR spectroscopy of 9 voxels (2.5 mL each) from angulated axial image (17 mm thick) at supraventricular level (3 voxels in mesial cortex and 3 each in right and left centrum semiovale)	16 healthy volunteers 10 elderly (6 M, 4 F; 70 ± years), 6 young (4 M, 2 F; 32 ± years) No evidence of major medical, neurological, or psychiatric illness, and MMSE > 28	No difference between young and elderly groups in distribution or signal intensities of NAA, of Cho residues representing lipid metabolites, or of Cr-containing metabolites Interactions with gender or laterality not reported
Smith et al. 1995	MR (1.5 tesla) MR spectroscopy of voxel (50 mL) from anterosuperior frontal lobe	25 healthy volunteers 8 old (75 ± 7 years old); 5 M, 3 F 17 young (29 ± 9 years old); 9 M, 8 F No neurological illness and no psychoactive drugs for at least 2 weeks	Old group had higher ratio of PCr/Pi In young group, age correlated with a decrease in Pi mole percent and an increase in PCr/Pi ratio Interactions with gender not reported

(continued)

APPENDIX 9–4. Imaging studies of human aging and other brain changes (*continued*)

Study	Subjects	Imaging and measurement technique	Findings
Chang et al. 1996	36 healthy volunteers 19–78 years old (40.8 ± 2.9 years) No additional details provided	MR imaging (1.5 tesla) MR spectroscopy of voxels (2–4 mL) from mid-frontal gray matter or right frontal white matter	In gray matter, age associated with increased concentrations of total Cr, Cho-containing compounds, and *myo*-inositol, as well as increased percent age of CSF; no change in NAA compounds No age-related spectroscopic changes in white matter
Soher et al. 1996	16 healthy volunteers 5–74 years (39 ± 20) 11 M; 5 F All "free of any known neuropathological conditions"	MR imaging (1.5 tesla) MR spectroscopy of voxels from two oblique slices (15 mm thick, 2.5-mm gap) at levels of third ventricle and centrum semiovale	Age associated with increased concentrations of Cho in frontal white matter, thalamus, putamen, and genu of callosum, and of Cr in frontal white matter; no changes in forceps minor or major, centrum semiovale, posterior white matter, splenium of callosum, or frontoparietal gray matter
Fukuzako et al. 1997	36 healthy volunteers 24–78 years old (48.8 ± 14.6 years) 17 M; 19 F No history of psychiatric or neurological illness, no medications All right-handed	MR imaging (2.0 tesla) MR spectroscopy (STEAM) of voxels (3 mL) from left frontal lobe and left medial temporal lobe	No relation between age and ratios of NAA/Cho, NAA/Cr, and Cho/Cr (M = F)
Lim and Spielman 1997	10 healthy F volunteers 5 young (20–28 years), 5 old (65–75 years) All free of medical and psychiatric disorders	MR imaging (1.5 tesla) MR spectroscopy of two oblique axial slices (15 mm thick, 5-mm gap) at 30 mm and 50 mm above the AC-PC line	Ratio of NAA signal in gray matter to white matter was lower in the old group than in the young group
Brain iron			
Steffens et al. 1996	56 healthy volunteers 25–82 years old (57.4 ± 15.8 years) 27 M; 29 F No history of neurological or psychiatric illness 52 were right-handed, 3 were left-handed, 1 unknown	MR imaging (1.5 tesla) Global visual ratings of signal hypointensity in the putamen (5-point scale) made from T2-weighted axial films (slices 5 mm thick, 2.5-mm gap) by single rater (blind?)	Age associated with higher ratings of signal hypointensity in putamen consistent with increased iron deposition Interactions with gender not reported

Note.   *AC-PC line* = anterior commissure–posterior commissure line; Cho = choline; Cr = creatine; CSF = cerebrospinal fluid; F = female(s); M = male(s); MR = magnetic resonance; NAA = N-acetylaspartate; Pi = inorganic phosphate; PCr = phosphocreatine.

10

Functional Brain Imaging

Cerebral Blood Flow and Glucose Metabolism in Healthy Human Aging

Pietro Pietrini, M.D., Ph.D.

Stanley I. Rapoport, M.D.

Senectus enim insanabilis morbus est.

—Seneca, *Epistolae*

Getting older may be bad, but the alternative is worse.

—Anonymous older participant in
the Laboratory of Neurosciences
Research Program on Aging, 1997

▌ Introduction

That aging is invariably associated with changes in body and mind has been known since the ancient days. The Roman philosopher Seneca wrote, "aging in fact is an incurable disease." Although advances in health care during the last decades have improved the quality of life of older people and have softened Seneca's statement, it remains true that the human body and mind undergo inevitable modifications during aging, even in the absence of evident disease.

As far as the brain is concerned, many cognitive, neurochemical, histological, and morphological changes are known to accompany aging. Neuropsychological tests, for example, have shown that some cognitive features, referred to as "fluid intelligence," including perceptual

We wish to thank Giampiero Giovacchini, M.D., for his comments and assistance during the preparation of this manuscript.

speed, memory span, and associative memory, usually decline with age, whereas others, referred to as "crystallized intelligence," including verbal comprehension, general information, and arithmetic skills, remain intact (Horn 1975). This suggests that a large part of cognitive processing, related to the ability to cope with the environment, is preserved in older people (Creasey and Rapoport 1985). Long before the development of the cognitive sciences, the French essayist Montaigne (1580/1952), provided a clear description of the phenomenon: "Since I was 20 years of age, I am certain that my mind and body have deteriorated more than they have developed. It is likely that knowledge and experience increase with aging, but activity, alertness, strength and other important qualities nevertheless decline."

Different experimental approaches have been used to examine the functional neurobiological correlates of these alterations. In the past two decades, the introduction of sophisticated imaging techniques such as positron-emission tomography (PET) has made it possible to visualize cerebral metabolism and blood flow in vivo and to investigate metabolic and flow correlates of brain function and structure in relation to human aging. In this chapter, we describe these and earlier related techniques and examine how functional neuroimaging has helped to elucidate aging of the human brain.

Historical Background: Kety-Schmidt and Xenon-133 Techniques

Noninvasive measurements of brain function have been sought since the beginning of modern medicine. Normally, the brain produces the energy necessary for its functioning through oxidation of glucose. Although comprising only 2% of body weight in the adult, the human brain consumes about 20% of glucose used by the body as a whole (Sokoloff 1959). Neurons require energy in the form of adenosine triphosphate (ATP) to maintain their membrane potentials through activation of the Na^+/K^+ membrane pumps to support their electrical activity for signal transduction (Purdon and Rapoport 1998) and for synthetic processes. Accordingly, the regional cerebral metabolic rate for glucose (rCMRglc) will represent largely the functional and baseline metabolic activity of neurons in a given region (Rogers and Friedhoff 1998). Furthermore, because regional cerebral blood flow (rCBF) normally is coupled with rCMRglc (Roy and Sherrington 1890), the earliest clinical investigations by Kety and Schmidt (1948) were designed to determine in vivo average cerebral blood flow (CBF) in order to examine global brain functional activity. The technique chosen was based on the Fick principle, which relates arterial delivery of a chemically inert substance, its brain uptake, and its removal by the venous system. This method did not provide regional information, and it was invasive because it required a carotid artery injection and internal jugular sampling of nitrous oxide, a freely diffusible and nonmetabolizable substance. Initial studies with the Kety-Schmidt technique confirmed that global CBF and the cerebral metabolic rate for oxygen ($CMRO_2$) were correlated. Both rapidly decreased from childhood to adolescence, followed by a more gradual but progressive decline throughout the adult life span (Kety 1956).

Subsequent modifications of the original method led to the clearance technique that used the γ-emitting isotope xenon-133 (^{133}Xe) (Obrist et al. 1967, 1975; Risberg 1980). With this method, it was possible to quantify rCBF in regions of the cerebral cortex after inhalation or intracarotid artery injection of ^{133}Xe and, when using extracranial scintillation crystals, to record and localize radioactivity. Although the ^{133}Xe methods were an improvement over the Kety-Schmidt technique, their limited spatial resolution and inability to examine subcortical structures restricted investigations to large areas of the lateral surface of the cerebral cortex. Studies performed with ^{133}Xe consistently indicated an age-related decline in cortical blood flow.

In addition to technical limitations, methodological restrictions affected conclusions obtained with the Kety-Schmidt and ^{133}Xe clearance techniques. Most studies did not select optimally healthy subjects, blurring distinctions between effects of healthy aging and of age-related brain disease on CBF. Thus, subjects were recruited from hospitalized patients having "minor elective surgery" (Scheinberg et al. 1953) or "minor illness" (Schieve and Wilson 1953), or even from patients with a history of convulsive disorder (Kennedy, in Kety 1956). Patients with a history of psychosis, mental deterioration, or other degenerative processes often were included, and study conditions frequently were uncontrolled. With the exception of the study by Melamed et al. (1980), ^{133}Xe measurements were not performed with subjects in the "resting state," with eyes covered and ears plugged with cotton to minimize sensory stimulation. As vision and hearing acuities on average decline with age (Lehnert and Wuensche 1966), observed age-related flow reductions in subjects not studied in the "resting state" may be in part a result of these extrinsic changes, rather than a result of reduced intrinsic brain functional activity (see below) (Rapoport 1983).

Positron-Emission Tomography

During the last two decades, PET has facilitated the noninvasive investigation of brain functional activity in awake human subjects, not only in the cerebral cortex but also in subcortical structures, with progressively better spatial and temporal resolutions. A number of positron-emitting compounds have been employed to study various aspects of brain integrity and function, including neurotransmitter metabolism. It is now possible to determine rCBF, rCMRglc, and the regional cerebral metabolic rate for oxygen (rCMRO$_2$) in regions of the human brain smaller than 3 mm in diameter (Jagust et al. 1993). Radiolabeled transmitters (i.e., [^{18}F]fluoro-L-dopa) and transmitter receptors (i.e., serotonin or dopamine receptors) can also be studied with PET. More recently, measuring in vivo signal transduction with PET using [^{11}C]arachidonic acid has become feasible (Chang et al. 1997; Rapoport et al. 1997). PET scans can be repeated, thus allowing brain functional patterns to be evaluated in the same subject under different test conditions (resting state versus sensory stimulation), before and after drug administration, or in longitudinal studies of aging.

Basic Principles of Positron-Emission Tomography Technology

PET employs unstable nuclides that have an excess of protons in their nucleus and thus emit *positrons*, antimatter electrons with the same mass as an electron but with a positive charge. Once emitted, a positron has the kinetic energy to travel a few millimeters within tissue, until it meets an unbound electron. Because the two particles have opposite charge, they annihilate each other and, following the law of conservation of energy, emit two γ ray photons of 511 keV energy at 180° to each other (Horwitz 1990) (Figure 10–1). The γ photons are detected by rings of radiation detectors that surround the subject's head and measure the number of photons originating from all the angles within the brain. Through a computer reconstruction algorithm, it is possible to identify where the annihilation event took place and from where the positron was emitted (with an approximation of a few millimeters because of the distance traveled by the positron before the event of annihilation), as well as the quantity of radiation emitted from that site.

Regional cerebral blood flow. By employing PET and water labeled with oxygen-15 (^{15}O), rCBF can be assessed. Water is an excellent flow indicator because it is almost freely diffusible at physiological flow rates and can quickly equilibrate between brain and blood. Immediately after an intravenous injection of a bolus of 10–40 mCi of radiolabeled water (depending on the sensitivity of the tomograph employed), a dynamic acquisition PET scan is obtained to measure local cerebral radioactivity during the subsequent 1–4 minutes. Radioactivity concurrently is

monitored in the blood through an indwelling arterial line connected to an automatic counter. Using this method, it is possible to determine absolute rCBF values, expressed in mL/100 g tissue/minute.

In a variant of this procedure, the subject continuously inhales ^{15}O-labeled carbon dioxide, which in the lung gives rise to ^{15}O-labeled water. When a steady state is reached, and the rate of delivery of radioactive water to the brain equals its rate of removal by venous washout, measured brain radioactivity is directly proportional to the constant input function, which is a function of rCBF (Frackowiak and Lammertsma 1985).

Because the ^{15}O in water has a rapid radioactive decay (half-life = 2.02 minutes), multiple studies only 6–12 minutes apart can be performed sequentially in the same subject. This makes it possible to evaluate rCBF repeatedly in a single sitting, while the subject is in the resting state or performing any of several tasks. By subtracting baseline rCBF from task rCBF, regions that are specifically and significantly activated during the task can be identified. In such studies, global CBF frequently is corrected for arterial blood PaCO$_2$, which should be measured.

Cerebral glucose metabolism. By using PET with [^{18}F]fluoro-2-deoxy-D-glucose (FDG), an analogue of glucose labeled with ^{18}F, it is possible to visualize and measure the uptake of FDG by neural cells in different brain regions in an awake subject. FDG reaches the brain through blood flow and, like glucose, can be transported bidirectionally across cerebral capillaries by a monosaccharide transport system. Once inside brain cells, FDG is phosphorylated to FDG-6-phosphate (FDG-6-P) by the enzyme hexokinase. Unlike glucose-6-P, however, FDG-6-P cannot be transformed into fructose-6-P and is not further metabolized by glycolytic pathway enzymes. As brain phosphatase activity is low, FDG-6-P remains essentially trapped inside brain cells, virtually unchanged during the duration of the study (Sokoloff 1982) (Figure 10–2).

The quantity of FDG-6-P that has accumulated in a brain region during 45 minutes after FDG injection is measured by PET and is a function of the rate of phosphorylation of glucose to glucose-6-P by hexokinase, the first reaction in the glycolytic pathway, and the plasma integral of FDG to which the brain is exposed. At a steady state with regard to unlabeled concentrations, the net rate of any step in a pathway equals the net rate of the overall pathway; thus, the net rate of glucose phosphorylation estimated with FDG represents the net flux of glucose through the entire glycolytic pathway. Sokoloff et al. (1977) elaborated an operational equation to calculate rCMRglc from 1) the quantity of FDG-6-P within brain, 2) the ratio of the integrated

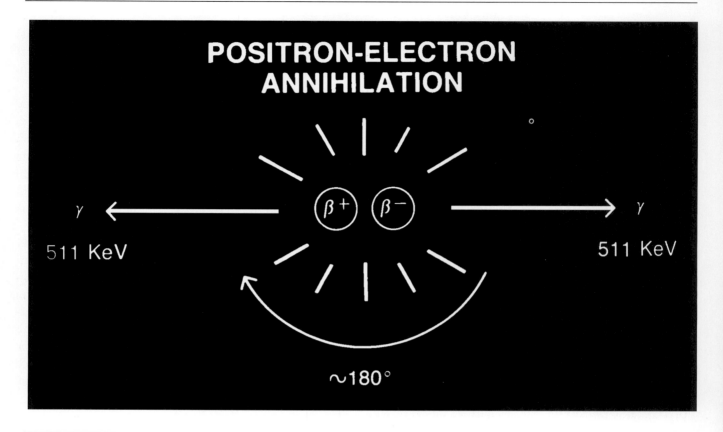

FIGURE 10–1. Positron-emission tomography (PET) detection. After the annihilation of a positron (β^+) with an electron (β^-), two γ rays are emitted in diametrically opposite directions. These γ rays are detected by the PET machine, and their local site of origin and intensity are reconstructed. KeV = kiloelectron volts.

plasma activity of FDG to cold plasma glucose concentration during 45 minutes, and 3) a "lumped constant" to correct for the use of FDG instead of the natural glucose ("isotope effect") (Huang et al. 1980).

A detailed description of the physical principles and the technical and methodological aspects of PET goes far beyond the aims of this review; the interested reader may refer to Herscovitch (1994), Holcomb et al. (1989), and Mazziotta and Phelps (1986).

Positron-Emission Tomography Studies in Healthy Aging

Regional Cerebral Blood Flow and Oxygen Consumption

PET has allowed researchers to overcome many of the limitations of earlier techniques and to obtain more reliable information about relations among regional cerebral metabolism, rCBF, and age. Results of human aging studies with regard to rCBF and rCMRO$_2$ are summarized in Table 10–1. The table shows that, in general, studies per-

formed in the resting state (reduced auditory and visual input) demonstrated lesser changes than those in which visual and/or auditory input was uncontrolled.

In accord with conclusions from a majority of studies performed with the ^{133}Xe technique, initial PET studies using the steady-state ^{15}O inhalation method supported a decrease of rCBF with aging. Frackowiak et al. (1983, 1984) found a 28% reduction in mean gray matter rCBF in a group of 14 older subjects compared with 18 young subjects, not studied in the resting state. The regression between rCBF and age was statistically significant and had a slope of –4.9 mL/100 g/minute/decade. rCMRO$_2$ in gray matter was significantly decreased by –19% in the older subjects, but failed to show a significant regression with age. White matter showed no rCBF group difference. The tendency of the oxygen extraction ratio (OER, the ratio of rCMRO$_2$ to rCBF) to be elevated in the elderly group (Frackowiak and Gibbs 1983), if confirmed, could be an early sign of hemodynamic decompensation increasing neuronal vulnerability and characterize subjects with cerebrovascular disease (Yao et al. 1990). An age-associated decline in rCBF in temporosylvian, medial frontal, and visual medial occipital areas also was demonstrated in 19

Capillary   Brain

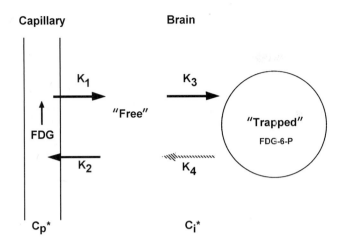

FIGURE 10–2. Fluorodeoxyglucose model.
[^{18}F]Fluoro-2-deoxy-D-glucose (FDG) reaches the brain via blood and is transferred across brain capillaries and into cells with an influx rate constant equal to K_1. Once inside cells, FDG is phosphorylated to FDG-6-P by the enzyme hexokinase, at a rate equal to K_3. FDG-6-P remains essentially trapped intracellularly because the rate of dephosphorylation, K_4, is quite slow as a result of a low brain activity of the enzyme glucose-6-P phosphatase. K_2 is the rate constant for efflux of FDG from cells to blood. $C_p{}^*$ is the concentration of FDG in plasma; $C_i{}^*$ is its concentration in brain.
Source. Reprinted from Grady CL, Rapoport SI: "Cerebral Metabolism in Aging and Dementia," in *Handbook of Mental Health and Aging.* Edited by Birren J, Sloane RB, Cohen G. San Diego, CA, Academic Press, 1992, pp. 201–228.

"hospitalized patients with nonacute illness," using low-resolution PET in subjects with eyes closed but ears unobstructed (Lebrun-Grandie et al. 1983).

In a later study, the same group (Pantano et al. 1984) examined 27 "healthy hospitalized patients" ages 19–76 years and found a significant linear decline with age of gray matter rCBF (3.2 mL/100 g/minute/decade) but not of rCMRO$_2$. When the younger (< 50 years old) and older (> 55 years old) subjects were compared, both mean rCBF and rCMRO$_2$ were decreased significantly in the older group (by –18% and –17%, respectively). Decreases were mostly in frontal, temporosylvian, and parieto-occipital cortical areas. White matter rCBF and rCMRO$_2$ did not differ between groups. Although the OER was age invariant, no correction for a possible difference in cerebral blood volume (CBV) was performed.

Takada et al. (1992) in an inadequately described study also reported a significant linear decline with age for CMRO$_2$ but not for rCBF, and only in the association neocortex of the left hemisphere. Significant age reductions of rCBF in the frontal cortex and insular gray matter and of rCMRO$_2$ and regional cerebral blood volume (rCBV) in white matter and in many cortical areas were reported in

healthy subjects between 22 and 82 years of age with eyes closed but ears unobstructed (Leenders et al. 1990). Rates of decline approximated 0.5%/year. OER significantly increased with age in some cortical regions.

In contrast to these results, no age difference in mean rCBF, OER, or CBV was noted in 22 healthy volunteers, whereas mean gray rCMRO$_2$ significantly decreased with age (Yamaguchi et al. 1986). A slight increase of PaCO$_2$ and a decrease of hematocrit observed in the older subjects could have tended to elevate rCBF in this study, masking an age-related decrease.

Structural changes, such as enlargement of the CSF spaces and cortical atrophy, have been claimed to be responsible for intrinsic (by reducing the number of neurons in the gray matter) and apparent (by increasing partial volume effects of cerebrospinal fluid or white matter) age declines in rCBF. However, despite evidence of progressive cortical atrophy by X-ray computed tomography (CT), no significant decrease in rCBF or rCMRO$_2$ was detected in healthy subjects between 50 and 85 years of age (Itoh et al. 1990). High-resolution morphometric measurements of brain structures, which can now be obtained by using magnetic resonance imaging (MRI), can be co-registered with functional PET images. As we discuss later, this methodology has begun to be applied to correct for brain atrophy rCMRglc data obtained in neurodegenerative disorders, and it could be employed also to demonstrate to what extent atrophy influences PET-rCBF measurements in the elderly.

With high-resolution PET and a sophisticated method of anatomical localization, statistical parametric mapping (Friston et al. 1990, 1995), Martin et al. (1991) recently reported a significant age-related decline in rCBF in limbic regions and in bilateral temporal, parietal, and frontal association cortices, more in the left than right hemisphere. These changes in subjects studied with eyes closed and ears unobstructed were unrelated to differences in global CBF and thus were thought to represent an age-related redistribution of rCBF (Martin et al. 1991).

As illustrated in Table 10–1, PET studies relating rCBF and rCMRO$_2$ to age have differed technically and methodologically, and it is not surprising therefore that results have been inconsistent and have not led to firm conclusions. Early PET studies employed low-resolution scanners, with limited anatomical definition of cortical and subcortical structures and significant error as a result of "partial voluming" (see below). Subjects ranged from "healthy hospitalized patients" (Pantano et al. 1984) or "hospitalized patients with nonacute illness" (Lebrun-Grandie et al. 1983) to carefully screened healthy volunteers (Eustache et al. 1995; Marchal et al. 1992), and cogni-

TABLE 10–1. Summary of principal studies and methods and techniques used with positron-emission tomography (PET), relating regional cerebral blood flow (rCBF) and regional cerebral metabolic rate for oxygen ($rCMRO_2$) in human subjects to age

Study	Subjects	PET procedure	Results and comment
Lebrun-Grandie et al. 1983	14 M, 5 F (19–76 yr) Hospitalized patients with nonacute illness	Oxygen-15 Steady state ECAT (FWHM 19 mm) Eyes closed; ears open Measured attenuation	rCBF declined with age in temporosylvian, medial frontal, and medial occipitovisual regions. No age effect on $CMRO_2$.
Frackowiak and Gibbs 1983	18 young (24–43 yr) 14 older (49–74 yr)	Oxygen-15 Steady state ECAT II (FWHM 17 mm)	Gray matter: 19% $CMRO_2$ and 28% rCBF reductions; −0.5 mL/100 mL/min/year.
Pantano et al. 1984	19 M, 8 F (19–76 yr) Healthy hospitalized patients	Oxygen-15 Steady state ECAT II (FWHM 17 mm)	$CMRO_2$ significantly reduced in the older group; rCBF: −0.32 mL/100 mL/min/year.
Yamaguchi et al. 1986	17 M, 5 F (26–64 yr) (14 < 50 yr; 8 > 50 yr) Healthy, no medications	Oxygen-15 Steady state HEADTOME III (FWHM 8.2 mm)	Gray matter $CMRO_2$: linear negative correlation with age. No difference in rCBF, OER, CBV.
Itoh et al. 1990	17 M, 11 F (50–85 yr) Healthy volunteers	Oxygen-15 Steady state ECAT II (FWHM 17 mm) Calculated attenuation	No change with age; $CMRO_2$, and rCBF were not related to brain atrophy as measured by CT scan.
Leenders et al. 1990	18 M; 16 F (22–82 yr) Patient relatives and hospital staff No CT or MRI scan	Oxygen-15 Steady state ECAT II (FWHM 17 mm) Eyes closed; ears open No face mask Measured attenuation	rCBF, CBV, and $CMRO_2$ decreased significantly in the frontal cortex and insular matter. OER increased in some areas.
Martin et al. 1991	15 M, 15 F (30–85 yr) Healthy, no medications	Oxygen-15 Steady state ECAT 931/8/12 Eyes closed; ears open Measured attenuation	No change in global CBF; decrease in limbic and association areas.

Study	Subjects	Methods	Findings
Takada et al. 1992	15 M, 17 F (27–67 yr) Healthy volunteers	Oxygen-15 Steady state PET scanner: ? Eyes closed; sensory stimulation or deprivation	CMRO$_2$ significantly decreased in bilateral putamen and left temporal, frontal, and parietal cortices. rCBF decreased only in the left superior temporal cortex. Methodology poorly described.
Burns and Tyrrell 1992	6 M, 8 F (51–85 yr) Patients' healthy relatives No careful medical screening	Oxygen-15 Steady state ECAT 931/8/12	CMRO$_2$ significantly decreased in the parietal lobe.
Marchal et al. 1992	14 M, 11 F (20–68 yr) Healthy volunteers Careful medical screening At least 7-year education	Oxygen-15 Steady state LETI TTV03 (FWHM 8 mm) stereotactic frame Eyes closed; ears open Measured attenuation	CMRO$_2$ decreased in 24/31 cortical gyri (–6% per decade); rCBF decreased in 10/31 gyri.
Eustache et al. 1995	14 M, 11 F (20–68 yr) Healthy volunteers Careful medical screening	Oxygen-15 Steady state LETI TTV03 (FWHM 8 mm) stereotactic frame Eyes closed; ears open Measured attenuation	CMRO$_2$ values, normalized to cerebellum, decreased significantly with age in all the neocortical regions and in left thalamus.

Note. CBV = cerebral blood volume; CT = computed tomography; F = female; FWHM = full width at half maximum, millimeter; M = male; MRI = magnetic resonance imaging; OER = oxygen extraction rate; yr = age in years.
[a]Mean ± SD. ECAT, ECAT II, HEADTOME III, LETI TTV03, and Scanditronix PC1024-7B are different PET scanners, whose properties are described in original references.

tive evaluation was rarely carried out. Dementing processes, such as Alzheimer's disease, can have an insidious onset and progress for years before becoming clinically evident. For example, in early stages of Alzheimer's disease, in subjects with only a memory deficit, abnormal rCMRglc has been demonstrated in association neocortices and precedes additional cognitive deficits that later appear (Grady et al. 1988; Haxby et al. 1990). To date, all aging studies have been cross-sectional, and the possibility cannot be ruled out that some reported age-related differences reflected sampling bias from surviving subjects (Martin et al. 1991).

Marchal et al. (1992) attempted to control for some of these variables by examining 25 optimally healthy, carefully screened volunteers between the ages of 20 and 68 years studied with eyes closed and ears unobstructed. High-resolution PET and stereotactic positioning of the head were employed. A significant decline in rCBF was detected only in two frontal gyri, perhaps because of the large coefficient of variation in the other regions (up to 32%). However, a significant age-related decrease of $rCMRO_2$ was seen throughout the cerebral cortex, except for the orbitofrontal gyrus, hippocampal, and lateral occipital regions. $rCMRO_2$ declined by 6%/decade. No significant relation was shown between whole-cortex $rCMRO_2$ and gender, cortical atrophy, or head size; subcortical structures, the cerebellum, and white matter showed no significant age-dependent change. An age-related linear decline in global brain oxygen consumption (normalized to cerebellum) also was found in a group of 25 health-screened subjects (examined with their eyes closed but ears open) who were part of a larger sample in a neuropsychological study (Eustache et al. 1995). The reduction in oxygen consumption reached statistical significance in all the neocortical areas and in the left thalamus. An age-associated decline was observed in some cognitive abilities, including working memory and verbal episodic and explicit memory; other cognitive skills remained unaffected by age.

In summary, data from numerous studies relating rCBF and $rCMRO_2$ to age are somewhat contradictory. In studies of subjects not in the resting state, age-dependent reductions are of the order of 20%–25%. The functional significance of these changes is not clear. In some studies, largest reductions were reported in cortical association regions, which subserve cognitive functions that decline even in the healthy elderly. These association areas appeared relatively recently during primate evolution, usually are the latest to myelinate, and may be selectively vulnerable to age-related degenerative processes such as Alzheimer's disease (Rapoport 1988, 1990). In subjects not studied in the resting state, age reductions could have been affected by re-

duced visual and auditory acuities (Creasey and Rapoport 1985; Grady et al. 1984), as the majority of the studies did not screen for ocular or auditory age-related pathologies, including cataract, glaucoma, or hearing loss (see earlier). A reduced rCBF in older people also might be caused by subclinical cerebrovascular disease, as atherosclerotic brain lesions are more frequent in the elderly and 50% of brains show such lesions after 50 years of age (Moossy 1971). Atherosclerotic vascular disease (Dastur et al. 1963) and hypertension (Meyer et al. 1985; Salerno et al. 1995), whose prevalence also increases with age, have been shown to be accompanied by reduced rCBF and/or rCMRglc.

Regional Cerebral Metabolic Rate for Glucose

PET studies of rCMRglc and human aging also have led to conflicting results, but, in general, studies outside of the resting state have demonstrated greater declines than those within it (Table 10–2). Kuhl et al. (1982) found a gradual age decline in rCMRglc in 40 healthy subjects between 18 and 78 years old, who were studied with eyes open and ears unplugged. The rate of decline was 0.43%/year (a net of 26% in the above age range), with no hemispheric preference. The ratio of rCMRglc in the frontal cortex to rCMRglc in the parietal cortex, an index of "hyperfrontality" (Ingvar 1979), fell with age, suggesting a selective effect on the frontal lobe. Chawluk et al. (1987) reported a comparable 0.26%/year decline in rCMRglc in healthy subjects studied outside of the "resting state." In contrast, other studies found no significant age-associated reduction in rCMRglc both in subjects studied in the resting state (eyes covered, ears plugged with cotton) (Duara et al. 1983, 1984) and in subjects with eyes closed and ears unobstructed (de Leon et al. 1983). In a relatively large sample of subjects, significantly lower absolute rCMRglc was seen in frontal, temporal, and parietal regions in the older group ($\geq$ 50 years old) as compared with the young subjects (< 50 years old). These reductions were no longer significant when rCMRglc was corrected for brain volume and atrophy (Yoshii et al. 1988). It should be noted, however, that a global correction method was applied that did not take into account any regional variability in atrophy-related brain changes (see discussion on atrophy correction later).

In the last few years, additional sophisticated methods of analysis have been developed to explore the effects of healthy aging on the brain metabolic data obtained in relatively large samples. Moeller et al. (1996) applied a statistical model of regional covariation to two large independently studied groups of subjects between 21 and 90 years in age. The main topographic profile identified by this

TABLE 10–2. Summary of principal studies and of methods and techniques employed with positron-emission tomography (PET), relating regional cerebral metabolic rate for glucose (rCMRglc) in human subjects to age

Study	Subjects	PET procedure	Results and comment
Kuhl et al. 1982	17 M, 23 F; 18–78 yr	ECAT II (FWHM 17 mm) Eyes and ears open Calculated attenuation	Generalized decrease in rCMRglc (0.43%/yr); frontal cortex more affected.
de Leon et al. 1983	14 young M (26 ± 5 yr) 21 older M (67 ± 7 yr)	PETT III (FWHM 15 mm) Eyes closed; ears open No attenuation correction	No change with age.
Hawkins et al. 1983	7 M, 1 F (18–68 yr)	NeuroECAT (FWHM 12 mm) Eyes and ears open	FDG rate constants do not change with age; no rCMRglc change with age.
Duara et al. 1983, 1984	40 M (21–83 yr) Healthy volunteers Careful medical screening	ECAT II (FWHM 17 mm) Eyes and ears covered Measured attenuation	No change with age.
Horwitz et al. 1986	15 young M (20–32 yr) 15 older M (64–83 yr) (Data from Duara 1984)	ECAT II (FWHM 17 mm) Eyes and ears covered Analysis of cerebral functional intercorrelations	No change with age. Decreased number of correlations between frontal and parietal areas and within the parietal lobes bilaterally in the older subjects.
Chawluk et al. 1987	21 young (mean age 27 yr) 23 older (mean age 63 yr) Subjects with medical illness included	PETT V (FWHM 16.5 mm) Eyes and ears open Calculated attenuation	rCMRglc was reduced in frontal, parietal, and temporal regions. No difference between subjects with and without cardiovascular or minor noncardiovascular disease.
Schlageter et al. 1987	49 M (21–83) Healthy volunteers	ECAT II (FWHM 17 mm) Eyes and ears covered CT scan for cerebral atrophy correction	No change with age; cerebral atrophy negatively correlates with rCMRglc.
Hoffman et al. 1988	22 M, 14 F (21–74 yr) Healthy volunteers	NeuroECAT (FWHM 12 mm) Eyes and ears open	Significant rCMRglc reductions only in some frontal areas. No effects of handedness or gender.
Yoshii et al. 1988	39 M/37 F (21–84 yr) Healthy volunteers Careful medical screening	PETT V (FWHM 15 mm) Eyes patched; ears open "Arterialized" venous blood	Absolute rCMRglc lower in older (≥ 50 yr) than in young (< 50 yr) subjects in frontal, temporal, and parietal lobes. Age difference no longer significant after taking into account brain volume and atrophy.
Grady et al. 1990	23 M, 37 F (20–90 yr) Healthy volunteers Careful medical screening	Scanditronix PC1024-7B (FWHM 6 mm) Eyes and ears covered Measured attenuation	12% decline in global CMRglc over 60-yr age range.
Salmon et al. 1991	14 young (mean age 26 yr) 11 older (mean age 27 yr) Healthy volunteers	NeuroECAT (FWHM 12.4 mm)	No age-related reduction in absolute rCMRglc. Age-related reduction in normalized rCMRglc in frontal lobe and increase in normalized rCMRglc in cerebellum.

(continued)

TABLE 10–2. Summary of principal studies and of methods and techniques employed with positron emission tomography (PET), relating regional cerebral metabolic rate for glucose (rCMRglc) in human subjects to age (*continued*)

Study	Subjects	PET procedure	Results and comment
Loessner et al. 1995	64 M, 56 F (19–79 yr) Some medical conditions in the elderly	PENN-PET (FWHM 5.5 mm) Eyes open; ears unoccluded Qualitative inspection of scans	Decreased cortical glucose metabolism particularly in the frontal lobes. Preservation of subcortical structures, cerebellum, posterior cingulate, and visual cortical areas.
DeSanti et al. 1995	40 young (mean age 28 yr) 32 older (mean age 68 yr) Partial medical screening	Siemens CTI-931 (FWHM 6.2 mm) Eyes open; ears unoccluded Measured attenuation	Reduced frontal and temporal rCMRglc, with stronger effect (24% decline in rCMRglc over 40-yr age range) in the frontal lobes.
Eberling et al. 1995	6 M, 3 F young (mean age 27 yr) 4 M, 4 F older (mean age 66 yr) Healthy volunteers Some medical screening	PET 600 (FWHM 2.6 mm) Eyes open; ears unoccluded	Reduced temporal lobe rCMRglc in older subjects (up to 27% in anterior temporal cortex).
Moeller et al. 1996	Group 1 62 M, 68 F (21–90 yr) Group 2 10 M, 10 F (24–78 yr)	Scanditronix PC 1024-7B (FWHM 6 mm) Measured attenuation Eyes patched; ears occluded Scanditronix Superpett 3000 (FWHM 8 mm) Eyes open and ears unoccluded in a dimly lit room Analysis of cerebral functional intercorrelations	12.5% decline in global CMRglc over 60-yr age range relative frontal hypometabolism associated with covariate normalized metabolic increases in parieto-occipital association areas, basal ganglia, cerebellum.
Murphy et al. 1996	55 M, 65 F (21–91 years) Healthy volunteers Careful medical screening	Scanditronix PC 1024-7B (FWHM 6 mm) Measured attenuation Eyes patched; ears occluded	Significant age-related rCMRglc decline in global CMRglc and in frontal, temporal, and parietal regions. Metabolic reductions differed between males and females.
Blesa et al. 1997	9 M, 8 F (20–74 years) Healthy volunteers Partial medical screening	Scanditronix PC 2048-15B (FWHM 6.5 mm) Measured attenuation Eyes patched; ears occluded	8% decline in global CMRglc per decade; decline more pronounced in limbic structures.
Petit-Taboué et al. 1998	15 M, 9 F (20–67 yr) Healthy volunteers Careful medical screening	LETI TTV03 (FWHM 8 mm) Eyes closed; ears partially blocked; pixel by pixel analysis (SPM)	6% decline in global CMRglc per decade; decline most pronounced in frontal, temporal, and anterior cingulate cortical areas.

Note. CT = computed tomography; F = female; FDG = [^{18}F]fluorodeoxy-D-glucose; FWHM = full width at half maximum, millimeter; yr = age in years; M = male; SPM = statistical parametric mapping.
[a] Mean ± SD. ECAT, ECAT II, HEADTOME III, LETI TTV03, and Scanditronix PC1024–7B are different PET scanners, whose properties are described in original references.

principal component analysis was characterized by relative frontal glucose hypometabolism with covariate metabolic increases in parieto-occipital association areas, basal ganglia, midbrain, and cerebellum. A more selective effect of aging on frontal lobe glucose metabolism also was found in a study by DeSanti et al. (1995), with less pronounced reductions in the temporal lobes of the elderly subjects, whereas Eberling et al. (1995) found cerebral metabolic rates lower only in the temporal lobes in older subjects compared with rates in younger subjects.

All the previous studies discussed above employed a regions of interest approach for the metabolic analyses. Recently, a systematic voxel by voxel analysis performed by using the statistical parametric mapping software (Friston 1995) demonstrated a global CMRglc decrease of 6%/decade (Petit-Taboué et al. 1998). Decreases in rCMRglc were bilateral and symmetrical, with some areas (frontal inferior and posterior lateral areas; anterior cingulate, anterior temporal, and parietotemporal junction cortices; left caudate; anterior thalamus) affected more than others.

Factors Influencing Positron-Emission Tomography Studies of Aging

As in the cases of rCBF and rCMRO$_2$ (see earlier), the question of whether and to what extent rCMRglc declines with age is not settled. Methodological issues and technical limitations noted above probably contributed to discrepancies in the different studies (Table 10–3). This chapter is not the place to discuss these issues in detail (for an excellent review, see Horwitz 1990), but it may be useful to discuss some of them in order to better interpret the findings in the literature.

What we measure with PET, using the FDG or ^{15}O-labeled water isotopes, are absolute values and correlated patterns of regional cerebral glucose metabolism and blood flow. Unlike morphometric measurements of dimensions of brain structures obtained with CT or MRI, which are invariant over years in adult subjects except with progressive neurodegenerative or cerebrovascular disease (Luxenberg et al. 1987), PET examines variable and often uncontrolled states of cerebral functional activity (Gur et al. 1987). Differences in sensory input during a scan can induce dramatic variations in rCMRglc or rCBF. Indeed, hemispheric CMRglc was shown to be approximately 20% higher in young subjects scanned with their eyes open and ears plugged, compared with subjects studied in the condition of eyes closed and ears plugged (resting state) (Mazziotta et al. 1982). Progressive increases in the complexity of visual stimulation resulted in parallel elevations of rCMRglc in visual association areas, with an average

TABLE 10–3. Factors that may contribute to variability of data obtained in different PET studies measuring rCBF, rCMRO$_2$, or rCMRglc in relation to age in human subjects

PET technique

Low-resolution (17-mm) versus high-resolution (6-mm) PET scanners

Up to 25% coefficient of variation with low-resolution PET scanners to measure a potential 15%–30% change in rCMRglc over an adult age span of 60 years.

Brain atrophy

"Partial volume effect" may artificially reduce rCBF and rCMRglc values.

Health screening

Selection of "too healthy" elderly subjects ("supernormals").

Inclusion of subjects with (sub)clinical vascular disorders or with subtle cognitive deterioration.

Medications with potential effects on brain metabolism and function.

Experimental procedure

Sensory input: eyes covered and ears plugged (resting state) versus eyes closed and ears open versus eyes and ears open.

Resting state versus cognitive activation (e.g., performing a neuropsychological task).

Calculated versus individually measured radiation attenuation by head tissues and skull.

Semiautomated regions of interest on individual brains versus automated pixel-by-pixel on stereotaxically normalized brains methods of image analysis.

Anxiety and stress during PET examination

High levels of stress or anxiety may affect frontal lobe metabolism.

"Familiarity" with PET scanning: first versus repeated scan examination

Gender

Differences in time course and topographical distribution of the brain areas primarily affected by the aging process between men and women.

Effect of hormone cycle in female subjects at the time of the PET scan examination.

Note. PET = positron-emission tomography; rCBF = regional cerebral blood flow; rCMRO$_2$ = regional cerebral metabolic rate for oxygen; rCMRglc = regional cerebral metabolic rate for glucose.

60% rCMRglc difference between subjects who were at rest and subjects who looked at a landscape of a park during the uptake period of FDG (Phelps et al. 1981).

Metabolic and flow responses to different sensory stimuli are unlikely to be age invariant, as visual and auditory acuities, and even proprioception, decline with age (Creasey and Rapoport 1985; Grady et al. 1984; Lehnert and Wuensche 1966). Thus, reported age differences in PET measures in subjects not in the sensory-deprived resting state could partially reflect reduced sensory acuity rather than only intrinsic age-related reduced activity. To date, resting state studies such as those by Duara et al. (1983, 1984) and Murphy et al. (1996) on optimally healthy subjects provide the best estimate of the actual age decline in intrinsic (sensory independent) brain functional activity.

Other factors, such as anxiety and stress during a scan or simply the novelty of the experimental setting, may affect cerebral metabolism and should be taken into consideration. Although minimally invasive, PET is stressful to some subjects because it involves arterial and venous catheterization, frequent blood sampling, a restraint to minimize head movement, resting in place for perhaps longer than 1 hour, and some sensory deprivation. Gur et al. (1987) reported an inverted U-shaped relation between rCBF and anxiety; rCBF increased with increasing anxiety up to a point and then decreased with additional anxiety. Swedo et al. (1989) also reported a direct correlation between anxiety during PET and rCMRglc in prefrontal areas. Healthy male volunteer subjects with high anxiety showed significantly greater right/left hemisphere metabolic ratios than low-anxiety people (Stapleton et al. 1997). Moreover, in the low-anxiety subjects, cerebral metabolism was lower in the second PET session compared with that in the first examination, whereas no changes occurred in the high-anxiety group, suggesting that metabolic changes may be related simply to becoming familiar with the procedure. This finding would warrant that subjects be trained before undergoing the actual PET scan examination to minimize this "novelty" effect and ensure more homogenous conditions across experimental sessions (something similar to the adaptation night used in sleep research). Training was used in our laboratory to maximize compliance in PET studies of young and older individuals with Down's syndrome (Dani et al. 1996; Pietrini et al. 1997). Furthermore, these findings highlight the necessity that the order of presentation of different experimental conditions be counterbalanced when one wishes to examine brain functional activity associated with distinct sensory or cognitive stimulation states (Pietrini et al. 1997).

Subject selection is particularly important in studies of functional activity and human aging. In many such PET studies, no attempt was made to exclude subjects with cardiovascular risk factors or clinical disorders that might affect the brain. Only a few studies (e.g., Duara et al. 1983, 1984; Marchal et al. 1992; Murphy et al. 1996) performed careful clinical, laboratory, and neuropsychological testing to rule out organic or mental abnormalities that might interfere with functional measurements. Although careful screening has been criticized as selecting for "supernormals" who, especially in the elderly, may not represent a "normally distributed" population, for the issue at hand we believe that such selection is appropriate. Less restrictive selection to obtain a sample more representative of the "normal population" might be adopted if many hundreds of subjects of both sexes and of different ages could be studied in the same PET facility with the same procedure. Then, one would have enough subjects to statistically partial out effects of confounding variables and risk factors (such as cardiovascular risk factors, history of psychiatric or medical disorders, mental status during examination) on the results. Additional variability may derive from gender differences and, in women, from fluctuations in plasma levels of sex hormones linked to the menstrual cycle. In a small sample of young women, Reiman et al. (1996a) showed that glucose metabolism was significantly higher in thalamic, prefrontal, temporal, and parietal areas in the mid-follicular phase (low plasma concentrations of estradiol and progesterone) and in superior temporal, anterior temporal, occipital, cerebellar, and limbic regions in the mid-luteal phase (high plasma concentrations of estradiol and progesterone). When using MRI and PET in a large population of carefully screened healthy subjects, we reported significant gender-related differences in aging of brain areas that are essential to higher cognitive functions, including temporal and parietal lobes, Broca's area, thalamus, and hippocampus (Murphy et al. 1996). This evidence of gender-specific morphometric and metabolic profiles in brain aging may underlie some of the reported differences between men and women in age-related cognitive decline.

Finally, technical aspects related to PET instrumentation have contributed to variability between PET centers. Tomographs with different spatial resolutions ranging from 6 to 17 mm full width at half maximum (FWHM) have been used to measure cerebral metabolism and blood flow. The degree of recovery of radioactivity in a brain region depends on the relation between regional volume and scanner resolution, and only high-resolution PET machines are appropriate for examining small regions.

In our laboratory, initial PET studies of aging (Duara et al. 1983, 1984) used a low-resolution PET tomograph (ECAT II; FWHM = 17 mm) for subjects in the resting state (see above). Global gray CMRglc, assessed in 77 healthy men between 20 and 70 years of age, showed a nonsignificant 7% decrease over this age range (Grady et al. 1990) (Figure 10–3, *panel A*). When we later used a Scanditronix PC 1024-7B scanner (6 mm in-plane resolution), under the same resting state conditions to study 60 healthy men, a statistically significant –12% age decline in global gray rCMRglc was evident (Figure 10–3, *panel B*). The slope of the regression lines in Figure 10–3 do not differ significantly (0.01 versus 0.02 mg glucose/100 g/minute/year), but because the slope with the high-resolution Scanditronix scanner had a much smaller coefficient of variation than with the lower resolution ECAT scanner, the former reached statistical significance. The –12% decline obtained with the high-resolution scanner likely represents a maximum rate of change because it was not corrected for partial voluming and brain atrophy.

In this regard, age-associated brain atrophy (de Leon et al. 1984; Schwartz et al. 1985; Zatz et al. 1982) is an additional complication. Resulting from partial voluming, atrophy can reduce recovery by the scanner of radioactivity from a given region. Recently, Ibanez et al. (1998) developed a segmented MRI-based method to correct rCMRglc data from patients with Alzheimer's disease and age-matched older healthy control subjects for the effects of partial voluming as a result of brain atrophy. This correction increased global CMRglc by approximately 12% in the control subjects and 20% in the patients with Alzheimer's disease, with the largest corrections being in the frontal and insular areas. Nevertheless, the initial uncorrected rCMRglc differences between the two groups remained statistically significant after correction. Thus, rCMRglc reductions obtained by PET in Alzheimer's disease reflect intrinsic metabolic reductions per gram tissue and are not artifacts of partial voluming. They represent neuronal/synaptic dysfunction in the affected regions (Pietrini et al. 1997, 1999). The Ibanez correction algorithm is now being applied to our other PET data involving age, gender, and disease group differences.

In some studies, attempts were made to correct PET data for brain atrophy by correcting with regard to dilation of lateral ventricles, measured using CT or MRI (Alavi et al. 1985; Herscovitch et al. 1986; Schlageter et al. 1987). Schlageter et al. (1987) used CT and PET to study 49 healthy men between 21 and 83 years old. When global CMRglc (which included gray and white matter and ventricular cerebrospinal fluid spaces) was corrected for age changes in lateral ventricular volume, the correlation coefficient with age changed from –0.29 to –0.04, indicating that the calculated uncorrected decline with age in resting glucose utilization largely was reflected by atrophy.

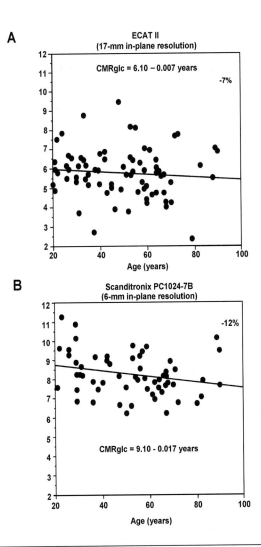

FIGURE 10–3. Global gray matter cerebral metabolic rate for glucose (CMRglc) as a function of age in 77 healthy men studied with a low-resolution ECAT II positron-emission tomography (PET) scanner (*panel A*) and in 60 healthy men studied with a high-resolution Scanditronix PC 1024-7B machine (*panel B*). Regression analyses demonstrated an insignificant –7% decrease in CMRglc over a 70-year range in *panel A*, but a statistically significant –12% decline in *panel B*. Data from the high-resolution scanner had a smaller coefficient of variation than data obtained with the low-resolution scanner. *Source.* Reprinted from Grady CL, Rapoport SI: "Cerebral Metabolism in Aging and Dementia," in *Handbook of Mental Health and Aging.* Edited by Birren J, Sloane RB, Cohen G. San Diego, CA, Academic Press, 1992, pp. 201–228.

In summary, despite the many studies that have been carried out to ascertain the effects of age on rCMRglc, the exact relation is not yet known. As in the cases of rCBF and rCMRO$_2$, most evidence suggests that an age-dependent reduction in rCMRglc, if present, is modest and of the order of –12% for a 60-year range, despite some isolated reports of much more dramatic reductions (Petit-Taboué et al. 1998). In view of the many possible confounding factors that can affect measurements, and given that several technical advances have recently been introduced, a renewed effort to quantify age-related in vivo measures of brain functional activity, and to understand how these measures reflect changes in cognition and behavior, should prove fruitful.

Can Functional Imaging Tell Us More About Brain Function and Brain Aging?

In the last few years, our ability to understand and characterize brain metabolism and functional activity in vivo has been greatly expanded by the rapid development of sophisticated experimental paradigms that combine neuroimaging techniques with cognitive, sensory, or pharmacological stimulation paradigms. Furthermore, new ways to interpret PET data, using powerful methods of analysis, have allowed us to identify specific patterns of functional interrelationship among different brain regions. Finally, new functional imaging methodologies, particularly functional magnetic resonance imaging, have become available to investigate functional activity in the living human brain with high spatial and temporal resolutions.

Brain functional correlations. With the exception of the study by Moeller and collaborators (1996), the PET studies that are summarized above simply reported differences in mean values for cerebral blood flow or glucose metabolism between young and older subjects or the regression of these values with age. However, another way to examine age-related differences in functional activity with PET is to use correlational or multivariate analysis to determine pattern of brain glucose metabolism and blood flow in the resting state or during activation. Indeed, despite that the subjects studied in the resting state by Duara et al. (1983, 1984) showed no age-related declines in rCMRglc, they did demonstrate clear age differences in their correlation patterns (Horwitz et al. 1986).

Correlation coefficients between pairs of rCMRglc values are thought to indicate functional associations between the two brain regions (Clark et al. 1984; Horwitz et al. 1984; Metter et al. 1984). The fundamental assumption of the correlation method is that if two brain regions (A and B) are functionally coupled, so that neuronal activity in one region depends on activity in the other, a plot of rCMRglc in region A against rCMRglc in region B across subjects, using normalized parameters such as rCMRglc/CMRglc, will demonstrate a statistically significant correlation. Conversely, if two regions show a significant correlation between their normalized rCMRglc parameters, these two

regions are assumed to be functionally coupled. Two regions may have a significant correlation in activity if they are anatomically linked and that link is functional in the resting state or during a specific task. However, the regions also could have a large correlation if they are not directly connected, but rather receive concomitant inputs from a third region, for example, a thalamic nucleus. Or, one could have a combination of both direct and indirect effects going on at the same time. Horwitz et al. (1986) compared pairwise correlations of normalized resting state metabolic rates between a group of 15 young healthy subjects (20–32 years old) and a group of 15 elderly optimally healthy subjects (64–83 years old). In the young group, many statistically significant positive correlations were demonstrated within and between the frontal and parietal lobes, a smaller number were demonstrated within and between the temporal and occipital lobes, and only a few such correlations were found between the frontal-parietal and the temporal-occipital domains. The older group, although demonstrating the same general pattern of correlations, had fewer significant correlations between frontal and parietal areas and between regions within the parietal lobes than did the younger group. This evidence of loss of functional integration among regions of the parietal lobe corresponded to measured deficits in cognitive performance subserved by parietal structures (Grady et al. 1990). Even more complex mathematical models, including discriminant function analysis and structural equation modeling (often referred to as path analysis), have been elaborated and applied successfully to identify subtle changes in brain metabolic functions indicative of disease or even in asymptomatic subjects at risk for developing brain disorders, including Alzheimer's disease (Azari and Pietrini 1995; Horwitz et al. 1995).

Cognitive and sensory stimulation paradigms. In addition to measuring brain metabolism and blood flow in the resting state, several experimental paradigms have been developed to examine brain activity during cognitive tasks or sensory stimulation conditions in healthy subjects at different ages. Most of these studies have been conducted using the ^{15}O-labeled water PET methodology to determine rCBF in distinct conditions of brain activity. The short half-life of ^{15}O makes it possible to perform a number of sequential studies during the same PET scan session. With the PET scanners of the last generation, which exhibit an excellent sensitivity and thus require the injection of very small amounts of radioactive water, more than two dozen of these short studies (called *runs*) can be performed during the same PET session while subjects alternate among different experimental paradigms. Given that neuropsychological studies and clinical observations indicate that several cognitive abilities decline with aging (Creasey and Rapoport 1985; Horn 1975), functional PET studies have been designed to investigate brain activation, as revealed by rCBF changes, during visuospatial and object recognition tasks, memory tasks, abstract reasoning, and sensory stimulation (Table 10–4).

In our laboratory, Grady et al. (1992) used ^{15}O-labeled water to show that healthy elderly (9 subjects, mean age 72 ± 7 (SD) years), compared with healthy young subjects (11 subjects, mean age 27 ± 4 years), while performing certain visual tasks during PET with equivalent mean accuracies and reaction times, activated different network components within their brain. In the young subjects, the occipitotemporal cortex was selectively activated during an object recognition task (face matching) compared with a sensorimotor control task, whereas the occipitoparietal cortex was activated during a spatial location task (dot location) (Figure 10–4). In the elderly subjects, the same regions were activated as in the young, but, in addition, rCBF increased significantly in the occipitotemporal cortex during the spatial task and in the superior parietal cortex during the object recognition task.

Age-related differences in activation were found also when subjects were tested on encoding and recognition processes during memory tasks. Young subjects showed rCBF increases in the right hippocampus and the left prefrontal and temporal cortical areas during encoding of novel faces and in the right prefrontal and parietal cortex during recognition (Grady et al. 1995). In contrast, the older subjects failed to show significant activation in the areas activated in the young during encoding, but they did have rCBF increases in the right prefrontal cortex during recognition (Figure 10–5). The lack of activation of hippocampal and frontal cortex during encoding suggests that memory decline in the elderly is a result of a failure to encode the stimuli properly.

Other studies of memory processes provide further support to age-associated changes in brain activity (Table 10–4). Elderly people show not only reduced or absent activation in many regions activated in young subjects, but also show significant activation of different regions. Additionally, several studies indicate that young subjects have a lateralized pattern of activation, with the left frontal cortex involved during encoding and the right frontal cortex involved during recall (hemispheric encoding/retrieval asymmetry model; Tulving et al. 1994). In the older subjects, in contrast, this lateralization appears to be disrupted as they show a more bilateral activation of the frontal cortex (Cabeza et al. 1997; Madden et al. 1999). These areas of increased activity in the elderly may be recruited for alternative strategies to maintain performance (Cabeza et al. 1997).

Taken together, the resting state correlation analyses of Horwitz et al. (1986) and the results of the visual and memory activation studies (Cabeza et al. 1997; Grady et al. 1992, 1994, 1995, 1998) suggest that healthy aging is accompanied by reorganization of network integrity and network processing efficiency in the brain, and that such reorganization can be elucidated with methods of functional imaging and multivariate data analyses, during tasks related to vision, audition, memory, attention, language, and other cognitive processes.

As the cognitive paradigms described above require that subjects actively perform on a given task, interpretation of the results would be biased if subjects perform poorly or not at all. The issue of compliance with the task requirements becomes critical when one wishes to compare effects of healthy aging with effects of a neurodegenerative disorder of the elderly, such as Alzheimer's disease (see below). Patients with moderate to severe dementia (Folstein et al. 1975) may be unable to understand or follow the instructions of even simple cognitive tasks testing visual recognition or memory. To address these limitations, our laboratory developed a passive audiovisual stimulation paradigm that makes it possible to assess brain responses to widespread audiovisual stimulation that does not require active performance by subjects. Using this experimental paradigm in combination with PET, we examined brain metabolic responses in young and middle-aged subjects with Down's syndrome and in patients with Alzheimer's disease with mild to severe dementia.

Employing a "double FDG injection technique" (Brooks et al. 1987) with blood flow measurements using ^{15}O-labeled water, two sequential measures of both rCBF and rCMRglc were obtained during the same PET session while a subject is in the resting state and during audiovisual stimulation (seeing and hearing a simple and colorful movie). As the two sets of studies were performed less than 1 hour apart, with the subject remaining in the tomograph, variance arising from differences in mental status, head positioning, or experimental procedure is minimized. Resting state and audiovisual stimulation were alternated randomly, and young and elderly subjects and patients and control subjects were studied alternately as well. Anxiety during PET was rated by a subjective measure (ranging from 0 = absent to 3 = severe) (Duara et al. 1983) and by administering a State Anxiety Questionnaire (Spielberger 1968) after the scan. Subjects were instructed to remain awake and were confirmed to be awake by the attending physician during the resting state measurements and were told that they would be given a questionnaire on the content of the movie at the end of the study. Subjects who had no previous experience of PET scan examination were

TABLE 10–4. Summary of principal studies that have used positron-emission tomography (PET) in combination with sensory or cognitive stimulation paradigms to examine brain activity in human subjects at different ages

Reference	Subjects	PET procedure	Results and comment
Grady et al. 1992	11 young M (27 ± 4 yr) 9 older M (72 ± 7 yr) Healthy volunteers Careful medical screening	Oxygen-15 water iv bolus Scanditronix PC 1024-7B (FWHM 6 mm) Object and spatial vision task Statistical parametric mapping	Less functional separation of the dorsal and ventral visual pathways in the older subjects.
Grady et al. 1994	15 young (26 ± 4 yr) 17 older (67 ± 6 yr) Healthy volunteers Careful medical screening	Oxygen-15 water iv bolus Scanditronix PC 1024-7B and Scanditronix PC2048-15B Faces and location visual task Statistical parametric mapping	Young and older subjects have different patterns of activation during face-matching and spatial location visual tasks, suggestive of reduced efficiency of occipital visual areas in the elderly.
Tempel and Perlmutter 1992	14 M, 12 F (20–72 yr) Healthy volunteers Careful medical screening	Oxygen-15 water iv bolus PETT VI; low-resolution mode Vibrotactile stimulation to one hand (130 Hz) Pixel-by-pixel subtraction	rCBF responses to vibrotactile stimulation in contralateral primary sensorimotor and supplementary motor areas do not change with normal aging.
Grady et al. 1995	10 young (8 M, 2 F) (25 ± 2 yr) 10 older (7 M, 3 F) (70 ± 6 yr) Healthy volunteers Careful medical screening	Oxygen-15 water iv bolus Scanditronix PC 2048-15B (FWHM 6.5 mm) Memory for faces task Statistical parametric mapping	Medial temporal cortex (including hippocampus) was activated in young but not in older subjects during encoding of faces.
Madden et al. 1996	10 young M (18–27 yr) 10 older M (63–75 yr) Healthy volunteers Careful medical screening	Oxygen-15 water iv bolus GE 4096-Plus Visual word identification Statistical parametric mapping	Older subjects have, in comparison with young subjects, reduced increase of rCBF during visual word identification in ventral occipitotemporal pathway.
Schacter et al. 1996	8 young (mean age = 21 yr) 8 older (mean age = 68 yr) Healthy volunteers	Oxygen-15 steady state GE-Scanditronix PC 4096 (FWHM 6 mm) Retrieval of episodic memories Statistical parametric mapping	Young and older subjects had similar hippocampal activations during recollection of a studied word. Young subjects showed bilateral activations in anterior prefrontal cortex during retrieval attempts, whereas in older subjects activations were more posterior.
Cabeza et al. 1997	12 young (6 M, 6 F) (19–31 yr) 12 older (5 M, 7 F) (67–75 yr) Healthy volunteers Careful medical screening	Oxygen-15 water iv bolus Scanditronix PC 2048-15B Memory task: encoding and retrieval of word pairs Statistical parametric mapping	Young and older subjects showed different patterns of activation during encoding, recognition, and recall suggestive of age-related deficits and neuroplastic compensatory mechanisms.

Study	Subjects	Method	Results
Nagahama et al. 1997	6 young (6 M) (21–24 yr) 6 older (4 M, 2 F) (66–71 yr) Healthy volunteers	Oxygen-15 water iv bolus PCT-3600W (FWHM 7.5 mm) Modified Card Sorting Test Statistical parametric mapping	Older subjects had, in comparison with young subjects, reduced rCBF increases during a Card Sorting Test in left dorsolateral prefrontal cortex and inferior parietal lobule, striate, and prestriate cortices.
Grady et al. 1998	13 young (10 M, 3 F) (25 ± 3 yr) 16 older (11 M, 5 F) (66 ± 4 yr) Healthy volunteers Careful medical screening	Oxygen-15 water iv bolus Scanditronix PC 2048-15B (FWHM 6.5 mm) Working memory for faces Statistical parametric mapping	Older subjects showed reduced activation in right ventrolateral prefrontal cortex and greater activation in left dorsolateral prefrontal cortex during working memory for faces as compared with that of young subjects.
Madden et al. 1999	12 young (6 M, 6 F) (20–29 yr) 12 older (5 M, 7 F) (62–79 yr) Healthy volunteers Partial medical screening	Oxygen-15 water iv bolus GE Advance (FWHM 5 mm) Verbal Recognition Memory Task	Age-related slowing of encoding and retrieval processes. During retrieval, young subjects had activation in right prefrontal cortex, whereas older subjects had bilateral prefrontal activation.

Note: F = female; FWHM = full width at half maximum; iv = intravenous; M = male; rCBF = regional cerebral blood flow; yr = age in years.

trained to increase compliance during the actual PET session and minimize the effects of novelty (Stapleton et al. 1997) on brain metabolism. The results of the first studies in patients with Alzheimer's disease or at risk for developing Alzheimer's disease are presented below.

◼ Positron-Emission Tomography in Geriatric Neuropsychiatry

Although our focus in this chapter is the aging process in healthy humans, it may be useful to mention briefly some PET studies of neuropsychiatric disorders that may affect the elderly, such as Alzheimer's disease and depression, which are discussed extensively elsewhere in this textbook.

Alzheimer's disease, the most common cause of dementia, accounts for up to 80% of all cases of dementia, followed by vascular diseases (4%–10%) and other diseases, including Pick's dementia (Chui 1989). Alzheimer's disease is characterized by a progressive, global, and irreversible deterioration of cognitive functions, which initially presents with memory problems and, later in the course of the disease, with language, mathematical, visuospatial, and personality decline. Many studies have been conducted with PET to investigate cerebral glucose metabolism in the different stages of Alzheimer's disease. In agreement with autopsy studies that demonstrated an unequal distribution of neurofibrillary tangles in the Alzheimer's disease brain, PET with FDG in the resting state showed reduced rCMRglc values mostly in the association neocortical areas, with a relative sparing of primary neocortical and subcortical regions, at least until the latest stages of the disease (DeCarli et al. 1992; Duara et al. 1986; Grady and Rapoport 1992; Kumar et al. 1991; Pietrini et al. 1996).

As shown in Figure 10–6, the reduction in rCMRglc in patients with Alzheimer's disease usually first appears in parietal and temporal neocortical areas and then later in the remainder of the neocortical mantle (severe stage), with only a relative preservation of the sensorimotor and primary visual cortices (Duara et al. 1986; Grady and Rapoport 1992; Kumar et al. 1991). The pattern of reduced rCMRglc may be different in individual patients, that is, some patients may show a greater involvement of the left side, whereas others may show more reductions in the right hemisphere. Interestingly, these heterogeneous reductions in neocortical rCMRglc may precede and predict later nonmemory impairments of cognitive functions thought to involve the neocortex and are correlated with heterogeneous patterns of nonmemory impairments in individual patients (Grady et al. 1988; Haxby et al. 1990). In other words, patients with predominant left hemisphere

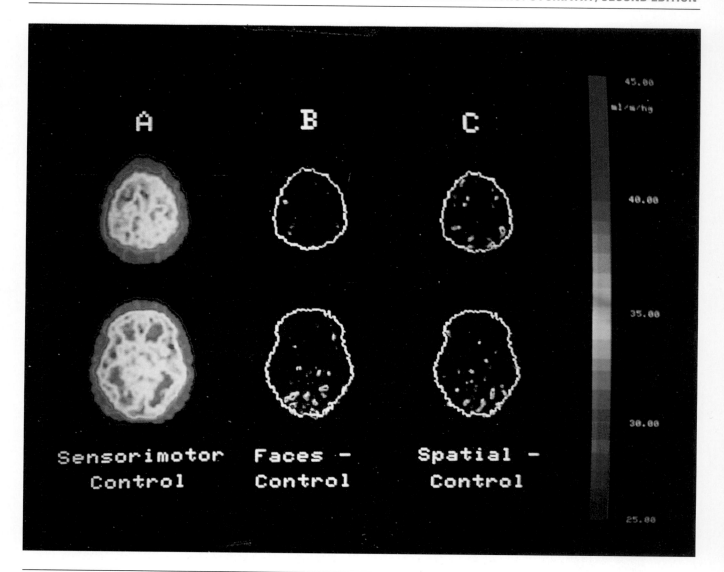

FIGURE 10–4.   Positron-emission tomography (PET) scan images from a young healthy subject, obtained using oxygen-15 water during different neuropsychological tasks. Pictures are taken parallel and 45 mm (*bottom*) and 90 mm (*top*) above the inferior orbitomeatal line. The pictures in *column A* show the pattern of regional cerebral blood flow (rCBF) during a sensorimotor control task. Pictures in *column B* and *column C* are obtained by subtracting the sensorimotor control task rCBF pattern from the rCBF pattern obtained during a faces-matching task and a spatial-location task, respectively. Thus only the areas selectively activated during either task are shown. During face matching, there was a selective activation of the occipitotemporal regions (*column B*), whereas during a spatial location task the occipitoparietal cortex was activated (*column C*). (See text for further explanation.) The color bar on the right side shows rCBF in mL/100 g tissue per minute. For each individual picture, the right side corresponds to the right side of the brain, and the left to the left side.

hypometabolism will have a greater language impairment compared with visuospatial function, and those with disproportionate right hemisphere hypometabolism will show a greater impairment of visuoconstructive abilities (Haxby et al. 1985).

Depression is common in older individuals, probably also because of age-related decrease in the serotoninergic system (Meltzer et al. 1998). Depression in the elderly often represents a clinical dilemma because its symptoms may resemble those of a dementia process. The term "de-

pressive pseudo-dementia" was proposed to indicate cases of depression that, because of the coexistence of cognitive impairment, were mistakenly diagnosed as dementia (Kiloh 1961). Early diagnostic differentiation between the two conditions is important because some antidepressant treatments may actually worsen cognitive impairment as a result of their anticholinergic effects and because an undiagnosed depression can be life-threatening (Dolan et al. 1992). PET can help to distinguish these two conditions. Baxter et al. (1989) found that patients with depres-

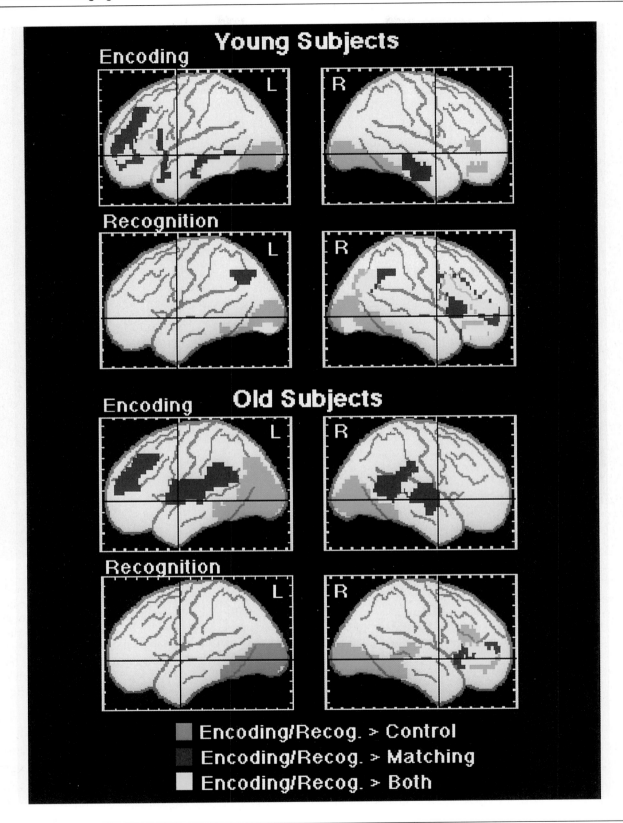

FIGURE 10–5. Graphical representation of the cortical areas that showed regional cerebral blood flow increases during encoding and recognition (*Recog.*) in a face-memory task in young (*top*) and older (*bottom*) healthy subjects. All areas in *color* showed significant activation when the encoding and the retrieval conditions were compared with the sensorimotor control task (*green*), with a forced-choice match-to-sample task (*red*; in this condition a sample face and two choice faces were presented simultaneously), or both (*yellow*).

Source. Adapted from Grady et al. 1995.

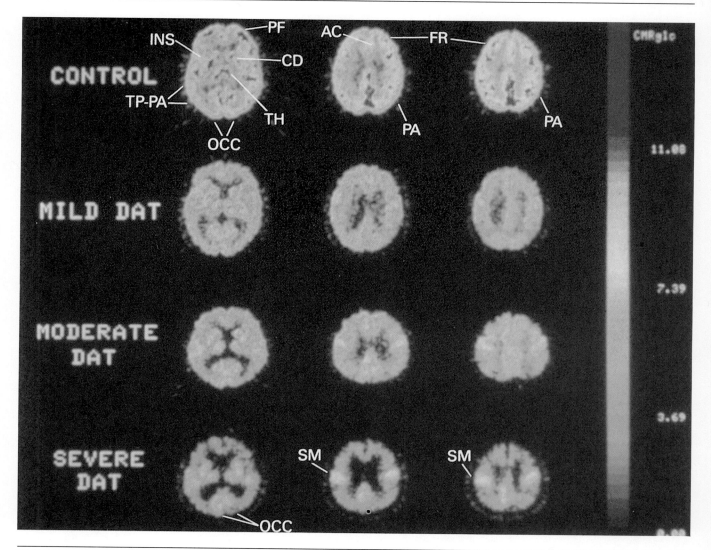

FIGURE 10–6. Positron-emission tomography (PET) images from a healthy control subject (age 69 years), a patient with mild dementia (age 53), a patient with moderate dementia (age 63), and a patient with severe dementia (age 72). All subjects were women. Scans were obtained using a Scanditronix PC 1024-7B positron tomograph (full width at half maximum [FWHM] 6 mm). For each subject, three horizontal brain slices taken parallel and above the inferior orbitomeatal line are shown: 45 mm (*left*), 70 mm (*middle*), and 90 mm (*right*). For each individual picture, the right side corresponds to the right side of the brain; the left, to the left side of the brain. In comparison to the healthy control subject, reduction of regional cerebral metabolic rate for glucose (rCMRglc) can be appreciated in the association cortical areas of the patients with dementia. In the early stages of disease, primary cortical areas and subcortical structure are not affected. With the progression of disease, the deficit becomes gradually worse, and in the patient with severe dementia of the Alzheimer type (DAT), only primary sensorimotor areas show a relative sparing. The *color scale* indicates rCMRglc in milligrams per 100 grams of tissue per minute. AC = anterior cingulate; CD = caudate nucleus; FR = frontal cortex; INS = insula; OCC = occipital cortex; PA = parietal cortex; PF = prefrontal cortex; SM = sensorimotor cortex; TH = thalamus; TP-PA = temporoparietal cortex.
Source. Adapted from Grady and Rapoport 1992.

sion had decreased lateral left prefrontal lobe rCMRglc compared with matched healthy control subjects. In addition, patients with bipolar depression and those with unipolar depression had significantly lower normalized caudate rCMRglc. Reduced rCMRglc values became normal values when patients returned to the euthymic state. The finding of a reduced rCMRglc in prefrontal areas and in the caudate nucleus of patients with depression is of par-

ticular interest because an independent study in patients with Parkinson's disease showed reduced inferior orbitofrontal and caudate rCMRglc only when depression was evident, whereas metabolism was normal in those with motor symptoms only (Mayberg et al. 1990). These regions usually are not affected in early Alzheimer's disease, and thus their involvement could help to differentiate the two processes.

In the last few years, as new drugs are being developed, the search for early changes in brain metabolism that could be used for a preclinical diagnosis of Alzheimer's disease has become a major focus of the researchers working in this field. This is particularly important because the early metabolic changes in Alzheimer's disease are potentially reversible, whereas the later ones are irreversible (Rapoport, in press). Using distinct PET approaches, different groups have examined populations at risk for developing Alzheimer's disease, such as individuals with family history of autosomal dominant Alzheimer's disease, those who are homozygous for the APOEε4 allele, or older subjects with Down's syndrome (Pietrini et al. 1993, 1997; Reiman et al. 1996b; Small et al. 1995). For example, we conducted neuropsychological and neuroimaging studies in young and middle-aged subjects with Down's syndrome. All subjects with Down's syndrome who are over 40 years of age show some neuropathological and neurochemical changes of Alzheimer's disease, and some 90% develop dementia after 60 years of age. Thus, subjects with Down's syndrome can be used to investigate the preclinical and clinical stages of Alzheimer's disease.

A longitudinal study in older nondemented and otherwise healthy subjects with Down's syndrome showed that cognitive measures and resting state brain metabolism remained stable until the onset of dementia, at which point the subjects began to rapidly decline. This suggested that dementia and metabolic dysfunction appear only after a threshold level of neuropathology is attained (Dani et al. 1996). On the other hand, the accumulation of Alzheimer's neuropathology in the years preceding clinical onset of dementia may impair the neuronal capability to respond to an increase in functional load or stress. To test this hypothesis, we measured rCMRglc in conjunction with the audiovisual stimulation paradigm described above, in young and older nondemented adults with Down's syndrome. Supporting our hypothesis, we found that the brain of older compared with younger nondemented subjects with Down's syndrome showed reduced metabolic increments in response to audiovisual stimulation in brain regions known to be affected by Alzheimer's disease, particularly temporal and parietal cortical regions (see above) (Figure 10–7, *panel B*). In the resting state, in contrast, glucose metabolism between the two groups did not differ in any cortical area (Figure 10–7, *panel A*). Although in need of being replicated in other at-risk groups without Down's syndrome, these results indicate that a paradigm that increases the functional demand on the brain can reveal neuronal/synaptic dysfunction that is not evident in the resting state before the onset of dementia.

This audiovisual paradigm also has been used to investigate neuronal/synaptic efficiency as a function of dementia severity in patients with Alzheimer's disease. In 15 otherwise healthy patients with Alzheimer's disease with mild to severe dementia (Folstein et al. 1975), we demonstrated that brain responsiveness to stimulation declined with worsening of dementia, to a point where no metabolic response could be elicited by audiovisual stimulation (Pietrini et al. 1999; Pietrini et al., in press). Reduced synaptic integrity in patients with moderate to severe dementia may contribute to unsuccessful responses to pharmacological treatment to enhance synaptic transmission in such patients (Rogers and Friedhoff 1998). As most drugs act by enhancing (cholinergic) neurotransmission, these agents require that synapses be functional in order for them to exert their pharmacological effects.

Summary

The rapid development of increasingly more sophisticated techniques for functional neuroimaging and of accompanying mathematical and statistical models to analyze multivariate imaging data have made it possible to quantify, localize, and interpret in vivo measures of brain functional activity. The majority of the studies to date indicate that absolute and normalized values of rCBF, rCMRglc, and rCMRO$_2$ are modestly affected by the aging process and that the net decline in intrinsic brain functional activity between 20 and 70 years of age for these parameters does not exceed approximately – 12% in the resting state, with the largest changes affecting the frontal lobes. Furthermore, partial voluming as a result of age-related brain atrophy and morphological changes may have inflated the magnitude of the reported metabolic reductions. Larger declines reported in the literature, when obtained under uncontrolled conditions of sensory stimulation, in part may also be biased by age-related reductions in visual and auditory acuities. In the absence of systematic screening, declines could also be in part a result of age-related brain disease such as hypertension.

Age differences in cognition and behavior may be better related to demonstrable and clear differences in integration of brain functional activity, rather than to differences in absolute or normalized values of rCBF, rCMRglc, and rCMRO$_2$. Such differences deserve to be explored in more detail by employing multivariate correlation or path analysis approaches. Horwitz et al. (1986) demonstrated clear age differences in correlated metabolic activity obtained in the resting state, which are more robust than the observed differences in absolute or normalized metabolic values. Finally, the stimulation approach initiated by

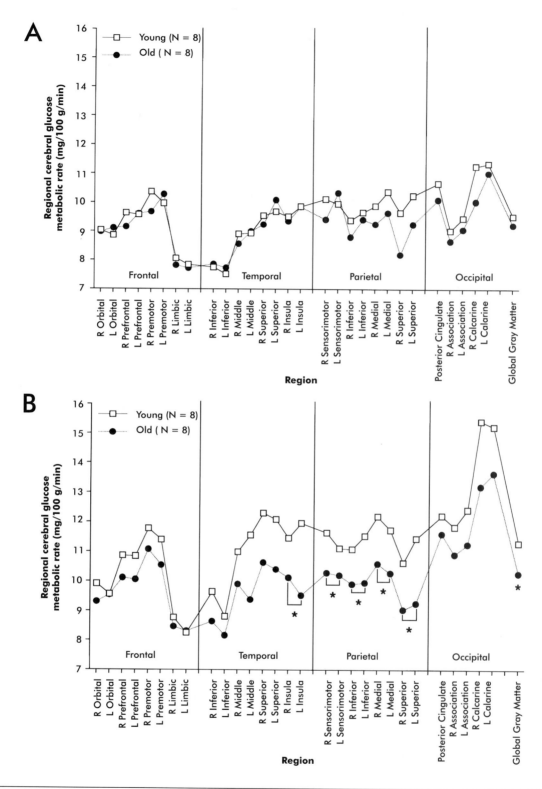

FIGURE 10–7. Brain glucose metabolism in young and older subjects with Down's syndrome without dementia at rest (*panel A*) and during passive audiovisual stimulation (*panel B*). *Asterisks* indicate significantly lower regional cerebral metabolic rate for glucose (rCMRglc) (*P* <.05) in the older compared with the young subjects with Down's syndrome. Despite no differences in brain metabolism in the resting state between older and young subjects with Down's syndrome (*top*), during audiovisual stimulation (*bottom*) significant rCMRglc reductions in parietal and temporal cortical areas are observed in the older group. R = right; L = left.

Source. Adapted from Pietrini et al. 1997.

Grady et al. (1992) and Pietrini et al. (1997, 1999), especially if it is used parametrically with tasks of continuously varying difficulty (Rapoport and Grady 1993), should prove useful for examining which brain networks actually are used during a given cognitive process and how network strategies may change with age.

■ References

Alavi A, Leonard JC, Chawluk J, et al: Correlative studies of the brain with positron emission tomography, nuclear magnetic resonance, and x-ray computed tomography, in Cerebral Blood Flow and Metabolism Measurement. Edited by Hartmann A, Hoyer S. Berlin, Springer-Verlag, 1985, pp 523–538

Azari NP, Pietrini P: Preclinical stages in subjects at risk for neurological disorders: can PET-FDG tell us more? J Neurol 242:112–114, 1995

Baxter LR, Schwartz JC, Mazziotta JC, et al: Reduction of prefrontal cortex glucose metabolism common to three types of depression. Arch Gen Psychiatry 46:243–250, 1989

Blesa R, Mohr E, Miletich RS, et al: Changes in glucose metabolism with normal aging. European Journal of Neurology 4:8–14, 1997

Brooks RA, Di Chiro G, Zukerberg BW, et al: Test-retest studies of cerebral glucose metabolism using fluorine-18 deoxyglucose: validation of method. J Nucl Med 28:53–59, 1987

Burns A, Tyrrell P: Association of age with regional cerebral oxygen utilization: a positron emission tomography study. Age Ageing 21:316–320, 1992

Cabeza R, Grady CL, Nyberg L, et al: Age-related differences in neural activity during memory encoding and retrieval: a positron emission tomography study. J Neurosci 17:391–400, 1997

Chang MC, Arai T, Freed LM, et al: Brain incorporation of [1-^{11}C]arachidonate in normocapnic and hypercapnic monkeys, measured with positron emission tomography. Brain Res 755:74–83, 1997

Chawluk JB, Alavi A, Jamieson DG, et al: Changes in local cerebral metabolism with normal aging: the effects of cardiovascular and systemic health factors (abstract). J Cereb Blood Flow Metab 7 (suppl 1):S411, 1987

Chui HC: Dementia. A review emphasizing clinicopathologic correlation and brain-behavior relationships. Arch Neurol 46:806–814, 1989

Clark CM, Kessler R, Buchsbaum MS, et al: Correlational methods for determining regional coupling of cerebral glucose metabolism: a pilot study. Biol Psychiatry 19:663–678, 1984

Creasey H, Rapoport SI: The aging human brain. Ann Neurol 17:2–10, 1985

Dani A, Pietrini P, Furey ML, et al: Brain cognition and metabolism in Down syndrome adults in association with development of dementia. Neuroreport 7:2933–2936, 1996

Dastur DK, Lane MH, Hansen DB, et al: Effects of aging on cerebral circulation and metabolism in man, in Human Aging—A Biological and Behavioral Study (Publ No 986). Edited by Birren JE, Butler RN, Greenhouse SW, et al. Bethesda, MD, U.S. Department of Health, Education and Welfare, 1963, pp 59–76

de Leon MJ, Ferris SH, George AE, et al: Computed tomography and positron emission transaxial evaluations of normal aging and Alzheimer's disease. J Cereb Blood Flow Metab 3:391–394, 1983

de Leon MJ, George AE, Ferris SH, et al: Positron emission tomography and computed tomography assessments of the aging human brain. J Comput Assist Tomogr 8:88–94, 1984

DeCarli CS, Atack JR, Ball MJ, et al: Post-mortem regional neurofibrillary tangle densities but not senile plaque densities are related to regional cerebral metabolic rates for glucose during life in Alzheimer's disease patients. Neurodegeneration 1:113–121, 1992

DeSanti S, de Leon MJ, Convit A, et al: Age related changes in brain, II: positron emission tomography of frontal and temporal lobe glucose metabolism in normal subjects. Psychiatr Q 66:357–370, 1995

Dolan RJ, Bench CJ, Brown RG, et al: Regional cerebral blood flow abnormalities in depressed patients with cognitive impairment. J Neurol Neurosurg Psychiatry 55:768–773, 1992

Duara R, Margolin RA, Robertson-Tchabo EA, et al: Cerebral glucose utilization, as measured with positron emission tomography in 21 healthy men between the ages of 21 and 83 years. Brain 106:761–775, 1983

Duara R, Grady CL, Haxby JV, et al: Human brain glucose utilization and cognitive function in relation to age. Ann Neurol 16:702–713, 1984

Duara R, Grady CL, Haxby JV, et al: Positron emission tomography in Alzheimer's disease. Neurology 36:879–887, 1986

Eberling JL, Nordahl TE, Kusubov N, et al: Reduced temporal lobe glucose metabolism in aging. J Neuroimaging 5:178–182, 1995

Eustache F, Rioux P, Desgranges B, et al: Healthy aging, memory subsystems and regional cerebral oxygen consumption. Neuropsychologia 33:867–887, 1995

Folstein MF, Folstein SE, McHugh PR: Mini-Mental State: a practical method for grading the cognitive state of patients for the clinician. J Psychiatr Res 12:189–198, 1975

Frackowiak RSJ, Gibbs JM: Cerebral metabolism and blood flow in normal and pathologic aging, in Functional Radionuclide Imaging of the Brain. Edited by Magistretti PL. New York, Raven, 1983, pp 305–309

Frackowiak RSJ, Lammertsma AA: Clinical measurement of cerebral blood flow and oxygen consumption, in Positron Emission Tomography. Edited by Reivich M, Alavi A. New York, Alan R Liss, 1985, pp 153–181

Frackowiak RSJ, Wise RJS, Gibbs JM, et al: Positron emission tomographic studies in aging and cerebrovascular disease at Hammersmith Hospital. Ann Neurol 15 (suppl): S112–S118, 1984

Friston KJ: Commentary and opinion, II: statistical parametric mapping: ontology and current issues. J Cereb Blood Flow Metab 15:361–370, 1995

Friston KJ, Frith CD, Liddle PF, et al: The relationship between global and local changes in PET scans. J Cereb Blood Flow Metab 10:458–466, 1990

Grady CL, Rapoport SI: Cerebral metabolism in aging and dementia, in Handbook of Mental Health and Aging. Edited by Birren J, Sloane RB, Cohen G. San Diego, CA, Academic Press, 1992, pp 201–228

Grady CL, Grimes AM, Pikus A, et al: Alterations in auditory processing of speech stimuli during aging in healthy subjects. Cortex 20:101–110, 1984

Grady CL, Sonies B, Haxby J, et al: Cerebral metabolic asymmetries predict decline in language performance in dementia of the Alzheimer type (DAT). J Clin Exp Neuropsychol 10:576–596, 1988

Grady CL, Horwitz B, Schapiro MB, et al: Changes in the integrated activity of the brain with healthy aging and dementia of the Alzheimer's type, in Aging Brain and Dementia. New Trends in Diagnosis and Therapy. Edited by Battistin L, Gerstenbrand F. New York, Wiley-Liss, 1990, pp 355–370

Grady CL, Haxby JV, Horwitz B, et al: Dissociation of object and spatial vision in human extrastriate cortex: age-related changes in activation of regional cerebral blood flow measured with [15-O] water and positron emission tomography. J Cogn Neurosci 4:23–34, 1992

Grady CL, Maisog JM, Horwitz B, et al: Age-related changes in cortical blood flow activation during visual processing of faces and location. J Neurosci 14:1450–1462, 1994

Grady CL, McIntosh AR, Horwitz B, et al: Age-related reductions in human recognition memory due to impaired encoding. Science 269:218–221, 1995

Grady CL, McIntosh AR, Bookstein F, et al: Age-related changes in regional cerebral blood flow during working memory for faces. Neuroimage 8:409–425, 1998

Gur RC, Gur RE, Resnick SM, et al: The effect of anxiety on cortical cerebral blood flow and metabolism. J Cereb Blood Flow Metab 7:173–177, 1987

Hawkins RA, Mazziotta JC, Phelps ME, et al: Cerebral glucose metabolism as a function of age in man: influence of rate constants in the fluorodeoxyglucose method. J Cereb Blood Flow Metab 3:250–253, 1983

Haxby JV, Duara R, Grady CL, et al: Relations between neuropsychological and cerebral metabolic asymmetries in early Alzheimer's disease. J Cereb Blood Flow Metab 5:193–200, 1985

Haxby JV, Grady CL, Koss E, et al: Longitudinal study of cerebral metabolic asymmetries and associated neuropsychological patterns in early dementia of the Alzheimer type. Arch Neurol 47:753–760, 1990

Herscovitch P: Radiotracer techniques for functional neuroimaging with positron emission tomography, in Functional Neuroimaging. Edited by Thatcher RW, Hallet M, Zeffiro T, et al. San Diego, CA, Academic Press, 1994, pp 29–46

Herscovitch P, Auchus AP, Gado M, et al: Correction of positron emission tomography data for cerebral atrophy. J Cereb Blood Flow Metab 6:120–124, 1986

Hoffman JM, Guze BH, Hawk TC, et al: Cerebral glucose metabolism in normal individuals: effects of aging, sex and handedness. Neurology 38 (suppl 1):371, 1988

Holcomb HH, Links J, Smith C, et al: Positron emission tomography: measuring the metabolic and neurochemical characteristics of the living human nervous system, in Brain Imaging: Applications in Psychiatry. Edited by Andreasen N. Washington, DC, American Psychiatric Press, 1989, pp 235–370

Horn JL: Psychometric studies of aging and intelligence, in Genesis and Treatment of Psychologic Disorders in the Elderly. Aging, Vol 2. Edited by Gershon S, Raskin A. New York, Raven, 1975, pp 19–23

Horwitz B: Quantification and analysis of positron emission tomography metabolic data, in Positron Emission Tomography in Dementia. Edited by Duara R. New York, Wiley-Liss, 1990, pp 13–70

Horwitz B, Duara R, Rapoport SI: Intercorrelations of glucose metabolic rates between brain regions: applications to healthy males in a state of reduced sensory input. J Cereb Blood Flow Metab 4:484–499, 1984

Horwitz B, Duara R, Rapoport SI: Age differences in intercorrelations between regional cerebral metabolic rates for glucose. Ann Neurol 19:60–67, 1986

Horwitz B, McIntosh AR, Haxby JV, et al: Network analysis of PET-mapped visual pathways in Alzheimer type dementia. Neuroreport 6:2287–2292, 1995

Huang SC, Phelps ME, Hoffman EJ, et al: Non-invasive determination of local cerebral metabolic rate of glucose in man. Am J Physiol 238:E69–E82, 1980

Ibanez V, Pietrini P, Alexander GE, et al: Regional glucose metabolic abnormalities are not the result of atrophy in Alzheimer's disease. Neurology 50:1585–1593, 1998

Ingvar DH: "Hyperfrontal" distribution of the cerebral grey matter flow in resting wakefulness; on the functional anatomy of the conscious state. Acta Neurol Scand 60:12–25, 1979

Itoh M, Hatazawa J, Miyazawa H, et al: Stability of cerebral blood flow and oxygen metabolism during normal aging. Gerontology 36:43–48, 1990

Jagust WJ, Eberling JL, Richardson BC, et al: The cortical topography of temporal lobe hypometabolism in early Alzheimer's disease. Brain Res 629:189–198, 1993

Kety SS: Human cerebral blood flow and oxygen consumption as related to aging. Research Publication of the Association for Research in Nervous Mental Disorders 35:31–45, 1956

Kety SS, Schmidt CF: The nitrous oxide method for quantitative determination of cerebral blood flow in man: theory, procedure and normal values. J Clin Invest 27:475–483, 1948

Kiloh LG: Pseudo-dementia. Acta Psychiatr Scand 37:336–350, 1961

Kuhl DE, Metter EJ, Riege WH, et al: Effects of human aging on patterns of local glucose utilization determined by the [18F]fluorodeoxyglucose method. J Cereb Blood Flow Metab 2:163–171, 1982

Kumar A, Schapiro MB, Grady CL, et al: High-resolution PET studies in Alzheimer's disease. Neuropsychopharmacology 4:35–46, 1991

Lebrun-Grandie P, Baron JC, Soussaline F, et al: Coupling between regional blood flow and oxygen utilization in the normal human brain. A study with positron emission tomography and oxygen 15. Arch Neurol 40:230–236, 1983

Leenders KL, Perani D, Lammertsma AA, et al: Cerebral blood flow, blood volume and oxygen utilization. Normal values and effect of age. Brain 113:27–47, 1990

Lehnert W, Wuensche H: Das Electroretinogramm in verschiedenen Lebensaltern. Graefes Arch Clin Exp Ophthalmol 170:147–155, 1966

Loessner A, Alavi A, Lewandrowski K-U, et al: Regional cerebral function determined by FDG-PET in healthy volunteers: normal patterns and changes with age. J Nucl Med 36:1141–1149, 1995

Luxenberg JS, Haxby JV, Creasey H, et al: Rate of ventricular enlargement in dementia of the Alzheimer type correlates with rate of neuropsychological deterioration. Neurology 37:1135–1140, 1987

Madden DJ, Turkington TG, Coleman RE, et al: Adult age differences in regional cerebral blood flow during visual world identification: evidence from H2 15O PET. Neuroimage 3:127–142, 1996

Madden DJ, Turkington TG, Provenzale JM, et al: Adult age differences in the functional neuroanatomy of verbal recognition memory. Hum Brain Mapp 7:115–135, 1999

Marchal G, Rioux P, Petit-Taboué MC, et al: Regional cerebral oxygen consumption, blood flow, and blood volume in healthy human aging. Arch Neurol 49:1013–1020, 1992

Martin AJ, Friston KJ, Colebatch JG, et al: Decreases in regional cerebral blood flow with normal aging. J Cereb Blood Flow Metab 11:684–689, 1991

Mazziotta JC, Phelps ME: Positron emission tomography studies of the brain, in Positron Emission Tomography and Autoradiography: Principles and Applications for the Brain and Heart. Edited by Phelps ME, Mazziotta JC, Schelbert HR. New York, Raven, 1986, pp 493–580

Mazziotta JC, Phelps ME, Carson RE, et al: Tomographic mapping of human cerebral metabolism: sensory deprivation. Ann Neurol 12:435–444, 1982

Mayberg HS, Starkstein SE, Sadotz B, et al: Selective hypometabolism in the inferior frontal lobe in depressed patients with Parkinson's disease. Ann Neurol 28:57–64, 1990

Melamed E, Lavy S, Bentin S, et al: Reduction in regional cerebral blood flow during normal aging in man. Stroke 11:31–35, 1980

Meltzer CC, Smith G, DeKosky ST, et al: Serotonin in aging, late-life depression, and Alzheimer's disease: the emerging role of functional imaging. Neuropsychopharmacology 18:407–430, 1998

Metter EJ, Riege WH, Kuhl DE, et al: Cerebral metabolic relationships for selected brain regions in healthy adults. J Cereb Blood Flow Metab 4:1–7, 1984

Meyer JS, Rogers RL, Mortel KT: Prospective analysis of long-term control of mild hypertension on cerebral blood flow. Stroke 16:985–990, 1985

Moeller JR, Ishikawa T, Dhawan V, et al: The metabolic topography of normal aging. J Cereb Blood Flow Metab 16:385–398, 1996

Montaigne ME de: De l'age (1580), in Les Essais, Vol 1. Paris, Editions Garnier, 1952, pp 360–363

Moossy J: Cerebral atherosclerosis: intracranial and extracranial lesions, in Pathology of the Nervous System, Vol 1. Edited by Minckler J. New York, McGraw-Hill, 1971, pp 1423–1432

Murphy DGM, DeCarli C, McIntosh AR, et al: Sex differences in human brain morphometry and metabolism: an in vivo quantitative magnetic resonance imaging and positron emission tomography study on the effect of aging. Arch Gen Psychiatry 53:585–594, 1996

Nagahama Y, Fukuyama H, Yamauchi H, et al: Age-related changes in cerebral blood flow activation during a card sorting test. Exp Brain Res 114:571–577, 1997

Obrist WD, Thompson HK, King CH, et al: Determination of regional cerebral blood flow by inhalation of 133-xenon. Circ Res 20:124–135, 1967

Obrist WD, Thompson HK Jr, Wang HS, et al: Regional cerebral blood flow estimated by 133-xenon inhalation. Stroke 6:245–256, 1975

Pantano P, Baron JC, Lebrun-Grandie P, et al: Regional cerebral blood flow and oxygen consumption in human aging. Stroke 4:635–641, 1984

Petit-Taboué MC, Landeau B, Desson JF, et al: Effects of healthy aging on the regional cerebral metabolic rate of glucose assessed with statistical parametric mapping. Neuroimage 7:176–184, 1998

Phelps ME, Mazziotta JC, Kuhl DE, et al: Tomographic mapping of human cerebral metabolism: visual stimulation and deprivation. Neurology 31:517–529, 1981

Pietrini P, Azari NP, Grady CL, et al: Pattern of cerebral metabolic interactions in a subject at risk for Alzheimer's disease. Dementia 4:94–101, 1993

Pietrini P, Furey ML, Graff-Radford N, et al: Preferential metabolic involvement of visual cortical areas in a subtype of Alzheimer's disease: clinical implications. Am J Psychiatry 153:1261–1268, 1996

Pietrini P, Dani A, Furey M, et al: Brain stimulation reveals reduced glucose metabolism in Down's syndrome subjects at risk for Alzheimer's disease prior to dementia. Am J Psychiatry 154:1063–1069, 1997

Pietrini P, Furey ML, Alexander GE, et al: Association between brain functional failure and dementia severity in Alzheimer's disease: resting versus stimulation PET study. Am J Psychiatry 158:470–473, 1999

Pietrini P, Alexander GE, Furey ML, et al: Cerebral metabolic response to passive audiovisual stimulation in Alzheimer's disease patients and healthy controls assessed by positron emission tomography. J Nucl Med (in press)

Purdon AD, Rapoport SI: Energy requirements for two aspects of phospholipid metabolism. Biochem J 335:313–318, 1998

Rapoport SI: Brain metabolism in aging and dementia (Publ No 83-2625), in Medicine for the Laymen Series. National Institutes of Health Publication. Bethesda, MD, U.S. Department of Health and Human Services, 1983

Rapoport SI: Brain evolution and Alzheimer's disease. Rev Neurol (Paris) 144:79–90, 1988

Rapoport SI: Integrated phylogeny of the primate brain, with special reference to humans and their diseases. Brain Res Brain Res Rev 15:267–294, 1990

Rapoport SI: In vivo PET imaging and postmortem studies suggest potentially reversible and irreversible stages of brain metabolic failure in Alzheimer disease. Eur Arch Psychiatry Clin Neurosci (in press)

Rapoport SI, Grady CL: Parametric in vivo brain imaging during activation to examine pathological mechanisms of functional failure in Alzheimer disease. Int J Neurosci 70:39–56, 1993

Rapoport SI, Chang MC, Connolly K, et al: In vivo imaging of fatty acid incorporation into brain to examine signal transduction and neuroplasticity involving phospholipids. Ann N Y Acad Sci 820:56–74, 1997

Reiman EM, Armstrong SM, Matt KS, et al: The application of positron emission tomography to the study of the normal menstrual cycle. Hum Reprod 11:2799–2805, 1996a

Reiman EM, Caselli RJ, Yun LS, et al: Preclinical evidence of Alzheimer's disease in persons homozygous for the e4 allele for apolipoprotein E. N Engl J Med 334:752–758, 1996b

Risberg J: Regional cerebral blood flow measurements by 133-Xe-inhalation: methodology and application in neuropsychology and psychiatry. Brain Lang 9:9–34, 1980

Rogers SL, Friedhoff LT: Long-term efficacy and safety of donepezil in the treatment of Alzheimer's disease: an interim analysis of the results of a U.S. multicentre open label extension study. Eur Neuropsychopharmacol 8:67–75, 1998

Roy CS, Sherrington CS: On the regulation of blood supply of the brain. J Physiol (Lond) 11:85–108, 1890

Salerno JA, Grady CL, Mentis MJ, et al: Brain metabolic function in older men with chronic essential hypertension. J Gerontol A Biol Sci Med Sci 50:M147–M154, 1995

Salmon E, Maquet P, Sadzot B, et al: Decrease of frontal metabolism demonstrated by positron emission tomography in a population of healthy elderly volunteers. Acta Neurol Belg 91:288–295, 1991

Schacter DL, Savage CR, Alpert NM, et al: The role of the hippocampus and frontal cortex in age-related memory changes: a PET study. Neuroreport 7:1165–1169, 1996

Scheinberg P, Blackburn I, Rich M, et al: Effects of aging on cerebral circulation and metabolism. Arch Neurol Psych 70:77–85, 1953

Schieve JF, Wilson WP: The influence of age, anesthesia and cerebral arteriosclerosis on cerebral vascular activity to CO_2. Am J Med 15:171–174, 1953

Schlageter NL, Horwitz B, Creasey H, et al: Relation of measured brain glucose utilization and cerebral atrophy in man. J Neurol Neurosurg Psychiatry 50:779–785, 1987

Schwartz M, Creasey H, Grady CL, et al: CT analysis of brain morphometrics in 30 healthy men, aged 21 to 81 years. Ann Neurol 17:146–157, 1985

Small GW, Mazziotta JC, Collins MT, et al: Apolipoprotein E type 4 allele and cerebral glucose metabolism in relatives at risk for familial Alzheimer disease. JAMA 273:942–947, 1995

Sokoloff L: The action of drugs on the cerebral circulation. Pharmacol Rev 11:1–85, 1959

Sokoloff L: The radioactive deoxyglucose method, theory, procedure and application for the measurement of local cerebral glucose utilization in the central nervous system, in Advances in Neurochemistry, Vol 4. Edited by Agranoff BW, Aprison MH. New York, Plenum, 1982, pp 1–82

Sokoloff L, Reivich M, Kennedy C, et al: The [^{14}C]-deoxyglucose method for the measurement of local cerebral glucose utilization: theory, procedure and normal values in the conscious and anesthetized albino rat. J Neurochem 28:897–916, 1977

Spielberger CD: 20-Item State Anxiety Questionnaire—Manual. Palo Alto, CA, Consulting Psychologist Press, 1968

Stapleton JM, Morgan MJ, Liu X, et al: Cerebral glucose utilization is reduced in second test session. J Cereb Blood Flow Metab 17:704–712, 1997

Swedo SE, Schapiro MB, Grady CL, et al: Cerebral glucose metabolism in childhood-onset obsessive compulsive disorder. Arch Gen Psychiatry 45:518–523, 1989

Takada H, Nagata K, Hirata Y, et al: Age-related decline of cerebral oxygen metabolism in normal population detected with positron emission tomography. Neurol Res 14 (suppl 2):128–131, 1992

Tempel LW, Perlmutter JS: Vibration-induced regional cerebral blood flow responses in normal aging. J Cereb Blood Flow Metab 12:554–561, 1992

Tulving E, Kapur S, Craik FIM, et al: Hemispheric encoding/retrieval asymmetry in episodic memory: positron emission tomography findings. Proc Natl Acad Sci U S A 91:2012–2015, 1994

Yamaguchi T, Kanno I, Uemura K, et al: Reduction in regional cerebral metabolic rate of oxygen during human aging. Stroke 6:1220–1228, 1986

Yao H, Sadoshima S, Kuwabara Y, et al: Cerebral blood flow and oxygen metabolism in patients with vascular dementia of the Binswanger type. Stroke 21:1694–1699, 1990

Yoshii F, Barker WW, Chang JY, et al: Sensitivity of cerebral glucose metabolism to age, gender, brain, volume, brain atrophy, and cerebrovascular risk factors. J Cereb Blood Flow Metab 8:654–661, 1988

Zatz LM, Jernigan TL, Ahumada AJ Jr: Changes on computed cranial tomography with aging: intracranial fluid volume. AJNR Am J Neuroradiol 3:1–11, 1982

11

Functional Brain Imaging

Functional Magnetic Resonance Imaging and
Magnetic Resonance Spectroscopy

Mark S. George, M.D., Kathleen A. McConnell

Jeffrey P. Lorberbaum, M.D., Andrew Greenshields

Daryl E. Bohning, Ph.D., Jacobo Mintzer, M.D.

Advances in neuroimaging are transforming basic and clinical neuroscience. Technological developments first in computed tomography (CT) and then magnetic resonance imaging (MRI) have provided noninvasive methods of directly examining brain structure. For years, however, the only ways to examine brain *function* included electroencephalograms (EEGs) (with poor spatial resolution) or radiotracer-based methods such as single photon emission computed tomography (SPECT) and positron-emission tomography (PET) (also with relatively poor spatial resolution and requiring the injection of radioactive tracers). Recently, researchers have devised several methods to use conventional MRI scanners to obtain images of brain function. By varying the ways in which the magnetic signal is acquired, researchers can now use MRI to not only image brain structure and pathology in exquisite detail, but they can also image regional brain oxygen use, blood perfusion, and diffusion of water through and across membranes. Additionally, by using MR spectroscopy, they can directly image brain neurochemical activity as well.

These new applications using MRI to image brain function rather than structure are collectively referred to as *functional MRI*, or *fMRI*. These exciting developments are still in early stages and do not have many direct clinical applications yet, but they hold the enormous promise of one day having a single examination that will yield information about both brain structure and function. Such innovations directly allow for the development of MR scanning protocols that would facilitate diagnosis and monitor treatment. For example, in the diagnosis and treatment of multiple sclerosis, structural MRI is crucial for initial diagnosis and is a sensitive evaluator of changes in disease activity, even better than a detailed physical examination (Khoury and Weiner 1998). Eventually, fMRI will likely assume a similarly important role in many other areas of geriatric neuropsychiatry. Perhaps most important for the future clinical utility and application of fMRI is that it involves only minor upgrading of conventional MRI machines (see Table 11–1).

Despite this enormous promise, MRI presents several problems specific to imaging in aging individuals. MRI involves the patient's lying relatively motionless in the bore of a scanner that is generally 3–4 feet in diameter and long enough to extend from one's thighs past the head. Many patients find this situation frightening and claustrophobic, especially those who are already agitated or who are cognitively impaired with delirium or dementia. Additionally, when the magnetic gradients inside the scanner disturb the magnetic field in the process of producing an image, they generate a loud rhythmic noise. The combination of confinement and noise can result in up to 20% of the general population being unable to remain still enough for a quality examination.

Technicians are working to circumvent this problem. Newer MRI scanners are being designed with shorter

TABLE 11–1. **Advantages of functional magnetic resonance imaging (MRI) compared with advantages of positron-emission tomography (PET) and single photon emission computed tomography (SPECT), especially in geriatrics**

Advantages

Has potential for high temporal and spatial resolution

Lacks radioactivity, and most techniques are noninvasive

Can be repeated multiple times

Is performed on upgraded, common MRI scanners

Disadvantages

Is extremely sensitive to head movement

Is awkward environment for complex functional imaging paradigms

Has contraindications:

Irremovable magnetic devices

Extreme claustrophobia

Cannot perform receptor-ligand studies as with PET and SPECT

Is new technique with less track record than PET and SPECT

bores that are less confining, and some MRI machines are "open," that is, they wrap around rather than encompass the patient. Other, more easily applicable, techniques for reducing anxiety include using prism glasses, goggles, and earphones to minimize the feelings of confinement. These measures do help in some cases. In an agitated patient with dementia, however, one must often resort to pharmacological sedation, which directly affects the functional image. On another front, more rapid MRI sequences are now able to image the entire brain in much shorter time (3 seconds), decreasing the amount of time that a subject must remain still. Nevertheless, problems of motion sensitivity and a relatively confining environment will likely continue to be of particular concern in using MRI in the elderly for many years to come, despite the wealth of clinical information that MR scanning can provide.

Previous chapters review the use of MRI to image brain structure in geriatrics, as well as the use of PET and SPECT. In this chapter, we briefly describe the new fMRI techniques and then highlight many of the initial geriatric applications.

Magnetic Resonance Spectroscopy

Nuclear magnetic resonance (NMR), discovered in 1946, describes the fact that certain molecules are magnetic and resonate to specific radio frequencies depending on the molecule's magnetic elements and the chemical bonding of these elements (Kato et al. 1998). Magnetic resonance spectroscopy (MRS) exploits this phenomenon to detect the presence of various molecules in millimolar concentrations. Since 1946, MRS has been used mostly in chemistry research to analyze molecular structure. In 1978, Chance et al. first used in vivo ^{31}P MRS in mouse brain, but it was not until the much more recent development of MRI that spectroscopic analysis became applicable for use in the human brain because the two techniques require basically the same hardware (Kato et al. 1998). Some of the molecules resolvable by MRS are involved in high-energy phosphate or membrane phospholipid metabolism, so a particular advantage of MRS is that it allows the noninvasive, in vivo measurement of tissue metabolites and steady-state metabolic processes (see Table 11–2).

Basic Principles of Magnetic Resonance Spectroscopy

As mentioned above and discussed in the previous chapter on structural MRI, the isotopes of certain atoms are magnetic and spin about their axes. In a uniform magnetic field

TABLE 11–2. Some general features of magnetic resonance imaging (MRI) spectroscopy

Noninvasively measures tissue biochemistry

Relies on flipping nonwater hydrogen atoms or other magnetic atoms

Magnetic compounds identified by spectrographic peaks

Single voxel and metabolic spatial techniques available

Common types:

^{1}H spectroscopy

^{31}P spectroscopy

^{7}Li spectroscopy

^{19}F spectroscopy (i.e., fluorinated compounds such as fluoxetine hydrochloride [Prozac] and trifluoperazine hydrochloride [Stelazine])

Restricted to the study of mobile magnetic compounds

Receptor-ligand studies not currently possible

Limited spatial and temporal resolution

Resolution may improve with introduction of stronger MRI magnets

such as that produced by an MRI scanner, each magnetic isotope aligns in the direction of the magnetic field and spins at a rate specific to its type and chemical bonding pattern. In response to a magnetic pulse of specific frequency (Larmor frequency), a nucleus spinning at its Larmor frequency resonates; that is, it absorbs the energy of the pulse, and temporarily flips out of alignment with the magnetic field. As the flipped nucleus gradually relaxes back to its aligned state, it emits absorbed energy in the form of electromagnetic waves called free induction decay (FID). The concentration of the target nucleus is related to the intensity of its observed decay. The Larmor frequency for each nucleus depends not only on the identity of the isotope itself but also on that nucleus's local molecular magnetic environment as determined by its chemical bonding. Depending on this local environment, the resonant or Larmor frequency for a particular nucleus will shift (chemical shift) and produce a slightly different signal, thus allowing one to distinguish the presence of the same nucleus in different molecules.

The results of a spectrographic assay appear as a spectrograph of several peaks, each representing a particular molecule. Figure 11–1 illustrates an idealized ^{1}H MRS spectrograph and Figure 11–2, an actual spectrograph with accompanying structural MRI. The location of each peak corresponds to a specific molecule's Larmor frequency, and the area under each peak is proportional to the concentration of the metabolites in the target tissue.

Generally the concentrations of these molecules are so

small that many samples must be acquired and averaged to obtain enough signals for quantitative analysis. To achieve this repetition, one uses a spin-echo method, in which the radiofrequency signal is pulsed a second time after a period called the echo time (TE), and a second decay signal, the echo, is observed. One repeats this process over a period called the repetition time (TR) and averages the values of observed decay times (FID), or echoes.

Spectrographic assays can be localized to certain regions of the brain. The simplest and oldest method is to use a surface coil, which roughly targets cortical regions under the area of the scalp covered by the body of the coil itself (Charles et al. 1997). At least three techniques are used for targeting more focal, single-voxel regions such as a tumor or stroke: depth-resolved surface coil spectroscopy (DRESS), stimulated-echo method (STEAM), and image selected in vivo spectroscopy (ISIS) (Kato et al. 1998). For analyzing several regions of the brain simultaneously, one uses a method of multiple voxel localization called magnetic resonance spectroscopic imaging (MRSI) or chemical shift imaging (CSI) (Charles et al. 1997; Kato et al. 1998). With this method, one can even reformat the data to

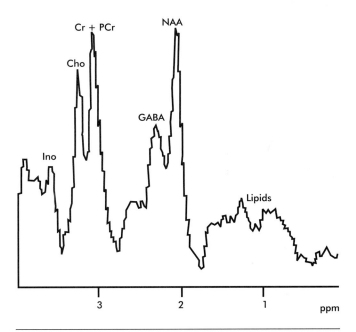

FIGURE 11–1. Idealized examples of a proton magnetic resonance imaging spectra.

Cho = choline; Cr = creatine; GABA = γ-aminobutyric acid; Ino = inositol; NAA = *N*-acetyl-L-aspartate; PCr = phosphocreatine; ppm = parts per million.

Source. Reprinted with permission from Moore CM, Renshaw PF: "Magnetic Resonance Spectroscopy Studies of Affective Disorders," in *Brain Imaging in Clinical Psychiatry.* Edited by Krishnan KRR, Doraiswarmy PM. New York, Marcel-Dekker, 1997, pp. 185–213.

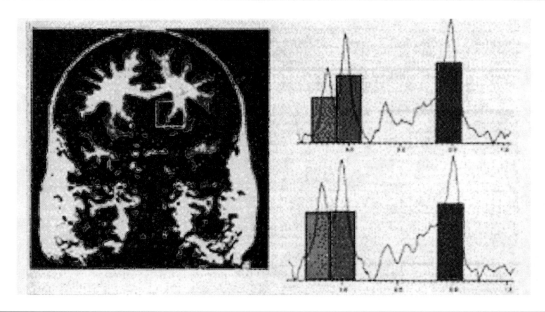

FIGURE 11–2. Magnetic resonance imaging scan and actual proton spectra from primary psychiatry.

Source. Reprinted with permission from Cohen BM, Renshaw PF, Stoll AL, et al.: "Decreased Brain Choline Uptake in Older Adults: An In Vivo Proton Magnetic Resonance Spectroscopy Study." *JAMA* 274:902–907, 1995.

produce an image of the spatial distribution of a particular metabolite in the brain.

Complications of Magnetic Resonance Spectroscopy Data Analysis

Several inherent features of MRS make it difficult to obtain accurate measures of absolute concentrations. For example, signal peaks sometimes overlap, making it difficult to define an area under a specific peak. Differences in hardware conditions, even within the same scanner, such as the magnetic field drifting with time, mean that any MR analyses are relative and not absolute. In an attempt to correct for these complications, most spectrographic data on molecular concentrations are normalized to an internal (usually H_2O) or external signal and/or expressed in terms of ratios to a metabolite whose concentration remains relatively constant in the brain, such as creatine. Finally, because research in neurochemistry has tended to focus on neurotransmitters and neuroreceptors at the expense of the neurometabolites detectable by MRS, and because the technical capabilities of in vivo MRS in humans are so new, MRS is still in its infancy. Many of the techniques for both data acquisition and data analysis have yet to be standardized. All of the issues above contribute to the considerable discrepancies in the results of many MRS studies. The highest hope for MRS in geriatric medicine seems to be its development as a diagnostic tool for differentiating early stages of Alzheimer's disease (AD) from other kinds of de-

mentia such as vascular dementia or Parkinson's dementia. These diagnoses are particularly difficult for the practitioner, and in fact, to date, AD can be definitively proven only by biopsy and postmortem pathological examination. A less invasive and more reliable in vivo diagnosis would guide both the differential treatment of these dementias and the development of drugs that could combat them in their early stages. For this reason, most MRS studies in the geriatric population have focused on comparisons between AD and other forms of dementia. After a cursory description of the main spectra and the metabolites they resolve, we proceed to a discussion of these studies.

Different Magnetic Resonance Spectra and Their Neurochemical Correlates

[31]P magnetic resonance spectroscopy. In a phosphorus-31 magnetic resonance spectrograph of human brain, seven peaks typically appear, representing the seven most abundant nuclei in metabolites containing phosphorus: phosphomonoester (PME), inorganic phosphate (Pi), phosphodiester (PDE), phosphocreatine (PCr), adenosine diphosphate (ADP), and adenosine triphosphate (ATP), and nucleoside triphosphate (NTP).

■ Phosphomonoester: The PME peak includes metabolites involved in membrane phospholipid synthesis such as phosphatidylcholine or phosphoethanolamine. The concentration of PME normally decreases with age but is elevated in early AD (Lorberbaum et al. 1998; Pettegrew et al. 1988).

- Inorganic phosphate (Pi): The Pi peak includes both PO_4^- and PO_4^{-2} from the dynamic equilibrium reaction $H_2PO_4^- \rightarrow HPO_4^{-2} + H^+$. Based on this reaction, one can calculate the intracellular pH of the target voxel from the specific chemical shift of this peak. pH has been found to increase in cases of chronic infarction, possibly because of the high pH of macrophages that gravitate to the site of a lesion (Ross and Michaelis 1994; Vion-Dury et al. 1994).

- Phosphodiester (PDE): The PDE peak, alternately, represents metabolites produced in membrane phospholipid degeneration such as glycerophosphotidylcholine and glycerophosphoethanolamine. It was once thought that the PME/PDE ratio represented membrane phospholipid turnover, but because of the complexities of determining the specific source of the PDE signal, this is no longer the case (Kato et al. 1998). The concentration of PDE normally increases with age.

- Phosphocreatine (PCr): PCr is a high-energy phosphate found in both brain and muscle. PCr can donate its phosphate group to ADP, thus helping replenish a cell's ATP. This probably explains the observed decrease in PCr levels in response to increased energy demand, such as with photic stimulation.

- Adenosine triphosphate (ATP): Concentration of ATP remains relatively constant in response to stimulation, but the chemical shift of these peaks can be affected by magnesium and lithium and has allowed assays of these nuclei (Gupta et al. 1984; Iotti et al. 1996; Kato et al. 1998; Ramasamy and Mota de Freitas 1989).

^{1}H magnetic resonance spectroscopy. Because H_2O is the most abundant molecule in the body, its spectrographic peak normally obliterates the signals of those molecules containing hydrogen that appear in lesser concentrations. After one suppresses the huge signal for H_2O, five peaks generally appear: *N*-acetyl-L-aspartate (NAA), creatine (Cr)/phosphocreatine (PCr), choline (Cho), inositol, and lactate.

- *N*-acetyl-L-aspartate (NAA): NAA is a component of neurons but not glial cells. It is thought to be a marker of viable or functional neurons, and its concentration has been observed to decrease in conditions of neuronal death and degeneration such as stroke and AD (Charles et al. 1997; Kato et al. 1998).

- Creatine (Cr)/phosphocreatine (PCr): The Cr peak contains both Cr and PCr. The sum of these molecules (Cr + PCr) was thought to remain relatively constant in the brain and has been used as an internal concentration standard for expressing concentrations of other metabolites as ratios (Kato et al. 1998; Lorberbaum et al. 1998).

- Choline (Cho): The choline peak includes signals from choline containing compounds such as phosphocholine and glycerophosphocholine, which are involved in membrane synthesis and breakdown, and to a lesser degree the neurotransmitter acetylcholine and its precursor choline.

- Inositol: The inositol peak contains *myo*-inositol, which is important in phospholipid metabolism and second messenger systems (Belmaker et al. 1990).

- Others: The excitatory neurotransmitters glutamate and aspartate and the inhibitory neurotransmitter γ-aminobutyric acid can be resolved by ^{1}H MRS, as can lipids. Because the fat surrounding the brain contains high concentrations of lipids, however, signals from these lipids outside the brain can easily contaminate the lipid peak in a spectrum.

Lithium-7 and fluorine-19 spectra. Because lithium and fluorine do not naturally appear in the human body but are components of many psychotropic drugs, spectra of these isotopes can be used for pharmacokinetic studies in patients treated with such drugs (Komoroski et al. 1994). Tables 11–3 and 11–4 provide chronological lists of ^{31}P MRS and ^{1}H MRS studies relevant to the field of geriatric neuropsychiatry.

Normal Aging

In an $_1$H MRS study of age-related changes in NAA, Cr + PCr, and Cho, Christiansen et al. (1993) examined four different brain regions: occipital, temporal and frontal lobes, and the basal ganglia, in eight healthy volunteers between the ages of 20 and 30 and eight healthy volunteers between the ages of 60 and 80. The researchers had expected elevated levels of NAA in the basal ganglia because this region has the highest density of neurons. Between brain regions of both groups, the only significant difference in metabolite concentrations was an increase in NAA in the occipital region of the younger group.

In a 1994 $_1$H MRS study of age- and gender-related changes, Charles et al. examined 34 healthy volunteers (15 men, 19 women) between the ages of 21 and 75. They found no differences between men and women and generally lower levels of Cho, Cr, NAA, Cho/NAA, and Cho/Cr in white matter compared to levels in gray matter in all

TABLE 11–3. Chronological table of phosphorus ^{31}P magnetic resonance spectroscopy (MRS) studies relevant to geriatric neuropsychiatry (starting in 1989)

Study	Subjects	Purpose	Results
Brown et al. 1989	17 control 17 AD 10 MSID	To examine phosphorus metabolism in groups with different dementias	% PME and PME/PDE increased in temporo-parietal area of brains of patients with AD. Pi increased in AD. PCr/Pi increased in MSID.
Bottomley et al. 1992	11 AD 14 control	To see if phosphorus metabolism is altered in AD To combine MRI and MRS to attempt to get absolute values for volumes of brain	After correcting for atrophy, study found no change in any metabolites across groups.
Sappey-Marinier et al. 1992a	30 subjects with WMSH and no other significant neuro-logical disease	To characterize cerebral oxidative phospholipid metabolism in WMSH	No change in PCr, PME, and PDE levels or ratios. Decrease in ATP/Pi in WMSH, inconclusive if this relates to ischemia.
Brown et al. 1993	18 MSID 21 control 19 AD	To test whether ^{31}P MRS can distinguish among patients with AD, those with vascular dementia, and control subjects	Patients with MSID had higher high-energy phosphate levels than did either those with AD or control subjects.
Longo et al. 1993	2 case studies of AD 6 control	To attempt to find objective marker of AD	PDE/ATP and PCr/ATP were elevated for patients with AD, but these results might be the result of noise effects or even normal aging. ^{1}H MRS on one patient with AD found lower NAA levels and increased Cho.
Murphy et al. 1993	9 AD 8 control	To examine differences in phosphorus metabolism between patients with AD and control subjects To see if that difference correlates with severity of AD Using PET, to examine how glucose metabolism is related to above changes To use MRI to correct for atrophy	Glucose metabolism decreased in patients with AD, but no change in Pi ratios or con-centration between those with AD and control subjects or with severity of the disease.
Cuenod et al. 1995	24 mild AD 15 control	To look for changes in PME and PDE levels in early stages of AD	Increased levels of PME/Pi found in frontal regions of AD.
Pettegrew et al. 1995	7 AD active 5 AD placebo 21 control	To see if acetyl-L-carnitine helps symptoms, membrane phospholipid, and high-energy phosphate metabolism	Active treatment showed less symptomatic decline than with placebo. Baseline PME levels were lower in both AD groups than in control subjects. PME levels for the active treatment group increased. ATP and PCr increased in group given placebo.

(continued)

TABLE 11–3. Chronological table of phosphorus ^{31}P magnetic resonance spectroscopy (MRS) studies relevant to geriatric neuropsychiatry (starting in 1989) *(continued)*

Study	Subjects	Purpose	Results
Smith et al. 1995	17 mild-moderate AD elderly and young control	To examine differences between patients with AD and control subjects	PCr/Pi levels elevated in patients with AD compared with both groups of control subjects.
			No change found in PME nor PDE except as a feature of gender.
			PME and PME/PDE decreased in women patients with AD.
			PCr/Pi levels correlated with age in patients with AD and in young control subjects.
			Decreased PCr/Pi found in frontal lobe of patients with AD and control subjects.
Gonzaléz et al. 1996	16 mild-moderate AD 8 control	To find neuronal abnormalities early in course of AD	NTP and PCr found normal.
			Decreased levels of PDE/NTP in patients with AD.
			PME/PDE increased in patients with AD because of decrease in PDE.

Note. AD = Alzheimer's disease; Cho = choline; MRI = magnetic resonance imaging; MSID = multiple subcortical ischemic dementia; NAA = *N*-acetyl-L-aspartate; NTP = nucleoside triphosphate; PCr = phosphocreatine; PDE = phosphodiester; PET = positron-emission tomography; Pi = inorganic phosphate; PME = phosphomonoester; WMSH = white matter signal hyperintensities.

ages. They did find that the Cho, Cr, and NAA levels in the cortical and subcortical gray matter containing the caudate and putamen decreased with age. The authors point out that the reduction in metabolite concentrations in this region corresponds with previously reported age-related morphometric changes here also. Charles et al. address here an issue that is central to MRS data analysis, that is, the need to correlate "volumetric observations in MRI with metabolic observations in MRS" or more generally, correcting for the general atrophy of our brains as we age.

^{31}P magnetic resonance spectroscopy studies of brains of patients with Alzheimer's disease. As mentioned above, most MRS studies in the geriatric population have sought to find alterations in metabolite concentrations specific to the most common types of dementia with the intention of 1) *understanding* the metabolic processes in each disease, 2) *diagnosing* dementia causes, and 3) *tracking disease progression and response to treatment.* One of the more promising findings so far involves alterations in PME and PDE levels in the brains of patients with AD that might distinguish AD from normal aging (Pettegrew et al. 1988). In a series of in vitro studies, Pettegrew et al. found that, in normal aging, PME levels decreased while PDE levels increased (Pettegrew et al. 1987, 1990), but that, in early AD, PME levels increased.

Because PME and PDE are involved in membrane phospholipid synthesis and breakdown, alterations of these metabolites suggest increased membrane turnover.

Brown et al. in 1989 replicated Pettegrew's finding in vivo. They observed elevations in percentage of PME and PME/PDE in the temporoparietal region significant enough to differentiate patients with AD from control subjects and those with multi-infarct dementia (MID). But, in 1992, Bottomley et al. found no such alterations in any metabolites (PCr/NTP, PCr/Pi, PDE/NTP, PME/NTP, Pi/NTP, PDE/PME) after correcting for the atrophy of the brains of their patients with AD, as measured by MRI. Murphy et al. in 1993 also found no changes in PME and PDE levels in patients with AD as compared with control subjects after correcting for atrophy. Later, in 1993, Brown et al. again found elevated PME levels in the frontal regions of brains of patients with AD compared with brains of control subjects and subjects with MID, but no change in the temporoparietal regions of all three groups. In 1995, Cuénod found increased levels of PME in the brains of patients with early AD, in agreement with Brown et al. and in disagreement with Bottomley et al., even after correcting for brain atrophy. Cuénod suggests that differences in the techniques of acquiring spectrographic data might actually account for the different results. Smith et al. in 1995 found no significant differences in PME or PDE between pa-

TABLE 11–4. Chronological table of proton ^{1}H magnetic resonance spectroscopy (MRS) studies relevant to geriatric neuropsychiatry

Study	Subjects	Purpose	Results
Sappey-Marinier et al. 1992b	7 control 7 stroke 7 WMSH	To test hypothesis of coexistent ischemia in brain infarcts and WMSH as evidenced by increased lactate levels To test hypothesis that brain infarct and WMSH are associated with greater loss of neurons than other cells as evidenced by decrease in NAA	In patients with stroke, increased lactate and decreased NAA. For patients with WMSH, no changes in proton metabolites except Cho, which was increased.
Ford et al. 1992	8 cerebral infarction 5 control	To investigate the time course and distribution of bio-chemical changes after stroke	6 patients had decreased NAA/PCr and NAA/Cr. Greater decreases correlated with least recovery of function. Lactate was observed in infarcted region 9 and 11 days after stroke.
Christiansen et al. 1993	Healthy volunteers 8 in 20s and 30s 8 in 60s and 70s	To observe differences in NAA, Cr + PCr, and Cho in different brain regions (occipital, basal ganglia, temporal, frontal) in two different age groups	Within younger group, NAA was higher in occipital than other areas. No other significant regional variations. NAA levels were higher in occipital area in younger group compared with that in older. No significant regional or age-related variation in T1 and T2 relaxation times.
Shiino et al. 1993	9 PDD 3 NPH 21 control, age 21–72	To investigate metabolic changes associated with dementia	No age-related changes in NAA/Cr in volunteer control subjects. NAA/Cr reduced in PDD. No reduction in NAA/Cr in NPH.
Charles et al. 1994	34 healthy volunteers (15 men, 19 women) between the ages of 21 and 75	To assess the effect of age and gender on brain metabolites	No differences between men and women. NAA, Cho, Cr, Cho/NAA, and Cho/Cr were lower in white matter than in gray matter. Cho, Cr, and NAA were lower in cortical and subcortical gray matter of older individuals.
Meyerhoff et al. 1994	8 AD 10 healthy control	To survey large sections of brains of patients with AD to see if cortical loss in AD measured in vitro is also detectable in vivo To see if alterations in NAA levels in brains of patients with AD correlate with atrophy as estimated from structural MRI	NAA was lower throughout the white matter of brains of patients with AD. NAA/Cho was lower and the Cho/Cr higher in mesial gray matter of subjects with AD compared with that of control subjects. Posterior section of centrum semiovale of brains of patients with AD showed increased Cho/Cr and Cho/NAA ratios with NAA/Cr unchanged between patients with AD and control subjects.
Christiansen et al. 1995	12 AD 8 control	To survey absolute differences in metabolite levels using the unsaturated water signal as an internal standard; also, with varied echo times and repetition times, to estimate the T1 and T2 relaxation times of the three metabolites	NAA concentration lower in patients with AD than in control subjects. No significant difference found for any other metabolite ratios. The only significant difference in signal ratios was that, at TE = 92 msec and TR = 1.6 seconds, the NAA/Cho ratio was lower in patients with AD.

(continued)

TABLE 11–4. Chronological table of proton ^{1}H magnetic resonance spectroscopy (MRS) studies relevant to geriatric neuropsychiatry *(continued)*

Study	Subjects	Purpose	Results
Bowen et al. 1995	14 Parkinson's disease 13 healthy control	To determine whether the proton spectra from patients with clinically diagnosed Parkinson's disease differ from that of control subjects with respect to major cerebral metabolite resonances as well as lactate	No significant difference in NAA/Cr or NAA/Cho between patients with Parkinson's disease and control subjects. A significant increase was found in lactate/NAA for patients with Parkinson's disease compared with that for control subjects.
Shonk et al. 1995	65 AD 39 other dementias 10 FLD 98 medical patients without dementia 32 healthy control subjects	To distinguish patients with AD from those with other dementias and from the elderly without dementia	Reduced levels of NAA and increased levels of MI characterized AD. Patients with other dementias had reduced NAA, but normal MI. Using MI/NAA, patients with AD differed from normals, with 83% sensitivity and 98% specificity. Using MI/Cr, patients with other dementias were distinguished from those with AD and FLD with negative predictive rate of 80%, sensitivity of 82%, and specificity of 64%.
Constans et al. 1995	21 elderly control 8 WMSH 11 probable AD with WMSH 8 IVD with WMSH	To investigate the association of WMSH with changes in ^{1}H metabolites	Differences in regional metabolite levels were found within supraventricular brain of elderly control subjects. In patients with AD, extensive WMSHs showed a lower percentage of NAA and a higher percentage of Cho compared with contralateral normal-appearing white matter. In patients with IVD, extensive and large WMSHs were associated with a higher percentage of Cho and a lower percentage of Cr compared with contralateral normal-appearing white matter.
MacKay et al. 1996	14 AD 8 SIVD 18 elderly control	To study differences in neuron density (NAA), membrane phospholipid metabolites (Cho), and creatine-containing metabolites (Cr + PCr) in subjects with AD (SIVD) and elderly control subjects	Lower levels of NAA/Cho and NAA/Cr and higher levels of Cho/Cr in both gray and white matter in subjects with AD. Lower levels of NAA/Cho and higher levels of Cho/Cr in posterior gray matter of subjects with AD. Subjects with SIVD had lower gray and white matter NAA/Cr levels. NAA/Cr level was lower in frontal white matter of subjects with SIVD compared with control subjects.

(continued)

TABLE 11–4. Chronological table of proton ^{1}H magnetic resonance spectroscopy (MRS) studies relevant to geriatric neuropsychiatry *(continued)*

Study	Subjects	Purpose	Results
Parnetti et al. 1996	6 DAT 6 AAMI 6 cognitively healthy control	To examine neuroanatomical (MRI), perfusional (SPECT), and neurochemical (^{1}H MRS) differences among groups	Lower NAA concentration in brains of patients with DAT and AAMI compared with that in control subjects. Mean inositol concentration was higher in brains of patients with DAT than in brains of control subjects. MRI showed reduced hippocampal formation in patients with DAT and those with AAMI. SPECT showed frontal, temporoparietal, and occipital hypoperfusion only in patients with DAT.
Kattapong et al. 1996	10 DAT 8 vascular dementia	To identify biochemical differences in brain tissue between patients with DAT and those with vascular dementia	NAA/Cr and NAA/Cho were lower in regions of subcortical white matter in patients with vascular dementia compared with those with DAT.
Frederick et al. 1997	47 AD 16 control	To test the hypothesis that differences in MRS metabolite resonance ratios are more pronounced in the temporal lobe than in the parietal lobe	No significant differences in parietal lobe metabolite ratios between patients with AD and control subjects, but a decrease was found in NAA/Cr in temporal lobe of the AD group compared with control subjects.
Parnetti et al. 1997	13 AD 7 control	To evaluate the pattern of ^{1}H MRS in the gray and white matter of patients with AD compared with that of control subjects	In patients with AD, NAA levels decreased in both gray and white matter, and MI increased in gray matter. The gray matter NAA/MI ratio clearly separated the two groups.

Note. AAMI = age-associated memory impairment; AD = Alzheimer's disease; Cho = choline; Cr = creatine; DAT = dementia of the Alzheimer type; FLD = frontal lobe dementia; IVD = ischemic vascular dementia; MI = *myo*-inositol; MRI = magnetic resonance imaging; NAA = *N*-acetyl-L-aspartate; NPH = normal pressure hydrocephalus; PCr = phosphocreatine; PDD = primary degenerative dementia; SIVD = subcortical ischemic vascular dementia; SPECT = single photon emission computed tomography; TE = echo time; TR = repetition time; WMSH = white matter signal hyperintensities.

tients with AD and elderly control subjects but surprisingly did find decreased levels of PME and increased levels of PDE in women with AD as compared with men with AD. They found similar but not as pronounced differences in the elderly control group. In 1996, Gonzaléz et al. found no changes in absolute PME and PDE levels between patients with AD and control subjects but did find significantly decreased levels of PME/PDE, probably as a result of decreases in overall level of PDE. Gonzaléz et al. also point out that the discrepancies between their study and previous ones might be attributable to technical issues of data acquisition or analysis.

Conclusions of magnetic resonance spectroscopy and aging. Obviously, the field of MRS con-

tinues to evolve as researchers further develop techniques of data acquisition and interpretation. Spectroscopy offers the enormous potential of providing noninvasive information about brain neurochemistry in a host of diseases involving a geriatric population. Most MRS studies in the geriatric population have sought to find alterations in metabolite concentrations specific to the most common types of dementia with the intention of 1) *understanding* the metabolic processes in each disease, 2) *diagnosing* dementia causes, and 3) *tracking disease progression and response to treatment.* To date, no firm conclusions have been reached in any of these three areas, although progress is rapid in all. MRS cannot at this time be used to diagnose a dementia. Ongoing studies will soon reveal whether MRS has utility as a marker for disease progression, which would supplement clinical ratings. The next few years should see many studies assessing the sensitivity and repeatability of spectroscopy in understanding, diagnosing, and following neuropsychiatric diseases of the elderly.

Functional Magnetic Resonance Imaging

Blood Oxygen Level–Dependent Functional Magnetic Resonance Imaging

Blood oxygen level–dependent (BOLD)-fMRI is currently the most commonly used fMRI technique (Table 11–5). For BOLD imaging, the MRI scanner is tuned to resonate and image hydrogen atoms as in conventional MRI; however, T2*-weighted images are performed, which take advantage of the fact that deoxygenated hemoglobin is magnetic, whereas oxygenated hemoglobin is not (Kwong et al. 1992; Turner et al. 1991). Because of the magnetic properties of the unflipped magnetic deoxyhemoglobin molecule, which causes rapid dephasing, T2* signal is retained longer in a region when it has more oxygenated blood compared with when there is less oxygenated blood. An activated brain region has relatively more oxygenated blood compared with when it is resting. Thus, an area with more oxygenated blood will show up more intense on T2*-weighted images compared to when there is less oxygenated blood around. With this technique, it is assumed that when a brain region is active, arterial oxygenated blood will redistribute and increase to this area (Sokoloff 1977, 1978). Importantly, there is a time lag of 2–6 seconds between when a brain region is activated and when blood flow increases (Kwong et al. 1992; Turner et al. 1991). During the initial fraction of a second after increased neuronal activity, the activated areas experience a relative decrease in oxygenated blood as oxygen is extracted by the active regional neurons. Afterward, the amount of blood flowing to the entire area far outweighs the amount of oxygen that is extracted so that the level of oxygenated blood is now higher. Some have said that the brain floods the entire garden (region) for want of one thirsty flower (a small group of active neurons). Although new MRI machines can acquire images every 100 msec with echoplanar imaging, a type of rapid acquisition, this predictable but time-varied delayed onset of the BOLD response limits the immediate temporal resolution to several seconds instead of the 100-msec potential. In the future, researchers may be able to improve the temporal resolution of fMRI by measuring the initial decrease in oxygenated blood rather than the later flood of oxygen (Menon et al. 1995). Additionally, many researchers are us-

ing BOLD fMRI to look at brain changes after a single event rather than a repeated task over several seconds. Single-event MRI may offer improved temporal resolution.

BOLD fMRI is a relative technique in that it must compare images taken during one mental state to another to create a meaningful picture. Because images are acquired very rapidly (e.g., a set of 30 coronal brain slices every 3 seconds is commonly done at the Medical University of South Carolina [MUSC]), one can acquire enough images to measure the relative differences between two states to perform a statistical analysis within a single individual. Ideally, these states would differ in only one aspect so that everything is controlled for except the behavior in question. BOLD fMRI paradigms generally have several periods of rest alternating with several periods of activation. Images are then compared over the entire activation to the rest periods. Images obtained over the first 3–6 seconds of each period are generally discarded because of the delay in hemodynamic response. Alternating paradigms are used because the signal intensity generated by the MRI scanner drifts with time. Typically, one compares activity between task and rest and then generates a statistical map of regions that are significantly changed during the task. This statistical map is then merged onto a structural MRI scan obtained in the same slices (see Figure 11–3).

With current technology, BOLD fMRI is best used for studying processes that can be rapidly turned on and off, such as language, vision, movement, hearing, and memory.

TABLE 11–5. Blood oxygen level–dependent (BOLD) functional MRI (fMRI)

Based on

- Differential magnetic properties of deoxyhemoglobin and oxyhemoglobin
- Coupling of oxygenated blood flow and neuronal activity

High spatial and temporal resolution

2- to 6-second delay in blood flow response limits optimal temporal resolution

With rapid scanning, one compares images taken during active and rest states within an individual within a single session

Inferior frontal and temporal areas vulnerable to air-tissue artifacts

Very sensitive to movement and thus has not been used much so far in geriatric populations

Technique has good potential to

- Show brain activity during memory tasks
- Help understand pathophysiology
- Perhaps be used in diagnosis and treatment monitoring

1.5 Tesa PICKER MRI-whole body high performance gradients

Image analysis

1. Motion check—MEDx (discard if > 5mm)

2. Coregistration—Automatic Image Registration

3. Student's T-Tests across comparisons-T-Map

4. Particle analysis (conservative double screen)

- Convert to z, with degrees of freedom

- Threshold z at $p < 0.001$ (3.09)

- Assign new weighting based on clusters ($P < 0.05$)

5. Merge particle map onto structure images

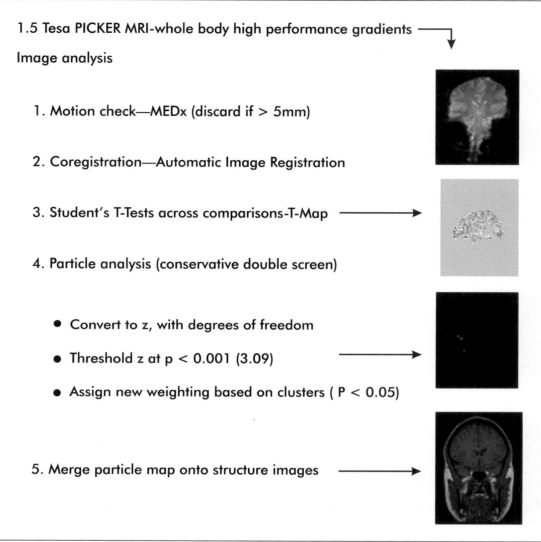

FIGURE 11–3.   An outline of the image analysis steps used in blood oxygen level–dependent functional magnetic resonance imaging analysis.

The true power of BOLD fMRI for examining subtle mental processes was demonstrated in the study by Whalen and colleagues (1998). They used a backward masking procedure to present three alternating conditions to 10 subjects: 1) a baseline condition, in which subjects would see a "+" sign; 2) a "happy" (H) condition, in which subjects would see repeated presentations of 33 msec of a happy face followed by 167 msec of a neutral face; and 3) a "fear" (F) condition, in which subjects would see repeated presentations of 33 msec of a fearful face followed by 167 msec of a neutral face. Here, fearful and happy faces were presented in such a way that 8 of the 10 participants could not identify them. Despite their lack of conscious awareness of the emotive faces, subjects had relatively increased amygdala activation with fearful faces and relatively decreased amygdala activation with the happy faces, indicating that they must have processed the information at an unconscious level.

Unfortunately, BOLD fMRI is sensitive to movement so that tasks are limited to those without head movement, including speaking, which, of course, also severely limits its use in patients with dementia or those who are agitated. (With single-event fMRI, however, one cannot image during movement [speech], but because there is a 3–6 second delay in blood flow to the region, instead one must image after the task, when movement stops.) Another limitation of BOLD fMRI is that artifacts often appear on scans in brain regions that are close to air (i.e., sinuses), which cause problems in observing regions at the base of the brain such as the orbitofrontal and mediotemporal cortices. Sometimes observed areas of activation may be located more in large draining veins rather than directly at a capillary bed near the site of neuronal activation, which also complicates the interpretation of these scans (Moseley et al. 1996).

Neurologists and neurosurgeons are beginning to use

this technique clinically to noninvasively map language, motor, and memory function in patients undergoing neurosurgery (Binder 1997; Binder et al. 1996; Bookheimer 1996; Jack et al. 1994). Currently, there are no indications for BOLD fMRI in clinical psychiatry, although this technique holds considerable promise for unraveling the neuroanatomical basis of neuropsychiatric diseases. BOLD fMRI may be of potential help in sorting out diagnostic heterogeneity and treatment planning in the future.

A large literature documents that brain blood flow at rest and in response to cortical tasks declines with age. Several PET studies have reported that brain blood flow activation is reduced in elderly subjects who are shown a checkerboard or asked to move their fingers (Melamed et al. 1980). Ross and colleagues used fMRI to test this hypothesis that blood flow response to tasks declines with increasing age (Ross et al. 1997). They used echoplanar BOLD fMRI imaging of changes as a result of photic stimulation in 9 elderly subjects (average age 71) and 17 young control subjects (average age 24). The magnitude of the BOLD response was reduced in the elderly subjects (2.5% increase in the elderly compared with an average 4% increase in the younger group).

All of these activation studies employ some aspect of the peripheral nervous system to elicit brain changes. Our group at MUSC has recently been able to stimulate the brain directly and noninvasively with transcranial magnetic stimulation (TMS), thus bypassing the peripheral nervous system, while also acquiring BOLD fMRI responses. Although this work is still in progress, there does not appear to be a decline with age (Figure 11–4). An important confound is that the distance from the coil to cortex matters a great deal in TMS (the magnetic field falls off logarithmically), and this distance does increase with age. More work is necessary with this novel combination method before it can be reliably used to test the generally accepted notion that a mild decline in blood flow response to activation does occur as people age.

Perfusion Functional Magnetic Resonance Imaging

Two fMRI methods have been developed for directly measuring cerebral blood flow. The first method, called intravenous bolus tracking, relies on the intravenous injection of a magnetic compound such as a gadolinium-containing contrast agent and measuring its T2*-weighted signal as it perfuses through the brain over a short period of time (Belliveau et al. 1991; Rosen et al. 1991). Areas perfused with the magnetic compound show less signal intensity as the compound creates a magnetic inhomogeneity that de-

creases the T2* signal. The magnetic compound may be injected once during the control and once during the activation task, and relative differences in blood flow between the two states may be determined to develop a perfusion image; alternatively, one can measure changes in blood flow over time after a single injection to generate a perfusion map. Belliveau et al. (1991) used the technique to create the first functional magnetic resonance maps of human task activation using a visual stimulation paradigm. They imaged the occipital lobe after injecting gadolinium–diethylenetriamine pentaacetic acid once during darkness and again during a flashing light to map the visual response. They made a statistical comparison between images obtained during visual stimulation versus those obtained during darkness to generate an image.

Although gadolinium-based contrasts are not radioactive, the number of boluses that can be given to an individual is limited by the potential for kidney toxicity with repeated tracer administration. Also, this technique generates a map of only relative cerebral blood flow, not absolute flow, as in the technique described below. Several groups have used gadolinium bolus perfusion MRI in elderly subjects, with promising initial results. González and colleagues (1995) performed fluorodeoxyglucose PET (measuring glucose metabolism) and then in the same 10 subjects assessed relative regional perfusion using fMRI. The subjects had a range of diagnoses from AD (6) to Pick's disease (1) and primary progressive aphasia (1). These researchers found that abnormal areas of metabolism also had abnormal flow as measured by the new fMRI technique.

Mattay and colleagues (1996) performed an exploratory perfusion fMRI study in 4 young control subjects, 6 psychiatrically healthy elderly control subjects (average age 71 years), and 6 matched elderly patients with senile dementia, Alzheimer type. All subjects also received perfusion SPECT. The perfusion fMRI scans were of good quality with little motion artifact (motion artifact was seen in the SPECT studies and was likely a result of a longer acquisition time). All subjects with senile dementia, Alzheimer type, showed decreased perfusion in the temporoparietal cortex. Unfortunately, the perfusion fMRI also showed decreased cortical activity in 2 elderly healthy control subjects (false-positives). In a more formal study, Harris and colleagues (1996) used bolus fMRI to study 13 patients with AD and 13 matched control subjects. Relative activity in temporoparietal cortex was decreased in the group with AD. Relative motor cortex activity did not differ. These two studies demonstrate that bolus perfusion MRI likely can be used to differentiate brain activity in patients with AD compared with that in control subjects. Larger pro-

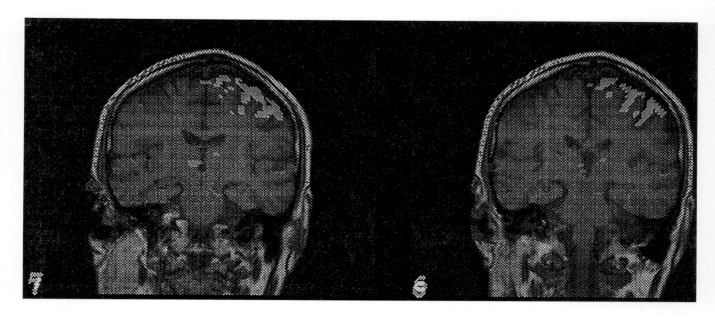

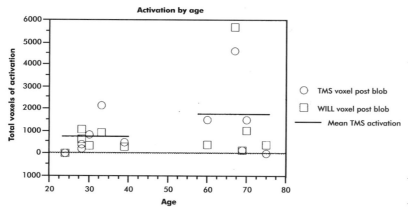

FIGURE 11–4.   Brain activity during transcranial magnetic stimulation (TMS)/functional magnetic resonance imaging over motor cortex from work done at the Medical University of South Carolina. Note in the graph on the *bottom* no significant decline with increased age across a small cohort. This is contrary to other studies, which have found that blood flow response to stimulation declines with increasing age. "WILL" denotes activity during volitional or willful movement.

spective studies in a more heterogeneous clinical sample are needed before making a final conclusion about the ultimate clinical utility of this form of MRI to diagnose and monitor AD.

Arterial spin labeling is a T1-weighted noninvasive technique in which intrinsic hydrogen atoms in arterial water outside of the slice of interest are magnetically tagged ("flipped") as they course through the blood and are then imaged as they enter the slice of interest (Table 11–6) (Bohning et al. 1996a, 1996b; Warach et al. 1994). In contrast to the gadolinium bolus perfusion method described above, arterial spin labeling is noninvasive, does not involve an intravenous bolus injection, and can thus be repeatedly performed in individual subjects. Also, absolute regional blood flow can be measured, which cannot be eas-

TABLE 11–6.   Arterial spin-labeling functional magnetic resonance imaging (fMRI)

Provides for magnetic tagging of hydrogen atoms as they course through the blood and imaging them as they course through the slice of interest

Measures absolute blood flow

Directly compares data taken in different imaging sessions

Is suited to measuring state differences between groups (e.g., patients with Alzheimer's disease versus psychiatrically healthy control subjects)

ily measured with SPECT or BOLD fMRI and which requires an arterial line with PET. Because absolute information is obtained, cerebral blood flow can be serially measured over separate imaging sessions, such as measuring blood flow in subjects with bipolar disorder as they course through different disease states (Speer et al. 1997). Absolute blood flow information may be important in imaging such processes as anxiety, which may be hard to turn on and off. For instance, in patients with AD, a medication-free cognitive task may be imaged on one day, and performing the same task following a single dose of a medication may be imaged on the next day. Comparing these separate tasks in different imaging sessions would not be possible with BOLD fMRI. Figure 11–5 shows an example of the arterial spin-labeling technique from MUSC as applied to understanding the pathological changes in advanced AD.

Our group at MUSC has had difficulty implementing this arterial spin-labeling perfusion fMRI technique to diagnose AD as a result of the low signal-to-noise ratio of this tool, although we are hopeful that better analysis of the time curves will improve our data (Mirski et al. 1998). Sandson and colleagues recently successfully demonstrated that their version of this technique revealed differences in blood flow in 11 patients with AD compared with 8 psychiatrically healthy age-matched control subjects (Sandson et al. 1996). Further, they found that parieto-occipital hypoperfusion correlated with dementia (i.e., the more severe the dementia, the less blood flow in this region). It thus now remains for research groups to refine this technique and see if it can detect more subtle brain changes in early AD or even before symptoms manifest. This technique thus offers much promise in dementia diagnosis and follow-up because during one MRI scanning session one can accurately detect blood flow changes resulting from ischemia and measure brain volume in key structures such

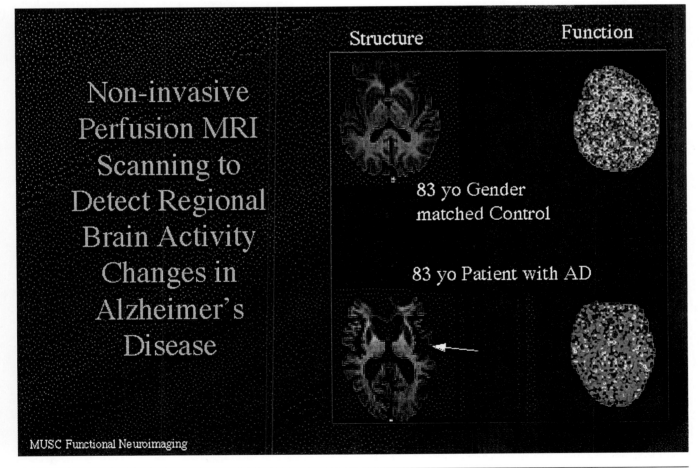

FIGURE 11–5. A transverse structural magnetic resonance imaging (MRI) scan (*left*) and spin-labeled perfusion functional MRI (*right*) from a psychiatrically healthy control subject (*top*) and patient with Alzheimer's disease (AD) (*bottom*). Note the atrophy in the brain of the patient with AD as well as the decreased perfusion both globally and in parietal cortex. yo = year old.
Source. From Mirski D, Greenshields AJ, Mintzer J, et al.: "Perfusion Studies of Patients with Alzheimer's Disease." Abstract presented at the Annual Meeting of the American Association of Geriatric Psychiatry, San Diego, CA, June 1998.

as the hippocampus, while at the same time detecting perfusion defects associated with classical AD, all with the elegance of 1-mm resolution. Although there is currently no clinical indication for this MRI perfusion technique, it may soon be used clinically to help characterize the different stages of acute ischemic stroke (Fisher et al. 1995).

Summary

Functional MRI scanning is an area in its infancy. However, already it is apparent that fMRI can noninvasively provide several types of information that will undoubtedly be helpful in understanding and treating neuropsychiatric diseases in later life. MRS is still unproven but promises to serve as a noninvasive marker of disease progression in AD. An explosion of BOLD fMRI studies is mapping which brain regions are involved in performing different cognitive tasks. Most of this work is initially focusing on healthy young adults. Work in the next few years will likely begin addressing how the brain changes over time and whether the general conclusions about brain mapping drawn from young cohorts also apply to the elderly. Perfusion MRI has already been shown to distinguish subjects with AD from those with other forms of dementia. Widespread adoption of this tool in diagnosing and monitoring treatment awaits larger studies showing clinical utility and cost-effectiveness.

Although these advanced techniques have a limited role now, over the next few years these methods likely will become increasingly more a part of general clinical practice, provided that minor technical hurdles are overcome and that the early studies show that MRI can truly make a cost-effective difference in clinical care.

References

Belliveau JW, Kennedy DN, McKinstry RC, et al: Functional mapping of the human visual cortex by magnetic resonance imaging. Science 254:716–719, 1991

Belmaker RH, Livne A, Agam G, et al: Role of inositol-1-phosphatase inhibition in the mechanism of action of lithium. Pharmacol Toxicol 66 (suppl 3):76–83, 1990

Binder JR: Neuroanatomy of language processing studies with functional MRI. Clin Neurosci 4:87–94, 1997

Binder JR, Swanson SJ, Hammeke TA, et al: Determination of language dominance using functional MRI: a comparison with the Wada test. Neurology 46:978–984, 1996

Bohning DE, Wright AC, Pecheny AP, et al: Perfusion phantom for quantitative spin labelling and Gd tracer-based perfusion measurements (abstract). American Association of Physicists in Medicine, 1996a

Bohning DE, Wright AC, Pecheny AP, et al: Repeatability of spin label-based in vivo perfusion maps (abstract). Neuroimage 3:S128, 1996b

Bookheimer SY: Functional MRI applications in clinical epilepsy. Neuroimage 4:S139–S146, 1996

Bottomley PA, Cousins JP, Pendrey DL, et al: Alzheimer dementia: quantification of energy metabolism and mobile phosphoesters with P-31 NMR spectroscopy. Radiology 183:695–699, 1992

Bowen BC, Block RE, Sanchez-Ramos J, et al: Proton MR spectroscopy of the brain in 14 patients with Parkinson disease. AJNR Am J Neuroradiol 16:61–68, 1995

Brown GG, Levine SR, Gorell JM, et al: In vivo P31 NMR profiles of Alzheimer's disease and multiple subcortical infarct dementia. Neurology 39:1423–1427, 1989

Brown GG, Garcia JH, Gdowski JW, et al: Altered brain energy metabolism in demented patients with multiple subcortical ischemic lesions. Arch Neurol 50:384–388, 1993

Chance B, Nakase Y, Bond M, et al: Detection of ^{31}P nuclear magnetic resonance signals in brain by in vivo and freeze-trapped assays. Proc Natl Acad Sci U S A 75:4925–4929, 1978

Charles HC, Lazeyras F, Krishnan KR, et al: Proton spectroscopy of human brain: effects of age and sex. Prog Neuropsychopharmacol Biol Psychiatry 18:995–1004, 1994

Charles HC, Snyderman TB, Ahearn E: Magnetic resonance spectroscopy, in Brain Imaging in Clinical Psychiatry. Edited by Krishnan KRR, Doraiswarmy PM. New York, Marcel Dekker, 1997, pp 13–21

Christiansen P, Toft P, Larsson HB, et al: The concentration of N-acetyl aspartate, creatine + phosphocreatine, and choline in different parts of the brain in adulthood and senium. Magn Reson Imaging 11:799–806, 1993

Christiansen P, Schlosser A, Henriksen O: Reduced N-acetylaspartate content in the frontal part of the brain in patients with probable Alzheimer's disease. Magn Reson Imaging 13:457–462, 1995

Cohen BM, Renshaw PF, Stoll AL, et al: Decreased brain choline uptake in older adults: an in vivo proton magnetic resonance spectroscopy study. JAMA 274:902–907, 1995

Constans JM, Meyerhoff DJ, Gerson J, et al: H-1 MR spectroscopic imaging of white matter signal hyperintensities: Alzheimer disease and ischemic vascular dementia. Radiology 197:517–523, 1995

Cuenod CA, Kaplan DB, Michot JL, et al: Phospholipid abnormalities in early Alzheimer's disease: in vivo phosphorus 31 magnetic resonance spectroscopy. Arch Neurol 52:89–94, 1995

Fisher M, Prichard JW, Warach S: New magnetic resonance techniques for acute ischemic stroke. JAMA 274:908–911, 1995

Ford CC, Griffey RH, Matwiyoff NA, et al: Multivoxel H1-MRS of stroke. Neurology 42:1408–1412, 1992

Frederick B, Satlin A, Yurgelun-Todd DA, et al: In vivo proton magnetic resonance spectroscopy of Alzheimer's disease in the parietal and temporal lobes. Biol Psychiatry 42:147–150, 1997

González RG, Fischman AJ, Guimaraes AR, et al: Functional MR in the evaluation of dementia: correlations of abnormal dynamic cerebral blood volume measurements with changes in cerebral metabolism on positron emission tomography with fluorodeoxyglucose F 18. AJR Am J Neuroradiol 16:1763–1770, 1995

González RG, Guimaraes AR, Moore GJ, et al: Quantitative in vivo ^{31}P magnetic resonance spectroscopy of Alzheimer disease. Alzheimer Dis Assoc Disord 10:46–52, 1996

Gupta RK, Gupta P, Moore RD: NMR studies of intracellular metal ions in intact cells and tissues. Annual Review of Biophysics and Bioengineering 13:221–246, 1984

Harris GJ, Lewis RF, Satlin A, et al: Dynamic susceptibility contrast MRI of regional cerebral blood volume in Alzheimer's disease. Am J Psychiatry 153:721–724, 1996

Iotti S, Frassineti C, Alderighi L: In vivo assessment of free magnesium concentration in human brain by 31P MRS: a new calibration curve based on a mathematical algorithm. NMR Biomed 9:24–32, 1996

Jack CR, Thompson RM, Butts RK, et al: Sensory motor cortex: correlation of presurgical mapping with functional MR imaging and invasive cortical mapping. Radiology 190:85–92, 1994

Kato T, Inubushi T, Kato N: Magnetic resonance spectroscopy in affective disorders. J Neuropsychiatry Clin Neurosci 10:133–147, 1998

Kattapong VJ, Brooks WM, Wesley MH, et al: Proton magnetic resonance spectroscopy of vascular- and Alzheimer-type dementia. Arch Neurol 53:678–680, 1996

Khoury SJ, Weiner HL: Multiple sclerosis: what have we learned from magnetic resonance imaging studies? Arch Intern Med 158:565–573, 1998

Komoroski RA, Newton JE, Cardwell D, et al: In vivo 19F spin relaxation and localized spectroscopy of fluoxetine in human brain. Magn Reson Med 31:204–211, 1994

Kwong KK, Belliveau JW, Chesler DA, et al: Dynamic magnetic resonance imaging of human brain activity during primary sensory stimulation. Proc Natl Acad Sci U S A 89:5675–5679, 1992

Longo R, Giorgini A, Magnali S, et al: Alzheimer's disease histologically proven studied by MRI and MRS: two cases. Magn Reson Imaging 11:1209–1215, 1993

Lorberbaum JP, Bohning DE, Shastri A, et al: Functional magnetic resonance imaging (fMRI) for the psychiatrist. Primary Psychiatry 5:60–66, 1998

MacKay S, Meyerhoff DJ, Constans JM, et al: Regional gray and white matter metabolite differences in subjects with AD, with subcortical ischemic vascular dementia, and elderly controls with ^{1}H magnetic resonance spectroscopic imaging. Arch Neurol 53:167–174, 1996

Mattay VS, Frank JA, Duyn JH, et al: Three-dimensional "BURST" functional magnetic resonance imaging: initial clinical applications. Acad Radiol 3:S379–S383, 1996

Melamed E, Lavy S, Bentin S, et al: Reduction in regional cerebral blood flow during normal aging in man. Stroke 11:31–35, 1980

Menon RS, Ogawa S, Hu X, et al: BOLD based functional MRI at 4 Tesla includes a capillary bed contribution: echo-planar imaging correlates with previous optical imaging using intrinsic signals. Magn Reson Med 33:453–459, 1995

Meyerhoff DJ, MacKay S, Constans JM, et al: Axonal injury and membrane alterations in Alzheimer's disease suggested by in vivo proton magnetic resonance spectroscopic imaging. Ann Neurol 36:40–47, 1994

Mirski D, Greenshields AJ, Mintzer J, et al: Perfusion studies of patients with Alzheimer's disease. Abstract presented at the Annual Meeting of the American Association of Geriatric Psychiatry, San Diego, CA, June 1998

Moore CM, Renshaw PF: Magnetic resonance spectroscopy studies of affective disorders, in Brain Imaging in Clinical Psychiatry. Edited by Krishnan KRR, Doraiswarmy PM. New York, Marcel Dekker, 1997, pp 185–213

Moseley ME, deCrespigny A, Spielman DM: Magnetic resonance imaging of human brain function. Surgical Neurology 45:385–391, 1996

Murphy DGM, Bottomley PA, Salerno JA, et al: An in vivo study of phosphorus and glucose metabolism in Alzheimer's disease using magnetic resonance spectroscopy and PET. Arch Gen Psychiatry 50:341–349, 1993

Parnetti L, Lowenthal DT, Presciutti O, et al: 1H-MRS, MRI-based hippocampal volumetry, and ^{99m}Tc-HMPAO-SPECT in normal aging, age-associated memory impairment, and probable Alzheimer's disease. J Am Geriatr Soc 44:133–138, 1996

Parnetti L, Tarducci R, Presciutti O, et al: Proton magnetic resonance spectroscopy can differentiate Alzheimer's disease from normal aging. Mech Ageing Dev 97:9–14, 1997

Pettegrew JW, Withers G, Panchalingam K, et al: ^{31}P nuclear magnetic resonance (NMR) spectroscopy of brain in aging and Alzheimer's disease. J Neural Transm 24 (suppl):261–268, 1987

Pettegrew JW, Panchalingam K, Moossy J, et al: Correlation of phosphorus-31 magnetic resonance spectroscopy and morphological findings in Alzheimer's disease. Arch Neurol 45:1093–1096, 1988

Pettegrew JW, Panchalingam K, Withers G, et al: Changes in brain energy and phospholipid metabolism during development and aging in the Fischer 344 rat. J Neuropathol Exp Neurol 49:237–249, 1990

Pettegrew JW, Klunk WE, Panchalingam K, et al: Clinical and neurochemical effects of acetyl-L-carnitine in Alzheimer's disease. Neurobiol Aging 16:1–4, 1995

Ramasamy R, Mota de Freitas DM: Competition between Li$^+$ and Mg^{2+} for ATP in human erythrocytes. FEBS Lett 244:223–226, 1989

Rosen BR, Belliveau JW, Aronen HJ, et al: Susceptibility contrast imaging of cerebral blood volume: human experience. Magn Reson Med 22:293–299, 1991

Ross B, Michaelis T: Clinical applications of magnetic resonance spectroscopy. Magnetic Resonance Quarterly 10: 191–247, 1994

Ross MH, Yurgelun-Todd DA, Renshaw PF, et al: Age-related reduction in functional MRI response to photic stimulation. Neurology 48:173–176, 1997

Sandson TA, O'Connor M, Sperling RA, et al: Noninvasive perfusion MRI in Alzheimer's disease: a preliminary report. Neurology 47:1339–1342, 1996

Sappey-Marinier DS, Deicken RF, Fein G, et al: Alterations in brain phosphorus metabolite concentrations associated with areas of high signal intensity in white matter at MR imaging. Radiology 183:247–256, 1992a

Sappey-Marinier DS, Calabrese G, Hetherington HP, et al: Proton magnetic resonance spectroscopy of human brain: applications to normal white matter, chronic infarction, and MRI white matter signal hyperintensities. Magn Reson Med 26:313–327, 1992b

Shiino A, Matsuda M, Morikawa S, et al: Proton magnetic resonance spectroscopy with dementia. Surg Neurol 39: 143–147, 1993

Shonk TK, Moats RA, Gifford P, et al: Probable Alzheimer's disease: diagnosis with proton MR spectroscopy. Radiology 195:65–72, 1995

Smith CD, Pettigrew LC, Avison MJ, et al: Frontal lobe phosphorus metabolism and neuropsychological function in aging and Alzheimer's disease. Ann Neurol 38:194–201, 1995

Sokoloff L: Relation between physiological function and energy metabolism in the central nervous system. J Neurochem 29:13–26, 1977

Sokoloff L: Local energy metabolism: its relationship to local functional activity and blood flow, in Cerebral Vascular Smooth Muscle and Its Control. Edited by Purves MJ, Elliott L. Amsterdam, Elsevier, 1978, pp 171–197

Speer AM, Upadhyaya VH, Bohning DE, et al: New windows into bipolar illness: serial perfusion MRI scanning in rapid-cycling bipolar patients. Abstract presented at the Annual Meeting of the American Psychiatric Association, San Diego, CA, May 1997

Turner R, Le Bihan D, Moonen CT, et al: Echo-planar time course MRI of cat brain oxygenation changes. Magn Reson Med 22:159–166, 1991

Vion-Dury J, Meyerhoff DJ, Cozzone PJ: What might be the impact in neurobiology of the analysis of brain metabolism by in vivo magnetic resonance spectroscopy? J Neurol 241:354–371, 1994

Warach S, Sievert B, Darby D, et al: EPISTAR perfusion echo-planar imaging of human brain tumors. J Magn Reson Imaging 4:S8, 1994

Whalen PJ, Rauch SL, Etcoff NL, et al: Masked presentations of emotional facial expressions modulate amygdala activity without explicit knowledge. J Neurosci 18:411–418, 1998

12

Quantitative Electroencephalography

Neurophysiological Alterations in Normal Aging and Geriatric Neuropsychiatric Disorders

Daniel P. Holschneider, M.D.

Andrew F. Leuchter, M.D.

Electroencephalography (EEG) is the oldest form of functional brain imaging. It has several advantages over newer forms of functional imaging, such as positron-emission tomography (PET) or single photon emission computed tomography (SPECT): EEG is noninvasive, inexpensive, and portable, and it can provide images based on less than 1 second of data. It also provides direct information about the functional integrity of fiber tracts, without the risk of exposure to ionizing radiation.

The central limitation of EEG has been the difficulty in relating potentials measured at the scalp surface to underlying brain physiology. Although most of the brain's energy metabolism is devoted to the production of electrical gradients and signals, brain electrical activity traditionally has been only a dim reflection of brain perfusion, metabolism, or structural integrity.

Over the past several years, significant advances have been made in our understanding of the relationship among

We thank John Mazziotta, M.D., Ph.D., and Michael Phelps, Ph.D., of the Division of Nuclear Medicine, Department of Radiology, as well as Lewis Baxter, M.D., Barry Guze, M.D., and Gary Small, M.D., of the Department of Psychiatry, UCLA School of Medicine, who supplied the PET image. We also thank Kelly Shaw, who provided expert assistance in the preparation of the manuscript and figures. This work was supported by Mentored Clinical Science Development Program Award 5-K12-AG-00521 (to D. P. H.), research grant MH40705 and Research Scientist Development Award MH01165 from the National Institute of Mental Health (to A. F. L.), and the UCLA Alzheimer's Disease Center from the National Institute on Aging (Grant P30 AG10123-05, to A. F. L.).

brain energy metabolism, structure, and electrical signal production. Driven by widespread availability of inexpensive microcomputers, quantitative EEG (QEEG) has supplanted conventional EEG in research laboratories and many clinical settings. Studies correlating alterations in electrical activity with changes in perfusion and metabolism, or with structural disease, have significantly advanced methods for QEEG signal analysis. New algorithms have established QEEG as a reliable, noninvasive method of brain imaging with significant clinical utility. In this chapter, we review the history of EEG and QEEG and discuss their potential uses in geriatric neuropsychiatry.

History of Electroencephalography

EEG was popularized in the early 20th century by a psychiatrist, Dr. Hans Berger, who demonstrated changes in the EEG with arousal, anxiety, and other emotions and activities. Enthusiasm for EEG was supported by Berger's study of the EEGs of institutionalized patients (Berger 1937), many of whom showed distinct abnormalities (particularly diffuse slowing).

Berger's suppositions about the information contained in brain electrical activity were correct, but his technology was inadequate to decode the complex information embedded in the EEG signal. Berger used a double-coil galvanometer whose oscillations moved a mirror, thereby deflecting a beam of light, which traced the EEG signal on photographic paper (Gloor 1969). Grass and Gibbs performed the first QEEG analysis in 1938, but their mechanical Fourier transform (using a rotating drum) was too cumbersome and unreliable to process large volumes of data or multiple channels simultaneously. The development of techniques through pen-and-ink recorders, and then mechanical frequency analyzers, did not provide the tools necessary to decode the complex information contained in the EEG. As a result, researchers struggled with a central irony: although most of the brain's energy metabolism was devoted to the production of electrical potentials, researchers could not realize Berger's dream of studying brain processes, and particularly cognitive functions, using EEG. As a result, the applications for EEG in neuropsychiatry have traditionally been limited.

Conventional Electroencephalography

Indications for Conventional Electroencephalography

Conventional EEG has several clinical applications in psychiatric practice, primarily in the evaluation of disorders at the interface between psychiatry and neurology. First, EEG is useful for distinguishing psychiatrically healthy elderly from those with possible dementia. The EEG of a psychiatrically healthy elderly subject may differ little from that of a psychiatrically healthy young adult (Hubbard et al. 1976; Hughes and Cayaffa 1977; Katz and Horowitz 1982). Most reports, however, suggest that, beginning in the fifth or sixth decade, one observes a decrease of 0.5–1.0 Hz in the mean frequency of the posterior dominant ("alpha") rhythm (Busse 1983; Kanowski 1971; Obrist and Busse 1965; Roubicek 1977), decreased reactivity of posterior dominant rhythm to eye opening (decreased alpha blocking) (Andermann and Stoller 1961), increased theta slow-wave activity (F. A. Gibbs and Gibbs 1951; Obrist 1979), and focal slowing, primarily in the left anterotemporal region. Focal slowing has been reported in 17%–59% of psychiatrically healthy elderly subjects (Helmchen et al. 1967; Hughes and Cayaffa 1977; Katz and Horowitz 1982; Obrist and Busse 1965; Otomo and Tsubaki 1966; Soininen et al. 1982; Torres et al. 1983; Visser et al. 1987), but, if normal, it should be intermittent and never exceed 25% of the EEG recording. Similarly, although the posterior dominant rhythm may slow somewhat, it should remain above 8 Hz in the waking state (Obrist 1979; Oken and Kaye 1992). Some researchers have noted a slight increase in high frequency (beta) activity with aging (E. Gibbs et al. 1950; Matousek et al. 1967; Mundy-Castle 1951; Obrist 1954), whereas others have found a decline in beta activity in psychiatrically healthy elderly after the sixth decade (Busse and Obrist 1965; Obrist 1976; Schlagenhauff 1973; Wang and Busse 1969).

These findings contrast with those from patients with dementia. EEG abnormalities in dementia were first reported by Berger (Berger 1937), who described gross slowing of the dominant frequency. For almost 40 years after Berger's initial reports, EEG studies of dementia described decreases in the frequency, quantity (Stoller 1949), and reactivity of the alpha rhythm (Andermann and Stoller 1961; Dejaiffe et al. 1964), as well as an excess of theta and delta slow-wave activity (McAdam and Robinson 1956; Weiner and Schuster 1956). Early reports suggested that only patients with moderately advanced dementia could be distinguished from psychiatrically healthy elderly subjects because normal EEGs were the rule in patients with the early stages of dementia (Gordon and Sim 1967; Loeb 1980; Weiner and Schuster 1956). More recently, however, it has been shown that a majority of patients with dementia have abnormal EEGs, and that fully half of individuals with equivocal impairment (Mini-Mental State Exam [MMSE] scores ≥ 24) show abnormalities (Folstein et al. 1975; Leuchter et al. 1993a). The high prevalence of abnormalities even in the early stages of the illness increases the diagnostic usefulness of the test.

Conventional EEG is a nonspecific indicator of the type of dementia. Focal abnormalities are reported to be more common in patients with vascular dementia (74% of patients) than in those with primary degenerative dementia (19% of patients) (Dejaiffe et al. 1964; Harrison et al. 1979; Logar et al. 1987; Roberts et al. 1978), but this finding is of limited diagnostic usefulness. Furthermore, some patients will have both illnesses, and their coexistence can be difficult to detect (Ettlin et al. 1989). Bilateral paroxysmal activity occurs in approximately 25% of patients with either vascular or primary degenerative dementia (Dejaiffe et al. 1964; Fortin 1966; Liddell 1958). Bifrontal, repetitive sharp waves or triphasic waves are seen in a majority of patients with Creutzfeldt-Jakob disease in early stages of the illness (Aguglia et al. 1997; Burger et al. 1972; Chiofalo et al. 1980; Steinhoff et al. 1996) but also are seen in a variety of toxic or metabolic dementias. The increase in focal abnormalities seen in vascular dementias, the low-amplitude background activity of Huntington's disease (Margerison and Scott 1965; Oltman and Friedman 1961; Scott et al. 1972), and the well-preserved posterior dominant background rhythm of Pick's disease (Groen and Endtz 1982; Johannesson et al. 1977; Tissot et al. 1975) are characteristic for groups of patients but have not proven sufficiently specific to allow confident diagnostic classification of individual subjects.

The abnormalities found in patients with dementia have not only diagnostic but also prognostic significance. These abnormalities identify the subgroup of patients who are at greatest risk for functional decline (Leuchter et al. 1994d, 1994e), and the degree of EEG slowing is the single best predictor of 1-year mortality in patients with dementia (Kaszniak et al. 1978).

A second illness in which EEG has a useful diagnostic role is delirium. Excessive slowing is seen almost universally in patients with delirium (G. Engel and Romano 1959), making EEG a useful physiological tool to support the diagnosis. More importantly, EEG may be used to monitor recovery because the degree of slowing is an indicator of the severity of the encephalopathy, and slowing resolves in response to effective interventions (Brenner 1991; Romano and Engel 1944). In cases in which mental status examination is equivocal, or difficult to perform (such as in a patient on a ventilator or with aphasia), such physiological testing can be useful for monitoring the resolution of the delirium. Distinguishing patients with depression or the changes of normal aging from those with delirium has been reported not to be problematic because of the severity of the abnormalities commonly seen in delirium (Brenner 1991; G. Engel and Romano 1959; Rabins and Folstein 1982).

The evaluation of late-onset seizures is not uncommon: the elderly may account for one-quarter of the cases of new-onset epilepsy (Sander et al. 1990), most commonly in association with stroke, trauma, mass lesions, and toxic metabolic disorders (Ettinger and Shinnar 1993; Luhdorf et al. 1986a, 1986b; Sung and Chu 1990). The prevalence of seizures in patients with Alzheimer's disease (AD) has been estimated at 3%–17% (Burns et al. 1991; Hauser et al. 1986; Mendez et al. 1994). The EEG may be used to confirm the presence of epileptiform discharges and to help establish the type of seizure disorder. It cannot, however, rule out a seizure disorder because a significant proportion of patients with late-onset seizure disorders have normal EEGs (estimated at 10%–47%, depending on etiology of the seizure and the time of recording on follow-up) (Ahuja and Mohanta 1982; Carney et al. 1969; da Silva et al. 1992; Luhdorf et al. 1986a, 1986b). Even when epileptiform abnormalities (i.e., spikes or spike-and-wave complexes) are detected, a diagnosis of a seizure disorder is not certain because these abnormalities generally are *interictal* in nature (i.e., not contemporaneous with an actual seizure). In some brain areas (such as occipital cortex), interictal abnormalities may have a low correlation with clinical seizures (Niedermeyer and Lopes da Silva 1987). In other cases, renal failure or degenerative brain disease can lead to the development of generalized sharp waves or spike foci that have a low association with clinical seizures. To be certain of the diagnosis, long-term observation with ambulatory or telemetered EEG with video monitoring may be necessary to capture an episode of behavioral disturbance and the attendant changes in brain electrical activity. In all cases, seizures are diagnosed on the basis of clinical presentation (Thomas 1997).

Conventional EEG has been found to be normal in a large proportion of subjects with depression (60%–76%) (Heyman et al. 1991; Leuchter et al. 1993a). Abnormalities, when they are found, are usually mild. A normal EEG may be useful in distinguishing patients with pseudodementia from those with advanced dementia. However, conventional EEG is of limited use in distinguishing among depression, early dementia, and states of depression superimposed on an underlying dementia. In fact, many patients who have cognitive complaints and a primary diagnosis of depression also have abnormal conventional EEGs (Leuchter et al. 1993a).

Limitations of Conventional Electroencephalography

At least three factors limit the applications of conventional EEG in psychiatric practice. First, the EEG is a complex test that is not readily subject to interpretation by most physicians. A significant degree of training is necessary to develop proficiency at identification of abnormalities and in distinguishing abnormalities from artifact. Second, even among skilled interpreters, there is an inherent problem of the limited reliability of qualitative interpretation. Different electroencephalographers (or a single electroencephalographer on different occasions) yield different interpretations of the same test a disturbingly high proportion of the time (Woody 1966, 1968). Third, for certain types of EEG activity, no consensus has been reached on the definitions of the upper and lower limits of normality. For example, excessive slow-wave activity in the EEG is a common finding in the elderly who are organically impaired and suggests the presence of either dementia or delirium. No well-established guidelines exist, however, for determining when slow-wave activity is excessive. Electroencephalographers may differ on how much slow-wave activity is acceptable at any given age. Even with general agreement, it is difficult to standardize such agreement among physicians (particularly those who do not work in the same facility) and to determine the sensitivity and specificity of the qualitative finding of "excessive slowing" in detecting brain disease. This lack of standardization also has hampered research efforts.

Quantitative Electroencephalography

QEEG analysis minimizes or even eliminates some of the limitations of conventional EEG. After a brief discussion of the technical aspect of QEEG, the clinical applications of the technique are discussed below.

Description of the Quantitative Electroencephalography Technique

Conventional EEG is rapidly yielding to QEEG, in which on-line digitization of the signal and recordings onto magnetic or optical media replace analogue pen-and-ink recordings. As short a time as 15 years ago, quantitation commonly was performed with a roomful of costly minicomputers. Starting in the mid-1980s, coincident with the wide availability of low-cost microcomputers, QEEG began to flourish and now is performed by academic and community-based physicians.

QEEG data are sampled at rates of at least 100 points per channel per second, and the analogue waveforms may be displayed in real time from these digital data either through a polygraph interface on paper or on a high-resolution video display terminal. Either of these display methods allows for conventional EEG interpretation of the digital recording.

Once digital data are recorded, the data can be transformed from the domain of amplitude versus frequency, in which they are recorded, to the domain of energy (or "power") versus frequency band (Figure 12–1). The process of this transformation is known as spectral analysis and commonly is achieved by processing the data through an algorithm known as Fourier transform. This algorithm is based upon the assumption that the complex waveform of the EEG may be modeled as the summation of a series of sinusoidal waveforms of different amplitudes and frequencies. A segment (or epoch) is decomposed into a series of simpler sine wave components, and the power at each frequency band for that epoch can be calculated from the characteristics of the sine wave at that frequency. Power (or amplitude^2) can be calculated for frequencies up to half the value of the sampling rate (the so-called Nyquist frequency).

Power estimates can be calculated for a second of data or even less, although the representative nature of such a small epoch for that individual's resting brain electrical activity is questionable. Commonly, the power in a series of frequency bands (the so-called power spectrum) is calculated for 20–30 seconds of data, either as discrete smaller

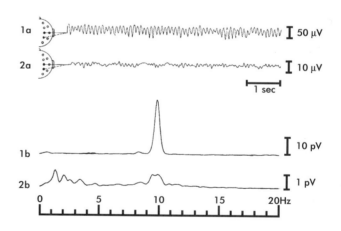

FIGURE 12–1. *Panel 1a:* Posterior dominant rhythm from a psychiatrically healthy subject, showing a sinusoidal 10-Hz rhythm. *Panel 1b:* Spectral analysis of this signal showing a peak of power at 10 Hz. *Panel 2a:* Posterior dominant rhythm such as that seen in a patient with dementia. Although some retained 10-Hz activity is seen, a number of intermixed slow waves are also present. *Panel 2b:* Spectral analysis of this more complex signal, showing peaks of power in the delta (0–4 Hz), theta (4–8 Hz), and alpha range.
sOURCE. Reprinted with permission from Spehlmann R: *EEG Primer.* New York, Elsevier Science, 1981, pp. 124. Copyright 1981 by Elsevier Biomedical Press.

epochs averaged together or as a single epoch.

QEEG overcomes several of the limitations of conventional EEG. Because it yields quantitative measurements of the frequency content of any segment of EEG, it provides much more reliable information regarding the amount of slow-wave activity in a record. These quantitative estimates not only minimize errors in judgment but also yield reproducible estimates that can be compared over time in a single individual.

The QEEG procedure also provides information that is not accessible from the visual inspection of the conventional recording. For example, QEEG can reliably measure the proportion of the total power that is in any given frequency band (so-called relative power, measured as a percent of total power). This measure is particularly useful because it normalizes for the wide fluctuations in total power across individuals and can detect subtle shifts in brain function in an individual over time.

Another product of the Fourier transform is *coherence*. Coherence quantifies the phase consistency of two signals, that is, the extent to which EEG signals from different brain regions have common, time-locked frequency components. Coherence is analogous to a correlation coefficient between the signals recorded at two locations and is computed from the formula:

$$ C_{xy}(\lambda) = \frac{|\,Sxy\,(\lambda)\,|^{\,2}}{Sx\,(\lambda) * Sy\,(\lambda)} $$

in which the square of the cross-spectrum is divided by the product of the spectra of the individual channels (Bendat and Piersol 1986). Values vary between 0 and 1. A value near 1 indicates extensive shared activity; a value near 0 indicates little shared activity. Coherence has been used as an indirect measure of functional connectivity and intactness of neuronal fiber tracts.

Evoked Potentials

In an attempt to standardize QEEG information, some investigators have controlled variability by recording electrical activity while the subjects are exposed to standardized visual, auditory, or other stimuli. These so-called evoked potentials (EPs), or event-related potentials (ERPs), are multicomponent waves of positive and negative potentials that result when the EEG signal from the scalp is averaged across numerous trials for a specified time interval after a stimulus. ERP components are labeled usually according to their polarities ("P" for positive, "N" for negative) and according to their latency from time of the stimulus (in milliseconds); some components are labeled according to their presumed function (e.g., contingent negative variation).

ERPs are classified as to the type of triggering physical stimuli used. Visual evoked potentials (VEPs) commonly are generated in response to simple flashes of light or to reversal of background and foreground colors in complex patterns (such as a checkerboard). Auditory evoked potentials (AEPs) are generated in response to a series of clicks or tones that may be constant or vary unpredictably over time. Somatosensory evoked potentials (SSEPs) are generated as a result of the electrical stimulation of a peripheral nerve.

After stimulation of a sense organ, it takes approximately 20 msec for the electrical signal to reach the cortex. ERPs recorded with short latencies of 20–80 msec are termed *stimulus bound* or *exogenous*, as they are believed to represent obligate responses of the nervous system generated in spinal cord or brainstem structures. Perhaps of greater interest for geriatric neuropsychiatry are ERPs with medium to long latencies, termed *endogenous* or *cognitive* potentials, thought to represent responses of higher centers (including primary or association cortex). These potentials are more sensitive to psychological variables, such as the subject's motivation, attention, or intention, and less sensitive to characteristics of the eliciting stimulus. Certain endogenous ERPs are indicative of the subject's "cognitive set" or preparation for a motor response or cognitive task and may be recorded even in the absence of an associated physical stimulus. The main advantage of ERPs is their fine temporal resolution, which is fast enough to monitor the multiple, sequential stages of human sensory and cognitive processes.

Quantitative electroencephalography and event-related potential changes with normal aging. QEEG studies of normal aging reveal some differences from conventional EEG studies. It is agreed that there is a slight slowing of the posterior dominant rhythm by 0.5–1.0 Hz, although by definition it must remain above 8 Hz (Busse 1983; Duffy et al. 1984a; Oken and Kaye 1992), and decreased alpha blocking (Duffy et al. 1984a). There is disagreement, however, regarding increases in slow-wave power, with several studies finding that delta and theta power do not increase with normal aging (Duffy et al. 1984a; Katz and Horowitz 1982; Leuchter et al. 1993b; Matejcek et al. 1979; Williamson et al. 1990). Factors associated with aging such as hypertension (Visser 1991), atherosclerosis (Obrist et al. 1963), and diabetes (Mooradian et al. 1988; Pramming et al. 1988) can cause subclinical cerebrovascular insufficiency and structural and functional brain changes (Giaquinto and Nolfe 1988; Obrist et al. 1963; Visser 1991; Visser et al. 1987). The finding in some QEEG studies that slow-wave power does not increase with aging probably reflects a superior health status of the subjects (Oken and Kaye 1992). QEEG studies further indicate that increased temporal slow-wave power with aging may reflect underlying pathology because it is inversely related to performance on memory testing (Rice et al. 1991).

Studies of beta power suggest that it increases with aging until the seventh decade, when decreases can occur (Duffy et al. 1984a; Holschneider and Leuchter 1995; Williamson et al. 1990). The effects of health status on beta power have not been addressed, but augmented beta power has been seen during cognitive tasks including states of focused arousal (Sheer 1975, 1976, 1984) and performance on problem-solving tasks (Loring et al. 1985; Spydell and Sheer 1982). Retained beta activity may be an indicator in the elderly of preserved cognitive function.

Investigators have reported consistent changes in long-latency ERPs with aging. During development, the P300 decreases in latency until approximately the second decade. Using auditory stimuli, Goodin and colleagues (1978a) were the first to describe increased P300 latency in the elderly. Since then, similar observations have been by made by others using AEPs, VEPs, and SSEPs (Beck et al. 1980; Brown et al. 1983; Pfefferbaum et al. 1984a; Picton et al. 1984, 1986; Syndulko et al. 1982). It now is widely accepted that P300 latency increases between 0.9 and 1.8 msec/year (Hillyard and Picton 1987; Polich 1991); this increase is believed to occur independently of any change in motor reaction time. Some investigators have found that the relationship between P300 latency and age is best described by a linear function (Pfefferbaum et al. 1984a; Picton et al. 1984; Polich et al. 1985; Squires et al. 1980; Syndulko et al. 1982), whereas others (Brown et al. 1983; Mullis et al. 1985) report a curvilinear relationship with greater annual latency increases for elderly subjects. Some have described increasing frontal distribution of the P300 (Pfefferbaum et al. 1984a; Smith et al. 1980). Others have been unable to replicate this finding (Maurer et al. 1988; Picton et al. 1984) with increasing age (Figure 12–2, *panel A*).

Detection of dementia.

It is generally agreed that QEEG is useful for detecting the presence of a dementing illness (Duffy et al. 1984b; Nuwer 1997; Prichep et al. 1994). Few studies, however, have systematically compared conventional EEG interpretation with QEEG for the detection of dementing illness. Brenner and colleagues (1998) compared 35 patients with clinically diagnosed dementia of the Alzheimer type (DAT), 23 with major depressive episodes, and 61 psychiatrically healthy control subjects. They found that QEEG offered "modest gains" in sensitivity over conventional EEG for the detection of moderate dementia (an increase from 57% to 66%), with

essentially equal specificity (95% and 93%, respectively). This improved sensitivity using QEEG methods was found despite collecting data from only four pooled QEEG channels from the parasagittal regions and relying upon mean frequency as the sole parameter studied. Furthermore, the fact that minutes of QEEG data could achieve greater sensitivity than conventional EEG, with equal specificity and using less physician time for test interpretation, suggests an advantage of QEEG over conventional EEG for routine evaluations.

Most studies use several types of QEEG measures (absolute power, relative power, spectral ratios) and linear combinations of these to discriminate subjects with de-

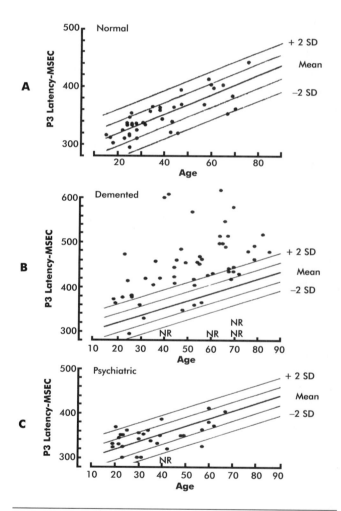

FIGURE 12–2. P300 (*P3*) latencies from the rare-tone evoked potential waveforms as a function of age for individual psychiatrically healthy subjects (*panel A*); individual patients with dementia (*panel B*); and individual psychiatric patients without dementia (*panel C*). Also shown are regression lines 1 and 2 SD from the mean, derived from the data for psychiatrically healthy subjects.

Source. Adapted from Squires et al. 1980.

mentia from those without dementia. These measures are complementary: they are additive in detection of abnormality and yield different regional information regarding the distribution of the abnormalities (Leuchter et al. 1993b). A number of studies have shown increased delta and theta power and decreased alpha and beta power, as well as decreased mean frequency in dementia (Brenner et al. 1986; Breslau et al. 1989; Coben et al. 1985; Giaquinto and Nolfe 1986; Pentillä et al. 1985; Stigsby et al. 1981; Visser et al. 1985; Vitiello and Prinz 1987). Such brain electrical changes are seen usually in a generalized distribution, though recent work suggests that, in DAT, increases in cortical slow-wave activity and decreases in high-frequency activity appear most prominent in the temporoparietal region (Albert et al. 1990; Buchan et al. 1997; Duffy et al. 1995; Holschneider and Leuchter 1995; Kwa et al. 1993; Pozzi et al. 1996; Saletu et al. 1991; Schreiter-Gasser et al. 1993).

In comparing patients with early- and late-onset DAT, Duffy and colleagues (1984b) found that increases in theta and/or delta activity and decreases in beta activity were maximal in temporal regions in subjects with early-onset DAT and in the frontal regions in subjects with late-onset DAT. Retrospective subject classification by discriminant function analysis using a combination of evoked response and electroencephalographic features correctly discriminated 95.8% of patients with early-onset DAT and 90% of patients with late-onset DAT from their respective control subjects. Leuchter and colleagues (1987) found large differences among subjects with DAT, those with vascular dementia (VaD), and control subjects in spectral ratios, which combine high-frequency and low-frequency power in a single measure. Using spectral ratios, as well as coherence variables, these researchers accurately classified more than 90% of subjects into their correct diagnostic group.

Most studies suggest that a positive linear relationship exists between the degree of cognitive impairment in dementia and increases in slow-wave power and decreases in high-frequency power (Brenner et al. 1986; Erkinjuntti et al. 1988; Holschneider and Leuchter 1995; Hughes et al. 1989; Johannesson et al. 1979; Rae-Grant et al. 1987; Soininen et al. 1982). It has been considerably uncertain, however, how early in the course of dementia QEEG may be useful for detecting disease. The answer to this question depends, to a great extent, on which measures are assessed. Gordon and Sim (Gordon 1968; Gordon and Sim 1967) reported that changes in alpha power preceded increased slow-wave power as a manifestation of disease, whereas others have reported that either increases in theta power or decreases in beta power were the earliest changes (Berg et al. 1984; Coben et al. 1983a; Jelic et al. 1996; Prichep et al.

1994). Sensitivities ranging from 20% to 36% and specificities ranging from 93% to 100% have been reported by others using a combination of EEG measures in varying scalp locations (Brenner et al. 1998; John et al. 1988; Prichep et al. 1994). The highest sensitivity (24%) and specificity (100%) for any single QEEG variable have been reported with percentage theta (Coben et al. 1990). Recently, Jelic and colleagues reported in subjects with AD, with average MMSE scores of 21, that when temporoparietal coherence appears as a discriminant variable together with alpha and theta relative power, sensitivity increases to 78%, while retaining a specificity of 100% (Jelic et al. 1996).

QEEG appears to be of greater use for distinguishing depression from dementia than is conventional EEG. Pollock and Schneider (1990) reviewed studies performed over the preceding decade and found that more than half found increases in both alpha and beta power in depression; these investigators themselves (Pollock and Schneider 1989) found that increased alpha activity persisted after recovery from depression. Other specific QEEG findings in depression have included right temporal slowing, increased frontal beta (Schatzberg et al. 1986), and increased left frontal alpha power (Davidson 1988). The increased delta (Brenner et al. 1986; John et al. 1988; Visser et al. 1985) and decreased beta power in dementia (Brenner et al. 1986; Visser et al. 1985) appear particularly helpful in separating those with dementia from those with depression alone. Because no single feature appears to be robust for the diagnosis of depression, several investigators have used a multivariate statistical approach to the diagnosis of depression (John et al. 1977, 1988; Shagass et al. 1984) and have reported overall accuracy in classification of 60%–90%. The stability of these multivariate methods for diagnosis remains to be verified.

An abnormal EEG may identify a subgroup of depressed patients with structural brain disease. These structural changes (as defined by hyperintensity on T2-weighted magnetic resonance imaging [MRI] scans) have been associated both with late-life depression (Leuchter et al. 1997) and EEG abnormalities (Oken and Kaye 1992). The high prevalence of these changes is of clinical significance because elderly subjects with abnormal EEGs show functional decline regardless of their diagnostic group (Leuchter et al. 1994d, 1994e). In some instances, these abnormalities may portend the development of a dementing illness (Liston 1979). Although an abnormal EEG in subjects with depression is not specific for dementia, it does identify the patients at greatest risk for functional decline and therefore is a useful part of the evaluation for dementia.

QEEG is an excellent tool for monitoring the effect of manipulations of the cholinergic system and thus may be a useful adjunct in monitoring response to cholinomimetic treatment in patients with dementia. Administration of cholinergic antagonists increases slow-wave power and decreases high-frequency power, whereas cholinergic agonists result in a reversal of this phenomenon (Vanderwolf 1992). The topography of such brain electrical changes has in animal models been shown to directly correlate with regional cortical changes of choline acetyltransferase (Holschneider et al. 1997a; Ray and Jackson 1991). Serial brain mapping studies in subjects with DAT who have been administered the cholinergic agonist bethanechol have demonstrated a dose-dependent decrease in slow-wave power (Leuchter et al. 1991). Decreases in slow-wave power and increases in high-frequency power have been shown also after the administration of the acetylcholinesterase inhibitor tetrahydroaminoacridine (tacrine) (Minthon et al. 1993; Perryman and Fitten 1991; Riekkinen et al. 1991; Shigeta et al. 1993), the acetylcholine-releasing agent DuP 996 (Saletu et al. 1989), as well as nerve growth factor (NGF), a cholinergic neurotrophin (Holschneider et al. 1997a; Olson et al. 1992). Though QEEG appears sensitive in monitoring response to cognitive enhancers, changes in brain electrical activity may not be specific for alterations of cholinergic function. Decreases in slow-wave power and increases in high-frequency power have been reported also after the use of estrogen (Ohkura et al. 1994) and ergoloid mesylates (Hydergine) (Matejcek et al. 1979; Saletu et al. 1990). A greater understanding of neurochemical correlates of individual QEEG parameters is needed.

Several investigators have attempted to use short-latency ERPs for the diagnosis of dementia (Coben et al. 1983b; Harkins 1981; Visser et al. 1976). Prolonged flash VEP latency and increased amplitude (Coben et al. 1983b; Visser et al. 1976; Wright et al. 1984), as well as some changes in brainstem AEPs (Harkins 1981) and SSEPs (Huisman et al. 1985), have been reported in patients with dementia. However, the differences in the exogenous potentials between subjects with dementia and psychiatrically healthy control subjects are too small or inconsistent to permit definitive classification.

Most of the research on the late components of ERPs in dementia has focused on the P300 peak. It has been established that the P300 latency is prolonged in dementia in excess of that seen during normal aging. Goodin and co-workers (1978b) first reported an abnormally large increase in the P300 latency in a group of patients with dementia of different etiologies; they also noted that the increase in latency correlated with severity of dementia as

assessed by the MMSE. Although these findings have been confirmed by several laboratories, prevalence of reported "abnormal" latency varies from 13% to 83%, with most studies reporting that 70%–80% of patients with dementia have prolonged P300 latency (Brown et al. 1982, 1983; Gordon et al. 1986; Patterson et al. 1988; Squires et al. 1980; Syndulko et al. 1982) (Figure 12–2, *panel B*).

The usefulness of the P300 latency alone is limited for several reasons. First, there is the wide variability in the prevalence of the abnormality. Pfefferbaum and colleagues (1984a, 1984b) used both auditory and visual ERP paradigms to compare 77 subjects with dementia of different etiologies (MMSE < 25) with 66 normal control subjects. They reported that fewer than 30% of the patients with dementia had P300 latencies that were at least 2 SDs greater than that expected for age. Although this low specificity reflects in part the particular paradigm used to elicit the P300 component, as well as the variability in normal P300 latency in the control subjects, the increases in P300 latency in mild dementia have been reported to be too small to be clinically useful (Leppler and Greenberg 1984; Polich et al. 1986; Syndulko et al. 1984).

Second, the P300 latency has been shown to be prolonged in other conditions and has been reported in up to 12% of patients with depression and 13% of patients with schizophrenia (Gordon et al. 1986; O'Donnell et al. 1995). Furthermore, an increased P300 latency is seen with dementia in a variety of conditions such as alcohol abuse, Huntington's disease, Parkinson's disease, Down's syndrome, scopolamine-induced "dementia," and geriatric depression (Calloway et al. 1985; Hansch et al. 1982; Kalayam et al. 1998; Lukas et al. 1990; Pfefferbaum et al. 1979; Rosenberg et al. 1985; St. Clair and Blackwood 1985). Patients with DAT cannot be distinguished from patients with other dementias on the basis of P300 amplitude or latency (Brown et al. 1982; Polich et al. 1986).

P300 latency measures are useful in certain clinical situations and as a component of a broader neurophysiological evaluation. Measurement of P300 latency can be useful as a component of an overall evaluation when there is a specific diagnostic question of dementia versus depression or delirium (Goodin 1990; Pfefferbaum et al. 1990), although it probably is of little use for specifying the type of dementia (Pfefferbaum et al. 1990). In combination with measures of power and/or coherence, this ERP measure can add greater sensitivity to the QEEG evaluation of dementia.

Diagnosis and assessment of delirium.   QEEG offers substantial advantages over conventional EEG in the examination of subjects with delirium. Although Engel and

Romano (G. Engel and Romano 1959; Romano and Engel 1944) demonstrated that EEG slowing is almost invariably present in delirium, and grossly excessive slowing suggests the presence of delirium instead of, or in addition to, dementia (Brenner 1991; Rabins and Folstein 1982), it is difficult to determine the severity of slowing by visual inspection.

Examination of subjects with delirium indicates that QEEG can be used to successfully quantitate the magnitude of slow-wave power. QEEG detects significant changes in the amount of slow-wave power in the course of a delirium when the conventional EEG shows equivocal change, and decreases in slow-wave power may actually precede improvements in mental status (Leuchter and Jacobson 1991). QEEG indices are strongly correlated with not only the severity of delirium but also the length of delirium and hospitalization (Koponen 1991; Koponen et al. 1989).

Although it has been suggested that the severity of slowing may differ between subjects with delirium and those with dementia, studies indicate that it may be practical to differentiate these two groups based upon QEEG. Koponen and colleagues (1989) found that subjects with delirium with concomitant dementia had more severe slowing than those without dementia. Jacobson and colleagues (1993a) reported that several QEEG indices were useful for distinguishing delirium from dementia. Follow-up work from this group indicates that distinct QEEG measures of absolute and relative power indices are sensitive to the progression of dementia or the development of delirium, suggesting that QEEG may be particularly helpful for identifying the onset of delirium as a complication of dementia (Jacobson et al. 1993b).

ERPs also have been used in the assessment of delirium, primarily in patients with hepatic or renal encephalopathy (some of whom are elderly). Some investigators have reported abnormal latencies of brainstem auditory evoked potentials (Chu and Yang 1987; Pierelli et al. 1985; Rossini et al. 1984), whereas others have not (Trzepacz et al. 1989; Yang et al. 1986). More consistent results have been obtained with VEPs (Casellas et al. 1985; Kuba et al. 1983; Levy and Bolton 1986; Levy et al. 1990; Pierelli et al. 1985; Rossini et al. 1981; Zeneroli et al. 1984) and SSEPs, in which changes in latency correlate with severity of encephalopathy (Trzepacz et al. 1989; Yen and Liaw 1990).

In hepatic encephalopathy, changes occur in both VEP and SSEP latency during progressive stages of encephalopathy (Davies et al. 1991). In a review of the clinical usefulness of QEEG methods, including spectral analysis, EEG, SSEPs, brainstem auditory evoked potentials, VEPs, and

P300, van der Rijt and Schalm (1992) found that the highest percentage of abnormalities in patients with subclinical hepatic encephalopathy was detected by flash VEPs (25%–46%, 95% confidence interval). The auditory and pattern-reversal P300 shows an increase in latency and may be used for the detection of milder disease, although its applications are limited because it requires more patient participation than short-latency ERPs (Sandford and Saul 1988).

Little work has been done using ERP topographic mapping in hepatic encephalopathy. This area holds considerable promise for the future. Researchers led by Matos and Paiva (Matos et al. 1988; Paiva et al. 1988) have reported that 73%–75% of patients with liver disease without clinical signs of encephalopathy show abnormal VEP topographic maps.

Limitations of Quantitative Electroencephalography

Quantitation of the power in different frequency bands has been touted as more "objective" and as minimizing variability in interpretation. It is true that QEEG yields more reliable and reproducible measurements of brain activity and is more likely to detect subtle focal or generalized alterations in brain function (Jerrett and Corsak 1988; Nuwer et al. 1987). Quantitation alone does not, however, indicate whether activity is normal or abnormal; traditionally, these determinations are made based upon statistical comparison of data from an individual to a normal base value and determination of whether the individual is beyond the "cutoff" for normality. Thus, QEEG does not eliminate the confounding problem that slowing increases both with age and emergence of organic brain disease. It does, however, allow the clinician to be more precise in measuring the amount of slowing and determining whether this appears to be excessive for the patient's age. The most common method for establishing base values is building a *normative database* by collecting data from individuals who are in good health and not receiving any medications that might influence brain electrical activity. Stratification of normative data by age and gender may be additionally helpful in determining whether changes in an individual's record are indicative of abnormality. Commonly, when the amount of slow-wave power at a given site is 2 SDs from the mean of a group of psychiatrically healthy subjects, this is interpreted as abnormal.

This statistical database approach can be useful for the interpretation of an individual's data but has significant limitations. First, it is not clear how much deviation from a group of age-matched psychiatrically healthy control subjects is acceptable for any given EEG measure. Some patterns of brain activity are very different from the patterns seen on most EEGs, and would be 2 SDs from a normal mean, but are a recognized *normal variant* (such as the low-voltage fast recording without any posterior dominant rhythm). Second, there are instances in which a persistent focal increase in slow-wave power is significant and indicative of abnormality but may be less than 2 SDs from the mean for that subject's age group. Such a focal increase can be especially significant if it is progressive over time. Third, a small but consistent deviation at many or all recording sites could be highly significant clinically and indicative of brain dysfunction, even if less than 2 SDs. Finally, a highly significant difference (i.e., 4 SDs) at a single recording site may need to be interpreted with caution because with multiple tests at multiple recording sites in multiple frequency bands, false-positive results can occur.

Several different approaches can be used to increase confidence in the comparisons between a patient's data and a normative database. Some researchers have proposed looking at multiple independent segments of data from within a recording session (Duffy et al. 1990, 1992). Another alternative is to examine a subject by using multiple modalities, such as resting EEG and evoked potentials. If a brain area appears abnormal in multiple independent samples of data, obtained under different recording paradigms, this could increase confidence that a finding is valid (Duffy 1998). Of course, if the abnormality is not detected on all occasions or under all conditions, this does not necessarily mean that it is not "real"; it simply may be episodic or state-dependent.

An alternative to the normative database model is to compare a given individual to his or her own baseline. When the first recording is performed in the premorbid condition, this may be the ideal method for assessment of brain electrical activity. Both the absolute intensity of power in any given frequency band, as well as the proportional distribution of power across frequency bands, may be examined and a determination made if there has been a change from the individual's baseline. This method is particularly applicable to the study of patients with delirium, in whom multiple studies over a short period of time may be indicated, or for the long-term follow-up of patients with dementia. Unfortunately, normal baseline studies rarely are available, so this method is of little help in interpreting the initial study of a patient with possible dementia or delirium. Furthermore, significant fluctuations can occur in patients' brain electrical activity with changes in state, so that it still is difficult to determine if subtle changes are indicative of abnormality or are within the normal range.

At present, QEEG is considered an adjunct to conventional EEG in the study of psychiatric illnesses (American Psychiatric Association Task Force on Quantitative Electrophysiological Assessment 1991). This is understandable because, in some clinical situations, conventional EEG offers some advantages over QEEG. Very fast transient EEG activity lasting only milliseconds is not easily detected through quantitative analysis because it accounts for a very low proportion of the total power in a recording epoch. Therefore, an area of focal damage that is producing transient disturbances, such as rare epileptiform spikes, will not be detected by spectral analysis unless it also is producing a disproportionate amount of slow- or fast-wave power. Computer programs are currently available to scan QEEG data for the presence of epileptiform spikes or other specific abnormalities, but these are not yet widely accepted.

QEEG is sensitive to the proportion of energy in any given frequency band but is much less sensitive to specific wave morphology; in other words, it is less sophisticated at pattern recognition. Therefore, rhythmic triphasic waves would not be readily distinguished from frontally predominant intermittent rhythmic delta activity (FIRDA) or from continuous polymorphic delta activity in the frontal region. Although pattern recognition might lead the electroencephalographer to suspect either a particular metabolic encephalopathy or focal structural lesion with one or the other of these patterns, the frequency spectra might look remarkably similar.

The unique advantages of visual pattern interpretation indicate that there always will be a role for conventional electroencephalography, although as artificial intelligence algorithms for pattern recognition develop, conventional EEG may evolve into "computer-assisted EEG."

New Methods for Interpreting Quantitative Electroencephalography

Neurophysiology of Electroencephalography Abnormalities

Ample evidence from studies of both animals and humans indicates that pathological slow waves in the EEG are caused by partial deafferentation of pyramidal cells of the cerebral cortex (Steriade et al. 1990). Complete destruction of cortex does not cause excessive slowing but instead leads to electrical silence; only through partial deafferentation of the cortex or nonlethal damage to cortical neurons do pathological slow waves develop (Gloor et al. 1977) (Figure 12–3). One of the strengths of QEEG is its ability to monitor the activity and integrity of afferent and efferent fibers that are responsible for integrating electrical activity of different brain areas. Deafferentation can be the result of primary neuronal disease or of a brain insult (such as a stroke) secondarily affecting nerve function. Deafferentation can occur at any level: direct damage to the cortex, undercutting of the cortex by white matter lesions, and damage to the cortically projecting basal forebrain neurons all can cause an increase in cortically recorded slow waves. Research suggests that deafferentation can be structural or functional (such as through reversible toxic damage) (Steriade et al. 1990). This finding explains the similar patterns of increased slowing resulting from either DAT or administration of atropine: the former process causes loss of the origins of cortically projecting cholinergic afferents from the basal forebrain, whereas the latter inhibits firing of the cortically projecting afferent cells (Buzsaki et al. 1988; Detari and Vanderwolf 1987; Schaul et al. 1981; Steriade et al. 1990). The mechanism of slow waves that accompany metabolic derangements such as hypoxia, hypoglycemia, or other toxic states has not been established, but these also may represent dysfunction of cells projecting to the cortex or of the cortical pyramidal cells themselves.

Detection of deafferented cortex: the cordance method. A specific measure of cortical deafferentation could be useful clinically. Such a measure could potentially indicate which slow waves were pathological and even in the absence of grossly excessive slowing suggest that pathology exists. Based on the knowledge that surface-recorded EEG should be sensitive to cortical deafferentation, we studied subjects with large white matter lesions that presumably undercut and partially deafferented cerebral cortex (Leuchter et al. 1994a, 1994b). These areas appeared to be hypoperfused on SPECT scanning and hypometabolic on PET, findings consistent with deafferentation. Such areas showed a characteristic QEEG pattern: although the deafferented cortex produced less slow-wave power on an absolute basis than did other cortical areas, it produced greater slow-wave power on a relative basis compared with that of other brain areas.

This finding of decreased absolute but increased relative slow-wave power over white matter lesions was termed *discordance*. Though not all white matter lesions were sufficient to cause discordance, the presence of discordance was associated reliably with areas that were found to be hypoperfused as a result of stroke or the presence of brain degeneration (i.e., DAT). The opposite indicator state, called *concordance*, was associated reliably with states of high perfusion and appears to be an indicator of cortex that is

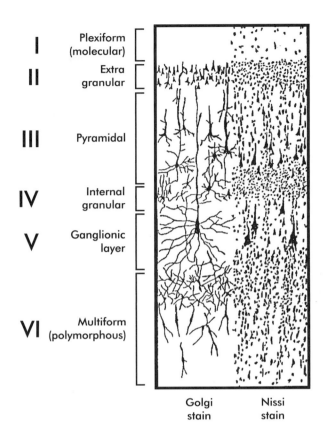

FIGURE 12–3. Schematic representation of the layers of the cerebral cortex (showing association cortex; from Cummings and Coffey, in this volume). Partial deafferentation of the large pyramidal cells in layers II and III is the cause of pathological slow waves in the electroencephalogram.
Source. Reprinted with permission from Carpenter MB: *Core Text of Neuroanatomy*, 4th Edition. Philadelphia, PA, Williams & Wilkins, 1991, p 391.

functioning normally. For example, in patients with DAT, discordance is seen over the parietal regions and other areas that are hypometabolic on PET (Figure 12–4). These areas are known to be deafferented by the degenerative processes of DAT, in which the pyramidal cells of laminae II and III that project corticocortical afferents die selectively (Morrison et al. 1986). Concordance is seen over the central brain areas, particularly the area of the motor strip, which is known to be relatively spared by the neuropathological changes of DAT.

The concordance and discordance indicators (known jointly as *cordance*) show promise for detecting pathological changes, even in cognitively intact subjects. We recently examined cordance in six psychiatrically healthy subjects who underwent simultaneous $H_2{}^{15}O$ PET scanning and cordance studies, both in the resting state and while they performed motor tasks. A moderately strong association was found among their levels of perfusion, and PET and

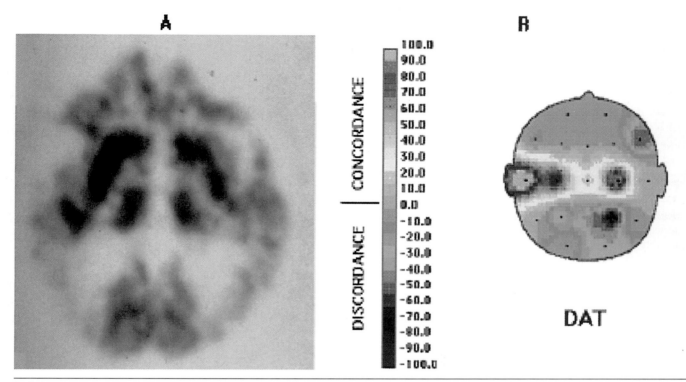

FIGURE 12–4. Brain scans of an 88-year-old man with progressive confusion, memory loss, social withdrawal, and agitation, who was diagnosed with dementia of the Alzheimer type (*DAT*). His positron emission tomography (PET) scan showed biparietal hypometabolism as well as focal left temporal hypometabolism (*panel A*). The cordance map shows three prominent areas of discordance, at the right and left parietal and left temporal electrodes, that have a strong spatial association with the three areas of hypometabolism (*panel B*). Significant alpha concordance is seen over the frontocentral region bilaterally, in the general area of the motor strip; this area commonly has the highest metabolism in subjects with DAT. PET scan shows the brain as viewed from below, whereas cordance map shows it viewed from above (i.e., right and left are reversed in the two pictures).

cordance were equally effective detecting the lateralized activation that accompanied motor tasks (Leuchter et al. 1999). This suggests that cordance is sensitive to even modest changes in perfusion and can be used to monitor brain function in subjects with relatively normal brain function.

We recently have applied cordance to the study of subjects with depression and have found that cordance is sensitive both to the brain dysfunction of depression and to the effects of antidepressant medication. Cook and colleagues (1998) studied 27 subjects with late-life depression and found that those with depression showed significantly more discordance than did psychiatrically healthy subjects. Interestingly, subjects who were undergoing treatment with antidepressant medication had *further* decreases in cordance in the prefrontal region. This finding is consistent with the work of Drevets and Raichle (1992), Sackeim (Sackeim and Prohovnik 1993; Sackeim et al. 1990), and others, showing that antidepressant treatment leads to further decreases in cerebral perfusion, particularly in the frontal regions.

We recently studied prospectively over 8 weeks 24 subjects with current unipolar major depression who were receiving fluoxetine (Cook et al. 1999; Leuchter et al. 1997). In this double-blind study, subjects demonstrating concordance prior to treatment has a more robust response to the antidepressant than did subjects with a pretreament discordant pattern. This suggests that cordance may be useful in predicting treatment response to fluoxetine. An example of these changes is shown in Figure 12–5. This subject, who underwent treatment with venlefaxine, showed a significant, sustained bilateral reduction in frontal cordance during antidepressant treatment (Figure 12–5, *panels B and C*).

This decrease appears to be specific for a stable and lasting antidepressant response. A subject with depression (Figure 12–6) showed a decrease in frontal cordance in response to the first antidepressant she received, but this decrease was only mild and asymmetrical (Figure 12–6, *panel B*). Within a few months, the patient suffered a relapse of her symptoms and, despite an increase in dose, there was no remission (Figure 12–6, *panel C*). The patient was changed

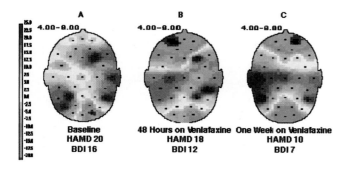

FIGURE 12–5. A series of cordance maps from a 32-year-old woman, recorded during the first week of venlafaxine treatment. *Panel A* shows the baseline image. Subject started to show resolution of depressed cordance pattern as early as 2 days after medication was started (*panel B*), before clinical symptoms improved. The cordance continued to decrease over the next week as depression scores (*panel C*) decreased. BDI = Beck Depression Inventory (Beck 1978); HAMD = Hamilton Rating Scale for Depression (Hamilton 1960).

to a second antidepressant, but without response (Figure 12–6, *panel D*). Finally, she was changed to a third antidepressant to which she had a robust and lasting response. Only at this time did the patient show a marked, bilateral reduction in frontal cordance, which is indicative of successful antidepressant treatment (Figure 12–6, *panel E*).

Cordance may have wide applicability for the assessment and treatment of mental disorders. Additional studies of subjects undergoing treatment for depression, AD, and other conditions will help to determine if this technique could be used to guide treatment.

Disconnection between brain areas: the role of coherence. Another example of the usefulness of the deafferentation model of QEEG lies in the ability of this model to detect damage to afferent and efferent fibers linking two brain regions. As discussed above, coherence is a measure of synchronization of brain electrical activity between regions. Coherence appears to be a reliable measure of the functional connections between brain areas, monitoring interactions between cortical areas while subjects are at rest or engaged in a relevant cognitive task (Busk and Galbraith 1975; Davis and Wada 1974; O'Connor and Shaw 1978; Shaw et al. 1977, 1978; Tucker et al. 1986). In subjects with dementia, coherence measures have been shown to correlate with measures of cognitive function (Dunkin et al. 1995; Jelic et al. 1996), as well as functional outcome (Leuchter et al. 1994d, 1994e), consistent with the notion that the extent of neuronal deafferentation determines the severity of a dementia.

Deafferentation as measured through QEEG coherence has proved useful in detecting differences between subjects with DAT and those with VaD. In the past, differential diagnosis between these disorders using conventional EEG has relied upon detection of focal abnormalities, which reportedly are more common among subjects with VaD. This finding is not sufficiently prevalent, however, to be of diagnostic usefulness (Dejaiffe et al. 1964; Harrison et al. 1979; Logar et al. 1987; Roberts et al. 1978). Likewise, although measures of brain electrical power or spectral ratios have proved useful at differentiating between DAT and VaD in the research setting (Leuchter et al. 1993b; Logar et al. 1987), such measures have not been sufficiently robust to be used clinically.

Electrographic coherence has been used with greater success to distinguish patients with DAT from those with VaD. It has been helpful in understanding differences in the specific types of disconnections that characterize these neurodegenerative disorders. DAT and VaD have been hypothesized, on the basis of neuropathological data, to effect different types of brain connections: DAT causes selective disconnection of long corticocortical fibers, whereas VaD causes more diffuse disconnection of corticosubcortical white matter networks. Leuchter and colleagues (1992), as well as others (O'Connor et al. 1979), have shown that coherence detects these different types of disconnection and may be used to successfully distinguish high proportions of subjects with DAT or VaD (Figures 12–7 and 12–8).

Morrison and colleagues (Hof et al. 1990; Morrison et al. 1991) have highlighted the heterogeneity in types of disconnection among patients with DAT and have found that those with greater visuospatial difficulty (Balint's syndrome) show greater neuropathological disruption of the visual association pathways. The strong associations between performance on neuropsychological tests and coherence in relevant brain regions (particularly visuospatial function and visual system coherence) (Dunkin et al. 1995) suggest that coherence may be useful for characterizing the distribution of pathology among patients with dementia.

Given the ubiquitous nature of white matter disease in geriatric patients with depression or dementia or those without illness, the concept of disconnection may have applications for the study of other groups of elderly subjects. An area that is particularly vulnerable to white matter changes is the periventricular region (Bowen et al. 1990), where high-signal lesions may be seen in 60%–100% of asymptomatic control subjects (Leuchter et al. 1994c). These periventricular fibers are critical components of the networks that subserve higher cortical functions, containing the projections of the prefrontal cortical neurons and the visual association pathways. Leuchter and colleagues

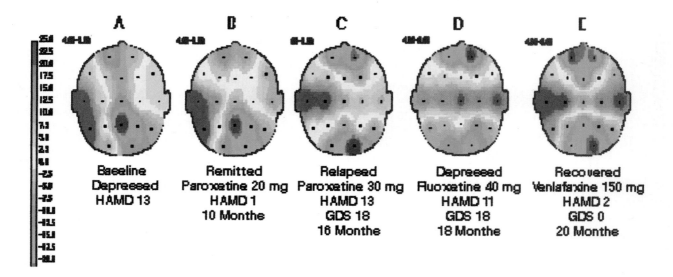

FIGURE 12–6.   A series of cordance maps from a subject undergoing treatment for depression. At baseline (*panel A*), the subject had low cordance over the frontal regions and the right temporal region. Although symptoms resolved after treatment with paroxetine (*panel B*), the frontal cordance did not decrease further, and the temporal cordance did not increase. The subject relapsed, and an increased dose of paroxetine did not resolve the depression (*panel C*). Fluoxetine in a dosage up to 40 mg also was ineffective (*panel D*). Finally, the subject was treated with venlafaxine, which led to a complete remission of symptoms. The cordance map showed a large bilateral decrease in frontal cordance and a bilateral increase in temporal cordance, consistent with effective treatment (*panel E*). GDS = Yesavage Geriatric Depression Scale (Yesavage 1998); HAMD = Hamilton Rating Scale for Depression (Hamilton 1960).
Source.   Reprinted with permission from Leuchter AF, Cook IA, Vijtdehaage SHU, et al: "Brain Structure and Function and the Outcomes of Treatment for Depression." *Journal of Clinical Psychiatry* 58:22–31, 1997.

(1994c) have shown that there is an association between the presence of periventricular damage seen on MRI and decreased coherence in the frontal and visual networks of connections. The association between these two measures is stronger than the association between white matter disease and clinical diagnosis, suggesting that the degree and type of disconnection may be a useful model for categorizing cognitive impairment among elderly subjects, even those who do not meet all criteria for dementia.

Recent work suggests that the cholinergic system is an important determinant of the synchronization of brain electrical activity. Indirect cholinergic agonists such as physostigmine or eserine enhance the synchronization in specific frequency bands, whereas antagonists such as atropine diminish it (Dickson et al. 1994; Leung et al. 1994). Animal studies have shown that electrocortical coherence decreases after deafferentation of cholinergic fiber tracts projecting from the basal forebrain (Holschneider et al. 1998, 1999). Losses in coherence are restored, in part, by the administration of NGF, a cholinergic neurotrophin. Increases in coherence associated with NGF are largely seen for coherences within a hemisphere, but not between hemispheres. Such observations are consistent with findings that cholinergic projections from the basal forebrain to the cortex remain largely ipsilateral, whereas virtually all fibers connecting the hemispheres through the corpus callosum or hippocampal commissures are noncholinergic, employing glutamate, aspartate, or γ-aminobutyric acid as their transmitters (Conti and Manzoni 1994). Studies such as these represent a first step in the elucidation of the neurochemical correlates of brain electrical coherence.

Unmasking cortical deafferentation during pharmacological activation.   As described above, generalized reductions of beta frequencies have been consistently reported in patients with dementia. Despite a high specificity, however, the low sensitivity of beta activity obtained with patients in the resting state has constrained the clinical utility of this measure in distinguishing pathological changes from those of normal aging (Coben et al. 1990). Although it has not been extensively studied in subjects with dementia, it appears that pharmacological activation of the brain may unmask the inability of diseased neurons to mount an adequate electrophysiological response. In the brain of a psychiatrically healthy human, prenarcotic dosages of barbiturates produce an abrupt onset of fast activity (20–28 Hz) (Bickford 1953; Brazier and Finesinger 1945; Kiersey et al. 1951; Pampiglione 1952). As early as 1950, Alema and Sinisi (1950) and later Pampiglione (1952) found that these barbiturate-induced rhythms were re-

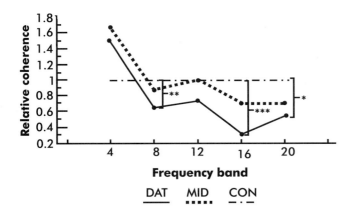

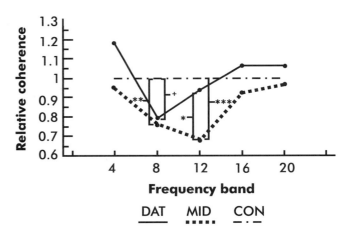

FIGURE 12–7. Frequency spectrum of coherence mediated by long corticocortical connections (called *FASCICLE-PA measure* because it is similar to the distribution of fibers of the superior longitudinal fasciculus). Coherence is displayed for the subjects with dementia of the Alzheimer type (*DAT*) and subjects with multiinfarct dementia (*MID*) as a proportion of the mean value for the control (*CON*) group. Mean value for the control group is standardized to 1 in each frequency band and indicated by the *dotted line* across the middle of the figure. Frequency bands are displayed across the bottom of the figure, with numbers representing the center frequency of each band (e.g., *4* represents the 2- to 6-Hz band, *8* represents the 6- to 10-Hz band).
*Difference between subjects with DAT and control subjects, $P < .05$.
**Difference between subjects with DAT and control subjects, $P < .01$.
***Difference between subjects with DAT and control subjects, $P < .005$.
Source. Reprinted with permission from Leuchter AF, Newton TF, Cook IA, et al.: "Changes in Brain Functional Connectivity in Alzheimer-Type and Multi-Infarct Dementia." *Brain* 115:1543–1561, 1992. Copyright 1992 by Oxford University Press.

FIGURE 12–8. Frequency spectrum of coherence mediated by networks of short corticocortical and corticosubcortical connections (called *VISUAL measure* because it is similar to the projectors of the visual pathway). Coherence is displayed for the subjects with dementia of the Alzheimer type (*DAT*) and those with multiinfarct dementia (*MID*) groups as a proportion of the mean value for the control (*CON*) group. Mean value for the control group is standardized to 1 in each frequency band and indicated by the *dotted line* across the middle of the figure. Frequency bands are displayed across the bottom of the figure, with numbers representing the center frequency of each band (i.e., *4* represents the 2- to 6-Hz band, *8* represents the 6- to 10-Hz band, etc.).
*Difference between subjects with DAT and MID subjects, $P < .05$.
**Difference between subjects with MID and control subjects, $P < .01$.
***Difference between subjects with MID and control subjects, $P < .005$.
*Difference between subjects with DAT and control subjects.
Source. Reprinted with permission from Leuchter AF, Newton TF, Cook IA, et al.: "Changes in Brain Functional Connectivity in Alzheimer-Type and Multi-Infarct Dementia." *Brain* 115:1543–1561, 1992. Copyright 1992 by Oxford University Press.

duced over areas of damage and aided in localizing lesions. Using QEEG, our laboratory has examined high-frequency power in patients with DAT, those with VaD, and psychiatrically healthy elderly control subjects after an intravenous bolus of thiopental. Compared with both control subjects and patients with VaD, subjects with DAT showed a marked loss of high-frequency power elicited across the cortex, with largest differences noted in the frontal region (Holschneider et al. 1997b) (Figure 12–9). Barbiturate challenge revealed differences in high-frequency activity not seen at baseline between subjects with DAT and those with VaD. Such an attenuation in the brain electrical response can be seen even in the early stages of DAT (average MMSE 26) (Holschneider and Leuchter, in press).

The etiology of a decrease in the barbiturate-induced high-frequency response is not clearly understood. Depth

recordings of the EEG during light pentothal anesthesia suggest that the generators of fast waves are cortical in location (unlike the activity recorded at deeper anesthetic levels) (Brazier et al. 1956; J. J. Engel et al. 1982). Histopathological studies in subjects with DAT strongly suggest a selective loss of large pyramidal cells whose axons form corticocortical connections between higher order association areas. This deafferentation, which has been described as a neocortical disconnection syndrome (Leuchter et al. 1992; Morrison et al. 1990), may play a role in the decreased beta activity seen in DAT. By comparison, in subjects with VaD, the thiopental response is less affected, perhaps because this dementia is characterized by greater deep–white matter ischemic disease and subcortical dys-

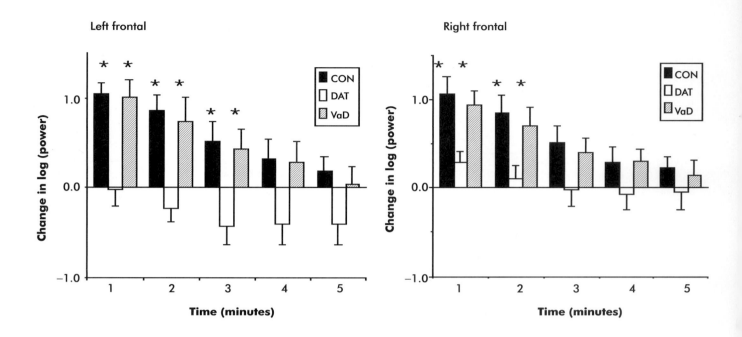

FIGURE 12–9. Changes in $\log_{10}$ (power) (mV^2, 20–28 Hz) over time in the left and right frontal regions after thiopental administration for psychiatrically healthy elderly control subjects (*CON*) (*solid bars*), subjects with dementia of the Alzheimer type (*DAT*) (*open bars*), and subjects with vascular dementia (*VaD*) (*cross-hatched bars*). Error bars represent 1 standard error.
* represents significant differences with respect to subjects with DAT, $P < .01$.
Source. Reprinted with permission from Holschneider DP, Leuchter AF, Uijtdehaage SHJ, et al.: "Loss of High Frequency EEG Response to Thiopental in Alzheimer's Dementia." *Neuropsychopharmacology* 20:1–7, 1997. Copyright 1997 by American College of Neuropsychopharmacology.

function. A thiopental challenge may be well suited for the in vivo assessment of brain function in dementias characterized by prominent cortical pathology.

Deafferentation in ascending pathways: the role of evoked potentials. Another type of afferent connection that can successfully be characterized with QEEG comprises the sensory input pathways. Results suggest that many of the changes observed in ERPs reflect changes in afferent fiber function and structure. Some of the most compelling evidence for ERPs changing in response to afferent damage has been seen in patients with dementia. Several researchers (Abbruzzese et al. 1984; Kato et al. 1990) have shown a delayed central conduction time for somatosensory evoked potentials in patients with VaD, but not in those with DAT. This finding is consistent with the fact that subjects with VaD have central white matter demyelination (which delays conduction of impulses), whereas subjects with DAT do not have such demyelination.

Using the deafferentation model, investigators have used ERPs to localize damage to brain structures. Mauguiere and Ibanez (1990) studied a series of patients with strokes in a variety of subcortical (either thalamus or subcortical white matter) and cortical locations, to determine if lesion location explained losses of specific somatosensory ERPs. These investigators found that damage to specific afferent pathways (confirmed by MRI) was associated with loss of specific ERP components and with the particular symptoms that patients reported. These investigators concluded that alterations in specific ERP components represented states of "hemispheric deafferentation." This finding may have implications for studies of sensory gating using ERPs in psychiatric patients.

Of greater direct relevance to geriatric neuropsychiatry are the changes in latency and amplitude of the P300 and other long-latency ERPs that are now well established in schizophrenia (Barrett et al. 1986; Morstyn et al. 1983). These also have been reported in children with schizophrenia (Erwin et al. 1986) and relatives of subjects with schizophrenia (Blackwood et al. 1991; Saitoh et al. 1984). Some evidence suggested significant P300 asymmetry, with lower amplitude potentials specifically over the left temporal region (McCarley et al. 1993; Morstyn et al. 1983); other investigators, however, were unable to confirm this asymmetry and suggested that it might represent a medication effect (Pfefferbaum et al. 1984b). Work by McCarley et al. (1993), however, indicates that these ERP abnormalities are associated with specific damage to the left supertemporal gyrus and that left-sided abnormalities are associated not only with reduced P300 amplitude over the left hemisphere but also with positive symptoms. McCarley and his colleagues (1991) have hypothesized that the P300 abnormalities seen in patients with schizophrenia may represent the results of neuronal excitotoxicity on the pyramidal cells of the left hippocampus. They propose that both psychotic symptoms and neuroleptic responsiveness reflect alteration in response in efferent fibers from the hippocampus, once again emphasizing the potential usefulness of the afferent fiber model of neurophysiology.

Future of Quantitative Electroencephalography

QEEG offers a unique contribution to the armamentarium of imaging technologies. Several powerful imaging technologies, such as PET or SPECT, directly measure the metabolism or perfusion of brain tissue; these techniques provide little or no information about damage to pathways that bring information into the central nervous system or that transfer information among critical brain areas. QEEG complements these techniques by assessing fiber system function. In some situations, QEEG using the cordance method may be the preferred method for assessing perfusion and metabolism. Because it is noninvasive, does not expose the patient to ionizing radiation, and does not require costly equipment, cordance would be ideal for patients who require long-term, frequent, or even bedside monitoring.

For similar reasons, QEEG has a variety of uses in the research setting. Researchers can observe brain function to assess drug effects, monitor the course of illness, determine prognosis, or screen novel treatments in a cost-effective manner. Multivariate analysis of QEEG measures, using several sensory modalities of ERPs or cognitive activation tasks, may improve diagnostic accuracy. The correlation of anatomical and physiological measures of brain function obtained from MRI, SPECT, and PET, with QEEG measurements, holds great promise for the future.

In the next few years, conventional EEG and QEEG probably will evolve into independent and complementary diagnostic tests. The clinician interested in detecting epileptiform abnormalities, or some other transient brain electrical activity, will request a conventional EEG. Clinicians interested in assessing global brain function, detecting focal brain dysfunction, or assessing cerebral perfusion or metabolism will request QEEG alone.

A conventional EEG in addition to a QEEG study will yield marginally more information than the quantitative study alone, at least until computer-assisted pattern recognition algorithms develop further. As pressures for medical cost containment mount, however, clinicians in all specialties likely will more heavily use diagnostic tests that are computer-based and that therefore require less physician time. Just as computers have reduced the physician time required for electrocardiogram interpretation, QEEG will eventually eliminate much of the physician time required for EEG interpretation. QEEG in many places still is a relatively costly procedure. As computer prices decline and QEEG systems become more widely available, however, QEEG will become a highly cost-effective means of imaging the brain.

Summary

EEG is an important tool in the evaluation of cerebral function and brain disease in geriatric patients. EEG findings rarely are pathognomonic for a specific diagnosis but provide information that is consistent with (e.g., slowing in DAT or delirium), supportive of (e.g., triphasic waves in Creutzfeldt-Jakob disease), or highly suggestive of the presence of a particular illness (e.g., anterotemporal spike-and-wave foci in a seizure disorder).

In the clinical practice of geriatric neuropsychiatry, the conventional EEG is very sensitive to the presence of an encephalopathy, but it remains a nonspecific indicator of the type of dysfunction. EEG is a useful physiological tool to confirm the diagnosis and severity of delirium and for monitoring response to treatment, but it lacks specificity in differentiating between dementia and mild-to-moderate states of delirium.

QEEG overcomes many of the limitations of conventional EEG. It yields more reliable and reproducible measurements of brain activity and is more sensitive for detecting subtle focal or generalized alterations in brain function. QEEG measures such as absolute power, relative power, and spectral ratios provide information that is not accessible from visual inspection of the conventional recording. These measures yield different functional and regional information regarding abnormality and thus are complementary and additive in the detection of brain dysfunction. QEEG measures are sensitive to changes in cholinergic tone. Hence, QEEG may be a useful adjunct in monitoring response to acetylcholinesterase inhibitors and other cognitive enhancers in patients with dementia.

Another product of quantitative EEG analysis is

ERPs. These are multicomponent waves of positive and negative potentials that result when the EEG signal from the scalp is averaged for a specified time interval after a repetitive stimulus. ERPs may be useful as supportive evidence in the diagnosis of dementia, depression, or delirium, but they probably are of little use for specifying the type of dementia.

Quantitation of the power in different frequency bands is more "objective" than conventional EEG interpretation and therefore minimizes variability in test interpretation. Standard QEEG does not, however, overcome all the limitations of conventional EEG. For example, despite the greater precision of QEEG in power determinations, the nature of the power changes observed with normal aging still shares some of the features of emerging organic brain disease. Normative databases of age-matched control subjects are useful for describing the range of normality but are of limited use for determining that a clinically significant abnormality exists in patients with mild excesses of slowing. In the absence of a consensus definition of what constitutes a statistically significant excess of slowing, comparison of serial studies from a patient over time remains the most reliable method for determining if abnormalities exist.

Recent research suggests that QEEG can provide information that is specific for the detection and diagnosis of different organic mental syndromes. New algorithms appear to be sensitive and specific for the detection of cortical deafferentation through monitoring dysfunction in different types of white matter fiber tracts. Coherence, a measure of the synchronization of electrical activity between different cortical regions, has proved useful in distinguishing subjects with DAT from those with VaD and in detecting cholinergic deafferentation, as well as fiber tract dysfunction associated with periventricular white matter changes on MRI. Cordance, a measure of cortical deafferentation in a single brain region, has strong associations with direct measures of perfusion or metabolism. Cordance appears to reliably detect areas of hypoperfusion resulting from stroke or brain degeneration (i.e., AD). Unmasking the inability of diseased neurons to mount an adequate electrophysiological response during pharmacological activation holds significant promise for examination of patterns of neuronal deafferentation in different dementias. ERPs also have been useful in examining deafferentation of ascending sensory pathways. Future research elucidating the neurophysiological and neurochemical correlates of such findings may permit the use of QEEG in the direct assessment of deafferentation within specific neuronal circuits.

Currently, QEEG is considered an adjunct to conventional EEG. Conventional EEG remains more sensitive for detecting very fast transient EEG activity as well as specific wave morphology and is the modality of choice for the evaluation of possible seizure disorders. As more sophisticated algorithms for interpreting neurophysiological signals are developed and validated, conventional EEG and QEEG may evolve into independent clinical tests.

References

Abbruzzese G, Reni L, Cocito L, et al: Short-latency somatosensory evoked potentials in degenerative and vascular dementia. J Neurol Neurosurg Psychiatry 47:1034–1037, 1984

Aguglia U, Gambardella A, Le Piane E, et al: Disappearance of periodic sharp wave complexes in Creutzfeldt-Jakob disease. Neurophysiol Clin 27:277–282, 1997

Ahuja GK, Mohanta A: Late onset epilepsy. A prospective study. Acta Neurol Scand 66:216–226, 1982

Albert MS, Duffy FH, McAnulty GR, et al: Electrophysiologic comparisons between two groups of patients with Alzheimer's disease. Arch Neurol 47:857–863, 1990

Alema G, Sinisi L: Il comportamento EEG dei soggetti affetti da tumor cerebri durante la narcosi da tiobarbiturici. Archivio di Psicologia, Neurologia e Psichiatria 11:390, 1950

American Psychiatric Association Task Force on Quantitative Electrophysiological Assessment: Quantitative electroencephalography: a report on the present state of computerized EEG techniques. Am J Psychiatry 148:961–964, 1991

Andermann K, Stoller A: EEG patterns in hospitalized and nonhospitalized aged. Electroencephalogr Clin Neurophysiol 13:319, 1961

Barrett K, McCallum WC, Pocock PV: Brain indicators of altered attention and information processing in schizophrenic patients. Br J Psychiatry 148:414–420, 1986

Beck AT: Depression Inventory. Philadelphia, PA, Philadelphia Center for Cognitive Therapy, 1978

Beck EC, Swanson C, Dustman RE: Long latency components of the visually evoked potential in man: effects of aging. Exp Aging Res 6:523–545, 1980

Bendat JS, Piersol AG: Random Data: Analysis and Measurement Procedures. New York, Wiley, 1986

Berg L, Danziger WL, Storandt M, et al: Predictive features in mild senile dementia of the Alzheimer type. Neurology 34:563–569, 1984

Berger H: On the electroencephalogram of man: twelfth report. Archiv fur Psychiatrie und Nervenkrankheiten 106: 165–187, 1937

Bickford R: Some effects of barbiturate anesthesia on the depth electroencephalogram. Proceedings of the Staff Meetings at the Mayo Clinic 28:162–170, 1953

Blackwood DH, St Clair DM, Muir WJ, et al: Auditory P300 and eye tracking dysfunction in schizophrenic pedigrees. Arch Gen Psychiatry 48:899–909, 1991

Bowen BC, Barker WW, Lowenstein D, et al: MR signal abnormalities in memory disorder and dementia. AJNR Am J Neuroradiol 11:283–290, 1990

Brazier MAB, Finesinger JE: Action of barbiturates on the cerebral cortex. Archives of Neurology and Psychiatry 53:51–58, 1945

Brazier MA, Hamlin H, Delgado JMR, et al: The persistence of electroencephalogram effects of pentothal. Anesthesiology 17:95–102, 1956

Brenner RP: Utility of EEG in delirium: past views and current practice. Int Psychogeriatr 3:211–229, 1991

Brenner RP, Ulrich RF, Spiker DG, et al: Computerized EEG spectral analysis in elderly normal, demented and depressed subjects. Electroencephalogr Clin Neurophysiol 64:483–492, 1986

Brenner RP, Reynolds CF, Ulrich RF: Diagnostic efficacy of computerized spectral versus visual EEG analysis in elderly normal, demented and depressed subjects. Electroencephalogr Clin Neurophysiol 69:110–117, 1998

Breslau J, Starr A, Sicotte N, et al: Topographic EEG changes with normal aging and SDAT. Electroencephalogr Clin Neurophysiol 72:281–289, 1989

Brown WS, Marsh JT, La Rue A: Event-related potentials in psychiatry: differentiating depression and dementia in the elderly. Bulletin of the Los Angeles Neurological Societies 47:91–107, 1982

Brown WS, Marsh JT, La Rue A: Exponential electrophysiological aging: P300 latency. Electroencephalogr Clin Neurophysiol 55:277–285, 1983

Buchan RJ, Nagata K, Yokoyama E, et al: Regional correlations between the EEG and oxygen metabolism in dementia of Alzheimer's type. Electroencephalogr Clin Neurophysiol 103:409–417, 1997

Burger LJ, Rowan J, Goldenshon E, et al: Creutzfeldt-Jakob disease. Arch Neurol 26:428–433, 1972

Burns A, Jacoby R, Levy R: Neurological signs in Alzheimer's disease. Age Ageing 20:45–51, 1991

Busk J, Galbraith G: EEG correlates of visual-motor practice in man. Electroencephalogr Clin Neurophysiol 38:415–422, 1975

Busse EW: Electroencephalography, in Alzheimer's Disease. Edited by Reisberg B. New York, Free Press, 1983, pp 231–236

Busse EW, Obrist WD: Pre-senescent electroencephalographic changes in normal subjects. J Gerontol A Biol Sci Med Sci 20:315–320, 1965

Buzsaki G, Bickford RG, Ponomareff G, et al: Nucleus basalis and thalamic control of neocortical activity in the freely moving rat. J Neurosci 8:4007–4026, 1988

Calloway E, Halliday R, Naylor H, et al: Effects of oral scopolamine on human stimulus evaluation. Psychopharmacology 85:133–138, 1985

Carney LR, Hudgins RL, Espinosa SE, et al: Seizures beginning after the age of 60. Arch Intern Med 124:707–709, 1969

Casellas F, Sagalés T, Calzada MD, et al: Visual evoked potentials in hepatic encephalopathy. Lancet 1:394–395, 1985

Chiofalo N, Fuentes A, Galves S: Serial EEG findings in 27 cases of Creutzfeldt-Jakob disease. Arch Neurol 37:143–145, 1980

Chu NS, Yang SS: Brainstem auditory evoked potentials in different types of hepatic diseases. Electroencephalogr Clin Neurophysiol 67:337–339, 1987

Coben LA, Danziger WL, Berg L: Frequency analysis of the resting awake EEG in mild senile dementia of Alzheimer type. Electroencephalogr Clin Neurophysiol 55:372–380, 1983a

Coben LA, Danziger WL, Hughes CP: Visual evoked potentials in mild senile dementia of the Alzheimer's type. Electroencephalogr Clin Neurophysiol 55:121–130, 1983b

Coben LA, Danziger W, Storandt M: A longitudinal EEG study of mild senile dementia of Alzheimer type: changes at 1 year and at 2.5 years. Electroencephalogr Clin Neurophysiol 61:101–112, 1985

Coben LA, Chi D, Snyder AZ, et al: Replication of a study of frequency analysis of the resting awake EEG in mild probable Alzheimer's disease. Electroencephalogr Clin Neurophysiol 75:148–154, 1990

Conti F, Manzoni T: The neurotransmitters and postsynaptic actions of callosally projecting neurons. Behav Brain Res 64:37–53, 1994

Cook IA, Leuchter AF, Vijtdehaage SH, et al: Altered cerebral energy utilization in late life depression. J Affect Disord 49:89–99, 1998

Cook IA, Leuchter AF, Wittle E, et al: Neurophysiologic predictors of treatment response to fluoxetine in major depression. Psychiatry Res 85:263–273, 1999

da Silva AM, Nunes B, Vaz AR, et al: Posttraumatic epilepsy in civilians: clinical and electroencephalographic studies. Acta Neurochir Suppl 55:56–63, 1992

Davidson RJ: EEG measures of cerebral asymmetry: conceptual and methodological issues. Int J Neurosci 39:71–89, 1988

Davies MG, Rowan MJ, Feely J: EEG and event related potentials in hepatic encephalopathy. Metab Brain Dis 6:175–186, 1991

Davis A, Wada J: Hemispheric asymmetry: frequency analysis of visual and auditory evoked responses to non-verbal stimuli. Electroencephalogr Clin Neurophysiol 37:1–9, 1974

Dejaiffe G, Constantinidis J, Ret-Bellet J, et al: Corrélations électrocliniques dans les démences de l'age avancé. Acta Neurol Belg 64:677–707, 1964

Detari LC, Vanderwolf H: Activity of identified cortically projecting and other basal forebrain neurones during large slow waves and cortical activation in anaesthetized rats. Brain Res 437:1–8, 1987

Dickson CT, Trepel C, Dickson BH: Extrinsic modulation of theta field activity in the entorhinal cortex of the anesthetized rat. Hippocampus 4(1):37–51, 1994

Drevets WC, Raichle ME: Neuroanatomical circuits in depression: implications for treatment mechanisms. Psychopharmacol Bull 28(3):261–274, 1992

Duffy F: Clinical decision making in quantified electroencephalographic analysis, in Statistics and Topography in Quantitative EEG. Edited by Samson-Dollfus D. Rouen, France, Elsevier, 1998, pp 9–26

Duffy FH, Albert MS, McAnulty G, et al: Age-related differences in brain electrical activity in healthy subjects. Ann Neurol 16:430–438, 1984a

Duffy FH, Albert MS, McAnulty G: Brain electrical activity in patients with presenile and senile dementia of the Alzheimer type. Ann Neurol 16:439–448, 1984b

Duffy FH, Jones K, Bartels P, et al: Quantified neurophysiology with mapping: statistical inference, exploratory and confirmatory data analysis. Brain Topogr 3:3–12, 1990

Duffy FH, Jones K, Bartels P, et al: Unrestricted principal components analysis of brain electrical activity: issues of data dimensionality, artifact, and utility. Brain Topogr 4:291–307, 1992

Duffy FH, McAnulty GB, Albert MS: Temporoparietal electrophysiological differences characterize patients with Alzheimer's disease: a split-half replication study. Cereb Cortex 5:215–221, 1995

Dunkin JJ, Osato S, Leuchter AF: Relationships between EEG coherence and neuropsychological tests in dementia. Clin Electroencephalogr 26:47–59, 1995

Engel G, Romano J: Delirium, a syndrome of cerebral insufficiency. Journal of Chronic Diseases 9:260–277, 1959

Engel JJ, Kuhl DE, Phelps ME, et al: Comparative localization of epileptic foci in partial epilepsy by PCT and EEG. Ann Neurol 12:529–537, 1982

Erkinjuntti T, Larsen T, Sulkava R, et al: EEG in the differential diagnosis between Alzheimer's disease and vascular dementia. Acta Neurol Scand 77:36–43, 1988

Erwin RJ, Edward R, Tanguay PE, et al: Abnormal P300 responses in schizophrenic children. J Am Acad Child Adolesc Psychiatry 25:615–622, 1986

Ettinger AB, Shinnar S: New-onset seizures in an elderly hospitalized population. Neurology 43:489–492, 1993

Ettlin T, Staehelin T, Kischka U, et al: Computed tomography, electroencephalography, and clinical features in the differential diagnosis of senile dementia. Arch Neurol 46:1217–1220, 1989

Folstein MF, Folstein SE, McHugh PR: Mini-Mental State: a practical method for grading the cognitive state of patients for the clinician. J Psychiatr Res 12:189–198, 1975

Fortin A: La signification clinique du tracé EEG de la maladie de Alzheimer. Acta Neurologica et Psychiatrica Belgica 66:106–115, 1966

Giaquinto S, Nolfe G: The EEG in the normal elderly: a contribution to the interpretation of aging and dementia. Electroencephalogr Clin Neurophysiol 63:540–546, 1986

Giaquinto S, Nolfe G: The electroencephalogram in the elderly: discrimination from demented patients and correlation with CT scan and neuropsychological data: a review, in The EEG of Mental Activities. Edited by Giannitrapani M. Basel, Karger, 1988, pp 50–65

Gibbs E, Lorimer F, Lennox W: Clinical correlates of exceedingly fast activity in the electroencephalogram. Disorders of the Nervous System 11:323–326, 1950

Gibbs FA, Gibbs EL: Changes with age awake, in Atlas of Electroencephalography, Vol 1. Reading, MA, Addison-Wesley, 1951, pp 82–88

Gloor P: Hans Berger and the discovery of the electroencephalogram. Electroencephalogr Clin Neurophysiol Suppl 28:1–36, 1969

Gloor P, Ball G, Schaul N: Brain lesions that produce delta waves in the EEG. Neurology 27:326–333, 1977

Goodin DS: Clinical utility of long latency 'cognitive' event-related potentials (P3): the pros. Electroencephalogr Clin Neurophysiol 76:2–5; discussion 1, 1990

Goodin D, Squires K, Henderson B, et al: Age-related variations in evoked potentials to auditory stimuli in normal human subjects. Electroencephalogr Clin Neurophysiol 44:447–458, 1978a

Goodin DS, Squires KC, Starr A: Long latency event-related components of the auditory evoked potential in dementia. Brain 101:635–648, 1978b

Gordon EB: Serial EEG studies in presenile dementia. Br J Psychiatry 114:779–780, 1968

Gordon EB, Sim M: The EEG in presenile dementia. J Neurol Neurosurg Psychiatry 30:285–291, 1967

Gordon E, Kraiuhin C, Harris A, et al: The differential diagnosis of dementia using P300 latency. Biol Psychiatry 21:1123–1132, 1986

Grass AM, Gibbs FA: A Fourier transform of the electroencephalogram. J Neurophysiol 1:521–526, 1938

Groen JJ, Endtz LJ: Hereditary Pick's disease, second re-examination of a large family and discussion of other hereditary cases with particular reference to electroencephalography and computerized tomography. Brain 105:443–459, 1982

Hamilton M: A rating scale for depression. J Neurol Neurosurg Psychiatry 23:56–62, 1960

Hansch EC, Syndulko K, Cohen SN, et al: Cognition in Parkinson disease: an event-related potential perspective. Ann Neurol 11:599–607, 1982

Harkins SW: Effects of presenile dementia of the Alzheimer's type on brainstem transmission time. Int J Neurosci 15:165–170, 1981

Harrison MJ, Thomas DJ, Du-Boulay GM, et al: Multi-infarct dementia. J Neurol Sci 40:97–103, 1979

Hauser WA, Morris ML, Heston LL, et al: Seizures and myoclonus in patients with Alzheimer's disease. Neurology 36:1226–1230, 1986

Helmchen H, Kanowski S, Künkel H: Die Altersabhängigkeit der Lokalisation von EEG-Herden. Archiv für Psychiatrie und Nervenkrankheiten 209:474–483, 1967

Heyman RA, Brenner RP, Reynolds CF, et al: Age at initial onset of depression and waking EEG variables in the elderly. Biol Psychiatry 29:994–1000, 1991

Hillyard SA, Picton TW: Electrophysiology of cognition, in Handbook of Physiology, Vol 5. Edited by Mountcastle VB, Plum F, Geiger SR. Bethesda, MD, American Physiology Society, 1987, pp 519–584

Hof PR, Bouras C, Constantinidis J, et al: Selective disconnection of specific visual association pathways in cases of Alzheimer's disease presenting with Balint's syndrome. J Neuropathol Exp Neurol 49:168–184, 1990

Holschneider DP, Leuchter AF: Beta activity in aging and dementia. Brain Topogr 8:169–180, 1995

Holschneider DP, Leuchter AF: Attenuation of brain high frequency response after thiopental in early stages of Alzheimer's dementia. Psychopharmacology (in press)

Holschneider DP, Leuchter AF, Walton NY, et al: Changes in cortical EEG and cholinergic function in response to NGF in rats with nucleus basalis lesions. Brain Res 765:228–237, 1997a

Holschneider DP, Leuchter AF, Vijtdehaage SH, et al: Loss of high frequency EEG response to thiopental in Alzheimer's dementia. Neuropsychopharmacology 20:1–7, 1997b

Holschneider DP, Leuchter AF, Scremin OU, et al: Effects of cholinergic deafferentation and NGF on brain electrical coherence. Brain Res Bull 45:531–541, 1998

Holschneider DP, Waite J, Leuchter AF, et al: Changes in electrocortical power and coherence in response to the cholinergic toxin [192]IgG-Saporin. Exp Brain Res 126:270–280, 1999

Hubbard O, Sunde D, Goldensohn ES: The EEG in centenarians. Electroencephalogr Clin Neurophysiol 40:407–417, 1976

Hughes JR, Cayaffa JJ: The EEG in patients at different ages without organic cerebral disease. Electroencephalogr Clin Neurophysiol 42:776–84l, 1977

Hughes JR, Shanmugham S, Wetzel LC, et al: The relationship between EEG changes and cognitive functions in dementia: a study in a VA population. Clin Electroencephalogr 20:77–85, 1989

Huisman UW, Posthuma J, Visser SL, et al: The influence of attention on visual evoked potentials in normal adults and dementia. Clin Neurol Neurosurg 87:11–16, 1985

Jacobson SA, Leuchter AF, Walter D: Conventional and quantitative EEG in the diagnosis of delirium among the elderly [see comments]. J Neurol Neurosurg Psychiatry 56:153–158, 1993a

Jacobson SA, Leuchter AF, Walter D, et al: Serial quantitative EEG among elderly subjects with delirium. Biol Psychiatry 34:135–140, 1993b

Jelic V, Shigeta M, Julin P, et al: Quantitative electroencephalography power and coherence in Alzheimer's disease and mild cognitive impairment. Dementia 7(6):314–323, 1996

Jerrett SA, Corsak J: Clinical utility of topographic EEG brain mapping. Clin Electroencephalogr 19:134–143, 1988

Johannesson G, Brun A, Gustafson I, et al: EEG in pre-senile dementia related to cerebral blood flow and autopsy findings. Acta Neurol Scand 56:89–103, 1977

Johannesson G, Hagberg B, Gustafson L, et al: EEG and cognitive impairment in presenile dementia. Acta Neurol Scand 59:225–240, 1979

John ER, Karmel BZ, Corning WC, et al: Neurometrics. Science 196(4297):1393–1410, 1977

John ER, Prichep LS, Fridman J, et al: Neurometrics: computer-assisted differential diagnosis of brain dysfunctions. Science 239:162–169, 1988

Kalayam B, Alexopoulos GS, Kindermann S, et al: P300 latency in geriatric depression. Am J Psychiatry 155:425–427, 1998

Kanowski S: EEG und Alterpsychiatrie. Nervenarzt 42:347–355, 1971

Kaszniak AW, Fox J, Gandell DL, et al: Predictors of mortality in presenile and senile dementia. Ann Neurol 3:246–252, 1978

Kato H, Sugawara Y, Ito H, et al: White matter lucencies in multi-infarct dementia: a somatosensory evoked potentials and CT study. Acta Neurol Scand 81:181–183, 1990

Katz RI, Horowitz GR: Electroencephalogram in the septuagenarian: studies in a normal geriatric population. J Am Geriatr Soc 3:273–275, 1982

Kiersey DK, Bickford RG, Faulconer A: Electro-encephalographic patterns produced by thiopental sodium during surgical operations: description and classification. Br J Anaesth 23:141–152, 1951

Koponen H: Delirium in the elderly: a brief overview. Int Psychogeriatr 3:177–179, 1991

Koponen H, Partanen J, Paakkonnen A, et al: EEG spectral analysis in delirium. J Neurol Neurosurg Psychiatry 52:980–985, 1989

Kuba M, Peregrin J, Vit F, et al: Pattern-reversal visual evoked potentials in patients with chronic renal insufficiency. Electroencephalogr Clin Neurophysiol 56:438–442, 1983

Kwa VI, Weinstein HC, Meyjes EF, et al: Spectral analysis of the EEG and 99m-Tc-HMPAO SPECT-scan in Alzheimer's disease. Biol Psychiatry 33:100–107, 1993

Leppler JG, Greenberg HJ: The P3 potential and its clinical usefulness in the objective classification of dementia. Cortex 20:427–433, 1984

Leuchter AF, Jacobson SA: Quantitative measurement of brain electrical activity in delirium. Int Psychogeriatr 3:231–247, 1991

Leuchter A, Spar J, Walter D, et al: Electroencephalographic spectra and coherence in the diagnosis of Alzheimer's-type and multi-infarct dementia. Arch Gen Psychiatry 44:993–998, 1987

Leuchter AF, Read SL, Shapira J, et al: Stable bimodal response to cholinomimetic drugs in Alzheimer's disease. Brain mapping correlates. Neuropsychopharmacology 4:165–173, 1991

Leuchter AF, Newton TF, Cook IA, et al: Changes in brain functional connectivity in Alzheimer-type and multi-infarct dementia. Brain 115:1543–1561, 1992

Leuchter AF, Daly KA, Rosenberg-Thompson S, et al: Prevalence and significance of electroencephalographic abnormalities in patients with suspected organic mental syndromes. J Am Geriatr Soc 41:605–611, 1993a

Leuchter AF, Cook IA, Newton TF, et al: Regional differences in brain electrical activity in dementia: use of spectral power and spectral ratio measures. Electroencephalogr Clin Neurophysiol 87:385–393, 1993b

Leuchter AF, Cook IA, Mena I, et al: Assessment of cerebral perfusion using quantitative EEG cordance. Psychiatry Res Neuroimaging 55:141–152, 1994a

Leuchter AF, Cook IA, Lufkin RB, et al: Cordance: a new method for assessment of cerebral perfusion and metabolism using quantitative electroencephalography. Neuroimage 1:208–219, 1994b

Leuchter AF, Dunkin JJ, Lufkin RB, et al: Effect of white matter disease on functional connections in the aging brain. J Neurol Neurosurg Psychiatry 57:1347–1354, 1994c

Leuchter AF, Simon SL, Daly KA, et al: Quantitative EEG correlates of outcome in older psychiatric patients, Part I: cross-sectional and longitudinal assessment of patients with dementia. Am J Geriatr Psychiatry 2:200–209, 1994d

Leuchter AF, Simon SL, Daly KA, et al: Quantitative EEG correlates of outcome in older psychiatric patients, Part II: two-year follow-up of patients with depression. Am J Geriatr Psychiatry 2:290–299, 1994e

Leuchter AF, Cook IA, Vijtdehaage SH, et al: Brain structure and function and the outcomes of treatment for depression. J Clin Psychiatry 58(suppl 16):22–31, 1997

Leuchter AF, Cook IA, Vijtdehaage SH, et al: Relationship between brain electrical activity and cortical perfusion in normal subjects, Psychiatry Research Neuroimaging 90:125140, 1999

Leung LS, Martin LA, Stewart DJ, et al: Hippocampal theta rhythm in behaving rats following ibotenic acid lesion of the septum. Hippocampus 4:136–147, 1994

Levy LJ, Bolton RP: Visual evoked potentials in hepatic encephalopathy. J Hepatol 3:7P, 1986

Levy LJ, Bolton RP, Losowsky MS: The visual evoked potential in clinical hepatic encephalopathy in acute and chronic liver disease. Hepatogastroenterology 37(suppl 2):66–73, 1990

Liddell DW: Investigations of EEG findings in presenile dementia. J Neurol Neurosurg Psychiatry 21:173–176, 1958

Liston EH: Clinical findings in presenile dementia. A report of 50 cases. J Nerv Ment Dis 167:337–342, 1979

Loeb C: Clinical diagnosis of multi-infarct dementia, in Aging of the Brain and Dementia. Edited by Amaducci L, Davison AN, Antuono P. New York, Raven, 1980, pp 251–260

Logar C, Grabmair W, Schneider G, et al: EEG-Veränderungen bei seniler Demenz vom Alzheimer Typ. Zeitschrift fur EEG-EMG 18:214–216, 1987

Loring DW, Sheer DE, Largen JW, et al: Forty hertz EEG activity in dementia of the Alzheimer's type and multi-infarct dementia. Psychophysiology 22:116–121, 1985

Luhdorf K, Jensen LK, Plesner AM: Epilepsy in the elderly: incidence, social function, and disability. Epilepsia 27:135–141, 1986a

Luhdorf K, Jensen LK, Plesner AM: Etiology of seizures in the elderly. Epilepsia 27:458–463, 1986b

Lukas SE, Mendelson JH, Khourii E, et al: Ethanol-induced alterations in EEG alpha activity and apparent source of the auditory P300 evoked response potential. Alcohol 7:471–477, 1990

Margerison JH, Scott DF: Huntington's chorea: clinical EEG and neuropathological findings (abstract). Electroencephalogr Clin Neurophysiol 19:314, 1965

Matejcek M, Knor K, Piguet PV, et al: Electroencephalographic and clinical changes as correlated in geriatric patients treated three months with an ergot alkaloid preparation. J Am Geriatr Soc 27:198–202, 1979

Matos L, Paiva T, Cravo M: Multimodal evoked potentials in subclinical hepatic encephalopathy, in Advances in Ammonia Metabolism and Hepatic Encephalopathy. Edited by Soeters PB, Wilson JHP, Meijer AJ, et al. Amsterdam, Elsevier, 1988, pp 373–381

Matousek M, Volavka J, Roubicek J, et al: EEG frequency analysis related to age in normal adults. Electroencephalogr Clin Neurophysiol 23:162–167, 1967

Mauguiere F, Ibanez V: Loss of parietal and frontal somatosensory evoked potentials in hemispheric deafferentation, in New Trends and Advanced Techniques in Clinical Neurophysiology. Edited by Rossini P, Mauguiere F. New York, Elsevier, 1990, pp 274–285

Maurer K, Ihl R, Dierks T: Topographie der P300 in der psychiatrie. II. Kognitive P300-felder bei Demenz. Zeitschrift fur EEG-EMG 19:26–29, 1988

McAdam W, Robinson RA: Senile intellectual deterioration and the electroencephalogram: a quantitative correlation. Mental Science 102:819–825, 1956

McCarley RW, Faux SF, Shenton ME, et al: Event-related potentials in schizophrenia: their biological and clinical correlates and a new model of schizophrenic pathophysiology. Schizophr Res 4:209–231, 1991

McCarley RW, Shenton ME, O'Donnell B, et al: Auditory P300 abnormalities and left posterior superior temporal gyrus volume reduction in schizophrenia. Arch Gen Psychiatry 50:190–197, 1993

Mendez MF, Catanzaro P, Doss RC, et al: Seizures in Alzheimer's disease: clinicopathologic study. J Geriatr Psychiatry Neurol 7:230–233, 1994

Minthon L, Gustafson L, Dalfelt G, et al: Oral tetrahydroaminoacridine treatment of Alzheimer's disease evaluated clinically and by regional cerebral blood flow and EEG. Dementia 4:32–42, 1993

Mooradian AD, Perryman K, Fitten J, et al: Cortical function in elderly non-insulin dependent diabetic patients. Behavioral and electrophysiologic studies. Arch Intern Med 148:2369–2372, 1988

Morrison J, Scherr S, Lewis D, et al: The laminar and regional distribution of neocortical somatostatin and neuritic plaques: implications for Alzheimer's disease, in The Biological Substrates of Alzheimer's Disease. Edited by Scheibel A, Wechsler A, Brazier M. Orlando, FL, Academic Press, 1986

Morrison JH, Hof PR, Campbell MJ, et al: Cellular pathology in Alzheimer's disease: implications for corticocortical disconnection and differential vulnerability, in Imaging, Cerebral Topography and Alzheimer's Disease. Edited by Rapoport S, Petit H, Leys D, Christen Y. New York, Springer, 1990, pp 19–40

Morrison JH, Hof PR, Bouras C: An anatomic substrate for visual disconnection in Alzheimer's disease. Ann N Y Acad Sci 640:36–43, 1991

Morstyn R, Duffy HF, McCarley RW: Altered P300 topography in schizophrenia. Arch Gen Psychiatry 40:729–734, 1983

Mullis RJ, Holcomb PJ, Diner BC, et al: The effects of aging on the P3 component of the visual event-related potential. Electroencephalogr Clin Neurophysiol 62:141–149, 1985

Mundy-Castle A: Theta and beta rhythm in the electroencephalograms of normal adult. Electroencephalogr Clin Neurophysiol 3:477–486, 1951

Niedermeyer E, Lopes da Silva F: Electroencephalography: Basic Principles, Clinical Applications, and Related Fields. Baltimore, MD, Urban & Schwarzenberg, 1987

Nuwer M: Assessment of digital EEG, quantitative EEG, and EEG brain mapping: report of the American Academy of Neurology and the American Clinical Neurophysiology Society. Neurology 49:277–292, 1997

Nuwer MR, Jordan SE, Ahn SS: Evaluation of stroke using EEG frequency analysis and topographic mapping. Neurology 37:1153–1159, 1987

Obrist W: The electroencephalogram of normal aged adults. Electroencephalogr Clin Neurophysiol 6:235–244, 1954

Obrist WD: Problems of aging, in Handbook of Electroencephalography and Clinical Neurophysiology, Vol 6, Part A. Edited by Rémond A. Amsterdam, Elsevier, 1976, pp 275–292

Obrist WD: Electroencephalographic changes in normal aging and dementia, in Brain Function in Old Age, Bayer Symposium VII. Edited by Hoffmeister F, Müller C. Berlin, Springer-Verlag, 1979, pp 102–111

Obrist WD, Busse EW: The electroencephalogram in old age, in Applications of Electroencephalography in Psychiatry. Edited by Wilson WP. Durham, NC, Duke University Press, 1965, pp 185–205

Obrist WD, Sokoloff L, Lassen NA, et al: Relation of EEG to cerebral blood flow and metabolism in old age. Electroencephalogr Clin Neurophysiol 15:610–619, 1963

O'Connor K, Shaw J: Field dependence, laterality and the EEG. Biol Psychol 6:93–109, 1978

O'Connor KP, Shaw JC, Ongley CO: The EEG and differential diagnosis in psychogeriatrics. Br J Psychiatry 135:156–162, 1979

O'Donnell BF, Faux SF, McCartney RW, et al: Increased rate of P300 latency prolongation with age in schizophrenia. Electrophysiological evidence for a neurodegenerative process. Arch Gen Psychiatry 52:544–549, 1995

Ohkura T, Isse K, Akazawa K, et al: Evaluation of estrogen treatment in female patients with dementia of the Alzheimer type. Endocr J 41:361–371, 1994

Oken BS, Kaye JA: Electrophysiologic function in the healthy, extremely old. Neurology 42:519–526, 1992

Olson L, Nordberg A, von Holst H, et al: Nerve growth factor affects ^{11}C-nicotine binding, blood flow, EEG, and verbal episodic memory in an Alzheimer patient (case report). J Neural Transm 4:79–95, 1992

Oltman JE, Friedman S: Comments on Huntington's chorea. J Med Genet 3:298–314, 1961

Otomo E, Tsubaki T: Electroencephalography in subjects sixty years and over. Electroencephalogr Clin Neurophysiol 20:77–82, 1966

Paiva T, Fred A, Nunes-Leitao J: EEG and VER mapping in some metabolic disease, in Statistics and Topography in Quantitative EEG. Paris, Elsevier, 1988, pp 237–241

Pampiglione G: Induced fast activity in the EEG as an aid in the location of cerebral lesions. Electroencephalogr Clin Neurophysiol 1:79–82, 1952

Patterson JV, Michalewski HJ, Starr A: Latency variability of the components of auditory event-related potentials to infrequent stimuli in aging, Alzheimer type dementia, and depression. Electroencephalogr Clin Neurophysiol 71:450–460, 1988

Pentillä M, Partanen J, Soininen H, et al: Quantitative analysis of occipital EEG in different stages of Alzheimer's disease. Electroencephalogr Clin Neurophysiol 60:1–6, 1985

Perryman KM, Fitten LJ: Quantitative EEG during a double-blind trial of THA and lecithin in patients with Alzheimer's disease. J Geriatr Psychiatry Neurol 4:127–133, 1991

Pfefferbaum A, Horvath TB, Roth WT, et al: Event-related potential changes in chronic alcoholics. Electroencephalogr Clin Neurophysiol 47:637–647, 1979

Pfefferbaum A, Ford JM, Wenegrat BG, et al: Clinical application of P3 component of event-related potentials. I. Normal aging. Electroencephalogr Clin Neurophysiol 59:85–103, 1984a

Pfefferbaum A, Wenegrat BG, Ford JM, et al: Clinical application of the P3 component of event-related potentials. II. Dementia, depression and schizophrenia. Electroencephalogr Clin Neurophysiol 59:104–124, 1984b

Pfefferbaum A, Ford JM, Kraemer C: Clinical utility of long latency "cognitive" event-related potentials (P3): the cons. Electroencephalogr Clin Neurophysiol 76:6–12; discussion 1, 1990

Picton TW, Stuss DT, Champagne SC, et al: The effects of age on human event-related potentials. Psychophysiology 21:312–325, 1984

Picton TW, Cherri AM, Champagne SC, et al: The effects of age and task difficulty on the late positive component of the auditory evoked potential. Electroencephalogr Clin Neurophysiol 38:132–133, 1986

Pierelli F, Pozzessere C, Sanarelli L, et al: Electrophysiological study in patients with chronic hepatic insufficiency. Acta Neurol Belg 85:284–291, 1985

Polich J: P300 in the evaluation of aging and dementia. Electroencephalogr Clin Neurophysiol Suppl 42:304–323, 1991

Polich J, Howard L, Starr A: Aging effects on the P300 component of the event-related potential from auditory stimuli: peak definition, variation, and measurement. J Gerontol 40:721–726, 1985

Polich J, Ehlers CL, Otis S, et al: P300 latency reflects the degree of cognitive decline in dementing illness. Electroencephalogr Clin Neurophysiol 63:138–144, 1986

Pollock VE, Schneider LS: Topographic electroencephalographic alpha in recovered depressed elderly. J Abnorm Psychol 98:268–273, 1989

Pollock VE, Schneider LS: Quantitative, waking EEG research on depression. Biol Psychiatry 27:757–780, 1990

Pozzi D, Vazquez S, Petracchi M, et al: Quantified electroencephalographic correlates of relative frontal or parietal hypoperfusion in dementia. J Neuropsychiatry Clin Neurosci 8:26–32, 1996

Pramming S, Thorsteinsson B, Stigsby B, et al: Glycaemic threshold for changes in electroencephalograms during hypoglycaemia in patients with insulin dependent diabetes. BMJ 296:665–667, 1988

Prichep LS, John ER, Ferris SH, et al: Quantitative EEG correlates of cognitive deterioration in the elderly. Neurobiol Aging 15:85–90, 1994

Rabins PV, Folstein MF: Delirium and dementia: diagnostic criteria and fatality rates. Br J Psychiatry 140:149–153, 1982

Rae-Grant A, Blume W, Lau C, et al: The electroencephalogram in Alzheimer-type dementia: a sequential study correlating the electroencephalogram with psychometric and quantitative pathologic data. Arch Neurol 44:50–54, 1987

Ray PG, Jackson WJ: Lesions of nucleus basalis alter ChAT activity and EEG in rat frontal neocortex. Electroencephalogr Clin Neurophysiol 79:62–68, 1991

Rice DM, Buchsbaum MS, Hardy D, et al: Focal left temporal slow EEG activity is related to a verbal recent memory deficit in a non-demented elderly population. J Gerontol 46:144–151, 1991

Riekkinen P Jr, Jakala P, Sirvio V, et al: The effects of THA on scopolamine and nucleus basalis lesion-induced EEG slowing. Brain Res Bull 26:633–637, 1991

Roberts M, McGeorge AP, Caird FI: Electroencephalography and computerized tomography in vascular and nonvascular dementia in old age. J Neurol Neurosurg Psychiatry 41:903–906, 1978

Romano J, Engel G: Delirium, I: electroencephalographic data. Arch Neurol Psychiatry 51:356–377, 1944

Rosenberg C, Nudleman K, Starr A: Cognitive evoked potentials (P300) in early Huntington's disease. Arch Neurol 42:984987, 1985

Rossini PM, Pirchio M, Treviso M, et al: Checkerboard reversal pattern and flash VEPs in dialyzed and nondialyzed subjects. Electroencephalogr Clin Neurophysiol 52:435–444, 1981

Rossini PM, diStefano E, Febbo A, et al: Brainstem auditory evoked responses in patients with chronic renal failure. Electroencephalogr Clin Neurophysiol 57:507–514, 1984

Roubicek J: The electroencephalogram in the middle-aged and elderly. J Am Geriatr Soc 25:145–152, 1977

Sackeim HA, Prohovnik I: Studies of brain imaging in mood disorders, in Biology of Depressive Disorders. Part A: A Systems Perspective. Edited by Mann JJ, Kupfer DJ. New York, Plenum, 1993, pp 205–258

Sackeim HA, Prohovnik I, Moeller JR, et al: Regional cerebral blood flow in mood disorders, I: comparison of major depressives and normal controls at rest. Arch Gen Psychiatry 47:60–70, 1990

Saitoh O, Niwa S, Hiramatsu K, et al: Abnormalities in late positive components of event-related potentials may reflect a genetic predisposition to schizophrenia. Biol Psychiatry 19:293–303, 1984

Saletu B, Darragh A, Salmon P, et al: EEG brain mapping in evaluating the time-course of the central action of DUP 996—a new acetylcholine releasing drug. Br J Clin Pharmacol 28:1–16, 1989

Saletu B, Grunberger J, Anderer R: On brain protection of co-dergocrine mesylate (Hydergine) against hypoxic hypoxidosis of different severity: double-blind placebo-controlled quantitative EEG and psychometric studies. International Journal of Clinical Pharmacology, Therapy, and Toxicology 28:510–524, 1990

Saletu B, Anderer P, Paulos E, et al: EEG brain mapping in diagnostic and therapeutic assessment of dementia. Alzheimer Dis Assoc Disord 5(suppl 1):S57–S75, 1991

Sander JW, Hart YM, Johnson AL, et al: National General Practice Study of Epilepsy: newly diagnosed epileptic seizures in a general population. Lancet 336:1267–1271, 1990

Sandford NL, Saul RE: Assessment of hepatic encephalopathy with visual evoked potentials compared with conventional methods. Hepatology 8:1094–1098, 1988

Schatzberg AF, Elliot GR, Lerbinger JE, et al: Topographic mapping in depressed patients, in Topographic Mapping of Brain Electrical Activity. Edited by Duffy FH. Boston, MA, Butterworths, 1986, pp 389–391

Schaul N, Lueders H, Sachdev K, et al: Generalized, bilaterally synchronous bursts of slow waves in the EEG. Arch Neurol 38:690–692, 1981

Schlagenhauff RE: Electroencephalogram in gerontology. Clin Electroencephalogr 4:163–168, 1973

Schreiter-Gasser U, Gasser T, Ziegler P: Quantitative EEG analysis in early onset Alzheimer's disease: a controlled study. Electroencephalogr Clin Neurophysiol 86:15–22, 1993

Scott DF, Heathfield KWG, Toone B, et al: The EEG in Huntington's chorea: a clinical and neuropathological study. J Neurol Neurosurg Psychiatry 35:97–102, 1972

Shagass C, Roemer RA, Straumanis JJ, et al: Psychiatric diagnostic discriminations with combinations of quantitative EEG variables. Br J Psychiatry 144:581–592, 1984

Shaw J, O'Connor K, Ongley C: The EEG as a measure of cerebral functional organization. Br J Psychiatry 130:260–264, 1977

Shaw JC, O'Connor K, Ongley C: EEG coherence as a measure of cerebral functional organization, in Architectonics of the Cerebral Cortex. Edited by Brazier MAB, Petsche H. New York, Raven, 1978, pp 245–255

Sheer DE: Biofeedback training of 40 Hz EEG activity and behavior, in Behavior and Brain Electrical Activity. Edited by Burch N, Altschuler H. New York, Plenum, 1975, pp 325–362

Sheer DE: Focused arousal and 40 Hz EEG, in The Neuropsychology of Learning Disabilities. Edited by Knight RM. Baltimore, MD, University Park Press, 1976, pp 71–87

Sheer DE: Focused arousal, 40 Hz EEG, and dysfunction, in Self-Regulation of the Brain and Behavior. Edited by Elbert T, Rockstroh B, Lutzenberger W, Birbaumer N. New York, Springer-Verlag, 1984, pp 64–84

Shigeta M, Persson A, Viitanen M, et al: EEG regional changes during long-term treatment with tetrahydroaminoacridine (THA) in Alzheimer's disease. Acta Neurol Scand Suppl 149:58–61, 1993

Smith DB, Michalewski HJ, Brent GA, Thompson LW: Auditory averaged evoked potentials and aging: factors of stimulus, task and topography. Biol Psychol 11:135–151, 1980

Soininen H, Partanen VJ, Helkala EL, et al: EEG findings in senile dementia and normal aging. Acta Neurol Scand 65:59–70, 1982

Spehlmann R: EEG Primer. New York, Elsevier, 1981

Spydell JD, Sheer DE: Forty hertz EEG activity in Alzheimer's type dementia. Psychophysiology 20:313–319, 1982

Squires KC, Chippendale TJ, Wrege KS, et al: Electrophysiological assessment of mental function in aging and dementia, in Aging in the 1980s: Selected Contemporary Issues in the Psychology of Aging. Edited by Poon LW. Washington, DC, American Psychological Association, 1980, pp 125–134

St. Clair D, Blackwood D: Premature senility in Down's syndrome (letter). Lancet 2:34, 1985

Steinhoff BJ, Racker S, Herrendorf G, et al: Accuracy and reliability of periodic sharp wave complexes in Creutzfeldt-Jakob disease. Arch Neurol 53:162–166, 1996

Steriade M, Gloor P, Llinas R, et al: Report of IFCN Committee on Basic Mechanisms. Basic mechanisms of cerebral rhythmic activities. Electroencephalogr Clin Neurophysiol 76:481–508, 1990

Stigsby B, Jóhannesson G, Ingvar DH: Regional EEG analysis and regional cerebral blood flow in Alzheimer's and Pick's diseases. Electroencephalogr Clin Neurophysiol 51:537–547, 1981

Stoller A: Slowing of the alpha-rhythm of the electroencephalogram and its association with mental deterioration and epilepsy. Journal of Mental Science 95:972–984, 1949

Sung CY, Chu NS: Epileptic seizures in elderly people: aetiology and seizure type. Age Ageing 19:25–30, 1990

Syndulko K, Hansch MA, Cohen SN, et al: Long-latency event related potentials in normal aging and dementia, in Clinical Applications of Evoked Potentials in Neurology (Advances in Neurology, Vol 32). Edited by Courjon J, Maugiere F, Revol M. New York, Raven, 1982, pp 279–286

Syndulko K, Cohen SN, Pettler-Jennings P, et al: P300 and neurocognitive function in neurologic patients, in Evoked Potentials, II. The Second International Evoked Potentials Symposium. Edited by Nodar RH, Barber C. Boston, MA, Butterworth, 1984, pp 441–445

Thomas RJ: Seizures and epilepsy in the elderly. Arch Intern Med 157:605–617, 1997

Tissot R, Constantinidis J, Richard J: La Maladie de Pick. Paris, Masson, 1975

Torres F, Faoro A, Loewenson R, et al: The electroencephalogram of elderly subjects revisited. Electroencephalogr Clin Neurophysiol 56:391–398, 1983

Trzepacz PT, Sclabassi RJ, Van Thiel DH: Delirium: a subcortical phenomenon? J Neuropsychiatry 1:283–290, 1989

Tucker D, Roth D, Bair T: Functional connections among cortical regions: topography of EEG coherence. Electroencephalogr Clin Neurophysiol 63:242–250, 1986

van der Rijt CCD, Schalm SW: Quantitative EEG analysis and evoked potentials to measure (latent) hepatic encephalopathy. J Hepatol 14:141–142, 1992

Vanderwolf C: The electrocorticogram in relation to physiology and behavior: a new analysis. Electroencephalogr Clin Neurophysiol 82:165–175, 1992

Visser SL: The electroencephalogram and evoked potentials in normal aging and dementia, in Event-Related Brain Research. Edited by Brunia CHM, Mulder G, Verbaten MV. New York, Elsevier, 1991, pp 289–303

Visser SL, Stan FC, Van Tilburg W, et al: Visual evoked response in senile and presenile dementia. Electroencephalogr Clin Neurophysiol 40:385–392, 1976

Visser SL, Van Tilburg W, Hooijer C, et al: Visual evoked potentials (VEPs) in senile dementia (Alzheimer's type) and in non-organic behavioural disorders in the elderly; comparison with EEG parameters. Electroencephalogr Clin Neurophysiol 60:115–121, 1985

Visser SL, Hooijer C, Jonker C, et al: Anterior temporal focal abnormalities in EEG in normal aged subjects: correlations with psychopathological and CT brain scan findings. Electroencephalogr Clin Neurophysiol 66:1–7, 1987

Vitiello MV, Prinz PN: Sleep and EEG studies in Alzheimer's disease, in Alzheimer's Disease: Advances in Basic Research and Therapies. Edited by Wurtman RJ, Corkin SJ, Growdon JH. Cambridge, MA, Center for Brain Sciences and Metabolism Charitable Trust, 1987, pp 625–634

Wang H, Busse E: EEG of healthy old persons—a longitudinal study. I. Dominant background activity and occipital rhythm. J Gerontol 24:419–426, 1969

Weiner H, Schuster DB: The electroencephalogram in dementia. Some preliminary observations and correlations. Electroencephalogr Clin Neurophysiol 8:479–488, 1956

Williamson PC, Merskey H, Morrison S, et al: Quantitative electroencephalographic correlates of cognitive decline in normal elderly subjects. Arch Neurol 47:1185–1188, 1990

Woody RH: Intra-judge reliability in clinical electroencephalography. J Clin Psychol 22:150–154, 1966

Woody RH: Inter-judge reliability in clinical electroencephalography. J Clin Psychol 24:251–256, 1968

Wright CE, Harding GFA, Orwin A: Presenile dementia—the use of the flash and pattern VEP in diagnosis. Electroencephalogr Clin Neurophysiol 57:405–415, 1984

Yang SS, Chu NS, Liaw YF: Brainstem auditory evoked potentials in hepatic encephalopathy. Hepatology 6:1352–1355, 1986

Yen CL, Liaw YF: Somatosensory evoked potentials and number connection test in the detection of subclinical hepatic encephalopathy. Hepatogastroenterology 37:332–334, 1990

Yesavage JA: Geriatric Depression Scale. Psychopharm Bull 24:709–711, 1988

Zeneroli ML, Pinelli G, Gollini G, et al: Visual evoked potential: a diagnostic tool for the assessment of hepatic encephalopathy. Gut 25:291–299, 1984

SECTION III

Neuropsychiatric Aspects of Psychiatric Disorders in the Elderly

Godfrey D. Pearlson, M.D., Section Editor

Mood Disorders

Carl Salzman, M.D.

Symptomatic Differences in the Elderly

Mood disorders, divided into depressive disorders and bipolar disorder, are relatively common in the elderly. Although diagnostic criteria for either major depressive disorder, unipolar type, or bipolar disorder are not different for the elderly than for young and middle-aged adults, symptom expression can be age-dependent. For example, some elderly patients with depression may display typical vegetative symptoms of diminished sleep, appetite, and energy, as well as persistently altered mood, motivation, and pleasure-seeking behaviors. In other elderly patients, however, symptoms of affective disorders may be atypical and quite different from symptoms in young and middle-aged adults. For example, some older patients with depression, particularly those who are frail and above the age of 80, may not appear sad or use the term "depressed" to describe their inner affective state. Rather, they are irritable and socially withdrawn. Older patients in a manic episode may also be more irritable and paranoid rather than displaying or expe-

riencing elation and euphoria. The terms *masked depression* and *depressive equivalents* are sometimes used to describe older patients who do not appear depressed but manifest physical symptoms such as chronic pain, fatigue, or hypochondriasis. Current DSM-IV (American Psychiatric Association 1994) diagnostic terminology includes these patients in the category of major depressive episode (Katz et al. 1998).

Not only may the clinical pattern of late-life depression vary from older person to older person, and from young-old to old-old, it may vary depending on prior episodes of depression in the older person's life. Studies suggest that elderly patients with early-onset depression, as compared with those who have a first episode in late life, have more first-degree relatives with depression. In contrast, those whose depression first appears in late life have more chronic physical illness. Patients with late-onset depression are also more likely to have brain imaging findings suggestive of dementia, respond less well to treatment, and have an increased mortality (Alexopoulos 1998; Baldwin and Tomenson 1995; Coffey 1996; Coffey et al. 1990; Katz et al. 1998; Nelson 1998).

I have divided this chapter on late-life affective disorders into two general diagnostic categories: depressive disorder and bipolar disorder.

▌Depressive Disorder

Types of Depressive Disorder

Major Depressive Disorder

Major depressive disorder in elderly adults is diagnosed by the same DSM criteria that are used for young and middle-aged adults. However, disturbances in sleep, sexual functioning, and appetite are not always reliable indicators of depression in older people because these functions can be affected by normal aging, by medications, and by numerous physical illnesses. Subtypes of major depression include melancholia, delusional depression, and seasonal affective disorder.

Nonmajor Depressive Disorders

Older people experience a significant rate of nonmajor depression, including dysthymic disorder and subclinical depressions (characterized by depressed mood or markedly diminished interest or pleasure in activities). Depression also commonly occurs together with symptoms of personality disorder, especially in older people whose onset of depressive illness was earlier in life.

Depression and Medical Illness

A complex relationship exists between depression in late life and medical illness. Major depression has been found in as many as 20%–25% of older patients with medical illness (Katon and Sullivan 1990; Rodin and Voshart 1986), and nearly 90% of older patients with unipolar major depression had at least one medical illness (Conwell et al. 1989). Depression increases the morbidity and mortality of patients with medical illness in all ages, but the deleterious effect of depression may be greater in the elderly. For example, mortality rates of patients with depression admitted to a nursing home is higher than that for patients without depression who are admitted (Rovner et al. 1991) (see also Chapter 37 in this volume). Medical illness also may be a common precipitant for the development of a major depression in elderly people (Nelson 1998).

Relationship of Late-Life Depression to Neuropsychiatric Disorders

Depression and Dementia

Depression and dementia are commonly associated in older patients (see also Chapters 23 and 24 in this volume). Depression may occur in as many as 23% of patients with dementia, and dementia may occur in 14% of patients with depression (Alexopoulos 1998). The dementia syndrome of depression is well known in all ages but may be more severe in the elderly. Interestingly, older patients who are depressed do not complain more of cognitive impairment than do middle-aged populations (Alexopoulos 1998).

It may be helpful to divide the dementia syndrome associated with depression into two categories: dementia in the elderly patient with depression whose dementia improves upon resolution of the depression (*reversible dementia*) and dementia in those older patients with depression whose dementia does not improve (*irreversible dementia*). Many older patients with depression and an initial reversible dementia begin to develop an irreversible dementia approximately 2 years after the initial recovery from depression and dementia (Alexopoulos 1998; Alexopoulos et al. 1993).

Depression may be the manifestation of a dementia (Alexopoulos 1998). Approximately one-third of patients with Alzheimer's disease and depression have a history of previous psychiatric illness, especially depression (Agbayewa 1986; Rovner et al. 1989). The possibility that the cognitive impairment of an elderly patient with depression may be reversible with adequate treatment of the depression indicates that clinicians should treat the elderly patient with depression with cognitive impairment in an effort to improve the cognitive disturbance as well as the depressive disorder itself.

Depression and Alzheimer's Disease

Depression is quite common in patients with Alzheimer's dementia, the comorbidity rate ranging from 17% to 50% (Alexopoulos 1991; Rovner et al. 1989; Sano et al. 1989; Wragg and Jeste 1989). Depressive symptoms are more likely to occur in patients with Alzheimer's disease than is the full syndrome of major depression (Alexopoulos 1998; Lazarus et al. 1987).

Imaging studies of elderly patients with depression consistently show structural changes that would also be apparent in persons with diminished cognitive function, although not necessarily with a diagnosis of true Alzheimer's dementia (Campbell et al., in press; Coffey 1996; Coffey et al. 1990, 1993). These imaging changes are shown in Table 13–1. Some patients with Alzheimer's disease and major depression have also been found to have brainstem lesions (Pearlson et al. 1989; Zubenko and Moossy 1988). Also, a clear relationship exists between depression and the presence of vascular (multiple-infarct) dementia as well as stroke (see below).

Depression and Neurological Disorders Other Than Dementia

Parkinson's disease. Depression is associated with Parkinson's disease in at least two ways (see Chapter 26 in this volume). It is likely that some older people who develop Parkinson's disease may experience a *secondary depression* about having the disorder. But depression can also be an integral part of the disease itself and occurs in at least half of all patients (Cummings 1992; Dooneief et al. 1992; Mayeux 1982). Clinical diagnosis of depression, however, can be difficult in some cases because the masklike, akinetic facies of patients with the disorder may look like depression, and the depressed facies of some older people may look parkinsonian. Difficulties in diagnosis also occur because of the "on-off" experiences associated with treatment of Parkinson's disease. Characteristically, the "off" period (the period when the bradykinetic symptoms are intense) is associated with significantly increased depression, hopelessness, and suicidal thinking. Despair, lack of initiative, marked anergia, and loss of appetite are common during the off period. In contrast, during an "on" period, the

older patient with Parkinson's disease may look, behave, and feel like a completely different person. With the patient being lively, optimistic, and engaged, it can be difficult to recall that a short time earlier the patient had all the characteristics of a patient with a severe major depressive disorder.

Depression may be more common among patients with right hemisphere parkinsonism (Starkstein et al. 1990). However, there appears to be no relationship between the degree of motor impairment and the degree of depression (Thiagarajan and Anand 1994). Disturbances in a number of neurotransmitter systems are probably related to the depressive component of Parkinson's disease. The disturbance in dopamine function characteristic of Parkinson's disease has been hypothesized as an etiology for the depression as well as the motor disorder (Brown and Gershon 1993; Willner 1995). Serotonin function also can be disturbed in patients with Parkinson's disease who are depressed (Sussman 1998).

Poststroke depression. Although the characteristics of depression after a stroke are similar to those of a major depressive disorder without stroke, a number of its symptoms may vary depending on the location of the lesion. Left hemisphere lesions are significantly associated with major depression as compared with right hemisphere lesions (Robinson et al. 1988). Major as well as minor depressive disorders have been associated with stroke or cerebral ischemia—20% of patients develop a major depression (Robinson and Price 1982), and another 20% develop a minor depression (dysthymia) (Robinson et al. 1998). With

TABLE 13–1. Imaging studies of depressed patients

Scan	Study
Computed tomography	• Enlarged lateral ventricles in depressed geriatric patients
	• Greater ventricular enlargement in late-onset than in early-onset geriatric depression
	• Enlarged ventricles associated with poor response to nortriptyline
Magnetic resonance imaging	• Significant white and gray matter hyperintensity ("leukoariosis") in elderly depressed patients; associated with late onset of first episode, suicidal ideation, delusions, DST nonsuppression, poor response to antidepressant treatment
	• Widening of cortical sulci, temporal lobe sulci, temporal horns, sylvian fissures, lateral and third ventricles
	• Widespread cortical and subcortical atrophy and basal ganglia lacunae inversely correlated with ^{3}IMI binding
Positron-emission tomography	• In depressed patients, decreased cerebral glucose metabolism most prominent in frontal lobe and right hemisphere; contrasts with Alzheimer's disease, in which glucose metabolism decrements are most prominent in parietal lobe

Source. Reprinted from Katz IR, Miller D, Oslin D: "Diagnosis of Late-Life Depression," in *Clinical Geriatric Psychopharmacology*, 3rd Edition. Edited by Salzman C. Baltimore, MD, Williams & Wilkins, 1998, pp. 153–183.

the exception of early morning awakening, the symptoms of poststroke major depressive disorder resemble late-life major depressive disorder that was not preceded by stroke (Robinson et al. 1998).

The relationship between impaired speech and comprehension in patients with depression is complex. Patients with Broca's aphasia (nonfluent aphasia) have more severe depressive symptoms than do patients with mild comprehension deficit and Wernicke's (fluent) aphasia or global aphasia (Robinson and Benson 1981). It appears that, although depression and language impairment tend to occur together, they are not related in a causal fashion to one another (Robinson et al. 1998). The frequency of depression among patients without aphasia is not different than the frequency of depression among those with aphasia (Starkstein and Robinson 1988), and it does not appear that depression is common in those patients with mild comprehension deficits (Robinson and Benson 1981; Robinson et al. 1998).

Understanding the relationship between the site of the lesion, the function of the brain area affected, and the appearance or lack of appearance of depression has been helpful in understanding the role of different brain centers in the regulation of mood. Lesions in left cortical and subcortical nuclei are associated with depression significantly greater than similar lesions on the right side, especially for major depression (Figure 13–1).

Patients with left hemisphere lesions have been shown to have decrements in serotonin binding in the left temporal cortex, suggesting that the left hemisphere may be more vulnerable to dysregulation of monoaminergic projections through the central cortex (Robinson et al. 1984, 1998). (For more on the neuropsychiatric aspects of stroke, see Chapter 27 in this volume.)

Vascular depression.   Vascular depression is depression related to multiple infarcts damaging the striato-pallado-thalamo-cortical pathways in the brain (Krishnan 1993; Krishnan et al. 1997). Depression that appears late (or very late) in life is more likely to be associated with these vascular lesions than is depression with an onset earlier in life (Campbell et al., in press; Coffey 1996; Coffey et al. 1990; Krishnan et al. 1997). This depression is characterized by a lower risk of family history of mental disorder or suicide and by a higher presence of anhedonia and functional disability. As in vascular dementia, the vascular changes seen in the brain may be related to carotid atherosclerosis, hypertension, and a history of myocardial infarcts (Bots et al. 1993; Manolio et al. 1994). Patients with vascular depression have a greater cognitive impairment than do those with nonvascular depression and have more

psychomotor retardation and less agitation (Alexopoulos et al. 1997).

Although it is not yet clear whether vascular depression requires a different pharmacological or other (e.g., electroconvulsive therapy [ECT]) treatment approach than that for nonvascular depression, prevention and treatment of cerebrovascular disease may play an important role in this syndrome.

Etiology of Late-Life Depression

There may be numerous pathways to the development of late-life depression. As discussed above, medical illness, neurological illnesses, and early-onset depression can all precede and play a role in the development of late-life depression. Additional factors include cerebral ischemia, the effects of commonly taken medications, and the numerous losses of function, friends, and health that older people must bear. No studies suggest that the neurochemical pathophysiology of depression is different in older people than in younger people when these other factors are excluded. However, virtually all markers of noradrenergic function, such as 3-methoxy-4-hydroxyphenylglycol, and α_2 binding tend to be diminished with age (Table 13–2), suggesting a correlation between reduced noradrenergic functioning (Sunderland 1998) and late-life depression (see Chapter 4 in this volume). Similarly, many (although not all) markers of serotonin function, such as tritiated imipramine binding, indicate a decreased function and sensitivity of serotonin receptors (Sunderland 1998) (Table 13–3) (also see Chapter 4 in this volume).

A search for biological markers that would help distinguish the elderly patient with depression as distinct from the older patient with dementia or the older patient with the normal mood variations of advanced age has been the subject of numerous studies that have not been fruitful. A summary of these studies is shown in Table 13–4. Unfortunately, none of these tests are currently useful in clinical practice.

Treatment of Major Unipolar Depressive Disorder in the Elderly

Treatment guidelines for an older patient with depression follow those for younger and middle-aged individuals, with a few notable exceptions. As a general principle, it is reasonable to assume that most (although not all) older patients are likely to be more sensitive to both the therapeutic as well as side effects of antidepressant drugs (see Chapter 34 in this volume). Older patients with depression who also have structural and functional brain disorders such as

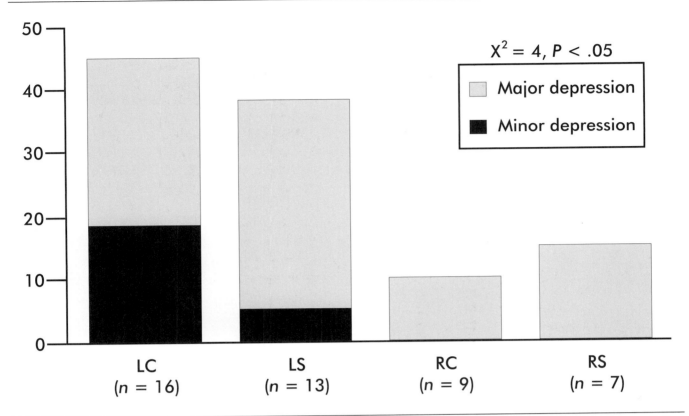

FIGURE 13–1. Percent of patients with single-stroke lesions visualized on CT scan and localized to left cerebral cortex (LC), right cerebral cortex (RC), left subcortical nuclei (LS), or right subcortical nuclei (RS) who have major or minor depression. There was a significant increase in the frequency of major depression among patients with LC or LS lesions compared with patients with RC or RS lesions.
Source. Reprinted from Robinson RG, Schultz SK, Paradiso S: "Treatment of Poststroke Psychiatric Disorders," in *Geriatric Psychopharmacology.* Edited by Nelson JC. New York, Marcel Dekker, 1998, pp. 61–186.

dementia, stroke, or Parkinson's disease also may be especially sensitive to the brain toxic properties of antidepressant drugs. Older patients who are taking multiple medications are also at greater risk for side effects and drug interactions.

Regardless of the selection of antidepressant, increased vulnerability of the older person to the unwanted effects of antidepressant medication has led to the following prescribing principles for antidepressant medication (McDonald and Salzman 1994; Salzman 1995, 1997, 1998; Salzman et al. 1995).

- "Start low and go slow" (i.e., start with low doses and use only gradual dosage increments).
- Select medications with the least likelihood to produce anticholinergic and orthostatic hypotensive side effects.
- Patience is a virtue: it may take longer for the older patient to respond to an antidepressant medication, especially if they have had many previous depressions.

- Older patients may not have a complete response to antidepressant medications but may be left with significant residual symptoms.
- As with younger patients, maintenance antidepressant medication may be essential for recovered older patients who have had numerous prior depressive episodes.

And lastly, two additional guidelines are

- Special treatments may be necessary for the older patient whose depression includes delusions.
- Special caution must be taken when treating the older patient with depression who has a dementing illness.

Relatively few studies have used a double-blind placebo-controlled design to examine treatment of mood disorders (depression) in individuals with brain diseases of known pathology. Rummans et al. (in press) note that subject numbers in such controlled treatment trials are very

TABLE 13–2. Age-related changes in the noradrenergic system

Noradrenergic markers	Location	Techniques	Findings
Adrenergic neurons			
Mann 1991	Locus coeruleus	Cell counts	Decreased
G-protein coupling			
Insel 1993	Animal cortex	Forskolin	Decreased
α_2-receptor			
Sastre and Garcia-Sevilla 1994; Surpiano and Hogikyan 1993	Cortex, platelets	^{3}H-yohimbine	Decreased
Pascual et al. 1992	Cortex, platelets	Autoradiography	Decreased
Kalaria and Andorn 1991	Hypothalamus	^{3}H-clonidine	Decreased
β-receptors			
β_1	Cortex	Autoradiography	
Arango et al. 1990; Kalaria et al. 1989			Decreased
β_2	Cortex	Autoradiography	
Mendelson and Paxinos 1991			Decreased
Kalaria et al. 1989			Unchanged
MHPG			
Hartikainen et al. 1991	Selected brain areas	Biochemical assay	Unchanged
Gottfries 1990	Cerebrospinal fluid	Biochemical assay	Increased

Please refer to the original publication for full reference citations listed in this table.
Source.   Reprinted from Sunderland T: "Neurotransmission in the Aging Central Nervous System," in *Clinical Geriatric Psychopharmacology*, 3rd Edition. Edited by Salzman C. Baltimore, MD, Williams & Wilkins, 1998, pp. 51–69.

small for any one such group, making it difficult to endorse any one approach in treating depression in these samples. For example, only three such studies reporting significant improvement in active drug over placebo in the treatment of depression in people with neurological illness contained more than 10 subjects. These studies include one using citalopram in patients with depression occurring in Alzheimer's disease (Nyth et al. 1992), another with citalopram in patients with poststroke depression (G. Andersen et al. 1994), and a third using desipramine in patients with depression occurring in multiple sclerosis (Schiffer and Wineman 1990). Studies showing beneficial effects of nortriptyline in patients with Parkinson's disease (J. Andersen et al. 1980) were complicated by significant problems with the patients' low blood pressure; likewise, delirium and cardiovascular morbidity occurred in patients taking nortriptyline for poststroke depression (Lipsey et al. 1984).

It has become commonplace to discuss the use of antidepressant medications for older patients by grouping the medications according to their common chemical properties. For convenience, there is also a disparate category of antidepressants known as "atypical antidepressants." This antidepressant classification yields

- Tricyclic antidepressants (TCAs);
- Selective serotonin reuptake inhibitors (SSRIs);

- Monoamine oxidase (MAO) inhibitors; and
- Atypical antidepressants.

Studies demonstrate no significant therapeutic differences between compounds in these four classes (Alexopoulos and Salzman 1998; Nelson 1998). Therefore, clinicians tend to select antidepressant medications based on side-effect profile, on the patient's prior experience and response, and on their own personal prescribing preferences based on experience with other patients. Prescribing patterns of antidepressants for late-life depression also vary according to age, training, experience, and locality within the United States of the prescribing clinician, as well as with nationwide fluctuating patterns of drug-prescribing preferences. Nevertheless, at present, clinicians appear to be using antidepressants to treat late-life depression (Salzman 1998; Salzman et al. 1998) as follows:

1. SSRIs are the typical first-choice antidepressants for all except the most severely depressed elderly patients.
2. TCAs, especially nortriptyline and desipramine, appear to be used either to augment SSRI antidepressants or to replace SSRIs when they are not producing an adequate therapeutic response. Nortriptyline and desipramine also tend to be preferred

TABLE 13-3. Age-related changes in the serotonergic system

Serotonergic markers	Location	Techniques	Findings
5-HT transporter			
Marcussen et al. 1987	Neocortex	$^{123}\beta$-CIT SPECT	Decreased
5-HT$_{1A}$-receptor			
Burnet et al. 1994	Hippocampus	mRNA	Increased
Marcussen et al. 1984, 1987	Striatum	^{3}H-IMI binding	No change
Middlemiss et al. 1986	Frontal cortex	^{3}H-8-OH-DPAT	Decreased
5-HT$_{2A}$-receptor			
Wang et al. 1995; Sparks 1989	Frontal, occipital	^{18}F-NMS PET	Decreased
Burnet et al. 1994	Hippocampus	mRNA	Unchanged
Tryptophan hydroxylase			
Meck 1977	Selected brain areas		Decreased
Serotonergic levels			
Severson et al. 1995;	Selected brain areas	Cell count	Decreased
Gottfries et al. 1979			
5-HIAA			
Bareggi et al. 1985	Cerebrospinal fluid	Biochemical assay	Increased

Please refer to the original publication for full reference citations listed in this table.
Source. Reprinted from Sunderland T: "Neurotransmission in the Aging Central Nervous System," in *Clinical Geriatric Psychopharmacology*, 3rd Edition. Edited by Salzman C. Baltimore, MD, Williams & Wilkins, 1998, pp. 51–69.

for the most severely depressed elderly patients (usually inpatients).

3. The miscellaneous group of atypical antidepressants are also widely used for the treatment of depression, and in many cases their effects are equal to or even superior to SSRIs and TCAs. The patterns of their use are difficult to discern.

4. MAO inhibitors are used significantly less frequently than the other three classes of antidepressants. They may be useful for carefully selected elderly patients (see below).

Selective Serotonin Antidepressants

To date, approximately 1,500 elderly patients with a major depression have participated in studies of SSRI antidepressants. There appears to be little difference in the efficacy among SSRI antidepressants. The magnitude of therapeutic response with SSRIs is modest, interindividual variability of response is large, and significant residual symptoms are found at the end of the treatment period (Small and Salzman 1998). Although differences in pharmacokinetics exist among the four available SSRI medications, it is not clear that they significantly influence either the therapeutic response or the side-effect profile. It is likely that variations in drug response among older persons is greater than meaningful differences among the SSRIs antidepressants

(Salzman 1996). The pharmacokinetics of these drugs are also shown in Table 13–5.

Because of their relatively favorable side-effect profile, SSRIs are often the drugs of first choice, especially for the mildly to moderately ill patient with depression. The use of SSRIs for the treatment of the elderly patient with depression follows the usual geriatric guidelines of "start low and go slow." Even though side effects from these medications are less likely to interfere with the older person's function than are TCA side effects, doses that are too high may still cause unwanted side effects and treatment noncompliance. For example, traditional starting doses may produce unwanted agitation, sedation, or gastrointestinal upset. Average therapeutic daily doses are shown in Table 13–5.

SSRI antidepressants are metabolized through a number of cytochrome P450 isoenzymes and are subject to blood level fluctuation when the activity of these enzymes is altered by other medications. However, fluoxetine and paroxetine themselves significantly inhibit the 2D6 isoenzyme of this hepatic enzyme family. Because the 2D6 isoenzyme is primarily responsible for metabolizing TCAs, the combined use of tricyclic and SSRI antidepressants for therapeutic augmentation purposes may result in unsafe and unwanted high levels of TCA blood levels. Fluvoxamine is a potent inhibitor of the 1A2 isoenzyme, which metabolizes certain psychotropic drugs, such as tacrine (Cognex), that may be taken by elderly patients.

Although SSRIs may cause agitation, insomnia, or dis-

TABLE 13–4.   Studies of biological markers in late-life depression

Biological markers	Study results	References
MHPG	• Plasma MHPG increases with age; decrease may be associated with onset of late-life depression	Karege 1989; Koslow 1983
α_2 binding	• Poorly correlated with depression; may correlate with late age of onset	Kafka 1988; Doyle 1985; Sachetti 1985
Platelet MAO	• Higher in elderly patients with depression and reversible dementia (pseudodementia); associated with anhedonia, anxiety, and medical illness in depressed elderly outpatients	Fischer 1994; Schneider 1988; Veith 1988; Alexopoulos 1987; George 1986; Alexopoulos 1984a
^{3}IMI	• Decreased binding in elderly patients	Nemeroff 1988; Schneider 1988; Schneider 1986; Suranyi-Cadotte 1985
	• No decreased binding in elderly patients	Georgotas 1987
	• Binding may be lower in geriatric depressed patients than in younger depressed patients	Nemeroff 1988; Schneider 1988
	• High specificity; binding does not decrease in dementia	Nemeroff 1988; Schneider 1988
	• Associated with poor response to antidepressant treatments	Schneider 1986
DST	• Nonsuppression more frequent in geriatric than in younger depressed patients; occurs in one-third of demented patients; low specificity	APA 1987; Gieri 1987; Georgotas 1986; Greenwald 1986; Alexopoulos 1985a; Sunderland 1985; Alexopoulos 1984b; Davis 1984; Rosenbaum 1984; Oxenkrug 1983; Tourigny-Rivard 1981
TRH-TSH	• Low specificity; blunted response in depressed geriatric patients and in patients with Alzheimer's disease	Tsuboyama 1992; Molchan 1991; Sunderland 1986; Alexopoulos 1985b
Altered sleep architecture	• Similar to midlife depressed patients; shorter REM latency; prolonged first REM period; shift of EEG delta activity from first to second REM period; early morning awakening	Reynolds 1988; Hoch 1986; Reynolds 1983

Please refer to the original publication for full reference citations listed in this table.
Source.   Reprinted from Katz IR, Miller D, Oslin D: "Diagnosis of Late-Life Depression," in Clinical Geriatric Psychopharmacology, 3rd Edition. Edited by Salzman C. Baltimore, MD, Williams & Wilkins, 1998, pp. 153–183.

turbed gastrointestinal function, these side effects are usually mild and often transient. SSRIs do not cause cognitive impairment, although their use has been associated with confusion in some elderly patients, depending on the dose (Tourjman and Fontaine 1992).

SSRI treatment of the neurologically impaired patient.   SSRIs have been used for the treatment of elderly patients with depression and dementia because of their relatively benign side-effect profile, in particular the low anticholinergic side effects. SSRIs may be used safely in this population of older patients, and, in some patients, reduction of depressive symptoms may be accompanied by a mild improvement in cognitive impairment (Nyth et al. 1992). Starting doses of SSRIs should be low for the dementia patient with depression because the usual

starting doses can be associated with an increased appearance of unwanted side effects, especially agitation. Paroxetine, alone among the SSRIs, has anticholinergic properties, although they tend to be mild. No data as yet, however, suggest that these anticholinergic properties interfere with the cognitive function of the older dementia patient with depression. In one study of paroxetine in nursing home residents over the age of 80, treatment with 20 mg/day for 8 weeks was not associated with impaired cognition (Burrows et al., unpublished data, July 1999).

It is likely that the efficacy of SSRIs in enhancing cognitive function in the older patient with depression and dementia will depend partly on the severity of the dementia. In early stages of dementia, in which most cognitive and behavioral function is preserved, these medications may be quite helpful for cognition as well as for mood. In the later

TABLE 13–5. Clinical pharmacology of serotonin reuptake inhibitors

Drug	Elimination half-life (hr)	Active metabolites	Metabolite elimination half-life	Recommended elderly daily dose (mg)
Paroxetine	12–20	No	—	5–40
Fluvoxamine	15	No	15	25–200
Sertraline	25	No	—	125–1500
Fluoxetine	85	Yes	330	5–60

Source. Reprinted from Small GW, Salzman C: "Treatment of Depression With New and Atypical Antidepressants," in *Clinical Geriatric Psychopharmacology*, 3rd Edition. Edited by Salzman C. Baltimore, MD, Williams & Wilkins, 1998, pp. 245–261.

stages of the illness, when there is more pervasive and behavioral impairment, SSRIs may have little effect on cognition.

Fluoxetine has been studied for the treatment of poststroke major and minor depression and, like the comparative drug nortriptyline, its use was associated with improved Mini-Mental State Exam scores compared with those scores with placebo (Folstein and McHugh 1978; Gonzalez-Torrecillas et al., in press).

Reports are conflicting on the usefulness of SSRIs in depressed patients with Parkinson's disease. The SSRIs may worsen motor symptoms in Parkinson's disease (Sussman 1998). However, in one case report, a patient with Parkinson's disease who was depressed responded to fluvoxamine (McCance-Katz et al. 1992). It appears that the beneficial effects of SSRIs do not necessarily outweigh the possibility of worsening motor symptoms in depressed elderly patients with Parkinson's disease. Because SSRIs may diminish central nervous system dopamine (Salzman et al. 1993), and potentially worsen motor symptoms, they probably should not be used as antidepressants of first choice for these patients.

Tricyclic Antidepressants

Most geriatric clinicians tend to avoid using tertiary TCAs in elderly patients because of the relatively frequent appearance of anticholinergic and orthostatic hypotensive side effects. Side-effect profile favors the use of the secondary amines, nortriptyline or desipramine. Elderly patients treated with either of these TCAs respond to the same plasma levels as younger and middle-aged individuals. However, the response to TCAs may be influenced by a number of factors that are more common in older people than in younger and middle-aged adults. For example, a large ventricular/brain ratio predicts poor response to nortriptyline (Young et al. 1990), and low serum albumin along with poor self-care also predicts poor response to nortriptyline in very old nursing home residents (Katz et al. 1990).

Treatment with TCAs also follows the "start low and go slow" principle. Clinicians, therefore, commonly start with doses of 10–25 mg for either drug and gradually increase into the therapeutic range, using plasma levels for monitoring, although the plasma level of nortriptyline may not correlate with the therapeutic response (Young et al. 1990, 1991). A pretreatment electrocardiogram (ECG) is essential because these TCAs can cause serious conduction difficulties. Repeat ECGs during the treatment period provide information that is also helpful to the clinician in determining the dose. There is no risk of cardiotoxicity if the QRS (or QT interval) does not widen. Using the ECG in conjunction with drug plasma levels and clinical status of the patient provides useful guidelines for treatment. Average starting and therapeutic doses are shown in Table 13–6.

Nortriptyline and desipramine produce anticholinergic side effects and orthostatic hypotension, although less severely than tertiary amine antidepressants, such as imipramine or amitriptyline. Brain anticholinergic side effects include delirium (disorientation, memory loss, confusion, and increased forgetfulness; see Chapter 19 in this volume). At low therapeutic doses, these side effects are little more than an annoyance for older patients (although for the very frail and very elderly person they may significantly interfere with daily activities). At higher doses, however, or when TCAs are given in conjunction with other medications that have anticholinergic side effects, the intensity of

TABLE 13–6. Starting and therapeutic doses of recommended tricyclic antidepressants

Drug	Starting dose	Average daily dose	Blood level
Nortriptyline	10 mg	25–100 mg	50–150 ng/mL
Desipramine	10 mg	25–100 mg	>115 ng/mL

brain anticholinergic toxicity may increase to the point of a delirium (see Chapter 19 in this volume). In the anticholinergic delirious state, the older person is very confused, very disoriented, and has impaired short-term memory. Symptoms are much worse in the evening, and the delirious picture may include paranoid delusions, visual hallucinations, assaultiveness, and agitation. Anticholinergic side effects are particularly disastrous for the depressed older patient who already has a dementia. At high doses, or even sometimes at the usual therapeutic doses used for young and middle-aged adults, depressed older individuals with moderately severe dementia become more cognitively impaired. Clinical experience suggests that patients with Alzheimer's disease may also become more agitated by TCAs. For these reasons, doses of TCAs need to be kept as low as possible to produce a therapeutic response, and the older person must be monitored closely.

Nortriptyline and desipramine are metabolized by several hepatic enzymes of the CP450 family. The primary metabolizing enzyme, IID6, responsible for hydroxylating TCAs into water-soluble compounds, may be inhibited by a variety of other medications, particularly fluoxetine and paroxetine. When these SSRIs are given to augment TCA response (or vice versa, see below), substantial risk of TCA toxicity occurs because of markedly elevated blood levels.

Because hydroxymetabolites are water soluble, their clearance may be impaired by age-related diminished renal function in the very elderly, or as a consequence of impaired renal clearance as a result of medications such as nonsteroidal anti-inflammatory drugs (see Chapter 34 in this volume). Hydroxymetabolites are cardiotoxic (Young et al. 1990, 1991) and, as they gradually accumulate, cardiac conduction abnormalities can develop. This toxicity is reflected in QRS widening, indicating a further need to employ follow-up ECGs during treatment.

Tricyclic antidepressant treatment of the patient with neurological illness. A substantial body of literature demonstrates that patients with dementia who are depressed, as well as depressed patients with dementia, can be successfully treated with TCAs (Rummans et al., in press). Virtually all studies also indicate that there may be a favorable effect on cognitive performance with resolution of the depression (Reifler et al. 1989). At least four clinical trials have demonstrated response to antidepressant treatment in elderly patients with depression and cognitive impairment (Gottfries et al. 1992; Rabins 1989; Reifler et al. 1989; Reynolds et al. 1987). The subject has been well reviewed by Jones and Reifler (1994), who cite, in particular, a study showing an improvement in Mini-Mental State Exam scores of nearly 7 points in those elderly

patients with dementia whose depression responded to treatment (Folstein and McHugh 1978).

Five clinical trials have been published, each demonstrating improvement in mood in the depressed elderly patient with Parkinson's disease (J. Andersen et al. 1980; Boer et al. 1976; Indaco and Carrieri 1988; Laitinen 1969; Strang 1965). The anticholinergic properties of TCAs may also slightly help the motor impairment as well, although significant anticholinergic blockade will exacerbate some of the dementing symptoms that sometimes occur in well-advanced Parkinson's disease.

Two studies of nortriptyline in patients poststroke have demonstrated antidepressant efficacy in patients with depression (Balunov and Alemasova 1990; Lipsey et al. 1984). When stroke has resulted in cognitive impairment, treatment of a patient with poststroke depression with TCAs may result in an improvement in cognitive functioning (Lipsey et al. 1984), although anticholinergic side effects may be more prominent, resulting in disorientation, confusion, dysarthria, incoherent speech, and anxiety (Robinson et al. 1998).

Treatment of Depression With Miscellaneous "Atypical" Antidepressants

This group of medications includes bupropion, venlafaxine, nefazodone, and mirtazapine. Each has demonstrated efficacy as an antidepressant, although the number of clinical trials data supporting their efficacy in older individuals is considerably fewer than that for the other groups of antidepressants. When clinicians follow the prescribing maxim of "start low and go slow" and use low starting doses with gradual dosage increments, the benign side-effect profiles of each of these drugs may make them useful for older patients. The starting doses, effective geriatric daily dose range, and side effects are shown in Table 13–7.

Bupropion tends to be used for its activating properties, whereas nefazodone has sedating properties. Venlafaxine is increasingly popular because it has many of the properties of TCAs but lacks significant anticholinergic side effects. Mirtazapine has not yet been assigned a specific prescribing niche for older depressed patients.

Another advantage of this group of drugs is the relative lack of significant interactions with other psychotropic drugs. Bupropion, venlafaxine, and mirtazapine appear to be relatively free of enzymatic interactions affecting the metabolism of other drugs. Nefazodone is an inhibitor of the 3A4 isoenzyme, which metabolizes numerous medications, including triazolam and alprazolam.

TABLE 13–7. Miscellaneous antidepressants

Drug	Starting dose (mg)	Geriatric daily dose range	Side effects
Bupropion	37.5	37.5–300	Agitation, insomnia
Venlafaxine	12.5	25–100	Nausea, vomiting, headache, hypertension
Nefazodone	50	50–300	Sedation
Mirtazapine	7.5	Insufficient information	Sedation, weight gain

Monoamine Oxidase Inhibitors

MAO inhibitors are effective antidepressants and sometimes produce a remarkable reversal of depressive symptoms in some elderly patients. Their use for the general geriatric population of patients with depression, however, is limited by two factors: 1) the risk of noncompliance leading to potentially toxic combinations with other medications or tyramine-containing food substances; and 2) side effects, especially orthostatic hypotension and the potential for serious hypertensive crises.

Despite potential problems using MAO inhibitors, these medications may provide enhanced energy, optimism, and the return of zest to the lives of selected elderly patients with depression, particularly the younger depressed patients who are cognitively intact and physically healthy.

MAO inhibitor treatment of the patient with neurological illness. No clinical trials of MAO inhibitors have been performed in patients with neurological illness. MAO inhibitors have been reported to be effective in activating and improving the mood of elderly patients with depression (Ashford and Ford 1979), although they also have been noted to cause severe agitation and insomnia in the same sample of patients. A family member, spouse, or caregiver must be in charge of the MAO inhibitor administration, supervise the administration of the MAO inhibitor, and guard against potential drug and food interactions. This further limits the usefulness of these medications in this population.

No studies or clinical reports of the use of MAO inhibitors exist for elderly patients with poststroke depression. Because of the possibility of MAO inhibitor interactions with tyramine in foods or with blood pressure increase from medications causing a stroke, these drugs probably should not be used in this population of elderly patients with depression.

Treatment of Delusional Depression

Psychotic (delusional) depression is relatively frequent in the elderly population and ranges from a prevalence of 3.6% of community residents to as much as 20%–45% of hospitalized patients (Alexopoulos and Salzman 1998). In elderly people, psychotic depression is a severe and potentially lethal illness, usually requiring inpatient treatment. Evidence suggests that elderly patients with psychotic depression respond poorly to treatment with all forms of antidepressants when used alone (Alexopoulos and Salzman 1998). When TCAs are combined with neuroleptics, however, therapeutic response has been noted (Alexopoulos and Abrams 1991; Baldwin 1988). Because of the life-threatening nature of psychotic depression, many clinicians prefer to use ECT rather than antidepressant medication (see Chapter 35 in this volume).

ECT has demonstrated efficacy for the treatment of severe depressions in elderly patients with psychotic depression (Sackeim 1998), although its use has been questioned because it induces memory impairment. The magnitude of cognitive impairment produced by ECT in the elderly differs among individuals. For some patients, the anterograde and retrograde amnesia caused by the treatment may be partially offset by the improved attention and concentration that results from reduction of depressive symptoms. For those who may be at greatest risk of memory loss (e.g., elderly patients with severe preexisting cognitive impairment), unilateral nondominant treatment carefully spaced out may mitigate the possible worsening of preexisting cognitive impairment (Sackeim 1998).

Treatment Resistance and Augmentation Strategies

It appears that older patients, particularly those over 75, may have a less robust response to antidepressant treatment, even at appropriate dosages and blood levels. This lack of response is particularly true for TCAs (Agency for Health Policy and Research 1993), but is not as dramatic for the SSRIs. The elderly may take longer to respond to adequate treatment (Georgotas and McCue 1989; Nelson 1998). For these reasons, clinicians sometimes add a second antidepressant to bolster or accelerate the therapeutic response from the first drug. Although these augmentation strategies are sometimes successful in young and middle-aged patients, their efficacy in the elderly is not as convincing. Adding a second antidepressant is also likely to increase side effects.

Studies of lithium augmentation in the elderly have shown only a modest improvement in therapeutic response and a higher likelihood of neuropsychiatric side effects (Alexopoulos and Salzman 1998; Nelson 1998). Mixing antidepressants together (typically adding low dose of a TCA to an SSRI) has demonstrated efficacy in the elderly as well, although side effects are increased, and drug interactions may produce toxic TCA blood levels (Nelson et al. 1991; Seth et al. 1992). Stimulants in low doses are sometimes effective when added to other antidepressants. Methylphenidate, the most commonly used of the psychomotor stimulants, when used alone, may increase motivation, attention, and a sense of well-being, even at low doses of 2.5–20 mg/day. In conjunction with other antidepressants, methylphenidate may enhance energy and motivation. Doses must be very low to avoid unwanted agitation and insomnia. (For more information on geriatric neuropsychopharmacology, see Chapter 34 in this volume.)

Diagnosis and Treatment of Mania (Bipolar Disorder) in the Elderly

Types of Late-Life Mania

Mania is not unusual in the elderly, although it rarely appears for the first time in late life. The clinical picture of mania differs in the elderly from patterns seen in young and middle-aged adults. Euphoria and elation are less common in the older patients with mania. More typically, features of late-life mania include confusion, paranoia, irritability, dysphoria, and distractibility. Onset of bipolar illness earlier in life, if untreated, becomes more severe and mood alterations more frequent in late life, both for the mania and the depressive component of the bipolar illness (Dhingra and Rabins 1991).

Manic symptoms can be caused also by a variety of physical disorders as well as medications. For example, vitamin B_{12} deficiency, hypothyroidism, and infections can cause mania. The use of medications such as corticosteroids, anticholinergics, L-dopa, psychostimulants, and sympathomimetics, as well as hemodialysis, can cause late-life mania.

Mania in late life can be associated with neuropsychiatric disorders (Satlin and Liptzin 1998). Symptoms that suggest mania secondary to a medical condition as opposed to late-life onset of bipolar disorder include

- Distractibility, reduced attention span, impaired concentration, and disorientation resembling dementia or delirium;
- A first onset of affective symptoms in late life;
- A long latency period between the first episode of depression and the appearance of mania;
- A history of frequent mood cycles (rapid cycling);
- Chronic course;
- Absence of a family history of bipolar disorder; and
- Poor response to lithium or the development of neurotoxicity at low therapeutic lithium levels.

Although depression is more common after stroke than is mania, the appearance of manic symptoms after stroke is not uncommon (Robinson et al. 1998). As opposed to depression, the development of poststroke mania may be associated with right-sided lesions rather than left-sided lesions (Robinson et al. 1988; Starkstein et al. 1991). Poststroke mania may persist as poststroke bipolar depression. Patients with this disorder have greater cognitive impairment than those with just depression (Starkstein et al. 1991).

Treatment of Late-Life Mania

The treatment of late-life mania follows general geriatric prescribing principles, using the same medications that are available for treating young and middle-aged adults. Mood-stabilizing medications, including lithium, valproate, and carbamazepine, are all useful in managing late-life mania. As for all other medications, however, older patients are more sensitive to the side effects of these medications. Starting doses, average daily doses, and side effects are shown in Table 13–8.

As with younger patients, maintenance treatment with mood stabilizers is an important part of the overall treatment program of elders with bipolar disorder. However, because older patients are more sensitive to the side effects of mood-stabilizing drugs, and may become progressively even more sensitive as they age, the maintenance doses may need to be readjusted frequently.

Neuropsychiatric Side Effects of Mood-Stabilizing Medication

Neuropsychiatric and neurological side effects of mood-stabilizing medications are common in the elderly. In some cases, these side effects may appear even before other side effects, such as gastrointestinal distress, that usually appear as the first side effects in younger adults.

Lithium.   Diminished memory loss, cognitive dulling, and apathy are common lithium side effects in the elderly.

TABLE 13–8. Mood stabilizers

Drug	Starting dose (mg)	Daily dose (mg)	Side effects
Lithium	75–300	300–900 (BL 0.3–0.7)	Neurological, cardiovascular, renal, thyroid, gastrointestinal disturbances
Valproic acid	125	250–1000 (BL 50–100)	Neurological disturbances, alopecia, weight gain, gastrointestinal disturbance
Carbamazepine	100	200–800 (BL 4–8)	Cardiac arrhythmia, confusion, unsteadiness

Mild confusion and forgetfulness may cause lithium non-compliance. At higher doses and blood levels, however, lithium-induced delirium characterized by confusion, forgetfulness, disorientation, and impaired consciousness is common. Other signs of lithium toxicity include tremor, lethargy, ataxia, slurred speech, and eventually coma. These toxic effects may be evident at therapeutic dosages even when lithium blood levels are within the usual therapeutic range. As many as 60% of elderly patients appear to have prolonged periods of lithium-induced neurotoxicity lasting up to 10 weeks after the discontinuation of treatment (Satlin and Liptzin 1998). Hypothesized reasons for this prolonged neurotoxicity include increased brain vulnerability as a result of late-life brain diseases such as parkinsonism, stroke, or dementia.

Valproic acid. Valproic acid can cause neurological symptoms in older patients. Tremor, sedation, and ataxia are not unusual. Some older patients may experience a cognitive impairment, although not as frequently as with lithium.

Carbamazepine. Neurotoxicity is produced by carbamazepine, resulting in confusion, sedation, disorientation, ataxia, and memory loss.

Treatment of Poststroke Mania

Although no controlled studies of the treatment of poststroke mania have been undertaken, clinical experience suggests that secondary manic states after stroke are more difficult to treat than primary mania (Evans et al. 1995). A single case report found carbamazepine to be ineffective, but clonidine (600 mg/day) rapidly reversed manic symptoms (Bakchine et al. 1989). Lithium may be useful, as may other mood stabilizers, although research studies are needed for these treatments. Valproate and carbamazepine may be particularly useful in patients with poststroke mania because of the risk of seizures in this population (Robinson et al. 1998).

Other medications to treat mania, such as clonazepam and calcium channel blockers, have not been adequately studied in the elderly. Similarly, use of new anticonvulsant mood stabilizers, such as lamotrigine and gabapentin, in the elderly has not been reported in the literature to date.

Conclusion

Affective disturbances in the elderly range in severity from mild to severe. Present clinical and research experience suggests that assertive, but careful, pharmacological treatment can bring substantial relief from the suffering of affective illness in late life. Following the prescribing principles of low starting doses, with gradual dose increments ("start low and go slow"), with frequent evaluations, many elderly people may have significant improvement in the quality of their life.

References

Agbayewa MO: Earlier psychiatric morbidity in patients with Alzheimer's disease. J Am Geriatr Soc 34:561–564, 1986

Agency for Health Policy and Research: Clinical Practice Guideline: Depression in Primary Care: Treatment of Major Depression, Vol 2. Rockville, MD, U.S. Government Printing Office, 1993

Alexopoulos GS: Heterogeneity and comorbidity in dementia-depression syndromes. Int J Geriatr Psychiatry 6:125–127, 1991

Alexopoulos GS: The assessment and treatment of depressed-demented patients, in Geriatric Psychopharmacology. Edited by Nelson JC. New York, Marcel Dekker, 1998, pp 223–244

Alexopoulos GS, Abrams RC: Depression in Alzheimer's disease. Psychiatr Clin North Am 14:327–340, 1991

Alexopoulos GS, Salzman C: Treatment of depression with heterocyclic antidepressants, monoamine oxidase inhibitors, and psychomotor stimulants, in Clinical Geriatric Psychopharmacology, 3rd Edition. Edited by Salzman C. Baltimore, MD, Williams & Wilkins, 1998, pp 184–244

Alexopoulos GS, Meyers BS, Young RC, et al: The course of geriatric depression with "reversible dementia": a controlled study. Am J Psychiatry 150:1693–1699, 1993

Alexopoulos GS, Barnett S, Meyers MD, et al: Clinically defined vascular depression. Am J Psychiatry 154:562–565, 1997

American Psychiatric Association: Diagnostic and Statistical Manual of Mental Disorders, 4th Edition. Washington, DC, American Psychiatric Association, 1994

Andersen G, Vestergaard K, Lauritzen L: Effective treatment of poststroke depression with the selective serotonin reuptake inhibitor citalopram. Stroke 25:1099–1104, 1994

Andersen J, Aabro E, Gulmann N, et al: Anti-depressive treatment in Parkinson's disease. A controlled trial of the effect of nortriptyline in patients with Parkinson's disease treated with L-DOPA. Acta Neurol Scand 62:210–219, 1980

Ashford JW, Ford CV: Use of MAO inhibitors in elderly patients. Am J Psychiatry 136:1466–1467, 1979

Bakchine S, Lacomblez L, Benoit N, et al: Manic-like state after orbitofrontal and right temporoparietal injury: efficacy of clonidine. Neurology 39:777–781, 1989

Baldwin RC: Delusional and non-delusional depression in late life. Evidence for distinct subtypes. Br J Psychiatry 152:39–44, 1988

Baldwin RC, Tomenson B: Depression in later life: a comparison of symptoms and risk factors in early and late onset cases. Br J Psychiatry 167:649–652, 1995

Balunov OA, Alemasova AY: Therapy of depression in post-stroke patients. Alaska Med 32:20–29, 1990

Boer BH, Erdman RAM, Onstenk HJVC, et al: Clomipramine, depresie en de ziekte van Parkinson. Tijdschrift voor Psychiatrie 28:499–509, 1976

Bots ML, van Swieten JC, Breteler MM, et al: Cerebral white matter lesions and atherosclerosis in the Rotterdam Study. Lancet 341:1232–1237, 1993

Brown AS, Gershon S: Dopamine and depression. J Neural Transm Gen Sect 91:75–109, 1993

Campbell JJ, Duffy JD, Coffey CE: The neuropsychiatry of depression. Psychiatric Annals (in press)

Coffey CE: Brain morphology in primary mood disorders: implications for ECT. Psychiatric Annals 26:713–716, 1996

Coffey CE, Figiel GS, Djang WT, et al: Subcortical hyperintensity on magnetic resonance imaging: a comparison of normal and depressed elderly subjects. Am J Psychiatry 147:187–189, 1990

Coffey CE, Wilkinson WE, Weiner RD, et al: Quantitative cerebral anatomy in depression: a controlled magnetic resonance imaging study. Arch Gen Psychiatry 50:7–16, 1993

Conwell Y, Nelson C, Kim KM, et al: Elderly patients admitted to the psychiatric unit of a general hospital. J Am Geriatr Soc 37:35–41, 1989

Cummings JL: Depression and Parkinson's disease: a review. Am J Psychiatry 149:443–454, 1992

Dhingra U, Rabins PV: Mania in the elderly: a 5–7 year follow-up. J Am Geriatr Soc 39:581–583, 1991

Dooneief G, Mirabello E, Bell K, et al: An estimate of the incidence of depression in idiopathic Parkinson's disease. Arch Neurol 49:305–307, 1992

Evans DL, Byer LYM, Greer R: Secondary mania: diagnosis and treatment. J Clin Psychiatry 56 (suppl 3):31–37, 1995

Folstein MF, McHugh PR: Dementia syndrome of depression, in Alzheimer's Disease and Related Disorders. Edited by Katzman R, Terry RD, Bick KL. New York, Raven, 1978, pp 45–63

Georgotas A, McCue RE: The additional benefit of extending an antidepressant trial past seven weeks in the depressed elderly. Int J Geriatr Psychiatry 4:191–195, 1989

Gonzalez-Torrecillas JL, Mendlewicz J, Lobo A: Repercussion of early treatment of post-stroke depression on neurophysiological rehabilitation. Int Psychogeriatr (in press)

Gottfries C-G, Karlsson I, Nyth AL: Treatment of depression in elderly patients with and without demential disorders. Int Clin Psychopharmacol 6 (suppl 5):55–64, 1992

Indaco A, Carrieri PD: Amitriptyline in the treatment of headache in patients with Parkinson's disease. Neurology 38:1720–1722, 1988

Jones BN, Reifler BV: Depression coexisting with dementia. Med Clin North Am 78:823–839, 1994

Katon W, Sullivan MD: Depression and chronic medical illness. J Clin Psychiatry 51 (suppl 6):3–11, 1990

Katz IR, Simpson GM, Curlik SM, et al: Pharmacologic treatment of major depression for elderly patients in residential care settings. J Clin Psychiatry 51:41–47, 1990

Katz IR, Miller D, Oslin D: Diagnosis of late-life depression, in Clinical Geriatric Psychopharmacology, 3rd Edition. Edited by Salzman C. Baltimore, MD, Williams & Wilkins, 1998, pp 153–183

Krishnan KRR: Neuroanatomic substrates of depression in the elderly. J Geriatr Psychiatry Neurol 1:39–58, 1993

Krishnan KRR, Hays JC, Blazer DG: MRI-defined vascular depression. Am J Psychiatry 154:497–501, 1997

Laitinen L: Desipramine in treatment of Parkinson's disease. Acta Neurol Scand 45:109–113, 1969

Lazarus LW, Newton N, Cohler B, et al: Frequency and presentation of depressive symptoms in patients with primary degenerative dementia. Am J Psychiatry 144:41–45, 1987

Lipsey JR, Robinson RG, Pearlson GD, et al: Nortriptyline treatment of post-stroke depression: a double-blind study. Lancet 1:297–300, 1984

Manolio TA, Kronmal RA, Burke GL, et al: Magnetic resonance abnormalities and cardiovascular disease in older adults: the Cardiovascular Health Study. Stroke 25:318–327, 1994

Mayeux R: Depression and dementia in Parkinson's disease, in Movement Disorders. Edited by Marsden CO, Fahey S. London, Butterworth, 1982, pp 75–95

McCance-Katz EF, Marek KL, Price LH: Serotonergic dysfunction in depression associated with Parkinson's disease. Neurology 42:1813–1814, 1992

McDonald WM, Salzman C: Geriatric psychopharmacology, in Psychiatry, Revised Edition, Vol 2. Edited by Michels R, Cooper AM, et al. Philadelphia, PA, JB Lippincott, 1994, pp 1–23

Nelson JC: Treatment of major depression in the elderly, in Geriatric Psychopharmacology. Edited by Nelson JC. New York, Marcel Dekker, 1998, pp 61–98

Nelson JC, Mazure CM, Bowers MB, et al: A preliminary, open study of the combination of fluoxetine and desipramine for rapid treatment of major depression. Arch Gen Psychiatry 48:303–307, 1991

Nyth AL, Gottfries CG, Lyby K, et al: A controlled multicenter clinical study of citalopram and placebo in elderly depressed patients with and without concomitant dementia. Acta Psychiatr Scand 86:138–145, 1992

Pearlson GS, Rabins PV, Kims WS, et al: Structural brain CT changes and cognitive deficits in elderly depressives with and without reversible dementia ("pseudodementia"). Psychol Med 19:573–584, 1989

Rabins PV: Coexisting depression and dementia. J Geriatr Psychiatry 22:17–24, 1989

Reifler BV, Teri L, Raskind M, et al: Double-blind trial of imipramine in Alzheimer's disease patients with and without depression. Am J Psychiatry 146:45–49, 1989

Reynolds CF, Perel JM, Kupfer DJ, et al: Open-trial response to antidepressant treatment in elderly patients with mixed depression and cognitive impairment. Psychiatry Res 21:111–122, 1987

Robinson RG, Benson DF: Depression in aphasic patients: frequency, severity and clinical-pathological correlations. Brain Lang 14:282–291, 1981

Robinson RG, Price TR: Post-stroke depressive disorders: a follow-up study of 103 outpatients. Stroke 13:635–641, 1982

Robinson RG, Kubos KL, Starr LB, et al: Mood disorders in stroke patients: importance of location of lesion. Brain 107:81–93, 1984

Robinson RG, Boston JD, Starkstein SE, et al: Comparison of mania and depression after brain injury: causal factors. Am J Psychiatry 145:172–178, 1988

Robinson RG, Schultz SK, Paradiso S: Treatment of poststroke psychiatric disorders, in Geriatric Psychopharmacology. Edited by Nelson JC. New York, Marcel Dekker, 1998, pp 161–186

Rodin G, Voshart K: Depression in the medically ill: an overview. Am J Psychiatry 143:696–705, 1986

Rovner BW, Broadhead J, Spencer M, et al: Depression and Alzheimer's disease. Am J Psychiatry 146:350–363, 1989

Rovner BW, German PS, Brant LJ, et al: Depression and mortality in nursing homes. JAMA 265:993–996, 1991

Rummans TA, Lauterbach EC, Coffey CE, et al: Pharmacologic efficacy in neuropsychiatry: a review of placebo-controlled treatment trials. J Neuropsychiatry (in press)

Sackeim HA: Electroconvulsive therapy in late-life depression, in Clinical Geriatric Psychopharmacology, 3rd Edition. Edited by Salzman C. Baltimore, MD, Williams & Wilkins, 1998, pp 262–309

Salzman C: Psychopharmacology, in Core Readings in Psychiatry. Edited by Sacks MH, Sledge WH, Warren C. Washington, DC, American Psychiatric Press, 1995, pp 461–482

Salzman C: Heterogeneity of SSRI response. Harv Rev Psychiatry 4:215–217, 1996

Salzman C: Depressive disorders and other emotional issues in the elderly: current issues. Int Clin Psychopharmacol 12 (suppl 7):S37–S42, 1997

Salzman C: Geriatric psychopharmacology, in The Practitioner's Guide to Psychoactive Drugs, 4th Edition. Edited by Gelenberg AJ, Bassuk EL. New York, Plenum, 1998, pp 367–384

Salzman C, Jimerson D, Vasile R, et al: Response to SSRI antidepressants correlates with reduction in plasma HVA: pilot study. Biol Psychiatry 34:569–571, 1993

Salzman C, Satlin A, Burrows AB: Geriatric psychopharmacology, in Textbook of Psychopharmacology. Edited by Schatzberg AF, Nemeroff CB. Washington, DC, American Psychiatric Press, 1995, pp 803–821

Salzman C, Satlin A, Burrows AB: Geriatric psychopharmacology, in Textbook of Psychopharmacology, 2nd Edition. Edited by Schatzberg AF, Nemeroff CB. Washington, DC, American Psychiatric Press, 1998, pp 961–977

Sano M, Stern Y, Williams J, et al: Coexisting dementia and depression in Alzheimer's disease. Arch Neurol 46:1284–1285, 1989

Satlin A, Liptzin B: Diagnosis and treatment of mania, in Clinical Geriatric Psychopharmacology, 3rd Edition. Edited by Salzman C. Baltimore, MD, Williams & Wilkins, 1998, pp 310–330

Schiffer RB, Wineman NM: Antidepressant pharmacotherapy of depression associated with multiple sclerosis. Am J Psychiatry 147:1493–1497, 1990

Seth R, Jennings AL, Bindman J, et al: Combination treatment with noradrenalin and serotonin reuptake inhibitors in resistant depression. Br J Psychiatry 161:562–565, 1992

Small GW, Salzman C: Treatment of depression with new and atypical antidepressants, in Clinical Geriatric Psychopharmacology, 3rd Edition. Edited by Salzman C. Baltimore, MD, Williams & Wilkins, 1998, pp 245–261

Starkstein SE, Robinson RG: Aphasia and depression. Aphasiology 2:1–20, 1988

Starkstein SE, Preziosi TJ, Bolduc PL, et al: Depression in Parkinson's disease. J Nerv Ment Dis 178:27–31, 1990

Starkstein SE, Federoff JP, Berthea MD, et al: Manic depressive and pure manic states after brain lesions. Biol Psychiatry 29:149–158, 1991

Strang RR: Imipramine in treatment of Parkinsonism. A double-blind placebo study. BMJ 2:33–34, 1965

Sunderland T: Neurotransmission in the aging central nervous system, in Clinical Geriatric Psychopharmacology, 3rd Edition. Edited by Salzman C. Baltimore, MD, Williams & Wilkins, 1998, pp 51–69

Sussman N: Depression and Parkinson's disease, in Geriatric Psychopharmacology. Edited by Nelson JC. New York, Marcel Dekker, 1998, pp 199–222

Thiagarajan A, Anand KS: Parkinson's disease: incidence of depression, correlation of stages of depression to clinical staging and disability (abstract). Neurology 44 (suppl 2):A254, 1994

Tourjman S, Fontaine R: Fluvoxamine can induce confusion in the elderly (letter). J Clin Psychopharmacol 12:293, 1992

Willner P: Sensitization of dopamine D2- or D3-type receptors as final common pathway in antidepressant drug action. Clin Neuropharmacol 18 (suppl 1):S49–S56, 1995

Wragg RE, Jeste DV: Overview of depression and psychosis in Alzheimer's disease. Am J Psychiatry 146:577–587, 1989

Young RC, Mattis S, Alexopoulos GS, et al: Affective state, cognitive performance, and plasma concentrations in elderly depressives treated with nortriptyline, in Abstracts of the 29th meeting of the American College of Neuropsychopharmacology, San Juan, Puerto Rico, 1990

Young RC, Mattis S, Alexopoulos GS, et al: Verbal memory and plasma drug considerations in elderly depressives treated with nortriptyline. Psychopharmacol Bull 27:291–294, 1991

Zubenko GS, Moossy J: Major depression in primary dementia: clinical and neuropathologic correlates. Arch Neurol 45:1182–1186, 1988

14

Late-Life–Onset Psychoses

Godfrey D. Pearlson, M.D.

Late-life–onset psychosis is a fascinating but heterogeneous and insufficiently explored syndrome. To examine it objectively, one should put aside commonly held notions, such as that most cases of late-life–onset psychosis represent coarse brain disease (e.g., Alzheimer's disease or microvascular pathology) or that early- and late-life–onset schizophrenia merely represent opposite tails of age distribution of the same syndrome.

Late-life–onset psychosis is a common condition, accounting for up to 10% of admissions to psychiatric hospitals for patients over age 60 (Bridge and Wyatt 1980a, 1980b; Kay and Roth 1961; Roth 1955; Siegel and Goodman 1987). It is feasible that all psychoses, including late-life–onset forms, represent a final common expression of diverse etiopathologies. This diversity is likely to be especially marked in late-life–onset conditions, a viewpoint argued by Holden (1987) and Post (1966). In part, this diversity may be related to a general increase in age-related biological heterogeneity (Jeste and Caligiuri 1991), as well as to the emergence in late life of several neurodegenerative disorders in which psychotic symptoms are common.

Late-life–onset psychosis is a disorder classically defined on the basis of clinical phenomenology, but clinicians also define cases, somewhat inconsistently, on the basis of pathological entities (e.g., Alzheimer's disease) and etio-logical descriptions (e.g., amphetamine psychosis). Two useful, but competing, approaches to defining the syndrome of late-life psychosis are 1) to cast the net broadly (i.e., include all patients with onset of delusions and hallucinations for the first time in late life) and 2) to examine a more narrowly defined group of patients who have late-life–onset delusions and hallucinations, but in the clear absence of an affective syndrome, progressive cognitive impairment, or obvious "organic" cause (i.e., as a result of a discrete brain pathology). This more restricted syndrome is closer to what has been termed *late-life–onset schizophrenia*, or *late paraphrenia*.

Depending on which of these approaches is chosen and which age at onset is used, mixtures of patients will emerge with differing etiopathologies, genetics, brain changes, and responses to treatment (Jeste et al. 1988a, 1988b, 1991). The emergence of such heterogeneous patient mixtures is precisely what has occurred in studies of such patients, resulting in a lack of clarity. As late-life–onset psychosis likely comprises a heterogeneous group of etiopathologies, even the narrowly defined subgroup referred to above, which has been assumed by many to be most similar to early-onset schizophrenia, may well exhibit significantly more heterogeneity than would be found among a comparable group of patients with early-onset schizophrenia (Rabins and Pearlson 1994). (The full range of conditions commonly included under the broad umbrella of "late-life–onset psychosis" is discussed in the section "Diagnostic Diversity and Classification of Late-Life–Onset Psychosis" below.)

Historical Background

Use of the term *paraphrenia* (or *late paraphrenia*) is potentially problematic because of the weight of historical debates dragged in its wake. Kraepelin (1919/1971) used the former term to describe a group of chronic paranoid psychoses distinguished not by age at onset, but clinically by preservation of personality with lack of long-term deterioration and cross-sectionally by prominent elaborate delusions and hallucinations occurring in clear consciousness. Mayer (1921) followed up a large series of Kraepelin's patients and demonstrated that deterioration occurred over the long term in most such patients. The use of the term *paraphrenia* was, therefore, deleted from the subsequent edition of Kraepelin's textbook (Kraepelin 1926). Both Bleuler (1943) and Kraepelin (1903–1904) felt that late-life–onset cases of schizophrenia closely resembled, phenomenologically, more typical early-onset cases.

Roth revived and redefined the term in his descriptions of patients with "late paraphrenia." He studied elderly patients with vivid and paranoid delusions and multiple hallucinations occurring in clear consciousness, with maintenance of emotional responsiveness over time (Roth 1955; Roth and Morrisey 1952). He demonstrated that the clinical course of "late paraphrenia" was different from that of both affective disorder and dementia with onset in late life in its cross-sectional symptomatic presentation, response to treatment, and outcome; in later studies (Tomlinson et al. 1968), he demonstrated that it differed neuropathologically from dementia. Patients with "senile psychoses" (mainly Alzheimer's disease), delirious states, and arteriosclerotic psychoses (presumably multi-infarct dementia) showed a 30%–50% death rate at 6-month follow-up. Patients with late paraphrenia, who constituted approximately 10% of Roth's total group of elderly, hospitalized psychotic patients, showed a 6-month follow-up death rate of less than 5%.

Confusingly, though some authors have remained faithful to Roth's (1955) definition of *late paraphrenia*, others have retained the term but significantly broadened the concept to include patients with earlier onset (e.g., after age 45) or all late-life–onset psychoses. Some have also removed the qualifier "late," further confounding the issue.

Epidemiology and Prevalence

In a review of the literature, Harris and Jeste (1988) estimated that 13% of hospitalized patients with schizophrenia have onset of the syndrome in their 50s, 7% in their 60s, and 3% in their 70s or later. Prevalence rates of late-life–onset schizophrenia in previous studies are frequently complicated by the unselected nature of the patient samples (see Harris and Jeste 1988). Social isolation and suspiciousness associated with the syndrome may also tend to minimize the true prevalence of the disorder. Reviews by Almeida et al. (1994) and Naguib and Levy (1991) show that prior epidemiological surveys of schizophrenia in the elderly have mainly surveyed hospital samples. For example, the studies of Roth and Morrisey (1952), Kay and Roth (1961), and Blessed and Wilson (1982) showed that approximately 10% of elderly patients admitted to psychiatric hospitals have a later-life–onset schizophrenic syndrome. A small number of community-based studies in the United States and United Kingdom have depicted late-life–onset schizophrenia rates varying from 1% to 4% in elderly individuals. Holden's study (1987) of a community case register in the United Kingdom showed rates of 17–25 per 100,000 surveyed. Obviously, prevalence rates vary depending on the inclusion or exclusion criteria, perhaps most significantly the issue of possible organic etiology.

Clinical Picture and Phenomenology: Old Versus Young Patients With Schizophrenia

The best documented clinical descriptions of patients with late-life–onset schizophrenia remain the classic summaries of Kay and Roth (1961). The phenomenology of late-life–onset psychosis and its relationship to "classic" early-onset cases have engendered debates for nearly a century. As mentioned above, Kraepelin stated in the 7th edition of his textbook (Kraepelin 1903–1904) that late-life–onset schizophrenia "cannot be at all separated from juvenile forms of schizophrenia" (p. 213). However, some contrasts in phenomenological features and course between early- and late-life–onset cases have also frequently been commented on (e.g., Harris and Jeste 1988; Harris et al. 1988; Kolle 1931; Mayer-Gross 1932; Pearlson et al. 1989). Some of these differences are summarized in Table 14–1.

Phenomenologically, in cases of "late paraphrenia" (i.e., more narrowly defined late-life–onset schizophrenia), persecutory delusions are the most common, but delu-

TABLE 14–1. Comparison of symptoms among young patients with early-onset, patients with late-life–onset, and elderly patients with early-onset schizophrenia

Symptoms	Young patients with early-onset schizophrenia	Patients with late-life–onset schizophrenia	Elderly patients with early-onset schizophrenia
Hallucinations	80% (Pearlson et al. 1989)	Present in 94%; more vivid in multiple modalities (Kay and Roth 1961; Pearlson et al. 1989)	100% (Pearlson et al. 1989)
Delusions	69% (Pearlson et al. 1989)	98% (Pearlson et al. 1989), especially persecutory (also Kay and Roth 1961)	100% (Pearlson et al. 1989)
Schneiderian first-rank symptoms	50% (Pearlson et al. 1989)	35% (Pearlson et al. 1989); thought insertion and withdrawal rarer than that in early-onset schizophrenia (Grahame 1984; Holden 1987)	41% (Pearlson et al. 1989)
Formal thought disorder	52% (Pearlson et al. 1989)	Rare (5.6%) (Pearlson et al. 1989); similar (Bleuler 1943; Gabriel 1978; Huber et al. 1975)	55% (Pearlson et al. 1989)
Negative symptoms	22% (Pearlson et al. 1989)	Rarer (e.g., Bleuler 1943; Castle and Howard 1992; Pearlson et al. 1989)	23% (Pearlson et al. 1989)

sions of multiple types are often seen. Auditory hallucinations are most commonly seen, but hallucinations in multiple modalities are frequently reported, as are Schneiderian first-rank symptoms (Marneros and Deister 1984; Pearlson et al. 1989). Thought disorder and negative symptoms are relatively rare (Bleuler 1943; Castle and Howard 1992; Pearlson and Rabins 1988; Pearlson et al. 1989).

Pathoplastic age-associated features can mold the symptomatic expression. For example, "partition" delusions (i.e., delusions that people, gas, electricity, or some other force enters the patient's home through the walls [partitions] from a neighbor's apartment), which are said to be common in late-life–onset schizophrenia, can be influenced in content rather than form by the isolation and homeboundness commonly seen in elderly people. Castle and Murray (1991) argued that the schizophrenia-like illness occurring for the first time in elderly people, predominantly women, represents a variant of affective disorder. Although interesting (and further discussed in Chapter 13 in this volume), this assertion remains essentially unproven. However, few studies have contrasted patients with late-life–onset schizophrenia with groups of patients with affective disorder or with other relevant comparison samples, such as patients with early-onset schizophrenia who have grown old and young patients with early-onset schizophrenia (some exceptions being Pearlson et al. 1989; Rabins et al. 1984).

Until recently, clinical phenomenology has been the major classificatory tool for schizophrenia researchers. This limitation has put psychiatrists at a disadvantage

(comparable to that of cardiologists before electrocardiograms, chest X rays, nuclear medicine cardiac scans, and enzyme studies). Interpreting reasons behind the phenomenological differences between early- and late-life–onset schizophrenia, especially the differences in thought disorder and negative symptoms, is difficult. Is this, for example, a completely different illness, the same illness occurring in an older person, or only a case of similar clinical abnormalities occurring in an older brain assailed by neurodegenerative changes and mimicking what is most usually a neurodevelopmental disorder? (After reviewing further evidence, we attempt to address such questions in the "Conclusions" section below.)

Diagnostic Diversity and Classification of Late-Life–Onset Psychosis

Scope of the Disorder

If, as noted at the beginning of this chapter, one uses a broad definition of patients with late-life–onset psychosis, the following mixture of patient groups is likely to be included (Table 14–2):

1. **Elderly patients with early-onset schizophrenia.** Such patients are frequently encountered, as schizophrenia is not a fatal illness. Because it is unresolved whether early- and late-life–onset cases represent the same disorder, verification of age at onset must

TABLE 14–2. Groups included in a broad classification of patients with late-life–onset psychosis

Elderly patients with early-onset schizophrenia

Patients with late-life–onset schizophrenia ("late paraphrenia")

Patients with paranoid psychoses without hallucinations

Patients with psychotic affective disorder

Patients with cerebrovascular disease:
  Classic multi-infarct dementia with psychotic symptoms
  "Multi-infarct disease"

Patients with Alzheimer's disease with psychotic symptoms

Patients with psychoses of miscellaneous causes with and without defined neuropathology

Patients in delirious and toxic states

Patients with extremes of paranoid or schizoid personality types

be carefully sought from available relatives or other informants and by examination of prior medical records.

2. **Patients with late-life–onset schizophrenia ("late paraphrenia").** As discussed at the beginning of this chapter, nomenclature for this group has been especially confusing. In general, the term *late paraphrenia* (Roth 1955) has been applied to a more circumscribed group consisting of patients who have the onset in late life (i.e., over age 60) of a syndrome that clinically closely resembles early-onset schizophrenia. There is a long debate in the British literature (e.g., Almeida et al. 1992) between those psychiatrists who view these patients as having late-life–onset classic schizophrenia (e.g., Grahame 1984) and those who have emphasized its heterogeneity (e.g., Holden 1987). DSM-IV (American Psychiatric Association 1994) omits age criteria for schizophrenia onset.

3. **Patients with paranoid psychoses without hallucinations.** Unlike those with late-life–onset schizophrenia, in which hallucinations are vivid and often in multiple modalities, these patients correspond to those with "persistent delusional disorders" with late onset, as described by DSM-IV, and to earlier descriptions in the literature by researchers such as Kay and Roth (1961) and Holden (1987). Anecdotally, such patients do not later develop hallucinations, and they tend to respond poorly to neuroleptic medications. If such is the case, this disorder seems rather remote from late-life–onset schizophrenia.

4. **Patients with psychotic affective symptoms.** El-

derly patients with both affective symptoms and mood-incongruent delusions and hallucinations are often encountered (Kay et al. 1976). They correspond to individuals with the late-life onset of psychosis described as the "affective group" by Holden (1987), and, as discussed in Chapter 12 in this volume, family history and phenomenology of prior episodes may aid differential diagnosis.

5. **Patients with cerebrovascular disease.** *Classic multi-infarct dementia* is not infrequently accompanied by psychotic symptoms. Cummings (1985) reported that approximately 50% of patients with multi-infarct dementia have delusions. We propose below that the number of patients with *"multi-infarct disease"* (see below) is significantly larger than previously estimated, with the larger prevalence now revealed through the increasing clinical application of magnetic resonance imaging (MRI) and single photon emission computed tomography (SPECT). It is becoming clear that an unknown, but significant, percentage of patients with late-life–onset psychosis manifests imaging changes consistent with cerebrovascular disease, not necessarily accompanied by cognitive deficits and hence not meeting criteria for multi-infarct dementia. This finding accounts for our use of the more inclusive term *multi-infarct disease.* Case series have been described by Miller et al. (1991, 1992) and Lesser et al. (1992).

6. **Patients with Alzheimer's disease and psychotic symptoms.** Patients with Alzheimer's disease often manifest secondary delusions and hallucinations (e.g., Rubin 1992). The patient described in Alzheimer's original case report had delusional beliefs. The characteristics of hallucinating and delusional patients with Alzheimer's disease have been described in review articles by Wragg and Jeste (1989) and Burns et al. (1990a, 1990b). Delusions in Alzheimer's disease tend to be rather fragmentary and impersistent. Careful follow-up of all patients with late-life–onset psychosis is therefore necessary to identify those with emerging dementia syndromes.

7. **Patients with psychoses of miscellaneous causes with and without defined neuropathology.** Cerebral infections (Chapter 30), tumors (Chapter 30), Parkinson's disease (Chapter 26), stroke (Chapter 27), head injury (Chapter 28, all in this volume), and other causes can all be associated with late-life emergence of hallucinations and delusions in clear consciousness (e.g., Signer 1992). *Delirious and toxic states* (e.g., anticholinergic delirium, alcohol withdrawal, hypothyroidism, and amphetamine psycho-

sis) can manifest with similar symptomatology. Finally, *extremes of paranoid or schizoid personality types* (Chapter 20 in this volume) (e.g., those described by Post [1966] and Holden [1987]) can be mistaken for cases of late-life–onset psychosis if only cross-sectional information is available.

A Classificatory and Investigational Scheme

With so many possible syndromes encompassing diverse etiopathologies, yet sharing common clinical features, it is clear that prior studies have often been alluding to diverse patient groups. We (Rabins and Pearlson 1994) have used a multiaxial approach to classification using genetics, epidemiology, risk factors, phenomenology, course, treatment response, neuropathology, and biological markers. To evaluate patients thoroughly, to proceed from a common reference point, and to rule out other diagnoses, for a particular patient the information in Table 14–3 should ideally be gathered.

TABLE 14–3. Information (both clinical and laboratory) to be gathered in cases of late-life–onset psychosis

Family history (e.g., of early- or late-onset schizophrenia, affective disorder, and Alzheimer's disease)

Complete psychiatric history (especially prior affective episodes)

Medical history, including history of stroke and transient ischemic attacks, and an assessment of vascular risk factors, using standardized instruments

Premorbid level of functioning and intelligence

Premorbid personality

Current medications

Current detailed cognitive functioning

Current social supports

Sensory screening examination

History of present illness, especially age at onset of psychosis, relative to other known comorbid states (e.g., Alzheimer's disease)

Complete physical and neurological examination

Routine laboratory tests for reversible causes of dementia (e.g., B_{12} and folate levels and syphilis serology)

Standardized neuroimaging studies, especially magnetic resonance imaging (MRI) and single photon emission computed tomography (SPECT), both to rule out coarse brain disease (e.g., obvious strokes and tumors) and to assess extent of nonspecific changes (e.g., subcortical white matter hyperintensities)

Risk Factors for Late-Life–Onset Schizophrenia

As shown in many review articles (Almeida et al. 1994; Harris and Jeste 1988; Pearlson and Rabins 1988; Pearlson et al. 1989), multiple risk factors associated with more narrowly defined late-life–onset schizophrenia have been enumerated (Table 14–4).

Genetic Factors

As regards family history of schizophrenia, Kay (1972) showed that the percentage of affected first-degree relatives for patients with late-life–onset schizophrenia (3.4%) was intermediate between that of patients with early-onset schizophrenia (5.8%) and that of the known risk (1%) in the general population. As reviewed by Castle and Howard (1992) and by us (Pearlson and Rabins 1988), the assessment of family history rates presents problems, however. Prior studies have often not used standardized instruments such as family history, research diagnostic criteria, or strategies such as an adoption study design. Informants for late-life–onset diseases are often dead or unavailable and potential cases who are relatives may have died before the age of clinical risk, if the illness "breeds true" as has been suggested by some authors. The evidence overall is consistent with the notion that late-life–onset psychosis may be partly genetically determined; however, much remains to be clarified. This issue will be settled only when risk genes for schizophrenia are discovered.

Gender

Female gender appears to be a very robust risk factor, even when the relative excess of older women is corrected for. The excess of women patients in late-life–onset cases has variously been reported as 6- to 20-fold (Herbert and Jacobson 1967; Kay and Roth 1961). Although some authors

TABLE 14–4. Risk factors associated with late-life–onset schizophrenia

Family history of schizophrenia

Female gender

Sensory deficits (primarily auditory and visual)

Social isolation

Abnormal premorbid personality

Never married/no children

Human leukocyte antigen (HLA) subtypes

Lower social class

(e.g., Pearlson and Rabins 1988) believe that this gender effect represents a shift in the female incidence of schizophrenia to late life (Lewine 1981, 1985), others (e.g., Castle and Murray 1991) have argued otherwise. Similar changes in gender preponderance are not seen with early versus late-life affective disorder (e.g., Weisman 1987).

Wong et al. (1984), using positron-emission tomography (PET) to measure dopamine, subtype 2 (D_2), receptors, showed age-related decreases in the estimated number of D_2 receptors, in agreement with postmortem studies (e.g., Seeman et al. 1987) (also see Chapter 10 in this volume). These PET data suggested that physically and mentally healthy men possess more D_2 receptors but lose them at an accelerated rate with normal aging, compared with that of women. Hence, older women are left with a relative excess of D_2 receptors compared with that of men of the same age. If, as some (e.g., Pearlson and Coyle 1983) have suggested, schizophrenia is indeed related to an excess of D_2 receptors, the relative excess of D_2 receptors in young men and in elderly women may explain the classic age-related gender expression differences for schizophrenia (i.e., that schizophrenia is usually expressed by men at a significantly earlier age than it is by women). Seeman (1981, 1986) has speculated that estrogens have "neuroleptic-like" or neuroprotective effects on D_2 receptors, which would be lost after menopause. A PET study (Pearlson et al. 1993) offered preliminary support for D_2 receptor increases in late-life–onset schizophrenia.

Sensory Deficits

Sensory deficits, especially auditory and visual declines, which are more common in late life, have been reported in many studies to be a relative risk factor for late-life–onset schizophrenia. Cataracts and conductive deafness are the most common causes. Findings related to sensory deficits have been reported by multiple authors (e.g., Cooper and Porter 1976; Cooper et al. 1974; Naguib and Levy 1987; Pearlson et al. 1989; Post 1966). Conductive deafness seems to be a risk factor rather specific to late-life–onset schizophrenia, with prevalence being significantly higher than that in patients with late-life–onset affective disorder (e.g., Cooper et al. 1974). Some authors (e.g., Eastwood et al. 1981) have stated that, among the hearing impaired, psychotic symptoms respond favorably to treatment of the deafness. As reviewed by us (Pearlson and Rabins 1988), sensory impairment can be associated with reduced social contact and lead plausibly, therefore, to social isolation, suspiciousness, and liability to misinterpret environmental events. In an individual who is already predisposed to develop late-life–onset schizophrenia, sensory impairment may therefore encourage symptom formation. Sensory deficits may thus in part account for the higher rates of social isolation reported in patients with late-life–onset schizophrenia. Kay and Roth (1961) reported sensory impairment rates three times higher among patients with late-life–onset schizophrenia than rates among elderly patients with affective disorder.

Premorbid Personality

Another factor undoubtedly contributing to social isolation is the abnormal premorbid personality (mainly paranoid or schizoid) identified by multiple researchers as preceding late-life–onset psychosis (Herbert and Jacobson 1967; Kay 1972; Kay and Roth 1961; Pearlson et al. 1989; Post 1966). Kay and Roth (1961) and Post (1966), but not our group (Pearlson et al. 1989), found that women with late-life–onset schizophrenia were significantly more likely to have never married or had children. This observation has been reported less often in United States studies. If the finding is valid, low marriage rates may be related to the abnormal premorbid personalities seen in such patients.

It remains to be determined whether the abnormal premorbid personality traits described in late-life–onset schizophrenia represent a forme fruste of a schizophrenic disorder of a long-standing nature, significantly predating emergence of overt clinical symptoms, or a "risk factor" as classically understood. Other, miscellaneous factors have been explored, such as association with human leukocyte antigens (Naguib et al. 1987). Post (1966) showed that many patients with late-life–onset schizophrenia tended to have lower socioeconomic status premorbidly.

Brain Changes in Late-Life–Onset Psychosis

Compared with their respectively age-matched healthy control groups, individuals with late-life–onset psychosis have a significantly higher prevalence of identifiable brain abnormalities than do young individuals with similar symptoms (Miller et al. 1991). This observation is a rather general one, however. Many patients with late-life–onset psychosis do not have a specific lesion or an etiology for their brain change, and lesions reported in many studies do not share common localization or represent a single well-defined pathology. The reported prevalence of such brain changes varies, as might be expected for such a heterogeneous syndrome as late-life–onset psychosis. Some studies have carefully excluded all patients with probable organic pathology (e.g., Krull et al. 1991; Naguib and Levy

1987). Such series of screened patients have generally reported a smaller number of nonspecific brain changes (e.g., white matter hyperintensities) on MRI scans. Others (Lesser et al. 1989, 1992; Miller et al. 1992) included cases of probable vascular dementia. Nevertheless, given the above caveat, new and potentially important information has emerged from structural and functional brain imaging study of patients with late-life–onset psychosis (Table 14–5). It is clear that demonstrably altered brain structure or function is a predisposing factor in a proportion of such cases and that this proportion is higher than was suspected before modern neuroimaging methods became available. Reported changes fall into three broad categories: global structural changes, white matter hyperintensities on MRI, and cerebral blood flow changes documented on SPECT scans.

Structural Changes

Several studies have demonstrated increased ventricular-to-brain ratio (VBR) in patients with late-life–onset schizophrenia compared with that in age-matched psychiatrically healthy control subjects. For computed tomography (CT), such studies include Burns et al. (1989), Naguib and Levy (1987), Rabins et al. (1987), and ourselves (Pearlson et al. 1987). Howard et al. (1992a, 1992b) found lateral VBR (as well as third ventricular changes) to be no different from that for control subjects. Rabins et al. (1987) found patients with late-life–onset schizophrenia to have VBRs greater than those of control subjects, but smaller than those of patients with Alzheimer's disease with psychotic symptoms. Similarly, Krull et al. (1991), assessing VBRs on MRI scans, found values in late-life–onset schizophrenia to be intermediate between those of control subjects and patients with Alzheimer's disease. Howard et al. (1992a; see also Almeida et al. 1992) found patients with late-life–onset schizophrenia without Schneiderian first-rank symptoms to have ventricular and sulcal enlargement more comparable to that seen in patients with Alzheimer's disease; in contrast,

TABLE 14–5. Structural and functional abnormalities reported in early-onset and late-life–onset psychosis patients

Abnormality	Patients with early-onset schizophrenia	Patients with late-life–onset schizophrenia	Patients with late-life–onset depression
Increased ventricular/brain ratio on CT or MRI	Johnstone et al. 1976; Pearlson et al. 1987; Weinberger et al. 1979	Howard et al. 1992a, 1992b, 1994; Naguib and Levy 1987; Rabins et al. 1987	Pearlson et al. 1987; Rabins et al. 1991
Third ventricular enlargement	Boronow et al. 1985	Howard et al. 1994; Pearlson et al. 1989	
White matter abnormalities on MRI		Breitner et al. 1990; Flint et al. 1991; Kohlmeyer 1988; Miller et al. 1986, 1989 (not Howard et al. 1995b; Krull et al. 1991; or Symonds et al. 1997)	Coffey et al. 1989, 1990; Krishnan et al. 1988; Zubenko et al. 1990
Cortical atrophy on CT or MRI	Gur et al. 1991; Pfefferbaum et al. 1988	Howard et al. 1992a, 1992b (not Burns et al. 1989; Pearlson et al. 1993 [as CSF %])	Pearlson et al. 1987
Smaller superior temporal gyrus	Barta et al. 1990; Shenton et al. 1992	Barta et al. 1997 (not Howard et al. 1995a)	
Blood flow abnormalities on SPECT	Gur et al. 1985; Matthew et al. 1988	Miller et al. 1992	
Increased dopamine, subtype 2, receptor B_{max} on PET	Wong et al. 1986a, 1986b, 1986c	Pearlson et al. 1993	
rCBF abnormalities during provocative tasks	Weinberger et al. 1988		

Note. B_{max} = measure of receptor density; CSF = cerebrospinal fluid; CT = computed tomography; MRI = magnetic resonance imaging; PET = positron-emission tomography; rCBF = regional cerebral blood flow; SPECT = single photon emission computed tomography.

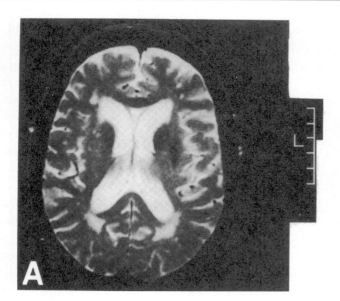
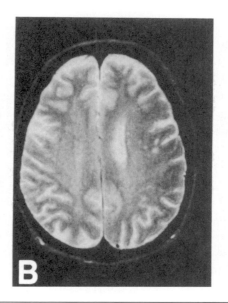

FIGURE 14–1. T2-weighted 5-mm axial magnetic resonance images of a 71-year-old woman with first onset of schizophrenic syndrome at age 69 (*panel A:* widest portion of lateral ventricles; *panel B:* centrum semiovale). Periventricular, subcortical, and cortical hyperintensities are visible. Ventricular enlargement is also evident (in *panel A*).

patients with late-life–onset schizophrenia with first-rank symptoms were more comparable to elderly control subjects.

MRI studies in general have been less convincing than those of CT in showing ventricular enlargement in subjects with late-life–onset psychosis. For example, Miller et al. (1991) found no differences between patients and control subjects; we reported a similar finding (Pearlson et al. 1991). We (Pearlson et al. 1993) also reported significant third ventricular enlargement in late-life–onset psychosis in an MRI study, whereas Burns et al. (1989) found no cortical atrophy compared with that in control subjects using CT. Table 14–5 lists other abnormalities noted in early- and late-life–onset schizophrenia. Overall, there is some evidence for moderate cortical and subcortical changes in late-life–onset psychosis, but less so for patients with "late paraphrenia" and in MRI studies. These latter emphasize the heterogeneity of late-life psychoses (e.g., see Howard et al. 1995a).

Several studies report an excess of white matter abnormalities or *unidentified bright objects* (UBOs) in patients with late-life–onset schizophrenia compared with that found in psychiatrically healthy control subjects (Figure 14–1). Such studies include Miller et al. (1986), Miller and Lesser (1988), Breitner et al. (1990), Lesser et al. (1991, 1992), and Miller et al. (1991), but not other workers (Table 14–5). Although some suggestions of localized patterns have been reported in such studies, a general review of the changes reported (including periventricular white matter hyper-

intensities, probable subcortical vascular lesions, and white matter hyperintensities) does not convince one that they are either uniform in nature or clearly localized to particular brain regions.

For example, Breitner et al. (1990) reported on 8 patients with late-life–onset paranoia, all of whom had significant white matter hyperintensities and 7 of whom had vascular lesions in pons or basal ganglia. Lesser et al. (1992) reported that 6 of 12 geriatric patients with DSM-III-R psychotic disorder not otherwise specified (American Psychiatric Association 1987) had large confluent white matter lesions. Miller et al. (1991) examined 24 patients with late-life–onset psychosis. Temporal lobe white matter hyperintensities occurred six times more frequently among these patients than in control subjects, whereas frontal and occipital hyperintensities were found four times more frequently. Significant excess of basal ganglia and cortical abnormalities was also reported in these subjects. Flint et al. (1991) examined 16 patients with late-life–onset paranoia or paraphrenia. Five of the 16 subjects had "silent cerebral infarction," especially those with paranoia (i.e., delusional patients without hallucinations). Krull et al. (1991) carefully screened their population of 11 patients with late-life–onset psychosis to attempt to eliminate those most likely to have a diagnosis of organic cerebral disorder. In 9 remaining patients, they found no increase in white matter disease compared with patients with Alzheimer's disease or psychiatrically healthy control subjects.

Howard et al. (1995b) pursued a similar screening strategy and also found no excess of white matter hyperintensities.

Functional Changes

Single photon emission computed tomography cerebral blood flow studies. Several SPECT studies now agree in showing a relative excess of multiple areas of reduced cerebral blood flow in patients with late-life–onset psychosis. For example, in a diagnostically mixed group of such patients, Lesser et al. (1993) showed that approximately 75% had SPECT scan abnormalities of this type. Miller et al. (1992) also demonstrated cerebral blood flow abnormalities suggestive of cerebrovascular disease in a proportion of patients with late-life–onset psychosis. Further, 83% of the patients with late-life–onset psychosis versus 27% of the control subjects had one or more small temporal or frontal areas of hypoperfusion.

Positron-emission tomography neuroreceptor studies. We (Pearlson et al. 1993) compared 13 neuroleptic-naive patients with late-life–onset schizophrenia (clinical onset after age 55) to 17 control subjects. Two PET scans were obtained in each subject to estimate caudate D_2 receptor density using the method previously described by Wong et al. (1986a, 1986b, 1986c). The second scan was preceded by the administration of unlabeled haloperidol to demonstrate binding under conditions of D_2 receptor blockade (Figure 14–2), and D_2 receptor B_{max} (receptor density) values were calculated using a four-compartment model.

To account for variation in B_{max} values with age and gender (the control subjects were younger), a regression equation was calculated in the control subjects, and a predicted B_{max} based on the control regression equation was then computed for each subject with schizophrenia. Residual values were then determined by subtraction of the observed B_{max} minus the predicted B_{max}. Standardized residual B_{max} values for subjects with schizophrenia showed significant increases from zero, suggesting that B_{max} values were elevated in this group of subjects with schizophrenia, even when age and gender were taken into account. This finding is similar to reports of elevated B_{max} values for D_2 receptors in drug-naive patients with early-onset schizophrenia reported by the same group using the same method (Wong et al. 1986a), although not by others using a different method (Farde et al. 1987).

Caveats come with many of the above neuroimaging studies. First, a proportion of patients in many of the reports had clinical evidence of cerebrovascular disease and would unequivocally be diagnosed as having organic psychiatric syndromes. The Flint et al. (1991) and Miller et al. (1986) studies in fact identified a proportion of patients whose stroke was first diagnosed by the neuroimaging studies. Many of the changes described in the structural and blood flow studies above are nonspecific—in the sense of being unlocalized in the brain and occurring in association with other late-life disorders, such as late-life–onset depression (e.g., Coffey et al. 1990)—and are not clearly associated with a particular neuropathology. Most of the reported series are small, and usually there was no follow-up to determine whether or not these patients later clinically expressed dementia syndromes. Neuropathological confirmation was lacking for most of the cases scanned. Patients with late-life–onset psychosis in the studies reviewed generally represent an unselected series, possibly representing a referral bias in which more cases are likely to have organic factors. Most of the imaging carried out has been semiquantitative or nonquantitative. Samples have generally been diagnostically heterogeneous, including not only patients with late-life-onset schizophrenia but also those with late-life-onset delusional disorder and late-life–onset psychosis not otherwise specified, and control subjects have not always been appropriately screened or matched to patients on age, gender, race, IQ, or community of origin. Nevertheless, much useful information is emerging, and study designs are gradually improving.

Neuropathology

Tomlinson et al. (1968) found no excess of plaques and tangles at autopsy in patients with late-life–onset schizophrenia compared with age-matched control subjects. Kay and Roth (1961) found limited cerebral lesions (mainly consisting of small strokes) in a percentage of patients with late-life–onset schizophrenia. These researchers interpreted these lesions as having often been present years before the onset of psychotic symptoms. This interpretation contrasts with the studies of Bleuler (1943) who found cerebral lesions in a proportion of patients with late-life–onset schizophrenia, lesions that he believed had appeared years after the onset of the psychotic symptoms. This vascular neuropathology, however, is in accord with several neuroimaging studies (Flint et al. 1991; Holden 1987; Miller et al. 1986) that have reported on association between stroke and the onset of psychotic symptoms in elderly patients. Such cases appear to be associated with mild cognitive loss, a greater propensity to manifesting visual hallucinations, fewer overall hallucinations, and fewer schneiderian first-rank symptoms and are thus less typi-

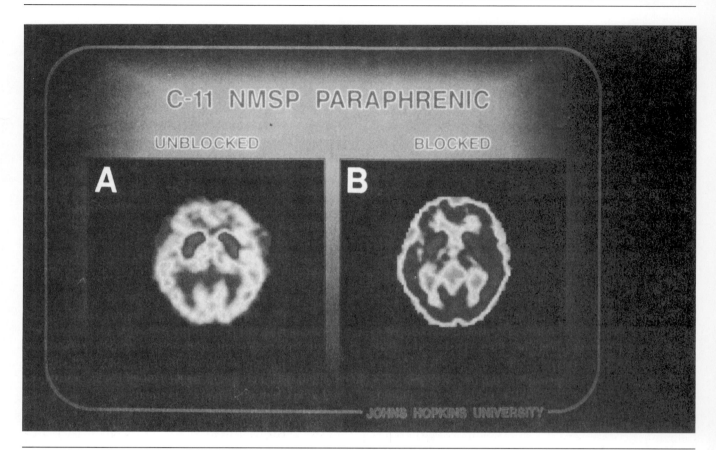

FIGURE 14–2. Transaxial positron-emission tomography (PET) images through basal ganglia in a never-medicated patient with late-life–onset schizophrenia (paraphrenia). *Panel A:* Uptake before blockade with oral neuroleptic, with high basal ganglia uptake relative to cortex. *Panel B:* A second scan in same subject, taken 4 hours after pretreatment with unlabeled oral haloperidol. Dopamine, subtype 2 (D_2), receptors are blocked by the cold ligand, revealing consequently lower basal ganglia activity. C-11 NMSP = carbon-11 labeled *N*-methyl spiperone, a PET receptor ligand.
Source. Photograph courtesy of D. Wong, Department of Radiology, Johns Hopkins University, Baltimore, Maryland.

cally "schizophrenic." Overall, neuropathological studies are few, and clear conclusions are hard to draw. Imaging studies and neuropathology suggest a role for cerebrovascular disease in some patients—a theme expanded in the "Conclusions" section below.

Neuropsychological Testing in Late-Life–Onset Psychosis

Miller et al. (1991) compared 21 patients with late-life–onset psychosis (over age 45) with an equal number of individually matched (on education, age, and gender) psychiatrically healthy control subjects. The patients showed an overall decrement in cognitive functioning. After correction for multiple comparisons, several frontal measures and a verbal memory task showed significant impairment of the patients. The authors felt that this pattern was similar to that identified by previous researchers in early-onset

schizophrenia. Naguib and Levy (1987) tested 43 subjects with late-onset paraphrenia and found cognitive differences from psychiatrically healthy control subjects. These patients were later followed by Hymas et al. (1989), who tested 42 patients with "late paraphrenia" and attempted to exclude those with obvious early dementias. Mild neuropsychological deficits were present at the onset of illness and tended to progress somewhat with time, but not to frank dementia.

Overall, patients seen in our own clinic tend to be poorly educated and from rural backgrounds, with low average estimated premorbid IQ. It is especially hard in such cases to document deterioration from an uncertain but low premorbid level of functioning. Our review of the literature suggests that patients with late-life–onset psychosis tend to perform worse on standardized tests than do matched control subjects, but if patients with obvious organic factors are excluded, the remaining patients do not have obvious dementia and most do not develop diagnosable dementing illnesses at follow-up.

■ Diagnosis, Treatment, and Treatment Response

Diagnosis

Differential diagnosis needs first to be reviewed. Our own experience is similar to that of Webster and Grossberg (1998). Those authors retrospectively evaluated the etiology and clinical findings of patients with first manifestations of psychotic symptoms (mostly delusions and hallucinations), arising after the age of 65 in more than 1,700 consecutive admissions to an inpatient psychogeriatric unit. Nearly 10% had late-life–onset psychotic symptoms, of which Alzheimer's disease was the most common cause, followed by major depression, medical or toxic causes or delirium, bipolar disorder, delusional disorder, schizophrenia, and schizoaffective disorder.

The differential diagnosis of psychotic symptoms occurring in late life begins with history and current symptomatology. When was the first onset of psychotic symptoms? Have they been present for many years or emerged only recently? Age at onset may have to be verified from old records and informants other than the patient. This information will, for example, help distinguish between late-life–onset and persisting early-life–onset schizophrenia. Next, determine what additional symptoms are occurring with the hallucinations and delusions. As schizophrenia at any age is always a diagnosis of exclusion, dementia, delirium, and affective disorder are the most important common primary neuropsychiatric entities to consider. Structural brain imaging is helpful to rule out coarse brain disease (e.g., stroke, tumors, bleeds, multiple sclerosis).

A useful rule is to consider the overall symptomatic context in which the psychotic symptoms occur. For example, are the psychotic symptoms present as the accompaniment to a dementing illness (see Gormley and Rizwan 1998)? Assessing current cognitive function and an estimate of premorbid ability (for the latter, using an instrument such as the National Adult Reading Test [NART, Blaine and Spreen 1989]) are helpful. It is also profitable to see whether cognitive impairment, if it exists, fits a typical pattern, for example, that of a cortical dementia. If clear cognitive decline has taken place, then an appropriate diagnostic work-up must be pursued (see Chapters 23 and 24 in this volume). Blood tests (e.g., Venereal Disease Research Laboratory [VDRL] test) are taken to rule out treatable causes of dementia, and other procedures (e.g., SPECT, apolipoprotein E subtyping) may be useful to help confirm a particular diagnosis. The presence of concomitant affective disorder symptoms must be assessed (refer to Chapter 13 in this volume). Are there clear-cut primary changes in mood, self-attitude, vital sense, or vegetative symptoms?

Is there a change in the patient's level of consciousness? A typical waxing and waning course with an abnormal, variable level of consciousness (refer to Chapter 19 in this volume) may be seen. If so, typical electroencephalogram disturbances may be detectable. Does the patient have marked extrapyramidal symptoms in the absence of current or prior treatment with neuroleptic drugs? If so, this may represent psychotic symptoms either occurring spontaneously in untreated Lewy body dementia or Parkinson's disease or secondary to L-dopa or carbidopa treatment in Parkinson's disease.

Treatment

Recent reviews of treatment of late-life–onset psychosis are to be found in Zayas and Grossberg (1998) and Mazure et al. (1998). Elderly cases of early-onset schizophrenia should be treated as for the late-life–onset disorder, that is, with a typical or atypical neuroleptic. Psychosis occurring in the context of a dementing illness involves both the treatment of the primary dementia (see Chapter 24 in this volume), for example, an acetylcholinesterase inhibitor for Alzheimer's disease (see Raskind 1997), which may help ameliorate the psychotic as well as the cognitive symptoms. The physician should generally avoid prescribing neuroleptics with marked anticholinergic side effects, for example, chlorpromazine, as these may exacerbate cognitive symptoms and increase risk for delirium. "Classic" high-potency neuroleptics such as haloperidol or fluphenazine are more likely to be associated with extrapyramidal side effects (EPS) and tardive dyskinesia in individuals with dementia. EPS in turn may lead to the need for treatment with undesirable anticholinergic compounds. There is thus an argument for atypical neuroleptic drugs as the compounds of choice for psychosis occurring in a dementing illness. Risperidone is the best documented of the atypical neuroleptics for this use (e.g., see Citrome 1997; Lavretsky and Sultzer 1998).

If the patient is suffering from a primary depressive illness, selective serotonin reuptake inhibitors are equally effective as classic tricyclic antidepressants (see Chapter 13 in this volume), with the advantage of fewer cardiac side effects and more safety in the case of overdose, both of which are important considerations in older patients. Psychotic affective symptoms may in some cases need to be treated with a neuroleptic drug in addition to the antidepressant. If so, atypical neuroleptic compounds may be preferable, for reasons cited above. Electroconvulsive therapy is also useful in patients with psychotic depressive symptoms (see Chapter 35 in this volume).

When a patient suffers from psychotic symptoms in the context of a delirious state, then the primary cause of the delirium must be addressed (see Chapter 19 in this volume). If neuroleptics need to be added for short-term behavioral control, then use the principles outlined for Alzheimer's disease above.

Psychotic symptoms in idiopathic Parkinson's disease that are a result of secondary effects of treatment of the Parkinson's disease are most often seen with L-dopa/carbidopa combinations and less likely to be seen with dopamine agonist treatments. Treatment with classic neuroleptic compounds will likely exacerbate parkinsonian symptoms. Some authors have advised treatment with ondansetron hydrochloride (Zofran), to avoid worsening EPS (Eichlorn et al. 1996; Zoldan et al. 1995); however, this medication is very expensive. Others (e.g., Friedman 1999) suggest treatment with clozapine; but clozapine is anticholinergic and entails weekly monitoring of white blood cell counts. Treatment with clozapine in the context of Parkinson's disease can still lead to exacerbations of parkinsonian symptoms (e.g., Wolters et al. 1990), as noted in the only placebo-controlled trial. Olanzapine may also be helpful (Wolters et al. 1996), as may risperidone (Workman et al. 1997), but both of these drugs, especially the latter, can still exacerbate the Parkinson's disease (although the risk is less than for high-potency dopamine D_2 receptor–blocking compounds). Note that remarkably few double-blind treatment trials of neuroleptics for psychotic symptoms appear in the above conditions (Rummans et al., in press).

Treatment of classic late-life–onset schizophrenia with "classic" neuroleptics such as haloperidol offers the advantage that these compounds are much cheaper. Disadvantages are the relatively greater frequency of EPS and a likely greater long-term risk of tardive dyskinesia. The usual caveats also apply to the older, high-potency D_2 receptor–blocking drugs, as well as to those with anticholinergic side effects; that is, in the elderly they are likely to exacerbate glaucoma and benign prostatic hypertrophy and have secondary effects on blood pressure that may increase the risk of falls. Double-blind placebo-controlled trials to demonstrate efficacy of atypical neuroleptics in late-life–onset schizophrenia are needed. Potential (if unproven) advantages of these drugs include likely fewer EPS and less ultimate risk of tardive dyskinesia, although EPS can certainly still occur with these medicines. Disadvantages include expense, although patient assistance programs from most pharmaceutical manufacturers are now available for indigent patients. The usual adage of "start low, go slow, but continue" in older people applies to all treatment groups.

The mainstay of treatment of late-life–onset psychosis has been neuroleptic medication, but the patient's lack of insight into illness and patient suspiciousness can result in variable medication compliance. Patients with late-life–onset psychosis tend not to seek treatment. The psychiatrist is often involved late in the illness, offering treatment to an uncooperative patient (e.g., see Almeida et al. 1994; Post 1984). As might be expected, medication compliance, depot medication, and use of a community psychiatric nurse for outpatients all favorably affect treatment response (Howard and Levy 1992).

Although well-organized, double-blind crossover treatment trials are scarce, several open trials of neuroleptics have shown substantial improvement in a subgroup of patients with well-characterized, late-life–onset psychosis. Four studies over a 25-year period are summarized in Table 14–6.

Clinical improvement overall seems most likely to occur in patients with late-life–onset psychosis whose phenomenology most resembles that of early-onset schizophrenia. We (Pearlson et al. 1989) found that patients with poor medication response tend to be characterized by schizoid premorbid traits; we also found no effect on response of presence of first-rank symptoms, positive family history of schizophrenia, or gender. Holden (1987) found that patients with poor clinical response were characterized by an absence of auditory hallucinations or affective features. This finding is similar to the situation in younger people with schizophrenia in which florid hallucinations, prominent affective features, and an acute onset (especially if associated with some precipitating event) are all associated with a good prognosis. Flint et al. (1991) similarly found patients with paranoid delusions alone to respond poorly to neuroleptic agents.

Although both early- and late-life-onset schizophrenia tend to respond to neuroleptics with amelioration of positive symptoms, factors affecting interpretation of studies in patients with late-life–onset illness include differential

TABLE 14–6.   Results of neuroleptic treatment in late-life–onset psychosis

Study	Complete remission	Partial remission	No improvement	N patients
Post 1966	60.5%	31%	8.5%	71
Rabins et al. 1984	57%	28.5%	14.5%	34
Pearlson et al. 1989	48%	28%	24%	54
Howard and Levy 1992	27%	31%	42%	64

symptom patterns in late-onset versus early-onset forms of schizophrenia and different pharmacodynamics in young versus old patients. Treatment with neuroleptic medications in elderly patients must be tempered by knowledge of differential responsiveness, which depends in part on age-related changes in body size and composition (e.g., increased proportion of adipose tissue and decreased renal function) (for a review, see Tran-Johnson et al. 1992; also see Chapter 34 in this volume). There are also pharmacokinetic changes (e.g., trend for higher plasma neuroleptic levels at same doses compared with that for younger patients) and pharmacodynamic changes, including increased sensitivity to therapeutic and toxic effects (possibly as a result of altered density and affinity of relevant cerebral receptors) (see Branchey et al. 1978). Overall, many patients with late-onset psychosis are adequately treated with very low drug doses. The differential side-effect profile of older patients includes higher risk of tardive dyskinesia, falls, anticholinergic side effects with low-potency neuroleptics (including delirium, worsening of glaucoma, cardiac abnormalities, and urinary outflow obstructions), and worsening of preexisting parkinsonian syndromes. Knowledge of individual patients' existing medical illness and other medications is therefore necessary (Table 14–2). Treatment with newer atypical agents (risperidone, olanzapine, quetiapine) may be preferable.

Course and Prognosis

Although more long-term follow-up studies are still needed, investigators agree that the course of late-life–onset schizophrenia is a chronic one (Herbert and Jacobson 1967; Kay and Roth 1961). Fish (1960) emphasized the poor prognosis of the condition, but Roth (1955) offered more optimism, stating that mortality was much less than that in patients of comparable ages who had dementia or depression. It is clear, however, that some patients with late-life–onset psychosis do develop dementia. This outcome is to be expected in any elderly population; the key fact is whether the proportion exceeds that predicted. Again, because heterogeneous samples have been followed in many studies, the relative proportions of subjects with clear-cut dementing illnesses initially presenting with psychotic symptoms are unknown.

Based on chart review only, Kay and Roth (1961) found that 12% of their patients with late-life–onset paraphrenia had developed dementing illnesses at 10-year follow-up. Holden (1987) found that 35% of his patient group had dementia at 3-year follow-up. Craig and Bregman (1988) followed a select group of patients with treatment-resistant,

late-life–onset psychosis and found that 10 of 15 had dementia. Lesser et al. (1989) and Miller et al. (1991) found that, as a group, their 24 patients with late-life–onset psychosis had mild cognitive abnormalities when initially evaluated; on follow-up, many of these patients had developed classic dementia syndromes such as Alzheimer's or Pick's disease. Finally, Hymas et al. (1989) found that nearly half of their 42 patients with late-life–onset psychosis showed evidence of cognitive decline at 4-year follow-up, especially those with low cognitive scores at entry. Only 2 of the patients, however, met diagnostic criteria for dementia.

The inconsistency of results obtained in different studies is difficult to explain but probably relates to ascertainment bias. The key point is that all studies report a significantly higher incidence of dementia in patients found to have late-life–onset psychosis than would be found in a comparable population of elderly individuals. Overall, predicting the long-term outcome of late-life–onset psychosis depends on a clearer division of these patients into diagnostic subgroups as suggested above.

Multi-Infarct Disease and Its Relationship to Late-Life–Onset Psychosis

Our hypothesis concerning multi-infarct disease and its relationship to late-life–onset psychosis is a straightforward one: that microvascular disease in elderly patients can be associated with new onset of major psychiatric disorders, including schizophrenia, in the absence of dementia. Thus we draw a distinction between multi-infarct *disease* and multi-infarct *dementia*.

Evidence for this conjecture derives from several sources. The observed excess of UBOs in both late-life–onset depression (most convincing) and late-life–onset schizophrenia (less convincing) on MRI and the patchy areas of reduced cerebral blood flow on SPECT suggest vascular pathology in patients with these syndromes. It appears from several studies (e.g., Breitner et al. 1990; Miller and Lesser 1988; Miller et al. 1986) that patients with white matter lesions on MRI tend to have higher numbers of vascular risk factors. However, several studies found no excess of white matter lesions in late-onset psychosis (Table 14–5). Various hypotheses can be generated from these observations. The most nonspecific is that any form of "brain damage" in late life renders an individual more likely to express major psychiatric syndromes and such "damage" subsumes a collection of common etiologies for several late-life–onset major psychiatric illnesses. Alternatively, and far more specifically, the observed white matter abnormalities on MRI and SPECT may represent a single pathophysiological outcome (i.e., cerebral microvascular disease) that is a highly specific risk factor for late-life–onset schizophrenia. This hypothesis seems unlikely, however, as similar changes are reported for late-life–onset depressive syndromes (Coffey et al. 1988). In addition, confirmation of the vascular etiology and/or pathology of the changes seen on cerebral imaging studies is still lacking.

From a consideration of the same observations, Guze and Szuba (1992) offered an alternative interpretation. They suggested that these neuroimaging findings are a function of normal age-related brain changes, but "beyond a critical threshold, they may increase vulnerability" to late-life–onset major psychiatric illnesses, in combination with other risk factors. Such additional risk factors could include family history of a particular disorder and the anatomic site of the brain findings (e.g., Rabins et al. 1991). These combined vulnerabilities determine the final form of the illness (e.g., late-life–onset schizophrenia, late-life–onset depression, multi-infarct dementia, or a senile-onset movement disorder). If UBOs and white matter lesions are of vascular origin, the above suggestions taken to their logical conclusion would place at least some cases of late-life–onset psychosis and depression in a continuum of pathology with multi-infarct dementia.

Conclusions

Late-life–onset psychosis is clearly a heterogeneous and understudied syndrome. Much that is vital to comprehend is still unknown, for example, how best to subdivide the condition meaningfully and, for each resulting separate syndrome, how to determine its precise prevalence and find its important pathophysiological underpinnings. Also remaining obscure are the syndrome's precise relationship to early-onset schizophrenia, response to treatment, and long-term outcome.

Although neuroimaging has the potential to provide important insights into the underlying pathophysiology, the numbers of subjects studied in most recent studies have been small, and a great need exists for large-scale longitudinal studies with suitable comparison patients (e.g., patients with late-life–onset affective disorders or elderly patients with early-onset schizophrenia). Finally, neuropathological examination is ultimately needed to clarify the nature of the underlying brain processes.

More narrowly defined cases of late-life–onset schizophrenia (or late paraphrenia) appear both more clinically homogeneous and most phenomenologically similar to early-onset schizophrenia. Even when more narrowly defined, late-life–onset psychosis appears to be a more diverse syndrome than early-onset schizophrenia, and neurodegenerative changes probably play a larger etiological role than formerly envisioned. Evidence suggests that neurodegenerative and neurodevelopmental changes likely contribute to late-life–onset psychosis, but because the relative importance of each is unknown in most cases, it is too soon to settle the question of whether early- and late-life–onset schizophrenia are essentially the same condition (a theme discussed by both Almeida et al. [1994] and us [Rabins and Pearlson 1994]). Perhaps the clearest parallel is with late-life–onset depressive illness (see Chapter 12 in this volume). There, too, one finds a genetic risk for the appropriate illness (albeit a diminished one compared with early-onset forms of the disease), evidence in some subjects of nonspecific brain changes (identified by neuroimaging techniques), and a likely heterogeneous mixture of delayed "true" cases and "organic phenocopies." Neuroimaging clearly has the potential to help "biotype" the syndrome and to clarify the question of diversity. However, documenting the choice of index and comparison patients, as well as of control subjects, is critical in this endeavor, as some neuroimaging studies have cast their recruitment net broadly, whereas others have excluded cases with likely "organic" associations.

Returning to the theme of affective illness, we believe that Castle and Murray's viewpoint (1991) that late-life-onset cases of schizophrenia in fact represent affective disorder is unlikely. Our opinion is based on observations that comparison patients with late-life–onset schizophrenia and affective disorder have different patterns of atrophy on the CERAD (Consortium to Establish a Registry for Alzheimer's Disease) (Morris et al. 1989) MRI rating scale (Aylward et al. 1993; Rabins et al., in press) and differ phenomenologically (Rabins et al. 1984). Also the types of abnormal premorbid personality reported in late-life–onset schizophrenia and affective disorder differ; the risks of family members being affected with affective disorder versus schizophrenia appear to be different in the two groups, and the syndromes respond to different types of treatment.

So far, interactions between the various risk factors reported for late-life–onset schizophrenia, as well as the ability to separate necessary from sufficient associations, lack the development of an encompassing theory. As we have stated (Pearlson et al. 1993), the etiology and timing of the structural changes in late-life–onset schizophrenia are unknown. They could be primarily initiated in late life or, alternatively, depend on age-related brain changes unmasking a preexisting (perhaps genetic) vulnerability. If a developmental origin, similar to that proposed for early-onset cases (Weinberger 1987), is also applicable to some cases of late-life–onset schizophrenia (e.g., as we have suggested [Pearlson and Rabins 1988]), a vital point to address is why symptomatic onset has been delayed to the senium. In this chapter, we review evidence that such possible precipitants for late-life–onset psychosis could include neuronal loss as a result of usual aging and vascular or age-related functional changes, especially those affecting women, such as postmenopausal estrogen loss and thus alterations in the relative balance of dopamine D_2 receptors in basal ganglia. The role of late-life brain abnormalities and the relative contributions of neurodegenerative processes versus brain damage secondary to stroke or microvascular disease remain to be elucidated. Cerebrovascular pathology is likely to prove an important etiological factor for at least some proportion of late-life–onset major psychiatric illnesses, including psychosis. The etiological evidence for late life-onset psychosis is less compelling than that for late-life depression, however.

References

Almeida OP, Howard R, Förstl H, et al: Should the diagnosis of late paraphrenia be abandoned? (editorial). Psychol Med 2:11–14, 1992

Almeida OP, Howard R, Förstl H, et al: Late onset paranoid disorders, Part I: coming to terms with late paraphrenia, in Functional Psychiatric Disorders in the Elderly. Edited by Edmond C, David A. New York, Cambridge University Press, 1994, pp 303–316

American Psychiatric Association: Diagnostic and Statistical Manual of Mental Disorders, 3rd Edition, Revised. Washington, DC, American Psychiatric Association, 1987

American Psychiatric Association: Diagnostic and Statistical Manual of Mental Disorders, 4th Edition. Washington, DC, American Psychiatric Association, 1994

Aylward EH, Pearlson GD, Rabins PV: Differences in early and late onset schizophrenia (letter). Am J Psychiatry 150:846–849, 1993

Barta PE, Pearlson GD, Powers RE, et al: Reduced superior temporal gyrus volume in schizophrenia. Am J Psychiatry 147:1457–1462, 1990

Barta PE, Powers RE, Aylward EH, et al: Quantitative MRI volume changes in late onset schizophrenia and Alzheimer's disease compared to normal controls. Psychiatry Res 68:65–75, 1997

Blair PE, Spreen O: Predicting premorbid IQ: a revision of the National Adult Reading Test. Clin Neuropsychol 3:129–136, 1989

Blessed G, Wilson D: The contemporary natural history of mental disorder in old age. Br J Psychiatry 141:59–67, 1982

Bleuler M: Late schizophrenic clinical pictures [in German]. Fortschr Neurol Psychiatr 15:259–290, 1943

Boronow J, Pickar D, Ninan PT: Atrophy limited to third ventricle only in chronic schizophrenic patients: report of a controlled series. Arch Gen Psychiatry 40:266–271, 1985

Branchey M, Lee J, Amen R, et al: High and low-potency neuroleptics in elderly psychiatric patients. JAMA 239:1860–1862, 1978

Breitner JCS, Husain MM, Figiel GS, et al: Cerebral white matter disease in late-onset paranoid psychosis. Biol Psychiatry 28:266–274, 1990

Bridge TP, Wyatt RJ: Paraphrenia: paranoid states of late life, I: European research. J Am Geriatr Soc 27:193–200, 1980a

Bridge TP, Wyatt RJ: Paraphrenia: paranoid states of late life, II: American research. J Am Geriatr Soc 27:201–205, 1980b

Burns A, Carrick J, Ames D, et al: The cerebral cortical appearance in late paraphrenia. Int J Geriatr Psychiatry 4:31–34, 1989

Burns A, Jacoby R, Levy R: Psychiatric phenomena in Alzheimer's disease, I: disorders of thought content. Br J Psychiatry 157:72–76, 1990a

Burns A, Jacoby R, Levy R: Psychiatric phenomena in Alzheimer's disease, II: disorders of perception. Br J Psychiatry 157:76–81, 1990b

Castle DJ, Howard R: What do we know about the aetiology of late-onset schizophrenia? European Psychiatry 7:99–108, 1992

Castle DJ, Murray RM: The neurodevelopmental basis of sex differences in schizophrenia. Psychol Med 21:565–575, 1991

Citrome L: New antipsychotic medications: what advantages do they offer? Postgrad Med 101:207–210, 213–214, 1997

Coffey CE, Figiel GS, Djang WT, et al: Leukoencephalopathy in elderly depressed patients referred for ECT. Biol Psychiatry 24:143–161, 1988

Coffey CE, Figiel GS, Djang WT, et al: White matter hyperintensity on magnetic resonance imaging: clinical and neuroanatomic correlates in the depressed elderly. J Neuropsychiatry Clin Neurosci 1:135–144, 1989

Coffey CE, Figiel GS, Djang WT, et al: Subcortical hyperintensity on magnetic resonance imaging: a comparison of normal and depressed elderly subjects. Am J Psychiatry 47:187–189, 1990

Cooper AF, Porter R: Visual acuity and ocular pathology in the paranoid and affective psychoses of later life. J Psychosom Res 20:107–114, 1976

Cooper AF, Kay DWK, Curry AR, et al: Hearing loss in paranoid and affective psychoses of the elderly. Lancet 2:851–861, 1974

Craig TJ, Bregman Z: Late onset schizophrenia-like illness. J Am Geriatr Soc 36:104–107, 1988

Cummings J: Organic delusions: phenomenology, anatomical correlations and review. Br J Psychiatry 145:184–197, 1985

Eastwood MR, Corbin S, Reed M: Hearing impairment and paraphrenia. J Otolaryngol 10:306–308, 1981

Eichhorn TE, Brunt E, Oertel WH: Ondansetron treatment of L-dopa-induced psychosis. Neurology 47:1608–1609, 1996

Farde L, Wiesel FA, Hall H, et al: No D_2 receptor increase in PET study of schizophrenia. Arch Gen Psychiatry 44:671–672, 1987

Fish F: Senile schizophrenia. Journal of Mental Science 106:938–946, 1960

Flint AJ, Rifat SL, Eastwood MR: Late-onset paranoia: distinct from paraphrenia? Int J Geriatr Psychiatry 6:103–109, 1991

Friedman J, the Parkinson Study Group: Low-dose clozapine for the treatment of drug-induced psychosis in Parkinson's disease. N Engl J Med 340:757–763, 1999

Gabriel D: Die Langfristige Entwicklung der Spatchziophrenien. Basel, Karger, 1978

Gormley N, Rizwan MR: Prevalence and clinical correlates of psychotic symptoms in Alzheimer's disease. Int J Geriatr Psychiatry 13:410–414, 1998

Grahame PS: Schizophrenia in old age (late paraphrenia). Br J Psychiatry 145:493–495, 1984

Gur RE, Bur RC, Skolnik BE, et al: Brain function in psychiatric disorders, III: regional cerebral blood flow in unmedicated schizophrenics. Arch Gen Psychiatry 42:329–334, 1985

Gur RE, Mozley PD, Resnick SM, et al: Magnetic resonance imaging in schizophrenia, I: volumetric analysis of brain and cerebrospinal fluid. Arch Gen Psychiatry 48:407–412, 1991

Guze BH, Szuba MP: Leukoencephalopathy and major depression: a preliminary report. Psychiatry Res 45:169–175, 1992

Harris MJ, Jeste DV: Late-onset schizophrenia: an overview. Schizophr Bull 14:39–55, 1988

Harris MJ, Cullum CM, Jeste DV: Clinical presentation of late-onset schizophrenia. J Clin Psychiatry 49:356–360, 1988

Herbert ME, Jacobson S: Late paraphrenia. Br J Psychiatry 113:461–469, 1967

Holden NL: Late paraphrenia or the paraphrenias? a descriptive study with a 10 year follow-up. Br J Psychiatry 150:635–639, 1987

Howard R, Levy R: Which factors affect treatment response in late paraphrenia? Int J Geriatr Psychiatry 7:667–672, 1992

Howard RJ, Förstl H, Almeida O, et al: Computer-assisted CT measurements in late paraphrenics with and without Schneiderian first-rank symptoms: a preliminary report. Int J Geriatr Psychiatry 7:35–38, 1992a

Howard RJ, Förstl H, Almeida O, et al: First-rank symptoms of Schneider in late paraphrenia: cortical structural correlates. Br J Psychiatry 160:108–109, 1992b

Howard RJ, Almeida O, Levy R, et al: Quantitative magnetic resonance imaging volumetry distinguishes delusional disorder from late-onset schizophrenia. Br J Psychiatry 165:474–480, 1994

Howard R, Mellers J, Petty R, et al: Magnetic resonance imaging volumetric measurements of the superior temporal gyrus, hippocampus, parahippocampal gyrus, frontal and temporal lobes in late paraphrenia. Psychol Med 25:495–503, 1995a

Howard R, Cox T, Almeida O, et al: White matter signal hyperintensities in the brains of patients with late paraphrenia and the normal, community-living elderly. Biol Psychiatry 38:86–91, 1995b

Huber G, Gross A, Schuttler R: Late schizophrenia. Archiv Psychaitrische Nervenkranken 221:53–66, 1975

Hymas N, Naguib M, Levy R: Late paraphrenia: a follow-up study. Int J Geriatr Psychiatry 4:23–29, 1989

Jeste DV, Caligiuri MP: Biological research in geriatric psychiatry (editorial). Biol Psychiatry 30:855–856, 1991

Jeste DV, Harris JM, Zweifach M: Late-onset schizophrenia. Psychiatry 56:1–8, 1988a

Jeste DV, Harris MJ, Pearlson GD, et al: Late-onset schizophrenia: studying clinical validity. Psychosis and Depression in the Elderly 11:1–13, 1988b

Jeste DV, Manley M, Harris MJ: Psychoses, in Comprehensive Review of Geriatric Psychiatry. Edited by Sadavoy J, Lazarus L, Jarvik L. Washington, DC, American Psychiatric Press, 1991, pp 353–368

Johnstone E, Crow T, Frith C, et al: Cerebral ventricular size and cognitive impairment in chronic schizophrenia. Lancet 2:924–926, 1976

Kay DWK: Schizophrenia and schizophrenia-like states in the elderly. British Journal of Hospital Medicine 8:369–379, 1972

Kay DWK, Roth M: Environmental and hereditary factors in the schizophrenias of old age ("late paraphrenia") and their bearing on the general problem of causation in schizophrenia. Journal of Mental Science 107:649–686, 1961

Kay DWK, Cooper AF, Garside RF, et al: The differentiation of paranoid from affective psychoses by patients' premorbid characteristics. Br J Psychiatry 129:207–215, 1976

Kohlmeyer K: Periventrikuläre Dichteminderungen des Grosshirnhemispherenmarks in Computertomogrammen von neuropsychiatrischen Patienten in der zweiten Lebenshälfte: diagnostische Bedeutung und Pathogenese. Fortschr Neurol Psychiat 56:279–287, 1988

Kolle K: Die Primare Veruckltheit. Leipzig, Thieme, 1931

Kraepelin G: Psychiatrie: Ein Lehrbuch für Studierende und Artzte, 7th Edition. Leipzig, Barth, 1903–1904

Kraepelin G: Dementia praecox and paraphrenia (1919), in Text-Book of Psychiatry, 8th Edition. Translated from the German by Barclay RM. Edited by Robertson GM. Huntington, NY, Krieger, 1971, pp 18–81

Kraeplin G: Psychiatrie: Ein Lehrbuch für Studierende und Artzte, 9th Edition. Leipzig, Barth, 1926

Krishnan KRR, Goli V, Ellinwood EH, et al: Leukoencephalopathy in patients diagnosed as major depressive. Biol Psychiatry 23:519–522, 1988

Krull AJ, Press G, Dupont R, et al: Brain imaging in late-onset schizophrenia and related psychoses. Int J Geriatr Psychiatry 6:651–658, 1991

Lavretsky H, Sultzer D: A structured trial of risperidone for the treatment of agitation in dementia. Am J Geriatr Psychiatry 6:127–135, 1998

Lesser IM, Miller BL, Boone KB, et al: Psychosis as the first manifestation of degenerative dementia. Bulletin of Clinical Neurosciences 54:59–63, 1989

Lesser IM, Miller BL, Boone KB, et al: Brain injury and cognitive function in late-onset psychotic depression. J Neuropsychiatry Clin Neurosci 3:33–40, 1991

Lesser IM, Jeste DV, Boone KB, et al: Late-onset psychotic disorder, not otherwise specified: clinical and neuroimaging findings. Biol Psychiatry 31:419–423, 1992

Lesser IM, Miller BL, Swartz JR, et al: Brain imaging in late-life schizophrenia and related psychoses. Schizophr Bull 19:773–782, 1993

Lewine RJ: Sex differences in schizophrenia: timing or subtypes? Psychol Bull 90:432–444, 1981

Lewine RJ: Schizophrenia: an amotivational syndrome in men. Can J Psychiatry 30:316–318, 1985

Marneros A, Deister A: The psychopathology of "late schizophrenia." Psychopathology 17:264–274, 1984

Matthew RJ, Wilson WH, Tant SR, et al: Abnormal resting regional cerebral blood flow patterns and their correlates in schizophrenia. Arch Gen Psychiatry 45:542–549, 1988

Mayer W: On paraphrenic psychoses. Zeitschrift für die Gesamte Neurologie und Psychiatrie 71:187–206, 1921

Mayer-Gross W: Die Schizophrenie. Berlin, Springer, 1932

Mazure CM, Nelson JC, Jatlow PI, et al: Acute neuroleptic treatment in elderly patients without dementia. Am J Geriatr Psychiatry 6:221–229, 1998

Miller BL, Lesser IM: Late-life psychosis and modern neuroimaging. Psychiatr Clin North Am 11:33–46, 1988

Miller BL, Benson FD, Cummings JL, et al: Late-life paraphrenia: an organic delusional system. J Clin Psychiatry 47:204–207, 1986

Miller BL, Lesser IM, Boone K, et al: Brain white-matter lesions and psychosis. Br J Psychiatry 155:73–78, 1989

Miller BL, Lesser IM, Boone KB, et al: Brain lesions and cognitive function in late-life psychosis. Br J Psychiatry 158:76–82, 1991

Miller BL, Lesser IM, Mena I, et al: Regional cerebral blood flow in late-life–onset psychosis. Neuropsychiatry Neuropsychol Behav Neurol 5:132–137, 1992

Morris JC, Heyman A, Mohs RC, et al: The consortium to establish a registry for Alzheimer's disease (CERAD), part I: clinical and neuropsychological assessment of Alzheimer's disease. Neurology 39:1159–1165, 1989

Naguib M, Levy R: Late paraphrenia: neuropsychological impairment and structural brain abnormalities on computed tomography. Int J Geriatr Psychiatry 2:83–90, 1987

Naguib M, Levy R: Paraphrenia, in Psychiatry in the Elderly. Edited by Jacoby R, Oppenheimer C. Oxford, England, Oxford University Press, 1991, pp 758–778

Naguib M, McGuffin P, Levy R, et al: Genetic markers in late paraphrenia: a study of HLA antigens. Br J Psychiatry 150:124–127, 1987

Pearlson GD, Coyle JT: The dopamine hypothesis and schizophrenia, in Neuroleptics: Neurochemical, Behavioral and Clinical Perspectives, Vol 3: CNS Pharmacology. Edited by Coyle JT, Enna S. New York, Raven, 1983, pp 297–327

Pearlson GD, Rabins PV: The late onset psychoses: possible risk factors. Psychiatr Clin North Am 11:15–33, 1988

Pearlson GD, Garbacz DJ, Tompkins RH, et al: Lateral cerebral ventricular size in late onset schizophrenia, in Schizophrenia and Aging. Edited by Miller NE, Cohen GD. New York, Guilford, 1987, pp 246–248

Pearlson GD, Kreger L, Rabins PV, et al: A chart review study of late-onset and early onset schizophrenia. Am J Psychiatry 146:1568–1574, 1989

Pearlson GD, Barta PE, Tune LE, et al: Quantitative MRI and PET in late life onset schizophrenia, in American College of Neuropsychopharmacology, Abstracts of Panels and Posters, 30th Annual Meeting, Caribe Hilton, San Juan, Puerto Rico. Nashville, TN, ACNP Secretariat, 1991, p 56

Pearlson GD, Tune LE, Wong DF, et al: Quantitative D2 dopamine receptor PET and structural MRI changes in late onset schizophrenia: a preliminary report. Schizophr Bull 19:783–795, 1993

Pfefferbaum A, Zipursky RB, Lim KO, et al: Computed tomographic evidence for generalized sulcal and ventricular enlargement in schizophrenia. Arch Gen Psychiatry 45:633–640, 1988

Post F: Persistent Persecutory States of the Elderly. London, Pergamon, 1966

Post F: Schizophrenic and paranoid psychoses, in Handbook of Studies on Psychiatry and Old Age. Edited by Kay DWK, Burrows W. Amsterdam, Elsevier, 1984, pp 291–302

Rabins PV, Pearlson GD: Late onset paranoid disorders, Part II: Paraphrenia, schizophrenia or ? in Functional Psychiatric Disorders in the Elderly. Edited by Edmond C, David A. New York, Cambridge University Press, 1994, pp 316–325

Rabins P, Pauker S, Thomas J: Can schizophrenia begin after age 44? Compr Psychiatry 25:290–295, 1984

Rabins PV, Pearlson GD, Jayaram G, et al: Elevated VBR in late-onset schizophrenia. Am J Psychiatry 144:1216–1218, 1987

Rabins PV, Pearlson GD, Aylward EH, et al: Cortical magnetic resonance imaging changes in elderly inpatients with major depression. Am J Psychiatry 148:617–620, 1991

Rabins PV, Aylward EH, Lavrisha M, et al: MRI measures using the CERAD scale in elderly depressed and schizophrenic patients. Psychiatry Res (in press)

Roth M: The natural history of mental disorder in old age. Journal of Mental Science 101:281–301, 1955

Roth M, Morrissey J: Problems in the diagnosis and classification of mental disorders in old age. Journal of Mental Science 98:66–80, 1952

Rubin EH: Delusions as part of Alzheimer's disease. Neuropsychiatry Neuropsychol Behav Neurol 5:108–113, 1992

Rummans TA, Lauterbach EC, Coffey CE, et al: Pharmacologic efficacy in neuropsychiatry: a review of placebo-controlled treatment trials. J Neuropsychiatry (in press)

Seeman MV: Gender and the onset of schizophrenia: neurohumoral influences. Psychiatry Journal of the University of Ottawa 6:136–137, 1981

Seeman MV: Current outcome in schizophrenia: women vs. men. Acta Psychiatr Scand 73:609–617, 1986

Seeman PF, Bzowej NH, Guan HC, et al: Human brain dopamine receptors in children and aging adults. Synapse 1:399–404, 1987

Siegel CE, Goodman AB: Mental illness among the elderly in a large state psychiatric facility: a comparison with other age groups, in Schizophrenia and Aging. Edited by Miller NE, Cohen GD. New York, Guilford, 1987, pp 23–34

Signer SF: Psychosis in neurologic diseases: Capgras symptom and delusions of reduplication in neurologic disorders. Neuropsychiatry Neuropsychol Behav Neurol 5:138–143, 1992

Symonds LL, Olichney JM, Jernigan TL, et al: Lack of clinically significant gross structural abnormalities in MRIs of older patients with schizophrenia and related psychoses. J Neuropsychiatry Clin Neurosci 9:251–258, 1997

Tomlinson BE, Blessed G, Roth M: Observations on the brains of non-demented old people. J Neurol Sci 7:331–343, 1968

Tran-Johnson TK, Krull AJ, Jeste DV: Late life schizophrenia and its treatment: pharmacologic issues in older schizophrenic patients. Clin Geriatr Med 8:401–410, 1992

Tune LE, Wong DF, Pearlson GD, et al: Elevated dopamine D_2 receptor density in schizophrenia: a PET study with 11C-N-methylspiperone. Psychiatry Res 49:219–237, 1993

Webster J, Grossberg GT: Late-life onset of psychotic symptoms. Am J Geriatr Psychiatry 6:196–202, 1998

Weinberger DR: Implications of normal brain development for the pathogenesis of schizophrenia. Arch Gen Psychiatry 44:660–669, 1987

Weinberger DR, Torrey EF, Neophytides AN, et al: Lateral cerebral ventricular enlargement in chronic schizophrenia. Arch Gen Psychiatry 36:735–739, 1979

Weinberger DR, Berman KF, Illowsky BP: Physiological dysfunction of dorsolateral prefrontal cortex in schizophrenia. Arch Gen Psychiatry 45:609–615, 1988

Weisman MM: Advances in psychiatric epidemiology: rates and risks for major depression. Am J Public Health 77:445–451, 1987

Wolters EC, Hurwitz TA, Mak E, et al: Clozapine in the treatment of parkinsonian patients with dopaminomimetic psychosis. Neurology 40:832–834, 1990

Wolters EC, Jansen EN, Tuynman-Qua HG, et al: Olanzapine in the treatment of dopaminomimetic psychosis in patients with Parkinson's disease. Neurology 47:1085–1087, 1996

Wong DF, Wagner HN, Dannals RF, et al: Effects of age on dopamine and serotonin receptors measured by positron emission tomography in the living human brain. Science 226:1393–1396, 1984

Wong DF, Wagner HN Jr, Tune LE, et al: Positron emission tomography reveals elevated D_2 dopamine receptors in drug-naive schizophrenics. Science 234:1558–1563, 1986a

Wong DF, Gjedde J, Wagner HN Jr: Quantification of neuroreceptors in the living human brain, I: irreversible binding of ligands. J Cereb Blood Flow Metab 6:177–176, 1986b

Wong DF, Gjedde J, Wagner HN Jr, et al: Quantification of neuroreceptors in the living human brain, II: assessment of receptor density and affinity using inhibition studies. J Cereb Blood Flow Metab 6:147–153, 1986c

Workman RH Jr, Orengo CA, Bakey AA, et al: The use of risperidone for psychosis and agitation in demented patients with Parkinson's disease. J Neuropsychiatry Clin Neurosci 9(4):594–597, 1997

Wragg R, Jeste DV: An overview of depression and psychosis in Alzheimer's disease. Am J Psychiatry 146:577–587, 1989

Zayas EM, Grossberg GT: The treatment of psychosis in late life. J Clin Psychiatry 59(suppl 1):5–10, 1998

Zoldan J, Friedberg G, Livneh M, et al: Psychosis in advanced Parkinson's disease: treatment with ondansetron, a 5-HT3 receptor antagonist. Neurology 45:1305–1308, 1995

Zubenko GS, Sullivan P, Nelson JP, et al: Brain imaging abnormalities in mental disorders of late life. Arch Neurol 47:1107–1111, 1990

15

Anxiety Disorders

Javaid I. Sheikh, M.D.

Anxiety in the elderly, as in the young, is a normal human emotion with adaptive value that helps one anticipate and prepare for noxious events. This normal emotion, however, can be considered pathological when it becomes unjustifiably excessive and maladaptive, as in morbid anxiety in clinical situations. This morbid anxiety usually manifests itself in the form of a multitude of cognitive, behavioral, and physiological symptoms, whereas the mental content of such anxiety can range from excessive worrying about everyday concerns regarding job and relationships to episodes of intense anxiety and fear (panic attacks). The term *anxiety* is used in this chapter to refer to such clinically significant or morbid anxiety, unless specified otherwise. Anxiety disorders are diagnostic entities comprising various constellations of signs and symptoms of anxiety combined with criteria regarding their intensity and duration, as described in DSM-IV (American Psychiatric Association 1994). Table 15–1 lists some examples of multidimensional symptoms that might be experienced by patients with various anxiety disorders.

As in younger adults, in elderly patients anxiety disorders are among the most frequent psychiatric illnesses (Blazer et al. 1991). However, unlike in younger populations, in whom these disorders have attracted considerable attention from investigators over the last two decades, anxiety disorders remain among the least studied of psychiatric illnesses in the elderly. In this chapter, I begin with classification of anxiety disorders based on DSM-IV, summarize findings of phenomenology of anxiety disorders in the elderly from the literature, discuss manifestations of anxiety in certain medical and neuropsychiatric illnesses, present a systematic way of assessing anxiety in the elderly and differentiating it from depression, and summarize treatment methods particularly suited to geriatric anxiety.

Classification of Anxiety Disorders

DSM-IV describes operationally defined, phenomenologically oriented diagnostic criteria for various anxiety disorders. A list of anxiety disorders based on DSM-IV classification appears in Table 15–2. A detailed description of the diagnostic characteristics of each disorder can be found in DSM-IV.

Epidemiological Studies

Epidemiological studies of anxiety disorders in the elderly are scant and data somewhat conflicting depending on the methodology used. Data from the Epidemiologic Catch-

347

TABLE 15–1. Multidimensional symptoms of anxiety

Cognitive	Behavioral	Physiological
Nervousness	Hyperkinesis	Tachycardia
Apprehension	Repetitive	Palpitations
Racing thoughts	motor acts	Chest tightness
Worry	Stiffness	Dry mouth
Fearfulness	Phobias	Hyperventilation
Irritability	Pressured speech	Paresthesias
Distractibility	Startle response	Lightheadedness
		Sweating
		Urinary frequency

Source. Reprinted with permission from Sheikh JI, "Clinical Features of Anxiety Disorders" in *Principles and Practice of Geriatric Psychiatry.* Edited by Copeland JM, Abou-Saleh MT, Blazer DG. London, Wiley, 1994, p. 725.

TABLE 15–2. DSM-IV anxiety disorders

Panic disorder
    With agoraphobia
    Without agoraphobia
Agoraphobia without history of panic disorder
Social phobia
Simple phobia
Generalized anxiety disorder
Obsessive-compulsive disorder
Posttraumatic stress disorder
Organic anxiety syndrome
Anxiety disorder not otherwise specified

Source. Adapted from American Psychiatric Association 1994.

ment Area (ECA) study (Myers et al. 1984) suggest that phobias are the most common psychiatric disorder in elderly women and the second most common in elderly men, ages 65 and above. In an age comparison of the Duke community sample of the ECA data between age groups of 45–64 (middle-aged) and 65 or older (older-aged), Blazer et al. (1991) show that prevalence of all anxiety disorders declines somewhat from the middle-aged to the older-aged group, although a formidable combined prevalence of 19.7% was found for the 6-month period when persons were not excluded as a result of a comorbid psychiatric disorder. Some other studies have reported lower point prevalence rates. For example, using a computerized program, AGECAT, which is an algorithm for assembling information at interview, Kay (1988) found a rate of anxiety disorders of around 2% in the United Kingdom. It appears, however, that 50%–75% of elderly cases with clinical levels of anxiety were diagnosed as depression. Kay (1988) suggests that, if diagnosed independently, the prevalence of anxiety disorders would be doubled. Similarly, lower prevalence rates of diagnosis of anxiety disorders were found in community samples in which depression was diagnosed first in samples presenting with a mixed picture of anxiety-depression (Copeland et al. 1987). Blazer et al. (1991) also suggest the possibility of underreporting as a result of a higher threshold for reporting generalized anxiety symptoms in the older-aged group and a tendency to seek assistance when that threshold is reached.

Earlier epidemiological studies investigating symptomatology of anxiety as opposed to distinct disorders have also suggested high prevalence of clinically significant symptomatology. For example, Himmelfarb and Murrell (1984) found clinically significant symptomatology of anx-

iety among 22% of women and 7% of men among a sample of more than 2,000 community persons in Kentucky, ages 55 and older. Evidence also shows that patients with chronic medical disorders are especially prone to developing anxiety. In a community survey based on data from the National Institute of Mental Health (NIMH) ECA Program, more than 11% of people with a chronic medical illness were found to have had a recent anxiety disorder (Wells et al. 1988). Because more than 80% of people in the United States older than 65 report at least one chronic medical condition (National Center for Health Statistics 1987), geriatric patients are at increased risk for developing anxiety.

In conclusion, it appears that anxiety symptoms and disorders are among the most common psychiatric ailments experienced by older adults, particularly when a mixed-symptom picture of anxiety-depression is also considered.

Phenomenology of Anxiety Disorders in the Elderly

As noted above, empirical studies of the phenomenology of late-life anxiety disorders are scant. However, recent data shed some light on panic disorder (Sheikh and Swales 1998), phobias (Lindesay 1991), and posttraumatic stress disorder (PTSD) (Goenjian et al. 1994) in late life. Panic disorder is usually a chronic syndrome with frequent recurrences and remissions. Preliminary investigations suggest that many older patients with onset of panic attacks in early life seem to continue with their symptomatology in later life, with many of them receiving inadequate or no treatment over the years (Sheikh et al. 1991). It is less common for panic disorder to appear de novo in old age (Luchins and Rose 1989; Sheikh et al. 1988).

We have previously reported data from ongoing research in our program suggesting phenomenological differences in patients with early-onset panic disorder (EOPD) with onset before the age of 55 versus patients with late-onset panic disorder (LOPD) (at or after the age of 55). Specifically, preliminary analysis of our data indicated that patients with LOPD commonly report less severe symptomatology during panic attacks, experience less severe catastrophic cognitions related to attacks, and have less avoidance behavior (Sheikh et al. 1991). In a more recent attempt to replicate our initial findings, we analyzed data from 171 self-referred patients with panic disorder (Sheikh and Swales 1998). Of this sample, 99 belonged to the EOPD group (mean age = 62.07); 26, to the LOPD group (mean age = 64.81); and 45, to the younger panic disorder (YPD) group (mean age = 38.82). After informed consent was obtained, participants were administered the Structured Clinical Interview for DSM-III-R (Spitzer et al. 1987), and a psychiatric and medical history was taken. Additional measures that assessed panic-associated domains included: cognitions, physiological symptoms, behaviors, and global functioning. Data from this larger sample replicate and confirm our earlier findings that patients with LOPD tend to have a less severe form of panic disorder and report less cognitive distress, fewer avoidance behaviors, less overall physiological arousal, and higher overall (global) functioning compared with that of either the EOPD or YPD group. This group difference may imply different causative mechanisms, risk factors, clinical course, and prognosis for patients with LOPD. Our group is investigating these issues by identifying possible risk factors (e.g., family history, life stressors, medical and psychiatric comorbidity) as well as studying the clinical course and any differential treatment response of these groups.

Epidemiological data (Blazer et al. 1991) indicate that phobic disorders are in general chronic and persisting in old age. Clinical experience suggests that public speaking may seem less frightening and eating in public more bothersome to the elderly compared with those tasks for younger people. Fear of crime seems to be particularly prevalent in the elderly population, especially in an urban setting. In a survey of elderly people in an English urban setting, Clarke and Lewis (1982) reported that 66% of their sample stated that they did not go out after dark for fear of victimization and 15% reported that this fear was a primary concern. There is also a suggestion of nocturnal neurosis in the elderly as a result of fear of crime (Cohen 1976). The elderly thus appear to be the group most anxious about crime, though they are apparently the least likely to be victimized

(Clarke and Lewis 1982). Another study (Lindesay 1991) indicates that phobic disorders in the elderly are associated with considerably higher psychiatric and medical morbidity compared with that in case controls. Further, 17 of the 28 agoraphobics described the onset of their symptomatology after the age of 65, and despite increased rates of contact with primary care services, none was receiving any specific treatment for his or her phobic disorders.

Reports of PTSD in elderly Holocaust survivors (Kuch and Cox 1992) and among elders who were prisoners of war during World War II (Speed et al. 1989) indicate that PTSD can be a chronic disorder continuing into old age. A report also documents development of PTSD for the first time in old age among survivors of the 1988 Armenian earthquake (Goenjian et al. 1994). It appears that although the overall severity of PTSD seemed similar among both young and elderly survivors of the earthquake, the elderly reported less reexperiencing but more symptoms of hyperarousal compared with that reported by the younger people. It may be premature to assign any significance to these differences before further replication of these findings.

In summary, from the limited available data, it appears that panic disorder starting earlier in life typically tends to run a chronic course with continuation into old age. New onset of panic disorder in late life is rare and when it does occur, it tends to be of milder severity. Data on phobias and PTSD are too scant and preliminary to draw any conclusions, whereas empirical data on phenomenological manifestations of other anxiety disorders in late life are nonexistent.

Neurobiology of Anxiety in the Elderly

Most recent work investigating neurobiology of anxiety has been performed in younger populations, and its relevance to the elderly remains unknown at present. In this section, I summarize literature on the neurobiology of anxiety and discuss the relevance of age-related changes in various neurotransmitter systems to phenomena of anxiety and fear in the elderly.

Attempts to discern neurobiology of anxiety date back to empirical work by Cannon (1929) in cats and suggested that central discharges, possibly thalamic in origin, are the harbinger of fear and anxiety. Increasing evidence accumulated during the last several years points to the locus ceruleus in the midbrain, containing approximately half of central norepinephrine neurons, as the harbinger of states of fear and panic. For example, Redmond and Huang (1979) document central noradrenergic activation in anxiety and fear states and suggest that the locus ceruleus is implicated in such emotions. Charney et al. (1985) report a greater number of yohimbine-induced anxiety symptoms in patients with panic disorder compared with that in control subjects as well as a blunting of yohimbine response after treatment with alprazolam, supporting the hypothesis of noradrenergic activation as a result of locus ceruleus discharge of norepinephrine in panic attacks. Simson and Weiss (1988) also suggest that locus ceruleus plays a key role in the "fight or flight" response mediated via activation of the central noradrenergic system. As for the normal age-related changes in noradrenergic functioning in older populations, Sunderland et al. (1991) summarize findings from several studies suggesting that such function in old age declines and includes a decrease in the number of locus ceruleus neurons, a decrease in norepinephrine content in many brain areas, and an increase in monoamine oxidase (type B) levels (also see Chapter 3 in this volume). These findings support the phenomenological research documenting a milder symptomatology in late-onset panic disorder (Sheikh et al. 1991). Unlike studies of the noradrenergic system, those of the serotonergic system in younger patients with anxiety disorder as well as in nonanxious elderly have yielded mixed and nonconclusive results (Sunderland et al. 1991).

Since the report by Pitts and McClure (1967) that an infusion of 10 mg/kg of 0.5 M racemic sodium lactate produced panic symptoms in 13 of 14 patients who were neurotically anxious (that is, had panic disorder by present criteria) and in only 2 of 16 psychiatrically healthy control subjects, various investigators have reproduced this finding (Kelly et al. 1971; Liebowitz et al. 1984). It is now well accepted that lactate infusion produces panic attacks in approximately 70% of patients with panic disorder. The underlying mechanism for induction of panic attacks with sodium lactate remains unclear, though various postulates include sodium lactate being a nonspecific stimulant producing uncomfortable somatic sensations or a conversion of lactate to bicarbonate and CO_2, with CO_2 crossing the blood-brain barrier and producing a transient intracerebral hypercapnia leading to stimulation of brainstem chemoreceptors. Other techniques for successful induction of panic include administration of caffeine, which may block adenosine receptors (Boulenger et al. 1984); administration of yohimbine, which may challenge locus ceruleus activation as a result of its α_2-adrenergic antagonism (Charney et al. 1982); and inhalation of 5% CO_2 (Gorman et al. 1989). No reports of panic induction in the elderly are described in the literature, and it is not clear whether such

methods will be safe to use in this population. Availability of neuroimaging techniques has provided an impetus for carrying out more specific studies to delineate neurobiological basis of anxiety disorders. For example, Reiman et al. (1989) have documented increased parahippocampal activity during panic attacks provoked by lactic acid as well as significant blood flow increases bilaterally in the temporal poles.

Of the various theoretical models of anxiety based on neurobiological findings, three seem to be the most popular at present. The first, espoused by Gray (1982), is a complex schema of the central role of a "Behavioral Inhibition System" in the manifestations of anxiety, which involves neuroanatomical structures of the septohippocampal system and the noradrenergic, serotonergic, and GABAergic[1] neurotransmitter systems in a rather complicated relationship. The second model is that of Gorman et al. (1989), who have proposed a neuroanatomical hypothesis for panic disorder locating the acute panic attack in the brainstem, anticipatory anxiety in the limbic system, and phobic avoidance in the prefrontal cortex. The third and most recent model of an integrated neurobiology of panic has been espoused by Goddard and Charney (1997). In this model, the amygdala is at the center of fear and anxiety responses, with extensive afferent and efferent connections to many other fear-related neuronal structures including hippocampus, locus ceruleus, hypothalamus, and orbitofrontal cortex. This more complex model has explanatory potential for several features of panic disorder including spontaneous panic attacks, anticipatory anxiety, and avoidance behavior, among others.

In summary, whereas the relevance of the above-mentioned theoretical models of anxiety to the elderly is unknown at present, a decline in central noradrenergic activity with aging may explain the milder symptomatology of LOPD.

Anxiety and Medical Illness

Anxiety is commonly associated with medical illness for several reasons. First, being the most common psychiatric conditions, anxiety symptoms and syndromes can present as coincidental comorbid conditions. In such cases, a long-standing history of an anxiety disorder is typically forthcoming. Second, anxiety could manifest as an expected response to a physical stressor, and a temporal association with the onset of a particular medical disorder is usually present. Third, anxiety can be a manifestation of

---

[1] γ-aminobutyric acid.

physiological changes occurring as a result of a medical illness (e.g., Parkinson's disease) or a medication (e.g., theophylline). Finally, sudden onset of anxiety can also signal a rapidly deteriorating medical condition in patients with or without a chronic medical illness (Wise and Griffies 1995). Common medical conditions associated with anxiety are briefly described below.

Cardiovascular Illness

Panic attack symptoms, consisting of palpitations, dyspnea, chest tightness, sweating, and tingling sensations in the arms, can simulate both angina pectoris and myocardial infarction. For example, between 30% and 50% of patients presenting with recurrent chest pain and no evidence of cardiovascular disease may have panic disorder (Beitman et al. 1990; Carter et al. 1997). Such episodes in older age group patients should, however, always prompt a thorough investigation of the cardiac status of the patient, except perhaps in patients in whom a diagnosis of panic disorder is well established. The relationship of panic disorder and mitral valve prolapse remains unclear, with some of the studies suggesting a higher rate of association than that in control subjects (Gorman et al. 1988; Kantor et al. 1980) and others questioning such evidence (Margraf et al. 1988; Mazza et al. 1986). Such studies have focused on generally younger patients, and data on such association or lack thereof in older patients are lacking.

Pulmonary Causes

Elderly patients at bed rest remain at risk for pulmonary embolism, which might be the most common pulmonary cause of sudden anxiety in such patients. A ventilation-perfusion scan and a phlebogram can be diagnostic. Some reports also suggest an unusually high number of panic disorder cases among patients with chronic obstructive pulmonary disease (Karajgi et al. 1990; Yellowlees et al. 1987). More recently, in another study, 40% of mostly geriatric patients with chronic obstructive pulmonary disease reported significant anxiety (White et al. 1997).

Dietary Causes

Caffeine intake in the form of coffee, tea, and soda can produce anxiety-like symptoms in doses as little as 200 mg (one cup = 150 mg) (Victor et al. 1981). Caffeine has also been implicated in precipitating full-blown panic attacks (Charney et al. 1985; Lee 1985; Uhde et al. 1984). A history of caffeine use should be obtained in patients with symptoms of anxiety to rule out any temporal relationship. A decrease in daily caffeine consumption in some cases can be a simple and effective intervention.

Drugs

For common cold and allergic conditions, the elderly commonly use over-the-counter preparations, which can produce anxiety-like symptoms as a result of their content of adrenergic agents such as ephedrine or pseudoephedrine. Prescription drugs that can produce anxiety include amphetamines, bronchodilators such as isoproterenol and theophylline, and some calcium channel blockers such as verapamil, nifedipine, and diltiazem. A careful history of drug intake should thus be a part of the clinical assessment of anxiety in the elderly. Akathisia, a common side effect of neuroleptics, is a subjective sense of restlessness often indistinguishable from anxiety. Akathisia can also closely resemble agitation because of a tendency in patients with both conditions to pace around. Inquiring about drug history can give a clue into its temporal relationship with drug intake. Alcohol withdrawal is a well-recognized cause of anxiety and agitation among hospitalized patients (Lerner and Fallen 1985). Sedative-hypnotic withdrawal, however, might be somewhat underestimated as a cause of anxiety syndromes in older populations, in whom hypnotic use is frequent (Schweizer et al. 1989). At the beginning of the hospitalization, clinicians should inquire about any such drug use and treat with appropriate medications.

Endocrine Causes

Unlike younger populations, in whom two-thirds or more of patients with hyperthyroidism may meet DSM-III criteria for an anxiety disorder (American Psychiatric Association 1980; Kathol et al. 1986), patients over 60 have hyperthyroidism more insidious in presentation, sometimes labeled as "apathetic" as opposed to "anxious or agitated" hyperthyroidism of younger people (Hurley 1983). Hypoparathyroidism and hyperparathyroidism, hypopituitarism and hyperpituitarism, hypoglycemia, diabetes mellitus, and Cushing's syndrome can also be associated with anxiety-like symptoms (Popkin and Mackenzie 1980).

In summary, older patients with medical illnesses commonly experience concomitant anxiety. Such comorbidity may confound the clinical picture for both the primary care physician and the neuropsychiatrist, and thus a systematic approach to proper evaluation of anxiety in such patients is needed and described below in the section on evaluation.

Neurological Disorders Associated With Anxiety

Many neurological disorders are associated with symptoms of anxiety or a diagnosable anxiety disorder. In a comprehensive review of psychiatric presentations of medical illnesses, Hall (1980) suggests that neurological disorders are among major contributors to medical causes of anxiety and contends that cerebral vascular insufficiency may be the most common neurological cause of anxiety. Below, I briefly review the literature describing association of anxiety with various neurological disorders, with particular focus on Parkinson's disease, dementia, and stroke.

Although association of depression with Parkinson's disease is now considered a generally accepted fact, presence of anxiety in this illness has received attention from researchers only relatively recently (see also Chapter 26 in this volume). In one study, 9 (38%) of 24 subjects (mean age = 58) with idiopathic Parkinson's disease had a clinically significant anxiety disorder (Stein et al. 1990). Another report describes 12 of 16 patients with Parkinson's disease meeting the criteria of a present or past diagnosis of either panic disorder or generalized anxiety disorder (Schiffer et al. 1988). Another study (Henderson et al. 1992) documents a picture of mixed anxiety-depression in 38% of 164 patients with Parkinson's disease (mean age = 67) compared with 8% in 150 age-matched psychiatrically healthy spouse control subjects. It also appears that left-sided Parkinson's disease may be associated with a greater degree of anxiety and depression (Fleminger 1991). There is some suggestion that high prevalence of anxiety disorders in patients with Parkinson's disease may be a result of a loss of normally existing dopaminergic inhibition of locus ceruleus (Iruela et al. 1992). It is speculated further that early ceruleal or nigroceruleal dopaminergic pathway degeneration leading to disinhibition of locus ceruleus may be responsible for high rates of panic disorder preceding the onset of motor signs in patients with familial parkinsonism (Lauterbach 1993). Finally, one has to be mindful that the drug treatment of Parkinson's disease itself may produce symptoms of anxiety (Cummings 1991).

In the Perth Community Stroke Study (Burvill et al. 1995), in a sample of 294 patients at 4 months poststroke, prevalence of anxiety disorders was 12% in men and 28% in women. After subtracting those who had evidence of anxiety disorder before stroke, the latter prevalence was 9% in men and 20% in women. Similarly, in 80 patients with acute stroke (0–3 months), prevalence of generalized anxiety disorder (GAD) was found to be 28% (Astrom 1996). Of concern, only 23% of these patients had remission of their GAD symptoms at 12-month follow-up. Although both depression and anxiety can be common consequences of a stroke, Robinson and Starkstein (1990) reported that comorbid major depression and GAD are associated with cortical lesions, whereas depression alone is associated with subcortical lesions (see also Chapter 27 in this volume). There is also some suggestion that women and younger patients may be more prone to developing anxiety after stroke (Schultz et al. 1997).

Anxiety-like symptoms and agitated behaviors are also common in dementing disorders (Teri et al. 1988). In fact, as many as 85% of patients with dementia develop disruptive agitated behavior (Jeste and Krull 1991) (see also Chapters 23 and 24 in this volume). Wands and colleagues (1990) reported that 38% of patients with early dementia were found to have anxiety. It is also speculated that agitation at times may be a possible expression of GAD in patients with dementia (Mintzer and Brawman-Mintzer 1996). Neurobiological underpinnings of agitation in patients with dementia remain controversial at best, although noradrenergic, serotonergic, and dopaminergic deficits are implicated (Kirby and Lawlor 1995).

In summary, anxiety can be frequently associated with Parkinson's disease, dementias, and stroke. Neurotransmitter mechanisms underlying such symptomatology are rather complex and probably depend on a functional balance between dopaminergic, cholinergic, GABAergic, glutamatergic, and peptidergic neurotransmission (Hartmann et al. 1993).

Other neurological disorders described in the literature as sometimes associated with anxiety include multiple sclerosis, peripheral neuropathy, myasthenia gravis, Huntington's disease, Wilson's disease, closed head injury, and tumors of the brain (Hall 1980). Further, anxiety remains one of the most disturbing symptoms in a small percentage of patients with postconcussion syndrome (Leigh 1979) (also see Chapter 28 in this volume), and temporal lobe epilepsy can mimic panic disorder (Edlund et al. 1987).

Evaluation of Anxiety in the Elderly

Several factors can make proper assessment of anxiety potentially difficult. These include a confounding of symptom picture by high medical comorbidity, frequent use of multiple prescribed and over-the-counter medications, substance use, difficulty of differentiating anxiety from depression, and a tendency to resist psychiatric evaluation in older cohorts. With these caveats in mind, evaluation of anxiety in the elderly is usually accomplished in three major ways: clinical evaluation, assessment with rating scales, and laboratory investigations.

Clinical Evaluation

The clinical evaluation should include a history of presenting symptomatology, past illness (e.g., panic disorder can be characterized by remissions and relapses), a detailed history of current prescribed and over-the-counter medications (including analgesics, cold medications, anticholinergic medications, herbal and vitamin supplements), a history of alcohol or substance use, and a family history (may be helpful in panic disorder). A mental status examination can reveal many of the cognitive and behavioral signs and symptoms of anxiety including apprehension, fearfulness, distractibility, hyperkinesis, and startle response. Physiological signs and symptoms including increased pulse rate, rapid breathing, sweating, and trembling should be assessed during the physical examination.

Assessment With Rating Scales

Anxiety rating scales are useful adjuncts to the clinical evaluation of anxiety. These measures can serve as initial screening devices, can be helpful in assessing severity of symptoms, and can be used as instruments to document effectiveness of various psychological and pharmacological therapeutic interventions. These scales are primarily of two kinds: observer-rated and self-rated. The most commonly used observer-rated scale is the Hamilton Anxiety Rating Scale (HARS) (Hamilton 1959). HARS is a 14-item scale with each item rated on severity from none (0) to very severe (4). A rating of 18 or above is generally considered to be suggestive of clinically significant anxiety. Though HARS is presently the standard in the field as a measure of change in clinical situations and in pharmacological research, older published studies in geriatrics seemed to indicate limited sensitivity to change with active drug treatment (Kochansky 1979; Salzman 1977). A more recent study, however, seems to suggest that HARS can differentiate between older patients with GAD and control subjects (Beck et al. 1996). The most frequently used self-rated scales are the State-Trait Anxiety Inventory (STAI) (Spielberger et al. 1970), the Sympton Checklist-90–Revised (SCL-90-R; Derogatis 1975), and the Beck Anxiety Inventory (BAI) (Beck et al. 1988). Several recent studies have suggested that BAI can be useful in differentiating anxious elderly subjects from nonanxious control subjects and also useful as an instrument sensitive to measure change with treatment (Stanley et al. 1996; Steer et al. 1994; Wetherell and Arean 1997). BAI is a 21-item inventory with a rating on a severity scale of none (0) to severe (3). A rating of 21 or above on BAI is suggestive of clinically significant anxiety.

Laboratory Investigations

Laboratory tests can aid in diagnosing underlying medical conditions producing signs and symptoms of anxiety. A complete blood count, vitamin B_{12} and folate levels, electrocardiogram, thyroid function tests, blood sugar, blood gases, and drug and alcohol screening can be helpful when used appropriately to rule out more common medical conditions associated with anxiety as described earlier.

Anxiety and Depression

Debate about the complex relationship of anxiety and depression has raged in the psychiatric literature since the days of Sir Aubrey Lewis (1934) and continues to be a recurrent theme in the psychiatric literature (see also Chapter 13 in this volume). Traditionally, three major positions have been adhered to by various investigators: 1) anxiety and depression lie on the same continuum; 2) they are distinct conditions that are frequently comorbid as a result of their high prevalence; and 3) they are different expressions of the same biological diathesis. Despite recent advances in our knowledge about the phenomenology and biology of these conditions, we do not seem any closer to resolving this controversy. Comorbid depression and anxiety appear to be extremely common in older adults (Flint 1994). In a small sample of geriatric psychiatry outpatients, Alexopoulos (1991) reported that 38% of patients with depression also met criteria for an anxiety disorder according to DSM-III. The Guy's/Age Concern Survey reported that 39% of subjects with phobia had comorbid depression compared with only 11% of subjects without phobia (Lindesay et al. 1989). The presence and severity levels of GAO and depression were especially associated. Studying geriatric adults in South Africa who had been diagnosed with depression, Ben-Arie and colleagues found that 26% also had generalized anxiety and 5% had panic attacks (Ben-Arie et al. 1987). Comorbid anxiety and depression are also common in geriatric medical patients. For example, in a study of geriatric patients with cancer, Derogatis and colleagues reported that 13% evidenced mixed anxiety-depressive syndrome, whereas 8% evidenced an anxiety disorder exclusively (Derogatis et al. 1983).

Making a distinction between anxiety and depression clinically was considered to have pragmatic value previously because older antidepressants such as the tricyclics had many undesirable side effects for the elderly, whereas anxiolytics such as benzodiazepines and buspirone were relatively well tolerated. However, since the introduction of the serotonin selective reuptake inhibitors (SSRIs) and increasing evidence of their efficacy in the mixed-symptom picture of both anxiety and depression, this debate seems to have lost some of its intensity. Thus, a recent philosophical shift has led to acceptance of a mixed-symptom picture as reflected in the inclusion of mixed anxiety-depression syndrome as a special category in the DSM-IV. Though mixed anxiety-depression is included as a research category, clinically it is one of the most frequently encountered presentations in geriatric neuropsychiatric practice. A mixed picture of depression and anxiety in older patients may signify the presence of an anxiety disorder coexisting with a distinct depressive disorder, the presence of one disorder associated with symptoms of another, or, more commonly, a mixed anxiety-depressive disorder in which symptoms of neither anxiety nor depression reach diagnostic threshold for an established disorder. Although symptoms of mixed anxiety-depression syndrome may not reach criteria for an established disorder, some patients experience significant functional impairment and marked subjective distress. If symptoms progress and persist for more than a month at this level of functional impairment, treatment is indicated.

In summary, a mixed picture of anxiety and depression is common among older patients in both medical and psychiatric settings. Recent studies suggesting efficacy of antidepressants for both depression and anxiety may make the older (at times painstaking) attempts to separate anxiety and depression somewhat less relevant from a clinician's perspective.

Complications of Anxiety Disorders

Physical Illness

The issue of short- and long-term effects of anxiety on physical health remains unresolved. This question may be of particular relevance to the elderly population because of their relative increased susceptibility to developing physical illness and the possibility that they may accumulate adverse effects of anxiety over many years. A strong association of anxiety states with many medical conditions has been discussed in the literature in the past two decades. For example, researchers have documented association of anxiety with asthma (Alexander 1972), hypertension (Whitehead et al. 1977), and duodenal ulcer (Sandberg and Bliding 1976). Some authors have also contended that anxiety can give rise to potentially lethal arrhythmias (Jenkins 1971) and have suggested the use of diazepam in such cases. Also, evidence suggests that anxiety might act as a predictor of future morbidity in patients with cancer. For example, Carey and Burish (1985) found that in patients with cancer who were receiving chemotherapy, greater treatment gains were found in patients with lower pretreatment anxiety. Such associations cannot be considered causal, however, because the relationship between anxiety and physical

functioning is complicated. For example, anxiety seems to contribute to heart disease, whereas heart disease itself increases anxiety (Jenike 1985). Though knowledge about the specific mechanism by which anxiety and autonomic arousal can cause tissue damage is lacking, it is possible that the elderly accumulate deleterious effects of anxiety on the cardiovascular system over many years. Of relevance, Nowlin et al. (1973) reported in a prospective study that elevated levels of anxiety predicted the future occurrence of myocardial infarction in older men. Though this study can be considered only preliminary because of the small sample, it is of sufficient importance to warrant attempts at replication. In another survey of older adults, Himmelfarb and Murrell (1984) found a significant association of anxiety with the presence of some medical conditions including high blood pressure, kidney and bladder disease, cardiac disease, stomach ulcers, arteriosclerosis, stroke, and diabetes. It appears that patients with chronic medical disorders are especially prone to developing anxiety. For example, in a community survey based on data from the NIMH ECA Program, more than 11% of people with a chronic medical illness were found to have had a recent anxiety disorder (Wells et al. 1988). Because more than 80% of Americans older than 65 report at least one chronic medical condition (National Center for Health Statistics 1987), geriatric patients are at increased risk for developing anxiety.

Alcohol Abuse

Several reports have documented unusually high rates of comorbidity between anxiety disorders and alcohol abuse (Chambless et al. 1987; Hasselbrock et al. 1985; Kushner et al. 1990; Ross et al. 1988; Weissman 1988) (also see Chapter 16 in this volume). Boyd et al. (1984) have estimated that the risk of alcohol problems in patients with phobia is about two and a half times that of the general population, and the risk in patients with panic disorder is more than four times. Some evidence from family studies suggests that alcoholism and anxiety are on the same spectrum of disorders. For example, Munjack and Moss (1981) found alcohol abuse among 26.5% of the first-degree relatives of people with agoraphobia, 20% of the relatives of those with social phobia, and 8.6% of the relatives of those with mixed simple phobia. Harris et al. (1983) found that approximately 10% of the relatives of patients with panic disorder and 17.6% of the relatives of those with agoraphobia had alcoholism, as opposed to only 5.4% in the control group. Though a relationship as to the cause and effect between alcoholism and anxiety disorders is not clear at present, sufficient evidence from the literature (Kushner et al. 1990) suggests that, at least in cases of agoraphobia and social phobia, alcohol problems seem to be related to attempts at self-medication. It also appears that comorbidity is not uniform for all anxiety disorders; therefore, generalizations regarding alcoholism in anxiety states as a homogeneous group should be avoided.

Even though none of these studies have looked at this issue with particular reference to the elderly, one should keep in mind that similar comorbidity with alcoholism can exist in that population also. Considering that older people may be particularly vulnerable to effects of alcohol as a result of changes in hepatic metabolism and increased sensitivity of the central nervous system (Atkinson 1989; Liptzin 1991), clinicians need to be alert to inquire about such history in patients with anxiety. Finally, alcohol withdrawal can itself present as severe anxiety, as noted above.

Insomnia

Sleep disturbances are common in patients with anxiety (also see Chapter 17 in this volume). In a study assessing vegetative signs and symptoms of anxiety, Mathew and colleagues (1982) found that restless sleep was the only vegetative symptom consistently related to anxiety. On the other hand, anxiety appears to be a common finding in patients with chronic insomnia. Some investigators have looked at differential effects on sleep of various anxiety syndromes. For example, in a study conducted by Reynolds et al. (1983), patients with GAD were found to have difficulty similar to that of patients with depression in both initiating and maintaining sleep. However, these investigators also found that the shortened rapid eye movement (REM) latency and increased percentage of REM sleep found in patients with depression are missing in patients with anxiety. Other researchers (Insel et al. 1982) suggest similarities between the sleep of patients with obsessive-compulsive disorder (OCD) and that of patients with depression in that both groups seem to have short REM latency compared with subjects without OCD or depression. Like patients with GAD, those with panic disorder frequently complain of difficulty in initiating and maintaining sleep (Sheehan et al. 1980). However, it appears that their REM latencies, though shorter than those of control subjects as a group, still fall within the lower limit of normal, unlike that of patients with depression (Uhde et al. 1984). Finally, it appears that patients with PTSD show a reduced efficiency of sleep, with recurrent nightmares and a lower percentage of REM sleep.

It thus appears from the foregoing studies that anxiety disorders can create problems in initiating and maintaining sleep as well as significantly affect the quality of sleep. The implications of these findings are significant for about 5 million elders in the United States who have severe sleep problems (Moran et al. 1988). Inquiry into the duration and quality of sleep should be an integral component of any management plans for geriatric anxiety. Such inquiry should take into account the common clinical observation that older people tend to go to bed early and may nap during the day; a seemingly early wake-up time may not be so in reality, and the total amount of sleep, including nap time, may be sufficient for many. Taken together, anxiety and insomnia are among the most frequently encountered problems in geriatric patients (Folks and Fuller 1997). In cases where both anxiety and insomnia overlap, it would be prudent to consider treatments beneficial for both, be they nonpharmacological aids to sleep or sedative-hypnotics.

Increased Mortality of Cardiovascular Origin

In a series of long-term (30–50 years) follow-up studies, Coryell et al. (1982, 1986) have documented increased mortality as a result of cardiovascular disease among male but not female patients with panic disorder. Specifically, it appears that males with a panic disorder diagnosis were twice as likely to die compared with expected deaths based on age and gender matching. After a review of causes of death in his sample of men, Coryell (1988) attributed the excess mortality to chronic hyperarousal and exercise intolerance of patients with panic disorder and possibly to additional deleterious effects of associated smoking or alcohol abuse. Such findings suggest the need for proper control of panic attacks and associated chronic hyperarousal, as well as the management of the associated smoking or alcohol abuse if present.

In summary, chronic untreated anxiety can be associated with myriad complications including long-standing sleep problems, alcohol abuse, high blood pressure, stroke, and possibly increased mortality of cardiovascular origin.

▍ Management of Geriatric Anxiety

Effective management of geriatric anxiety can be accomplished by using pharmacological or psychological treatments, sometimes as monotherapies and at other times in conjunction with each other.

Pharmacological Treatments

Several factors can complicate psychopharmacological management of the older patient with anxiety. These factors include physiological changes associated with aging that affect pharmacokinetics and pharmacodynamics of drugs, presence of comorbid medical conditions, and polypharmacy (see Chapter 34 in this volume).

Age-related changes in pharmacokinetics put older patients at higher risk of adverse reactions from drugs. The most important of these changes are: 1) decreased absorption (with decreased gastric acidity, motility, blood flow, and gastrointestinal surface area); 2) decreased protein binding (with decreased albumin); 3) increased volume of distribution of lipophilic drugs; 4) decreased hepatic function (with decreased hepatic metabolism, first-pass effect, demethylation, and hydroxylation); and 5) decreased renal excretion (with decreased renal blood flow, glomerular filtration rate, and tubular excretory capacity). The overall effect of these changes is that many medications are absorbed and metabolized less efficiently and eliminated more slowly in older patients than in younger ones (von Moltke et al. 1995). Thus, the period of risk of side effects is prolonged in older patients because these drugs stay in the body longer. Even average dose ranges for the general population may be toxic for the elderly. In addition, pharmacodynamic changes in the aging nervous system make older patients more sensitive to the side effects of psychotropic medications (Salzman et al. 1995).

Older patients are more likely than younger people to have concurrent medical illnesses that may be exacerbated by the side effects of medications. In addition, the presence of chronic kidney, liver, or heart disease can further delay clearance of drugs, thus making adverse reactions more likely. Although the elderly constitute 12% of the population, they are prescribed 25% of all medications and as a group consume the majority of over-the-counter drugs (Kane et al. 1994). Not surprisingly, the average older person typically takes six to eight different medications per day. The risk of adverse drug interactions also increases substantially with such polypharmacy. Further, many of the commonly prescribed nonpsychotropic agents (e.g., digoxin, theophylline, prednisolone, cimetidine) have detectable anticholinergic levels when measured with radioreceptor assay, though these agents are not commonly viewed as anticholinergic (Tune et al. 1992). However, when taken in combination, such medications can adversely affect cognition in the elderly while increasing the risk of anticholinergic syndrome when taken in combination with commonly used anticholinergic psychotropics.

Several additional factors should be considered when selecting a medication for an older patient with an anxiety disorder. For example, prior treatment response, the nature of the targeted symptoms, concurrent medications, and the most tolerable side-effect profile should all be taken into account. To reach the optimal dose for an older patient without causing intolerable side effects, the old adage "Start low and go slow" is well worth remembering. Drugs may be given in divided doses throughout the day to minimize possible adverse side effects. However, with divided doses, noncompliance may be an issue of concern especially in medically ill older patients taking multiple medications. Liquid medications may be easier for some patients to take. Given the prevalence of polypharmacy in this age group, only one change at a time during medication adjustments is preferable. Finally, with any change in dose or medication, close monitoring is essential.

Over the years, numerous compounds have been used as anxiolytics, including alcohol, barbiturates, antihistamines, antidepressants, neuroleptics, β-blockers, and benzodiazepines. Though empirical studies of the efficacy of different anxiolytics have primarily been conducted in younger populations, such efficacy is inferred in clinical practice for older patients and modifications in dosing made accordingly. A brief description of different classes of compounds currently used as anxiolytics follows.

Benzodiazepines. Benzodiazepines have been the most frequently prescribed anxiolytics for the last three decades. The elderly are prescribed benzodiazepines at a rate disproportionately high to their percentage in the population (Moran et al. 1988). Table 15–3 lists the more commonly used benzodiazepines along with relevant information about their half-lives and the daily doses recommended for the elderly. Lower doses of benzodiazepines are recommended for older patients because the elderly are more sensitive to both the therapeutic and toxic effects of the drugs. Thus, doses that are therapeutic in younger patients may actually be toxic in geriatric patients (Meyer 1982).

Short half-life benzodiazepines such as lorazepam, oxazepam, and temazepam appear preferable in that they are metabolized by direct conjugation in the liver (phase II metabolism), a mechanism that does not seem to be affected by aging (Moran et al. 1988). In addition, these drugs are relatively less lipophilic and are thus less prone to accumulate in fatty tissues of the elderly compared with a more lipophilic drug such as diazepam. Most other benzodiazepines tend to be metabolized via oxidative pathways (phase I metabolism) into active metabolites that tend to linger on in the elderly for long periods of time. Several studies have documented in the elderly undesirable side effects of long-acting benzodiazepines (e.g., diazepam, clorazepate, chlordiazepoxide) including drowsiness, fatigue, psychomotor impairment, and cognitive impairment (Boston Collaborative Drug Surveillance Program 1973; Curran et al. 1987; Larson et al. 1987; Pomara et al. 1984, 1991). For example, Rosenbaum (1979) documents that the half-life

TABLE 15–3. Commonly used anxiolytic benzodiazepines: a summary of pharmacokinetics

Drug	Half-life (hr)	Active metabolites	Daily dose (mg)	
			Adult	Elderly
Alprazolam	12–15	Yes	0.25–2.0	0.125–1
Chlordiazepoxide	7–28	Yes	25–100	5–50
Clonazepam	18–56	Yes	1–8	0.5–4
Clorazepate	30–200	Yes	15–60	7.5–30
Diazepam	20–60	Yes	5–30	2–15
Lorazepam	10–20	None	1–6	0.5–3
Halazepam	15–50	Yes	20–160	20–80
Oxazepam	5–15	None	15–90	10–45
Prazepam	25–200	Yes	20–60	10–20

of diazepam's metabolites increases from 20 hours in a 20-year-old to 90 hours in an 80-year-old. Alprazolam, a commonly used, intermediate half-life, antipanic medication, has also been shown to have a half-life of more than 21 hours in the elderly compared with 11 hours in young people (Kroboth et al. 1990).

In summary, this review suggests that short-acting benzodiazepines such as oxazepam, lorazepam, and temazepam are preferable in the elderly, whereas long-acting benzodiazepines such as diazepam, clorazepate, and flurazepam appear less desirable in general. Given the probability that, if taken for long periods of time, even short-acting benzodiazepines will tend to accumulate in older people, any use of benzodiazepines in the elderly should be for specific indications and time-limited, preferably to less than 6 months. Table 15–4 documents potential complications of long-term use of benzodiazepines in the elderly.

Buspirone. Buspirone, an anxiolytic medication with partial serotonin-agonist properties, has demonstrated in double-blind studies efficacy comparable to that of diazepam in patients with GAO (Rickels and Schweizer 1987; Rickels et al. 1982). Its nonaddictive profile, absence of withdrawal symptoms when discontinued (Rickels et al. 1988), and lack of psychomotor impairment even with long-term usage (Smiley and Moskowitz 1986) seem to be an advantage over benzodiazepines in chronic anxiety conditions. Studies in geriatric samples indicate that buspirone is well tolerated, does not cause adverse interactions when co-prescribed with a variety of other medications (including antihypertensives, cardiac glycosides, and bronchodilators), and is effective for remediation of chronic anxiety symptoms in this population (Napoliello 1986). It also appears that in both acute and chronic dosing the pharmacokinetics of buspirone in the elderly are very similar to the pharmacokinetics in younger people (Gammans

et al. 1989). Unlike the benzodiazepines, which can cause respiratory depression, buspirone does not seem to affect respiration adversely and has been shown in animal studies to stimulate respiratory drive (Garner et al. 1989). Such a profile seems to suggest that buspirone may be a particularly desirable anxiolytic for chronic anxiety conditions of the elderly in cases in which long-term use might be indicated. However, in contrast to research data, clinical experience with this medication suggests that a therapeutic response is somewhat inconsistent. It is important to remember that buspirone can require up to 4 weeks before manifesting its therapeutic effects. It might be desirable to combine buspirone initially with a short-acting benzodiazepine that will provide rapid relief of symptoms but that can then be withdrawn after 2–4 weeks, once the therapeutic effects of buspirone have been established.

Antidepressants. Several researchers have documented the efficacy of antidepressants for panic disorder,

TABLE 15–4. Potential complications of long-term benzodiazepine use in older patients

Excessive daytime drowsiness

Paradoxical reactions

Cognitive impairment and confusion

Amnesic syndromes

Psychomotor impairment and a risk of falls

Respiratory problems

Depression

Abuse and dependence

Intoxication even on therapeutic dosages

Breakthrough withdrawal reactions

Source. Adapted from Sheikh 1992a.

OCD, GAD, and PTSD in younger patients. For example, the tricyclic imipramine and the monoamine oxidase inhibitor phenelzine have proven to be efficacious in younger patients with panic disorder (Mavissakalian and Michelson 1986; Sheehan et al. 1980; Zitrin et al. 1983). More recently the SSRIs have been shown in several randomized and controlled clinical trials to demonstrate superior efficacy to placebo and at least equal efficacy to tricyclic antidepressants for panic disorder and OCD in generally younger patients (Boyer 1995; Coplan et al. 1996; Oehrberg et al. 1995). Emerging evidence indicates that newer "atypical" antidepressants such as venlafaxine (Geracioti 1995) and nefazodone may also be efficacious in panic disorder (Fawcett et al. 1995).

Given these studies documenting their efficacy in younger patients and their generally favorable side-effect profile, the SSRIs should now be considered the first drugs of choice for panic disorder in older patients. These medications can be given in a single daily dose to maximize compliance. Two potential problems can decrease compliance with antidepressants: delayed onset of action and a feeling of jitters in the first 2 weeks of treatment. These problems can be minimized by patient education, addition of benzodiazepines in the first few weeks, and use of very small doses (e.g., sertraline 12.5 mg/day) at the beginning of treatment, which can then be increased gradually upward.

Similar to the findings in studies of SSRIs for panic disorder, fluoxetine, sertraline, it has been found that fluvoxamine, and paroxetine are all superior to placebo control groups for OCD patients (Greist et al. 1992; Gunasekara et al. 1998; McDougle et al. 1993). Comparisons also found fluvoxamine, sertraline, and paroxetine to be equal in efficacy to clomipramine (Koran et al. 1996), a well-established anti-OCD compound that is undesirable for use in older patients as a result of its strong anticholinergic profile. In addition, phenelzine was found to be equal in efficacy to clomipramine (Vallejo et al. 1992), but side effects and dietary restrictions that go along with the monoamine oxidase inhibitor make the use of this medication more problematic in older patients. As is the case of SSRIs with panic disorder, SSRIs are increasingly being recognized as the treatment of choice for the treatment of OCD because they are better tolerated than clomipramine (Stokes and Holtz 1997). This is even more the case when treating older patients because of their sensitivity to anticholinergic side effects of psychotropics and the potential for cumulative anticholinergic delirium when combined with commonly used medications for chronic medical illnesses (Tune et al. 1992).

Over the last decade, the role of antidepressants in the treatment of GAD has become more prominent. At least one study has shown superior efficacy of a tricyclic antidepressant compared with that of a benzodiazepine for GAD (Hoehn-Saric et al. 1988). More recently, a double-blind, placebo-controlled study of 377 patients with GAD demonstrated superior efficacy of venlafaxine compared with that of placebo (Aguiar et al. 1998). Clomipramine, the SSRIs, and nefazodone are being studied currently and may also prove efficacious in GAD.

Randomized controlled trials of PTSD have been few and infrequent (Solomon and Gerrity 1992). Though mixed results were seen in earlier studies of tricyclic antidepressants (Davidson et al. 1990), SSRIs (Nagy et al. 1993), and benzodiazepines (Feldman 1987) for PTSD, recent open-label studies show promise with nefazodone and SSRIs (Davidson 1998; Hertzberg et al. 1998). Randomized controlled trials of sertraline and nefazodone are presently under way. As is the case with studies of other anxiety disorders, these studies have been conducted in generally younger patients. Treatment of PTSD in older patients in clinical practice is thus guided by results from studies in younger patients.

In summary, it appears that SSRIs can be efficacious in most anxiety disorders, whereas evidence is also emerging that newer antidepressants may also be efficacious in PTSD and panic disorder (nefazodone) and in GAD (venlafaxine).

Antihistamines, β–blockers, and neuroleptics. Antihistamines such as hydroxyzine and diphenhydramine are used with varying degrees of success to sometimes manage mild anxiety, though empirical data are generally lacking regarding their efficacy. Some older reports have suggested that β-blockers such as propranolol and oxprenolol may be suitable for some geriatric patients with anxiety and agitation (Petrie 1983; Petrie and Ban 1981), particularly for agitation of individuals with dementia who are refractory to antipsychotic or benzodiazepine therapy (also see Chapters 22 and 24 in this volume). However, as a result of the hypotensive effects of β-blockers as well as the possible risk for developing congestive cardiac failure while taking these agents, they are rarely used in clinical situations. A meta-analysis of controlled trials of neuroleptics shows evidence of a moderate effect of traditional neuroleptics for management of agitation associated with dementia (Schneider et al. 1990). Some recent evidence from a randomized controlled trial supports superior efficacy of the atypical neuroleptic risperidone compared with placebo in the management of agitation associated with dementia (Katz et al. 1997). Because long-term use of neuroleptics increases the risk for developing tardive dyskinesia, any long-term use of these agents should probably be restricted to agitated patients with clear evidence of, or strong clinical impression of, underlying psychosis.

In conclusion, a variety of compounds including benzodiazepines, buspirone, and antidepressants seem to show effectiveness for various anxiety disorders of the elderly, whereas atypical neuroleptics can be useful in the management of agitation associated with dementia.

Psychological Treatments

Although medications are frequently the first-line treatment for late-life anxiety disorders, cognitive-behavior treatment (CBT), that is, therapies that integrate both cognitive and behavioral approaches, should be considered as an alternative in cases in which the possibility of side effects and drug interactions is high as a result of intercurrent medical problems and polypharmacy or in which compliance with a medication regimen is an issue (also see Chapter 36 in this volume). Further, current treatment strategies for panic disorder with agoraphobia and OCD usually involve the use of CBT as an adjunct to pharmacotherapy (Baer 1993; Ballenger 1993; Telch and Lucas 1993).

Substantial empirical research documents efficacy of CBT in anxiety disorders among younger populations. For example, several reports document efficacy of CBT in panic disorder (Barlow and Cerny 1988; Clark 1986; Clark et al. 1985), phobias (Marks 1981, 1987), and OCD (Marks 1981; Rachman and Hodgson 1980; Van Noppen et al. 1997) in the general population. Typically, such empirically supported therapies for anxiety disorders have applied relaxation, exposure therapy, and cognitive therapy as their components, either singly or in combination (DeRubeis and Crits-Christoph 1998).

Despite the substantial number of systematic studies documenting efficacious CBT treatments for younger patients, such studies are generally lacking for older patients. The efficacy of numerous therapies for older adults is often extrapolated from evidence with younger populations (Sheikh and Salzman 1995). Sometimes modifications are made to treatment protocols in an effort to make them more suitable for a geriatric population, yet these modifications have not been systematically investigated (Beck and Stanley 1997).

A few recent research studies and case reports support the efficacy of using CBT with older patients. For panic disorder, case studies support the use of CBT among older adults specifically (Rathus and Sanderson 1996). A recent study from our group (Swales et al. 1996) reported significant improvement among older adults with panic disorder using CBT and applied relaxation, and these gains were maintained at the 3-month follow-up. One controlled study has compared CBT and nondirective supportive psychotherapy in a group format for older adults with GAD (Stanley et al. 1996). Participants in both conditions manifested significantly lower worry, anxiety, and depression scores posttreatment and at 6-month follow-up. Table 15–5 summarizes strategies for effective management of anxiety disorders in the elderly, and Table 15–6 summarizes recommendations for treatment of anxiety associated with neurological disorders in late life.

▮ Conclusions and Future Directions

Despite increasing research interest in the area of anxiety in younger age groups, few systematic studies of the phe-

TABLE 15–5. Treatment strategies for anxiety disorders in late life

Disorder	First-line treatment(s)	Second-line treatment(s)
Panic disorder with or without agoraphobia	SSRIs and/or CBT	TCAs, MAOIs, and newer antidepressants
Generalized anxiety disorder	Benzodiazepines, buspirone, and/or CBT	SSRIs or nefazodone
Obsessive-compulsive disorder	SSRIs plus CBT	Clomipramine, combination pharmacotherapy
Social phobia		
Generalized	Phenelzine, SSRIs plus CBT	Benzodiazepines
Specific	β blockers plus CBT	Buspirone
Simple (specific) phobia	CBT or benzodiazepines	β blockers
Posttraumatic stress disorder	SSRIs or nefazodone	CBT
Mixed anxiety depression	SSRIs or nefazodone	CBT

Note. CBT = cognitive-behavior treatment; MAOIs = monoamine oxidase inhibitors; SSRIs = selective serotonin reuptake inhibitors; TCAs = tricyclic antidepressants.

TABLE 15–6. Recommendations for treatment of anxiety associated with neurological disorders common in late life

Disorder	Predominant manifestations of anxiety	Recommendation(s) for treatment
Parkinson's disease	Mixed anxiety and depression	Serotonergic drugs (e.g., buspirone, nefazodone, SSRIs)
	Agitation	Atypical neuroleptics
Alzheimer's disease	Mixed anxiety and depression	Serotonergic drugs
	Agitation	Atypical neuroleptics, anticonvulsants, serotonergic drugs
Stroke	Mixed anxiety and depression	Serotonergic drugs
	Posttraumatic stress disorder	SSRIs, nefazodone

Note. SSRIs = selective serotonin reuptake inhibitors.

nomenology and treatment of anxiety disorders in the elderly have been performed. Data from ECA studies suggest that anxiety disorders remain among the most prevalent of all psychiatric disorders in the elderly. Geriatric anxiety thus remains woefully underaddressed, with large gaps of knowledge and a relevant information base predictably inadequate. The following is a list of some of the knowledge gaps and suggested directions for future research.

1. More information is needed about the phenomenology and clinical course of anxiety disorders in late life, both in healthy and physically ill populations. This goal can be achieved by designing both cross-sectional and longitudinal surveys of the elderly in various settings, including community, outpatient clinics in general medical settings, outpatient mental health clinics, hospitals, and nursing homes. DSM-IV criteria should be used as the guiding principle, but not the limiting factor, in such surveys because the elderly may exhibit differences in phenomenology from that of the general population.

2. Conducting clinical trials is a priority in the field of late-life anxiety. Such studies need to include both pharmacological and psychological treatments. Lacking such investigations, both clinicians and researchers will continue to rely on assumptions based on investigations in younger patients.

3. We need to establish safe guidelines for anxiolytic drugs for older patients. As mentioned above, the standard practice is to use the antianxiety medications proven efficacious in younger patients. Though most clinicians tend to be cautious with dosing and mindful of the possibility of causing adverse reactions when working with the elderly, in the absence of research data, such caution may lead to underdosing at times. Thus, empirically derived guidelines are needed for dosing, safety, efficacy, and specificity of these drugs in the elderly.

4. As for younger patients, studies are needed to establish the unique efficacy of the combination of pharmacological and psychological treatments for several anxiety disorders in older adults. This need is particularly true for panic disorder and OCD, in which cases clinicians frequently consider combination treatment based on symptomatology. However, empirical validation of such practice is needed.

5. Studies are needed to examine the differential phenomenology, clinical course, and treatment responses of late-onset anxiety disorders compared with anxiety disorders with onset in earlier life.

6. We need to design anxiety rating instruments specific for the elderly. Data from even well-designed treatment studies may not accurately reflect the extent of patients' anxiety unless reliable and valid measuring tools are available. The existing rating scales for anxiety have in general not been validated in the elderly. Validation studies of the existing measures of anxiety in the elderly using structured diagnostic interviews as the external validation criteria are needed. Such studies may lead to the development of better instruments specifically geared to measure anxiety in the elderly, both to carry out assessments as well as to measure progress in treatment.

7. We need to conduct studies in patients who are medically ill. Medical comorbidity is common in older patients and can complicate both assessment and treatment of anxiety. Most older patients are on several medications concurrently, which can lead to unwanted or unexpected interactions. Such interactions can exaggerate or reduce the therapeutic effi-

cacy of pharmacological treatments. Treatment investigations in this subgroup of older patients are clearly needed. Such investigations can guide the field in creating algorithms for treating such patients.

References

Aguiar LM, Haskins T, Rudolph RL, et al: Double blind, placebo controlled study of once daily venlafaxine extended release in outpatients with GAD. Paper presented at the 151st Annual Meeting of the American Psychiatric Association, Toronto, Canada, June 1998

Alexander AB: Systematic relaxation and flow rates in asthmatic children: relationship to emotional precipitants and anxiety. J Psychosom Res 16:405–410, 1972

Alexopoulos GS: Anxiety and depression in the elderly, in Anxiety in the elderly: treatment and Research. Edited by Salzman C, Lebowitz BD. New York, Springer, 1991, pp 131–150

American Psychiatric Association: Diagnostic and Statistical Manual of Mental Disorders, 3rd Edition. Washington, DC, American Psychiatric Association, 1980

American Psychiatric Association: Diagnostic and Statistical Manual of Mental Disorders, 3rd Edition, Revised. Washington, DC, American Psychiatric Association, 1987

American Psychiatric Association: Diagnostic and Statistical Manual of Mental Disorders, 4th Edition. Washington, DC, American Psychiatric Association, 1994

Astrom M: Generalized anxiety disorder in stroke patients: a 3 year longitudinal study. Stroke 27:270–275, 1996

Atkinson R: Aging and alcohol use disorders: diagnostic issues in the elderly. Paper presented at the NIMH/APA DSM-IV Geriatric Workshop, San Francisco, CA, May 1989

Baer L: Behavior therapy for obsessive compulsive disorder in the office-based practice. J Clin Psychiatry 54 (suppl 6):10–15, 1993

Ballenger JC: Panic disorder: Efficacy of current treatments. Psychopharmacological Bulletin 29(4):477–486, 1993

Barlow DH, Cerny JA: Psychological Treatment of Panic (Treatment Manuals for Practitioners Series). New York, Guilford, 1988

Beck JG, Stanley MA: Anxiety disorders in the elderly: the emerging role of behavior therapy. Behavior Therapy 28:83–100, 1997

Beck AT, Epstein N, Brown G, et al: An inventory for measuring clinical anxiety: psychometric properties. J Consult Clin Psychol 56:893–897, 1988

Beck JG, Stanley MA, Zebb BJ: Characteristics of generalized anxiety disorder in older adults: a descriptive study. Behav Res Ther 34:225–234, 1996

Beitman BD, Mukerji V, Alpert M, et al: Panic disorder in cardiology patients. Psychiatric Medicine 8(2):67–81, 1990

Ben-Arie O, Swartz L, Dickman BJ: Depression in the elderly living in the community: its presentation and features. Br J Psychiatry 150:169–174, 1987

Blazer D, George LK, Hughes D: The epidemiology of anxiety disorders: an age comparison, in Anxiety in the Elderly. Edited by Salzman C, Lebowitz BD. New York, Springer, 1991, pp 17–30

Boston Collaborative Drug Surveillance Program: Clinical depression of the central nervous system due to diazepam and chlordiazepoxide in relation to cigarette smoking and age. N Engl J Med 288:277–280, 1973

Boulenger JP, Marangos PJ, Patel J, et al: Central adenosine receptors: possible involvement in the chronic effects of caffeine. Psychopharmacol Bull 20:431–435, 1984

Boyd JH, Burke JD, Greenberg E, et al: Exclusion criteria of DSM-III: a study of co-occurrence of hierarchy-free syndromes. Arch Gen Psychiatry 41:983–989, 1984

Boyer W: Serotonin uptake inhibitors are superior to imipramine and alprazolam in alleviating panic attacks: a meta-analysis. Int J Clin Psychopharm 10:45–49, 1995

Burvill PW, Johnson GA, Jamrozik KD, et al: Anxiety disorders after stroke: results from the Perth Community Stroke Study. Br J Psychiatry 166:328–332, 1995

Cannon WB: Bodily Changes in Pain, Hunger, Fear, and Rage: An Account of Recent Researches Into the Function of Emotional Excitement. New York, Appleton-Century-Crofts, 1929

Carey MP, Burish TG: Anxiety as a predictor of behavioral outcome for chemotherapy patients. J Consult Clin Psychol 53:860–865, 1985

Carter CS, Servan-Schreiber D, Perlstein WM: Anxiety disorders and the syndrome of chest pain with normal coronary arteries: prevalence and pathophysiology. J Clin Psychiatry 58(suppl 3):70–75, 1997

Chambless DL, Cherney J, Caputo GC, et al: Anxiety disorders and alcoholism: a study with inpatient alcoholics. J Anxiety Disord 1:29–40, 1987

Charney DS, Heninger GR, Sternberg DE: Assessment of α-2 adrenergic autoreceptor function in humans: effects of oral yohimbine. Life Sci 30:2033–2041, 1982

Charney DS, Heninger GR, Jatlow PL: Increased anxiogenic effects of caffeine in panic disorder. Arch Gen Psychiatry 42:233–243, 1985

Clark DM: A cognitive approach to panic. Behav Res Ther 24:461–470, 1986

Clark DM, Salkovskis PM, Chalkley AJ: Respiratory control as a treatment for panic attacks. J Behav Ther Exp Psychiatry 16:23–30, 1985

Clarke AH, Lewis MJ: Fear of crime among the elderly. British Journal of Criminology 232:49, 1982

Cohen CI: Nocturnal neurosis of the elderly: failure of agencies to cope with the problem. J Am Geriatr Soc 24:86, 1976

Copeland JR, Davidson LA, Dewey ME: The prevalence and outcome of anxious depression in elderly people aged 65 and over living in the community, in Anxious Depression—Assessment and Treatment. Edited by Racagnia G, Sneraldi E. New York, Raven, 1987, p 43

Coplan JD, Pine DS, Papp LA, et al: An algorithm-oriented treatment approach for panic disorder. Psychiatric Annals 26:192–201, 1996

Coryell W: Mortality of anxiety disorders, in Classification, Etiological Factors and Associated Disturbances, Handbook of Anxiety, Vol 2. Edited by Noyes R Jr, Roth M, Burrows GD. Amsterdam, Elsevier North Holland, 1988, pp 311–320

Coryell W, Noyes R, Clancy J: Excess mortality in panic disorder: a comparison with primary unipolar depression. Arch Gen Psychiatry 39:701–703, 1982

Coryell W, Noyes R, Hause JD: Mortality among outpatients with anxiety disorders. Am J Psychiatry 143:508, 1986

Cummings JL: Behavioral complications of drug treatment of Parkinson's disease. J Am Geriatr Soc 39:708–716, 1991

Curran HV, Allen D, Lader M: The effects of single doses of alprazolam and lorazepam on memory and psychomotor performance in normal humans. J Psychopharmacol 2:81–89, 1987

Davidson J, Kudler H, Smith R, et al: Treatment of posttraumatic stress disorder with amitriptyline and placebo. Arch Gen Psychiatry 47:259–266, 1990

Davidson JR: PTSD: who responds to what treatment? Symposium conducted at the 151st Annual Meeting of the American Psychiatric Association, Toronto, Canada, June 1998

Derogatis LR: The SCL-90R. Baltimore, MD, Clinical Psychometric Research, 1975

Derogatis LR, Morrow GR, Fetting J, et al: The prevalence of psychiatric disorders among cancer patients. J Am Med Association 249:751–757, 1983

DeRubeis RJ, Crits-Christoph P: Empirically supported individual and group psychological treatments for adult mental disorders. J Cons Clin Psychol 66:37–52, 1998

Edlund MJ, Swan AC, Clothier J: Patients with panic attacks and abnormal EEG results. Am J Psychiatry 144:508–509, 1987

Fawcett J, Marcus RN, Anton SF, et al: Response of anxiety and agitation symptoms during nefazodone treatment of major depression. J Clin Psychiatry 56 (suppl 6):37–42, 1995

Feldman TB: Alprazolam in the treatment of posttraumatic stress disorder (letter). J Clin Psychiatry 48:216–217,1987

Fleminger S: Left-sided Parkinson's disease is associated with greater anxiety and depression. Psychol Med 21:629–638, 1991

Flint AJ: Epidemiology and comorbidity of anxiety disorders in the elderly. Am J Psychiatry 151:640–649, 1994

Folks DG, Fuller WC: Anxiety disorders and insomnia in geriatric patients. Psychiatr Clin North Am 20:137–64, 1997

Gammans RE, Westrick ML, Shea JP, et al: Pharmacokinetics of buspirone in elderly subjects. J Clin Pharmacol 29:72–78, 1989

Garner SJ, Eldridge FL, Wagner PG, et al: Buspirone, an anxiolytic drug that stimulates respiration. Am Rev Respiratory Diseases 139:946–950, 1989

Geracioti TD: Venlafaxine treatment of panic disorder: a case series. J Clin Psychiatry 56:408–410, 1995

Goddard AW, Charney DS: Toward an integrated neurobiology of panic disorder. J Clin Psychiatry 58(suppl 2):4–11, 1997

Goenjian AK, Najarian LM, Pynoos RS, et al: Posttraumatic stress disorder in elderly and younger adults after the 1988 earthquake in Armenia. Am J Psychiatry 151:895–901, 1994

Gorman JM, Goetz RR, Fyer M, et al: The mitral value prolapse—panic disorder connection. Psychosom Med 50:114–22, 1988

Gorman JM, Liebowitz MR, Fyer AJ, et al: A neuroanatomical hypothesis for panic disorder. Am J Psychiatry 146(2):148–161, 1989

Gray JA: A theory of anxiety: the role of the limbic system. Encephale 9:161B–166B, 1983

Greist J, Chouinard G, DuBoff E, et al: Double-blind comparison of three doses of sertraline and placebo in the treatment of outpatients with obsessive-compulsive disorder. Poster presented at the 18th Collegium Internationale Neuro-Psychopharmacologicum Congress, Nice, France, June 1992

Gunasekara NS, Noble S, Benfield P: Paroxetine: an update of its pharmacology and therapeutic use in depression and a review of its use in other disorders. Drugs 55:85–120, 1998

Hall RCW (ed): Psychiatric Presentations of Medical Illness. New York, Spectrum, 1980

Hamilton M: The assessment of anxiety states by rating. Br J Med Psychol 32:50–55, 1959

Harris EL, Noyes R, Crowe RR, et al: Family study of agoraphobia: report of a pilot study. Arch Gen Psychiatry 40:1061–1064, 1983

Hartmann J, Kunig G, Riederer P: Involvement of transmitter systems in neuropsychiatric diseases. Acta Neurol Scand Suppl 146:18–21, 1993

Hasselbrock MN, Meyer RE, Keener JJ: Psychopathology in hospitalized alcoholics. Arch Gen Psychiatry 42:1050–1055, 1985

Henderson R, Kurlan R, Kersun JM, et al: Preliminary examination of the comorbidity of anxiety and depression in Parkinson's disease. J Neuropsychiatry Clin Neurosci 4:257–264, 1992

Hertzberg MA, Feldman ME, Beckman JC, et al: Open trial of nefazodone for combat-related posttraumatic stress disorder. J Clin Psychiatry 59:460–464, 1998

Himmelfarb S, Murrell SA: The prevalence and correlates of anxiety symptoms in older adults. J Psychol 116:159–167, 1984

Hoehn-Saric R, McLeod DR, Zimmerli WD: Differential effects of alprazolam and imipramine in generalized anxiety disorder: somatic versus psychiatric symptoms. J Clin Psychiatry 49:293–301, 1988

Hurley JR: Thyroid diseases in the elderly. Med Clin North Am 67:497–516, 1983

Insel TR, Gillin JC, Moore A, et al: The sleep of patients with obsessive-compulsive disorder. Arch Gen Psychiatry 39:1372–1377, 1982

Iruela LM, Ibanez-Rojo V, Palanca I, et al: Anxiety disorders and Parkinson's disease (letter). Am J Psychiatry 149:719–720, 1992

Jenike MA: Handbook of Geriatric Psychopharmacology. Littleton, MA, PSG Publishing, 1985

Jenkins CD: Psychological and social precursors of coronary disease. N Engl J Med 284:244–255, 1971

Jeste DV, Krull AJ: Behavioral problems associated with dementia: diagnosis and treatment. Geriatrics 46:28–34, 1991

Kane RL, Ouslander JG, Abrass IB (eds): Essentials of Clinical Geriatrics, 3rd Edition. McGraw-Hill, San Francisco, CA, 1994

Kantor JS, Zitrin CM, Zeldis SM: Mitral valve prolapse syndrome in agoraphobic patients. Am J Psychiatry 137:467–469, 1980

Karajgi B, Rifkin A, Doddi S, et al: The prevalence of anxiety disorders in patients with chronic obstructive pulmonary disease. Am J Psychiatry 147(2):200–201, 1990

Kathol RG, Turner R, Delahunt J: Depression and anxiety associated with hyperthyroidism: response to antithyroid therapy. Psychosomatics 27:501–505, 1986

Katz I, Brecher M, Clyde C: Risperidone in the treatment of psychosis and aggressive behavior in patients with dementia. Paper presented at the annual scientific meeting of the American College of Neuropsychopharmacology, Honolulu, Hawaii, December 1997

Kay DWK: Anxiety in the elderly, in Biological, Clinical and Cultural Perspectives, Handbook of Anxiety, Vol 1. Edited by Roth M, Noyes JR, Burrows GD. Amsterdam, Elsevier North Holland, 1988, pp 289–310

Kelly D, Mitchell-Heggs SD, Sherman D: Anxiety and the effects of sodium lactate assessed clinically and physiologically. Br J Psychiatry 119:129–141, 1971

Kirby M, Lawlor BA: Biologic markers and neurochemical correlates of agitation and psychosis in dementia. J Geriatr Psychiatry Neurol 8:S2–S7, 1995

Kochansky GE: Psychiatric rating scales for assessing psychopathology in the elderly: a critical review, in Psychiatric Symptoms and Cognitive Loss in the Elderly. Edited by Raskin A, Jarvik L. Washington, DC, Hemisphere, 1979, pp 125–156

Koran LM, McElroy SL, Davidson JR, et al: Fluvoxamine versus clomipramine for obsessive-compulsive disorder: a double blind comparison. J Clin Psychopharmacology 16:121–129, 1996

Kroboth PD, McAuley JW, Smith RB: Alprazolam in the elderly: pharmacokinetics and pharmacodynamics during multiple dosing. Psychopharmacology 100:477–484, 1990

Kuch K, Cox BJ: Symptoms of PTSD in 124 survivors of the Holocaust. Am J Psychiatry 149:337–340, 1992

Kushner MG, Sher KJ, Beitman BD: The relation between alcohol problems and the anxiety disorders. Am J Psychiatry 147(6):685–695, 1990

Larson EB, Kukull WA, Buchner D, et al: Adverse drug reactions associated with global cognitive impairment in elderly persons. Ann Intern Med 107:169–173, 1987

Lauterbach EC: The locus ceruleus and anxiety disorders in demented and nondemented familial parkinsonism. Am J Psychiatry 150:994, 1993

Lee MA: Anxiety and caffeine consumption in people with anxiety disorders. Psychiatry Res 15:211–217, 1985

Leigh D: Psychiatric aspects of head injury. Psychiatry Digest 40:21–32, 1979

Lerner WD, Fallen HJ: The alcohol withdrawal syndrome. N Engl J Med 313:511–515, 1985

Lewis AJ: Melancholia: A clinical study of depressive states. J Psychiatry 109:451–463, 1934

Liebowitz MR, Fyer AJ, Gorman JM, et al: Lactate provocation of panic attacks, I: clinical and behavioral findings. Arch Gen Psychiatry 41:764–770, 1984

Lindesay J: Phobic disorders in the elderly. Br J Psychiatry 159:531–541, 1991

Lindesay J, Briggs K, Murphy E: The Guy's/Age Concern survey: prevalence rates of cognitive impairment, depression and anxiety in an urban elderly community. Br J Psychiatry 155:317–329, 1989

Liptzin B: Masked anxiety—alcohol and drug use, in Anxiety in the Elderly. Edited by Salzman C, Lebowitz BD. New York, Springer, 1991, pp 87–101

Luchins DJ, Rose RP: Late-life onset of panic disorder with agoraphobia in three patients. Am J Psychiatry 146:920–921, 1989

Margraf J, Ehlers A, Roth WT: Mitral valve prolapse and panic disorder: a review of their relationship. Psychosom Med 50:93–113, 1988

Marks IM: Cure and Care of Neuroses: Theory and Practice of Behavioral Psychotherapy. New York, Wiley, 1981

Marks IM: Fears, Phobias, and Rituals: Panic, Anxiety, and Their Disorders. New York, Oxford University Press, 1987

Mathew RJ, Swihart AA, Weinman ML: Vegetative symptoms in anxiety and depression. Br J Psychiatry 141:162, 1982

Mavissakalian M, Michelson L: Agoraphobia: relative and combined effectiveness of therapist-assisted in vivo exposure and imipramine. J Clin Psychiatry 47:117–122, 1986

Mazza DL, Martin D, Spacavento L, et al: Prevalence of anxiety disorders in patients with mitral valve prolapse. Am J Psychiatry 143:349–352, 1986

McDougle CJ, Goodman, WK, Leckman JF, et al: The efficacy of fluvoxamine in obsessive compulsive disorder: effects of comorbid chronic tic disorder. J Clin Psychopharm 13: 354–358, 1993

Meyer BR: Benzodiazepines in the elderly. Med Clin North Am 66(5):1017–1035, 1982

Mintzer JE, Brawman-Mintzer O: Agitation as a possible expression of generalized anxiety disorder in demented elderly patients: toward a treatment approach. J Clin Psychiatry 57 (suppl 7):55–63, 1996

Moran MG, Thompson TL II, Nies AS: Sleep disorders in the elderly. Am J Psychiatry 145(11):1369–1378, 1988

Munjack KJ, Moss HB: Affective disorder and alcoholism in families of agoraphobics. Arch Gen Psychiatry 38:869–871, 1981

Myers JK, Weissman MM, Tischler GL, et al: Six-month prevalence of psychiatric disorders in three communities: 1980–1982. Arch Gen Psychiatry 41:959–967, 1984

Nagy LM, Krystal JH, Charney DS, et al: Long-term outcome of panic disorder after short-term imipramine and behavioral group treatment: 2.9 year naturalistic follow-up study. J Clin Psychopharm 13:16–24, 1993

Napoliello MJ: An interim multicenter report on 677 anxious geriatric outpatients treated with buspirone. British Journal of Clinical Practice 40:71–73, 1986

National Center for Health Statistics: CUrrent estimates from the National Health Interview Survey: Vital and Health Statistics No 10, in Aging America: Trends and Projections, Washington, DC, US Government Printing Office, 1986–1987, p 164

Nowlin JB, Williams R, Wilkie F: Prospective study of physical and psychological factors in elderly men who subsequently suffer acute myocardial infarction (AMI). Clinical Research 21:465, 1973

Oehrberg S, Christiansen PE, Behnke K, et al: Paroxetine in the treatment of panic disorder: a randomized, double-blind, placebo-controlled study. Br J Psychiatry 167(3):374–379, 1995

Petrie WM: Drug treatment of anxiety and agitation in the aged. Psychopharmacol Bull 19:238–246, 1983

Petrie WM, Ban TA: Propranolol in organic citation. Lancet 1(8215):324, 1981

Pitts FN Jr, McClure JN: Lactate metabolism in anxiety neurosis. N Engl J Med 227:1329–1336, 1967

Pomara N, Stanley B, Block R, et al: Diazepam impairs performance in normal elderly subjects. Psychopharmacol Bull 20(1):137–139, 1984

Pomara N, Deptula D, Singh R, et al: Cognitive toxicity of benzodiazepines in the elderly, in Anxiety in the Elderly. Edited by Salzman CL, Lebowitz BD. New York, Springer, 1991, pp 175–196

Popkin MK, Mackenzie TB: Psychiatric presentations of endocrine dysfunction, in Psychiatric Presentations of Medical Illness. Edited by Hall RCW. New York, Spectrum, 1980, pp 139–156

Rachman SJ, Hodgson R: Obsessions and Compulsions. Englewood Cliffs, NJ, Prentice-Hall, 1980

Rathus JH, Sanderson WC: Cognitive behavioral treatment of panic disorder in elderly adults: two case studies. J Cognitive Psychotherapy 10:271–280, 1996

Redmond DE, Huang HY: New evidence for a locus coeruleus norepinephrine connection with anxiety. Life Sci 25: 2149–2162, 1979

Reiman EM, Raichle ME, Robins E, et al: Neuroanatomical correlates of a lactate-induced anxiety attack. Arch Gen Psychiatry 46:493–500, 1989

Reynolds CF, Shaw DH, Newton TF, et al: EEG sleep in outpatients with generalized anxiety: a preliminary comparison with depressed outpatients. Psychiatry Res 8(2):81–89, 1983

Rickels K, Schweizer EE: Current pharmacotherapy of anxiety and panic, in Psychopharmacology: The Third Generation of Progress. Edited by Meltzer HA. New York, Raven, 1987, pp 1193–1203

Rickels K, Weisman K, Norstad N, et al: Buspirone and diazepam in anxiety: a controlled study. J Clin Psychiatry 43(12 sec 2):81–86, 1982

Rickels K, Schweizer EE, Csanalosi I, et al: Long-term treatment of anxiety and risk of withdrawal: prospective comparison of clorazepate and buspirone. Arch Gen Psychiatry 45:444–450, 1988

Robinson RG, Starkstein SE: Current research in affective disorders following stroke. J Neuropsychiatry Clin Neurosci 2:1–14, 1990

Rosenbaum J: Anxiety, in Outpatient Psychiatry. Edited by Lazare A. Baltimore, MD, Williams & Wilkins, 1979, pp 252–256

Ross HE, Glasser FB, Germanson T: The prevalence of psychiatric disorders in patients with alcohol and other drug problems. Arch Gen Psychiatry 45:1023–1031, 1988

Salzman C: Psychometric rating of anxiety in the elderly, in Proceedings of a Conference on Anxiety in the Elderly. Co-sponsored by Roche Laboratories, University of Arizona College of Medicine, Tucson, AZ, November 1977

Salzman C, Satlin A, Burrows AB: Geriatric psychopharmacology, in The American Psychiatric Press textbook of pharmacology, Edited by Schatzberg AF, Nemeroff CB. Washington, DC, American Psychiatric Press, 1995, pp 803–821

Sandberg B, Bliding A: Duodenal ulcer in army trainees during basic training. J Psychosom Res 20:61–74, 1976

Schiffer RB, Kurlan R, Rubin A, et al: Evidence for atypical depression in Parkinson's disease. Am J Psychiatry 145: 1020–1022, 1988

Schneider LS, Pollock VE, Lynes SA: Meta analysis of controlled trials of neuroleptics in dementia. J Am Geriatr Soc 38:553–563, 1990

Schultz SK, Castillo CS, Kosier JT, et al: Generalized anxiety and depression: assessment over 2 years after stroke. Am J Geriatr Psychiatry 5:229–237, 1997

Schweizer E, Case WG, Rickels K: Benzodiazepine dependence and withdrawal in elderly patients. Am J Psychiatry 146(4):529–531, 1989

Sheehan DV, Ballenger JC, Jacobsen G: Treatment of endogenous anxiety with phobic, hysterical, and hypochondriacal symptoms. Arch Gen Psychiatry 13:51, 1980

Sheikh J, Salzman C: Anxiety in the elderly: course and treatment. Psychiatric Clin North Am 18:871–883, 1995

Sheikh JI, Swales PJ: Late-onset panic disorder: a distinct syndrome, in Proceedings of the Annual Scientific Meeting of the American Association for Geriatric Psychiatry, San Diego, CA, March 1998

Sheikh JI, Taylor CB, King RJ, et al: Panic attacks and avoidance behavior in the elderly. Proceedings of the annual meeting of the American Psychiatric Association, Montreal, May 1988

Sheikh JI, King RJ, Taylor CB: Comparative phenomenology of early-onset versus late-onset panic attacks: a pilot survey. Am J Psychiatry 148(9):1231–1233, 1991

Simson PE, Weiss JM: Altered activity of locus coeruleus in an animal model of depression. Neuropsychopharmacology 1:287–295, 1988

Smiley A, Moskowitz H: Effects of long-term administration of buspirone and diazepam on driver steering control. Am J Med 80(3b):22–29, 1986

Solomon SD, Gerrity ET, Muff AM: Efficacy of treatments for posttraumatic stress disorder. JAMA 268:633–638, 1992

Speed N, Engdahl B, Schwartz J, et al: Posttraumatic stress disorder as a consequence of the POW experience. J Nerv Ment Dis 177:147–153, 1989

Spielberger C, Gorsuch R, Lushene R: STAI Manual for the State-Trait Anxiety Inventory. Palo Alto, CA. Consulting Psychologists Press, 1970

Spitzer RL, Williams JBW, Gibbon M: Structured Clinical Interview for DSM-III-R—Patient Version (SCID-P, 4/1/87). New York, New York State Psychiatric Institute, 1987

Stanley MA, Beck JG, Zebb BJ: Psychometric properties of four anxiety measures in older adults. Behav Res Ther 34(10):827–838, 1996

Stanley MA, Beck JG, Glassco JD: Treatment of generalized anxiety in older adults: a preliminary comparison of cognitive-behavioral and supportive approaches. Behavior Therapy 27(4):565–581, 1996

Steer RA, Willman M, Kay PAJ, et al: Differentiating elderly medical and psychiatric outpatients with the Beck Anxiety Inventory. Assessment 1(4):345–351, 1994

Stein MB, Heuser IJ, Juncos JL, et al: Anxiety disorders in patients with Parkinson's disease. Am J Psychiatry 147:217–220, 1990

Stokes PE, Holtz: A Fluoxetine tenth anniversary update: the progress continues. Clin Ther 19(5):1135–1150, 1997

Sunderland T, Lawlor B, Martinez R, et al: Anxiety in the elderly: neurobiological and clinical interface, in Anxiety in the Elderly. Edited by Salzman C, Lebowitz BD. New York, Springer, 1991

Swales PJ, Solfvin JF, Sheikh JI: Cognitive-behavioral therapy in older panic disorder patients. Am J Geriatr Psychiatry 4:46–60, 1996

Telch MJ, Lucas RA: Combined pharmacological and psychological treatment of panic disorder: current status and future directions, in Treatment of Panic Disorder: A Consensus Development Conference. Edited by Wolfe BE, Maser JD, Washington, DC, American Psychiatric Press, 1993, pp 51–84

Teri L, Larson EB, Reifler B: Behavioral disturbance in dementia of Alzheimer type. J Am Geriatr Soc 36:1–6, 1988

Tune L, Carr S, Hoag E, et al: Anticholinergic effects of drugs commonly prescribed for the elderly: potential means for assessing risk of delirium. Am J Psychiatry 149:1393–1394, 1992

Uhde TW, Roy-Byrne P, Gillin JC, et al: The sleep of patients with panic disorder: a preliminary report. Psychiatry Res 12(3):251–259, 1984

Vallejo J, Olivares J, Marcos T, et al: Clomipramine versus phenelzine in obsessive-compulsive disorder. Br J Psychiatry 161:665–670, 1992

Van Noppen B, Steketee G, McCorkle BH, et al: Group and multifamily behavioral treatment for obsessive compulsive disorder: a pilot study. J Anxiety Disorders 11(4):431–446, 1997

Victor BS, Lubersky M, Greden F: Somatic manifestations of caffeinism. J Clin Psychiatry 42:185–188, 1981

Von Moltke LL, Greenblatt DJ, Harmatz JS, et al: Psychotropic drug metabolism in old age: principles and problems of assessment, in Psychopharmacology: The Fourth Generation of Progress. Edited by Bloom FE, Kupfer DJ. New York, Raven, 1995, pp 1461–1469

Wands K, Merskey H, Hachinski VC, et al: A questionnaire investigation of anxiety and depression in early dementia. J Am Geriatr Soc 38(5):535–538, 1990

Weissman MM: Anxiety and alcoholism. J Clin Psychiatry 49 (10 suppl):17–19, 1988

Wells KB, Golding JM, Burnam MA: Psychiatric disorder and limitations in physical functioning in a sample of the Los Angeles general population. Am J Psychiatry 145(6):712–717, 1988

Wetherell JL, Arean PA: Psychometric evaluation of the Beck Anxiety Inventory with older medical patients. Psych Assessment 9(2):136–144, 1997

White RJ, Rudkin ST, Ashley J, et al: Outpatient pulmonary rehabilitation in severe chronic obstructive pulmonary disease. J R Coll Physicians Lond 31(5):541–545, 1997

Whitehead WE, Blackwell B, DeSilva H, et al: Anxiety and anger in hypertension. J Psychosom Res 21:383–389, 1977

Wise MG, Griffies WS: A combined treatment approach to anxiety in the medically ill. J Clin Psychiatry 56 (suppl 2): 14–9, 1995

Yellowlees PM, Alpers JH, Bowden JJ, et al: Psychiatric morbidity in patients with chronic airflow obstruction. Med J Aust 146:305–307, 1987

Zitrin CM, Klein DF, Woerner MG, et al: Treatment of phobias, I: comparison of imipramine hydrochloride and placebo. Arch Gen Psychiatry 40:125–138, 1983

16

Substance Abuse

Roland M. Atkinson, M.D.

Introduction

Significant substance abuse occurs in older persons, although for various reasons the scope of the problem has been appreciated only recently. The view, espoused in several influential papers in the 1960s, that substance abuse was seldom seen after middle age was not challenged for several decades (Atkinson et al. 1992). People with lifelong addictions to alcohol and drugs were presumed to have died prematurely or to have recovered spontaneously, and late-onset addiction was said to be rare. Trained to this view, clinicians often overlook these disorders in elderly persons. In addition, symptoms of substance abuse in older individuals may mimic symptoms of other medical and behavioral disorders, leading to misdiagnosis. Elderly persons, in particular, tend to underreport drinking problems, and clinicians also are less likely to record these problems and to make appropriate referrals in this population (Booth et al. 1992; Curtis et al. 1989; McInnes and Powell 1994; Moos et al. 1993). In this chapter, I address substance abuse in elderly individuals. I begin with an overview of the terms and concepts used in the field, as well as risk factors involved in substance abuse in late life. General principles of assessment and management are then discussed. Finally, special sections are presented on alcohol, benzodiazepines, tobacco, and other substance use and dependence.

General Terms and Concepts in the Field of Substance Abuse

Table 16–1 lists the definitions of substance abuse terms used in this chapter. Two currently used sets of criteria for the diagnosis of substance dependence, the fundamental behavior disorder underlying most substance-related problems, are listed in Table 16–2. Although similar, these criteria sets differ sufficiently that agreement between them on case classification is less than optimal (Caetano and Tam 1995). (For further general information on substance abuse, see Begleiter and Kissin 1996; Lowinson et al. 1997; and Schuckit 1995.)

Importance of Substance Abuse in the Elderly

Alcohol use disorders and subsyndromal drinking problems are common in aging persons until well into the

Linda Ganzini helped prepare an earlier version of this chapter.

TABLE 16–1. Definitions of some terms used in the substance abuse field

Psychoactive: Any chemical—alcohol, tobacco, therapeutic agent, industrial compound, or illicit drug—with important effects on the central nervous system.

Substance: A psychoactive that typically is associated with a substance use disorder. The term includes alcohol; opioids; sedative-hypnotics; antianxiety agents of the barbiturate and benzodiazepine types; psychomotor stimulants, especially amphetamines and cocaine; tobacco products; and certain over-the-counter psychoactives. The terms *chemical* and *drug* in this context are synonymous with *substance* (e.g., "chemical dependence," "drug abuse").

Drink: A standard drink of beverage alcohol is equivalent to a 12-ounce domestic beer (alcohol content approximately 4%), a 4-ounce glass of table wine (approximately 12% alcohol), or a mixed drink containing $1-1\frac{1}{2}$ ounces of hard liquor (about 40% alcohol).

Use: Appropriate medical or social consumption of a psychoactive in a manner that minimizes the potential for dependence or abuse.

Heavy use: Use of a substance in greater quantity than the usual norms, but without obvious negative social, behavioral, or health consequences. Heavy alcohol or tobacco users may be dependent upon the substance. *At-risk* or *risky* drinkers refer to heavy consumers of alcohol, usually at rates of more than 15–21 drinks per week for men, 10–14 for women, or binges in which more than 4–6 drinks are consumed on a single drinking occasion. Safe drinking levels for healthy elderly persons are recommended by the National Institute on Alcohol Abuse and Alcoholism and are not to exceed 7 drinks per week or 2 drinks on a single drinking occasion.

Misuse: Use of a prescribed drug in a manner other than as directed. The term can mean overuse, underuse, improper dose sequencing, and lending or borrowing another's medication, with or without harmful consequences.

Problem use: Use of a substance in a manner that induces negative social, behavioral, or health consequences.

A "problem" user may or may not meet criteria for substance dependence or abuse, although many do. Alcohol "problems" or drug "problems" are categories that often have been used by epidemiologists in community prevalence surveys.

Abuse: Abuse of a substance is defined in DSM-IV (American Psychiatric Association 1994) as a maladaptive pattern of substance use leading to clinically significant impairment or distress, as manifested by one or more of the following, occurring within a 12-month period: 1) recurrent substance use resulting in failure to fulfill major role obligations at work or home; 2) recurrent substance use in physically hazardous situations; 3) recurrent substance-related legal problems; 4) continued substance use despite having persistent or recurrent social or interpersonal problems caused or exacerbated by the effects of a substance (pp. 182–183). *Harmful use* (ICD-10; World Health Organization 1992) approximates abuse in definition. Both imply milder severity of substance involvement than that in substance dependence.

Dependence: Dependence upon a substance is defined by explicit diagnostic criteria, such as those listed in DSM-IV or ICD-10 (Table 16–2). Serious and persistent involvement in the heavy use of the substance is the rule. These approaches set aside the older distinction between *physical dependence* and *psychological dependence*, which are now viewed as differing manifestations of similar disorders. The terms *alcoholism* and *addiction* are usually used as synonyms for dependence on alcohol and other drugs, respectively.

Substance use disorder: A clinical condition in which substance abuse or substance dependence can be diagnosed.

Substance abuse, chemical dependence, and addictions: These terms are often used to refer to the entire professional or scientific field.

---

eighth decade of life, especially in men. In addition to the negative behavioral and social consequences of these disorders that are seen at any age, alcoholism in older persons confers special hazards by aggravating a number of physical and mental disorders and altering the metabolism of many prescribed medications. Older persons as a group respond favorably to treatment for problem drinking.

The elderly are the most likely age group to receive long-term prescribed benzodiazepines. In addition to inducing physical dependence in a substantial proportion of these patients, long-term benzodiazepine administration often impairs cognitive status and general functioning of elderly persons.

Tobacco dependence is the most common addictive problem in the older population and doubles the mortality rate from all diseases. When smoking cessation strategies are suitably tailored to the older smoker, quit rates are favorable, and within 1–2 years of quitting, measurable reduction in mortality is evident.

Risk Factors for Substance Use Disorders in Later Life

Biomedical manifestations of substance abuse are as important in older patients as the psychosocial manifestations that form the more familiar clinical picture of these disor-

TABLE 16–2. DSM-IV versus ICD-10 criteria for substance dependence

DSM-IV criteria	ICD-10 criteria

1. Tolerance, as defined by either of the following:
 	
  a. A need for markedly increased amounts of the substance to achieve intoxication or desired effect; or
 	
  b. Markedly diminished effect with continued use of the same amount of the substance.
 	
2. Withdrawal, as manifested by either of the following:
 	
  a. The characteristic withdrawal syndrome for the substance; or
 	
  b. The same (or a closely related) substance is taken to relieve or avoid withdrawal symptoms.
 	
3. The substance is often taken in larger amounts or over a longer period than was intended.
 	
4. There is a persistent desire or unsuccessful efforts to cut down or control substance use.
 	
5. A great deal of time is spent in activities necessary to obtain the substance (e.g., visiting multiple doctors or driving long distances), use the substance (e.g., chain smoking), or recover from its effects.
 	
6. Important social, occupational, or recreational activities are given up or reduced because of substance use.
 	
7. Substance use is continued despite knowledge of having a persistent or recurrent physical or psychological problem that is likely to have been caused or exacerbated by the substance (e.g., current cocaine use despite recognition of cocaine-induced depression; continued drinking despite a peptic ulcer made worse by alcohol consumption).
	1. Strong desire or sense of compulsion to take the substance.
	
	2. Difficulties in controlling substance-taking behavior in terms of its onset, termination, or levels of use.
	
	3. A physiological withdrawal state when substance use has ceased or been reduced, as evidenced by: the characteristic withdrawal syndrome for the substance; or use of the same (or a closely related) substance with the intention of relieving or avoiding withdrawal symptoms.
	
	4. Evidence of tolerance, such that increased doses of the psychoactive substance are required to achieve effects originally produced by lower doses (clear examples of this are found in alcohol- and opiate-dependent individuals who may take daily doses sufficient to incapacitate or kill nontolerant users).
	
	5. Progressive neglect of alternative pleasures or interests because of psychoactive substance use, increased amount of time necessary to obtain or take the substance, or to recover from its effects.
	
	6. Persisting with substance use despite clear evidence of overtly harmful consequences, such as harm to the liver through excessive drinking, depressive mood states consequent to periods of heavy substance use, or drug-related impairment of cognitive functioning; efforts should be made to determine that the user was actually, or could be expected to be, aware of the nature and extent of the harm.

Note. For either system, at least three of the listed criteria must be met in the same 12-month period in order to make the diagnosis of dependence on a substance.
Source. Adapted from American Psychiatric Association: *Diagnostic and Statistical Manual of Mental Disorders*, 4th Edition. Washington, DC, American Psychiatric Association, 1994, p. 181; World Health Organization: *International Classification of Diseases*, 10th Edition. Geneva, Switzerland, World Health Organization, 1992, pp. 75–76.

ders in younger patients. The risk factors listed in Table 16–3 reflect this perspective. Predisposing factors are similar at all ages. Factors that may increase substance exposure and consumption level and thus set the stage for abuse or dependence in some individuals include demographics, for example, gender and ethnicity (Helzer et al. 1991); chronic illnesses for which controlled substances are often prescribed on a regular basis (American Psychiatric Association 1990; Finlayson and Davis 1994); institutionalization in long-term care settings (Beardsley et al. 1989; Beers et al. 1988; Buck 1988); and several psychological and social factors, especially negative affects associated with loss and loneliness (Dupree and Schonfeld 1998). Factors that increase or prolong the effects of substances with age (e.g., pharmacokinetic and pharmacodynamic factors; see Chap-

ter 34 in this volume) may increase their dependence liability, although studies proving such an effect with regard to alcohol, benzodiazepines, or opioid analgesics are lacking (Ozdemir et al. 1996). Regular alcohol or psychoactive drug use can also increase functional impairment caused by a variety of illnesses that are more common in old age, for example, cognitive, cardiovascular, pulmonary, gastrointestinal, and metabolic disorders. Clinical complications can arise from adverse drug-drug interactions between psychoactive substances and other prescribed medications (W. L. Adams 1995; Korrapati and Vestal 1995). These alterations in biological sensitivity to drugs, comorbid medical illness, and medication interactions can lead to biomedical problems in the elderly at substance consumption rates that would have caused little or no difficulty earlier in life.

TABLE 16–3. Risk factors for substance abuse in the elderly

Predisposing factors

    Family history (alcohol)

    Previous substance abuse

    Previous pattern of substance consumption (individual and cohort effects)

    Personality traits (sedative-hypnotics and anxiolytics)

Factors that can increase substance exposure and consumption level

    Gender (men: alcohol and illicit drugs; women: sedative-hypnotics and anxiolytics)

    Chronic illness associated with pain (opioid analgesics), insomnia (hypnotic drugs), or anxiety (anxiolytics)

    Long-term prescribing (sedative-hypnotics and anxiolytics)

    Caregiver overuse of as-needed medication (institutionalized elderly)

    Life stress, loss, social isolation

    Negative affects (depression, grief, demoralization, and anger) (alcohol)

    Family collusion and drinking partners (alcohol)

    Discretionary time, money (alcohol)

Factors that can increase the effects and abuse potential of substances

    Age-associated drug sensitivity (pharmacokinetic and pharmacodynamic factors)

    Chronic medical illnesses

    Other medications (alcohol-drug and drug-drug interactions)

Principles of Assessment and Management

Assessment of Geriatric Substance Use Disorders

General approach. Use of alcohol, tobacco products, prescription and over-the-counter psychoactive agents, and illicit substances should routinely be surveyed during the initial evaluation of all older adults. Standardized screening measures are available for problem drinking in geriatric patients, although accuracy of self-reports varies. Denial of substance abuse is common in affected persons of all ages and may be exaggerated in elderly patients because of memory problems, pessimism about recovery,

and shame based on a belief that substance abuse is immoral. For these reasons, careful rapport building through repeated contacts; inquiry with relatives, caregivers, and others in the social network; reviews of medical and pharmacy records; and home visitation are especially useful case assessment methods. DSM-IV (American Psychiatric Association 1994) and ICD-10 (World Health Organization 1992) dependence criteria offer a reasonable framework for acquiring information to establish a clinical diagnosis (Table 16–2).

Special examinations. Physical and laboratory findings can help to establish a diagnosis of alcohol dependence. Toxicological examinations of urine and blood for other suspected substances can be useful to corroborate the history. Neuropsychological evaluation and brain imaging (computed tomography, magnetic resonance imaging [MRI]) may help identify complicating brain disorders. Primary dementias and dementias secondary to alcohol or drugs may produce similar initial cognitive or imaging deficits. Because substance-induced deficits either remain static or actually improve with abstinence (Brandt et al. 1983; I. Grant et al. 1984; Larson et al. 1984a; Muuronen et al. 1989; Pfefferbaum et al. 1995; Schroth et al. 1988), serial psychometric and brain imaging studies may be useful in differential diagnosis (Oslin et al. 1998).

Clinical Features

In old age, the signs and symptoms of substance use disorders can be subtle, be atypical, or mimic symptoms of other geriatric illness. In mild or circumscribed cases among community-dwelling elderly, episodic alcohol abuse or benzodiazepine dependence may not produce obvious physical signs or complaints and may be easily concealed from others. Some heavy drinkers may have a circumscribed clinical presentation of increasingly uncontrolled hypertension or diabetes mellitus, whereas moderate benzodiazepine or alcohol dependence may present with the complaint of forgetfulness. In more severe cases, substance abuse can produce or aggravate delirium or dementia (American Psychiatric Association 1990; Freund 1987; Ron 1983), which the clinician may erroneously attribute to other causes. Other serious but nonspecific presenting signs and symptoms (e.g., poor grooming, squalid living quarters, depression, erratic changes of mood or behavior, malnutrition, bladder and bowel incontinence, muscle weakness or frank myopathy, gait disorders, recurring falls, burns, or head trauma) may be caused by unsuspected alcohol or drug abuse. Other features that may be associated with alcohol or prescription drug dependence include heavy tobacco use, chronic pain syndromes or insomnia, persistent family discord, a course of inexplicable ups and downs in mood, a pattern of doing well in hospital but poorly at home, and patient or caregiver defensiveness when queried about substance use. When such features are noted, the clinician needs to be especially alert to the possibility of underlying substance dependence.

Case Management and Treatment

Brief interventions (e.g., physician advice to cease or cut down alcohol use, adjustment of prescribed medications, smoking cessation measures) can prevent or resolve some substance-related problems. More severe substance use disorders require further treatment. The goals of substance abuse treatment in the elderly are threefold: 1) stabilization, reduction, or cessation of substance consumption; 2) treatment of coexisting medical and psychiatric problems; and 3) arrangement of appropriate educational and social interventions to reduce the risk of relapse. Reducing consumption can be complicated and hazardous, requiring initial hospital care and a protracted outpatient course in cases of long-standing or high-dose dependence. Treatment of coexisting problems can be a crucial step in curbing substance consumption, especially when chronic pain, chronic insomnia, or a mood disorder has been a major factor sustaining the substance dependence or when serious medical complications of substance abuse are present. Cognitive-behavioral techniques teach patients to cope more effectively with circumstances that typically have triggered substance use (Dupree and Schonfeld 1998). Social interventions range from informal plans (e.g., arranging for increased visitation by loved ones or enrollment in a senior activity program or day center) to admission to a senior substance abuse program (Atkinson 1995).

▍ Alcohol Use Disorders and Alcohol-Associated Organic Mental Disorders

Epidemiology

Alcohol use and alcohol problems decline with age but still constitute a significant public health problem. Recent community surveys show that alcohol use in the United States is most prevalent in the age group 25–45 years and declines stepwise in older age cohorts to 12-month prevalence levels, among persons age 55 and older, of 46% who report any alcohol use (Ruchlin 1997) and 30% who report having consumed at least 12 drinks in the past 12 months

(B. F. Grant 1997). Rates of any recent alcohol use continue to decline after age 55 to 25% of persons age 85 and older (Ruchlin 1997). Rates of heavy alcohol use, problem use, and alcohol dependence also decline with age from peaks in middle life (B. F. Grant 1997). Community prevalence rates for heavy and problem use of alcohol by older persons vary widely depending upon the population sampled and definitions of use (Atkinson 1990). Because of associated health problems, older alcoholic patients are much more commonly encountered in clinical settings. Illustrative reports on the prevalence of active alcohol problems in elderly clinical cohorts are summarized in Table 16–4. For comparison, this table also notes the prevalence of at-risk drinkers (persons identified in clinical settings who report heavy alcohol consumption without current alcohol-related problems) and community prevalence of alcohol dependence from two large national surveys.

Older men are twice as likely to use alcohol as are older women (B. F. Grant 1997), and older men are two to six times more likely than women to be problem drinkers (Atkinson 1990; Callahan and Tierney 1995; B. F. Grant 1997). These patterns hold true across diverse ethnic and racial groups (Barker and Kramer 1996; Callahan and Tierney 1995; B. F. Grant 1997; Lowe et al. 1997). Once alcohol dependence develops, it is more likely to persist in older men—especially black and Hispanic men—than in women (Callahan and Tierney 1995; Gomberg and Nelson 1995; B. F. Grant 1997). Negative health and social consequences of drinking are more severe in older black men with alcoholism than in older white men (Gomberg and Nelson 1995). Older homeless persons are more likely than younger homeless to be men and to meet criteria for lifetime alcohol use disorders (DeMallie et al. 1997). Indeed, prevalence data support the conclusion that alcoholism constitutes a public health problem of moderate proportion in men in their 60s and 70s.

As noted above, cross-sectional studies show a decline in the prevalence of alcohol dependence with age (B. F. Grant 1997). Some decline is accounted for by premature deaths of those with early-onset alcoholism and by moderation or cessation of drinking over time by those surviving alcoholism (Liberto et al. 1992) and by social drinkers (W. L. Adams et al. 1990). But longitudinal studies show that many drinkers maintain steady consumption levels into later life (Glynn et al. 1985; Gordon and Kannel 1983). Because younger birth cohorts have demonstrated increasingly higher rates of alcohol consumption and alcoholism, especially after the end of Prohibition and World War II (Atkinson et al. 1992; B. F. Grant 1997; Heath et al. 1997), the prevalence of alcohol problems in old age may increase, especially among women, for birth cohorts entering their

TABLE 16–4. Prevalence of active alcohol problems (current or in past year) among older patients in selected clinical settings

Setting (source)	Age cutoff	Sample size	Gender	Frequency of active alcoholism	Frequency of at-risk drinking
General medical outpatient clinic, Omaha, NE (Jones et al. 1993)	≥ 65	154	Both	4%	NA
Acute medical inpatient wards, San Diego, CA (Schuckit et al. 1980)	≥ 65	222	Men	6%	NA
Community geriatric outreach mental health team, Seattle, WA (Reifler et al. 1982)	≥ 60	2,309	Both	9%	NA
Primary care medical clinic, Indianapolis, IN (Callahan and Tierney 1995)	≥ 60	3,954	Both	11%	NA
Emergency department visitors, Chapel Hill, NC (W. L. Adams et al. 1992)	≥ 65	205	Both	14%	NA
Nursing home admissions, Portland, OR (Joseph et al. 1995)	> 50[a]	117	Both[a]	18%	NA
Geriatric psychiatry residential treatment unit, Tampa, FL (Speer and Bates 1992)	≥ 55	128	Both	23%	NA
U.S. national community sample, 1992 (Grant 1997)	≥ 55	Several thousand[b]	Both	1%	NA
U.S. sample, five communities, 1980 (Helzer et al. 1991)	≥ 65	Several thousand[b]	Both	Men: 3.1% Women: 0.5%	NA
At-risk drinkers, primary care office practices, SE Wisconsin (W. L. Adams et al. 1996)	≥ 60	5,065	Both	NA	Men: 15%[c] Women: 12%
At-risk drinkers, medical wards, London (Bristow and Clare 1992)	≥ 65	650	Both	NA	Men: 9%[d] Women: 4%

Note. NA = not applicable.
[a]Mean age 69 years; SD = 8.6; 97% of sample male.
[b]Exact number not stated in report.
[c]Men > 14 drinks per week; women > 7 drinks per week.
[d]Men ≥ 20 drinks per week; women ≥ 10 drinks per week.

60s in the years ahead. Even if prevalence rates remain stable, the anticipated aging of the general population over the next several decades will increase the absolute numbers of older problem drinkers substantially (American Medical Association 1996).

Patterns of Alcohol Use and Abuse

Heavy versus problem drinking. For the minority of aging persons who consume more than modest amounts of alcohol, the pathophysiological effects of alcohol in many instances may have more serious clinical consequences because of increasing biological sensitivity to alcohol and because alcohol aggravates preexisting diseases that are more common in later life. When older people continue to drink despite feeling unwell or advice to stop, this meets the definition of abusive drinking, even though such drinking may not be associated with socially deviant behavior or the desire to feel intoxicated. Put another way, the distinction between heavy drinking and problem drinking narrows with age (Chermack et al. 1996b).

Reactive drinking. Some older alcoholic patients (people with late-onset alcoholism, those who have a late relapse in early-onset alcoholism after years of sobriety, or those who have had a recent increase in lifelong heavy drinking) report major losses and chronic strains and hassles as precipitants of increased drinking. On the other hand, the relationship among alcohol use, alcohol problems, and life stress in older adults is enigmatic and complex, and findings vary from study to study (Finney and Moos 1984; Welte and Mirand 1995). Community studies of older drinkers show that good health, cohabitation, and financial well-being, rather than adversity, tend to correlate with increased alcohol consumption (Barnes 1979; Busby et al. 1988; C. M. Nakamura et al. 1990; Ruchlin 1997), whereas financial strain and poor health can be associated with resolution of drinking problems or achievement of abstinence (Moos et al. 1991). Once a pattern of excessive alcohol use has been established, evanescent negative affect states (e.g., depression, sadness, boredom, anger, tension) and, far less often, positive affects (e.g., calmness, cheerfulness, friendliness) can trigger repeated drinking episodes (Dupree and Schonfeld 1998). Social reinforcement for heavy drinking is evident in some, but not all, congregate retirement settings (W. L. Adams and Cox 1995; Alexander and Duff 1988; Paganini-Hill et al. 1986).

Early- versus late-onset alcohol problems. Although onset of alcoholism after age 45 was long thought to be rare, findings from community (Eaton et al. 1989) and clinical samples (Atkinson 1994; Atkinson et al. 1990) offer evidence that late-onset alcoholism (i.e., onset after age 55, 60, or 65) is not uncommon. The notion that late-onset alcohol dependence usually occurs secondary to a mood or organic mental disorder also has not been upheld by recent systematic studies (Atkinson 1994). Cases in which persons with early-onset alcoholism achieved prolonged abstinence in middle life, but relapsed later, can be mistaken for late-onset alcoholism. Others with late-onset problems were social drinkers (Neve et al. 1997) or heavy or reactive drinkers (Schutte et al. 1998) in the past. Late-onset alcohol problems are typically milder and more circumscribed than those beginning earlier in life. Compared with those with early-onset problem drinking, those with late-onset problem drinking tend to have less alcoholism among relatives, less psychopathology, and higher socioeconomic status, and a larger proportion are women (Atkinson 1994; Liberto and Oslin 1995). Although clinical evidence supports the view that late-onset drinking problems often begin in reaction to life stress (e.g., Finlayson et al. 1988), it is not true that those with late-onset drinking problems exhibit more reactive drinking than those with early-onset drinking problems. Compared with alcoholism of long duration, late-onset drinking problems tend to resolve more often without formal treatment (Moos et al. 1991) and may be more amenable to treatment (Atkinson 1994, 1995; Atkinson et al. 1993; Schonfeld and Dupree 1991).

Therapeutic Use and Health Maintenance Value of Alcohol

Use for socialization and appetite. The use of small amounts of beverage alcohol has been advocated as a social adjuvant in elder residential care facilities (reviewed in Atkinson and Kofoed 1984). Similarly, alcohol is often touted as an appetite stimulant: in healthy elderly persons

caloric intake and blood levels of some micronutrients may increase with alcohol intake, though other micronutrient levels decrease (Jacques et al. 1989). Clinicians who advise outpatients to use alcohol should beware that in the residential studies mentioned above the quantity of alcohol consumed was regulated and its use within a social context was ensured. Iatrogenic alcohol use disorders do occur. Alcohol as an "aid" for sleep is discussed below.

Protective value of alcohol against coronary heart disease. Consumption of regular but moderate amounts of alcohol (up to two drinks per day) tends to be associated with lower morbidity and mortality from coronary artery disease (CAD), especially in men, compared with that in heavy alcohol users and abstainers. This "U"- or "J"-shaped relationship appears to be quite robust. Explanations for a protective effect of alcohol in CAD include that alcohol elevates plasma levels of high-density lipoprotein cholesterol, reduces blood platelet aggregation, and has other anticoagulant effects, although under some circumstances alcohol also increases selected hemostatic processes (Davidson 1989; Srivastava et al. 1994). The antioxidant effects of beverage alcohol might also play a role (Artaud-Wild et al. 1993; Soleas et al. 1997). The heterogeneous abstainer group might be expected to include subgroups at high risk for CAD, for example, former drinkers and others with poor health, which might also explain why abstainers fare worse than moderate drinkers. Unfortunately, a number of reported studies did not characterize their abstainer cohorts. These include two studies reporting a protective effect that focused exclusively on the elderly (Colditz et al. 1985; Scherr et al. 1992).

Protective value against other health problems. A more general apparent protective effect of moderate drinking on mortality from all causes has been demonstrated in several studies (e.g., Colditz et al. 1985; Mertens et al. 1996; Thun et al. 1997), even taking into account those diseases for which increasing alcohol consumption is clearly associated with higher mortality. In one study of 490,000 persons age 35–70, moderate drinking reduced overall mortality by about 20%, although much of this general effect on mortality may be related to cardiovascular disease (Thun et al. 1997). Recent reports that moderate alcohol intake (especially red table wine) may have a beneficial effect on cognitive status (Christian et al. 1995; Dufouil et al. 1997; Letenneur et al. 1993; Orgogozo et al. 1997) and a possible protective effect against development of age-related retinal macular degeneration (Obisesan et al. 1998) require further study. An unexpected finding in several studies of alcohol and mortality that focused on older persons is that, in contrast to findings in studies of younger and mixed-age cohorts, no significant increase in mortality risk was found among heavier-drinking older adults with regard to CAD (Klatsky et al. 1981, 1992), cardiovascular disease in general (Thun et al. 1997), or mortality from all causes (Mertens et al. 1996). Possible explanations for this finding have included a selective survival effect, that is, that only healthier heavy drinkers survive to older ages, or moderation or cessation of drinking with age, so that former heavy drinkers now appear in the abstainer and moderate-drinking categories (Mertens et al. 1996).

Safe drinking levels in old age. Although evidence is accumulating that modest regular drinking has protective effects on health, not all recent large surveys confirm this finding (Hanna et al. 1997). Clinicians advising patients whether to drink obviously must weigh the possible protective effects of alcohol in light of the health status of the individual patient. Patients who already have cardiovascular, hepatic, neoplastic, or organic mental diseases should not drink, nor should patients receiving complex medication regimens. Deaths from disorders made worse by alcohol clearly increase with an increase in alcohol consumption level (Thun et al. 1997). The National Institute on Alcohol Abuse and Alcoholism currently recommends that physically fit older adults drink an average of no more than one standard drink daily, or seven drinks per week, and no more than two drinks per drinking occasion (National Institute on Alcohol Abuse and Alcoholism 1995).

Clinical Features, Complications, and Course of Alcohol Use Disorders

Primary and associated features; screening and diagnosis. Little evidence suggests that the elderly population differs greatly from other age groups in the primary manifestations of alcohol dependence (Table 16–2), even though several of the criteria for alcohol dependence (i.e., those related to social consequences) have questionable relevance for some elderly persons (Atkinson 1990). However, differences have been found between older and younger alcoholic patients. Biomedical consequences and complications become more evident with age, as previously discussed. Older people with alcoholism, especially women, more often drink alone at home than do younger people with alcoholism, and they are more likely to drink in response to negative affects, such as depression or loneliness, whereas younger people with alcoholism drink in response to a wider variety of personal and social

circumstances (Schonfeld et al. 1995). People with late-onset alcoholism may show fairly mild impairment, evidence for abuse but not dependence, and little evidence of either physical or psychiatric comorbidity (Atkinson 1994; Atkinson et al. 1990; Liberto and Oslin 1995). The CAGE test is an effective screening device for alcoholism in the elderly (Buchsbaum et al. 1992; T. V. Jones et al. 1993; Joseph et al. 1995; Morton et al. 1996), as is the MAST-G, a version of the Michigan Alcoholism Screening Test designed for the elderly (Blow et al. 1992b; Joseph et al. 1995; Morton et al. 1996). Not all studies agree that these screening questionnaires are sufficiently sensitive and specific in the elderly (Luttrell et al. 1997), and the CAGE was shown in one large study to be inadequate to identify at-risk drinkers or binge drinkers (W. L. Adams et al. 1996). It is also necessary to inquire about quantity and frequency of drinking because alcohol consumption is not surveyed by either the CAGE, the MAST-G, or DSM-IV alcohol use disorder criteria. Several characteristic laboratory abnormalities accompanying many cases of alcohol dependence are listed in Table 16–5.

Medical complications. Older patients with alcoholism are at high risk for development of multiple medical problems (Piette et al. 1998); these have been reviewed extensively elsewhere (Gambert and Katsoyannis 1995; J. W. Smith 1995). Alcohol-related liver disease, when present, carries a poor prognosis if drinking continues (Woodhouse and James 1985). A number of cancers (mouth, esophagus, pharynx, larynx, liver, colorectal), hypoglycemia, hyperuricemia, hypertriglyceridemia, osteoporosis, anemias, congestive heart failure, aspiration pneumonia, and accidental injuries can also be caused or aggravated by alcohol dependence. Breast cancer in one large recent survey was 1.3 times more common in women who currently drink than in nondrinkers (Thun et al. 1997). Control of hypertension and diabetes mellitus is compromised by excessive drinking. Alcohol-associated mental disorders and psychiatric comorbidities are considered separately below.

Adverse drug reactions. Several varieties of problematic alcohol-drug interactions can occur. Acute doses of alcohol compete with many medications for hepatic drug-metabolizing enzymes in the cytochrome P450 system, which can produce higher than desired drug blood levels (Lieber 1991; see also Chapter 34 in this volume). Long-term alcohol dosing, on the other hand, induces the cytochrome P450 system and can lead to more rapid metabolism of the same medications, with resulting lower than desired drug blood levels. Drugs commonly prescribed for the elderly that may be affected include warfa-

TABLE 16–5. Frequency of laboratory abnormalities in elderly and younger inpatients with alcoholism

	Results			
	Patients ≥ 65 years[a]		Younger patients[b]	
Blood tests	Number	Percent	Number	Percent
MCH increased	213	71	123	57*
AST increased	214	56	123	42**
GGT increased	123	55	101	48
MCV increased	213	44	124	17*
Glucose increased	206	32	124	36
Uric acid increased	201	21	123	< 1*
Albumin decreased	186	17	115	3*
Alkaline phosphatase increased	213	11	123	15
Triglycerides increased	191	16	122	19
Phosphorus increased	198	9	124	11

Note. Number refers to the number of patients tested in each age group; percent is the percent of patients tested in the age group who had an abnormal value. AST = aspartate aminotransferase; GGT = γ-glutamyltransferase; MCH = mean corpuscular hemoglobin; MCV = mean corpuscular volume.

[a]Older patients: $N = 216$; mean age 69.6 years; age range 65–83 years.

[b]Younger patients: $N = 125$; mean age 44.3 years; age range 19–64 years.

*$P < .01$ using Wilcoxon two-sample rank sum test to compare age groups for proportion having an abnormal value.

**$P < .05$; for others, $P > .3$.

Source. Adapted from Hurt et al. 1988.

rin, phenytoin, most benzodiazepines, and propranolol. Inhibition of hepatic alcohol dehydrogenase by such drugs as chlorpromazine and isoniazid or inhibition of gastric alcohol dehydrogenase by histamine receptor antagonists (e.g., cimetidine, ranitidine, nizatidine) can reduce alcohol metabolism and lead to higher blood alcohol levels (W. L. Adams 1995). Alcohol acts in the brain to intensify the depressant effects of opioids and sedative-hypnotic agents (Korrapati and Vestal 1995). When regular heavy drinking accompanies use of nonsteroidal anti-inflammatory drugs, bleeding times may be increased and the risk of gastrointestinal hemorrhage is higher (W. L. Adams 1995). Details of these and other clinically hazardous alcohol-medication interactions have recently been reviewed elsewhere (W. L. Adams 1995; Korrapati and Vestal 1995).

Course. The span from onset of the first alcohol problem to date of entry into current treatment can be as long as 50 years, and over this course, drinking may have been steady, progressive, or fluctuating. In some cases, sober periods of 10 years or more occur between problem drinking episodes. People with late-onset problem drinking often resolve their problems without formal treatment (Moos et al. 1991), and many with early-onset alcoholism can and do achieve long-term abstinence or controlled, problem-free drinking, with or without treatment (Chermack et al. 1996a; Vaillant 1995). Older alcoholic patients who com-

plete treatment have variable outcomes: younger age, unmarried status, and psychiatric comorbidity predicted 4-year readmission for drinking relapse in one nationwide study (Moos et al. 1994). Although cross-sectional surveys that are further stratified for age after 60 indicate that as many as 25% of persons age 85 and older continue to use alcohol in modest amounts (Ruchlin 1997), rates of *problem* drinking after age 85 are negligible.

Alcohol-Associated Mental Disorders

Alcohol-associated mental disorders are listed in Table 16–6 and described in standard texts on neuropsychiatry (Lishman 1997; Yudofsky and Hales 1997). Selected features of these disorders are highlighted that have special relevance to geriatric alcoholism and geriatric neuropsychiatry.

Aging and alcohol neurotoxicity. Although one strongly supported perspective is that all alcohol-related brain damage is a consequence primarily of thiamine deficiency and thus related to the Wernicke-Korsakoff syndrome ("continuity theory") (Langlais 1995; Victor et al. 1989), alcohol itself is a potent neurotoxin that may cause central nervous system (CNS) pathology, especially cortical damage. Evidence for an age-associated increase in CNS sensitivity to alcohol has been demonstrated

TABLE 16–6. Alcohol-associated mental disorders

Disorders manifested primarily by altered mental status

Alcohol intoxication

    Simple intoxication

    Idiosyncratic intoxication

    Alcohol blackout

Alcohol withdrawal syndromes

    Uncomplicated alcohol withdrawal (tremulous
        syndrome)

    Alcohol hallucinosis

    Alcohol withdrawal seizures ("rum fits")

    Alcohol withdrawal delirium (delirium tremens, or
        "DTs")

Wernicke-Korsakoff syndrome

    Wernicke's encephalopathy

    Alcohol amnestic disorder (Korsakoff's psychosis)

Other cognitive disorders related to alcohol neurotoxicity

    Alcoholic dementia

    Focal alcoholic cognitive deficits

Alcohol-associated insomnia

Alcohol-associated mood disorder

**Disorders manifested primarily by focal neurological
findings**

Alcoholic peripheral polyneuropathy

Alcoholic cerebellar degeneration

Alcohol-related movement disorder (Parkinson's type)

**Rare neurological disorders associated with chronic
alcoholism**

Marchiafava-Bignami disease

Nutritional amblyopia

Central pontine myelinosis

**Disorders associated with chronic alcoholism, but not
with alcohol neurotoxicity**

Hepatic encephalopathy

Acquired hepatocerebral degeneration

Trauma-induced acute and chronic subdural hematoma

in studies of animals (York 1983) and in nonalcoholic human subjects on measures of subjective intoxication experience (Beresford and Lucey 1995; A. W. Jones and Neri 1985), memory (M. K. Jones and Jones 1980), performance on divided attention tasks (Collins and Mertens 1988), and body sway and hand dexterity (Vogel-Sprott and Barrett 1984) after single alcohol doses. Not all human studies demonstrate an increased pharmacodynamic effect of alcohol with age (Tupler et al. 1995); differences can depend on whether subjects ingest alcohol in a fasted (effect observed) or fed (little or no effect) state (Beresford and Lucey 1995; Lucey et al. 1999; Tupler et al. 1995). A molecular basis for altered pharmacodynamic effects of alcohol with age has

not been determined (Wood 1995). Cognitive performance also tends to be impaired in older social drinkers tested in the sober state, but only at relatively high consumption levels (i.e., more than 21 drinks per week) (Parsons and Nixon 1998). Regional cerebral blood flow is reduced proportionally to reported alcohol consumption level in otherwise healthy elderly volunteers (Meyer et al. 1984).

In mixed-age groups of patients with alcoholism but without an amnestic disorder, alcohol neurotoxicity is suggested by a number of deficits in neuropsychological performance (Parsons 1994; Parsons and Nixon 1993; Ryan and Butters 1986) and by evidence from brain imaging studies of atrophy of the cerebral cortex (Jernigan et al. 1991; Pfefferbaum et al. 1992), corpus callosum (Pfefferbaum et al. 1996), anterior hippocampus (E. V. Sullivan et al. 1995), diencephalon, caudate nucleus, and parts of the limbic system, including the mesial temporal lobe (Jernigan et al. 1991) and thalamus (Kril et al. 1997). Age, rather than duration of alcoholism, tends to be a critical factor in the manifestation of both the psychological and imaging findings. Cortical changes reflect loss of both gray and white matter, occur in older alcoholic individuals beginning about the fifth decade, and are in addition to the changes associated with normal aging (Jernigan et al. 1991; Pfefferbaum et al. 1992, 1997). These losses are especially evident in frontal areas (Kril et al. 1997; Pfefferbaum et al. 1997). Frontal cortical deficits have also been demonstrated in positron-emission tomographic studies in older alcoholic individuals (K. M. Adams et al. 1993; Gilman et al. 1990), as well as in studies of regional cerebral blood flow (Berglund and Ingvar 1976; Kril et al. 1997) and event-related potentials (Biggins et al. 1995).

Studies of mixed-age persons with chronic alcoholism suggest that these frontal cortical deficits are related to impairment in neuropsychological performance: indeed, the pattern of test performance deficits in patients with chronic alcoholism has in recent years prompted the "frontal lobe hypothesis" (Oscar-Berman and Hutner 1993). According to this view, the vulnerability of the frontal lobes to alcohol accounts for many of the neuropsychological deficits in patients with chronic alcoholism, including problem solving, abstraction, organization, judgment, and working memory (studies reviewed in Kril et al. 1997; Pfefferbaum et al. 1997). On the other hand, recent research also indicates widespread damage throughout the brain, and other models besides the frontal lobe hypothesis can explain a number of performance deficits in persons with chronic alcoholism who do not have an amnestic disorder (Evert and Oscar-Berman 1995). For example, deficits in visual-spatial-motor skills may instead be associated with tissue loss in the anterior parietal cortex (Pfefferbaum et al. 1997) or with ventricular dilation rather than cortical atrophy (DiSclafani et al. 1995). Furthermore, ample evidence indicates tissue loss in deeper diencephalic and limbic structures in nonamnesic patients (Jernigan et al. 1991), which might be the primary basis for cerebral dysfunction and even cortical tissue loss (in accord with the "continuity theory") (Langlais 1995).

Histopathological findings in older persons with alcoholism include neuron loss and damage (Samorajski et al. 1984) and reduced dendritic connections (Ryan and Butters 1986). Several studies point in particular to changes in the frontal cortex (e.g., neuron loss, shrinkage of the neuronal soma, and loss or shrinkage of large pyramidal cells from the superior frontal cortex) in people with chronic alcoholism (Harper and Kril 1989, 1990; Kril and Harper 1989). Such changes also occur with normal aging (Flood 1993; Terry et al. 1987), suggesting that age-related decline in brain structural integrity, especially in the frontal lobes, reduces the margin of safety and leaves the brains of old, relative to young, persons more susceptible to alcohol neurotoxicity (Pfefferbaum et al. 1997).

Alcohol intoxication and withdrawal. Elderly people show increased intoxication after a standard alcohol load compared with younger persons. One factor accounting for this phenomenon is age-associated increase in peak blood alcohol level, related to reduced volume of distribution (Beresford and Lucey 1995; Lucey at al. 1999; Vestal et al. 1977; Vogel-Sprott and Barrett 1984). Peak blood alcohol level in older men and women is about 20%–25% higher than that in younger subjects (Beresford and Lucey 1995; Vestal et al. 1977). Evidence also suggests age-associated increases in brain sensitivity to alcohol (see discussion above). Other factors that can cause greater intoxication in older patients include possible age-associated reduction in gastric (but not hepatic) metabolism of alcohol (Hahn and Burch 1983; Pedrosa et al. 1996), potentiation of alcohol effects on the brain by concurrently used medications, comorbid cognitive disorders, and comorbid medical disorders (e.g., those that influence circulation and hepatic function).

In a large series of patients 65 or older who were admitted to an inpatient alcohol treatment unit (Finlayson et al. 1988), major alcohol withdrawal disorders were equally common compared with those in younger cohorts reported elsewhere (Atkinson 1988). In two studies comparing older with younger alcoholic patients undergoing detoxification in a hospital setting, older patients demonstrated more severe and protracted withdrawal signs and symptoms (Brower et al. 1994; Liskow et al. 1989), even though recent alcohol intake was similar in older and younger patients. Rather than age, a longer duration of alcoholism might have explained these group differences in withdrawal severity, but age itself also can play a role. Animal studies have demonstrated age-associated increases in both dependence liability (Ritzmann and Melchior 1984) and alcohol withdrawal severity (Samorajski et al. 1984; Wood 1995), although evidence for increasing dependence liability with age in humans is lacking (Ozdemir et al. 1996).

Slowly resolving cognitive deficits after alcohol withdrawal. Cognition is often impaired in recently detoxified alcoholic individuals of all ages, but deficits are greater and more long-lasting in older patients (Brandt et al. 1983; I. Grant et al. 1984). Impairment immediately after prolonged drinking bouts is probably multifactorial, representing the effects of chronic alcohol neurotoxicity; residual alcohol intoxication; depressed mood; hepatic and metabolic dysfunction (Schafer et al. 1991); alcohol withdrawal itself, especially in older patients (Brower et al. 1994); and effects of sedative medication used to treat withdrawal (Liskow et al. 1989). The often dramatic improvement in cognitive functioning of individuals with chronic alcoholism that typically occurs during the first few weeks of sobriety is attributable to amelioration of all these factors. Improvements in depression and liver dysfunction may be especially important (Schafer et al. 1991). Age, however, is an important predictor of the extent of residual neuropsychological performance deficits after 3–4 weeks of sobriety (Schafer et al. 1991).

These lingering deficits can be focal or patchy (i.e., may affect only one or a few specific cognitive functions) or can be sufficiently widespread to fulfill diagnostic criteria for dementia (Ryan and Butters 1986). DSM-IV offers no diagnostic category for focal abnormalities (apart from the characteristic amnestic disorder of Korsakoff's syndrome). Because focal and even widespread dysfunction may be partially or completely reversible over years of sobriety (Brandt et al. 1983), workers uneasy about the use of the term "dementia" for such conditions have suggested terms such as "reversible alcoholic cognitive deterioration" (Lishman 1997).

Lingering deficits resulting in psychosocial dysfunction occur in younger sober alcoholic individuals, but they are more common in older patients tested beyond 1 month. In one series of 50 male alcoholic outpatients (age 60 and older) who were assessed clinically and neuropsychologically 1–6 months after their last drink, 16% showed focal cognitive deficits whereas another 6% met criteria for dementia (Atkinson and Tolson 1992). In another series, older patients (50–69 years old), who were tested between

1 and 59 months after their last drink, performed less well on several measures of memory and visuospatial tasks than did younger patients and age-matched control subjects (Brandt et al. 1983). Resolution of some deficits (e.g., psychomotor skills and short-term memory) can be demonstrated 5 years or more after initiation of abstinence (Brandt et al. 1983). On the other hand, long-term memory tended to remain impaired even after 7 years of abstinence. These differences suggest different mediating mechanisms for reversible and nonreversible functions (Butters 1985; Ryan and Butters 1986). Corresponding improvement in cortical atrophy has been demonstrated by serial MRI in abstinent older alcoholic patients (Carlen et al. 1986; Ishikawa et al. 1986; Muuronen et al. 1989; Pfefferbaum et al. 1995; Schroth et al. 1988). Regional cerebral blood flow (Ishikawa et al. 1986) also improves with abstinence.

Alcohol-associated dementia and Alzheimer's disease. Whether the dementia associated with chronic alcoholism is distinct from the Wernicke- Korsakoff syndrome or is a part of it is not debated here; this subject is well addressed in other sources (Heindel et al. 1991; Lishman 1997; Ryan and Butters 1986; Victor et al. 1989; Willenbring 1988). However, a clinical dilemma concerning the differential diagnosis of dementia in patients with heavy drinking histories merits discussion. This issue has practical significance for the clinician because the prognosis for alcohol-related dementia is different from that for Alzheimer's disease, provided abstinence can be maintained. For the researcher, paying greater attention in systematic dementia studies to the drinking history and clinical findings typically associated with alcoholism may also clarify the role of alcohol as a risk factor for dementing disorders more generally (Atkinson 1997; Oslin et al. 1998).

Confounding of precise dementia diagnosis by alcoholism and heavy drinking may be a more substantial problem than previously acknowledged. In a British community survey of psychiatric disorders in older adults (Saunders et al. 1991), men with heavy drinking histories were 4.6 times more likely to have a dementia diagnosis than other men. An association between past heavy alcohol consumption and current cognitive disorder was also found in the Epidemiologic Catchment Area study (George et al. 1991). In clinical case series, alcohol-related dementias have typically been reported in 4%–10% of dementias from all causes (e.g., Larson et al. 1984b; Renvoize et al. 1985; Wells 1979). However, in more recently established dementia registries, if patients with heavy drinking histories are included with those having histories of alcohol use disorders, the proportion of cases at least partially attributable to alcohol is considerably higher, having been reported in 14 of 65 patients (21.5%) in one series (King 1986) and in 26 of 120 patients (21.7%) in another (Atkinson and Ganzini 1994; D. M. Smith and Atkinson 1995). And in a study of patients with dementia in long-term care facilities, alcohol was linked to dementia in 31 of 130 patients (24%) (Carlen et al. 1994). Commonly used criteria for primary degenerative dementia of the Alzheimer type prohibit this diagnosis when alcoholism or a history of heavy alcohol consumption is present. On the other hand, nothing in DSM-IV criteria for alcohol-associated dementia, beyond the physician's judgment, distinguishes it from dementias of other etiologies: it is in fact a diagnosis of exclusion. Is alcoholism merely coincident to Alzheimer's dementia (Ryan and Butters 1986; Victor et al. 1989)? Does alcoholism act in a permissive sense to increase the vulnerability of the brain to the development of Alzheimer's dementia, as do such phenomena as repeated head trauma or stroke? Is there a true alcohol-induced dementia, or can alcohol act indirectly but specifically to cause a dementia, for example, by affecting vascular supply to particular brain structures (Fisman et al. 1996)? The answers to these questions are not reliably known (Atkinson 1997; Oslin et al. 1998; D. M. Smith and Atkinson 1995). Imaging of the cerebral cortex may not be helpful because changes of early Alzheimer's disease can be similar to those seen in chronic alcoholism. Short of postmortem brain study, no effective way to clarify the diagnosis has been determined.

Currently efforts are under way to improve differential diagnosis by specifying additional provisional features that appear to be regularly associated with alcoholic dementia (Oslin et al. 1998; Osuntokun et al. 1994; J. Saxton, personal communication, November 1996). Features favoring alcohol-related dementia include 1) history of prolonged heavy alcohol use; 2) presence of peripheral polyneuropathy and/or gait ataxia; 3) sparing of naming (i.e., absence of dysnomia or anomia); 4) presence of other alcohol-related disorders, for example, hepatic cirrhosis; 5) evidence on MRI of *cerebellar* atrophy, especially of the vermis; 6) normal (rather than elevated) cerebrospinal fluid tau protein level; and 7) evidence, after a period of abstinence, of stabilization or improvement in cognitive functioning or reversal of cerebral atrophy seen on MRI (Atkinson 1997; Atkinson and Ganzini 1994; Morikawa et al. 1999; Oslin et al. 1998; Osuntokun et al. 1994; D. M. Smith and Atkinson 1995). This approach to differential diagnosis, if affirmed by prospective studies, may help distinguish more precisely among alcohol-associated dementia, dementia of the Alzheimer type, and mixed cases.

Alcohol-associated insomnia. Insomnia is emphasized because aging and chronic alcohol consumption affect sleep architecture in similar ways: both elderly subjects and recently abstinent alcoholic subjects tend to show frequent awakenings, especially from deep slow-wave sleep, and reduced rapid-eye-movement (REM) sleep (Dustman 1984; see also Chapter 17 in this volume). Put another way, sleep of 40-year-old alcoholic subjects in one study (Dustman 1984) more closely resembled the sleep of healthy elderly individuals than did the sleep of age-matched healthy control subjects. Sleep in recovering alcoholic individuals improves with abstinence, but slow-wave sleep may not reach normal values even after 4 years of abstinence. Advising an older patient to take a drink near bedtime to aid sleep is not warranted; although sleep latency might be reduced by this practice, if continued over time, late-night drinking is likely to exaggerate age-associated alterations of sleep pattern.

Alcohol-associated mood disorder. Depressive symptoms are widespread in newly admitted alcoholic patients of all ages, including the elderly. For example, at entry to a treatment program for alcoholic male veterans 55 years or older, 54% of 135 patients scored 70 or higher (T score) on the Depression Scale of the Minnesota Multiphasic Personality Inventory (MMPI) (R. M. Atkinson, unpublished data, January 1990). Subsyndromal depressive symptoms are much more common than diagnosable depressive disorders, which occurred in 12% of a large series of hospitalized elderly alcoholic patients (Finlayson et al. 1988). These symptoms resolve without specific antidepressant therapy in a majority of alcoholic patients over the first 3–4 weeks of abstinence (Brown and Schuckit 1988). Residual depression after 3 weeks suggests a comorbid mood disorder (Brown et al. 1995). Some workers hypothesize that subclinical chronic depression or a potential depressive diathesis may be manifested by evanescent depressive symptoms in early sobriety or even by alcoholic drinking itself. This suggestion is the rationale for trials of antidepressant drug maintenance of alcoholic patients who do not have a diagnosable comorbid depressive disorder. However, no trial of antidepressant agents in alcoholic patients without clinical depression has demonstrated any effects on subsequent drinking behavior. The high prevalence of depressive symptoms in recently drinking alcoholic patients, evidence that the level and recency of prior alcohol consumption is correlated with depressive symptoms in early abstinence (M. M. Nakamura et al. 1983), and the spontaneous resolution of depressive symptoms with abstention all support the inference that evanescent depression after a drinking bout represents a secondary mood disorder, that is, depression induced by alcohol or alcohol withdrawal (Schuckit et al. 1997). Alcohol

neurotoxicity may itself be the sole cause, although associated alterations in nutrition, sleep, and other organ functions can act together with alcohol to induce depressed mood.

Alcohol-associated movement disorder (Parkinson type). A single report (Carlen et al. 1981) described seven older alcoholic patients (age 53–70) who developed transient parkinsonian symptoms and signs either during alcohol withdrawal or during chronic severe intoxication. Parkinsonism disappeared or improved significantly with reduced alcohol consumption alone. This association is plausible in the light of evidence that alcohol can disrupt striatal dopamine activity (reviewed in Wilcox 1984).

Neuropsychiatric and Substance Comorbidity in Alcohol Use Disorders

Active tobacco dependence is highly prevalent in elderly alcoholic subjects (approximately 60%–70%) (Atkinson and Tolson 1992; Finlayson et al. 1988); active dependence on prescribed sedatives, anxiolytics, and opioid analgesics varies (from 2% to 14%) depending on the cohort studied (Atkinson and Tolson 1992; Blow et al. 1992a; Finlayson and Davis 1994); and recent illicit drug abuse is uncommon. Nonsubstance-related neuropsychiatric comorbidities in clinical data sets vary even more, depending upon the cohort and clinical setting where studied. Data from five recent reports are summarized in Table 16–7. Mood and cognitive disorders are the most common comorbid psychiatric conditions in older patients. Determining in a particular case whether depression or cognitive deficits are secondary to recent alcohol use or represent a true comorbid disorder can be difficult within the usual time constraints of inpatient care or consultation (Atkinson 1998b; in press). A strong association between major depressive disorder and alcohol dependence exists at all ages (B. F. Grant and Harford 1995), and a history of heavy drinking can be a risk factor for the occurrence (Saunders et al. 1991) and severity (B. L. Cook et al. 1991) of subsequent depressive disorders in the elderly. Alcohol problems are found in a significant number of cases of older people who commit suicide (Blazer 1982; Conwell et al. 1990; Grabbe et al. 1997; Martin and Streissguth 1982), although the association of alcoholism with suicide may be stronger in late-middle–aged men than in women or elderly men (Conwell et al. 1990). Functional impairment caused by heavy drinking ranges from mild to very severe, presenting in extreme cases as "senile squalor" or "Diogenes syndrome" (Cooney and Hamid 1995; Kafetz and Cox 1982; MacMillan and Shaw 1966; Wrigley and Cooney 1992).

TABLE 16–7. Studies of psychiatric comorbidity in older patients with alcoholism

Comorbid disorder	Study: authors, year, setting,[a] age group, basis of diagnoses, N					
	Atkinson and Tolson 1992 OP, A, age ≥ 60 DSM-III-R, N = 50	Finlayson et al. 1988 IP, A, age ≥ 65 DSM-III, N = 216	Blow et al. 1992a OP, MH, age 60–69 DSM-III, N = 3,986	Blow et al. 1992a OP, MH, age ≥ 70 DSM-III, N = 543	Speer and Bates 1992 IP, MH, age ≥ 55 DSM-III-R, N = 29	Blixen et al. 1997 IP, MH, age ≥ 60 DSM-IIIR, N = 38
Any other disorder (one or more)	32%	Approximately 50%[b]	48%	55%	100%	100%
Mood disorder	14%	12%	21%	21%	58%	79%
Major depression	0%	8%	9%	12%	33%	(c)
Bipolar/cyclothymic disorder	4%	2%	5%	4%	19%	8%
Dysthymic disorder	10%	1%	8%	5%	7%	(c)
Dementia and cognitive disorders	6%	25%	9%	18%	0%	11%
Anxiety disorder	2%	< 1%	10%	10%	0%	5%
Posttraumatic stress disorder	2%	0%	4%	2%	0%	0%
Schizophrenia	0%	0%	9%	8%	11%	3%
Personality disorder	Not reported	3%	6%	4%	58%	3%

[a]Setting: A = alcohol treatment program; IP = inpatient; MH = mental health or psychiatric treatment program; OP = outpatient. All studies were from a single setting except for Blow et al., which was pooled data from 172 Veterans Administration facilities. [b]Not reported in paper; personal communication from senior author, R.E. Finlayson, 1994. [c]Cases reported as "depression" without distinguishing among major depression, dysthymia, and other types.

Management of Alcohol-Related Disorders in the Elderly

In mild cases (heavy drinking with only mild alcohol-related problems or none), success can often be achieved simply by offering advice to cut down or abstain, accompanied by informal social interventions as needed. The use of a *brief intervention* strategy (i.e., brief sessions of structured patient education, physician advice, and contracting to reduce alcohol intake) has been found to be effective in reducing alcohol consumption by 35% at 1-year follow-up (from 15.5 to 10 drinks per week versus no change in control subjects) in one study of elderly heavier drinkers in primary care settings (M. F. Fleming, K. L. Barry, W. Adams, L. B. Manwell, and M. L. Krecker, unpublished data, June 1997). Brief intervention for older risky drinkers is currently under further study (W. Adams, personal communication, June 1998; Blow 1998).

The person with more severe alcoholism should enter an outpatient geriatric alcoholism treatment program if possible. Successful programs have been set up within geriatric centers and general substance abuse programs (reviewed in Atkinson 1995). Group social treatment (Atkinson et al. 1998; Kofoed et al. 1987) and cognitive-behavioral treatment (Dupree and Schonfeld 1996, 1998) are the predominant models for psychosocial treatment. When a geriatric alcoholism treatment program is not available, individual case management can be effective. Family involvement in treatment improves compliance and outcome (Atkinson et al. 1993). Use of drinking-deterrent drugs must be carefully considered: disulfiram can be hazardous, whereas naltrexone was well tolerated in one study of older patients (Oslin et al. 1997a, 1997b). Acamprosate appears to have a low toxicity profile, but most studies reported to date have excluded patients older than 60 or 65 (e.g., Paille et al. 1995; Sass et al. 1996). Treatment of comorbid disorders (e.g., tobacco dependence; major depression; cardiovascular, hepatic, and musculoskeletal disorders) is essential. Other specific treatment principles have been discussed in detail elsewhere (Atkinson et al. 1998; Center for Substance Abuse Treatment 1998). It is helpful to reassure the patient and family that older alcoholic patients fare as well as, or better than, younger persons in a variety of alcohol treatment settings (Atkinson 1995, 1998a).

In the most complex cases, the patient should be referred to an alcoholism inpatient treatment unit, which is also indicated when outpatient efforts fail. If severe medical or psychiatric complications are present or major withdrawal is anticipated or is already occurring, initial treatment on an acute medical or general psychiatric inpatient unit is warranted. Patients with dementia or chronic psychosis are best managed in a psychiatric day treatment center or home visitation program. Patients with personality disorders and major mental illness can best be managed individually in a psychiatric outpatient clinic, preferably in conjunction with an alcoholism group. Intractable heavy drinking in the face of dementia or other coexisting major mental disorder may force placement in residential care, where, unfortunately, alcoholic patients are not always welcomed (see Chapter 37 in this volume). In a few locales, alcohol-free foster homes and other residential facilities have been established and are staffed by personnel trained to care for recovering alcoholic patients in an accepting manner.

Benzodiazepine Dependence

Among young polysubstance abusers, benzodiazepine abuse includes such behaviors as consumption of the drug outside of medical supervision, use for euphoriant effects, escalation of the dosage over time, and continued use despite adverse social, economic, or legal consequences. This pattern of abuse is distinctly rare among older people (Busto et al. 1986a; Pinsker and Suljaga-Petchel 1984). However, among elderly patients, long-term therapeutic prescribing of benzodiazepines can lead to physical dependence with characteristic symptoms when the drug is discontinued. Three forms of discontinuance phenomena are recognized: 1) *recurrence* symptoms that include reemergence and persistence of the anxiety symptoms for which the drug was originally prescribed; 2) *rebound* anxiety, that is, recurrence symptoms that are temporarily worse than before treatment; and 3) a true *withdrawal* syndrome, that is, signs and symptoms that are time-limited and unlike symptoms of the disorder for which the drug was originally prescribed (American Psychiatric Association 1990). Although discontinuance symptoms occur after stopping a variety of psychotropic agents, the recurrence, rebound, and withdrawal symptoms that follow benzodiazepine cessation are so unpleasant as to promote relapse to drug use in a significant proportion of patients (Roy-Byrne and Hommer 1988).

Epidemiology

Use of benzodiazepines by community-dwelling elderly persons. Benzodiazepines are commonly prescribed for elderly patients, and community-dwelling older persons receive a disproportionate share of

benzodiazepine prescriptions. In 1991, persons 65 or older represented 13% of the United States population but received 27% of all benzodiazepine prescriptions and 38% of prescriptions for benzodiazepine hypnotic agents (Woods and Winger 1995). A survey of all prescriptions for the entire elderly population of British Columbia in 1990 showed that 24% had received at least one benzodiazepine prescription (Thomson and Smith 1995). Moreover, epidemiological studies indicate that courses of therapy are considerably longer in elderly than in younger patients. A large United States survey reported that 44% of older patients, compared with 20% of younger patients, who were prescribed these drugs used them for 4 months or longer (Mellinger et al. 1984). A large community-based study from Great Britain found that nearly 95% of elderly benzodiazepine users, compared with only 43% of young and middle-aged benzodiazepine users, were treated for 4 months or more (Dunbar et al. 1989). Long-term use is more common in older patients whether the drugs are prescribed as anxiolytics or hypnotics (K. Morgan et al. 1988; Smart and Adlaf 1988). A prospective study confirmed that once a benzodiazepine was prescribed, old age, especially if associated with low educational level, was significantly associated with continued prescriptions (Mant et al. 1988).

A 1979 United States national survey found that 1.6% of the population had used benzodiazepines for longer than 1 year (Mellinger et al. 1984); 71% of these long-term users were more than 50 years old. They were more likely than nonusers to report physical health problems, and despite use of these psychotropic drugs they reported considerable residual anxiety and depression. A British study (Rodrigo et al. 1988) found that 41% of long-term users were over age 70 and had used benzodiazepines daily for a mean of 5 years. Most had poor physical health, and a third had depressive disorders. More recent reports (e.g., Isacson et al. 1992; Simon et al. 1996; Thomson and Smith 1995) suggest that this pattern of more frequent long-term prescribing of benzodiazepines for community-dwelling elderly patients has persisted, even in the health maintenance organization (HMO) setting (Simon et al. 1996). Despite many years of continued benzodiazepine prescription, elderly long-term users rarely exceed recommended dosages or escalate their dosage over time (Busto et al. 1986a; Pinsker and Suljaga-Petchel 1984; Salzman 1991). One United States study found that the average daily dose for elderly outpatients rarely exceeded 4 mg in diazepam equivalents (Pinsker and Suljaga-Petchel 1984). Compared with elderly men, elderly women are more likely to receive benzodiazepine prescriptions and are more likely to take these drugs long-term (Ancill and Carlyle 1993; Simon et al. 1996; C. F. Sullivan et al. 1988). In the Liverpool Longitudinal Study of continuing health of community elderly, the female/male ratio of the entire study sample of persons 65 and older was 1.6:1, whereas the gender ratio for benzodiazepine users was significantly higher, 2.5:1 and 4.1:1 in separate years (C. F. Sullivan et al. 1988).

Use of benzodiazepines by institutionalized elderly persons. Among institutionalized elderly persons, physician prescription of benzodiazepines is widespread (see Chapter 37 in this volume). A survey of one state's Medicaid recipients found that 24% of elderly nursing home residents were prescribed a benzodiazepine and that flurazepam, a long half-life hypnotic, was one of the most frequently prescribed psychotropic drugs (Buck 1988). Another survey reported that 28% of 850 residents of intermediate care facilities received a regularly scheduled sedative-hypnotic (Beers et al. 1988). Of those patients prescribed a benzodiazepine, 30% received a drug with a long half-life. These and other studies in nursing homes have documented poorly advised prescribing practices such as benzodiazepine prescription in the absence of a mental disorder for which these agents are indicated, use of benzodiazepines with a long half-life (which are more likely to cause toxicity in the elderly), and use of standing orders for hypnotics as opposed to as-needed prescribing (Beardsley et al. 1989; Beers et al. 1988).

Problematic psychoactive drug–prescribing practices were the target of federal regulations in the late 1980s intended to improve prescribing in nursing homes, but these regulations have produced mixed results with regard to benzodiazepine use. Use of hypnotics has tended to decrease (e.g., Borson and Doane 1997; Lantz et al. 1996), and in some settings benzodiazepine anxiolytic use and use in general have declined as well (e.g., Lantz et al. 1996; Siegler et al. 1997). Studies have demonstrated that strategies to rationalize prescribing can and do reduce benzodiazepine use (e.g., Avorn et al. 1992; Gilbert et al. 1993; Schmidt et al. 1998). However, in a number of recent reports it appears that although inappropriate use of antipsychotic and other psychoactive drug classes may have been curbed by federal regulations, the use of benzodiazepines, especially for anxiety (Borson and Doane 1997), is increasing in many settings—to levels of 30%–40% of nursing home residents regularly receiving these agents (Lasser and Sunderland 1998). Whether this increase indicates improved recognition of anxiety as a result of more rigorous psychiatric assessment also mandated by federal regulation, substitution of benzodiazepines for antipsychotic and other agents controlled by regulation, or other reasons, is uncertain.

Prevalence of benzodiazepine dependence. The prevalence of late-life drug dependence of all types in persons 65 and older reported in community epidemiological surveys is very low (well under 1%), but such data almost certainly do not reflect therapeutic-dose benzodiazepine dependence, which is typically not recognized as such by the patient and poorly measured by the usual criteria for drug dependence. Inferring prevalence of therapeutic-dose dependence from the frequency of discontinuance symptoms is difficult because only true withdrawal symptoms (not recurrence or rebound symptoms) suggest frank physical dependence. True withdrawal signs and symptoms have been reported to occur in 20%–50% of chronic users after discontinuation (Roy-Byrne and Hommer 1988; Schweizer et al. 1990). Clinical reports of sizable samples of prescription drug–dependent older adults are rare, and the few studies available describe cohorts that are not representative of typical older medical outpatients who make up a majority of users (American Psychiatric Association 1990). Two such surveys have shown that, among elderly patients dependent on prescription drugs, benzodiazepines are involved far more often than are opioid analgesics, the next most common class of prescribed agents associated with dependence in this age group (Finlayson and Davis 1994; Holroyd and Duryee 1997).

Adverse Effects of Benzodiazepine Use

Age-associated increase in the neurotoxicity of benzodiazepines. The most important adverse effects of benzodiazepines in the elderly include excess daytime sedation, ataxia, and cognitive impairment. Studies have demonstrated that elderly patients have more adverse effects than do young patients at similar doses of these medications (Greenblatt et al. 1991a, 1991b). After single and multiple doses of benzodiazepines, elderly patients experience substantial impairment in attention, memory, arousal, and psychomotor abilities (Pomara et al. 1991). Among healthy elderly patients, single doses of diazepam as low as 2.5 mg can impair immediate and long-term memory and psychomotor performance (Pomara et al. 1985). Cognitive impairment is also more prolonged in older compared with younger patients after single doses of a benzodiazepine (Nikaido et al. 1990). The major effect on memory of acute doses of benzodiazepines is dose-dependent impairment in the acquisition of newly learned information into long-term storage (reviewed in Barbee 1993). Decrements in recall produced by benzodiazepines in elderly persons may be no greater proportionally than those produced in younger persons (Greenblatt et al. 1991c; Hinrichs and Ghoneim 1987; Pomara et al. 1989). However, because of baseline deficits in recall in the elderly, the additional impairment produced by benzodiazepines can represent a more severe compromise (Woods and Winger 1995). Elderly medical and surgical in-patients show deterioration in daytime performance after several nightly doses of even short half-life benzodiazepines such as temazepam (P. J. Cook et al. 1983), and daytime hangover from hypnotics can be especially prominent in frail elderly patients with dementia, hypoalbuminemia, or chronic renal insufficiency (P. J. Cook 1986).

Compared with young patients, elderly patients have more daytime balance impairment after nightly hypnotic treatment (Bonnet and Kramer 1981). Most, but not all, studies of the relationship of benzodiazepine use to risk of falls and hip fractures have shown an association (reviewed in Woods and Winger 1995). Other factors (e.g., concurrent use of other psychoactive and nonpsychoactive medications and alcohol [Neutel et al. 1996]; comorbid neurological and other medical disorders) are important additional risk factors. A large HMO study of persons over 65 demonstrated that any benzodiazepine use was associated significantly with impairment of functional status, independent of comorbid medical disorders (Ried et al. 1998). Benzodiazepines impair the driving skills of many older drivers (American Psychiatric Association 1990; Ray et al. 1992; Salzman 1991). Whether, and to what extent, tolerance develops in older persons to these various adverse brain effects of benzodiazepines are issues that have not been studied adequately (Woods and Winger 1995).

Cognitive impairment and long-term use. Clinical evidence suggests excess cognitive disability and morbidity associated with chronic benzodiazepine use. Continual use of benzodiazepines can result in a dementia-like syndrome in mixed-age (Golombok et al. 1988) and elderly (Larson et al. 1987) patients. Among 35 patients with drug-induced major cognitive disorders, benzodiazepines were the offending agents in 22 (Larson et al. 1987). Memory and other cognitive functions improve after discontinuation of long-term benzodiazepine treatment in younger (Tonne et al. 1995) and older persons (Golombok et al. 1988; Salzman et al. 1992).

Mechanisms underlying age-associated changes in response to benzodiazepines. As a person's age increases, alterations occur in the volume of distribution,

elimination half-life, and clearance of metabolized benzodiazepines, producing higher steady-state plasma drug concentrations (Greenblatt et al. 1991a, 1991b; Ozdemir et al. 1996; see also Chapter 34 in this volume).

However, even when old and young patients have comparable plasma drug concentrations, the elderly develop more sedation, psychomotor impairment, and memory problems (Bertz et al. 1997; Castleden et al. 1977; P. J. Cook et al. 1984; Greenblatt et al. 1991a, 1991b; Swift et al. 1985), suggesting an increased pharmacodynamic effect with age. Basic mechanisms accounting for age-associated increased sensitivity to benzodiazepines have not been determined but may involve postreceptor mechanisms in GABAergic[1] neurons and second messenger systems (Ozdemir et al. 1996).

Discontinuation Phenomena

Types and frequency of symptoms. The reported incidence of benzodiazepine discontinuation symptoms in long-term users (persons who have taken benzodiazepines daily for more than 1 year) varies widely from none to 100%, reflecting heterogeneous characteristics of the patient populations and differing measurement and definition of discontinuance syndromes (Bowden and Fisher 1980; Golombok et al. 1987; Laughren et al. 1982; Noyes et al. 1988; Petursson and Lader 1981). Discontinuance symptoms increase substantially after 8–12 months of daily benzodiazepine use (Rickels et al. 1983) but have been reported in patients taking high-potency, short half-life agents whose duration of daily use was only 4–6 weeks (Higgitt et al. 1985; Murphy et al. 1984; Rickels et al. 1983). Rebound insomnia can occur after 1 week of therapy with a hypnotic (Kales et al. 1979).

Major discontinuance symptoms are listed in Table 16–8. Symptoms that frequently occur after cessation of long-term benzodiazepines are, for the most part, recurrence and rebound phenomena. In a series of studies of mixed-age patients, 90% undergoing gradual discontinuation and 100% undergoing abrupt discontinuation experienced at least mild discontinuance symptoms (Rickels et al. 1990; Schweizer et al. 1990). Milder true withdrawal signs and symptoms (e.g., nausea, anorexia, tinnitus, perceptual distortions, hyperacusis, depersonalization, and derealization) are less common than are recurrence or rebound symptoms, but they may develop in 20%–50% of long-term users after discontinuation (Roy-Byrne and Hommer 1988; Schweizer et al. 1990). Severe withdrawal symptoms

---

[1] γ-aminobutyric acid.

TABLE 16–8.   **Benzodiazepine discontinuance symptoms by frequency**

Frequent	Common	Uncommon[a]
Anxiety	Flulike symptoms (nausea, coryza, lethargy, diaphoresis)	Delirium
Insomnia	Sensitivity to sound, touch, or light	Seizures
Restlessness	Aches and pains	Persistent tinnitus
Agitation	Blurred vision	Depersonalization
Irritability	Depression	Derealization
Muscle tension	Nightmares	Paranoid delusions
	Hyperreflexia	Hallucinations
	Ataxia	Psychosis
	Autonomic hyperactivity	

[a]Typically, when present these represent true withdrawal symptoms.
Source.   Adapted from American Psychiatric Association 1990.

(e.g., delirium, psychosis, and seizures) occur far less often than do milder symptoms. Seizures are more common in patients taking higher than therapeutic doses of benzodiazepines, especially high-potency agents (American Psychiatric Association 1990; Noyes et al. 1988). Both rebound and withdrawal symptoms generally abate within 2–4 weeks of drug cessation, although persistence for months of isolated symptoms such as tinnitus and perceptual distortions has been reported (Busto et al. 1986b; Higgitt et al. 1990; Schweizer et al. 1990).

Presentation of benzodiazepine withdrawal in the elderly.   Benzodiazepine dependence and withdrawal may be overlooked initially in elderly patients who, for example, do not or cannot disclose their daily use of these agents when entering the hospital, and a deteriorating course may be misdiagnosed as myocardial infarction, hypertensive crisis, or infection (Whitcup and Miller 1987). Delirium can be a more common presentation of withdrawal in older patients and be misattributed to other causes (see Chapter 19 in this volume). Withdrawal delirium occurred in 13% (7 of 52) of elderly long-term benzodiazepine users withdrawing abruptly from a mean of 7.75 mg/day of diazepam in one study (Foy et al. 1986). In a study of 45 medical inpatients age 60 and older who developed delirium in the hospital, benzodiazepine use was implicated in 29% of the cases (Foy et al. 1995). In an analysis of 48 case reports of benzodiazepine withdrawal seizures, only nine patients were over age 60, suggesting that elderly patients are not disproportionately represented among patients suffering this adverse event (Fialip et al. 1987).

Age and other factors affecting severity of discontinuance symptoms.   Two studies (Cantopher et al. 1990; Schweizer et al. 1989) found that older pa-

tients reported significantly less severe discontinuance symptoms than did younger patients. Withdrawal and other discontinuance symptoms in the elderly may be attenuated because of lowered prevalence of panic disorders, decreased rate of decline of benzodiazepine plasma levels, altered functional capacity, or age-associated changes in neurotransmitter systems (Schweizer et al. 1989). Other studies have failed to show age-related differences in withdrawal severity, but most excluded patients over age 70 as well as patients with medical problems (Roy-Byrne and Hommer 1988). Several studies have reported on the correlates of withdrawal severity among long-term users, though none has focused on the elderly. The following variables were correlated with increased severity of withdrawal in some but not all studies of mixed-age patients: presence of panic disorder, abrupt drug withdrawal, high-dose dependence, short half-life agents, comorbid alcohol problems, and personality pathology (American Psychiatric Association 1990; Busto et al. 1986b; Noyes et al. 1988; Rickels et al. 1990; Roy-Byrne and Hommer 1988; Schweizer et al. 1990; Tyrer 1989).

Outcome and Management of Benzodiazepine Dependence

Outcome of benzodiazepine withdrawal in elderly patients.   Despite evidence that old age is not associated with more severe withdrawal, the elderly have a poorer outcome after therapeutic attempts to discontinue benzodiazepines. Studies indicate that approximately half of mixed-age patients who participate in a withdrawal protocol successfully complete the program (Busto et al. 1986b; Golombok et al. 1987; Schweizer et al. 1990). Of patients who complete a withdrawal protocol, 50%–70% remain benzodiazepine-free at follow-up ranging from 10 months to 5 years (Ashton 1987; Golombok et al. 1987; Rickels et al. 1991). However, investigators in one study (Holton et al. 1992)—in which abstinence was defined as complete nonuse of benzodiazepines throughout a 5-year period—independently validated the subject's claims of abstinence and reported that only 15% were completely benzodiazepine free during this time period. Older age was associated with both difficulty completing withdrawal protocols and increased likelihood of relapse to benzodiazepine use despite completion of a cessation program (Ashton 1987; Golombok et al. 1987; Holton et al. 1992; Rickels et al. 1991). The mean age of subjects in these follow-up studies was 40–50 years, and numbers of elderly persons were small. Besides older age, risk factors for relapse in studies of mixed-aged patients include casual efforts to discontinue (as opposed to participation in a formal protocol), personality pathology, dependence on agents with short half-lives, higher drug doses, higher caffeine intake, and continued psychiatric symptomatology (American Psychiatric Association 1990; Golombok et al. 1987; Holton et al. 1992; Rickels et al. 1991).

For long-term benzodiazepine users who do succeed in discontinuing use of these drugs, several studies indicate the possibility of at least some improvement in cognitive functioning (Golombok et al. 1988; Salzman et al. 1992; Tonne et al. 1995) and, in addition, improvement, or at least no deterioration, in symptoms of anxiety, depression, and insomnia (e.g., Rickels et al. 1990; Salzman et al. 1992; Schweizer et al. 1990). A study of 76 patients (mean age 62) who were successfully withdrawn from chronic benzodiazepine use found that medical and mental health visits fell from 25.4 per year before detoxification to 4.4 per year afterward (Burke et al. 1995). But other studies suggest that the majority of patients who successfully withdraw from benzodiazepines will continue to experience significant anxiety, depression, and insomnia and thus remain at risk for return to use of these agents (Ashton 1987; Golombok et al. 1987; Holton et al. 1992).

Management of benzodiazepine dependence. Several interventions may decrease the severity of benzodiazepine discontinuation and improve the ability to maintain abstinence. However, few studies have been performed to measure the effectiveness of these interventions in the elderly. Withdrawal severity may be lessened, though rarely completely avoided, by a taper schedule (Busto et al. 1986b). The rate of dose reduction should be based on what can be tolerated by the patient. Considerable slowing of the rate of decrease is often required for the second half of the taper (Higgitt et al. 1985). Several authors have suggested that taper schedules should last at least 4 weeks, with many patients requiring 2–4 months to tolerate complete withdrawal (Higgitt et al. 1985; Noyes et al. 1988; Schweizer et al. 1990). Patients who are dependent on short half-life agents may be more comfortable when tapered using a long half-life agent (Rickels et al. 1990). Adjuvant pharmacological drugs to attenuate discontinuance symptoms are of limited success (Roy-Byrne and Ballenger 1993). Carbamazepine may improve outcome but has not been studied in elderly patients (Schweizer et al. 1991). Some patients will be able to reduce or discontinue benzodiazepines requiring only encouragement and support from the prescribing physician (Cormack et al. 1989; Hopkins et al. 1982). Pharmacological treatment of the comorbid depression found in many benzodiazepine-dependent elderly is recommended. Antidepressants are also an alternative therapy for panic disorder (see Chapter 15 in this volume).

The effectiveness of alternative (nondrug) anxiety reduction techniques is uncertain. Several reports found that psychological approaches are no more likely to improve outcome of benzodiazepine withdrawal than a physician's advice to reduce drug consumption (Fraser et al. 1990; Hopkins et al. 1982; Onyett and Turpin 1988). But psychological therapies (Gilbert et al. 1993; Golombok and Higgitt 1993) and self-help groups (Tattersall 1993) have been shown to be useful adjuncts for some persons withdrawing from these agents. Treatment in an inpatient substance abuse program may be required when benzodiazepine dependence has persisted for many years or is associated with comorbid alcohol or opioid analgesic dependence (Finlayson and Davis 1994). Patients requiring hospital treatment have higher rates of comorbid psychiatric disorders (including somatoform and personality disorders) compared with the rates in elderly primary alcoholic inpatients (Finlayson and Davis 1994).

Benefits of Long-Term Benzodiazepine Use

The benefit of long-term benzodiazepine treatment has generated considerable debate. The long-term use of benzodiazepines as hypnotics has little support because hypnotic efficacy diminishes substantially after several weeks of treatment (American Psychiatric Association 1990; Grad 1995; see also Chapter 17 in this volume). Rebound insomnia after discontinuation of benzodiazepines is a significant clinical problem, especially with agents that have short half-lives (Kales et al. 1979). Patients most likely to receive continued benzodiazepine prescriptions are older people with chronic somatic illness and substantial psychological distress. However, no rigorously designed studies of the efficacy of long-term benzodiazepine prescribing in elderly patients have been published. Some prospective studies of younger patients with anxiety disorders demonstrate no difference in outcome between those treated with anxiolytic drugs and psychotherapy (Catalan et al. 1984). Low-dose dependence is apt to occur with long-term use of any agent in this class (Martinez-Cano et al. 1996). More research is needed on the appropriate indications for benzodiazepine treatment in the elderly.

Most patients do not develop tolerance to the anxiolytic effects of benzodiazepines (American Psychiatric Association 1990). Several authors have proposed that if these patients receive continued benefit from benzodiazepine treatment, ongoing prescription is appropriate (Uhlenhuth et al. 1988; Woods and Winger 1995). Deciding when to prescribe long-term can be difficult, requiring consideration of the patient's relief from morbid anxiety balanced against the hazards of chronic toxicity and physical dependence (Ancill and Carlyle 1993). Long-term, low-dose therapy may be justified especially in patients whose anxiety responds better to a benzodiazepine than to alternative therapies, and who are reliable, have no history of alcoholism or drug addiction, and can be well supervised medically (American Psychiatric Association 1990). In these circumstances, however, the physician should anticipate the likelihood of inducing physical dependence and seek the informed consent of patient and family in deciding how to proceed. Moreover, as in the case of the patient with epilepsy or diabetes mellitus, steps should be taken to protect the patient from inadvertent abrupt drug withdrawal, for example, by clearly documenting in the medical record the status of the patient as a long-term user of benzodiazepines and by educating patient and family never to stop the drug abruptly.

Tobacco (Nicotine) Dependence

Although older adults are less likely to smoke cigarettes than are younger adults, tobacco dependence is the most common of all substance use disorders in the elderly population; is entirely obvious, thus taking no special effort to establish a diagnosis; and arguably accounts for far more medical disability and mortality among elderly persons than dependence on all other substances combined. Because of its low behavioral toxicity, however, tobacco dependence has held little interest for neuropsychiatrists. Compulsive tobacco use is rooted, nonetheless, in an abnormal behavior pattern that is determined by powerful nicotine effects on brain processes.

Epidemiology

The prevalence of smoking declines with age and also has declined among older smokers in recent years. In 1994 national surveys among persons 65 and older, 13% of men and 11% of women reported regular daily cigarette smoking (Husten et al. 1997; National Center for Health Statistics 1996). These rates are considerably lower than those reported for middle-aged adults: in the age group 45–64, 28% of men and 23% of women were current smokers in 1994 (National Center for Health Statistics 1996). A survey of four large, geographically diverse areas in the United States reported the prevalence of current smoking among people over age 84 as ranging from 4.6% to 10.8% in men and from 1.1% to 4.0% in women (Colsher et al. 1990). Although prevalence in older adults has declined substantially over the years 1965–1994, the rate of decline has been slower among this older age group than among others and slower among women than men (Husten et al. 1997; National Center for Health Statistics 1996). In one large elderly cohort followed for 6 years, prevalence of smokers declined from 15% to 9%, reflecting an annual cessation rate of 10% and relapse rate of less than 1% (Salive et al. 1992). In another study, the rate of smoking cessation among older adults rose with increasing educational attainment and was consistently higher for men than for women and higher for whites than for blacks (Husten et al. 1997). A study of 339 current smokers age 50–102 found that they were more likely to be heavily addicted smokers, compared with former smokers (Rimer et al. 1990).

Nicotine-Dependence Disorder

Diagnosis and clinical features. Nicotine is the addictive substance in tobacco, and regular use of tobacco in any form produces a nicotine-dependence disorder. Similar to heroin or cocaine addiction, nicotine dependence is characterized by pursuit of pleasurable effects from nicotine use, a compulsive pattern of use despite knowledge of harmful effects, withdrawal symptoms, tolerance, craving, and relapse after abstinence (Department of Health and Human Services 1988; Hughes et al. 1987; Jarvik and Schneider 1992). Some of the usual criteria for substance dependence (Table 16–2) are not satisfactory because low behavioral toxicity and easy access to relatively cheap tobacco products make several of these criteria irrelevant. Nicotine has euphorigenic properties; smokers claim, and some objective evidence supports, that nicotine improves motor performance and mood and decreases anxiety (Jarvik and Schneider 1992). How the psychotropic effects of nicotine are modified by age has been little researched. When tobacco is discontinued, smokers experience a variety of unpleasant mood and physical symptoms that begin within hours of abstinence. Psychological symptoms include irritability, anxiety, depression, and craving. Physiological symptoms include low energy, concentration difficulties, headache, increase appetite, and nonspecific somatic complaints (American Psychiatric Association 1994; Hughes et al. 1986; Jarvik and Schneider 1992). Investigation into age-related changes in the prevalence or severity of these withdrawal symptoms has been minimal.

Neuropharmacology of tobacco dependence. Nicotine has many effects on the CNS, mediated via widely distributed nicotinic receptors on cholinergic neurons innervating various structures. These effects include increases in cerebral glucose uptake, epinephrine, norepinephrine, arginine, vasopressin, adrenocorticotropic hormone, cortisol, growth hormone, and prolactin; increase in the bioavailability of dopamine; and release of endogenous opioids (reviewed in Brautbar 1995). Of greatest importance from the standpoint of tobacco dependence are the well-established effects of nicotine on midbrain dopamine systems (reviewed in Jarvik and Schneider 1992; Nisell et al. 1995). Like a number of other drugs of abuse such as cocaine, nicotine stimulates these systems: the main effects include increased burst firing in mesolimbic dopamine neurons of the ventral tegmental (VT) area, release of dopamine from the nucleus accumbens, and, in chronic dosing, increased dopamine metabolism in the prefrontal cortex (Nisell et al. 1995). Such actions are known to be associated with reward and reinforcement of learning and cognitive behavior.

These effects not only afford an explanation for tobacco dependence but also may help to explain the high prevalence of cigarette smoking (about 90%) observed in patients with schizophrenia (reviewed in Nisell et al. 1995). Reduced functional activity in the prefrontal cortex ("hypofrontality") has been demonstrated in patients with chronic schizophrenia and is correlated with negative symptoms. The prefrontal cortex provides direct input to dopamine cells in the VT area, and impaired functional activity of the prefrontal cortex in the rat decreases burst firing in dopamine neurons of the VT area (Nisell et al. 1995). Thus high consumption of cigarettes by patients with chronic schizophrenia could be a form of attempted self-medication (Svensson et al. 1990). Cigarette smoking does help to normalize impaired auditory sensory gating in patients with schizophrenia (Adler et al. 1993). Hypofrontality in aging patients with chronic alcoholism is also strongly suggested by the neuropsychological, neuro-

imaging, metabolic, and histopathological data reviewed earlier in this chapter. Thus a compensatory or self-medication hypothesis may also help to explain the high prevalence of smoking (60%–70%) in older patients with alcoholism.

Complications and Comorbidities

Tobacco use is the leading preventable cause of death in adults. Smoking doubles the risk of death from combined causes in persons age 35–70 (Thun et al. 1997), and longevity is inversely associated with cigarette consumption (Goldberg et al. 1996). Smoking increases the risk of a variety of cancers, atherosclerosis, chronic obstructive lung disease, peptic ulcer disease, and osteoporosis (Agner 1985; Hollenbach et al. 1993; Mellstrom et al. 1982; Rundgren and Mellstrom 1984; Tresch and Aronow 1996). Smoking in late life is associated with loss of mobility and poorer physical function (LaCroix and Omenn 1992) and may contribute to malnutrition in frail elderly by promoting weight loss and impairing sense of taste and smell (Rimer 1988). The metabolism of many prescribed drugs is altered by smoking (Dawson and Vestal 1984). Elderly smokers are more likely to consume alcohol (Colsher et al. 1990), and most older alcoholic patients in treatment are current smokers (Atkinson and Tolson 1992; Finlayson et al. 1988). Concomitant smoking cessation should be strongly considered in patients undergoing treatment for alcoholism (Gulliver et al. 1995; Hurt et al. 1995, 1996). Elderly smokers also report higher levels of depressive symptoms than former or never smokers (Colsher et al. 1990). Compared with older current smokers, older smokers who quit have a reduced risk of death that becomes evident within 1–2 years after quitting, and their overall risk of death approaches that of never smokers after 15–20 years of abstinence (LaCroix and Omenn 1992). Risks of coronary events, cardiac death, and death from smoking-related cancer and chronic obstructive lung disease are reduced in smokers who quit, and improvement occurs in pulmonary function and hip bone mineral density after smoking cessation (Hollenbach et al. 1993; LaCroix and Omenn 1992).

Smoking Cessation

Readiness to quit. Ninety percent of all adult smokers who quit do so without a specialized treatment program, typically by stopping abruptly (Fiore et al. 1990). Evidence shows that many older persons who continue smoking want to quit (Rimer et al. 1990), but it is unclear whether they are more (Fiore et al. 1990) or less (Yudkin et al. 1996) successful in quitting when compared with younger smokers. Only a minority report being advised to quit by their physicians (Cox 1993; Rimer et al. 1990). One population-based study found that, among smokers 50 and older, those with adverse health consequences of smoking and those who perceived smoking as an addiction were more likely to be ready to quit (Clark et al. 1997). In a longitudinal epidemiological study of elderly persons in three communities, intercurrent development of myocardial infarction, stroke, or cancer increased subsequent smoking cessation but not relapse (Salive et al. 1992), and among elderly women, but not men, smokers in one community, those reporting clinically significant levels of depressive symptoms were nearly four times more likely to quit smoking than nondepressed women (Salive and Blazer 1993). Among healthy older adults, on the other hand, current smokers may be less likely than younger smokers to believe in the health hazards of smoking and more likely to view smoking as a positive habit to enhance coping, reduce stress, and control weight (Orleans et al. 1994a).

Cessation methods and outcomes in older persons. Some smoking cessation methods (e.g., rapid smoking aversion therapy or medicinal nicotine substitutes such as polacrilex gum or transdermal patches) may be contraindicated in older patients with coronary artery disease, cardiac arrhythmias, hypertension, or diabetes mellitus. Brief intervention in primary care medical settings and self-help guides can, when appropriately tailored to elderly individuals, produce 6-month or 1-year quit rates as high as 20% compared with spontaneous quit rates of 5%–10% (G. D. Morgan et al. 1996; Rimer and Orleans 1994). Transdermal nicotine patch therapy yielded a 6-month quit rate of 29% in one naturalistic study of elderly smokers (Orleans et al. 1994b). Quit rates by any method seem to be influenced favorably by more frequent contact with supervising personnel, although elderly patients voice a preference for minimal contact approaches, which, for economic reasons, should in most cases be tried first. Success in quitting as a result of participation in a smoking cessation program has been found to be associated with previous attempts to quit, desire to quit, confidence in quitting, perceived health benefits, lower nicotine consumption, being married to a nonsmoking spouse, and achieving abstinence from smoking during the first week of treatment (Dale et al. 1997; G. D. Morgan et al. 1996; Yudkin et al. 1996). Older smokers who relapse report the same reasons as younger smokers for their return to smoking: irritability, weight gain, fear of weight gain, friction with family members, and inability to concentrate (Orleans et al. 1994a).

Other Substance Problems in Older Adults

Prescription Narcotic (Opioid) Analgesic Dependence

Old age is associated with the development of a variety of nonmalignant but painful chronic conditions (e.g., arthritis, neuropathies) for which narcotics are frequently, though controversially, prescribed (see Chapter 18 in this volume). Few studies have been published on the prevalence and characteristics of elderly abusers of prescription narcotic analgesics. In one community survey, the 2-week prevalence of prescribed narcotic use was 2.1% in elderly women and 2.3% in elderly men (Chrischilles et al. 1990). Abuse of prescribed narcotics by the elderly appears to be rare (Portenoy and Payne 1992; Porter and Jick 1980) unless the patient was an opioid abuser when young (Jinks and Raschko 1990). Tolerance and physical dependence can occur even in the absence of abuse (Portenoy and Payne 1992). Case series of elderly patients hospitalized for prescription drug dependence indicate that opioid analgesic dependence was less common than dependence on anxiolytic and hypnotic agents (Finlayson and Davis 1994; Jinks and Raschko 1990; Whitcup and Miller 1987), although in one study 49 of 100 inpatients age 65 and older were dependent on opioids (Finlayson and Davis 1994). In a survey of 140 outpatients in a geriatric psychiatry clinic, 1.4% were dependent on prescribed opioids (Holroyd and Duryee 1997). These reports (Finlayson and Davis 1994; Holroyd and Duryee 1997) point to an association of high levels of psychopathology with vulnerability to dependence in older persons taking prescribed opioids.

The degree to which chronic narcotic use causes cognitive impairment remains unknown. One study of middle-aged persons found no evidence of cognitive impairment associated with long-term prescribed narcotics (Hendler et al. 1980). Whether dependence liability changes with age is uncertain (Ozdemir et al. 1996). Codeine and dihydrocodeine are agents frequently used in the elderly; their analgesic effect appears to be mediated by the metabolite morphine. After a single standard morphine dose, elderly subjects, when compared with younger subjects, show higher plasma concentrations and impaired drug clearance (Baillie et al. 1989). Further studies of the pharmacokinetics, CNS pharmacodynamics, and dependence liability of opioid analgesics in the elderly are needed.

Illicit Drug Use and Dependence

Use of illicit drugs is uncommon among the current aging population, and illicit drug use disorders in this age group are rare (Anthony and Helzer 1991; Atkinson et al. 1992). Rates of use and abuse are higher in particular elderly subgroups, for example, aging criminals, long-term heroin addicts, and alcoholic individuals (Atkinson et al. 1992; Miller et al. 1991; Myers et al. 1984).

Illicit opioid dependence. Opioid addicts are the best studied of elderly illicit drug abusers, but elderly individuals constitute a very small proportion of heroin addicts. For example, in 1985 only 2% of all methadone maintenance clients in New York City were older than 60 (Pascarelli 1985). Data from the Drug Abuse Warning Network (DAWN) in 1991 indicated that 1.8% of all reports of heroin/morphine abuse in United States urban emergency departments are in persons older than 55 (National Institute on Drug Abuse 1992a). Development of addiction after young adulthood is rare, and mortality over the course of addiction is high (Atkinson et al. 1992). One United States study that followed heroin addicts for 24 years reported that 27.7% died during this period (Hser et al. 1993). Medical examiner data from the DAWN in 1991 showed that 5.6% of deaths from heroin or morphine occurred in persons older than 55 (National Institute on Drug Abuse 1992b). Older addicts often have comorbid addictions, especially tobacco and alcohol, contributing to disability and early mortality. Besides premature death, another explanation proposed to account for the decrease in elderly opioid addicts was that over time they "matured out," that is, gradually became abstinent (Winick 1962). More recent studies do not support this theory that increasing proportions of addicts become abstinent over time, especially once addiction exceeds 5–10 years (Haastrup and Jepson 1988; Hser et al. 1993). Studies from the 1970s characterized elderly addicts as socially aloof, secretive about their addiction, not otherwise criminally involved, and likely to support their drug habit with part-time licit employment (reviewed in Atkinson et al. 1992), although a more recent study suggests greater involvement in criminal activities by addicts entering their 50s (Hser et al. 1993).

Psychiatric and medical illnesses cause considerable morbidity in elderly addicts. As in younger addicts, elderly addicts experience the medical effects of contaminated needles and impure drugs, which increase their risk of a variety of systemic infections including endocarditis, sepsis, skin and CNS abscesses, and hepatitis B (Novick 1992). Of all elderly individuals with acquired immunodeficiency syndrome, 3% contracted the human immunodeficiency virus through intravenous drug use (Moss and Miles 1987). To some degree, the risk of medical complications is mitigated by the tendency of elderly addicts to practice scrupulous hygiene regarding needles and syringes (Capel et al. 1972; Des Jarlais et al. 1985; Pascarelli and Fischer 1974). Long-term heroin addicts develop neuropsychological and neuroimaging abnormalities (caused by cerebral damage from infections or injected foreign substances) that are likely to further impair their functioning (Schuckit 1977; Strang and Gurling 1989). Aging opioid-dependent people frequently die from the consequences of alcohol and tobacco dependence (Des Jarlais et al. 1985). Lifelong heroin addicts appear to be better managed on methadone maintenance than by drug-free strategies (reviewed in Atkinson et al. 1992).

Other illicit drugs. Little information is available regarding the use of other illicit drugs by the elderly. Combined results of three national representative household surveys, conducted during 1991–1993 ($N = 87,915$), showed 1-year prevalence rates in persons age 50 and older of 0.6% for marijuana use (0.8% in men, 0.5% in women) and 0.1% for cocaine use (0.2% in men, 0.1% in women) (Kandel et al. 1997). Both recreational and medical marijuana users are represented among the older population (Sussman 1997). Recent use of marijuana and cocaine is reported sporadically by older patients (Abrams and Alexopoulos 1988), especially by patients who are alcohol dependent (Miller et al. 1991). Older persons tend to acquire these drugs from their adult children or from younger sexual partners (Atkinson et al. 1998). Virtually nothing is known about age-associated changes in drug-induced psychiatric syndromes or altered treatment needs of elderly illicit drug abusers.

Nonprescription (Over-the-Counter) Drug Use and Dependence

Elderly people commonly use over-the-counter preparations, including vitamins and herbal medicines, such as ginkgo biloba; their use of these substances has been reviewed recently (Ganzini and Atkinson 1996). A potential exists for medical and behavioral problems from habitual overuse of many available nostrums, especially those with sedative, anticholinergic, sympathomimetic, and anti-inflammatory effects, and these effects may be additive to prescribed medications and, in some instances, to the effects of alcohol. Anticholinergics may affect cognition (Ganzini and Atkinson 1996). Chronic salicylate toxicity increases with age and may produce a dementia-like syndrome associated with tinnitus and irritability (Bailey and Jones 1989; Grigor et al. 1987). No data exist about the true extent of dependence on nonprescription drugs in old age.

Summary

In this chapter, the leading substance abuse problems affecting the elderly population are discussed, with special emphasis on neuropsychiatric features of these disorders. Tobacco, alcohol, and controlled prescription drugs, especially the benzodiazepines, present the greatest substance abuse hazards in old age.

Several aspects of substance abuse in old age can be highlighted. Tobacco, the substance most widely abused by elderly people, does not have prominent deleterious neurotoxic effects, though morbid effects on other organ systems such as the vascular system may result in cognitive impairment. Elderly people are more sensitive than younger people are to neurotoxic effects of substances such as alcohol and benzodiazepines. These effects are manifested both as decrements in performance on cognitive testing and as functional decline common to frail elderly such as impairment in activities of daily living or falls.

Illicit drug use by elderly persons is uncommon, but poorly investigated. The recent decade has produced little new information on the demography, characteristics, and treatment of elderly persons who abuse illicit drugs. The increasing prevalence of illicit drug abuse in current middle-aged persons (Glantz and Sloboda 1995; Sussman 1997) suggests that illicit substance abuse among elderly people looms as a possible future public health problem. Information is especially scarce on the neuropsychiatric effects of both licit and illicit opiates.

Fatalism on the part of health care providers regarding substance abuse in old age is misplaced. Studies of alcohol, tobacco, and illicit opiate dependence suggest that if abstinence could not be achieved at a younger age, it may still be achieved at an older age. Significant health benefits occur. Substance abuse may account for the largest portion of treatable dementias, and treatment of substance abuse may result in either arresting or reversing neuropsychiatric dysfunction. Further research is needed on specialized age-appropriate treatment for the substance-abusing elderly person.

References

Abrams RC, Alexopoulos GS: Substance abuse in the elderly: over-the-counter and illegal drugs. Hospital and Community Psychiatry 39:822–823, 829, 1988

Adams KM, Gilman S, Koeppe RA, et al: Neuropsychological deficits are correlated with frontal hypometabolism in positron emission tomography studies of older alcoholic patients. Alcohol Clin Exp Res 17:205–210, 1993

Adams WL: Interactions between alcohol and other drugs. International Journal of the Addictions 30:1903–1923, 1995

Adams WL, Cox NS: Epidemiology of problem drinking among elderly people. International Journal of the Addictions 30:1693–1716, 1995

Adams WL, Garry PJ, Rhyne R, et al: Alcohol intake in the healthy elderly: changes with age in a cross-sectional and longitudinal study. J Am Geriatr Soc 38:211–216, 1990

Adams WL, Magruder-Habib K, Trued S, et al: Alcohol abuse in elderly emergency department patients. J Am Geriatr Soc 40:1236–1240, 1992

Adams WL, Barry KL, Fleming MF: Screening for problem drinking in older primary care patients. JAMA 276:1964–1967, 1996

Adler LE, Hoffer LD, Wiser A, et al: Normalization of auditory physiology by cigarette smoking in schizophrenic patients. Am J Psychiatry 150:1856–1861, 1993

Agner E: Smoking and health in old age: a ten-year follow-up study. Acta Medica Scandinavica 218:311–316, 1985

Alexander F, Duff RW: Social interaction and alcohol use in retirement communities. Gerontologist 28:632–638, 1988

American Medical Association, Council on Scientific Affairs: Alcoholism in the elderly. JAMA 275:797–801, 1996

American Psychiatric Association: Benzodiazepine Dependence, Toxicity, and Abuse. Washington, DC, American Psychiatric Press, 1990

American Psychiatric Association: Diagnostic and Statistical Manual of Mental Disorders, 4th Edition. Washington, DC, American Psychiatric Press, 1994

Ancill RJ, Carlyle WW: Benzodiazepine use and dependency in the elderly: striking a balance, in Benzodiazepine Dependence. Edited by Hallstrom C. New York, Oxford University Press, 1993, pp 238–251

Anthony JC, Helzer JE: Syndromes of drug abuse and dependence, in Psychiatric Disorders in America: The Epidemiologic Catchment Area Study. Edited by Robins LN, Regier DA. New York, Free Press, 1991, pp 116–154

Artaud-Wild SM, Sonnor SL, Sexton G, et al: Differences in coronary mortality can be explained by differences in cholesterol and saturated fat intake in 40 countries but not in France and Finland. Circulation 88:2771–2779, 1993

Ashton H: Benzodiazepine withdrawal: outcome in 50 patients. British Journal of Addiction 82:665–671, 1987

Atkinson RM: Alcoholism in the elderly population (editorial). Mayo Clin Proc 63:825–829, 1988

Atkinson RM: Aging and alcohol use disorders: diagnostic issues in the elderly. Int Psychogeriatr 2:55–72, 1990

Atkinson RM: Late onset problem drinking in older adults. Int J Geriatr Psychiatry 9:321–326, 1994

Atkinson RM: Treatment programs for aging alcoholics, in Alcohol and Aging. Edited by Beresford TP, Gomberg ESL. New York, Oxford University Press, 1995, pp 186–210

Atkinson RM: Alcohol and drug abuse in the elderly, in Psychiatry in the Elderly, 2nd Edition. Edited by Jacoby R, Oppenheimer C. New York, Oxford University Press, 1997, pp 661–686

Atkinson RM: Age-specific treatment for older adult alcoholics, in Alcohol Problems and Aging (NIAAA Research Monograph No 33). Edited by Gomberg ESL, Hegedus AM, Zucker RA. Rockville, MD, U.S. Department of Health and Human Services, 1998a

Atkinson RM: The psychosocial impact of alcoholism in older adults: consequences, complications and comorbidities. Southwest Journal of Aging 14:73–83, 1998b

Atkinson RM: Depression, alcoholism, and aging: a brief review. Int J Geriatr Psychiatry (in press)

Atkinson RM, Ganzini L: Substance abuse, in Textbook of Geriatric Neuropsychiatry, 1st Edition. Edited by Coffey CE, Cummings JL. Washington, DC, American Psychiatric Press, 1994, pp 297–321

Atkinson RM, Kofoed LL: Alcohol and drug abuse, in Geriatric Medicine, Vol 2: Fundamentals of Geriatric Care. Edited by Cassell CK, Walsh JR. New York, Springer-Verlag, 1984, pp 219–235

Atkinson RM, Tolson RL: Late onset alcohol use disorders in older men. Research poster presented at the annual meeting of the American Association for Geriatric Psychiatry, San Francisco, CA, February 1992

Atkinson RM, Tolson RL, Turner JA: Late versus early onset problem drinking in older men. Alcohol Clin Exp Res 14:574–579, 1990

Atkinson RM, Ganzini L, Bernstein MJ: Alcohol and substance-use disorders in the elderly, in Handbook of Mental Health and Aging, 2nd Edition. Edited by Birren JE, Sloane RB, Cohen GD. New York, Academic Press, 1992, pp 515–555

Atkinson RM, Tolson RL, Turner JA: Factors affecting outpatient treatment compliance of older male problem drinkers. J Stud Alcohol 54:102–106, 1993

Atkinson RM, Turner JA, Tolson RL: Treatment of older adult problem drinkers: lessons learned from "the Class of '45." Journal of Mental Health and Aging 4:197–214, 1998

Avorn J, Soumerai SB, Everitt DE, et al: A randomized trial of a program to reduce the use of psychoactive drugs in nursing homes. N Engl J Med 327:168–173, 1992

Bailey RB, Jones SR: Chronic salicylate intoxication: a common cause of morbidity in the elderly. J Am Geriatr Soc 37:556–561, 1989

Baillie SP, Bateman DN, Coates PE, et al: Age and the pharmacokinetics of morphine. Age Ageing 18:258–262, 1989

Barbee JG: Memory, benzodiazepines, and anxiety: integration of theoretical and clinical perspectives. J Clin Psychiatry 54 (10 suppl):86–97, 1993

Barker JC, Kramer BJ: Alcohol consumption among older urban American Indians. J Stud Alcohol 57:119–124, 1996

Barnes GM: Alcohol use among older persons: findings from a western New York State general population survey. J Am Geriatr Soc 27:244–250, 1979

Beardsley RS, Larson DB, Burns BJ, et al: Prescribing of psychotropics in elderly nursing home patients. J Am Geriatr Soc 37:327–330, 1989

Beers M, Avorn J, Soumerai SB, et al: Psychoactive medication use in intermediate-care facility residents. JAMA 260:3016–3020, 1988

Begleiter H, Kissin B (eds): The Pharmacology of Alcohol and Alcohol Dependence. New York, Oxford University Press, 1996

Beresford TP, Lucey MR: Ethanol metabolism and intoxication in the elderly, in Alcohol and Aging. Edited by Beresford TP, Gomberg ESL. New York, Oxford University Press, 1995, pp 117–127

Berglund M, Ingvar DH: Cerebral blood flow and its regional distribution in alcoholism and in Korsakoff's psychosis. J Stud Alcohol 37:386–397, 1976

Bertz RJ, Kroboth PD, Kroboth FJ, et al: Alprazolam in young and elderly men: sensitivity and tolerance to psychomotor, sedative and memory effects. J Pharmacol Exp Ther 281:1317–1329, 1997

Biggins CA, MacKay S, Poole N, et al: Delayed P3A in abstinent elderly male chronic alcoholics. Alcohol Clin Exp Res 19:1032–1042, 1995

Blazer DG: Depression in Late Life. St. Louis, CV Mosby, 1982

Blixen CE, McDougall GJ, Suen L-J: Dual diagnosis in elders discharged from a psychiatric hospital. Int J Geriatr Psychiatry 12:307–313, 1997

Blow FC: The spectrum of alcohol interventions for older adults, in Alcohol Problems and Aging (NIAAA Research Monograph No 33). Edited by Gomberg ESL, Hegedus AM, Zucker RA. Rockville, MD, U.S. Department of Health and Human Services, 1998

Blow FC, Cook CAL, Booth BM, et al: Age-related psychiatric comorbidities and level of functioning in alcoholic veterans seeking outpatient treatment. Hospital and Community Psychiatry 43:990–995, 1992a

Blow FC, Brower KJ, Schulenberg JE, et al: The Michigan Alcoholism Screening Test—Geriatric Version (MAST-G): a new elderly-specific screening instrument. Alcohol Clin Exp Res 16:372, 1992b

Bonnet MH, Kramer M: The interaction of age, performance and hypnotics in the sleep of insomniacs. J Am Geriatr Soc 29:508–512, 1981

Booth BM, Blow FC, Cook CAL, et al: Age and ethnicity among hospitalized alcoholics: a nationwide study. Alcohol Clin Exp Res 16:1029–1034, 1992

Borson S, Doane K: The impact of OBRA-87 on psychotropic drug prescribing in skilled nursing facilities. Psychiatr Serv 48:1289–1296, 1997

Bowden CL, Fisher JG: Safety and efficacy of long-term diazepam therapy. South Med J 73:1581–1584, 1980

Brandt J, Butters N, Ryan C, et al: Cognitive loss and recovery in long-term alcohol abusers. Arch Gen Psychiatry 40: 435–442, 1983

Brautbar N: Direct effects of nicotine on the brain: evidence for chemical addiction (editorial). Arch Environ Health 50: 263–266, 1995

Bristow MF, Clare AW: Prevalence and characteristics of at-risk drinkers among elderly acute medical in-patients. British Journal of Addiction 87:291–294, 1992

Brower KJ, Mudd S, Blow FC, et al: Severity and treatment of alcohol withdrawal in elderly versus younger patients. Alcohol Clin Exp Res 18:196–201, 1994

Brown SA, Schuckit MA: Changes in depression among abstinent alcoholics. J Stud Alcohol 49:412–417, 1988

Brown SA, Inaba RK, Gillin JC, et al: Alcoholism and affective disorder: clinical course of depressive symptoms. Am J Psychiatry 152:45–52, 1995

Buchsbaum DG, Buchanan RG, Welsh J, et al: Screening for drinking disorders in the elderly using the CAGE questionnaire. J Am Geriatr Soc 40:662–665, 1992

Buck JA: Psychotropic drug practice in nursing homes. J Am Geriatr Soc 36:409–418, 1988

Burke KC, Meek WJ, Krych R, et al: Medical services used by patients before and after detoxification from benzodiazepine dependence. Psychiatr Serv 46:157–160, 1995

Busby WJ, Campbell AJ, Borrie MJ, et al: Alcohol use in a community-based sample of subjects aged 70 years and older. J Am Geriatr Soc 36:301–305, 1988

Busto U, Sellers EM, Naranjo CA, et al: Patterns of benzodiazepine abuse and dependence. British Journal of Addiction 81:87–94, 1986a

Busto U, Sellers EM, Naranjo CA, et al: Withdrawal reaction after long-term therapeutic use of benzodiazepines. N Engl J Med 315:854–859, 1986b

Butters N: Alcoholic Korsakoff's syndrome: some unresolved issues concerning etiology, neuropathology, and cognitive deficits. J Clin Exp Neuropsychol 7:181–210, 1985

Caetano R, Tam TW: Prevalence and correlates of DSM-IV and ICD-10 alcohol dependence: 1990 US National Alcohol Survey. Alcohol Alcohol 30:177–186, 1995

Callahan CM, Tierney WM: Health services use and mortality among older primary care patients with alcoholism. J Am Geriatr Soc 43:1378–1383, 1995

Cantopher T, Olivieri S, Cleave N, et al: Chronic benzodiazepine dependence: a comparative study of abrupt withdrawal under propranolol cover versus gradual withdrawal. Br J Psychiatry 156:406–411, 1990

Capel WC, Goldsmith BM, Waddell KJ, et al: The aging narcotic addict: an increasing problem for the next decades. J Gerontol 27:102–106, 1972

Carlen PL, Lee MA, Jacob M, et al: Parkinsonism provoked by alcoholism. Ann Neurol 9:84–86, 1981

Carlen PL, Penn RD, Fornazzari L, et al: Computerized tomographic scan assessment of alcoholic brain damage and its potential reversibility. Alcohol Clin Exp Res 10: 226–232, 1986

Carlen PL, McAndrews MP, Weiss RT, et al: Alcohol-related dementia in the institutionalized elderly. Alcohol Clin Exp Res 18:1330–1334, 1994

Castleden CM, George CF, Marcer D, et al: Increased sensitivity to nitrazepam in old age. BMJ 1:10–12, 1977

Catalan J, Gath D, Edmonds G, et al: The effects of non-prescribing of anxiolytics in general practice, I: controlled evaluation of psychiatric and social outcome. Br J Psychiatry 144:593–602, 1984

Center for Substance Abuse Treatment: Substance Abuse Among Older Adults: Treatment Improvement Protocol No 26 (DHHS Publ No SMA-98-3179). Rockville, MD, U.S. Department of Health and Human Services, 1998

Chermack ST, Blow FC, Gomberg ES, et al: Older adult controlled drinkers and abstainers. J Subst Abuse 8:453–462, 1996a

Chermack ST, Blow FC, Hill EM, et al: The relationship between alcohol symptoms and consumption among older drinkers. Alcohol Clin Exp Res 20:1153–1158, 1996b

Chrischilles EA, Lemke JH, Wallace RB, et al: Prevalence and characteristics of multiple analgesic drug use in an elderly study group. J Am Geriatr Soc 38:979–984, 1990

Christian JC, Reed T, Carmelli D, et al: Self-reported alcohol intake and cognition in aging twins. J Stud Alcohol 56:414–416, 1995

Clark MA, Rakowski W, Kviz FJ, et al: Age and stage of readiness for smoking cessation. J Gerontol 52:S212–S221, 1997

Colditz GA, Branch LG, Lipnick RJ, et al: Moderate alcohol and decreased cardiovascular mortality in an elderly cohort. Am Heart J 109:886–889, 1985

Collins WE, Mertens HW: Age, alcohol, and simulated altitude: effects on performance and breathalyser scores. Aviat Space Environ Med 59:1026–1033, 1988

Colsher PL, Wallace RB, Pomrehn PR, et al: Demographic and health characteristics of elderly smokers: results from established populations for epidemiologic studies of the elderly. Am J Prev Med 6:61–70, 1990

Conwell Y, Rotenberg M, Caine ED: Completed suicide at age 50 and over. J Am Geriatr Soc 38:640–644, 1990

Cook BL, Winokur G, Garvey MJ, et al: Depression and previous alcoholism in the elderly. Br J Psychiatry 158:72–75, 1991

Cook PJ: Benzodiazepine hypnotics in the elderly. Acta Psychiatr Scand Suppl 332:149–158, 1986

Cook PJ, Higgett A, Graham-Pole R, et al: Hypnotic accumulation and hangover in elderly inpatients: a controlled double blind study of temazepam and nitrazepam. BMJ 286: 100–102, 1983

Cook PJ, Flanagan R, James IM: Diazepam tolerance: effect of age, regular sedation, and alcohol. BMJ 289:351–353, 1984

Cooney C, Hamid W: Review: Diogenes syndrome. Age Ageing 24:451–453, 1995

Cormack MA, Owens RG, Dewey ME: The effect of minimal interventions by general practitioners on long-term benzodiazepine use. Journal of the Royal College of General Practitioners 39:408–411, 1989

Cox JL: Smoking cessation in the elderly patient. Clin Chest Med 14:423–428, 1993

Curtis JR, Geller G, Stokes EJ, et al: Characteristics, diagnosis, and treatment of alcoholism in elderly patients. J Am Geriatr Soc 37:310–316, 1989

Dale LC, Olsen DA, Patten CA, et al: Predictors of smoking cessation among elderly smokers treated for nicotine dependence. Tob Control 6:181–187, 1997

Davidson DM: Cardiovascular effects of alcohol. West J Med 151:430–439, 1989

Dawson GW, Vestal RE: Smoking, age, and drug metabolism, in Smoking and Aging. Edited by Bosse R, Rose CL. Lexington, MA, Lexington Books, 1984, pp 131–156

DeMallie DA, North CS, Smith EM: Psychiatric disorders among the homeless: a comparison of older and younger groups. Gerontologist 37:61–66, 1997

Department of Health and Human Services: The Health Consequences of Smoking: Nicotine Addiction—A Report of the Surgeon General (DHHS Publ No CDC-88-8406). Washington, DC, U.S. Government Printing Office, 1988

Des Jarlais DC, Joseph H, Courtwright DT: Old age and addiction: a study of elderly patients in methadone maintenance treatment, in The Combined Problems of Alcoholism, Drug Addiction and Aging. Edited by Gottheil E, Druley KA, Skoloda TE, Waxman HM. Springfield, IL, Charles C Thomas, 1985, pp 201–209

DiSclafani V, Ezekial F, Meyerhoff DJ, et al: Brain atrophy and cognitive function in older abstinent alcoholic men. Alcohol Clin Exp Res 19:1121–1126, 1995

Dufouil C, Ducimetiere P, Alperovitch A: Sex differences in the association between alcohol consumption and cognitive performance. Am J Epidemiol 146:405–412, 1997

Dunbar GC, Perera MH, Jenner FA: Patterns of benzodiazepine use in Great Britain as measured by a general population survey. Br J Psychiatry 155:836–841, 1989

Dupree LW, Schonfeld L: Substance abuse, in Psychological Treatment of Older Adults: An Introductory Textbook. Edited by Hersen M, Van Hasselt VB. New York, Plenum, 1996, pp 281–297

Dupree LW, Schonfeld L: Cognitive-behavioral and self-management treatment of older problem drinkers. Journal of Mental Health and Aging 4:215–232, 1998

Dustman RE: Alcoholism and aging: electrophysiological parallels, in Alcoholism in the Elderly. Social and Biomedical Issues. Edited by Hartford JT, Samorajski T. New York, Raven, 1984, pp 201–225

Eaton WW, Kramer M, Anthony JC, et al: The incidence of specific DIS/DSM-III mental disorders: data from the NIMH Epidemiologic Catchment Area Program. Acta Psychiatr Scand 79:163–178, 1989

Evert DL, Oscar-Berman M: Alcohol-related cognitive impairments: an overview of how alcoholism may affect the workings of the brain. Alcohol Health Res World 19:89–96, 1995

Fialip J, Aumaitre O, Eschalier A, et al: Benzodiazepine withdrawal seizures: analysis of 48 case reports. Clin Neuropharmacol 10:538–544, 1987

Finlayson RE, Davis LJ Jr: Prescription drug dependence in the elderly population: demographic and clinical features of 100 inpatients. Mayo Clin Proc 69:1137–1145, 1994

Finlayson RE, Hurt RD, Davis LJ Jr, et al: Alcoholism in elderly persons: a study of the psychiatric and psychosocial features of 216 inpatients. Mayo Clin Proc 63:761–768, 1988

Finney JW, Moos RH: Life stressors and problem drinking among older persons, in Recent Developments in Alcoholism, Vol 2. Edited by Galanter M. New York, Plenum, 1984, pp 267–288

Fiore MC, Novotny TE, Pierce JP, et al: Methods used to quit smoking in the United States. JAMA 263:2760–2765, 1990

Fisman M, Ramsay D, Weiser M: Dementia in the elderly alcoholic—a retrospective clinico-pathological study. Int J Geriatr Psychiatry 11:209–218, 1996

Flood DG: Critical issues in the analysis of dendritic extent in aging humans, primates, and rodents. Neurobiol Aging 14:649–654, 1993

Foy A, Drinkwater V, March S, et al: Confusion after admission to hospital in elderly patients using benzodiazepines. BMJ 293:1072, 1986

Foy A, O'Connell D, Henry D, et al: Benzodiazepine use as a cause of cognitive impairment in elderly hospital inpatients. J Gerontol A Biol Sci Med Sci 50:M99–M106, 1995

Fraser D, Peterkin GSD, Gamsu CV, et al: Benzodiazepine withdrawal: a pilot comparison of three methods. Br J Clin Psychol 29:231–233, 1990

Freund G: Drug- and alcohol-induced dementias, in Geriatric Clinical Pharmacology. Edited by Wood WG, Strong R. New York, Raven, 1987, pp 95–105

Gambert SR, Katsoyannis KK: Alcohol-related medical disorders of older heavy drinkers, in Alcohol and Aging. Edited by Beresford TP, Gomberg ESL. New York, Oxford University Press, 1995, pp 70–81

Ganzini L, Atkinson RM: Substance abuse, in Comprehensive Review of Geriatric Psychiatry—II, 2nd Edition. Edited by Sadevoy J, Lazarus LW, Jarvik LF, Grossberg GT. Washington, DC, American Psychiatric Press, 1996, pp 659–692

George LK, Landerman R, Blazer DG, et al: Cognitive impairment, in Psychiatric Disorders in America: The Epidemiologic Catchment Area Study. Edited by Robins LN, Regier DA. New York, Free Press, 1991, pp 291–327

Gilbert A, Innes JM, Owen N, et al: Trial of an intervention to reduce chronic benzodiazepine use among residents of aged-care accomodation. Aust N Z J Med 23:343–347, 1993

Gilman S, Adams K, Koeppe RA, et al: Cerebellar and frontal hypometabolism in alcoholic cerebellar degeneration studied with positron emission tomography. Ann Neurol 28: 775–785, 1990

Glantz MD, Sloboda Z: The elderly, in Handbook on Drug Abuse Prevention. Edited by Coombs RH, Ziedonis D. Boston, MA, Allyn and Bacon, 1995

Glynn RJ, Bouchard GR, LoCastro JS, et al: Aging and generational effects on drinking behaviors in men: results from the Normative Aging Study. Am J Public Health 75: 1413–1419, 1985

Goldberg RJ, Larson M, Levy D: Factors associated with survival to 75 years of age in middle-aged men and women. The Framingham Study. Arch Intern Med 156:505–509, 1996

Golombok S, Higgitt A: Psychological treatments for benzodiazepine dependence, in Benzodiazepine Dependence. Edited by Hallstrom C. New York, Oxford University Press, 1993, pp 296–309

Golombok S, Higgitt A, Fonagy P, et al: A follow-up study of patients treated for benzodiazepine dependence. Br J Med Psychol 60:141–149, 1987

Golombok S, Moodley PJ, Lader M: Cognitive impairment in long-term benzodiazepine users. Psychol Med 18: 365–374, 1988

Gomberg ESL, Nelson BW: Black and white older men: alcohol use and abuse, in Alcohol and Aging. Edited by Beresford TP, Gomberg ESL. New York, Oxford University Press, 1995, pp 307–323

Gordon T, Kannel WB: Drinking and its relation to smoking, BP, blood lipids, and uric acid. Arch Intern Med 143: 1366–1374, 1983

Grabbe L, Demi A, Camann MA, et al: The health status of elderly persons in the last year of life: a comparison of deaths by suicide, injury, and natural causes. Am J Public Health 87:434–437, 1997

Grad RM: Benzodiazepines for insomnia in community-dwelling elderly: a review of benefit and risk. J Fam Pract 41:473–481, 1995

Grant BF: Prevalence and correlates of alcohol use and DSM-IV alcohol dependence in the United States: results of the National Longitudinal Alcohol Epidemiologic Survey. J Stud Alcohol 58:464–473, 1997

Grant BF, Harford TC: Comorbidity between DSM-IV alcohol use disorders and major depression: results of a national survey. Drug Alcohol Depend 39:197–206, 1995

Grant I, Adams KM, Reed R: Aging, abstinence, and medical risk factors in the prediction of neuropsychologic deficit among long-term alcoholics. Arch Gen Psychiatry 41: 710–718, 1984

Greenblatt DJ, Harmatz JS, Shader RI: Clinical pharmacokinetics of anxiolytics and hypnotics in the elderly: therapeutic considerations (Part I). Clin Pharmacokinet 21:165–177, 1991a

Greenblatt DJ, Harmatz JS, Shader RI: Clinical pharmacokinetics of anxiolytics and hypnotics in the elderly: therapeutic considerations (Part II). Clin Pharmacokinet 21:262–273, 1991b

Greenblatt DJ, Jerold SH, Shapiro L, et al: Sensitivity to triazolam in the elderly. N Engl J Med 324:1691–1698, 1991c

Grigor RR, Spitz PW, Furst DE: Salicylate toxicity in elderly patients with rheumatoid arthritis. J Rheumatol 14:60–66, 1987

Gulliver SB, Rohsenow DJ, Colby SM, et al: Interrelationship of smoking and alcohol dependence, use and urges to use. J Stud Alcohol 56:202–206, 1995

Haastrup S, Jepson PW: Eleven year follow-up of 300 young opioid addicts. Acta Psychiatr Scand 77:22–26, 1988

Hahn HKJ, Burch RE: Impaired ethanol metabolism with advancing age. Alcohol Clin Exp Res 7:299–301, 1983

Hanna EZ, Chou SP, Grant BF: The relationship between drinking and heart disease morbidity in the United States: results from the National Health Interview Survey. Alcohol Clin Exp Res 21:111–118, 1997

Harper C, Kril J: Patterns of neuronal loss in the cerebral cortex in chronic alcoholic patients. J Neurol Sci 92:81–89, 1989

Harper CG, Kril JJ: Neuropathology of alcoholism. Alcohol Alcohol 25:207–216, 1990

Heath AC, Bucholz KK, Madden PAF, et al: Genetic and environmental contributions to alcohol dependence risk in a national sample: consistency of findings in women and men. Psychol Med 27:1381–1396, 1997

Heindel WC, Salmon DP, Butters N: Alcoholic Korsakoff's syndrome, in Memory Disorders: Research and Clinical Practice. Edited by Yanagihara T, Petersen R. New York, Marcel Dekker, 1991, pp 227–253

Helzer JE, Burnam A, McEvoy LT: Alcohol abuse and dependence, in Psychiatric Disorders in America. The Epidemiologic Catchment Area Study. Edited by Robins LN, Regier DA. New York, Free Press, 1991, pp 81–115

Hendler N, Cimini C, Ma T, et al: A comparison of cognitive impairment due to benzodiazepines and to narcotics. Am J Psychiatry 137:828–830, 1980

Higgitt AC, Lader MH, Fonagy P: Clinical management of benzodiazepine dependence. BMJ 291:688–690, 1985

Higgitt A, Fonagy P, Toone B, et al: The prolonged benzodiazepine withdrawal syndrome: anxiety or hysteria? Acta Psychiatr Scand 82:165–168, 1990

Hinrichs JV, Ghoneim MM: Diazepam, behavior, and aging: increased sensitivity or lower baseline performance? Psychopharmacology 92:100–105, 1987

Hollenbach KA, Barrett-Connor E, Edelstein SL, et al: Cigarette smoking and bone mineral density in older men and women. Am J Public Health 83:1265–1270, 1993

Holroyd S, Duryee JJ: Substance use disorders in a geriatric psychiatry outpatient clinic: prevalence and epidemiologic characteristics. J Nerv Ment Dis 185:627–632, 1997

Holton A, Riley P, Tyrer P: Factors predicting long-term outcome after chronic benzodiazepine therapy. J Affect Disord 24:245–252, 1992

Hopkins DR, Sethi KBS, Mucklaw JC: Benzodiazepine withdrawal in general practice. Journal of the Royal College of General Practitioners 32:758–762, 1982

Hser Y-I, Anglin D, Powers K: A 24-year follow-up of California narcotics addicts. Arch Gen Psychiatry 50:577–584, 1993

Hughes JR, Hatsukami DK, Mitchell JE, et al: Prevalence of smoking among psychiatric outpatients. Am J Psychiatry 143:993–997, 1986

Hughes JR, Gust SW, Pechacek TF: Prevalence of tobacco dependence and withdrawal. Am J Psychiatry 144:205–208, 1987

Hurt RD, Finlayson RE, Morse RM, et al: Alcoholism in elderly persons: medical aspects and prognosis of 216 inpatients. Mayo Clin Proc 63:753–760, 1988

Hurt RD, Dale LC, Offord KP, et al: Nicotine patch therapy for smoking cessation in recovering alcoholics. Addiction 90:1541–1546, 1995

Hurt RD, Offord KP, Croghan IT, et al: Mortality following inpatient addictions treatment. Role of tobacco use in a community-based cohort. JAMA 275:1097–1103, 1996

Husten CG, Shelton DM, Chrismon JH, et al: Cigarette smoking and smoking cessation among older adults: United States, 1965–94. Tob Control 6:175–180, 1997

Isacson D, Carsjo K, Bergman U, et al: Long-term use of benzodiazepines in a Swedish community: an eight-year follow-up. J Clin Epidemiol 45:429–436, 1992

Ishikawa Y, Meyer JS, Tanahashi N, et al: Abstinence improves cerebral perfusion and brain volume in alcoholic neurotoxicity without Wernicke-Korsakoff syndrome. J Cereb Blood Flow Metab 6:86–94, 1986

Jacques PF, Sulsky S, Hartz SC, et al: Moderate alcohol intake and nutritional status in nonalcoholic elderly subjects. Am J Clin Nutr 50:875–883, 1989

Jarvik ME, Schneider NG: Nicotine, in Substance Abuse: A Comprehensive Textbook, 2nd Edition. Edited by Lowinson JH, Ruiz P, Millman RB, Langrod JG. Baltimore, MD, Williams & Wilkins, 1992, pp 334–356

Jernigan TL, Butters N, DiTraglia G, et al: Reduced cerebral grey matter observed in alcoholics using magnetic resonance imaging. Alcohol Clin Exp Res 15:418–427, 1991

Jinks MJ, Raschko RR: A profile of alcohol and prescription drug abuse in a high-risk community-based elderly population. DICP 24:971–975, 1990

Jones AW, Neri A: Age-related differences in blood ethanol parameters and subjective feelings of intoxication in healthy men. Alcohol Alcohol 20:45–52, 1985

Jones MK, Jones BM: The relationship of age and drinking habits to the effects of alcohol on memory in women. J Stud Alcohol 41:179–186, 1980

Jones TV, Lindsey BA, Yount P, et al: Alcoholism screening questionnaires: are they valid in elderly medical outpatients? J Gen Intern Med 8:674–678, 1993

Joseph C, Ganzini L, Atkinson R: Screening for alcohol use disorders in the nursing home. J Am Geriatr Soc 43:368–373, 1995

Kafetz K, Cox M: Alcohol excess and the senile squalor syndrome. J Am Geriatr Soc 30:706, 1982

Kales A, Scharf MB, Kales JD, et al: Rebound insomnia: a potential hazard following withdrawal of certain benzodiazepines. JAMA 241:1692–1695, 1979

Kandel D, Chen K, Warner LA, et al: Prevalence and demographic correlates of symptoms of last year dependence on alcohol, nicotine, marijuana and cocaine in the U.S. population. Drug Alcohol Depend 44:11–29, 1997

King MB: Alcohol abuse and dementia. Int J Geriatr Psychiatry 1:31–36, 1986

Klatsky AL, Friedman GD, Siegelaub AB: Alcohol and mortality: a ten-year Kaiser Permanente experience. Ann Intern Med 95:139–145, 1981

Klatsky AL, Armstrong MA, Friedman GD: Alcohol and mortality. Ann Intern Med 117:646–654, 1992

Kofoed LL, Tolson RL, Atkinson RM, et al: Treatment compliance of older alcoholics: an elder-specific approach is superior to "mainstreaming." J Stud Alcohol 48:47–51, 1987; Correction 48:183, 1987

Korrapati MR, Vestal RE: Alcohol and medications in the elderly: complex interactions, in Alcohol and Aging. Edited by Beresford TP, Gomberg ESL. New York, Oxford University Press, 1995, pp 42–55

Kril JJ, Harper CG: Neuronal counts from four cortical regions of the alcoholic brain. Acta Neuropathol 79:200–204, 1989

Kril JJ, Halliday GM, Svoboda MD, et al: The cerebral cortex is damaged in chronic alcoholics. Neuroscience 79:983–998, 1997

LaCroix AZ, Omenn GS: Older adults and smoking. Clin Geriatr Med 8:69–87, 1992

Langlais PJ: Alcohol-related thiamine deficiency: impact on cognitive and memory functioning. Alcohol Health Res World 19:113–121, 1995

Lantz MS, Giambanco V, Buchalter EN: A ten-year review of the effect of OBRA-87 on psychotropic prescribing practices in an academic nursing home. Psychiatr Serv 47:951–955, 1996

Larson EB, Reifler BV, Canfield C, et al: Evaluating elderly outpatients with symptoms of dementia. Hospital and Community Psychiatry 35:425–428, 1984a

Larson EB, Reifler BV, Featherstone HJ, et al: Dementia in elderly outpatients: a prospective study. Ann Intern Med 100:417–423, 1984b

Larson EB, Kukull WA, Buchner D, et al: Adverse drug reaction associated with global cognitive impairment in elderly persons. Ann Intern Med 107:169–173, 1987

Lasser RA, Sunderland T: Newer psychotropic medication use in nursing home residents. J Am Geriatr Soc 46:202–207, 1998

Laughren TP, Battey Y, Greenblatt DJ, et al: A controlled trial of diazepam withdrawal in chronically anxious outpatients. Acta Psychiatr Scand 65:171–179, 1982

Letenneur L, Dartigues JF, Orgogozo JM: Wine consumption in the elderly. Ann Intern Med 118:317–318, 1993

Liberto JG, Oslin DW: Early versus late onset of alcoholism in the elderly. International Journal of the Addictions 30: 1799–1818, 1995

Liberto JG, Oslin DW, Ruskin PE: Alcoholism in older persons: a review of the literature. Hospital and Community Psychiatry 43:975–984, 1992

Lieber CS: Hepatic, metabolic and toxic effects of ethanol: 1991 update. Alcohol Clin Exp Res 15:573–592, 1991

Lishman WA: Organic Psychiatry: The Psychological Consequences of Cerebral Disorder. Oxford, Blackwell, 1997

Liskow BI, Rinck C, Campbell J, et al: Alcohol withdrawal in the elderly. J Stud Alcohol 50:414–421, 1989

Lowe LP, Long CR, Wallace RB, et al: Epidemiology of alcohol use in a group of older American Indians. Ann Epidemiol 7:241–248, 1997

Lowinson JH, Ruiz P, Millman RB, et al (eds): Substance Abuse: A Comprehensive Textbook, 3rd Edition. Baltimore, MD, Williams & Wilkins, 1997

Lucey MR, Hill EM, Young JP, et al: The influences of age and gender on blood ethanol concentrations in healthy humans. J Stud Alcohol 60:103–110, 1999

Luttrell S, Watkin V, Livingston G, et al: Screening for alcohol misuse in older people. Int J Geriatr Psychiatry 12: 1151–1154, 1997

MacMillan D, Shaw P: Senile breakdown in standards of personal and environmental cleanliness. BMJ 2:1032–1037, 1966

Mant A, Duncan-Jones P, Saltman D, et al: Development of long term use of psychotropic drugs by general practice patients. BMJ 296:251–254, 1988

Martin JC, Streissguth AP: Alcoholism and the elderly: an overview, in Treatment of Psychopathology in the Aging. Edited by Eisdorfer C, Fann WE. New York, Springer, 1982, pp 242–280

Martinez-Cano H, Vela-Bueno A, DeIceta M, et al: Benzodiazepine types in high versus therapeutic dose dependence. Addiction 91:1179–1186, 1996

McInness E, Powell J: Drug and alcohol referrals: are elderly substance abuse diagnoses and referrals being missed? BMJ 308:444–446, 1994

Mellinger GD, Balter MB, Uhlenhuth EH: Prevalence and correlates of the long-term regular use of anxiolytics. JAMA 251:375–379, 1984

Mellstrom D, Rundgren A, Jagenburg R, et al: Tobacco smoking, ageing and health among the elderly: a longitudinal population study of 70-year-old men and an age cohort comparison. Age Ageing 11:45–58, 1982

Mertens JR, Moos RH, Brennan PL: Alcohol consumption, life context, and coping predict mortality among late-middle-aged drinkers and former drinkers. Alcohol Clin Exp Res 20:313–319, 1996

Meyer JS, Largen JW Jr, Shaw T, et al: Interaction of normal aging, senile dementia, multi-infarct dementia, and alcoholism in the elderly, in Alcoholism in the Elderly. Social and Biomedical Issues. Edited by Hartford JT, Samorajski T. New York, Raven, 1984, pp 227–251

Miller NS, Belkin BM, Gold MS: Alcohol and drug dependence among the elderly: epidemiology, diagnosis, and treatment. Compr Psychiatry 32:153–165, 1991

Moos RH, Brennan PL, Moos BS: Short-term processes of remission and nonremission among late-life problem drinkers. Alcohol Clin Exp Res 15:948–955, 1991

Moos RH, Mertens JR, Brennan PL: Patterns of diagnosis and treatment among late-middle-aged and older substance abuse patients. J Stud Alcohol 54:479–487, 1993

Moos RH, Mertens JR, Brennan PL: Rates and predictors of four-year readmission among late-middle-aged and older substance abuse patients. J Stud Alcohol 55:561–570, 1994

Morgan GD, Noll EL, Orleans CT, et al: Reaching midlife and older smokers: tailored interventions for routine medical care. Prev Med 25:346–354, 1996

Morgan K, Dallosso H, Ebrahim S, et al: Prevalence, frequency, and duration of hypnotic drug use among the elderly living at home. BMJ 296:601–602, 1988

Morikawa Y, Arai H, Matsushita S, et al: Cerebrospinal fluid tau protein levels in demented and non demented alcoholics. Alcohol Clin Exp Res 23:575–577, 1999

Morton JL, Jones TV, Manganaro MA: Performance of alcoholism screening questionnaires in elderly veterans. Am J Med 101:153–159, 1996

Moss RJ, Miles SH: AIDS and the geriatrician. J Am Geriatr Soc 35:460–464, 1987

Murphy SM, Owen R, Tyrer PJ: Withdrawal symptoms after six weeks treatment with diazepam (letter). Lancet 2:1389, 1984

Muuronen A, Bergman H, Hindmarsh T, et al: Influence of improved drinking habits on brain atrophy and cognitive performance in alcoholic patients: a 5-year follow-up study. Alcohol Clin Exp Res 13:137–141, 1989

Myers JK, Weissman MM, Tischler GL, et al: Six-month prevalence of psychiatric disorder in three communities, 1980 to 1982. Arch Gen Psychiatry 41:959–967, 1984

Nakamura CM, Molgaard CA, Stanford EP, et al: A discriminant analysis of severe alcohol consumption among older persons. Alcohol Alcohol 25:75–80, 1990

Nakamura MM, Overall JE, Hollister LE, et al: Factors affecting outcome of depressive symptoms in alcoholics. Alcohol Clin Exp Res 7:188–193, 1983

National Center for Health Statistics: Cigarette smoking among adults—United States, 1994. MMWR Morb Mortal Wkly Rep 45:588–590, 1996

National Institute on Alcohol Abuse and Alcoholism: The Physician's Guide to Helping Patients With Alcohol Problems (NIH Publ No 95-3769). Rockville, MD, U.S. Department of Health and Human Services, 1995

National Institute on Drug Abuse: Annual Emergency Room Data 1991: Data From the Drug Abuse Warning Network (DAWN), Series 1, No 11-A (DHHS Publ No ADM-92-1955). Rockville, MD, U.S. Department of Health and Human Services, 1992a

National Institute on Drug Abuse: Annual Emergency Room Data 1991: Data From the Drug Abuse Warning Network (DAWN), Series 1, No 11-B (DHHS Publ No ADM-92-1956). Rockville, MD, U.S. Department of Health and Human Services, 1992b

Neutel CI, Hirdes JP, Maxwell CJ, et al: New evidence on benzodiazepine use and falls: the time factor. Age Ageing 25:273–278, 1996

Neve RJM, Lemmens PH, Drop MJ: Drinking careers of older male alcoholics in treatment as compared to younger alcoholics and to older social drinkers. J Stud Alcohol 58:303–311, 1997

Nikaido AM, Ellinwood EH Jr, Heatherly DG, et al: Age-related increase in CNS sensitivity to benzodiazepines as assessed by task difficulty. Psychopharmacology 100:90–97, 1990

Nisell M, Nomikos GG, Svensson TH: Nicotine dependence, midbrain dopamine systems and psychiatric disorders. Pharmacol Toxicol 76:157–162, 1995

Novick DM: The medically ill substance abuser, in Substance Abuse: A Comprehensive Textbook, 2nd Edition. Edited by Lowinson JH, Ruiz P, Millman RB, Langrod JG. Baltimore, MD, Williams & Wilkins, 1992, pp 647–657

Noyes R Jr, Garvey MJ, Cook BL, et al: Benzodiazepine withdrawal: a review of the evidence. J Clin Psychiatry 49:382–389, 1988

Obisesan TO, Hirsch R, Kosoko O, et al: Moderate wine consumption is associated with decreased odds of developing age-related macular degeneration in NHANES-1. J Am Geriatr Soc 46:1–7, 1998

Onyett SR, Turpin G: Benzodiazepine withdrawal in primary care: a comparison of behavioural group training and individual sessions. Behavioral Psychotherapy 16:297–312, 1988

Orgogozo JM, Dartigues JF, Lafont S, et al: Wine consumption and dementia in the elderly: a prospective community study in the Bordeaux area. Rev Neurol (Paris) 153:185–192, 1997

Orleans CT, Jepson C, Resch N, et al: Quitting motives and barriers among older smokers. Cancer 74:2055–2061, 1994a

Orleans CT, Resch N, Noll E, et al: Use of transdermal nicotine in a state-level prescription plan for the elderly. JAMA 271:601–607, 1994b

Oscar-Berman M, Hutner N: Frontal lobe changes after chronic alcohol ingestion, in Alcohol-Induced Brain Damage (NIAAA Research Monograph No 22). Edited by Hunt WA, Nixon SJ. Rockville, MD, U.S. Government Printing Office, 1993, pp 121–156

Oslin D, Liberto JG, O'Brien J, et al: Naltrexone as an adjunctive treatment for older patients with alcohol dependence. Am J Geriatr Psychiatry 5:324–332, 1997a

Oslin D, Liberto JG, O'Brien J, et al: The tolerability of naltrexone in treating older, alcohol dependent patients. Am J Addict 6:266–270, 1997b

Oslin D, Atkinson RM, Smith DM, et al: Alcohol related dementia: proposed clinical criteria. Int J Geriatr Psychiatry 13:203–212, 1998

Osuntokun BO, Hendrie HC, Fisher K, et al: The diagnosis of dementia associated with alcoholism: a preliminary report of a new approach. West Afr J Med 13:160–163, 1994

Ozdemir V, Fourie J, Busto U, et al: Pharmacokinetic changes in the elderly: do they contribute to drug abuse and dependence? Clin Pharmacokinet 31:372–385, 1996

Paganini-Hill A, Ross RK, Henderson BE: Prevalence of chronic disease and health practices in a retirement community. Journal of Chronic Diseases 39:699–707, 1986

Paille FM, Guelfi JD, Perkins AC, et al: Double-blind randomized multicentre trial of acamprosate in maintaining abstinence from alcohol. Alcohol Alcohol 30:239–247, 1995

Parsons OA: Determinants of cognitive deficits in alcoholics: the search continues. Clinical Neuropsychologist 8:39–58, 1994

Parsons OA, Nixon SJ: Neurobehavioral sequelae of alcoholism. Neurol Clin 11:205–218, 1993

Parsons OA, Nixon SJ: Cognitive functioning in sober social drinkers: a review of the research since 1986. J Stud Alcohol 59:180–190, 1998

Pascarelli EF: The elderly in methadone maintenance, in The Combined Problems of Alcoholism, Drug Addiction and Aging. Edited by Gottheil E, Druley KA, Skoloda TE, Waxman HM. Springfield, IL, Charles C Thomas, 1985, pp 210–214

Pascarelli EF, Fischer W: Drug dependence in the elderly. Int J Aging Hum Dev 5:347–356, 1974

Pedrosa MC, Russell RM, Saltzman JR, et al: Gastric emptying and first-pass metabolism of ethanol in elderly subjects with and without atrophic gastritis. Scand J Gastroenterol 31:671–677, 1996

Petursson H, Lader MH: Withdrawal from long-term benzodiazepine treatment. BMJ 283:643–645, 1981

Pfefferbaum A, Lim KO, Zipursky RB, et al: Brain gray and white matter volume loss accelerates with aging in chronic alcoholics: a quantitative MRI study. Alcohol Clin Exp Res 16:1078–1089, 1992

Pfefferbaum A, Sullivan EV, Mathalon DH, et al: Longitudinal changes in magnetic resonance imaging brain volumes in abstinent and relapsed alcoholics. Alcohol Clin Exp Res 19: 1177–1191, 1995

Pfefferbaum A, Lim KO, Desmond JE, et al: Thinning of the corpus callosum in older alcoholic men: a magnetic resonance imaging study. Alcohol Clin Exp Res 20:752–757, 1996

Pfefferbaum A, Sullivan EV, Mathalon DH, et al: Frontal lobe volume loss observed with magnetic resonance imaging in older chronic alcoholics. Alcohol Clin Exp Res 21: 521–529, 1997

Piette JD, Barnett PG, Moos RH: First-time admissions with alcohol-related medical problems: a 10-year follow-up of a national sample of alcoholic patients. J Stud Alcohol 59: 89–96, 1998

Pinsker H, Suljaga-Petchel K: Use of benzodiazepines in primary-care geriatric patients. J Am Geriatr Soc 32:595–597, 1984

Pomara N, Stanley B, Block R, et al: Increased sensitivity of the elderly to the central depressant effects of diazepam. J Clin Psychiatry 46:185–187, 1985

Pomara N, Deptula D, Medel M, et al: Effects of diazepam on recall memory: relationship to aging, dose, and duration of treatment. Psychopharmacol Bull 25:144–148, 1989

Pomara N, Deptula D, Singh R, et al: Cognitive toxicity of benzodiazepines in the elderly, in Anxiety in the Elderly: Treatment and Research. Edited by Salzman C, Lebowitz BD. New York, Springer, 1991, pp 175–196

Portenoy RK, Payne R: Acute and chronic pain, in Substance Abuse: A Comprehensive Textbook, 2nd Edition. Edited by Lowinson JH, Ruiz P, Millman RB, Langrod JG. Baltimore, MD, Williams & Wilkins, 1992, pp 691–721

Porter J, Jick H: Addiction rare in patients treated with narcotics (letter). N Engl J Med 302:123, 1980

Ray WA, Fought RL, Decker MD: Psychoactive drugs and the risk of injurious motor vehicle crashes in elderly drivers. Am J Epidemiol 136:873–883, 1992

Reifler B, Raskind M, Kethley A: Psychiatric diagnoses among geriatric patients seen in an outreach program. J Am Geriatr Soc 30:530–533, 1982

Renvoize EB, Gaskell RK, Klar HM: Results of investigations in 150 demented patients consecutively admitted to a psychiatric hospital. Br J Psychiatry 147:204–205, 1985

Rickels K, Case WG, Downing RW, et al: Long-term diazepam therapy and clinical outcome. JAMA 250:767–771, 1983

Rickels K, Schweizer E, Case WG, et al: Long-term therapeutic use of benzodiazepines, I: effects of abrupt discontinuation. Arch Gen Psychiatry 47:899–907, 1990

Rickels K, Case WG, Schweizer E, et al: Long-term benzodiazepine users 3 years after participation in a discontinuation program. Am J Psychiatry 148:757–761, 1991

Ried LD, Johnson RE, Gettman DA: Benzodiazepine exposure and functional status in older people. J Am Geriatr Soc 46:71–76, 1998

Rimer B: Smoking among older adults: the problem, consequences and possible solutions, in Surgeon General's Report on Health Promotion for Older Adults. Washington, DC, U.S. Department of Health and Human Services, 1988

Rimer BK, Orleans CT: Tailoring smoking cessation for older adults. Cancer 74:2051–2054, 1994

Rimer BK, Orleans CT, Keintz MK, et al: The older smoker. Status, challenges and opportunities for intervention. Chest 97:547–553, 1990

Ritzmann RF, Melchior CL: Age and development of tolerance to and physical dependence on alcohol, in Alcoholism in the Elderly. Social and Biomedical Issues. Edited by Hartford JT, Samorajski T. New York, Raven, 1984, pp 117–138

Rodrigo EK, King MB, Williams P: Health of long term benzodiazepine users. BMJ 296:603–606, 1988

Ron MA: The alcoholic brain: CT scan and psychological findings. Psychol Med 13(suppl):1–33, 1983

Roy-Byrne PP, Ballenger JC: Pharmacological treatments for benzodiazepine dependence, in Benzodiazepine Dependence. Edited by Hallstrom C. New York, Oxford University Press, 1993, pp 310–322

Roy-Byrne PP, Hommer D: Benzodiazepine withdrawal: overview and implications for treatment of anxiety. Am J Med 84:1041–1052, 1988

Ruchlin HS: Prevalence and correlates of alcohol use among older adults. Prev Med 26:651–657, 1997

Rundgren A, Mellstrom D: The effect of tobacco smoking on the bone mineral content of the ageing skeleton. Mech Ageing Dev 28:273–277, 1984

Ryan C, Butters N: The neuropsychology of alcoholism, in The Neuropsychology Handbook. Edited by Wedding D, Horton A, Webster J. New York, Springer, 1986, pp 376–409

Salive ME, Blazer DG: Depression and smoking cessation in older adults: a longitudinal study. J Am Geriatr Soc 41:1313–1316, 1993

Salive ME, Cornoni-Huntley J, LaCroix AZ, et al: Predictors of smoking cessation and relapse in older adults. Am J Public Health 82:1268–1271, 1992

Salzman C: Pharmacologic treatment of the anxious elderly patient, in Anxiety in the Elderly: Treatment and Research. Edited by Salzman C, Lebowitz BD. New York, Springer, 1991, pp 149–173

Salzman C, Fisher J, Nobel K, et al: Cognitive improvement following benzodiazepine discontinuation in elderly nursing home residents. Int J Geriatr Psychiatry 7:89–93, 1992

Samorajski T, Persson K, Bissell C, et al: Biology of alcoholism and aging in rodents: brain and liver, in Alcoholism in the Elderly. Social and Biomedical Issues. Edited by Hartford JT, Samorajski T. New York, Raven, 1984, pp 43–63

Sass H, Soyka M, Mann K, et al: Relapse prevention by acamprosate: results from a placebo-controlled study on alcohol dependence. Arch Gen Psychiatry 53:673–680, 1996

Saunders PA, Copeland JRM, Dewey ME, et al: Heavy drinking as a risk factor for depression and dementia in elderly men. Br J Psychiatry 159:213–216, 1991

Schafer K, Butters N, Smith T, et al: Cognitive performance of alcoholics: a longitudinal evaluation of the role of drinking history, depression, liver function, nutrition, and family history. Alcohol Clin Exp Res 15:653–660, 1991

Scherr PA, LaCroix AZ, Wallace RB, et al: Light to moderate alcohol consumption and mortality in the elderly. J Am Geriatr Soc 40:651–657, 1992

Schmidt I, Claesson CB, Westerholm B, et al: The impact of regular multidisciplinary team interventions on psychotropic prescribing in Swedish nursing homes. J Am Geriatr Soc 46:77–82, 1998

Schonfeld L, Dupree LW: Antecedents of drinking for early- and late-onset elderly alcohol abusers. J Stud Alcohol 52:587–592, 1991

Schonfeld L, Dupree LW, Rohrer GE: Age-specific differences between younger and older alcohol abusers. Journal of Clinical Geropsychology 1:219–227, 1995

Schroth G, Naegele T, Klose U, et al: Reversible brain shrinkage in abstinent alcoholics, measured by MRI. Neuroradiology 30:385–389, 1988

Schuckit MA: Geriatric alcoholism and drug abuse. Gerontologist 17:168–174, 1977

Schuckit MA: Drug and Alcohol Abuse, 4th Edition. New York, Plenum, 1995

Schuckit MA, Atkinson JH, Miller PL, et al: A three year follow-up of elderly alcoholics. J Clin Psychiatry 41:412–416, 1980

Schuckit MA, Tipp JE, Bergman M, et al: Comparison of induced and independent major depressive disorders in 2,945 alcoholics. Am J Psychiatry 154:948–957, 1997

Schutte KK, Brennan PL, Moos RH: Predicting the development of late-life late-onset drinking problems: a 7-year prospective study. Alcohol Clin Exp Res 22:1349–1358, 1998

Schweizer E, Case WG, Rickels K: Benzodiazepine dependence and withdrawal in elderly patients. Am J Psychiatry 146:529–531, 1989

Schweizer E, Rickels K, Case WG, et al: Long-term therapeutic use of benzodiazepines, II: effects of gradual taper. Arch Gen Psychiatry 47:908–915, 1990

Schweizer E, Rickels K, Case WG, et al: Carbamazepine treatment in patients discontinuing long-term benzodiazepine therapy: effects on withdrawal severity and outcome. Arch Gen Psychiatry 48:448–452, 1991

Siegler EL, Capezuti E, Maislin G, et al: Effects of a restraint reduction intervention and OBRA '87 regulations on psychoactive drug use in nursing homes. J Am Geriatr Soc 45:791–796, 1997

Simon GE, VanKorff M, Barlow W, et al: Predictors of chronic benzodiazepine use in a health maintenance organization sample. J Clin Epidemiol 49:1067–1073, 1996

Smart RG, Adlaf EM: Alcohol and drug use among the elderly: trends in use and characteristics of users. Can J Public Health 79:236–242, 1988

Smith DM, Atkinson RM: Alcoholism and dementia. International Journal of the Addictions 30:1843–1869, 1995

Smith JW: Medical manifestations of alcoholism in the elderly. International Journal of the Addictions 30:1749–1798, 1995

Soleas GJ, Diamandis EP, Goldberg DM: Resveratrol: a molecule whose time has come? And gone? Clin Biochem 30:91–113, 1997

Speer DC, Bates K: Comorbid mental and substance disorders among older psychiatric patients. J Am Geriatr Soc 40:886–890, 1992

Srivastava LM, Vasisht S, Agarwal DP, et al: Relation between alcohol intake, lipoproteins and coronary artery disease: the interest continues. Alcohol Alcohol 29:11–24, 1994

Strang J, Gurling H: Computerized tomography and neuropsychological assessment in long-term high-dose heroin addicts. British Journal of Addiction 84:1011–1019, 1989

Sullivan CF, Copeland JRM, Dewey ME, et al: Benzodiazepine usage amongst the elderly: findings of the Liverpool Community Survey. Int J Geriatr Psychiatry 3:289–292, 1988

Sullivan EV, Marsh L, Mathalon DH, et al: Anterior hippocampal volume deficits in nonamnestic, aging chronic alcoholics. Alcohol Clin Exp Res 19:110–122, 1995

Sussman S: Marijuana use in the elderly. Clinical Geriatrics 5(3):109–112, 117–119, 1997

Svensson TH, Grenhoff J, Engberg G: Effect of nicotine on dynamic function of brain catecholaminergic neurons, in The Biology of Nicotine Dependence (Ciba Foundation Symposium No 152). Edited by Bock G, Marsh J. Chichester, Wiley, 1990, pp 169–185

Swift CG, Ewen JM, Clarke P, et al: Responsiveness to oral diazepam in the elderly: relationship to total and free plasma concentrations. Br J Clin Pharmacol 20:111–118, 1985

Tattersall M: Self-help groups and benzodiazepine dependence, in Benzodiazepine Dependence. Edited by Hallstrom C. New York, Oxford University Press, 1993, pp 323–336

Terry RD, DeTeresa R, Hansen LA: Neocortical cell counts in normal human adult aging. Ann Neurol 21:530–539, 1987

Thomson M, Smith WA: Prescribing benzodiazepines for noninstitutionalized elderly. Can Fam Physician 41:792–798, 1995

Thun MJ, Peto R, Lopez AD, et al: Alcohol consumption and mortality among middle-aged and elderly U.S. adults. N Engl J Med 337:1705–1714, 1997

Tonne U, Hiltunen AJ, Vikander B, et al: Neuropsychological changes during steady-state drug use, withdrawal and abstinence in primary benzodiazepine-dependent patients. Acta Psychiatr Scand 91:299–304, 1995

Tresch DD, Aronow WS: Smoking and coronary artery disease. Clin Geriatr Med 12:23–32, 1996

Tupler LA, Hege S, Ellinwood EH Jr: Alcohol pharmacodynamics in young-elderly adults contrasted with young and middle-aged subjects. Psychopharmacology 118: 460–470, 1995

Tyrer P: Risks of dependence on benzodiazepine drugs: the importance of patient selection. BMJ 298:102, 104–105, 1989

Uhlenhuth EH, DeWit H, Balter MB, et al: Risks and benefits of long term benzodiazepine use. J Clin Psychopharmacol 8:161–167, 1988

Vaillant GE: The Natural History of Alcoholism Revisited. Cambridge, MA, Harvard University Press, 1995

Vestal RE, McGuire EA, Tobin JD, et al: Aging and ethanol metabolism in man. Clin Pharmacol Ther 21:343–354, 1977

Victor M, Adams RD, Collins GH: The Wernicke-Korsakoff Syndrome and Related Neurologic Disorders Due to Alcoholism and Malnutrition (Contemporary Neurology Series, Vol 3). Philadelphia, PA, FA Davis, 1989

Vogel-Sprott M, Barrett P: Age, drinking habits and the effects of alcohol. J Stud Alcohol 45:517–521, 1984

Wells CE: Diagnosis of dementia. Psychosomatics 20:517–522, 1979

Welte JW, Mirand AL: Drinking, problem drinking and life stressors in the elderly general population. J Stud Alcohol 56:67–73, 1995

Whitcup SM, Miller F: Unrecognized drug dependence in psychiatrically hospitalized elderly patients. J Am Geriatr Soc 35:297–301, 1987

Wilcox RE: Changes in biogenic amines and their metabolites with aging and alcoholism, in Alcoholism in the Elderly. Social and Biomedical Issues. Edited by Hartford JT, Samorajski T. New York, Raven, 1984, pp 85–115

Willenbring ML: Organic mental disorders associated with heavy drinking and alcohol dependence. Clin Geriatr Med 4:869–887, 1988

Winick C: Maturing out of narcotic addiction. United Nations Bulletin on Narcotics 14:1–7, 1962

Wood WG: Age differences in effects of alcohol on brain membrane structure, neurotransmitters, and receptors, in Alcohol and Aging. Edited by Beresford TP, Gomberg ESL. New York, Oxford University Press, 1995, pp 136–149

Woodhouse KW, James OFW: Alcoholic liver disease in the elderly: presentation and outcome. Age Ageing 14:113–118, 1985

Woods JH, Winger G: Current benzodiazepine issues. Psychopharmacology 118:107–115, 1995

World Health Organization: International Classification of Diseases, 10th Edition. Geneva, World Health Organization, 1992

Wrigley M, Cooney C: Diogenes syndrome. Irish Journal of Psychological Medicine 9:37–41, 1992

York JL: Increased responsiveness to ethanol with advancing age in rats. Pharmacol Biochem Behav 19:687–691, 1983

Yudkin PL, Jones L, Lancaster T, et al: Which smokers are helped to give up smoking using transdermal nicotine patches? Results from a randomized, double-blind, placebo-controlled trial. Br J Gen Pract 46:145–148, 1996

Yudofsky SC, Hales RE (eds): The American Psychiatric Press Textbook of Neuropsychiatry, 3rd Edition. Washington, DC, American Psychiatric Press, 1997

17

Sleep Disorders

Peter D. Nowell, M.D.

Carolyn C. Hoch, Ph.D.

Charles F. Reynolds III, M.D.

The primary challenge posed by the increasing proportion of elderly people in the United States is to increase active life expectancy and compress functional morbidity. Otherwise, increase in longevity is likely to be associated primarily with prolongation of dependency (Rosenwaike 1985). Changes in sleep, sleep quality, and daytime alertness in late life have enormous impact on quality of life, level of functioning, and ability to remain independent (Morin and Gramling 1989; Prinz et al. 1990; Wauquier et al. 1992). The prevalence of sleep disorders among the elderly ranges depending on the specific disorder, as discussed below, but approximately one in three community-dwelling older adults will report difficulties with poor sleep quality or daytime sleepiness (Ganguli et al. 1996; Newman et al. 1997). Hence, preserving the integrity of sleep for as long as possible is a major public health priority, as emphasized by the National Institutes of Health Consensus Development Conference on Sleep Disorders in Late Life (Consensus Development Conference 1990). Any understanding of how to attenuate the sleep changes and disturbances of usual and pathological aging that would reduce psychiatric morbidity, burden to families, and the rate of institutionalization, even by a single percentage point, would pay for itself many times over. Therefore, the benefits that would accrue from an understanding of how the successful functioning of the aging sleep/wake and circadian system can be preserved in the face of medical and psychosocial challenges would have an impact not only on elderly patients themselves but on society as a whole.

To facilitate understanding of this chapter, a brief review of important concepts from normal sleep physiology is useful. Two operating states of the central nervous system characterize sleep: rapid-eye-movement (REM) sleep and nonrapid-eye-movement (NREM) sleep. The deepest level of NREM sleep, slow-wave sleep, decreases greatly with age, whereas REM sleep tends to remain more stable. The continuity of sleep also tends to diminish with age, resulting in decreased "sleep efficiency" (the ratio of time spent asleep to total recording period). Sometimes, as noted below, decreased sleep efficiency with age may be the result of intrinsic sleep pathologies (e.g., sleep-disordered breathing), whereas at other times it may reflect psychopathological processes such as depression. The regular alteration of these operating states constitutes the essential ultradian rhythm of sleep, which in turn occurs within a circadian rhythm of sleep and wakefulness.

Self-reported symptoms of sleep cluster into domains of quantity, quality, and timing (including circadian aspects) of sleep and wakefulness. Symptoms of quantity and quality concern duration of sleep periods, time to sleep onset, number of awakenings, duration of wakefulness after sleep onset, perceived depth and satisfaction with sleep, and fatigue and sleepiness during the daytime. Symptoms related to the timing of sleep concern advances and delays in sleep-wake cycles, as well as symptoms related to shift work and jet lag. In addition to self-reported symptoms, signs and laboratory measures of sleep and wakefulness span sleep-specific measures such as polysomnography, multiple sleep latency tests (MSLTs), and circadian measures such as isolation studies under constant routines. Such procedures provide information on the "architecture" of sleep including the NREM-REM cycles, sleep stages, the quantification of levels of alertness-sleepiness, and rhythms of physiological activity such as body temperature and hormones. Supplementing these sleep-specific procedures is the full range of neuropsychological, neuroendocrine, neuroimaging, and other physiological test procedures.

In this chapter, we focus on sleep and aging and the symptoms and signs of sleep disorders in the elderly, particularly emphasizing empirical studies described since the first edition of this textbook. Generally, sleep disorders medicine is concerned with specific disorders of sleep and wakefulness as described in the *International Classification of Sleep Disorders* (Diagnostic Classification Steering Committee 1990) and more generally in DSM-IV (American Psychiatric Association 1994). As is discussed below, most disorders are not thought to be specific disorders of the elderly, though the epidemiology, expression of symptoms, comorbidity, treatment selection, and treatment outcome are modified for aging populations. This age effect has resulted in generalities such as an added emphasis on differential diagnosis in the elderly to identify general medical or medication-related etiologies of sleep complaints (Ancoli-Israel 1997; Folks and Burke 1998).

Likewise, treatment recommendations for the elderly typically caution about the potential for altered pharmacokinetics that may require dosage adjustments to reduce side effects or caution about interactions with other medications (see Chapter 34 in this volume). Specific relationships between sleep and aging would suggest strategies for prevention and intervention of sleep disorders in the elderly, thereby reducing morbidity and mortality and improving medical-related quality of life. (For general reviews of sleep and sleep disorders in the elderly, see

Ancoli-Israel 1997; Bachman 1992; Becker and Jamieson 1992; Gottlieb 1990; Moran et al. 1988; and Wooten 1992.)

A Conceptual Framework for Understanding Challenges to Sleep and Circadian Timekeeping in Late Life

We have formalized a model of the multiple factors that challenge successful circadian timekeeping (including sleep in elderly individuals). The model is based on the results of our own work, as well as other data in the literature, and is shown in Figure 17–1. The model explicitly shows important predictors of, as well as outcomes resulting from, the development of sleep and circadian function in very late life. Thus, changes in health and cognitive status and negative life events (particularly those associated with bereavement) are hypothesized to lead to "decay" in sleep and sleep quality. The model posits that the effect of these changes is mediated by two factors: changes in mood (negative shifts in affect balance) and worsening of sleep-disordered breathing. We also hypothesize that characteristics such as gender, stability of social rhythms, social support, nutrition, and physical fitness serve as important moderators, helping to buffer the subject from the effects of medical burden, negative life events, and their mediators. It is noteworthy that the model explicitly recognizes that sleep changes are also likely to influence subsequent adaptation to aging along physical and psychological dimensions. Thus, what appear as major predictors in the model can, over time, ultimately be influenced by the very outcomes that they have helped to produce.

Sleep Changes in Aging

Considerable data support the face validity and clinical utility of conceptualizing sleep, particularly sleep continuity, delta sleep, and REM sleep, as psychobiological markers or correlates of successful aging and adaptation in very late life (Reynolds et al. 1993). Pronounced alterations in sleep in aging consist primarily of reductions in subjective sleep quality, slow-wave and REM sleep, and a marked increase in the number and duration of awakenings interrupting sleep. Alterations in slow-wave sleep occur in young adulthood (30–40 years of age), whereas disturbances in amounts of REM and wake appear more later in life (Vancauter et al. 1998). In comparing the nocturnal

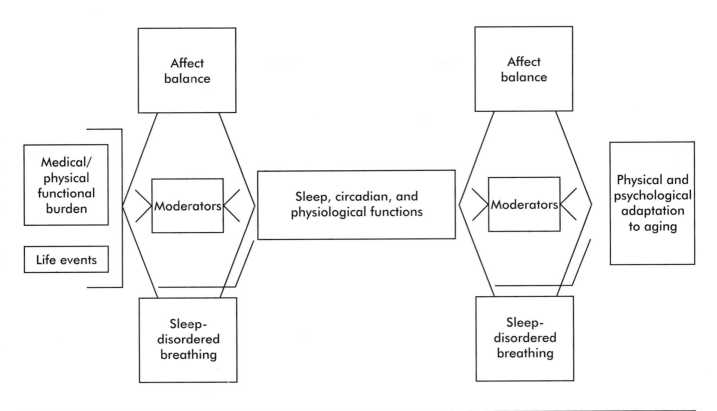

FIGURE 17–1. Model depicting relationships between potential factors linking the effects on sleep.

sleep of healthy subjects 80 years old or older with that of healthy 60- to 70-year-old subjects (i.e., "old old" versus "young old"), Reynolds et al. (1991) and Hoch et al. (1997) have reported the relative stability of sleep efficiency and REM sleep in the young old, but a decline of slow-wave sleep and sleep continuity in the old old. In a study using sleep deprivation as an experimental manipulation in 80- and 20-year-old subjects, Brendel et al. (1990) found that sleep continuity and delta sleep were enhanced in both groups on the first recovery night, indicating that sleep changes in very old subjects are at least partially reversible by this procedure. Surprisingly, mood and performance were disturbed by sleep loss to a significantly greater extent among the young subjects, suggesting that acute total sleep loss is a more disruptive procedure for the young than for the elderly.

Evidence is conflicting regarding changes in daytime alertness with aging. In some studies, the elderly are seen as physiologically more aroused or alert than are younger subjects (Hoch et al. 1992). In others studies, discrepancies are found between subjective and objective measures of alertness. For example, 19 elderly (mean age 65 years) and 19 young (mean age 21 years) subjects were tested by MSLTs and questionnaire. Elderly subjects were subjectively more alert than younger subjects were by question-

naire and rating scales, but MSLT results were equivalent (Kramer et al. 1998). Thus, despite changes in nighttime sleep consolidation and distribution of sleep stages in the elderly, the implications of these changes for daytime restedness and alertness remain unclear.

Successful adaptation in very late life may be associated with stable preservation of, or only modest changes in, REM sleep and sleep continuity. Failed adaptation, as discussed below, tends to be associated with decrements of sleep continuity and delta sleep and by either a relative increase of REM sleep (e.g., mood disorders) or decrease in REM sleep (e.g., neurodegenerative disorders). The latter, decreased REM sleep generation, has also been shown to be correlated with decreased survival time (Hoch et al. 1989). In contrast to healthy elderly patients, older patients with major depression comorbid with probable dementia of the Alzheimer type show less of the expected physiological hallmarks of recovery sleep after a night of total sleep deprivation (slow-wave sleep rebound and REM sleep rebound), attesting to diminished physiological resilience and plasticity (Reynolds et al. 1987). In the broader context provided by studies of sleep in aging, we concluded that the stability of REM sleep in aging suggests the utility and validity of REM sleep as a marker or correlate of successful adaptation in late life (Reynolds et al. 1993). The reversibility of age-dependent sleep changes needs to be further addressed by identifying factors that support or enhance successful aging.

Sleep in Aging: The Impact of Spousal Bereavement on Sleep in Late Life

Given the theoretical interest in negative life events and their potential to disrupt sleep via changes in mood, our own work, as well as that of others (e.g., N. G. Bliwise et al. 1985; Roehrs et al. 1982), provides evidence linking negative affect balance (i.e., depression) and sleep outcomes in late life. Sleep is frequently disturbed among recently bereaved elderly people who have a full depressive syndrome. Sleep efficiency is diminished, REM latency is short, and early slow-wave sleep generation is also reduced compared with those of nondepressed, recently bereaved subjects and compared with elderly control subjects (Reynolds et al. 1992). These findings are similar to those of Cartwright (1983) in depressed divorcing women. Depressed widows and widowers in our study carried a heavier burden of chronic medical illness than did the control subjects (Reynolds et al. 1992). Similar findings linking stress, depression, and electroencephalographic (EEG) sleep disturbances (including decreased delta sleep and shortened REM latency) were reported by Cartwright and Wood (1991) in a study of middle-aged divorcing spouses. Divorce, like the loss of a spouse through death, can be an occasion for grief. We were able to find one negative report, from Vitiello et al. (1990), who observed that sleep was undisturbed in elderly depressed individuals who have *not* sought health care.

We reported an investigation of EEG sleep measures in elderly, recently bereaved volunteers stratified by the presence or absence of syndromal major depression (Reynolds et al. 1992). As hypothesized, depressed bereaved subjects had significantly lower sleep efficiency and worse sleep quality, more early morning awakening, shorter REM latency, greater REM percent, and lower rates of delta wave generation in the first NREM sleep period (i.e., lower delta sleep ratio) compared with those characteristics in nondepressed, bereaved volunteers. Sleep in the latter group was similar to that of healthy control subjects. The relevance of these data to the proposed model of challenges to successful aging is that depression (or depressive symptoms) can be an important mediating variable that links negative life events with sleep-circadian outcomes, as well as with changes in perceived sleep qual-

ity. With respect to the role of hypothesized moderators (i.e., social support and stability of social rhythms), our data suggested greater stability of psychosocial rhythms and higher levels of perceived social support among nondepressed widows and widowers compared with their depressed counterparts. Testing of the proposed model would help elucidate antecedent-consequent relationships.

Similarly, the primary protective factor examined in previous research is social support, including the dimensions of social network, tangible support, and perceived social support. George (1989) concluded that "high levels of social support are associated with decreased risk of psychiatric morbidity and that perceived support is the dimension most strongly related to mental health outcomes" (p. 215). However, we do not know whether support exerts its effects directly on such outcomes or whether it serves primarily to buffer the impact of other stressors (see also Cohen and Wills 1985; George 1989; Kessler and McLeod 1985).

We have investigated the role of psychosocial factors in buffering the impact of major life events on depressive symptoms in our sample of elderly widows and widowers (Prigerson et al. 1993). Our results suggested the importance of subjects' sense of mastery—their feeling of competence in the face of stress—as a predictor of mood response after life stressors. Similar findings have been reported elsewhere in nonelderly samples (e.g., Dew et al. 1990), further supporting the selection of mastery as a potential buffer against the onset of disturbed mood and sleep.

General Medical Burden

Medical burden and increasing physical functional limitations represent chronic stressors in the presented model and are among the vulnerability factors most frequently addressed in previous research on the precursors of psychiatric symptoms and disorders (for a review, see George 1989). The specific chronic stressors that have received the most empirical scrutiny in mixed-age samples are job stress, chronic financial strain, and chronic physical illness, with all three being related to increased risk of psychiatric morbidity (George 1989). As reviewed by D. L. Bliwise (1993), considerable evidence now underscores the general effects (either direct or indirect) of medical illness in the poor sleep of old age (e.g., Ford and Kamerow 1989; Gislason and Almqvist 1987; Morgan et al. 1989). Specific clinical symptoms or disorders that have been shown to have negative effects on sleep quality in late life include nocturia (e.g., Zepelin and Morgan 1981), headache (Cook et al. 1989), gastrointestinal illness (Karacan et al. 1976; Mant and Eyland 1988), bronchitis and asthma (Mant and Eyland 1988), cardiovascular symptoms, and non–insulin-dependent diabetes mellitus (Hyyppa and Kronholm 1989). Chronic pain from conditions such as osteoarthritis also disrupts sleep in elderly individuals (Wittig et al. 1982). In addition, elevated autonomic activity (Prinz et al. 1979; Zepelin and McDonald 1987) and a greater susceptibility to external arousal (Roth et al. 1972; Zepelin et al. 1984) may be important predisposing factors to disturbed sleep in very late life. In general, the effects of these general medical conditions on sleep become issues in the elderly because they are more common conditions in older individuals. However, it is also possible that increased wakefulness at night or greater susceptibility to arousal may enhance the impact of these conditions on sleep in older individuals.

Among specific brain diseases in the elderly in which sleep and sleep disorders may play a role are Parkinson's disease and stroke. Patients with Parkinson's disease report decrements in sleep quality and demonstrate progressive deterioration in sleep continuity (Kostic et al. 1991; M. C. Smith et al. 1997). Some of the deterioration in sleep continuity and quality is attributed to muscle stiffness, dystonias, and nocturnal akinesia (Stocchi et al. 1998) separate from comorbid depression and anxiety (Kostic et al. 1991; Menza and Rosen 1995). Dopaminergic agonists have been demonstrated to improve sleep continuity disturbances in Parkinson's disease in some studies (Stocchi et al. 1998). However, dopaminergic agonists have also been shown to increase motor activity at night in some patients with Parkinson's disease (van Hilten et al. 1994). It may be that REM behavior disorder (see section below on Sleep Disorders) is an early feature in some patients who develop Parkinson's disease (Tan et al. 1996).

The issue of sleep and stroke has been studied primarily from the aspect of the possible increased risk of stroke that may be associated with sleep apnea. However, research has also been directed at the effects of specific stroke locations and their effects on sleep and breathing (Giubilei et al. 1992; Mohsenin and Valor 1995) and at the potential influence that circadian factors may have in the timing of stroke within the early morning. Whether obstructive sleep apnea increases the risk of cardiovascular morbidity, including myocardial infarct and stroke, when other risk factors common in sleep apnea such as hypertension and obesity are controlled has been much debated (Bassetti et al. 1996; Dyken et al. 1996). After a stroke, patients with sleep-disordered breathing may have a worse functional outcome than those who do not have sleep-disordered breathing (Good et al. 1996).

Sleep Disorders, Sleep Quality, and Aging

For a broad overview, see Monane (1992). Generally, subjective sleep quality deteriorates in later life. Such deterioration can be seen in the increasing sleep-related complaints and insomnia symptoms in the elderly. However, the extent to which subjective sleep quality deteriorates as a part of physiological aging as opposed to pathological conditions associated with aging remains unclear. For example, a prospective United States regional epidemiological study of an age-stratified, random, community sample of 1,050 seniors (mean age 74 years, 57% women) found that sleep complaints were common and persistent over a 2-year interval. The symptoms reported were difficulty falling asleep (37%), difficulty staying asleep (29%), and early morning awakening (19%) (Ganguli et al. 1996).

When associated medical symptoms and history are examined, the prevalence of sleep complaints varies with a number of other factors. For example, in a study of more than 9,000 seniors over the age of 65 years, more than half reported sleep difficulties most of the time (Foley et al. 1995). Twenty-four percent reported insomnia and 15% reported that they never felt rested. Multivariate analyses associated sleep complaints with respiratory symptoms, physical disabilities, nonprescription medication use, depressive symptoms, and poorer self-perceived health status. The authors concluded that sleep symptoms in older persons may often be secondary to coexisting diseases. They also drew attention to the difficulty in determining the prevalence of specific sleep disorders, independent of health status, and note that the development of more sophisticated and objective measures of sleep disturbance will be necessary to meet this objective (Foley et al. 1995).

In addition to general medical conditions, gender also plays a role in the reporting of sleep complaints in aging. In the Cardiovascular Health Study (Newman et al. 1997), 5,201 adults over the age of 65 years were identified in a random community sample. Women were found twice as likely as men to report difficulty falling asleep (30% versus 14%). Both difficulty falling asleep and frequently awakenings were found to increase in prevalence with age and were associated with poor health, depression, angina, limitations in activities of daily living, and the use of benzodiazepines. Female gender, depression, and regular use of hypnotics were also found to be associated with sleep complaints in the elderly in another community study (Maggi et al. 1998). In this study, depression symptoms were more strongly associated with nighttime complaints, and physical disability was more associated with feeling poorly rested upon awakening.

These studies are in contrast to a nonrandom survey-based study of 1,485 elderly patients over the age of 50 years (Middelkoop et al. 1996). In this study, the number of nighttime awakenings increased significantly only in males. No significant correlations were found between health status and gender, age, or subjective sleep quality. The most frequently reported causes of disturbed sleep onset and sleep maintenance were worries and nocturia, respectively. Subjective sleep quality was mostly associated with self-estimated sleep latency. Lastly, in a sample of patients between the ages of 50 and 65 who were carefully assessed for physical health status, the prevalence of difficulty falling asleep was only 1% in men and 2.6% in women, and difficulty maintaining sleep was only 4.4% in men and 3.3% in women (D. L. Bliwise et al. 1992). The authors concluded that when overall physical health factors are taken into account, a decline in sleep quality is not necessarily an inevitable component of aging specifically, but rather a result of processes that accompany aging. One methodological difference among these studies is the range of ages in each. Hoch et al. (1997) examined subjective and polysomnography-defined sleep quality over 3 years in 50 subjects between the ages of 60 and 87 years old who were carefully screened for medical and psychiatric status. Subjective sleep quality, sleep continuity, and slow-wave sleep diminished in the subjects 75 years and older, whereas these measures were relatively stable in the subjects younger than 75. Changes in medical status did not correlate with these declines in sleep outcomes. Thus, complaints of deterioration in sleep quality would appear to increase with age in the elderly and are associated with psychiatric and general medical symptoms.

Alcohol abuse or dependence in the elderly can lead to decreases in subjective sleep quality, increased number of nocturnal wakings, increased sleep apnea, and complaints of daytime sleepiness (J. W. Smith 1995; Wooten 1992). Thus, in addition to the evaluation of general medical conditions and psychiatric conditions, an evaluation of alcohol use in elderly patients with complaints of poor sleep quality or daytime sleepiness is indicated (see Chapter 17 in this volume).

Supplementing epidemiological studies of the prevalence of sleep complaints, more recent clinical studies of sleep symptoms have considered the clinical relevance of such symptoms. For example, nosological systems such as DSM-IV require that, in addition to symptom clusters, some level of clinically significant distress and impairment be present before a syndrome or disorder is considered to be present. This requirement has raised interesting questions about potential discrepancies between the deterioration of sleep quality with aging and the difficulty in measur-

ing daytime impairments presumably resulting from sleep loss in the context of chronic insomnias. For example, in a study of 239 women and 113 men (mean age 77 years), sleep disturbance was a significant predictor in multivariate analysis of perceived limitations in usual role activities (Kutner et al. 1994). However, in a related study, 124 retirement community residents were interviewed about sleep patterns and given neuropsychological assessments, but no correlations between sleep variables and neuropsychological performance were found. The authors conclude that in nonclinical populations nighttime sleep problems are not associated with neuropsychological deficits (Hayward et al. 1992). Thus, samples identified by epidemiological studies and those identified by help-seeking patients or from clinical populations can yield different results. We summarize principles of diagnosis in Figure 17–2.

Sleeping Pills, Behavioral Treatments, and the Elderly

The indications for the use of hypnotics and the optimal strategies to treat complaints of poor sleep quality in the elderly are still being developed. For a general review of the issues, see Folks and Burke (1998), who emphasize differential diagnosis and advocate combined nonpharmacological and pharmacological approaches. For a review of nonpharmacological interventions, see Morin et al. (1994), whose meta-analysis suggests that stimulus control and sleep restriction therapies may be the most efficacious behavioral interventions, though the studies reviewed were not specifically of the elderly. For specific studies of various behavioral interventions in aging populations, see D. L. Bliwise et al. 1995; Edinger et al. 1992; Engle-Friedman et al. 1992; Lichstein and Johnson 1993; Morin et al. 1993, 1999; Riedel et al. 1995; and Reynolds et al. 1999. For a review of pharmacological interventions in the elderly, see Shorr and Robin (1994) who advocate time-limited treatments of low-dose hypnotics, with regular and frequent assessment of side effects, and a planned taper schedule. As discussed by Bandera et al. (1984), hypnotics with short and intermediate half-lives are preferable in the elderly because of altered pharmacokinetics and the potential for next-day side effects.

It may be interesting to note a general trend in prescribing practices away from sedative-hypnotics to antidepressants, especially in the institutionalized elderly (Walsh and Engelhardt 1992) (see also Chapter 37 in this volume). In a study of 330 nonagenarians from the general popula-

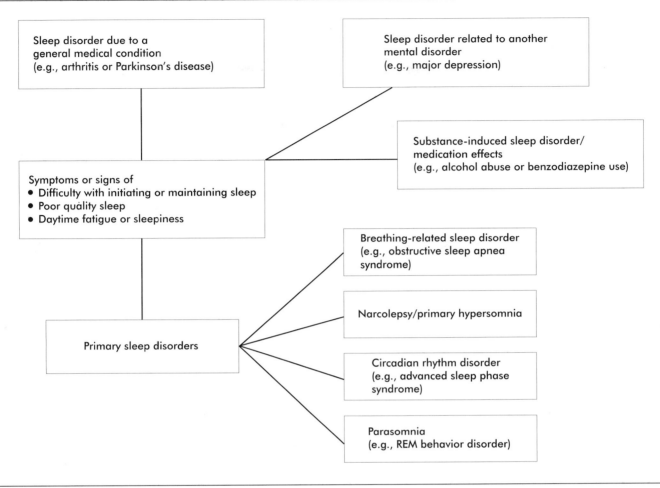

FIGURE 17–2. Principles of diagnosis chart. REM = rapid eye movement.

tion, half received some form of psychotropic medication, the most common being a hypnotic (Forsell and Winblad 1997). However, the authors noted that the rate of differential treatment after differential diagnosis was low. Little empirical evidence suggests that antidepressants are more effective than sedative-hypnotics in managing complaints of poor sleep quality in patients whose sleep disorder is not secondary to a primary psychiatric disorder. However, further studies are needed to evaluate the utility of using antidepressants in the place of sedative-hypnotics for primary insomnia (Nowell et al., in press). In at least one study of 262 residents admitted to nursing homes, psychotropic drugs, including hypnotics, were initiated within the first 2 weeks of admission, but the rate of use of such drugs was only slightly increased 6 months later (Wancata et al. 1997). The authors suggest that a large percentage of intake of psychotropic drugs is a result of new nursing home orders rather than continuation of medications that had been initiated in the community.

In a study of a stratified sample of 600 community-dwelling elderly subjects, use of hypnotics increased with age in both men and women (Seppala et al. 1997).

Multivariate analyses demonstrated that aging and poor health were independently associated with the use of hypnotics but, curiously, not with poor quality sleep or insomnia. In another study of a random sample of 516 community-living elderly over the age of 70 years, self-reported difficulties with falling asleep and global dissatisfaction with poor sleep were associated with the use of sleep medications (Englert and Linden 1998). In univariate and multivariate analyses, neither the duration of sleep time nor difficulties with sleeping through the night differentiated between those who did or did not take sleep medication. More studies are needed to identify factors that lead patients to seek treatment, as well as factors that lead providers to prescribe hypnotics in the elderly.

Sleepiness and Aging

Considerable attention has been paid in recent years to the impact of increasing shift work and restricted sleep schedules on the health of the national population. Considerably fewer studies, however, have addressed the prevalence and clinical significance of excessive daytime sleepiness in the elderly.

In Ganguli et al.'s 1996 study, described above, 19% of elderly subjects reported symptoms of daytime somnolence. In the Cardiovascular Health Study, described above, 20% of subjects demonstrated excessive daytime sleepiness as measured by the Epworth Sleepiness Scale (Newman et al. 1997; Whitney et al. 1998). Daytime sleepiness was related strongly to poor health and limitations in activities of daily living and was correlated with age. In a 4-year, multisite, prospective cohort study that included annual interviews, 3,962 subjects over the age of 65 years were evaluated for sleep-related symptoms and health status. The point prevalence of excessive daytime sleepiness was estimated at 25%. Daytime nappers were reported to more likely be male, urban, and heavier and have more depressive symptoms, more limited physical activity, and more functional impairments. The 4-year mortality rate was accelerated 1.73 times among older people who nap most of the time and make two or more errors on a cognitive status examination (Hays et al. 1996). Thus, excessive daytime sleepiness is a significant symptom associated with morbidity and mortality in the elderly. As with the symptom of poor sleep quality and insomnia, differential diagnosis of daytime sleepiness is important in the elderly. Among causes of daytime sleepiness in the elderly are narcolepsy, breathing-related sleep disorders, movement disorders in sleep, drug-related sedation and interactions, changes in circadian function, sleep deprivation from poor sleep habits, and sleepiness in the context of other general medical conditions (see Figure 17–2).

Narcolepsy

Although narcolepsy is generally believed to be a disorder arising in adolescence and early adulthood, patients with narcolepsy may present later in life. In one case series, 51% of retrospectively reviewed cases of narcolepsy seen in clinics were reported as presented by patients older than the age of 40 (Rye et al. 1998). Among the older patients, the diagnosis was delayed because of mild symptom severity, late-life expression of cataplexy, or absence of cataplexy with late-life expression of excessive daytime sleepiness. The authors concluded that narcolepsy should be considered in the differential diagnosis of sleepiness or transient loss of muscle tone in older patients.

Breathing-Related Sleep Disorders

It is generally held that breathing-related events in sleep increase with age. However, considerable controversy exists as to the clinical significance of such events. When breathing-related events occur frequently enough to fragment sleep and lead to excessive daytime sleepiness, then treatment to reduce daytime sleepiness is warranted. It remains unclear, however, whether sleep apnea syndromes, particularly mild or moderate sleep apnea, are risk factors for cardiovascular events in the elderly.

One way to measure the potential prevalence of breathing-related sleep disorders is to use home oximetry to gauge the frequency of oxygen desaturations. This method has the advantage of low cost and ease of application but can be limited by defining breathing-related disorders as desaturations rather than arousals from sleep. One such epidemiological study of nocturnal desaturations (defined in this study by a decrease in SaO_2 exceeding 4%) was conducted in 239 elderly subjects (mean age 76 years) from the general population (Philip et al. 1997). Twenty-seven percent had 10 or more episodes an hour of such desaturations, and 4.4% had 30 or more episodes per hour. Multivariate analysis demonstrated that snoring, male gender, body mass index, and advanced age in women were all correlated with 10 or more episodes per hour. However, no association was found between desaturations and daytime somnolence, difficulty with falling asleep, hypertension, or dysrhythmia. This finding led the authors to suggest that there is a high prevalence of sleep-related respiratory disturbance in elderly persons, but that there may be fewer consequences of such disturbance in the elderly than for younger groups.

Another method of trying to gauge the clinical impact of breathing-related sleep disorder in aging populations is to assess the frequency and subsequent correlates of snoring. In the Cardiovascular Health Study described above (Whitney et al. 1998), snoring, awakenings, awakening short of breath, depression, and limited activities of daily living were all independently associated with elevated Epworth scores, a self-report measure of situational sleepiness. The authors noted that neither cognitive function, magnetic resonance imaging evidence of brain atrophy or white matter abnormalities, nor cardiovascular disorders were independently associated with levels of daytime sleepiness. These findings were interpreted as calling into question the mediating role of hypersomnia on cognitive function or cardiovascular consequences in apnea.

In a two-stage random sample of the general population, both clinical screening and laboratory polysomnography were used to determine the prevalence and clinical significance of sleep apnea across the life span (Bixler et al. 1998). A total of 4,364 men (age 20–100 years) were screened by telephone, and a subset of 741 were evaluated in the sleep laboratory. Obstructive sleep apnea syndrome was found in 3.3% of the entire sample by using clinical criteria combined with an apnea-hypopnea index greater than 10. The maximum prevalence was found in the 45–64 age range. The prevalence of any type of sleep apnea increased monotonically with age. The severity of sleep apnea, as indicated by both number of events and minimum oxygen saturation, decreased with age when any sleep apnea criteria were used and when controlling for body mass index. The authors concluded that the prevalence of sleep apnea tends to increase with age, but that the clinical significance (severity) of apnea decreases. Based on these findings, the authors also suggested that the sleep laboratory criteria for diagnosis of sleep apnea should be adjusted for age.

In terms of the cognitive consequences of apnea in the elderly, Stone et al. (1994) administered neuropsychological tests to 45 older patients with insomnia (mean age 65 years) with and without sleep apnea. The results suggested that when the severity of sleep disruption was controlled for, minimal differences were found in neuropsychological functioning of older adults with mild to moderate sleep apnea compared with those without apnea. However, in a different study by Dealberto et al. (1996), 1,389 community-dwelling persons ages 60–70 years were evaluated with clinical scales and neuropsychological tests. In cross-sectional analyses, snoring and breathing pauses during sleep were found to be associated with daytime sleepiness and were risk factors for low cognitive performance in tests requiring visual attention skills.

Thus, the precise prevalence of breathing-related sleep disorder in elderly men and women and the health consequences of breathing-related sleep disorder in the elderly remain to be determined.

Movement Disorders

Periodic limb movements and the restless legs syndrome are syndromes that receive wide attention from the sleep disorders community (Williams 1996). Although research has been progressing, focus specifically in elderly populations remains limited. As with breathing-related sleep disorder, the prevalence of both periodic limb movements and restless legs syndrome is thought to increase with age, but the clinical significance of these syndromes in the elderly is unclear. Treatment is generally geared toward symptomatic reduction of restless legs syndrome or the excessive daytime sleepiness that is attributed to periodic limb movements during sleep (Williams 1996).

A different movement disorder, REM behavior disorder, is more properly considered a parasomnia. Yet, it can also be described as consisting of abnormal movements occurring during sleep (Schenck et al. 1986). These movements are believed to parallel the content of dreams ostensibly occurring in REM sleep. REM behavior disorder may be considered a sleep disorder somewhat more specific to the elderly. Although not well studied, the disorder is thought to arise in mid- to later life and to be associated with neurodegenerative disorders such as dementia (Schenck et al. 1987). Thus, differential diagnosis of new onset of abnormal movements in sleep becomes more important in the elderly because the presence of REM behavior disorder suggests that a more extensive assessment of the central nervous system be conducted before symptomatic treatment is instituted.

Circadian Rhythms in Aging

In older adults, many 24-hour rhythms are dampened and/or advanced. For review of circadian rhythms and psychiatric disorders in the elderly, see Myers and Badia (1995) and Sloan et al. (1996). The most marked change in circadian rhythms with age is an attenuation of amplitude. An advance of phase, a shortening of period, and a desynchronization of rhythms may also be evident. Examples of such rhythms are reflected in cortisol and growth hormone levels (reviewed by Vancauter et al. 1998). Amplitude reduction and phase advance of 24-hour rhythms may represent age-related changes in the central nervous system underlying circadian rhythmicity, for example, the suprachiasmatic nucleus and its afferents and efferents. On the other hand, age-related alterations in circadian function could also reflect decreased exposure or reactivity to photic and nonphotic information (Vancauter et al. 1998). Age-related changes in the retina, suprachiasmatic nucleus, and pineal gland, as well as behavioral changes such as a reduction in physical activity and exposure to light, can all interact to produce the changes in circadian rhythms observed in aging.

Changes in circadian rhythms are frequently associated with a reduction in nighttime sleep quality, a decrease in daytime alertness, and an attenuation in cognitive performance. In a study of young (19- to 29-year-old) and middle-aged (53- to 59-year-old) workers, three consecutive nights of shift work resulted in better phase adjustment (as measured by core body temperature) in younger subjects than in middle-aged subjects (Harma et al. 1994). The phase adjustment was correlated with subjective daytime recuperative sleep quality. In a series of studies examining circadian adjustment across the life span, Carrier and Monk (1997) and Monk et al. (1995) demonstrated that the declines in circadian phase adjustments apparent in middle age approach levels of severity similar to those observed in elderly samples (age 70 years and older). The question remains whether the changes in circadian rhythms result from changes in central nervous system functioning during aging or from changes in lifestyle such as daily activity and routines (Monk et al. 1997). Reversing such changes in circadian rhythms could enhance medical-related quality of life for a large and rapidly increasing percentage of the population (Myers and Badia 1995). Interventions to reverse such changes in circadian rhythms might include bright light therapy, melatonin, and scheduling of daily activities.

Bright Light Exposure and Sleep Quality in the Elderly

For an overview, see the Consensus Report for Light Treatment of Sleep Disorders (Campbell et al. 1995). The review describes the beneficial effects of bright light on sleep maintenance insomnia in the elderly. In addition, the review describes the effects of bright light on the behavioral disturbances that accompany dementia. For example, Campbell et al. (1993) examined 16 patients, ages 62–81 years, with sleep maintenance insomnia. Patients received 12 days of bright light exposure, which resulted in improvements in sleep quality and sleep efficiency. In another study (Satlin et al. 1992), 10 inpatients with Alzheimer's disease received 2 hours of exposure to bright light between 7:00 P.M. and 9:00 P.M. daily for 1 week. Patients wore activity monitors. Clinical ratings of sleep-wakefulness on the evening nursing shift improved with light treatment in 8 of the 10 patients. The proportion of total daily activity occurring during the nighttime decreased during the light-treatment week. The relative amplitude of the circadian locomotor activity rhythm, a measure of its stability, increased during the light-treatment week. In a more recent study by Cooke et al. (1998), 10 community-residing women between 67 and 87 years old who complained of poor sleep received bright light (2,000 lux) by visor for 30 minutes in the evening for 14 days in an unblinded, ABA design using self-report and home actigraphy as outcome measures. The authors reported improvements in sleep quality and sleep efficiency. Although the general results have been encouraging, bright light therapy has not received widespread acceptance as a medical intervention in the elderly, and more research is needed to define parameters such as dosing and duration of treatment.

Melatonin and Sleep Quality in the Elderly

Considerable controversy exists over the indications and physiological effects of melatonin. For an introduction to the debate, including issues related to the elderly, see

Kryger (1997). The issue of melatonin as a hypnotic is unresolved, despite the ease of acquiring this hormone from health food stores. In general, melatonin has not been shown to be a robust hypnotic. As discussed in the article cited above, it has been suggested that elderly patients with insomnia who are deficient in melatonin may benefit from "replacement" of melatonin by exogenous administration. However, there remains the question of optimal time of administration and the optimal dose necessary. In addition, some evidence suggests that younger patients with accumulated sleep debt may experience the strongest hypnotic effect to exogenous melatonin administration. In at least one recent study specific to the elderly (Youngstedt et al. 1998), neither self-reported sleep measures nor actigraphy outcomes were related to melatonin excretion. At present, research evidence is insufficient to guide clinicians in the use of melatonin in elderly patients with complaints of insomnia. No studies examine the use of melatonin to treat jet lag in the elderly.

■ Principles of Therapeutic Intervention

We believe that it is important to consider disturbed sleep in late life as symptomatic of underlying causes, with typically more than one factor operating in combination, and that therapy should address causes and related mediating factors (e.g., depression, as proposed in the model described above). Promising avenues of nonpharmacological intervention for persistent insomnia in late life usually address behaviors with a negative effect on sleep (e.g., sleep compression approaches to limit time in bed to enhance sleep efficiency and depth) or help to realign sleep and circadian rhythms with external time cues (e.g., via the use of bright light exposure). Useful pharmacological approaches tend to be simple, for example, monotherapy of depression, which uses a single antidepressant medication and avoids the premature use of adjunctive sleeping pills. Further research is strongly needed to address the utility of maintenance medication, such as low-dose antidepressants or intermittent benzodiazepines, for insomnia in late life.

■ References

American Psychiatric Association: Diagnostic and Statistical Manual of Mental Disorders, 4th Edition. Washington, DC, American Psychiatric Association, 1994

Ancoli-Israel S: Sleep problems in older adults: putting myths to bed. Geriatrics 52:20–30, 1997

Bachman DL: Sleep disorders with aging: evaluation and treatment. Geriatrics 47:53–56, 1992

Bandera R, Bollini P, Garattini S: Long-acting and short-acting benzodiazepines in the elderly: kinetic differences and clinical relevance. Curr Med Res Opin 8(suppl 4):94–107, 1984

Bassetti C, Aldrich MS, Chervin RD, et al: Sleep apnea in patients with transient ischemic attack and stroke: a prospective study of 59 patients. Neurology 47:1167–1173, 1996

Becker PM, Jamieson AO: Common sleep disorders in the elderly: diagnosis and treatment. Geriatrics 47:41–42, 1992

Bixler EO, Vgontzas AN, Ten HT, et al: Effects of age on sleep apnea in men, I: prevalence and severity. Am J Respir Crit Care Med 157:144–148, 1998

Bliwise DL: Sleep in normal aging and dementia. Sleep 16:40–81, 1993

Bliwise DL, King AC, Harris RB, et al: Prevalence of self-reported poor sleep in a healthy population aged 50–65. Soc Sci Med 34:49–55, 1992

Bliwise DL, Friedman L, Nekich JC, et al: Prediction of outcome in behaviorally based insomnia treatments. J Behav Ther Exp Psychiatry 26:17–23, 1995

Bliwise NG, Bliwise DL, Dement WC: Age and psychopathology in insomnia. Clinics in Gerontology 4:3–9, 1985

Brendel DH, Reynolds CF, Jennings JR, et al: Sleep-stage physiology, mood, and vigilance responses to total sleep deprivation in healthy eighty year olds and twenty year olds. Psychophysiology 27:677–686, 1990

Campbell SS, Dawson D, Anderson MW: Alleviation of sleep maintenance insomnia with timed exposure to bright light. J Am Geriatr Soc 41:829–836, 1993

Campbell SS, Terman M, Lewy AJ, et al: Light treatment for sleep disorders: consensus report, V: age-related disturbances. J Biol Rhythms 10:151–154, 1995

Carrier J, Monk TH: Estimating the endogenous circadian temperature rhythm without keeping people awake. J Biol Rhythms 12:266–277, 1997

Cartwright RD: REM sleep during and after mood-disturbing events. Arch Gen Psychiatry 40:197–201, 1983

Cartwright RD, Wood E: Adjustment disorders of sleep: the sleep effects of a major stressful event and its resolution. Psychiatry Res 39:199–209, 1991

Cohen S, Wills TA: Stress, social support, and the buffering hypothesis. Psychol Bull 98:310–357, 1985

Consensus Development Conference: Diagnosis and Treatment of Sleep Disorders in Late Life. Bethesda, MD, National Institutes of Health, 1990

Cook NR, Evans DA, Funkenstein H, et al: Correlates of headache in a population based cohort of elderly. Arch Neurol 46:1338–1344, 1989

Cooke KM, Kreydatus MA, Atherton A, et al: The effects of evening light exposure on the sleep of elderly women expressing sleep complaints. J Behav Med 21:103–114, 1998

Dealberto MJ, Pajot N, Courbon D, et al: Breathing disorders during sleep and cognitive performance in an older community sample: the EVA Study. J Am Geriatr Soc 44:1287–1294, 1996

Dew MA, Ragni MV, Nimorwicz P: Infection with human immunodeficiency virus and vulnerability to psychiatric distress. Arch Gen Psychiatry 47:737–744, 1990

Diagnostic Classification Steering Committee: International Classification of Sleep Disorders: Diagnostic and Coding Manual. Rochester, MN, American Sleep Disorders Association, 1990

Dyken ME, Somers VK, Yamada T, et al: Investigating the relationship between stroke and obstructive sleep apnea. Stroke 27:401–407, 1996

Edinger JD, Hoelscher TJ, Marsh GR, et al: A cognitive-behavioral therapy for sleep-maintenance insomnia in older adults. Psychol Aging 7:282–289, 1992

Engle-Friedman M, Bootzin RR, Hazlewood L, et al: An evaluation of behavioral treatments for insomnia in the older adult. J Clin Psychol 48:77–90, 1992

Englert S, Linden M: Differences in self-reported sleep complaints in elderly persons living in the community who do or do not take sleep medication. J Clin Psychiatry 59:137–144, 1998

Foley DJ, Monjan AA, Brown SL, et al: Sleep complaints among elderly persons: an epidemiologic study of three communities. Sleep 18:425–432, 1995

Folks DG, Burke WJ: Psychotherapeutic agents in older adults. Sedative hypnotics and sleep. Clin Geriatr Med 14:67–86, 1998

Ford DE, Kamerow DB: Epidemiologic study of sleep disturbances and psychiatric disorders: an opportunity for prevention? JAMA 262:1479–1488, 1989

Forsell Y, Winblad B: Psychiatric disturbances and the use of psychotropic drugs in a population of nonagenarians. Int J Geriatr Psychiatry 12:533–536, 1997

Ganguli M, Reynolds CF, Gilby JE: Prevalence and persistence of sleep complaints in a rural older community sample: the MoVIES project. J Am Geriatr Soc 44:778–784, 1996

George LK: Social and Economic Factors in Geriatric Psychiatry. Edited by Busse E, Blazer DG. Washington, DC, American Psychiatric Press, 1989, pp 203–234

Gislason T, Almqvist M: Somatic diseases and sleep complaints. Acta Medica Scandinavica 221:475–481, 1987

Giubilei F, Iannilli M, Vitale A, et al: Sleep patterns in acute ischemic stroke. Acta Neurol Scand 86:567–571, 1992

Good DC, Henkle JQ, Gelber D, et al: Sleep-disordered breathing and poor functional outcome after stroke. Stroke 27:252–259, 1996

Gottlieb GL: Sleep disorders and their management. Special considerations in the elderly. Am J Med 88:29S–33S, 1990

Harma MI, Hakola T, Akerstedt T, et al: Age and adjustment to night work. Occup Environ Med 51:568–573, 1994

Hays JC, Blazer DG, Foley DJ: Risk of napping: excessive daytime sleepiness and mortality in an older community population. J Am Geriatr Soc 44:693–698, 1996

Hayward LB, Mant A, Eyland EA, et al: Neuropsychological functioning and sleep patterns in the elderly. Med J Aust 157:51–52, 1992

Hoch CC, Reynolds CF, Houck PR, et al: Predicting mortality in mixed depression and dementia using EEG sleep variables. J Neuropsychiatry Clin Neurosci 1:366–371, 1989

Hoch CC, Reynolds CF, Jennings JR, et al: Daytime sleepiness and performance among healthy 80 and 20 year olds. Neurobiol Aging 13:353–356, 1992

Hoch CC, Dew MA, Reynolds CF, et al: Longitudinal changes in diary- and laboratory-based sleep measures in healthy "old old" and "young old" subjects: a three-year follow-up. Sleep 20:192–202, 1997

Hyyppa MT, Kronholm E: Quality of sleep and chronic illnesses. J Clin Epidemiol 42:633–638, 1989

Karacan I, Thornby JI, Anch M, et al: Prevalence of sleep disturbance in a primarily urban Florida county. Soc Sci Med 10:239–244, 1976

Kessler RC, McLeod JC: Social support and mental health in community samples, in Social Support and Health. Edited by Cohen S, Syme SL. New York, Academic Press, 1985, pp 219–240

Kostic VS, Susic V, Przedborski S, et al: Sleep EEG in depressed and nondepressed patients with Parkinson's disease. J Neuropsychiatry Clin Neurosci 3:176–179, 1991

Kramer CJ, Kerkhof GA, Hofman WF, et al: Transitions from wakefulness to sleep at different times of day—old vs. young subjects. Biological Rhythm Research 29:105–117, 1998

Kryger MH: Controversies in sleep medicine—melatonin. Sleep 20:898, 1997

Kutner NG, Schechtman KB, Ory MG, et al: Older adults' perceptions of their health and functioning in relation to sleep disturbance, falling, and urinary incontinence. FICSIT Group. J Am Geriatr Soc 42:757–762, 1994

Lichstein KL, Johnson RS: Relaxation for insomnia and hypnotic medication use in older women. Psychol Aging 8:103–111, 1993

Maggi S, Langlois JA, Minicuci N, et al: Sleep complaints in community-dwelling older persons—prevalence, associated factors, and reported causes. J Am Geriatr Soc 46:161–168, 1998

Mant A, Eyland EA: Sleep patterns and problems in elderly general practice attenders: an Australian survey. Community Health Studies 12:192–199, 1988

Menza MA, Rosen RC: Sleep in Parkinson's disease. The role of depression and anxiety. Psychosomatics 36:262–266, 1995

Middelkoop HA, Smilde-van DD, Neven AK, et al: Subjective sleep characteristics of 1,485 males and females aged 50–93: effects of sex and age, and factors related to self-evaluated quality of sleep. J Gerontol A Biol Sci Med Sci 51:M108–M115, 1996

Mohsenin V, Valor R: Sleep apnea in patients with hemispheric stroke. Arch Phys Med Rehabil 76:71–76, 1995

Monane M: Insomnia in the elderly. J Clin Psychiatry 53 (suppl):23–28, 1992

Monk TH, Buysse DJ, Reynolds CF, et al: Circadian temperature rhythms of older people. Exp Gerontol 30:455–474, 1995

Monk TH, Reynolds CF, Kupfer DJ, et al: Differences over the life span in daily life-style regularity. Chronobiol Int 14:295–306, 1997

Moran MG, Thompson TL, Nies AS: Sleep disorders in the elderly. Am J Psychiatry 145:1369–1378, 1988

Morgan K, Healey DW, Healey PJ: Factors influencing persistent subjective insomnia in old age: a follow-up study of good and poor sleepers aged 65–74. Age Ageing 18:117–122, 1989

Morin C, Gramling S: Sleep patterns and aging: comparison of older adults with and without insomnia complaints. Psychol Aging 4:290–294, 1989

Morin CM, Kowatch RA, Barry T, et al: Cognitive-behavior therapy for late-life insomnia. J Consult Clin Psychol 61:137–146, 1993

Morin CM, Culbert JP, Schwartz SM: Nonpharmacological interventions for insomnia: a meta-analysis of treatment efficacy. Am J Psychiatry 151:1172–1180, 1994

Morin CM, Colechi C, Stone J, et al: Behavioral and pharmacologic therapies for late-life insomnia: a randomized controlled trial. JAMA 281:991–999, 1999

Myers BL, Badia P: Changes in circadian rhythms and sleep quality with aging: mechanisms and interventions. Neurosci Biobehav Rev 19:553–571, 1995

Newman AB, Enright PL, Manolio TA, et al: Sleep disturbance, psychosocial correlates, and cardiovascular disease in 5201 older adults: the Cardiovascular Health Study. J Am Geriatr Soc 45:1–7, 1997

Nowell PD, Buysse DJ, Dew MA, et al: Paroxetine in the treatment of primary insomnia: preliminary clinical and EEG sleep data. J Clin Psychiatry 60:89–95, 1995

Philip P, Dealberto MJ, Dartigues JF, et al: Prevalence and correlates of nocturnal desaturations in a sample of elderly people. J Sleep Res 6:264–271, 1997

Prigerson HG, Frank E, Reynolds CF, et al: Protective psychosocial factors in depression among spousally bereaved elders. Am J Geriatr Psychiatry 1:296–309, 1993

Prinz PN, Halter J, Benedetti C, et al: Circadian variation of plasma catecholamines in young and old men: relation to rapid eye movements and slow wave sleep. J Clin Endocrinol Metab 49:300–304, 1979

Prinz PN, Vitiello MV, Raskind MA, et al: Geriatrics: sleep disorders and aging. N Engl J Med 323:520–526, 1990

Reynolds CF, Kupfer DJ, Hoch CC, et al: Sleep deprivation as a probe in the elderly. Arch Gen Psychiatry 44:982–990, 1987

Reynolds CF, Monk TH, Hoch CC, et al: EEG sleep in the healthy "old old": a comparison with the "young old" in visually scored and automated (period) measures. J Gerontol A Biol Med Sci 46:M39–M46, 1991

Reynolds CF, Hoch CC, Buysse DJ, et al: EEG sleep in spousal bereavement and bereavement-related depression of late life. Biol Psychiatry 31:69–82, 1992

Reynolds CF, Hoch CC, Buysse DJ, et al: REM sleep in successful, usual, and pathological aging: the Pittsburgh experience 1980–1991. J Sleep Res 2:203–210, 1993

Reynolds CF, Buysse DJ, Kupfer DJ: Treating insomnia in older adults: taking a long-term view. JAMA 281:1034–1035, 1999

Riedel BW, Lichstein KL, Dwyer WO: Sleep compression and sleep education for older insomniacs: self-help versus therapist guidance. Psychol Aging 10:54–63, 1995

Roehrs T, Lineback W, Zorick F, et al: Relationship of psychopathology to insomnia in the elderly. J Am Geriatr Soc 30:312–315, 1982

Rosenwaike I: A demographic portrait of the oldest old. Milbank Memorial Fund Quarterly 63:187–205, 1985

Roth T, Kramer M, Trinder J: The effect of noise during sleep on the sleep patterns of different age groups. Canadian Psychiatric Association Journal 1(17):ss197–ss201, 1972

Rye DB, Dihenia B, Weissman JD, et al: Presentation of narcolepsy after 40. Neurology 50:459–465, 1998

Satlin A, Volicer L, Ross V, et al: Bright light treatment of behavioral and sleep disturbances in patients with Alzheimer's disease. Am J Psychiatry 149:1028–1032, 1992

Schenck CH, Bundlie SR, Ettinger MG, et al: Chronic behavioral disorders of human REM sleep: a new category of parasomnia. Sleep 9:293–308, 1986

Schenck CH, Bundlie SR, Patterson AL, et al: Rapid eye movement sleep behavior disorder. A treatable parasomnia affecting older adults. JAMA 257:1786–1789, 1987

Seppala M, Hyyppa MT, Impivaara O, et al: Subjective quality of sleep and use of hypnotics in an elderly urban population. Aging (Milano) 9:327–334, 1997

Shorr RI, Robin DW: Rational use of benzodiazepines in the elderly. Drugs Aging 4:9–20, 1994

Sloan EP, Flint AJ, Reinish L, et al: Circadian rhythms and psychiatric disorders in the elderly. J Geriatr Psychiatry Neurol 9:164–170, 1996

Smith JW: Medical manifestations of alcoholism in the elderly. International Journal of the Addictions 30:1749–1798, 1995

Smith MC, Ellgring H, Oertel WH: Sleep disturbances in Parkinson's disease patients and spouses. J Am Geriatr Soc 45:194–199, 1997

Stocchi F, Barbato L, Nordera G: Sleep disorders in Parkinson's disease (review). J Neurol 245(suppl 1):S15–S18, 1998

Stone J, Morin CM, Hart RP, et al: Neuropsychological functioning in older insomniacs with or without obstructive sleep apnea. Psychol Aging 9:231–236, 1994

Tan A, Salgado M, Fahn S: Rapid eye movement sleep behavior disorder preceding Parkinson's disease with therapeutic response to levodopa. Mov Disord 11:214–216, 1996

van Hilten B, Hoff JI, Middelkoop HA, et al: Sleep disruption in Parkinson's disease. Assessment by continuous activity monitoring. Arch Neurol 51:922–928, 1994

Vancauter E, Plat L, Leproult R, et al: Alterations of circadian rhythmicity and sleep in aging—endocrine consequences. Horm Res 49:147–152, 1998

Vitiello MV, Prinz PN, Avery DH, et al: Sleep is undisturbed in elderly, depressed individuals who have not sought health care. Biol Psychiatry 27:431–440, 1990

Walsh JK, Engelhardt CL: Trends in the pharmacologic treatment of insomnia. J Clin Psychiatry 53(suppl):10–17, 1992

Wancata J, Benda N, Meise U, et al: Psychotropic drug intake in residents newly admitted to nursing homes. Psychopharmacology (Berl) 134:115–120, 1997

Wauquier A, van Sweden B, Lagaay AM, et al: Ambulatory monitoring of sleep-wakefulness in healthy elderly males and females (greater than 88 years): the "senieur" protocol. J Am Geriatr Soc 40:109–114, 1992

Whitney CW, Enright PL, Newman AB, et al: Correlates of daytime sleepiness in 4578 elderly persons—the cardiovascular health study. Sleep 21:27–36, 1998

Williams DC: Periodic limb movements of sleep and the restless legs syndrome. Va Med Q 123:260–265, 1996

Wittig RM, Zorick FJ, Blumer D, et al: Disturbed sleep in patients complaining of chronic pain. J Nerv Ment Dis 170:424–431, 1982

Wooten V: Sleep disorders in geriatric patients. Clin Geriatr Med 8:427–439, 1992

Youngstedt SD, Kripke DF, Elliott JA: Melatonin excretion is not related to sleep in the elderly. J Pineal Res 24:142–145, 1998

Zepelin H, McDonald CS: Age differences in autonomic variables during sleep. J Gerontol A Biol Sci Med Sci 42:142–146, 1987

Zepelin H, Morgan LE: Correlates of sleep disturbance in retirees. Sleep Research 10:120, 1981

Zepelin H, McDonald CS, Zammit GK: Effects of age on auditory awakening thresholds. J Gerontol A Biol Sci Med Sci 39:294–300, 1984

18

Pain

Michael R. Clark, M.D., M.P.H.

Definition and Assessment

Pain is a complex experience that integrates affective, cognitive, and behavioral factors with an extensive neurobiology (Turk et al. 1983). The formulation of pain simply as a disease of the body fails to appreciate the role of these factors and usually results in poor treatment outcome. Pain is not synonymous with a sensory event that is due to a nociceptive input resulting from injury or disease. Pain has been defined by the International Association for the Study of Pain as "an unpleasant sensory and emotional experience associated with actual or potential tissue damage, or described in terms of such damage" (Merskey et al. 1986). Pain is the most common reason a patient presents to a physician for evaluation (Kroenke and Mangelsdorff 1989; Kroenke et al. 1990). This physician is rarely a neuropsychiatrist. If the patient suffers from chronic pain, pain persisting on a daily basis for a month beyond what would be considered the usual time for healing of underlying pathology, then many specialists may be involved in the care of the patient (Bonica 1990).

Elderly patients with cancer pain are less likely to receive proper pain management than younger patients (Cleary and Carbone 1997). Unfortunately, elderly patients are often less likely to report pain or take opioids and other medications for pain because of fears of addiction, future tolerance coinciding with disease progression, and side effects and a belief that pain is an indicator of disease that may distract the doctor from primary and possibly curative treatment. Studies examining the use of patient-controlled analgesia in postoperative patients found that older patients "require" less opioids (Woodhouse and Mather 1997). However, it remains controversial whether older patients experience equivalent pain relief with less medication, are unable to report their pain, or continue to endure higher levels of pain despite medication being available to them. It would certainly be inappropriate and inaccurate to begin the evaluation of elderly patients believing that they experience less pain and suffering than younger patients (Ferrell 1991).

Although elderly patients may present to physicians with unusual complaints or lacking cardinal symptoms for a given illness, pain perception probably does not change with age (Harkins 1996). Pain is difficult to assess, especially in patients with terminal illnesses, cognitive impairments, and other chronic degenerative diseases of the brain (Nikolaus 1997; Parmelee 1996). Pain rating scales attempt to measure the severity and intensity of pain. Many factors can influence these ratings including disease states, mental disorders, distress, personality traits, and meaningful interpretations based on personal beliefs. Even the simplest self-report measures to record the presence of pain cannot be effectively used by many elderly individuals (Ferrell et al. 1995). The elderly often have deficits in abstract ability that make it difficult for them to rate pain by using a visual analogue scale (VAS) or a verbal descriptor scale (VDS) with terms such as "discomforting," "distressing," and "excruciating."

Increased age is associated with a greater frequency of incorrect responses to the VAS. In a comparison study of several pain rating scales, such as a vertical-oriented VAS, a VDS, a pain thermometer, and a numeric rating scale, the VDS was rated as the preferred, easiest, and best assessment tool for rating pain by the elderly (Herr and Mobily 1993). However, the ratings of pain intensity using these scales were poorly correlated with one another. Alternative tools for evaluating pain, such as pain drawings or maps and observations of pain behaviors, have been studied with positive results, but these methods are limited by reliance upon an outside observer to rate a patient's pain (Weiner et al. 1996, 1998). Animal studies also suggest that behavioral signs of pain are reduced in older rats with neuropathic pain (Chung et al. 1995). Different patient populations will probably require different pain rating instruments, depending on sensory, language, and neurological deficits. A comprehensive evaluation should be done for any patient who complains of pain, becomes agitated, or experiences deterioration in his or her functioning. This evaluation should incorporate simple standardized tools for rating pain severity, observations by others to determine the presence of pain-related behaviors including any problems with activities of daily living that would indicate the presence of pain, and clinical examination to elicit evidence of pain and the signs of possible etiologies.

Epidemiology

Pain is a common problem in the general population (Karlsten and Gordh 1997). The U.S. Center for Health Statistics conducted an 8-year follow-up survey and found that 32.8% of the general population suffered from chronic pain symptoms (Magni et al. 1993). A recent World Health Organization study of more than 25,000 primary care patients in 14 countries found that 22% of patients suffered from pain that was present for most of the time for at least 6 months (Gureje et al. 1998). In the community-dwelling elderly population, 25%–50% will suffer from pain (Gagliese and Melzack 1997; Gloth 1996). In a 24-year longitudinal study of chest, abdomen, and musculoskeletal pain, symptoms increased with aging, and women reported more persistent and severe pain (Brattberg et al. 1997). In people 65 years of age or older, musculoskeletal pain is associated with three times the likelihood of significant difficulty performing three or more physical activities (Scudds and Robertson 1998). In persons over the age of 75, more than two-thirds reported pain, almost half reported pain in multiple sites, and a third rated pain as severe in at least one location (Brattberg et al. 1996). Pain is even more common in residents of long-term care facilities and associated with significant decreases in function and quality of life. Sixty-six percent of nursing home residents over 65 reported chronic pain, which was not detected by physicians in 34% of residents (Stein and Ferrell 1996).

In patients surviving hospitalization for serious illness, those reporting moderately severe pain occurring most of the time or extremely severe pain occurring more than half of the time, 40% reported this pain up to 6 months after discharge from the hospital (Desbiens et al. 1997). The Study to Understand Prognoses and Preferences for Outcomes and Risks of Treatment (SUPPORT) has demonstrated that pain, dyspnea, and fatigue are the most prevalent symptoms experienced by patients with terminal illnesses at the end of life (Lynn et al. 1997). Sixty-three percent of patients at the end of life had difficulty tolerating physical or emotional symptoms.

Acute pain in the elderly is usually the result of trauma from a surgery, injury, or exacerbation of chronic disease, especially musculoskeletal conditions. Approximately 80% of the elderly suffer from some type of arthritis (Davis 1988). Treatment is focused on controlling inflammation and preventing tissue destruction. Recently, more emphasis has been placed on pain relief. Preliminary studies indicate that, compared with placebo, amitriptyline and fluoxetine significantly reduce pain (Rani et al. 1996). Older adults are likely to undergo surgery for degenerative problems, fractures, and cardiovascular disease (Ferrell 1996).

The approach to acute pain management in the elderly will usually be successful with straightforward strategies such as relaxation, immobilization, pharmacological agents (aspirin, acetaminophen, nonsteroidal anti-inflammatory drugs, opioids), massage, and transcutaneous electrical nerve stimulation (Acute Pain Management Guideline Panel 1992). To avoid delirium, side effects, and toxicity of the gastrointestinal, hepatic, and renal systems, the normal physiology of aging and presence of chronic diseases must be taken into consideration when using pharmacological treatments for pain. Although age and illness are risk factors for poor outcome, the elderly are more similar to the general population than they are different and benefit most when they receive excellent care rather than treatment by specialized algorithms.

Psychiatric Comorbidity

Patients with depression, anxiety, or psychological distress may experience increased pain or describe aspects of their suffering other than pain. Some patients cope with pain better than others, as reflected in their reports of pain, pain behaviors, and functional disabilities. In particular, elderly patients will often not report pain because they fear it means a deterioration of their condition, that it will distract practitioners from their underlying illness, or that it will upset others around them who are concerned about their well-being (Nishikawa and Ferrell 1993).

Pain Disorder

Pain "caused" by emotional factors was first classified in DSM-II under psychophysiological disorders (American Psychiatric Association 1968). DSM-III specifically addressed the problem of chronic pain with the introduction of psychogenic pain disorder, in which pathophysiology was either absent or insufficient to explain the severity and duration of pain (American Psychiatric Association 1980). In somatoform pain disorder (DSM-III-R), psychological factors were no longer required as an etiology of pain (American Psychiatric Association 1987). A preoccupation with pain instead of pain itself was established as the core criterion.

DSM-IV introduced pain disorder as a refinement of the DSM-III-R diagnosis of somatoform pain disorder (American Psychiatric Association 1994; S. A. King and Strain 1992). The primary criteria require 1) pain as the chief complaint, and 2) pain causing significant distress or functional impairment. In addition, psychological factors are recognized as having an important role in the pain, and the pain must not be the result of another mental disorder such as a factitious disorder, a mood disorder, or an anxiety disorder. If another mental disorder is present, the diagnosis of pain disorder cannot be given to a patient. It must be further specified if the pain disorder is acute or chronic and whether it is associated with just psychological factors or both psychological factors and a general medical condition. Unfortunately, the concept of psychological and physical dualism is still inherent in this diagnosis. Although it is difficult, the evaluation of a patient with pain should attempt to determine and enumerate all relevant diagnoses regardless of what specialty typically treats a particular diagnosis.

Somatization

Symptoms, not specific diseases, are the most common reason for seeking medical care (Brown et al. 1971; Koch 1978; Kroenke et al. 1990). Usually, a medical cause is never found for these "somatization" symptoms (Kroenke and Mangelsdorff 1989). As the number of medically unexplained symptoms increases, associated morbidity such as functional disability, increased health care utilization, inappropriate treatment with medications, excessive evaluations, and higher rates of psychiatric disorders increases (Katon et al. 1991; Kouyanou et al. 1998). These patients were more likely to exhibit catastrophic thinking and believe the cause of their pain to be a mystery. They often have feelings of losing control and that physicians believe their pain is imaginary. Patients with chronic pain and medically unexplained symptoms were also found to suffer iatrogenic consequences of their symptoms such as excessive medical evaluations and long-term treatment with inappropriate medications.

Although the actual diagnosis of somatization disorder is rare in patients with chronic pain, somatization is a common phenomenon in the practice of medicine, manifests itself along a spectrum of severity, and can emerge from and is shaped by many factors both in and around the patient. Somatization is conceptualized as at least three overlapping, distinct patterns of illness behavior "in which given symptoms may be differentially perceived, evaluated, and acted upon by different kinds of persons" (Mechanic 1962). These three forms have been operationalized and include 1) high levels of medically unexplained symptoms in multiple physiological systems; 2) levels of somatic preoccupation or illness worry beyond what is expected from demonstrable disease; and 3) the predominantly or exclusively somatic clinical presentation of psychiatric disorders, such as depression or anxiety (Atkinson et al. 1991; Katon et al. 1985; Kirmayer and Robbins 1991). Environmental forces such as the societal stigma of psychiatric disorders, history of physical and sexual abuse, and the reliance of physicians on the biomedical paradigm predispose to and reinforce somatization (Kroenke 1993; Walling et al. 1994).

Characterizing somatization as a psychophysiological process rather than a categorical psychiatric diagnosis or a psychological trait is probably more appropriate (Sullivan and Katon 1993). The process of somatization starts with symptom perception that varies along a continuum from minimization to amplification of sensory information. Once the symptom has been perceived, the individual attributes it to a cause, which could include a health problem. Finally, a decision is made about how to react to this symptom, and perhaps consultation with a health care professional will be sought. Fortunately, somatization can be managed effectively when the specific components of the process are addressed individually with understanding and rational treatments (Sullivan and Katon 1993).

Substance Use

Terms such as addiction, misuse, overuse, abuse, and dependence have been used inconsistently to describe various behaviors, making interpretation of many research studies difficult. The underreporting of medication use complicates accurate assessment of actual use patterns by patients with chronic pain (Ready et al. 1982). However, in patients with chronic pain who develop new substance use disorders, the problem most commonly involved the medications prescribed by their physicians (Long et al. 1988; Maruta et al. 1979). The mechanism of relapse to substance abuse in these patients is not well understood and probably involves multiple factors; however, a cycle of pain followed by relief after taking medications is an example of operant reinforcement of their future use (Fordyce et al. 1973).

In a study of patients attending a clinic specializing in pain, almost 90% of patients were taking medications (Kouyanou et al. 1997). Opioid analgesics were prescribed to 70%, whereas antidepressants and benzodiazepines were being taken by only 25% and 18%, respectively. In this population, 12% met DSM-III-R criteria for substance abuse or dependence; however, the misuse and abuse of medications was not limited to just psychoactive substances. In a review of 24 studies of drug/alcohol dependence/addiction in patients with chronic pain, only 7 studies met their standard of using acceptable criteria for these substance use disorders, and the prevalence ranged from 3.2% to 18.9% (Fishbain et al. 1992b). In a study of patients with chronic low back pain, 34% had a substance use disorder, yet in all cases such use was present before the onset of the chronic pain (Polatin et al. 1993). Those individuals with a history of substance abuse were found to be at increased risk for substance abuse during treatment for chronic pain, as well as increased risk of further physical injury (Savage 1993).

Substance abuse research has demonstrated abnormalities in pain perception and tolerance. In a study of persons who abused opiates and cocaine, cold pressor pain tolerance was significantly lower in individuals with current as opposed to former abuse (Compton 1994). Patients with alcoholism and nonalcoholic men with high familial-genetic risk for alcoholism demonstrate greater sensitivity to painful stimuli and pain reduction induced by alcohol (Stewart et al. 1995). These men rated an aversive shock as more painful, but differences from control subjects could be "normalized" with pharmacologically significant levels of ingested alcohol. This increased sensitivity to pain coupled with the relief experienced with substance use suggests at least one mechanism for the development of substance dependence in patients with chronic pain. (See also Chapter 16 in this volume.)

Depression

The National Health and Nutrition Study found that depression was more common in the elderly independent of the presence of pain (Harkins et al. 1984). However, the relationship between pain and depression remains controversial. Physical symptoms are common in patients suffering from major depression (Lipowski 1990). Approximately 60% of patients with depression report pain symptoms at the time of diagnosis (Magni et al. 1985; Von Knorring et al. 1983). The presence of a depressive disorder has been demonstrated to increase the risk of developing chronic musculoskeletal pain, headache, and chest pain 3 years later (Leino and Magni 1993; Magni et al. 1993, 1994; Von Korff et al. 1993). Older adults with depression were at increased risk for neck, back, and hip pain. Even after 8 years, previously depressed patients remained twice as likely to develop chronic pain as the nondepressed.

In 1,016 members of health maintenance organizations, the prevalence of depression was 12% in individuals with three or more pain complaints compared with only 1% in those with one or no pain complaints (Dworkin et al. 1990). The prevalence of major depression in patients with chronic low back pain is more than three times the rate in the general population (Sullivan et al. 1992). In groups of patients with medically unexplained symptoms such as back pain and dizziness, two-thirds of patients have a history of recurrent major depression compared with less than 20% of medically ill control groups (Atkinson et al. 1991; Katon and Sullivan 1990; Sullivan and Katon 1993). In patients with chronic pain referred to comprehensive pain programs for evaluation, 8%–50% have been reported to have a current major depression (Smith 1992). If pain resulted in a loss of independence or mobility that decreased an individual's participation in activities, the risk of depression was significantly increased (Williamson and Schulz 1992). Individuals with chronic physical complaints also have higher rates of lifetime major depression.

Depression is not simply a comorbid condition but interacts with chronic pain to increase morbidity and mortality. Patients with chronic pain and depression reported greater pain intensity, less life control, and more use of passive-avoidant coping strategies (Magni et al. 1985). They also described greater interference from pain and exhibited more pain behaviors than patients with chronic pain and without depression (Haythornthwaite et al. 1991; Weickgenant et al. 1993). The presence of preoperative depression in patients undergoing lumbar discectomy was predictive of poorer surgical outcome at 1-year follow-up (Junge et al. 1995). In patients with rheumatoid arthritis, depressive symptoms were significantly associated with negative health and functional outcomes as well as with increased health services utilization (Katz and Yelin 1993). Depression has been shown to be a significant predictor of pain persistence and the best predictor of application for early retirement (Hasenbring et al. 1994; Magni et al. 1993).

Patients with migraine, chronic abdominal pain, and orthopedic pain syndromes report increased rates of suicidal ideation and suicide attempts (Magni et al. 1998). In patients who attempted suicide, 52% had a somatic disease and 21% were taking analgesics on a daily basis for pain (Stenager et al. 1994). Patients with chronic pain completed suicide at two to three times the rate in the general population (Fishbain et al. 1991). Oncology patients with pain who also suffered from depression were significantly more likely to request assistance in committing suicide as well as to have taken steps to end their lives such as seeking information about suicide plans or hoarding medications. However, even if in pain, when depression was not present, they were unlikely to request the interventions of euthanasia and physician-assisted suicide (Emanuel et al. 1996). Depression should be treated aggressively and not simply "understood" as an expected outcome of having chronic pain. (See also Chapter 13 in this volume.)

Anxiety

Although anxiety is a common and expected component of acute pain, patients with chronic pain are also at increased risk for comorbid anxiety disorders. Patients with a variety of pain syndromes ranging from chronic low back pain, chronic neck pain after whiplash injury, and chronic pain from prostate cancer have increased rates of both anxiety symptoms and disorders (Heim and Oei 1993; Lee et al. 1993; Polatin et al. 1993; Weissman and Merikangas 1986). Almost 50% of patients report anxiety symptoms, and 19% of patients have an anxiety disorder such as panic disorder and generalized anxiety disorder (Devlen 1994; Fishbain et al. 1986; Katon et al. 1985). One prospective study of 1,007 young adults found that a baseline history of migraine was significantly associated with an increased risk (odds ratio = 12.8) of first-incidence panic disorder (Breslau and Davis 1993).

Conversely, anxiety disorders have been shown to be

associated with high levels of somatic preoccupation and physical symptoms. In a study of patients with panic disorder, almost 40% reported chronic pain symptoms and more than 7% were using analgesics on a daily basis (Kuch et al. 1991). When compared with the other patients with panic disorder, this subset had significantly higher rates of illness behaviors. The self-reported pain intensity of patients with rheumatoid arthritis was most significantly influenced by the presence of anxiety and depression even when controlling for disease activity (Smedstad et al. 1995). Other studies have argued that attentional focus and not anxiety exerts a more important influence on pain (Arntz et al. 1994). (See also Chapter 15 in this volume.)

Neurobiology

The neurobiology of pain is complex and described in numerous textbooks, chapters, and review articles (Borsook 1997; Cesaro and Ollat 1997; Wall and Melzack 1994). Ongoing nociceptive or neuropathic stimulation causes changes in peripheral nerves, spinal cord structures, and supraspinal structures (Siddal and Cousins 1995, 1998). Continuing neurobiological discoveries generate new ideas for the development of pharmacological agents to treat pain. Examples are N-methyl-D-aspartate (NMDA) receptor antagonists, adenosine receptor agonists, nitric oxide synthase inhibitors, and cyclo-oxygenase-2 inhibitors (Lane 1997; Lipman 1996).

Peripheral Mechanisms

Peripheral mechanisms of pain begin with the primary afferent nociceptors that respond to mechanical, thermal, and chemical stimuli (Meyer et al. 1994). The myelinated Aδ fibers transmit mechanothermal information (phasic pain with sharp, pricking quality), but unmyelinated C-fiber nociceptors are polymodal (tonic pain with burning, aching quality). The effect of age on the pain threshold is dependent on multiple factors such as sensory modality, location in the body, and experimental paradigm (Chakour et al. 1996; Heft et al. 1996; Lasch et al. 1997). The pain threshold may be raised in the elderly, as indicated by decreased reports of pain with esophageal distension and thermal stimulation to the skin, but unaffected in heat/cold pain sensation on the skin of the face or detection of electrical stimulation to the skin. In studies of heat nociception in leg skin, pain intensity ratings were not affected by age (Harkins et al. 1996). However, in the elderly, slow temporal summation (C fibers) failed to develop, and response times to pain (Aδ fibers) were delayed. In another study using a compression block of the superficial radial nerve, older adults exhibited an increase in pain threshold consistent with impaired Aδ-fiber function and not that of preserved C-fiber function (Chakour et al. 1996).

Usually, stimulation activates high-threshold nociceptors but, in conditions of inflammation or nerve injury, neurogenic inflammation occurs with the release of peptides from nociceptive afferents such as substance P and neurokinin A (Levine et al. 1993; Woolf and Chong 1993). As a result, nerve fibers become more excitable, vascular structures dilate, plasma proteins are extravasated, and inflammatory cells release a variety of chemical mediators (e.g., bradykinin, histamine, arachidonic acid metabolites). When these chemicals alter the response of high-threshold nociceptors, peripheral sensitization has occurred. Afterward, low-intensity stimuli can activate low-threshold Aβ-mechanoreceptors and produce pain. A zone of primary hyperalgesia is produced around the site of injury. The decrease in sensory nerve function with age may also be manifested by poor tissue healing, which can be reversed with the vasodilation produced by exogenous sensory peptides such as substance P and calcitonin gene-related peptide (Khalil and Helme 1996; Khalil et al. 1994; Merhi et al. 1998). High-frequency electrical stimulation of sensory nerves in aged rats produced an increased latency and decreased vasodilation response in injured tissues. The decrease in neurogenic inflammatory response that occurs with age as measured by the axon reflex flare response may be a result of decreased substance P content in skin (Helme and McKernan 1986).

When local tissues are injured, opioid receptors are produced in the dorsal root ganglion and transported to both the dorsal horn of the spinal cord and peripheral sites, where they become "unmasked" (Stein 1997). When a nerve is damaged, peptide production increases, the end of the nerve fiber sprouts, sensitivity to mechanical stimulation and noradrenaline increases, and the nerve fires spontaneously (Devor 1994). Similar changes occur at sites of demyelination and in the dorsal root ganglion of damaged nerves. Sympathetic efferent fibers release prostanoids during inflammation that sensitize primary nociceptive afferents, innervate the dorsal root ganglion, and excite primary afferents at α-adrenoceptors (Janig 1996). In studies of tissue inflammation in aging rat skin, the inhibitory modulation of sympathetic efferents is increased for high-frequency stimulation (Merhi et al. 1998). Silent nociceptors are a class of unmyelinated primary afferent neurons that respond only when sensitized by the chemical mediators of inflammation (McMahon and Koltzenburg 1990).

Dorsal Horn Mechanisms

The primary afferent nociceptors terminate in laminae I, II, and V of the dorsal horn (Willis and Coggeshall 1991). The second-order neurons can be classified into nociceptive-specific/high-threshold or wide dynamic range/convergent neurons. The nociceptive-specific neurons are located more superficially in the dorsal horn and respond only to noxious stimuli. In contrast, wide dynamic range neurons are more deeply located and respond to all types of stimuli. Allodynia, nonnoxious tactile stimuli perceived as painful, occurs when wide dynamic range neurons become sensitized and hyperexcitable and fire at increased frequency. The allodynia is manifested in a zone of secondary hyperalgesia in normal tissue adjacent to injured tissue. Local interneurons provide inhibitory modulation.

Central sensitization occurs in the dorsal horn, which is the site of action of many neurotransmitters and neuromodulators such as the excitatory amino acids (glutamate, aspartate) and peptides (Price et al. 1994). These act at several receptors including NMDA, kainate, metabotropic glutamate, opioid, neurokinin, α-adrenergic, serotonin, adenosine, and γ-aminobutyric acid (GABA) receptors. The prolonged activation of non-NMDA receptors (e.g., α-amino-3-hydroxy-5-methyl-4-isoxazolepropionic acid) readies the NMDA receptor to produce more long-term changes to the processing of sensory information (Dubner and Ren 1994; Woolf and Thompson 1991). These modifications include windup (progressive increases in neuronal activity throughout the stimulus duration), facilitation (magnification and prolongation of the duration of neuron response), action potential threshold reduction, receptive field expansion, oncogene induction, and long-term potentiation (strengthening of synaptic transmission efficacy after activity across the synapse). When calcium enters the cell with the activation of the NMDA receptor, second messengers such as protein kinase C, cGMP, and polyphosphoinositides are generated.

Approximately 75% of the opioid receptors in the dorsal horn are presynaptic and, when stimulated, reduce the release of neurotransmitters from primary nociceptive afferents. During inflammation and nerve injury, opioids increase NMDA activity promoting central sensitization and tolerance to opioids, cholecystokinin interferes with opioid analgesia, morphine-3-glucuronide antagonizes opioid analgesia, and presynaptic opioids are lost (Basbaum 1994). α-Adrenoceptors are activated by noradrenaline, which has a synergistic effect with opioid receptor agonists and is released by descending inhibitory pathways (Meert and DeKock 1994). GABA and glycine tonically inhibit nociception. When activated, $GABA_E$

receptors suppress the presynaptic release of excitatory amino acids from primary afferent terminals, whereas GABA$_A$ receptors have postsynaptic actions (Sivilotti and Woolf 1994).

Ascending Tract and Descending Inhibition Mechanisms

Second-order neurons project to supraspinal structures in the ascending tracts of the contralateral anterolateral spinal cord (spinothalamic, spinoreticular, spinomesencephalic) and a latent ipsilateral pathway. The ventroposterior nuclei of the thalamus represent the sensory-discriminative (temporal and spatial) aspects of pain, and the medial nuclei are involved with the affective-motivational features of pain. Increased thalamic activity has been associated with acute experimental pain in contrast with chronic pain states, which are associated with decreased thalamic activity on positron-emission tomography (Iadarola et al. 1995; Jones et al. 1991). Most of the other subcortical structures (e.g., basal ganglia, hypothalamus, amygdala, cerebellum) are postulated to function in the transmission of nociception and perception of pain.

The role of the cortical structures in pain and suffering is less well understood. The parietal lobes and somatosensory cortex probably contribute to the sensory-discriminative component, and the cingulate cortex, with the affective component of pain (Jannetta et al. 1990; Talbot et al. 1991). Pain can be decreased by descending inhibition as first postulated by the gate theory of Melzack and Wall (1965). Many structures (e.g., locus ceruleus, nucleus raphe magnus, periaqueductal gray matter, hypothalamus) and neurotransmitters (e.g., endogenous opioids, serotonin, noradrenaline, GABA) contribute to descending inhibition (Fields and Basbaum 1994). Serotonin and dopamine levels have been found to be decreased in studies of nociception in aged rats (Goicoechea et al. 1997). Treatment modalities involving electrical stimulation (e.g., deep brain stimulation, dorsal column stimulation, transcutaneous electrical nerve stimulation) attempt to activate descending inhibition to decrease chronic pain.

▌ Treatment

A large body of research now supports the use of traditional neuropsychiatric treatments in the management of chronic pain. Pharmacological, psychological, and multidisciplinary treatments have proven effective for many different pain syndromes. In the elderly, most chronic diseases are disproportionately represented, including cancer,

vascular disease, peripheral neuropathy, temporal arteritis, polymyalgia rheumatica, postherpetic neuralgia (PHN), stroke, and Parkinson's disease (Foley 1994; Gordon 1979). Several are described below to highlight a few of the more common conditions and the wide number of pathophysiological mechanisms that have been discovered.

For any specific disease, no single algorithm can dictate the modalities of treatment to be prescribed. Several classes of medications have proven efficacy for the treatment of neuropathic pain. However, the relief provided by these medications is usually incomplete and difficult to predict in advance. The selection of a particular medication will depend on multiple factors. The disease itself may change over time such that the efficacy of a treatment is altered, one treatment may be selected over another based on the response to previous treatments, and the patient's psychiatric comorbidity, temperament, coping skills, and personal history cannot be neglected.

Postherpetic Neuralgia

PHN is defined as pain persisting or recurring at the site of shingles at least 3 months after the onset of the acute varicella zoster viral rash (Bowsher 1997b). This condition is more likely to occur with age, and more than half of patients over 65 years old with shingles develop PHN. Patients with cancer, diabetes mellitus, and immunosuppression are more likely to develop PHN. Approximately 15% of referrals to pain clinics are for the treatment of PHN. Although degeneration and destruction of motor and sensory fibers of the mixed dorsal root ganglion characterize acute varicella zoster, other forms of neurological damage have been described. These changes include inflammation of the spinal cord, myelin disruption, axonal damage, and decreases in the number of nerve endings from the affected skin.

These same changes persist in patients with PHN, but the actual mechanism of pain is not well understood. Studies have suggested the role of both peripheral and central mechanisms, probably resulting from the loss of large-caliber neurons and subsequent central sensitization, but adrenergic receptor activation and alterations in C-fiber activity have also been reported (Fields et al. 1998). Early treatment of varicella zoster with low-dose amitriptyline has reduced the prevalence of pain at 6 months by 50% (Bowsher 1996, 1997a; Johnson 1997). A recent review of randomized controlled trials and meta-analysis concluded that tricyclic antidepressants (TCAs) are the most effective agents for the treatment of PHN (Volmink et al. 1996). Anticonvulsants and opioids are also under investigation.

Peripheral Neuropathy Pain

Sensory neurons are damaged by many diseases, both directly and indirectly (Scadding 1994). If C-fiber input is preserved but large-fiber input is lost, paresthesias and pain are the predominant sensory experiences. The pain of a peripheral neuropathy can range from a constant burning to episodic, paroxysmal, and lancinating in quality. These phenomena are primarily the manifestation of axonal degeneration and segmental demyelination. Sites of ectopic impulse generation can be found at any point along the peripheral nerve including the dorsal root ganglion regardless of where the nerve is actually damaged. Other changes can alter the magnitude and frequency of impulse generation such as sensitivity to mechanical or neurochemical stimuli. Ephaptic impulse transmission and crossed after-discharge have been described as models of peripheral neuropathic pain. Voltage-dependent sodium channels in the dorsal root ganglion undergo both upregulation and downregulation, depending on the subpopulation (Rizzo 1997). Many changes also occur in the central nervous system when a peripheral nerve is damaged. This central sensitization can amplify and sustain neuronal activity by a variety of mechanisms such as reduced inhibition of dorsal horn cells.

Parkinson's Disease

Pain is the most common sensory manifestation of Parkinson's disease and reported by half of patients (Goetz et al. 1986; Koller 1984; Starkstein et al. 1991). The pain is typically described as cramping and aching, located in the lower back and extremities, but not associated with muscle contraction or spasm. These pains often decrease when the patient is treated with levodopa, which suggests a central origin. The loss of dopaminergic input could explain how pain is produced. Specifically, studies of the rat rostral agranular insular cortex suggest a role in modulation of nociception probably through a loss of descending inhibition in the spinal cord (Burkey et al. 1996). The basal ganglia neurons in rats exhibit nociceptive-specific responses to noxious stimulation, and the marginal division of the neostriatum has high concentrations of substance P, metenkephalin, and dynorphin-B (Chudler and Dong 1995; Chudler et al. 1993).

Central Poststroke Pain

Approximately 5% of patients who have suffered a stroke experience intractable pain in addition to other neurological deficits (Bowsher 1995). Patients typically have hemibody sensory deficits and pain associated with dysesthesias, allodynia, and hyperalgesia. Radiographic lesions are present in the thalamus, although other sites are often involved. Excitatory amino acids may be involved in the development of this syndrome. Pharmacological treatment is usually not effective, and medications such as ketamine, an NMDA receptor antagonist, reduce pain in less than 50% of patients (Yamamoto et al. 1997). In contrast, patients with spinal cord injury experience reductions in continuous and evoked pain with ketamine and μ opioid receptor agonists, suggesting different mechanisms in different central pain states (Eide et al. 1995).

Migraine

The peak incidence of migraine occurs between the third and sixth decade of life and then decreases with age. However, over the life span, 18% of women and 6% of men will suffer from migraine (Lipton et al. 1997). The pathogenesis is still not well understood but probably involves the trigeminovascular system and plasma protein extravasation, antagonism of serotonin receptors, modulation of central aminergic control mechanisms, membrane-stabilizing effects through action at voltage-sensitive calcium channels, and substance P (Goadsby 1997; Solomon 1995). The common migraine is defined as a unilateral pulsatile headache, which may be associated with other symptoms such as nausea, vomiting, photophobia, and phonophobia (Szirmai 1997). The duration is usually up to several days. The classic form of migraine adds visual prodromal symptoms such as scintillating scotomata. The complicated migraine includes focal neurological signs such as cranial nerve palsies and is often described as the name of the primary deficit, for example, vestibular migraine, basilar migraine. The calcium channel blockers, antidepressants, and anticonvulsants are the treatments with best-documented efficacy.

Pharmacological Treatments

Opioids.   The use of opioids in nonmalignant chronic pain remains a subject of considerable debate (Chabal et al. 1992a). Until recently, opioids were reserved for use only in the treatment of acute and cancer pain syndromes. Nonmalignant chronic pain was considered to be unresponsive to opioids, which were associated with too many risks. Fears of regulatory pressure, medication abuse, and the development of tolerance create a reluctance to prescribe opioids, and many studies have documented this "underutilization" (Maruta et al. 1979; Morgan 1985; Schug et al. 1991). Studies investigating the risk of opioid abuse have been reassuring. In one study of 12,000 medical patients treated with opioids, only 4 patients without a history of substance abuse developed dependence on the medication (Porter and Jick 1980). Other studies of chronic opioid therapy found that patients who developed problems with their use of the medication all had a history of substance abuse (Portenoy and Foley 1986; Taub 1982). Even when the diagnosis of dependence is suspected in patients taking opioids for chronic pain, maladaptive behaviors such as stealing or forging prescriptions rarely occur (Fishbain et al. 1992b; Sees and Clark 1993). Fortunately, recent studies of physicians specializing in pain, as well as those who do not, have shown that prescription of long-term opioids is increasingly common (Turk et al. 1994). Surveys and open-label clinical trials support the safety and effectiveness of opioids in patients with chronic nonmalignant pain. Recently, several controlled trials have documented the effectiveness of opioids in the treatment of chronic nonmalignant pain.

A randomized double-blind crossover study of oral continuous-release morphine found a significant decrease in musculoskeletal pain compared with that found with placebo (Moulin et al. 1996). Although 9 weeks of therapy did not produce any evidence of addiction, patients did not experience significant psychological or functional improvement. Another randomized placebo-controlled clinical trial found that treatment with controlled-release codeine reduced reports of pain as well as pain-related disability (Arkinstall et al. 1995). Opioids are now being considered for the specific treatment of neuropathic pain. Recent studies of the treatments for neuropathic pain support the use of opioids to provide direct analgesic actions and not just to counteract the unpleasantness of pain (Dellemijn and Vanneste 1997; Watt et al. 1996). Other studies have documented the presence of opioid receptors in the peripheral tissues that become activated by inflammation (Stein et al. 1997). These findings suggest a role for opioids in the treatment of chronic inflammatory diseases.

Once the decision is made to prescribe opioids, several recommendations have been suggested to minimize the risks and optimize the potential benefits (Mendelson and Mendelson 1991; Schug 1991). The Agency for Health Care Policy and Research has produced guidelines for the treatment of acute and cancer pain (Acute Pain Management Guideline Panel 1992; Cancer Pain Management Guideline Panel 1994). The Federation of State Medical Boards (1998) has recently formulated guidelines for the treatment of chronic pain. The American Academy of Pain Medicine and the American Pain Society have produced a consensus statement (*The Use of Opioids for the Treatment of Chronic Pain*) to provide education and general principles for practitioners in this area. The American Geriatric Society (1998) has recently published clinical practice guidelines for the management of chronic pain in older persons.

Opioids with a short duration of analgesic activity generally create more problems than they solve. These medications must be taken multiple times a day, often interfering with the patient's daily activities, including sleep. But more importantly, opioids with short duration result in serum levels of considerable variability. Analgesia is difficult to achieve and side effects are more likely to occur. Controlled-release formulations of morphine, oxycodone, and fentanyl are now available. Multiple studies describe the more favorable pharmacokinetic and pharmacodynamic profiles of these medications. A recent study found comparable analgesia, with more vomiting occurring with controlled-release morphine and more constipation with controlled-release oxycodone (Heiskanen and Kalso 1997). Transdermal fentanyl is an effective analgesic with generally fewer side effects than oral medications and more than 90% of patients choosing to continue the medication after completion of a study trial (Donner et al. 1996). In the treatment of chronic low back pain, transdermal fentanyl significantly decreased pain and improved functional disability (Simpson et al. 1997). Tolerance leading to dosage escalation is generally not a problem in the management of patients taking long-term opioids (France et al. 1984; Portenoy 1990).

The most common side effect of chronic opioid therapy is decreased gastrointestinal motility, causing constipation (Portenoy and Foley 1987). However, concerns about potential cognitive impairment are more often the reason opioids are not prescribed. Again, the available research has not demonstrated these deleterious effects on neuropsychological testing or electroencephalography except in patients prescribed multiple types of medications, especially sedatives and hypnotics (Hendler et al. 1980; Lomardo et al. 1976; McNairy et al. 1984; Zielger 1994). Elderly patients are more susceptible to delirium than younger patients (see Chapter 19 in this volume). Although no studies have examined this risk of delirium in chronic pain syndromes treated with opioids, postoperative patients are less likely to develop cognitive impairment with fentanyl than with morphine (Herrick et al. 1996). Another similar study found that cognitive performance was poorer in patients receiving hydromorphone compared with those receiving morphine (Rapp et al. 1996). Many metabolites of opioids are excreted by the kidney and can cause toxicity in the elderly, especially those of methadone (Forman 1996). Creatinine clearance should be monitored to titrate dosing for adequate analgesia with minimal toxicity.

If treatment with opioids is unsuccessful in decreasing pain, discontinuation should be carefully monitored to minimize physiological withdrawal symptoms. The essential element for successful opioid detoxification is the gradual tapering of the dose of medication. Opioid withdrawal is generally not dangerous except with patients at risk from increased sympathetic tone, such as those with increased intracranial pressure or unstable angina. However, opioid withdrawal is very uncomfortable and distressing to patients. Tapering opioids often results in exacerbation of the patient's primary pain symptom (rebound pain). Increases in pain can occur even if the analgesic effects of opioid therapy had not been appreciable. Although it is generally not possible to avoid discomfort completely, the goal of detoxification is to ameliorate withdrawal.

Several nonopioid pharmacological agents are commonly used as adjunctive agents to provide patients additional relief from withdrawal symptoms. Clonidine, an α_2-adrenergic agonist that decreases adrenergic activity, is the most commonly prescribed (Fishbain et al. 1992a). Clonidine can help relieve many of the autonomic symptoms of opioid withdrawal such as nausea, cramps, sweating, tachycardia, and hypertension, which result from the loss of opioid suppression of the locus ceruleus during the withdrawal syndrome. Other adjunctive agents include nonsteroidal anti-inflammatory drugs for muscle aches, bismuth subsalicylate for diarrhea, anticholinergics for abdominal cramps, and antihistamines for insomnia and restlessness.

Antidepressants.   In 1960, the first report of imipramine used for trigeminal neuralgia was published (Paoli et al. 1960). Since then, the antidepressants, particularly the TCAs, have been commonly prescribed for the treatment of many chronic pain syndromes, especially neuropathic pain. Animal models have been established for the study of nociception and neuropathic pain (Ollat and Cesaro 1995). Current research suggests that antidepressant effects on pain are mediated by the blockade of norepinephrine and serotonin reuptake that increases the levels of these neurotransmitters and enhances the activation of descending inhibitory neurons (R. B. King 1981; Magni 1987). Other aspects of monoaminergic systems have been implicated in the analgesic action of antidepressants. β-Adrenoceptors have been demonstrated to mediate the analgesic effects of desipramine and nortriptyline (Mico et al. 1997). Imipramine demonstrated differential hypoalgesic effects depending on the experimental paradigm used to assess pain (Poulsen et al. 1995). TCAs may reduce hyperalgesia but not tactile allodynia because different neuronal mechanisms underlie different manifestations of neuropathic pain (Jett et al. 1997). Generally, amitriptyline or TCAs with a similar pharmacological profile are considered most

effective, but randomized controlled trials have not demonstrated consistent differences among the TCAs (Bryson and Wilde 1996).

In a review of 39 placebo-controlled studies, 80% found antidepressants superior to placebo (Magni 1991). These findings have been challenged because of poor study design and protocol criteria (Goodkin et al. 1995). A recent systematic review of randomized controlled trials and meta-analysis concluded that TCAs are the only agents proven to benefit PHN (Volmink et al. 1996). TCAs have been most effective in relieving neuropathic pain and headache syndromes, with the analgesic activity independent of effects on mood (Gruber et al. 1996; MacFarlane et al. 1997; Max et al. 1987; McQuay et al. 1996; Vrethem et al. 1997; Wesselmann and Reich 1996). A recent placebo-controlled, double-blinded, randomized clinical trial of nortriptyline for patients with chronic low back pain without depression demonstrated significant reduction in pain intensity scores (Atkinson et al. 1998).

A variety of treatment studies of PHN and painful diabetic peripheral neuropathy have used TCAs with mean daily doses ranging from 100 to 250 mg (Max 1994; Onghena and Van Houdenhove 1992). More than 60% of patients reported improvement usually beginning in the third week of treatment, with serum levels in the low end of the therapeutic range for the treatment of depression. The results of investigations of drug concentrations needed for pain relief remain contradictory, and no clear guidelines have been established (Kishore-Kumar et al. 1990; Sindrup et al. 1989). In a study of TCA utilization, 25% of patients in a multidisciplinary pain center were prescribed these medications. However, 73% of patients treated received only the equivalent of 50 mg or less of amitriptyline (Richeimer et al. 1997). Although tertiary amines have been used most commonly, they are metabolized to the secondary amines possessing fewer side effects such as decreased gastrointestinal motility and urinary retention. Desipramine and nortriptyline had significantly fewer side effects leading to discontinuation of the TCA than clomipramine, amitriptyline, and doxepin. Nortriptyline, the major metabolite of amitriptyline, causes less sedation, less orthostatic hypotension, and fewer falls than imipramine and has been demonstrated to be as effective as amitriptyline in treating chronic pain (Roose et al. 1981; Watson et al. 1988). The cost of TCAs for pain treatment is generally much lower (less than $5.00 per month) than other antidepressants and medications with analgesic activity such as β blockers and calcium channel blockers (Adelman and Von Seggern 1995).

The selective serotonin reuptake inhibitors produce weak antinociceptive effects in animal models of acute pain

(Gatch et al. 1998; Paul and Hornby 1995; Schreiber et al. 1996). This antinociception is blocked by serotonin receptor antagonists and enhanced by opioid receptor agonists. A large number of studies have investigated the role of serotonin receptor subtypes in both nociceptive and hyperalgesic mechanisms of pain; however, controversy remains and the relationships between various findings are complex (Belcheva et al. 1995; Tokunaga et al. 1998). The serotonin reuptake inhibitors have not been found to be as effective as the TCAs for many chronic pain conditions. For example, desipramine was superior to fluoxetine in the treatment of painful diabetic peripheral neuropathy (Max et al. 1992).

Inconsistencies still exist because another study of patients with diabetic neuropathy did find beneficial effects with paroxetine (Sindrup et al. 1990). Other studies indicate that fluoxetine significantly reduces pain in patients with rheumatoid arthritis and is comparable to amitriptyline (Rani et al. 1996). Recently, the serotonin reuptake inhibitors have demonstrated effectiveness in the treatment of headache, especially migraine, and were well tolerated by patients (Bank 1994; Foster and Bafaloukos 1994; Saper et al. 1994). In a study of chronic tension-type headache, amitriptyline significantly reduced the duration of headache, headache frequency, and the intake of analgesics, but citalopram, a serotonin reuptake inhibitor, did not (Bendtsen et al. 1996). Until the results with serotonin reuptake inhibitors are more consistent, they are not recommended as first-choice medications unless a specific contraindication exists for TCAs (Max et al. 1991).

The role of biogenic amines in the descending inhibition of pain suggests a potential efficacy for all antidepressants, despite their different pharmacological actions, in the treatment of chronic pain. Norepinephrine and dopamine reuptake inhibitors such as bupropion can produce antinociception in studies of thermal nociception (Gatch et al. 1998). Monoamine oxidase inhibitors have been found to decrease the frequency and severity of migraine headaches (Merikangas and Merikangas 1995). Buspirone has been found effective in the prophylaxis of chronic tension-type headache; however, patients used more drugs for short-term treatment of headache than those patients treated with amitriptyline (Mitsikostas et al. 1997). Protriptyline decreased chronic tension-type headache frequency by 86% in a study of women with this condition (Cohen 1997). Trazodone was ineffective in decreasing pain in a double-blind, placebo-controlled study of patients with chronic low back pain (Goodkin et al. 1990; Marek et al. 1992). Venlafaxine inhibits the reuptake of both serotonin and norepinephrine with fewer side effects. In an animal model of neuropathic pain, venlafaxine reversed hyperalgesia as well prevented its development (Lang et al. 1996). Nefazodone possesses both the actions of analgesia and potentiation of opioid analgesia in the mouse hot-plate assay (Pick et al. 1992). Other antidepressants that inhibit serotonin reuptake and block certain serotonin receptor subtypes such as mirtazapine will need to be studied in the treatment of pain (Galer 1995).

Anticonvulsants. Anticonvulsants are considered most effective in the treatment of trigeminal neuralgia, diabetic neuropathy, and migraine recurrence (McQuay et al. 1995). Many anticonvulsants block the activity of use-dependent sodium channels. This property stabilizes the presynaptic neuronal membrane, preventing the release of excitatory neurotransmitters, and decreases the spontaneous firing rate in damaged and regenerating nociceptive fibers. Subsequently, the activation of secondary spinal nociceptive neurons via NMDA receptors is prevented. Phenytoin was first reported as a successful treatment for trigeminal neuralgia in 1942 (Bergouignan 1942). Carbamazepine is the most widely studied anticonvulsant demonstrating effective treatment of neuropathic pain (Tanelian and Victory 1995).

However, anticonvulsants have many other pharmacological actions that may play a role in analgesia, making them potential treatments for a variety of chronic pain syndromes. Phenytoin regulates many aspects of nerve function such as ATPase activity, synaptic transmission, neurotransmitter release, and ion conductances, suggesting a large number of central nervous system effects (Lorenzo 1989). In spinal nerve–ligated rats with cooling and mechanical allodynia, carbamazepine has inhibitory effects on electrical C- and A-fiber neuronal responses (Chapman et al. 1998). Carbamazepine lowers the concentration of tryptophan bound to plasma proteins and subsequently elevates brain serotonin levels in rats (Pinelli et al. 1997). Carbamazepine has also been found to inhibit the development of different types of inflammation in the rat (Bianchi et al. 1995). In this model of inflammatory hyperalgesia, carbamazepine reduced the inflammatory exudate, prostaglandin E_2 activity, and substance P concentrations. Unfortunately, the use of carbamazepine can be limited by intolerable side effects such as sedation, ataxia, and aplastic anemia. Therapeutic serum levels have not been clearly established, with some evidence suggesting that lower levels may be effective in decreasing pain (Moosa et al. 1993).

Newer classes of anticonvulsants represent novel pharmacological actions that could potentially produce analgesia. Valproic acid is most commonly used in the prophylaxis of migraine but is also effective in the treatment of neuropathic pain (R. Jensen et al. 1994c). In studies of migraine, valproate was an effective prophylactic treatment in more than two-thirds of patients, with minimal side effects such as nausea, dizziness, and tremor (Mathew et al. 1995). Effectiveness is usually defined as improvement in a combination of variables such as frequency of headache, duration or headache-days per month, intensity of headache, use of other medications for acute treatment of headache, the patient's opinion of treatment, and ratings of depression and anxiety (Kaniecki 1997; Klapper 1997; Rothrock 1997).

The mechanism of action of valproate is probably related to increased GABA levels by the inhibition of GABA transaminase and enhanced GABA synthesis. Analgesia may result from the suppression of neuronal activity in the cortex, perivascular parasympathetic fibers, nociceptive trigeminal neurons innervating the meninges, or the trigeminal nucleus caudalis. However, other actions could include decreasing neurogenic inflammation via $GABA_A$ receptor–mediated mechanisms, altering levels of excitatory and inhibitory neurotransmitters, and having direct stabilizing effects on neuronal membranes (Cutrer et al. 1996, 1997). Valproate is generally well tolerated but requires regular monitoring because of potential hepatotoxicity and bone marrow suppression.

Gabapentin has been reported in open trials to reduce the pain of neuropathic states such as multiple sclerosis, migraine, PHN, and reflex sympathetic dystrophy (Houtchens et al. 1997; Wetzel and Connelly 1997). The mechanism of action of gabapentin may be related to binding with the $\alpha_2\delta$ subunit of voltage-dependent calcium channels (Field et al. 1997). Gabapentin selectively modulated the facilitation of spinal nociceptive processing generated by persistent small-fiber afferent input that resulted from tissue injury in an animal model of thermal hyperalgesia (Jun and Yaksh 1998). In the formalin test, gabapentin had antinociceptive activity (Shimoyama et al. 1997). Other studies have shown that gabapentin can reverse cold and tactile allodynia as well as heat hyperalgesia (Xiao and Bennett 1995).

Case reports indicate that lamotrigine may be effective in reducing the pain of phantom limbs, neuroma hypersensitivity, trigeminal neuralgia, causalgia, central poststroke pain, and PHN (Canavero and Bonicalzi 1996; Harbinson et al. 1997). Lamotrigine produced significant analgesia, as measured by the cold pressor test in healthy volunteers (Webb and Kamali 1998). Analgesia was correlated with serum drug concentrations and comparable to that obtained with phenytoin and dihydrocodeine. In contrast to gabapentin, lamotrigine reversed cold, but not tactile, allodynia (Hunter et al. 1997). The mechanism of action of lamotrigine may be a result of its ability to decrease

long-term excitatory effects of nociceptive glutaminergic transmission mediated by NMDA receptors, but it also blocks use-dependent voltage-gated sodium channels (Cheung et al. 1992; Leach et al. 1995; Lees and Leach 1993). Topiramate, tiagabine, vigabatrin, and zonisamide are new anticonvulsants with a spectrum of pharmacological actions that include enhancing neuronal inhibition, decreasing neuronal excitability, and protecting neurons from free radical damage (Marson et al. 1997).

Antiarrhythmics. The use-dependent sodium channel-binding properties of local anesthetics such as lidocaine and mexiletine have also proven effective in decreasing ectopic neural activity. Lidocaine and mexiletine reduce spontaneous and evoked neuronal activity in experimental neuroma models (Galer et al. 1996). However, mexiletine has also been shown to have an antinociceptive effect in the rat tail pinch model that was mediated by the delta 1-opioid receptor (Kamei et al. 1995). In a rat model of central sensitization and neuropathic pain, mexiletine decreased both the hyperalgesia and tactile allodynia (Jett et al. 1997). Mexiletine is structurally related to lidocaine and has similar electrophysiological properties, yet can be administered orally (Campbell 1987). Relief of pain with an intravenous infusion of lidocaine has been investigated as a predictive test of successful treatment with mexiletine (Galer et al. 1996; Zehender et al. 1988).

Current research supports mexiletine as an effective treatment for neuropathic pain such as painful diabetic neuropathy, peripheral nerve injury pain, alcoholic neuropathy, and phantom pain (Boulton 1993; Chabal et al. 1992b; Davis 1993; Nishiyama and Sakuta 1995). In one double-blind crossover study, mexiletine not only decreased reports of pain but also the accompanying paresthesias and dysesthesias (Dejgard et al. 1988). Another study found that mexiletine decreased pain and sleep disturbances associated with painful diabetic neuropathy (Oskarsson et al. 1997). No significant correlation was found between plasma concentrations of mexiletine and either therapeutic effect or adverse events.

Calcium channel blockers. Several classes of calcium channel blockers are available. Verapamil is the most commonly prescribed calcium channel blocker for chronic pain treatment and has proven effective in the treatment of migraine and cluster headaches (Lewis and Solomon 1996; Markley 1991). It is still unclear whether the mechanism of action is primarily related to cerebral artery vasodilation or interaction with serotonergic systems. In 922 subjects of the Hypertension Optimal Treatment study, intensive treatment to lower blood pressure also significantly reduced headaches and increased measures of well-being (Wiklund et al. 1997). In a rat model of peripheral neuropathy, repeated electroconvulsive treatments, which affect voltage-dependent calcium channels, reduced pain responses to heat stimulation (Shibata et al. 1998). Another possible mechanism of pain relief involves cortical L-type calcium channels as measured by ^{3}H-nitrendipine–binding sites (Antkiewicz-Michaluk et al. 1991). Chronic use of antidepressants has been shown to increase the density of cortical calcium channels, possibly limiting their analgesic effect and even contributing to hyperalgesia.

High-threshold, voltage-dependent P- and Q-type calcium channels are involved in neurotransmitter release. In animal studies of joint inflammation, the P-type calcium channels mediate the excitation of spinal cord neurons by mechanosensory input from inflamed tissue, resulting in pain generation (Nebe et al. 1997). Other studies of calcium channel subtypes have shown that L-, N-, and P-type channels are involved in the development of mechanical hyperalgesia and allodynia (Sluka 1997). On the other hand, calcium channel blockers have demonstrated μ opioid receptor agonistic activity in animals and augmentation of opioid analgesia in animals and humans (Hasegawa and Zacny 1997; Weizman et al. 1997). The L-type calcium channel blockers such as diltiazem and verapamil have also been found to potentiate morphine analgesia, but the results are inconsistent (Hodoglugil et al. 1996; Taniguchi et al. 1995). However, the neuron-specific, N-type, voltage-sensitive calcium channel blocker, ziconotide, possesses potent analgesic, antihyperesthesic, and antiallodynic activity (Bowersox et al. 1996; Brose et al. 1997; Xiao and Bennett 1995). Another action of calcium channel blockers may result in a reduction of neural nitric oxide synthase activity, with subsequent decreases in nitric oxide concentrations in perivascular nerves, limiting cerebral vasodilation (Ayajiki et al. 1997).

Benzodiazepines.   Benzodiazepines are commonly prescribed for insomnia and anxiety in patients with chronic pain (Holister et al. 1981; S. A. King and Strain 1990). No studies demonstrated any benefit for the target symptoms of insomnia and anxiety frequently reported by these patients. In an extensive review, only a limited number of chronic pain conditions such as trigeminal neuralgia, tension headache, and temporomandibular disorders were found to improve when treated with benzodiazepines (Dellemijn and Fields 1994). Clonazepam has been reported to provide long-term relief of the episodic lancinating variety of phantom limb pain (Bartusch et al. 1996). Benzodiazepines have been used for the detoxification of patients with chronic pain from sedative/hypnotic medications. Benzodiazepines were superior to barbiturates for minimizing symptoms of withdrawal (Sullivan et al. 1993).

Not only are the benefits of benzodiazepines difficult to document, but the negative effects are well studied and extend beyond the usual concerns of abuse, dependence, withdrawal, and secondary effects on mood. The elderly are particularly sensitive to the adverse effects of benzodiazepines such as sedation (Ganapathy et al. 1997; Max et al. 1988; Platten et al. 1998; Yosselson-Superstine et al. 1985). Benzodiazepines also cause cognitive impairment, as demonstrated by abnormalities found by neuropsychological testing and electroencephalography (Hendler et al. 1980). Benzodiazepines have been associated with exacerbation of pain and interference with opioid analgesia (France and Kirshman 1988; Sawynok 1985). These effects appear to be the result of activating supraspinal GABA$_A$ receptors known to antagonize opioid analgesia. Similarly, a study of the benzodiazepine antagonist, flumazenil, enhanced postoperative morphine analgesia in patients who received preoperative diazepam for sedation (Gear et al. 1997).

Psychological Treatments

Cognitive-behavior models.   Psychological treatment for chronic pain was pioneered by Fordyce using an operant conditioning behavioral model (Fordyce et al. 1973). The behavioral approach is based on an understanding of pain occurring in a social context. The behaviors of the patient with chronic pain not only reinforce the behaviors of others but also are reinforced by others. Pain behaviors such as grimacing, guarding, and taking pain medication have been found to be indicators of perceived pain severity and functional disability (Chapman et al. 1985; Fordyce et al. 1984; Keefe et al. 1986; Romano et al. 1988; Turk and Matyas 1992). In a study of medical practice patterns, only observed pain behaviors were predictive of whether opioid medications were prescribed to patients with chronic pain (Turk and Okifuji 1997). Other aspects of the patient's presentation to a health care practitioner such as reports of functional disability, distress, pain severity, objective physical pathology, duration of pain, and demographic variables were not predictive. If pain behaviors are reinforced, the behavioral model assumes that pain and disability will continue. In treatment, productive behaviors are targeted for reinforcement, and pain behaviors for extinction.

Many psychological interventions such as distraction, relaxation, biofeedback, and hypnosis have been useful in the reduction of pain and its associated distress (Turner 1982b; Turner and Chapman 1982). The cognitive-behavior model of chronic pain assumes that individual perceptions and evaluations of life experiences affect emotional and behavioral reactions to these experiences. Pain and the resultant pain behaviors are influenced by biomedical, psychological, and socioenvironmental variables (Keefe et al. 1996). If patients believe pain, depression, and disability are inevitable and uncontrollable, then they will experience more negative affective responses, increased pain, and even more impaired physical and psychosocial functioning. The components of cognitive-behavior therapy (CBT) such as relaxation, cognitive restructuring, and coping self-statement training interrupt this cycle of disability. Patients are taught to become active participants in the management of their pain through the utilization of methods that minimize distressing thoughts and feelings. Specifically, elderly patients benefit from CBT that presents information in concrete, well-organized, and brief formats (Manetto and McPherson 1996). Outcome studies of CBT in patients with a variety of chronic pain syndromes have demonstrated significant improvements in pain intensity, pain behaviors, distress, depression, and coping (Keefe et al. 1990a; Turner 1982a; Turner and Romano 1990). Pain reduction and improved physical function have been found to continue up to 6 months after the completion of active cognitive-behavior treatment (Keefe et al. 1990b).

Beliefs. The success of CBT in chronic pain treatment has led to focused attention on many elements of the chronic pain experience. The relationship between beliefs about pain and subsequent patient adjustment central to the cognitive-behavior model has been reviewed (M. P. Jensen et al. 1991a). Adjustment is defined as the ability to carry out normal physical and psychosocial activities. The three dimensions of adjustment have been defined as social functioning, morale, and somatic health (Lazarus and Folkman 1984). Examples of these dimensions include pain intensity, medication use, depression, anxiety, employment, health care utilization, and functional ability.

Beliefs are conceptualized as the thoughts of an individual about their personal pain problem and have been categorized in several different domains (M. P. Jensen et al. 1987; Morley and Wilkinson 1995). Psychosocial dysfunction has been correlated with solicitous responses from family, believing emotions are related to pain, and attributing the inability to function to pain (M. P. Jensen et al. 1994b). In contrast, although physical disability was also correlated with beliefs about pain interfering with function, patients also endorsed the belief that pain signifies in-

jury and, therefore, activity should be avoided.

Other related cognitive variables under study in patients with chronic pain include self-efficacy, outcome expectancies, and locus of control (Anderson et al. 1995; Keefe et al. 1992). A self-efficacy expectancy is a belief about one's ability to perform a specific behavior, whereas an outcome expectancy is a belief about the consequences of performing a behavior. These variables have been derived from social learning theory (M. P. Jensen et al. 1991b). Individuals are considered more likely to engage in coping efforts that they believe both are within their capabilities and will result in a positive outcome.

Patients with a variety of chronic pain syndromes who score higher on measures of self-efficacy or have an internal locus of control report lower levels of pain, higher pain thresholds, increased exercise performance, and more positive coping efforts. However, in one study of patients with chronic pain being treated with a procedure, expectations of pain relief were not correlated with actual changes in pain ratings (Galer et al. 1997). Interestingly, physician expectations of pain relief were significant predictors of patient pain relief ratings, supporting the important role of other persons in an individual's chronic pain experience. Similarly, acceptance of pain was found to be associated with reports of lower pain intensity, less pain-related anxiety and avoidance, less depression, less physical and psychosocial disability, more daily up time, and better work status (McCracken 1998).

Coping. Coping has been defined as "a person's cognitive and behavioral efforts to manage the internal and external demands of the person-environment transaction that is appraised as taxing or exceeding the person's resources" (Folkman and Lazarus 1986). The Coping Strategies Questionnaire defines seven specific coping strategies (Rosenstiel and Keefe 1983). A comprehensive review of the research in this area concluded that the coping strategies concept generally supported the cognitive-behavior model of chronic pain (M. P. Jensen et al. 1991a). Higher levels of disability were found in persons who remain passive or use coping strategies such as catastrophizing; ignoring or reinterpreting pain sensations; diverting attention from pain; and praying or hoping for relief. In a 6-month follow-up study of patients completing an inpatient pain program, improvement was associated with decreases in the use of passive coping strategies and beliefs about pain being an illness (M. P. Jensen et al. 1994a).

The effectiveness of particular coping strategies with improved adjustment to chronic pain is dependent on many aspects of a patient's experience with illness. For example, reinterpreting pain sensations as not being signs of ongoing injury has been typically formulated as useful for reducing the effects of experimentally induced pain. However, in a study of amputees with phantom limb pain, this coping strategy was not associated with reduced pain levels but instead with greater psychosocial dysfunction (Hill et al. 1995). Attempting to reinterpret pain sensations may not be an appropriate technique for individuals with persistent pain because it requires greater amounts of time spent focusing on pain and disability. This may prevent patients from engaging in social activities. Catastrophic thinking about pain has been attributed to the amplification of threatening information and interference with the attentional focus needed to facilitate patients remaining involved with productive instead of pain-related activities (Crombez et al. 1998).

Some evidence indicates that older patients with chronic pain utilize different patterns of coping strategies. Older patients were more likely to use passive strategies such as praying and hoping for relief from pain, less likely to ignore pain, and benefited most from coping self-statements that emphasize an ability to actively manage pain (Corran et al. 1994). In contrast, younger patients were more likely to get benefit from ignoring pain. Training older adults to use adaptive coping strategies resulted in lower levels of both pain and psychological disability (Keefe et al. 1987, 1990b). These results were achieved when patients perceived an increase in the effectiveness of their new skills and reduced their use of maladaptive coping strategies such as catastrophic thinking.

Patient classifications. Controversy over the type of psychological treatment most effective in the treatment of chronic pain still persists, as exemplified by a recent study finding no differences between the treatment effects of cognitive and behavior therapies in patients mildly disabled by chronic low back pain (Turner and Jensen 1993). As a result, attempts to define more homogeneous subgroups of patients with chronic pain have led to several empirical classifications based on factor analyses of the responses on a variety of instruments (Deardorff et al. 1993; Sanders and Brena 1993; Williams et al. 1995). In a cluster analysis of patients with chronic pain, a subgroup was defined in the elderly that combined high levels of depression and impact of pain on daily living despite low levels of pain intensity (Corran et al. 1997).

Three groups have been described based on a cluster analysis of responses on the Multidimensional Pain Inventory (Kerns et al. 1985; Turk and Rudy 1990). The "dysfunctional" group scored higher on pain severity, life interference as a result of pain, and psychological distress. This group also scored lower on perceptions of control and performance of daily activities. The "interpersonally distressed" group was characterized by the perception of poor support from others. The "adaptive copers" described lower ratings of pain severity, pain interference, affective distress, physical disability, and perceptions of being out of control. Differential patterns of improvement across subgroups in patients with temporomandibular disorders receiving an interocclusal appliance and biofeedback/stress management treatment protocol have been demonstrated (Rudy et al. 1995). The "dysfunctional" group showed the best response to multidisciplinary treatment, with greater improvements in pain intensity, interference, catastrophizing, depression, and negative thoughts when compared with the other groups.

Another classification of patients with chronic low back pain has been described based on responses to the McGill Pain Questionnaire (Melzack 1975), the Sickness Impact Profile (Bergner et al. 1976a, 1976b; Gilson et al. 1975; Pollard et al. 1976), and the Beck Depression Inventory (Beck 1978; Klapow et al. 1995). Again three groups were identified based on levels of pain, impairment, and depression. The group with higher levels of pain, impairment, and depression reported greater life adversity, more reliance on passive coping strategies, and less satisfaction with social support networks. The patients reporting lower levels in these domains were characterized by the opposite findings. The group with higher levels of pain but lower levels of impairment and depression reported less life adversity and more satisfactory social support, but continued reliance on passive coping strategies.

Multidisciplinary Treatment

Methodology. Patients with chronic pain suffer dramatic reductions in physical, psychological, and social well-being, with health-related quality of life rated lower than that for those with almost all other medical conditions (Becker et al. 1997; Skevington 1998). A study of sequential trials of different treatment modalities found that the success of nerve blocks was diminished when used later in the treatment sequence. These results suggest that early failures of a single modality treatment for chronic pain can have devastating consequences for future treatment attempts (Davies et al. 1997). In another study of more than 1,200 treated patients and 1,700 follow-up patients with low back or neuropathic pain, wide variations in medical practice changed significantly after feedback was given to the practitioners. This information simply informed practitioners about treatment modalities being used in the clinic and other options that were available for treatment (Davies et al. 1996). The multidisciplinary pain center offers the setting to provide the full range of treatments for the most difficult pain syndromes, including those of the elderly (Gibson et al. 1996; Helme et al. 1996).

A distinction between *multidisciplinary* and *interdisciplinary* pain centers has been described (Turk and Stieg 1987). A multidisciplinary approach is a serial evaluation by multiple specialists. Usually, this process leads to diagnoses by exclusion and implies a hierarchy of diagnostic importance. Neuropsychiatry is often the last specialty to evaluate the patient, reinforcing the belief that pain is truly mysterious and "just a figment of your imagination." Even attempts at simultaneous evaluation by multiple specialists including a neuropsychiatrist or psychologist can be misconstrued as trying to determine if symptoms are "real."

Interdisciplinary approaches are characterized by combining areas of expertise to form a shared view of chronic pain. The individual team members, although representatives of different fields of study, recognize that all symptoms can have a variety of causes. These etiologies are organized by specialty for clarity, but the classification structure does not invalidate certain diagnoses, such as psychiatric disorders, as a cause for the patient's symptoms. This approach emphasizes that all diagnoses are real and can be made by any number of specialists if properly trained. When a specific diagnosis cannot be made, an etiology for the patient's symptoms has simply not yet been discovered. As a result, the patient can remain in treatment to receive symptomatic interventions and the coordination of future evaluations. The patient is no longer stigmatized as having a "false" condition but instead recognized as having a legitimate problem with understandable distress.

Effectiveness. Substantial evidence indicates that multidisciplinary pain programs improve patient functioning in a number of areas (Cutler et al. 1994; Fishbain et al. 1993; Flavell et al. 1996). In one of the most comprehensive reviews to date, a meta-analysis of 65 studies evaluated the efficacy of treatments in patients who attended multidisciplinary pain clinics (Flor et al. 1992). Although significant limitations were found, the study concluded that multidisciplinary pain clinics are efficacious. Combination treatments were superior to unimodal treatments or no treatment, treatment effects were maintained over a period of up to 7 years, and improvements were found not only on subjective but also on objective measures of effectiveness such as return to work and decreased health care utilization.

The elderly with chronic pain are often considered more likely to fail treatment because they have more chronic medical conditions, take twice as many medications, and have four times the rate of health care utilization when compared with that of younger patients with chronic pain. It is argued that younger patients with more years of potential productivity should have preferential access to scarce medical resources. However, multidisciplinary outcome studies of elderly patients with chronic pain demonstrate a variety of benefits from treatment (Gibson et al. 1996; Middaugh et al. 1988). Types of improvement include increased activity, decreased magnitude of pain, reductions in the use of medical services, improvement in depression and anxiety, and decreased use of medications. In general, the elderly experience a level of improvement that is the same or even greater than that of younger patients. Therapeutic nihilism is not justified and should never be the treatment of choice for any patient suffering from chronic pain.

Ultimately, the goal of treating patients with chronic pain is to end disability and return people to work or other productive activities. In the longest follow-up study of an inpatient pain management program, patients with chronic pain did not demonstrate an increased risk of mortality 13 years after treatment (Maruta et al. 1998). Only half of the patients were unemployed compared with almost 90% of the patients at the time of their admission for treatment. In a 30-month follow-up study of patients with chronic pain receiving multidisciplinary treatment, employment status was predicted by the patient's voiced "intent" to return to work as well as the perception of a job's dangerousness and the patient's education level (Fishbain et al. 1997). Patients not intending to return to work were more likely to complain of their job's excessive physical demands and reported more job dissatisfaction and feelings of disability (Fishbain et al. 1995; Hildebrandt et al. 1997).

Summary

Chronic pain is a significant public health problem and frustrating to everyone affected by it, especially the elderly who believe that health care has failed them but who wish to remain in their own homes, live independently, and avoid becoming a burden to others (Anikeeff and Mueller 1998; Bendelow and Williams 1996). Neuropsychiatrists as medical specialists should take an active role in the care of these patients. Neuropsychiatrists offer skills with pharmacological and psychological treatments now recognized as effective in the management of chronic pain. Recent advances in the treatment of chronic pain include the diagnosis and treatment of psychiatric comorbidity, the application of neuropsychiatric treatments to chronic pain, and the development of interdisciplinary efforts to provide comprehensive health care to the patient suffering with chronic pain. Specifically, the neuropsychiatrist provides the expertise of examining mental life and behavior as well as understanding the individual person and the systems in which he or she interacts. And finally, neuropsychiatrists can facilitate the integration of the delivery of medical care with other health care professionals and medical specialists.

References

Acute Pain Management Guideline Panel: Acute pain management: operative or medical procedures and trauma. Clinical practice guideline (AHCPR Publ No 92-0032). Rockville, MD, Agency for Health Care Policy and Research, Public Health Service, U.S. Department of Health and Human Services, 1992

Adelman JU, Von Seggern R: Cost considerations in headache treatment, Part 1: prophylactic migraine treatment. Headache 35:479–487, 1995

American Geriatric Society Panel on Chronic Pain in Older Persons: The management of chronic pain in older persons. J Am Geriatr Soc 46:635–651, 1998

American Psychiatric Association: Diagnostic and Statistical Manual of Mental Disorders, 2nd Edition. Washington, DC, American Psychiatric Press, 1968, pp 46–48

American Psychiatric Association: Diagnostic and Statistical Manual of Mental Disorders, 3rd Edition. Washington, DC, American Psychiatric Press, 1980, pp 247–249

American Psychiatric Association: Diagnostic and Statistical Manual of Mental Disorders, 3rd Edition, Revised. Washington, DC, American Psychiatric Press, 1987, pp 264–266

American Psychiatric Association: Diagnostic and Statistical Manual of Mental Disorders, 4th Edition. Washington, DC, American Psychiatric Press, 1994, pp 458–462

Anderson KO, Dowds BN, Pelletz RE, et al: Development and initial validation of a scale to measure self-efficacy beliefs in patients with chronic pain. Pain 63:77–84, 1995

Anikeeff MA, Mueller GR (eds): Seniors Housing, National Investment Conference for the Senior Living and Long Term Care Industries and American Real Estate Society, Research Issues in Real Estate, Vol 4. Dordrecht, Netherlands, Kluwer Academic, 1998

Antkiewicz-Michaluk L, Romanska I, Michaluk J, et al: Role of calcium channels in effects of antidepressant drugs on responsiveness to pain. Psychopharmacology (Berl) 105: 269–274, 1991

Arkinstall W, Sandler A, Goughnour B, et al: Efficacy of controlled-release codeine in chronic non-malignant pain: a randomized, placebo-controlled clinical trial. Pain 62: 169–178, 1995

Arntz A, Dreessen L, De Jong P: The influence of anxiety on pain: attentional and attributional mediators. Pain 56:307–314, 1994

Atkinson JH, Slater MA, Patterson TL, et al: Prevalence, onset and risk of psychiatric disorders in men with chronic low back pain: a controlled study. Pain 45:111–121, 1991

Atkinson JH, Slater MA, Williams RA, et al: A placebo-controlled randomized clinical trial of nortriptyline for chronic low back pain. Pain 76:287–296, 1998

Ayajiki K, Okamura T, Toda N: Flunarizine, an anti-migraine agent, impairs nitroxidergic nerve function in cerebral arteries. Eur J Pharmacol 329:49–53, 1997

Bank J: A comparative study of amitriptyline and fluvoxamine in migraine prophylaxis. Headache 34:476–478, 1994

Bartusch SL, Sanders BJ, D'Alessio JG, et al: Clonazepam for the treatment of lancinating phantom limb pain. Clin J Pain 12:59–62, 1996

Basbaum AI: Mechanisms of substance P–mediated nociception and opioid-mediated antinociception, in Anesthesiology and Pain Management. Edited by Stanley TH, Ashburn MA. Dordrecht, Netherlands, Kluwer Academic, 1994, pp 1–17

Beck AT: Depression Inventory. Philadelphia, PA, Philadelphia Center for Cognitive Therapy, 1978

Becker N, Bondegaard Thomsen A, Olsen AK, et al: Pain epidemiology and health related quality of life in chronic non-malignant pain patients referred to a Danish multidisciplinary pain center. Pain 73:393–400, 1997

Belcheva S, Petkov VD, Konstantinova E, et al: Effects on nociception of the Ca_{2+} and 5-HT antagonist dotarizine and other 5-HT receptor agonists and antagonists. Acta Physiol Pharmacol Bulg 21:93–98, 1995

Bendelow GA, Williams SJ: The end of the road? Lay views on a pain-relief clinic. Soc Sci Med 43:1127–1136, 1996

Bendtsen L, Jensen R, Olesen J: A non-selective (amitriptyline), but not a selective (citalopram) serotonin reuptake inhibitor is effective in the prophylactic treatment of chronic tension-type headache. J Neurol Neurosurg Psychiatry 61: 285–290, 1996

Bergner M, Bobbitt RA, Kressel S, et al: The Sickness Impact Profile: conceptual formulation and methodology for the development of a health status measure. International Journal of Health Services 6:393–415, 1976a

Bergner M, Bobbitt RA, Pollard WE, et al: The Sickness Impact Profile: validation of a health status measure. Medical Care 14:57–67, 1976b

Bergouignan M: Cures heureuses de nevralgies faciaales essentielles par le diphenyl-hydantoinate de soude. Rev Laryngol Otol Rhinol (Bord) 63:34–41, 1942

Bianchi M, Rossoni G, Sacerdote P, et al: Carbamazepine exerts anti-inflammatory effects in the rat. Eur J Pharmacol 294:71–74, 1995

Bonica JJ: Definitions and taxonomy of pain, in The Management of Pain. Edited by Bonica JJ. Philadelphia, PA, Lea & Febiger, 1990, pp 18–27

Borsook D (ed): Molecular Neurobiology of Pain, Progress in Pain Research and Management, Vol 9. Seattle, WA, IASP Press, 1997

Boulton AJ: Causes of neuropathic pain. Diabet Med 10(suppl 2):87S–88S, 1993

Bowersox SS, Gadbois T, Singh T, et al: Selective N-type neuronal voltage-sensitive calcium channel blocker, SNX-111, produces spinal antinociception in rat models of acute, persistent and neuropathic pain. J Pharmacol Exp Ther 279:1243–1249, 1996

Bowsher D: The management of central post-stroke pain. Postgrad Med J 71:598–604, 1995

Bowsher D: Postherpetic neuralgia and its treatment: a retrospective survey of 191 patients. J Pain Symptom Manage 12:290–299, 1996

Bowsher D: The effects of pre-emptive treatment of postherpetic neuralgia with amitriptyline: a randomized, double-blind, placebo-controlled trial. J Pain Symptom Manage 13:327–331, 1997a

Bowsher D: The management of postherpetic neuralgia. Postgrad Med J 73:623–629, 1997b

Brattberg G, Parker MG, Thorslund M: The prevalence of pain among the oldest old in Sweden. Pain 67:29–34, 1996

Brattberg G, Parker MG, Thorslund M: A longitudinal study of pain: reported pain from middle age to old age. Clin J Pain 13:144–149, 1997

Breslau N, Davis GC: Migraine, physical health and psychiatric disorder: a prospective epidemiologic study in young adults. J Psychiatr Res 27:211–221, 1993

Brose WG, Gutlove DP, Luther RR, et al: Use of intrathecal SNX-111, a novel, N-type, voltage-sensitive, calcium channel blocker, in the management of intractable brachial plexus avulsion pain. Clin J Pain 13:256–259, 1997

Brown JW, Robertson LS, Kosa J, et al: A study of general practice in Massachusetts. JAMA 2216:301–306, 1971

Bryson HM, Wilde MI: Amitriptyline. A review of its pharmacological properties and therapeutic use in chronic pain states. Drugs Aging 8:459–476, 1996

Burkey AR, Carstens E, Wenniger JJ, et al: An opioidergic cortical antinociception triggering site in the agranular insular cortex of the rat that contributes to morphine antinociception. J Neurosci 16:6612–6623, 1996

Campbell RWF: Mexiletine. N Engl J Med 316:29–34, 1987

Canavero S, Bonicalzi V: Lamotrigine control of central pain. Pain 68:179–181, 1996

Cancer Pain Management Guideline Panel: Management of cancer pain. Clinical practice guideline (AHCPR Publ No 94-0592). Rockville, MD, Agency for Health Care Policy and Research, Public Health Service, U.S. Department of Health and Human Services, 1994

Cesaro P, Ollat H: Pain and its treatments. Eur Neurol 38: 209–215, 1997

Chabal C, Jacobson L, Chaney EF, et al: Narcotics for chronic pain: yes or no? A useless dichotomy. American Pain Society Journal 1:276–281, 1992a

Chabal C, Jacobson L, Mariano AJ, et al: The use of oral mexiletine for the treatment of pain after peripheral nerve injury. Anesthesiology 76:513–517, 1992b

Chakour MC, Gibson SJ, Bradbeer M, et al: The effect of age on Aδ- and C-fibre thermal pain perception. Pain 64:143–152, 1996

Chapman CR, Casey KL, Dubner R, et al: Pain measurement: an overview. Pain 22:1–31, 1985

Chapman V, Suzuki R, Chamarette HLC, et al: Effects of systemic carbamazepine and gabapentin on spinal neuronal responses in spinal nerve ligated rats. Pain 75:261–272, 1998

Cheung H, Kamp D, Harris E: An in vitro investigation of the action of lamotrigine on neuronal voltage-activated sodium channels. Epilepsy Res 13:107–112, 1992

Chudler EH, Dong WK: The role of the basal ganglia in nociception and pain. Pain 60:3–38, 1995

Chudler EH, Sugiyama K, Dong WK: Nociceptive responses of neurons in the neostriatum and globus pallidus of the rat. J Neurophysiol 69:1890–1903, 1993

Chung JM, Choi Y, Yoon YW, et al: Effects of age on behavioral signs of neuropathic pain in an experimental rat model. Neurosci Lett 183:54–57, 1995

Cleary JF, Carbone PP: Palliative medicine in the elderly. Cancer 80:1335–1347, 1997

Cohen GL: Protriptyline, chronic tension-type headaches, and weight loss in women. Headache 37:433–436, 1997

Compton MA: Cold-pressor pain tolerance in opiate and cocaine abusers: correlates of drug type and use status. J Pain Symptom Manage 9:462–473, 1994

Corran TM, Gibson SJ, Farrell MJ, et al: Comparison of chronic pain experience between young and elderly patients, in Proceedings of the 7th World Congress on Pain, Progress in Pain Research and Management, Vol 2. Seattle, WA, IASP Press, 1994, pp 895–906

Corran TM, Farrell MJ, Helme RD, et al: The classification of patients with chronic pain: age as a contributing factor. Clin J Pain 13:207–214, 1997

Crombez G, Eccleston C, Baeyens F, et al: When somatic information threatens, catastrophic thinking enhances attentional interference. Pain 75:187–198, 1998

Cutler BR, Fishbain DA, Rosomoff HL, et al: Does non-surgical pain center treatment of chronic pain return patients to work? a review and meta-analysis of the literature. Spine 19:643–652, 1994

Cutrer FM, Moskowitz MA, Wolff A: Wolff Award 1996: the actions of valproate and neurosteroids in a model of trigeminal pain. Headache 36:579–585, 1996

Cutrer FM, Limmroth V, Moskowitz MA: Possible mechanisms of valproate in migraine prophylaxis. Cephalalgia 17: 93–100, 1997

Davies HT, Crombie IK, Macrae WA, et al: Audit in pain clinics: changing the management of low-back and nerve-damage pain. Anaesthesia 51:641–646, 1996

Davies HT, Crombie IK, Brown JH, et al: Diminishing returns or appropriate treatment strategy?—an analysis of short-term outcomes after pain clinic treatment. Pain 70:203–208, 1997

Davis MA: Epidemiology of osteoarthritis. Clin Geriatric Med 4:241–255, 1988

Davis RW: Successful treatment for phantom pain. Orthopaedics 16:691–695, 1993

Deardorff WW, Chino AF, Scott DW: Characteristics of chronic pain patients: factor analysis of the MMPI-2. Pain 54:153–158, 1993

Dejgard A, Petersen P, Kastrup J: Mexiletine for treatment of chronic painful diabetic neuropathy. Lancet 1:9–11, 1988

Dellemijn PL, Fields HL: Do benzodiazepines have a role in chronic pain management? Pain 57:137–152, 1994

Dellemijn PL, Vanneste JA: Randomised double-blind active-placebo-controlled crossover trial of intravenous fentanyl in neuropathic pain. Lancet 349:753–758, 1997

Desbiens NA, Wu AW, Azola C, et al: Pain during hospitalization is associated with continued pain six months in survivors of serious illness. The SUPPORT Investigators. The Study to Understand Prognoses and Preferences for Outcomes and Risks of Treatment. Am J Med 102:269–276, 1997

Devlen J: Anxiety and depression in migraine. J R Soc Med 87:338–341, 1994

Devor M: The pathophysiology of damaged peripheral nerves, in Textbook of Pain, 3rd Edition. Edited by Wall PD, Melzack R. Edinburgh, Churchill Livingstone, 1994, pp 79–100

Donner B, Zenz M, Tryba M, et al: Direct conversion from oral morphine to transdermal fentanyl: a multicenter study in patients with cancer pain. Pain 64:527–534, 1996

Dubner R, Ren K: Central mechanisms of thermal and mechanical hyperalgesia following tissue inflammation, in Touch, Temperature, and Pain in Health and Disease: Mechanisms and Assessments, Vol 3. Edited by Boivie J, Hansson P, Lindblom U. Seattle, WA, IASP Press, 1994, pp 267–277

Dworkin SF, Von Korff M, LeResche L: Multiple pains and psychiatric disturbance: an epidemiologic investigation. Arch Gen Psychiatry 47:239–244, 1990

Eide PK, Stubhaug A, Stenehjem AE: Central dysesthesia pain after traumatic spinal cord injury is dependent on N-methyl-D-aspartate receptor activation. Neurosurgery 37:1080–1087, 1995

Emanuel EJ, Fairclough DL, Daniels ER, et al: Euthanasia and physician-assisted suicide: attitudes and experiences of oncology patients, oncologists, and the public. Lancet 347:1805–1810, 1996

Ferrell BA: Pain management in elderly people. J Am Geriatr Soc 39:64–73, 1991

Ferrell BA: Overview of aging and pain, in Pain in the Elderly. Edited by Ferrell BR, Ferrell BA. Seattle, WA, IASP Press, 1996, pp 1–10

Ferrell BA, Ferrell BR, Rivera L: Pain in cognitively impaired nursing home patients. J Pain Symptom Manage 10:591–598, 1995

Field MJ, Holloman EF, McCleary S, et al: Evaluation of gabapentin and S-(+)-3-isobutylgaba in a rat model of postoperative pain. J Pharmacol Exp Ther 282:1242–1246, 1997

Fields HL, Basbaum AI: Central nervous system mechanisms of pain modulation, in Textbook of Pain, 3rd Edition. Edited by Wall PD, Melzack R. Edinburgh, Churchill Livingstone, 1994, pp 243–257

Fields HL, Rowbotham M, Baron R: Postherpetic neuralgia: irritable nociceptors and deafferentation. Neurobiol Dis 5:209–227, 1998

Fishbain DA, Goldberg M, Meagher BR, et al: Male and female chronic pain patients characterized by DSM-III diagnostic criteria. Pain 26:181–187, 1986

Fishbain DA, Goldberg M, Rosomoff RS, et al: Completed suicide in chronic pain. Clin J Pain 7:29–36, 1991

Fishbain DA, Rosomoff HL, Rosomoff RS: Detoxification of nonopiate drugs in the chronic pain setting and clonidine opiate detoxification. Clin J Pain 8:191–203, 1992a

Fishbain DA, Rosomoff HL, Rosomoff RS: Drug abuse, dependence: addiction in chronic pain patients. Clin J Pain 8:77–85, 1992b

Fishbain DA, Rosomoff HL, Goldberg M, et al: The prediction of return to the workplace after multidisciplinary pain center treatment. Clin J Pain 9:3–15, 1993

Fishbain DA, Rosomoff HL, Cutler RB, et al: Do chronic pain patients' perceptions about their preinjury jobs determine their intent to return to the same type of job post-pain facility treatment. Clin J Pain 11:267–278, 1995

Fishbain DA, Cutler RB, Rosomoff HL, et al: Impact of chronic pain patients' job perception variables on actual return to work. Clin J Pain 13:197–206, 1997

Flavell HA, Carrafa GP, Thomas CH, et al: Managing chronic back pain: impact of an interdisciplinary team approach. Med J Aust 165:253–255, 1996

Flor H, Fydrich T, Turk DC: Efficacy of multidisciplinary pain treatment centers: a meta-analytic review. Pain 49:221–230, 1992

Foley K: Pain in the elderly, in Principles of Geriatric Medicine and Gerontology. Edited by Hazzard WR, Bierman EL, Blass JP, et al. New York, McGraw-Hill, 1994, pp 281–295

Folkman S, Lazarus RS, Gruen RJ, et al: Appraisal, coping, health status, and psychological symptoms. J Pers Soc Psychol 50:571–579, 1986

Fordyce W, Fowler R, Lehmann J, et al: Operant conditioning in the treatment of chronic pain. Arch Phys Med Rehabil 54:399–408, 1973

Fordyce WE, Lansky D, Calsyn DA, et al: Pain measurement and pain behavior. Pain 18:53–69, 1984

Forman WB: Opioid analgesic drugs in the elderly. Clin Geriatr Med 12:489–500, 1996

Foster CA, Bafaloukos J: Paroxetine in the treatment of chronic daily headache. Headache 34:587–589, 1994

France RD, Kirshman KRR: Psychotropic drugs in chronic pain, in Chronic Pain. Edited by France RD, Kirshman KRR. Washington, DC, American Psychiatric Press, 1988, pp 322–374

France RD, Ruban BJ, Keefe FJ: Long-term use of narcotic analgesics in chronic pain. Soc Sci Med 19:1379–1382, 1984

Gagliese L, Melzack R: Chronic pain in elderly people. Pain 70:3–14, 1997

Galer BS: Neuropathic pain of peripheral origin: advances in pharmacologic treatment. Neurology 45:S17–S25, 1995

Galer BS, Harle J, Rowbotham MC: Response to intravenous lidocaine infusion predicts subsequent response to oral mexiletine: a prospective study. J Pain Symptom Manage 12:161–167, 1996

Galer BS, Schwartz L, Turner JA: Do patient and physician expectations predict response to pain-relieving procedures? Clin J Pain 13:348–351, 1997

Ganapathy S, Herrick IA, Gelb AW, et al: Propofol patient-controlled sedation during hip or knee arthroplasty in elderly patients. Can J Anaesth 44:385–389, 1997

Gatch MB, Negus SS, Mello NK: Antinociceptive effects of monoamine reuptake inhibitors administered alone or in combination with mu opioid agonists in rhesus monkeys. Psychopharmacology (Berl) 135:99–106, 1998

Gear RW, Miaskowski C, Heller PH, et al: Benzodiazepine mediated antagonism of opioid analgesia. Pain 71:25–29, 1997

Gibson SJ, Farrell MJ, Katz B, et al: Multidisciplinary management of chronic nonmalignant pain in older adults, in Pain in the Elderly. Edited by Ferrell BR, Ferrell BA. Seattle, WA, IASP Press, 1996, pp 91–99

Gilson BS, Gilson JS, Bergner M, et al: The Sickness Impact Profile: development of an outcome measure of health status. American Journal of Public Health 65:1304–1310, 1975

Gloth RM III: Concerns with chronic analgesic therapy in elderly patients. Am J Med 101:19S–24S, 1996

Goadsby PJ: How do the currently used prophylactic agents work in migraine? Cephalalgia 17:85–92, 1997

Goetz CG, Tannen CM, Levy M, et al: Pain in Parkinson's disease. Mov Disord 10:541–549, 1986

Goicoechea C, Ormazabal MJ, Alfaro MJ, et al: Age-related changes in nociception, behavior, and monoamine levels in rats. Gen Pharmacol 28:331–336, 1997

Goodkin K, Gullion C, Agras WS: A randomized, double-blind, placebo-controlled trial of trazodone hydrochloride in chronic low back pain syndrome. J Clin Psychopharmacol 10:269–278, 1990

Goodkin K, Vrancken MAE, Feaster D: On the putative efficacy of the antidepressants in chronic, benign pain syndromes: an update. Pain Forum 4:237–247, 1995

Gordon RS: Pain in the elderly. JAMA 241:2191–2192, 1979

Gruber AJ, Hudson JI, Pope HG Jr: The management of treatment-resistant depression in disorders on the interface of psychiatry and medicine. Fibromyalgia, chronic fatigue syndrome, migraine, irritable bowel syndrome, atypical facial pain, and premenstrual dysphoric disorder. Psychiatr Clin North Am 19:351–369, 1996

Gureje O, Von Korff M, Simon GE, et al: Persistent pain and well-being: a World Health Organization study in primary care. JAMA 280:147–151, 1998

Harbinson J, Dennehy F, Keating D: Lamotrigine for pain with hyperalgesia. Ir Med J 90:56, 1997

Harkins SW: Geriatric pain. Pain perceptions in the old. Clin Geriatr Med 12:435–459, 1996

Harkins SW, Kwentus J, Price DD: Pain and the elderly, in Advances in Pain Research and Therapy, Vol 7. Edited by Benedetti C, Chapman CE, Moricca G. New York, Raven, 1984, pp 103–121

Harkins SW, Davis MD, Bush FM, et al: Suppression of first pain and slow temporal summation of second pain in relation to age. J Gerontol A Biol Sci Med Sci 51:M260–M265, 1996

Hasegawa AE, Zacny JP: The influence of three L-type calcium channel blockers on morphine effects in healthy volunteers. Anesth Analg 85:633–638, 1997

Hasenbring M, Marienfeld G, Kuhlendahl D, et al: Risk factors of chronicity in lumbar disc patients. A prospective investigation of biologic, psychologic, and social predictors of therapy outcome. Spine 19:2759–2765, 1994

Haythornthwaite JA, Sieber WJ, Kerns RD: Depression and the chronic pain experience. Pain 46:177–184, 1991

Heft MW, Cooper BY, O'Brien KK, et al: Aging effects on the perception of noxious and non-noxious thermal stimuli applied to the face. Aging (Milano) 8:35–41, 1996

Heim HM, Oei TPS: Comparison of prostate cancer patients with and without pain. Pain 53:159–162, 1993

Heiskanen T, Kalso E: Controlled-release oxycodone and morphine in cancer related pain. Pain 73:37–45, 1997

Helme RD, McKernan S: Effects of age on the axon reflex response to noxious chemical stimulation. Clin Exp Neurol 22:57–61, 1986

Helme RD, Katz B, Gibson SJ, et al: Multidisciplinary pain clinics for older people. Do they serve a role? Clin Geriatr Med 12:563–582, 1996

Hendler N, Cimini C, Ma T, et al: A comparison of cognitive impairment due to benzodiazepines and to narcotics. Am J Psychiatry 137:828–830, 1980

Herr KA, Mobily PR: Comparison of selected pain assessment tools for use with the elderly. Appl Nurs Res 6:39–46, 1993

Herrick IA, Ganapathy S, Komar W, et al: Postoperative cognitive impairment in the elderly. Choice of patient-controlled analgesia opioid. Anaesthesia 51:356–360, 1996

Hildebrandt J, Pfingsten M, Saur P, et al: Prediction of success from a multidisciplinary treatment program for chronic low back pain. Spine 22:990–1001, 1997

Hill A, Niven CA, Knussen C: The role of coping in adjustment to phantom limb pain. Pain 62:79–86, 1995

Hodoglugil U, Guney HZ, Savran B, et al: Temporal variation in the interaction between calcium channel blockers and morphine-induced analgesia. Chronobiol Int 13:227–234, 1996

Holister LE, Conley FK, Britt R, et al: Long-term use of diazepam. JAMA 246:1568–1570, 1981

Houtchens MK, Richert JR, Sami A, et al: Open label gabapentin treatment for pain in multiple sclerosis. Mult Scler 3:250–253, 1997

Hunter JC, Gogas KR, Hedley LR, et al: The effect of novel anti-epileptic drugs in rat experimental models of acute and chronic pain. Eur J Pharmacol 324:153–160, 1997

Iadarola MJ, Max MB, Berman KF, et al: Unilateral decrease in thalamic activity observed with positron emission tomography in patients with chronic neuropathic pain. Pain 63:55–64, 1995

Janig W: The puzzle of "relex sympathetic dystrophy": mechanisms, hypotheses, open questions, in Reflex Sympathetic Dystrophy: A Reappraisal. Edited by Janig W, Stanton-Hicks M. Seattle, WA, IASP Press, 1996, pp 1–24

Jannetta PJ, Gildenberg PL, Loeser JD, et al: Operations on the brain and brain stem for chronic pain, in The Management of Pain, Vol 2. Edited by Bonica JJ. Philadelphia, PA, Lea & Febiger, 1990, pp 2082–2103

Jensen MP, Karoly P, Huger R: The development and preliminary validation of an instrument to assess patients' attitudes toward pain. J Psychosom Res 31:393–400, 1987

Jensen MP, Turner JA, Romano JM, et al: Coping with chronic pain: a critical review of the literature. Pain 47:249–283, 1991a

Jensen MP, Turner JA, Romano JM: Self-efficacy and outcome expectancies: relationship to chronic pain coping strategies and adjustment. Pain 44:263–269, 1991b

Jensen MP, Turner JA, Romano JM: Correlates of improvement in multidisciplinary treatment of chronic pain. J Consult Clin Psychol 62:172–179, 1994a

Jensen MP, Turner JA, Romano JM, et al: Relationship of pain-specific beliefs to chronic pain adjustment. Pain 57:301–309, 1994b

Jensen R, Brinck T, Olesen J: Sodium valproate has a prophylactic effect in migraine without aura: a triple-blind, placebo-controlled crossover study. Neurology 44:647–651, 1994c

Jett MF, McGuirk J, Waligora D, et al: The effects of mexiletine, desipramine and fluoxetine in rat models involving central sensitization. Pain 69:161–169, 1997

Johnson RW: Herpes zoster and postherpetic neuralgia. Optimal treatment. Drugs Aging 10:80–94, 1997

Jones AKP, Brown WD, Friston KJ, et al: Cortical and subcortical localization of response to pain in man using positron emission tomography. Proc R Soc Lond B Biol Sci 244:39–44, 1991

Jun JH, Yaksh TL: The effect of intrathecal gabapentin and 3-isobutyl gamma-aminobutyric acid on the hyperalgesia observed after thermal injury in the rat. Anesth Analg 86:348–354, 1998

Junge A, Dvorak J, Ahrens S: Predictors of bad and good outcomes of lumbar disc surgery. A prospective clinical study with recommendations for screening to avoid bad outcomes. Spine 20:460–468, 1995

Kamei J, Saitoh A, Kasuya Y: Involvement of delta 1-opioid receptors in the antinociceptive effects of mexiletine in mice. Neurosci Lett 196:169–172, 1995

Kaniecki RG: A comparison of divalproex with propranolol and placebo for the prophylaxis of migraine without aura. Arch Neurol 54:1141–1145, 1997

Karlsten R, Gordh T: How do drugs relieve neurogenic pain? Drugs Aging 11:398–412, 1997

Katon W, Sullivan M: Depression and a chronic medical illness. J Clin Psychiatry 150(suppl):3–11, 1990

Katon W, Egan K, Miller D: Chronic pain: lifetime psychiatric diagnoses and family history. Am J Psychiatry 142:1156–1160, 1985

Katon W, Lin E, Von Korff M, et al: Somatization: a spectrum of severity. Am J Psychiatry 148:34–40, 1991

Katz PP, Yelin EH: Prevalence and correlates of depressive symptoms among persons with rheumatoid arthritis. J Rheumatol 20:790–796, 1993

Keefe FJ, Crisson JE, Maltbie A, et al: Illness behavior as a predictor of pain and overt behavior patterns in chronic low back pain patients. J Psychosom Res 30:543–551, 1986

Keefe FJ, Caldwell DS, Queen KT, et al: Pain coping strategies in osteoarthritis patients. J Consult Clin Psychol 55:208–212, 1987

Keefe FJ, Caldwell DS, Williams DA, et al: Pain coping skills training in the management of osteoarthritic knee pain: a comparative study. Behavior Therapy 21:49–62, 1990a

Keefe FJ, Caldwell DS, Williams DA, et al: Pain coping skills training in the management of osteoarthritic knee pain, II: follow-up results. Behavior Therapy 21:435–447, 1990b

Keefe FJ, Dunsmore J, Burnett R: Behavioral and cognitive-behavioral approaches to chronic pain: recent advances and future directions. J Consult Clin Psychol 60:528–536, 1992

Keefe FJ, Beaupre PM, Weiner DK, et al: Pain in older adults: a cognitive-behavioral perspective, in Pain in the Elderly. Edited by Ferrell BR, Ferrell BA. Seattle, WA, IASP Press, 1996, pp 11–19

Kerns R, Turk D, Rudy T: The West Haven–Yale Multidimensional Pain Inventory. Pain 23:345–356, 1985

Khalil Z, Helme R: Sensory peptides as neuromodulators of wound healing in aged rats. J Gerontol A Biol Sci Med Sci 51:B354–B361, 1996

Khalil Z, Ralevic V, Bassirat M, et al: Effects of ageing on sensory nerve function in rat skin. Brain Res 641:265–272, 1994

King RB: Neuropharmacology of depression, anxiety, and pain. Clin Neurosurg 28:116–136, 1981

King SA, Strain JJ: Benzodiazepine use by chronic pain patients. Clin J Pain 6:143–147, 1990

King SA, Strain JJ: Revising the category of somatoform pain disorder. Hospital and Community Psychiatry 43:217–219, 1992

Kirmayer LJ, Robbins JM: Three forms of somatization in primary care: prevalence, co-occurrence, and sociodemographic characteristics. J Nerv Ment Dis 179:647–655, 1991

Kishore-Kumar R, Max MB, Schafer SC, et al: Desipramine relieves post-herpetic neuralgia. Clin Pharmacol Ther 47:305–312, 1990

Klapow JC, Slater MA, Patterson TL, et al: Psychosocial factors discriminate multidimensional clinical groups of chronic low back pain patients. Pain 62:349–355, 1995

Klapper J: Divalproex sodium in migraine prophylaxis: a dose-controlled study. Cephalalgia 17:103–108, 1997

Koch HK: The National Ambulatory Medical Care Survey: 1975 Summary (DHHS Publ No PHS 78-1784). Hyattsville, MD, U.S. Department of Health, Education, and Welfare, 1978

Koller WC: Sensory symptoms in Parkinson's disease. Neurology 34:957–959, 1984

Kouyanou K, Pither CE, Wessely S: Medication misuse, abuse and dependence in chronic pain patients. J Psychosom Res 43:497–504, 1997

Kouyanou K, Pither CE, Rabe-Hesketh S, et al: A comparative study of iatrogenesis, medication abuse, and psychiatric morbidity in chronic pain patients with and without medically explained symptoms. Pain 76:417–426, 1998

Kroenke K: Somatization in primary care: an inclusive approach to the symptomatic patient. American Pain Society Journal 2:150–153, 1993

Kroenke K, Mangelsdorff A: Common symptoms in ambulatory care: incidence, evaluation, therapy, and outcome. Am J Med 86:262–266, 1989

Kroenke K, Arrington ME, Mangelsdorff AD: The prevalence of symptoms in medical outpatients and the adequacy of therapy. Arch Intern Med 150:1685–1689, 1990

Kuch K, Cox BJ, Woszczyna CB, et al: Chronic pain in panic disorder. J Behav Ther Exp Psychiatry 22:255–259, 1991

Lane NE: Pain management in osteoarthritis: the role of COX-2 inhibitors. J Rheumatol 24(suppl 49):20–24, 1997

Lang E, Hord AH, Denson D: Venlafaxine hydrochloride (Effexor) relieves thermal hyperalgesia in rats with an experimental mononeuropathy. Pain 68:151–155, 1996

Lasch H, Castell DO, Castell JA: Evidence for diminished visceral pain with aging: studies using graded intraesophageal balloon distension. Am J Physiol 272:G1–G3, 1997

Lazarus RA, Folkman S: Stress, Appraisal, and Coping. New York, Springer, 1984

Leach MJ, Lees G, Riddall DR: Lamotrigine: mechanisms of action, in Proceedings of the 7th World Congress on Pain, Progress in Pain Research and Treatment, Vol 2. Edited by Gebhart GF, Hammond DL, Jensen TS. Seattle, WA, IASP Press, 1995, pp 861–869

Lee J, Giles K, Drummond PD: Psychological disturbances and an exaggerated response to pain in patients with whiplash injury. J Psychosom Res 37:105–110, 1993

Lees G, Leach MJ: Studies on the mechanism of action of the novel anticonvulsant lamotrigine (Lamictal) using primary neuroglial cultures from rat cortex. Brain Res 612: 190–199, 1993

Leino P, Magni G: Depressive and distress symptoms as predictors of low back pain, neck-shoulder pain, and other musculoskeletal morbidity: a 10 year follow-up of metal industry employees. Pain 53:89–94, 1993

Levine JD, Fields HL, Basbaum AI: Peptides and the primary afferent nociceptor. J Neurosci 13:2273–2286, 1993

Lewis TA, Solomon GD: Advances in cluster headache management. Cleve Clin J Med 63:237–244, 1996

Lipman AG: Analgesic drugs for neuropathic and sympathetically maintained pain. Clin Geriatr Med 12:501–515, 1996

Lipowski ZJ: Somatization and depression. Psychosomatics 31:13–21, 1990

Lipton RB, Stewart WF, von Korff M: Burden of migraine: societal costs and therapeutic opportunities. Neurology 48 (suppl 3):S4–9, 1997

Lomardo WK, Lombardo B, Goldstein A: Cognitive functioning under moderate and low dosage methadone maintenance. International Journal of the Addictions 11:389–401, 1976

Long DM, Filtzer DL, BenDebba M, et al: Clinical features of the failed-back syndrome. J Neurosurg 69:6171, 1988

Lorenzo RJ: Mechanisms of action of phenytoin, in Antiepileptic Drugs, 3rd Edition. Edited by Levy RH, Dreifuss FE, Mattson RH. New York, Raven, 1989, pp 143–158

Lynn J, Teno JM, Phillips RS, et al: Perceptions by family members of the dying experience of older and seriously ill patients. SUPPORT Investigators. Study to Understand Prognoses and Preferences for Outcomes and Risks of Treatments. Ann Intern Med 1226:97–106, 1997

MacFarlane BV, Wright A, O'Callaghan J, et al: Chronic neuropathic pain and its control by drugs. Pharmacol Ther 75:1–19, 1997

Magni G: On the relationship between chronic pain and depression when there is no organic lesion. Pain 31:1–21, 1987

Magni G: The use of antidepressants in the treatment of chronic pain: a review of the current evidence. Drugs 42:730–748, 1991

Magni G, Schifano F, DeLeo D: Pain as a symptom in elderly depressed patients. Relationship to diagnostic subgroups. European Archives of Psychiatry and Neurological Sciences 235:143–145, 1985

Magni G, Marchetti M, Moreschi C, et al: Chronic musculoskeletal pain and depressive symptoms in the National Health and Nutrition Examination, I: epidemiologic follow-up study. Pain 53:163–168, 1993

Magni G, Moreschi C, Rigatti-Luchini S, et al: Prospective study on the relationship between depressive symptoms and chronic musculoskeletal pain. Pain 56:289–297, 1994

Magni G, Rigatti-Luchini S, Fracca F, et al: Suicidality in chronic abdominal pain: an analysis of the Hispanic Health and Nutrition Examination Survey (HHANES). Pain 76:137–144, 1998

Manetto C, McPherson SE: The behavioral-cognitive model of pain. Clin Geriatr Med 12:461–471, 1996

Marek GJ, McDougle CJ, Price LH, et al: A comparison of trazodone and fluoxetine: implications for a serotonergic mechanism of antidepressant action. Psychopharmacology (Berl) 109:2–11, 1992

Markley HG: Verapamil and migraine prophylaxis: mechanisms and efficacy. Am J Med 90:48S–53S, 1991

Marson AG, Kadir ZA, Hutton JL, et al: The new antiepileptic drugs: a systematic review of their efficacy and tolerability. Epilepsia 38:859–880, 1997

Maruta T, Swanson DW, Finlayson RE: Drug abuse and dependency in patients with chronic pain. Mayo Clin Proc 54:241–244, 1979

Maruta T, Malinchoc M, Offord KP, et al: Status of patients with chronic pain 13 years after treatment in a pain management center. Pain 74:199–204, 1998

Mathew NT, Saper JR, Silberstein SD, et al: Migraine prophylaxis with divalproex. Arch Neurol 52:281–286, 1995

Max MB: Treatment of post-herpetic neuralgia: antidepressants. Ann Neurol 35:850–853, 1994

Max MB, Culnane M, Schafer SC, et al: Amitriptyline relieves diabetic neuropathy pain in patients with normal or depressed mood. Neurology 37:589–596, 1987

Max MB, Schafer SC, Culnane M, et al: Amitriptyline, but not lorazepam, relieves postherpetic neuralgia. Neurology 38: 1427–1432, 1988

Max MB, Kishore-Kumar R, Schafer SC, et al: Efficacy of desipramine in painful diabetic neuropathy: a placebo controlled trial. Pain 45:3–9, 1991

Max M, Lynch S, Muir J, et al: Effects of desipramine, amitriptyline and fluoxetine on pain in diabetic neuropathy. N Engl J Med 326:1250–1256, 1992

McCracken LM: Learning to live with the pain: acceptance of pain predicts adjustment in persons with chronic pain. Pain 74:21–27, 1998

McMahon S, Koltzenburg M: The changing role of primary afferent neurones in pain. Pain 43:269–272, 1990

McNairy SI, Maruta T, Ivnik RJ, et al: Prescription medication dependence and neuropsychological function. Pain 18: 169–177, 1984

McQuay H, Carroll D, Jadad AR, et al: Anticonvulsant drugs for management of pain: a systematic review. BMJ 311: 1047–1052, 1995

McQuay HJ, Tramer M, Nye BA, et al: A systematic review of antidepressants in neuropathic pain. Pain 68:217–227, 1996

Mechanic D: The concept of illness behavior. Journal of Chronic Diseases 15:189–194, 1962

Meert TF, DeKock M: Potentiation of the analgesic properties of fentanyl-like opioids with alpha2-adrenoceptor agonists in rats. Anesthesiology 81:677–688, 1994

Melzack R, Wall PD: Pain mechanisms: a new theory. Science 150:971–979, 1965

Melzack R: The McGill Pain Questionnaire: major properties and scoring methods. Pain 1:277–299, 1975

Mendelson G, Mendelson D: Legal aspects of the management of chronic pain. Med J Aust 155:640–643, 1991

Merhi M, Helme RD, Khalil Z: Age-related changes in sympathetic modulation of sensory nerve activity in rat skin. Inflammation Research 47:239–244, 1998

Merikangas KR, Merikangas JR: Combination monoamine oxidase inhibitor and beta-blocker treatment of migraine, with anxiety and depression. Biol Psychiatry 38:603–610, 1995

Merskey H, Lindblom U, Mumford JM, et al: Pain terms: a current list with definitions and notes on usage. Pain (suppl 3): S215–S221, 1986

Meyer RA, Campbell JN, Raja SN: Peripheral neural mechanisms of nociception, in Textbook of Pain, 3rd Edition. Edited by Wall PD, Melzack R. Edinburgh, Churchill Livingstone, 1994, pp 13–44

Mico JA, Gibert-Rahola J, Casas J, et al: Implication of beta 1- and beta 2-adrenergic receptors in the antinociceptive effect of tricyclic antidepressants. Eur Neuropsychopharmacol 7:139–145, 1997

Middaugh SJ, Levin RB, Kee WG, et al: Chronic pain: its treatment in geriatric and younger patients. Arch Phys Med Rehabil 69:1021–1026, 1988

Mitsikostas DD, Gatzonis S, Thomas A, et al: Buspirone vs. amitriptyline in the treatment of chronic tension-type headache. Acta Neurol Scand 96:247–251, 1997

Model Guidelines for the Use of Controlled Substances for the Treatment of Pain. Policy documents of the Federation of State Medical Boards of the United States, Inc. Euless, TX, May 1998

Moosa RS, McFayden ML, Miller R, et al: Carbamazepine and its metabolites in neuralgias: concentration-effect relations. Eur J Clin Pharmacol 45:297–301, 1993

Morgan JP: American opiophobia: customary underutilization of opioid analgesics. Advances in Alcohol and Substance Abuse 5:163–173, 1985

Morley S, Wilkinson L: The pain beliefs and perceptions inventory: a British replication. Pain 61:427–433, 1995

Moulin DE, Iezzi A, Amireh R, et al: Randomised trial of oral morphine for chronic non-cancer pain. Lancet 347: 143–147, 1996

Nebe J, Vanegas H, Neugebauer V, et al: Omega-agatoxin IVA, a P-type calcium channel antagonist, reduces nociceptive processing in spinal cord neurons with input from the inflamed but not from the normal knee joint—an electrophysiological study in the rat in vivo. Eur J Neurosci 9:2193–2201, 1997

Nikolaus T: Assessment of chronic pain in elderly patients. Ther Umsch 54:340–344, 1997

Nishikawa ST, Ferrell BA: Pain assessment in the elderly. Clinics in Geriatric Issues in Long Term Care 1:15–28, 1993

Nishiyama K, Sakuta M: Mexiletine for painful alcoholic neuropathy. Intern Med 34:577–579, 1995

Ollat H, Cesaro P: Pharmacology of neuropathic pain. Clin Neuropharmacol 18:391–404, 1995

Onghena P, Van Houdenhove B: Antidepressant-induced analgesia in chronic non-malignant pain: a meta-analysis of 39 placebo-controlled studies. Pain 49:205–219, 1992

Oskarsson P, Ljunggren JG, Lins PE: Efficacy and safety of mexiletine in the treatment of painful diabetic neuropathy. Diabetes Care 20:1594–1597, 1997

Paoli F, Darcourt G, Corsa P: Note preliminaire su l'action de l'impramine dans les etats douloureux. Revue de Neurologie 2:503–504, 1960

Parmelee PA: Pain in cognitively impaired older persons. Clin Geriatr Med 12:473–487, 1996

Paul D, Hornby PJ: Potentiation of intrathecal DAMGO antinociception, but not gastrointestinal transit inhibition, by 5-hydroxytryptamine and norepinephrine uptake blockade. Life Sci 56:PL83–PL87, 1995

Pick CG, Paul D, Eison MS, et al: Potentiation of opioid analgesia by the antidepressant nefazodone. European Journal of Pharmacology 211:375–381, 1992

Platten HP, Schweizer E, Dilger K, et al: Pharmacokinetics and the pharmacodynamic action of midazolam in young and elderly patients undergoing tooth extraction. Clin Pharmacol Ther 63:552–560, 1998

Polatin PB, Kinney RK, Gatchel RJ, et al: Psychiatric illness and chronic low back pain. Spine 18:66–71, 1993

Pollard WE, Bobbitt RA, Bergner M, et al: The Sickness Impact Profile: reliability of a health status measure. Medical Care 14:146–155, 1976

Portenoy RK: Chronic opioid therapy in non-malignant pain. J Pain Symptom Manage 5(suppl 1):S46–S62, 1990

Portenoy RK, Foley KM: Chronic use of opioid analgesics in non-malignant pain: report of 38 cases. Pain 25:171–186, 1986

Portenoy RK, Foley KM: Constipation in the cancer patient. Med Clin North Am 71:303–312, 1987

Porter J, Jick H: Addiction rate in patients treated with narcotics. N Engl J Med 302:123, 1980

Poulsen L, Arendt-Nielsen L, Brosen K, et al: The hypoalgesic effect of imipramine in different human experimental pain models. Pain 60:287–293, 1995

Price DD, Mao JR, Mayer DJ: Central neural mechanisms of normal and abnormal pain states, in Pharmacological Approaches to the Treatment of Chronic Pain: New Concepts and Critical Issues. Progress in Pain Research and Management, Vol 1. Edited by Fields HL, Liebeskind JC. Seattle, WA, IASP Press, 1994, pp 61–84

Rani PU, Naidu MU, Prasad VB, et al: An evaluation of antidepressants in rheumatic pain conditions. Anesth Analg 83:371–375, 1996

Rapp SE, Egan KJ, Ross BK, et al: A multidimensional comparison of morphine and hydromorphone patient-controlled analgesia. Anesth Analg 82:1043–1048, 1996

Ready LB, Sarkis E, Turner JA: Self-reported vs. actual use of medications in chronic pain patients. Pain 12:285–294, 1982

Richeimer SH, Bajwa ZH, Kahraman SS, et al: Utilization patterns of tricyclic antidepressants in a multidisciplinary pain clinic: a survey. Clin J Pain 13:324–329, 1997

Rizzo MA: Successful treatment of painful traumatic mononeuropathy with carbamazepine: insights into a possible molecular pain mechanism. J Neurol Sci 152:103–106, 1997

Romano JM, Syrjala KL, Levy RL, et al: Overt pain behaviors: relationship to patient functioning and treatment outcome. Behavior Therapy 19:191–201, 1988

Roose SP, Glassman AH, Siris S: Comparison of imipramine and nortriptyline-induced orthostatic hypotension: a meaningful difference. J Clin Psychopharmacol 1:316–319, 1981

Rosenstiel AK, Keefe FJ: The use of coping strategies in chronic low back pain patients: relationship to patient characteristics and current adjustment. Pain 17:33–44, 1983

Rothrock JF: Clinical studies of valproate for migraine prophylaxis. Cephalalgia 17:81–83, 1997

Rudy TE, Turk DC, Kubinski JA, et al: Differential treatment responses of TMD patients as a function of psychological characteristics. Pain 61:103–112, 1995

Sanders SH, Brena SF: Empirically derived chronic pain patient subgroups: the utility of multidimensional clustering to identify differential treatment effects. Pain 54:51–56, 1993

Saper JR, Silberstein SD, Lake AE III, et al: Double-blind trial of fluoxetine: chronic daily headache and migraine. Headache 34:497–502, 1994

Savage SR: Addiction in the treatment of pain: significance, recognition and management. J Pain Symptom Manage 8:265–278, 1993

Sawynok J: GABAergic mechanisms of analgesia: an update. Pharmacol Biochem Behav 26:463–474, 1985

Scadding FW: Peripheral neuropathies, in Textbook of Pain, 3rd Edition. Edited by Wall PD, Melzack R. Edinburgh, Churchill Livingstone, 1994, pp 667–683

Schreiber S, Backer MM, Yanai J, et al: The antinociceptive effect of fluvoxamine. Eur Neuropsychopharmacol 6:281–284, 1996

Schug SA, Merry AF, Acland RH: Treatment principles for the use of opioids in pain of nonmalignant origin. Drugs 42:228–239, 1991

Scudds RJ, Robertson JM: Empirical evidence of the association between the presence of musculoskeletal pain and physical disability in community-dwelling senior citizens. Pain 75:229–235, 1998

Sees KL, Clark HW: Opioid use in the treatment of chronic pain: assessment of addiction. J Pain Symptom Manage 8:257–264, 1993

Shimoyama N, Shimoyama M, Davis AM, et al: Spinal gabapentin is antinociceptive in the rat formalin test. Neurosci Lett 222:65–67, 1997

Siddal PJ, Cousins MJ: Pain mechanisms and management: an update. Clin Exp Pharmacol Physiol 22:679–688, 1995

Siddal PJ, Cousins MJ: Introduction to pain mechanisms. Implications for neural blockade, in Neural Blockade in Clinical Anesthesia and Management of Pain, 3rd Edition. Edited by Cousins MJ, Bridenbaugh PO. Philadelphia, PA, Lippincott-Raven, 1998, pp 675–713

Simpson RK Jr, Edmondson EA, Constant CF, et al: Transdermal fentanyl as treatment for chronic low back pain. J Pain Symptom Manage 14:218–224, 1997

Sindrup SH, Ejlertsen B, Froland A, et al: Imipramine treatment in diabetic neuropathy: relief of subjective symptoms without changes in peripheral and autonomic nerve function. Eur J Clin Pharmacol 37:151–153, 1989

Sindrup SH, Gram LF, Brosen K, et al: The SSRI paroxetine is effective in the treatment of diabetic neuropathy symptoms. Pain 42:135–144, 1990

Sivilotti L, Woolf CJ: The contribution of GABA-A and glycine receptors to central sensitization: disinhibition and touch-evoked allodynia in the spinal cord. J Neurophysiol 72:169–179, 1994

Skevington SM: Investigating the relationship between pain and discomfort and quality of life, using the WHOQOL. Pain 76:395–406, 1998

Sluka KA: Blockade of calcium channels can prevent the onset of secondary hyperalgesia and allodynia induced by intradermal injection of capsaicin in rats. Pain 71:157–164, 1997

Smedstad LM, Vaglum P, Kvien TK, et al: The relationship between self-reported pain and sociodemographic variables, anxiety, and depressive symptoms in rheumatoid arthritis. J Rheumatol 22:514–520, 1995

Smith GR: The epidemiology and treatment of depression when it coexists with somatoform disorders, somatization, or pain. Gen Hosp Psychiatry 14:265–272, 1992

Solomon GD: The pharmacology of medications used in treating headache. Semin Pediatr Neurol 2:165–177, 1995

Starkstein SE, Preziosi TJ, Robinson RG: Sleep disorders, pain, and depression in Parkinson's disease. Eur Neurol 31:352–355, 1991

Stein C, Schafer M, Cabot PJ, et al: Opioids and inflammation, in Molecular Neurobiology of Pain, Progress in Pain Research and Management, Vol 9. Edited by Borsook D. Seattle, WA, IASP Press, 1997, pp 25–43

Stein WM, Ferrell BA: Pain in the nursing home. Clin Geriatr Med 12:601–613, 1996

Stenager EN, Stenager E, Jensen K: Attempted suicide, depression and physical diseases: a one-year follow-up study. Psychother Psychosom 61:65–73, 1994

Stewart SH, Finn PR, Pihl RO: A dose-response study of the effects of alcohol on the perceptions of pain and discomfort due to electric shock in men at high familial-genetic risk for alcoholism. Psychopharmacology 119:261–267, 1995

Sullivan M, Katon W: Somatization: the path between distress and somatic symptoms. American Pain Society Journal 2:141–149, 1993

Sullivan MJ, Reesor K, Mikail S, et al: The treatment of depression in chronic low back pain: review and recommendations. Pain 50:5–13, 1992

Sullivan M, Toshima M, Lynn P, et al: Phenobarbital versus clonazepam for sedative-hypnotic taper in chronic pain patients. A pilot study. Ann Clin Psychiatry 5:123–128, 1993

Szirmai A: Vestibular disorders in patients with migraine. Eur Arch Otorhinolaryngol Suppl 1:S55–S57, 1997

Talbot JD, Marrett S, Evans AC, et al: Multiple representations of pain in human cerebral cortex. Science 251:1355–1358, 1991

Tanelian DL, Victory RA: Sodium channel-blocking agents: their use in neuropathic pain conditions. Pain Forum 4:75–80, 1995

Taniguchi K, Miyagawa A, Mizutani A, et al: The effect of calcium channel antagonist administered by iontophoresis on the pain threshold. Acta Anaesthesiol Belg 46:69–73, 1995

Taub A: Opioid analgesics in the treatment of chronic intractable pain on non-neoplastic origin, in Narcotic Analgesics in Anesthesiology. Edited by Kitahata LM, Collins JG. Baltimore, MD, Williams & Wilkins, 1982, pp 199–208

Tokunaga A, Saika M, Senba E: 5-HT$_{2A}$ receptor subtype is involved in the thermal hyperalgesic mechanism of serotonin in the periphery. Pain 76:349–355, 1998

Turk DC, Matyas TA: Pain-related behaviors: communication of pain. American Pain Society Journal 1:109–111, 1992

Turk DC, Okifuji A: What features affect physicians' decisions to prescribe opioids for chronic noncancer pain patients? Clin J Pain 13:330–336, 1997

Turk DC, Rudy TE: The robustness of an empirically derived taxonomy of chronic pain patients. Pain 42:27–35, 1990

Turk DC, Stieg RL: Chronic pain: the necessity of interdisciplinary communication. Clin J Pain 3:163–167, 1987

Turk DC, Meichenbaum D, Genest M (eds): Pain and Behavioral Medicine: A Cognitive-Behavioral Perspective. New York, Guilford, 1983

Turk DC, Brody MC, Okifuji EA: Physicians' attitudes and practices regarding the long-term prescribing of opioids for non-cancer pain. Pain 59:201–208, 1994

Turner JA: Comparison of group progressive-relaxation training and cognitive-behavioral group therapy for chronic low back pain. J Consult Clin Psychol 50:757–765, 1982a

Turner JA: Psychological interventions for chronic pain: a critical review, II: operant conditioning, hypnosis, and cognitive-behavioral therapy. Pain 12:23–46, 1982b

Turner JA, Chapman CR: Psychological interventions for chronic pain: a critical review, I: relaxation training and biofeedback. Pain 12:1–21, 1982

Turner JA, Jensen MP: Efficacy of cognitive therapy for chronic low back pain. Pain 52:169–177, 1993

Turner JA, Romano JM: Psychological and psychosocial techniques: cognitive-behavioral therapy, in The Management of Pain. Edited by Bonica JJ. Philadelphia, PA, Lea & Febiger, 1990, pp 1711–1720

The Use of Opioids for the Treatment of Chronic Pain. Consensus statement from the American Academy of Pain Medicine and the American Paid Society. Glenview, IL, 1997

Volmink J, Lancaster T, Gray S, et al: Treatments for postherpetic neuralgia—a systematic review of randomized controlled trials. Fam Pract 13:84–91, 1996

Von Knorring L, Perris C, Eisemann M, et al: Pain as a symptom in depressive disorders, I: relationship to diagnostic subgroup and depressive symptomatology. Pain 15:19–26, 1983

Von Korff M, LeResche L, Dworkin SF: First onset of common pain symptoms: a prospective study of depression as a risk factor. Pain 55:251–258, 1993

Vrethem M, Boivie J, Arnqvist H, et al: A comparison of amitriptyline and maprotiline in the treatment of painful polyneuropathy in diabetics and nondiabetics. Clin J Pain 13:313–323, 1997

Wall PD, Melzack R (eds): Textbook of Pain, 3rd Edition. Edinburgh, Churchill Livingstone, 1994

Walling MK, O'Hara MW, Reiter RC, et al: Abuse history and chronic pain in women, II: a multivariate analysis of abuse and psychological morbidity. Obstet Gynecol 84:200–206, 1994

Watson CP, Evans RJ, Watt VR, et al: Postherpetic neuralgia: 208 causes. Pain 35:289–298, 1988

Watt JW, Wiles JR, Bowsher DR: Epidural morphine for postherpetic neuralgia. Anaesthesia 51:647–651, 1996

Webb J, Kamali F: Analgesic effects of lamotrigine and phenytoin on cold-induced pain: a crossover placebo-controlled study in healthy volunteers. Pain 357–363, 1998

Weickgenant AL, Slater MA, Patterson TL, et al: Coping activities in chronic low back pain: relationship with depression. Pain 53:95–103, 1993

Weiner D, Pieper C, McConnell E, et al: Pain measurement in elders with chronic low back pain: traditional and alternative approaches. Pain 67:461–467, 1996

Weiner D, Peterson B, Keefe F: Evaluating persistent pain in long term care residents: what role for pain maps? Pain 76:249–257, 1998

Weissman MM, Merikangas KR: The epidemiology of anxiety and panic disorders: an update. J Clin Psychiatry 47 (suppl):11–17, 1986

Weizman R, Pankova IA, Schreiber S, et al: Flunarizine analgesia is mediated by mu-opioid receptors. Physiol Behav 62:1193–1195, 1997

Wesselmann U, Reich SG: The dynias. Semin Neurol 16:63–74, 1996

Wetzel CH, Connelly JF: Use of gabapentin in pain management. Ann Pharmacother 31:1082–1083, 1997

Wiklund I, Halling K, Ryden-Bergsten T, et al: Does lowering the blood pressure improve the mood? quality-of-life results from the Hypertension Optimal Treatment (HOT) study. Blood Press 6:357–364, 1997

Williams DA, Urban B, Keefe FJ, et al: Cluster analyses of pain patients' responses to the SCL-90R. Pain 61:81–91, 1995

Williamson GM, Schulz R: Pain, activity restriction and symptoms of depression among community-residing elderly adults. J Gerontol A Biol Sci Med Sci 47:P367–P372, 1992

Willis WD, Coggeshall RE: Sensory Mechanisms of the Spinal Cord. New York, Plenum, 1991

Woodhouse A, Mather LE: The influence of age upon opioid analgesic use in the patient-controlled analgesia (PCA) environment. Anaesthesia 52:949–955, 1997

Woolf CJ, Chong MS: Pre-emptive analgesia-treating postoperative pain by preventing the establishment of central sensitization. Anesth Analg 77:362–379, 1993

Woolf CJ, Thompson SWN: The induction and maintenance of central sensitization is dependent on N-methyl-D-aspartic acid receptor activation; implications for the treatment of post-injury pain hypersensitivity states. Pain 44:293–299, 1991

Xiao WH, Bennett GJ: Synthetic omega-conopeptides applied to the site of nerve injury suppress neuropathic pains in rats. J Pharmacol Exp Ther 274:666–672, 1995

Yamamoto T, Katayama Y, Hirayama T, et al: Pharmacological classification of central post-stroke pain: comparison with the results of chronic motor cortex stimulation therapy. Pain 72:5–12, 1997

Yosselson-Superstine S, Lipman AG, Sanders SH: Adjunctive antianxiety agents in the management of chronic pain. Isr J Med Sci 21:113–117, 1985

Zehender M, Geibel A, Treese N, et al: Prediction of efficacy and tolerance of oral mexiletine by intravenous lidocaine application. Clin Pharmacol Ther 44:389–395, 1988

Zielger DK: Opiate and opioid use in patients with refractory headache. Cephalalgia 14:5–10, 1994

19

Delirium

Larry E. Tune, M.D.

Delirium is a serious and often undetected neuropsychiatric syndrome. Delirium is particularly common in elderly patients in hospitals, where as many as 32%–67% of all cases of delirium are undetected (Beresin 1988; Inouye et al. 1990). Failure to identify delirium can have serious consequences. Delirium is associated with increased morbidity and mortality. In-hospital mortality rates for elderly patients with delirium are 10%–65% (Gottlieb et al. 1991; Levkoff et al. 1986). Outcome studies of patients with delirium at 1 month and at 1 year postdischarge from hospital also show increased mortality rates (Rabins and Folstein 1982). A few studies have matched elderly patients both with and without delirium by severity of concomitant medical illnesses. Under this condition, delirium may be a risk for significantly increased morbidity and mortality independent of medical status (Flacker and Lipsitz 1998).

The financial impact of delirium is enormous. Approximately 35% of all Americans over the age of 65 were hospitalized in 1993 (accounting for 40% of all inpatient days). By using a 20% prevalence estimate for delirium in the elderly, it is estimated that 7% of all persons over the age of 65 become delirious annually. Delirium will complicate the hospital stay for over 2.2 million patients (for 17.5 million inpatient days). Based on these estimates, the cost of delirium exceeds $8 billion annually (Inouye 1998). Delirium in

the hospital is associated with increased morbidity, closer nursing surveillance, higher hospital costs per day, longer hospitalizations, and increased rates of nursing home placements (Inouye and Charpentier 1996; Thomas et al. 1986). Delirium in the nursing home is associated with significantly increased morbidity and mortality and with increased requirement for nursing time (Fries et al. 1993).

Because delirium is often treatable, early detection and aggressive medical treatment, including management of associated neuropsychiatric symptoms, should result in substantial reduction in morbidity and mortality.

Diagnostic Terminology

Detection of delirium has been hampered by the absence of reliable and valid diagnostic criteria, a dearth of rating instruments, and a wide array of terms applied to the condition. Table 19–1 lists a number of "diagnoses" that have been used synonymously with delirium. Most of these terms (with the exception of metabolic encephalopathy) have little or no explicit diagnostic criteria. When this wide array of terms is applied to patients in the same clinical setting, the magnitude of the unitary underlying problem is often unappreciated.

The later versions of the DSM (American Psychiatric

TABLE 19–1. Alternative diagnostic labels for delirium

Acute brain syndrome

Acute confusional state

Acute toxic psychosis

Metabolic encephalopathy

Subacute befuddlement

Toxic brain syndrome

Toxic encephalopathy

Association 1952) have provided more rigorous diagnostic criteria. DSM-IV criteria (Table 19–2) represent the most current criteria to date (American Psychiatric Association 1994).

Clinical Features

The essential clinical features of delirium are 1) relatively acute onset with fluctuating course, 2) disorganized thinking, 3) alteration in level of consciousness, and 4) inattention. Other symptoms are associated with delirium; for example, inappropriate behavior, disorientation, and psychosis (e.g., hallucinations, paranoid ideation) are common in cases of delirium (Gottlieb et al. 1991). However, these symptoms are not absolute requirements for the diagnosis.

Onset. The disturbance of consciousness usually evolves over hours to days and often fluctuates through the day. It is this disturbance of consciousness that distinguishes delirium from most cases of dementia and affective disturbance.

Although the onset of delirium is usually acute, it can present subacutely. Psychopathology tends to fluctuate through the day in most cases, although reliance on this clinical feature will likely lead to underdetection. It is common for a subsyndromal prodrome phase, lasting many days to (occasionally) weeks, to precede the onset of the full syndrome of delirium. During this prodrome, the most common symptoms are restlessness, sleep disturbance (insomnia and daytime sleeping), behavioral problems including anxiety and irritability, and subjective difficulty thinking (Inouye and Charpentier 1996).

Disturbance in attention and concentration. Many aspects of cognitive functioning are impaired in delirium, including orientation, memory, and information acquisition, processing, and retrieval. Specific impairments include diminished awareness of the environment, disorientation to time and place, and diminished capacity

TABLE 19–2. DSM-IV criteria for delirium

A. Disturbance of consciousness (i.e., reduced clarity of awareness of the environment) with reduced ability to focus, sustain, or shift attention.

B. A change in cognition (such as memory deficit, disorientation, language disturbance) or the development of a perceptual disturbance that is not better accounted for by a preexisting, established, or evolving dementia.

C. The disturbance develops over a short period of time (usually hours to days) and tends to fluctuate during the course of the day.

D. There is evidence from the history, physical examination, or laboratory findings that the disturbance is caused by the direct physiological consequences of a general medical condition.

to focus or sustain attention (e.g., in response to questions asked at the bedside). Part of a routine clinical examination of any patient suspected of having delirium should include questions about orientation to time and place, ability to recall several items after a few minutes, and ability to focus attention on a particular task (e.g., subtracting serial 7s or spelling "world" backwards). These types of questions are incorporated into a number of short screening instruments (Mini-Mental State Examination [Folstein et al. 1975], the Short Portable Mental Status Questionnaire [Pfeiffer 1975]).

Thinking is usually disorganized and often incoherent. The content of the patient's language may be either rich in imagery or impoverished. The ability to think in a logical, goal-directed manner is usually compromised. This disturbance will often include rambling, unpredictable switching from topic to topic, or responses that are irrelevant to questions asked of the patient.

Detection of disturbances in consciousness is often difficult, partly because the concept of "disturbance of consciousness" is inherently vague. This disturbance is nonetheless a critical feature of the syndrome. Disturbance of consciousness refers to impairments in attention and the ability to be aware of and sustain attention to the environment. The patient may sit in bed with his or her eyes open. Through the course of a routine clinical examination, it is clear that the patient's ability to mobilize and sustain attention for a reasonable period of time is seriously impaired. Her or his overall level of alertness is usually impaired (i.e., the patient is either hypervigilant or hypovigilant).

This disturbance in consciousness tends to fluctuate through the day. Patients will often "sundown" (much like that seen in patients with dementia), with their symptoms, including hallucinations and delusions, worsening at night.

The patient may have a "lucid interval," during which he or she becomes more aware of his or her situation. The explanation for these fluctuations is poorly understood. They have been attributed to fluctuations in disease state or to environmental or psychosocial factors (e.g., greater stimulation during the day, more environmental cues).

The practical result of these impairments is that the patient usually cannot 1) learn new information, 2) solve problems, or 3) engage in meaningful goal-directed behavior. It is for these reasons that even the patient who is mildly delirious is usually disabled.

Phenomenology.   Delusions and hallucinations occur in as many as 90% of patients with delirium. The most typical delusion is of persecution, but all types of delusions can be found. The delusions are often poorly articulated, are often related in some way to environmental stimuli, and tend to fluctuate through the day. At some point in the course of the syndrome, 40%–90% of patients have hallucinations, which are usually visual and less commonly auditory. The hallucinations may be dramatic and vivid, often threatening in nature. The patient, who is usually unable to appreciate that these hallucinations are unreal, often responds with fear and agitation. Hallucinations tend to fluctuate through the day, though many patients hallucinate only at night.

Clinical Subtypes

Attempts to distinguish subtypes of delirium according to etiology (e.g., infection, drug toxicity) have failed (Lipowski 1987; Wolf and Curran 1935). Generally, the two clinical subtypes of delirium are the hypervigilant and the somnolent. Hypervigilant delirium is more commonly found in drug or alcohol intoxication or withdrawal. It is also seen in delirium resulting from other causes. The typical hypervigilant patient is agitated, psychotic, and often uncooperative with medical therapy; the typical somnolent patient is lethargic or sluggish. A large number of etiologies have been associated with somnolent delirium, and it is this type of delirium that is most frequently undiagnosed.

Neurobiology of Arousal and Consciousness

The central features of delirium are alterations in arousal and attention and disorders of cognition. The normal physiology of arousal and attention is only partially under-stood, but pathway tracing techniques and chemical anatomical techniques have identified ascending systems likely to be involved in maintenance of normal arousal and attention (see Ross 1991; Saper 1986; Shute and Lewis 1974).

The classic picture of a central arousal system involves the reticular activating system diffusely distributed in the brainstem and projecting multisynaptically to the thalamic intralaminar nuclei (Chedru and Geschwind 1972; Lindsley et al. 1950; Moruzzi and Magoun 1949). Studies using modern anatomical techniques (for a review, see Saper 1986) have shown that the so-called nonspecific afferents to the superficial cortex, which are believed to be involved in maintenance of cortical arousal, do not arise exclusively from the thalamus. Critical sources of nonspecific cortical afferents may be extrathalamic regions such as basal forebrain, hypothalamus, and caudal brainstem. These extrathalamic cortical afferent systems contain several neurotransmitters (discussed below) that may relate to the pathophysiology of delirium.

Anatomical studies (see Saper 1986) suggest a differing organization of cortical nonspecific afferents within the thalamus. The diffuse innervation of superficial cortex may arise less from the intralaminar nuclei and more from the ventromedial thalamic nucleus, as well as the ventro-anterolateral nucleus, the lateral dorsal nucleus, and the posterior and lateral posterior nuclei (Herkenham 1980). Physiological studies of the role of the thalamus in sleep and arousal have yielded contradictory results. Ranson (1939) found little effect of large lesions of the thalamus on sleep and arousal from sleep in the monkey. However, a hereditary condition involving the selective degeneration of certain thalamic nuclei is associated with abnormalities of sleep and consciousness (Lugaresi et al. 1986), supporting other clinical observations. Little is known of the neurotransmitters involved in these thalamic projections.

Basal Forebrain Cholinergic Projections

Cholinergic neurons in the basal forebrain provide widespread topographically organized innervation of layers 1, 3, 5, and 6 of the cerebral cortex (Saper 1984, 1986). Application of acetylcholine within the cortex causes predominantly excitatory responses. These cholinergic projections may be involved in the generation of cortical and hippocampal electroencephalogram (EEG) rhythms. Basal forebrain cholinergic neurons degenerate in Alzheimer's disease (see Chapter 24 in this volume). Drugs with anticholinergic properties are important contributors to the problem of delirium in some hospitalized patients. It may be that disruption of the function of the basal forebrain cholinergic cortical afferents explains some of the features of anticholinergic delirium. This hypothesis would be consistent with the fact that patients with Alzheimer's disease, in whom these neurons are already compromised, are unusually sensitive to anticholinergics. Under most circumstances, patients with Alzheimer's disease do not have changes in consciousness, despite their loss of basal forebrain cholinergic neurons, suggesting that abnormalities of other cholinergic neurons (e.g., cholinergic neurons in the brainstem) may be more important in delirium.

Hypothalamic-Cortical Projections

Classic physiological experiments suggested an important role for the hypothalamus in the regulation of sleep and arousal (Nauta 1946). More recent experiments, such as those using injections of excitatory amino acid toxins (Jouvet 1988), have suggested a particular role for the posterolateral hypothalamus in regulation of sleep and waking. Although traditional views of the reticular formation assume that the hypothalamus projects through the thalamus to reach the cortex, modern pathway tracing techniques have demonstrated direct hypothalamic projections to the cerebral cortex (Kievet and Kuypers 1975; Saper 1985). The areas that project directly to the cortex are the fields of Forel, the posterior lateral hypothalamic area, and the tuberal lateral and tuberal mammary hypothalamic areas. The hypothalamus contains more neurons innervating the cerebral cortex than does the basal forebrain. Most suggestive for the pathophysiology of delirium are neurons in this region of hypothalamus containing γ-aminobutyric acid (GABA) and histamine.

Double-label retrograde transport immunocytochemical techniques have identified GABA-synthesizing neurons residing in the posterior hypothalamus and projecting to the cerebral cortex (Vincent et al. 1983). These systems may be involved in the pathophysiology of hepatic encephalopathy. Alterations of GABA or benzodiazepine-like systems in animal models with hepatic encephalopathy are suggested by reports of altered benzodiazepine receptor binding (Baraldi et al. 1984; Basile et al. 1991). Benzodiazepine antagonists can ameliorate hepatic encephalopathy in animal models and in patients (Bansky et al. 1985; Baraldi et al. 1984; Bassett et al. 1987). Clinical studies in humans have suggested that benzodiazepine antagonists may be helpful in treating hepatic encephalopathy.

Histamine-synthesizing hypothalamic neurons 1) are present in the posterior hypothalamus, 2) are concentrated in the magnocellular nuclei and the tuberal regions (Wada et al. 1991), and 3) project diffusely to the cerebral cortex. Jouvet (1988) suggested that histaminergic neurons in the

hypothalamus have a function in arousal. These neurons may be involved in the delirium caused by anticholinergic drugs because many drugs with anticholinergic properties are also antihistaminergics.

Brainstem Neuronal Groups

In addition to projections from the hypothalamus and basal forebrain, well-known monoaminergic nuclei in the pons and midbrain project diffusely to the cerebral cortex. These nuclei include midbrain dopaminergic groups in the midbrain ventral tegmentum, cholinergic neurons in the rostral pons, noradrenergic neurons in the locus ceruleus, and serotonergic neurons in the raphe complex. Dopaminergic systems appear to have no clearly identified role in the pathophysiology of delirium. Neurons in the locus ceruleus have been implicated in the control of attention and arousal (Foote et al. 1980). Serotonergic neurons have been linked to the visual hallucinations after ingestion of lysergic acid diethylamide (LSD)–like hallucinogenic drugs (Glennon et al. 1984). Hallucinogens induce an oneiroid state resembling delirium. Unlike the characteristic auditory hallucinations of schizophrenia or bipolar disorder, the hallucinations induced by hallucinogens and seen in delirium tend to be visual.

Pathophysiology of Delirium

Delirium has been investigated with animal models (Gibson et al. 1991; Posner and Plum 1960), human EEG studies (Romano and Engel 1944), and functional brain imaging studies (Gjedde et al. 1978). Several animal models of encephalopathy have identified a disturbance of cortical glucose metabolism. These models support an early pathophysiological hypothesis that cerebral metabolic insufficiency is the underlying mechanism or final common pathway in delirium. This mechanism is generally thought of as a threshold-related phenomenon: the cumulative effects of multiple cerebral insults lead to "depletion of cortical reserves" and then to an insufficiency in global metabolism. A few brain imaging studies of cerebral blood flow (in patients with delirium tremens and with traumatic brain injury) have also shown impairments in cerebral glucose metabolism.

EEG data support involvement of white matter generally and of thalamocortical projections particularly. The commonest EEG abnormality in somnolent delirium is diffuse, nonparoxysmal delta-wave slowing. This finding has been taken to suggest that the cortex is deafferentiated. In some cases of delirium, the posterior dominant rhythm is slowed, possibly implicating thalamocortical projections. Patients with hypervigilant delirium associated with alcohol withdrawal often have EEGs with low-voltage fast activity. This finding represents a global disturbance that may reflect a hyperactivity of catecholaminergic neurotransmission.

Of the possible neurotransmitters, disturbances in cholinergic transmission are the most consistently implicated in preclinical and clinical investigations. One animal model found dose-dependent effects of the cholinergic antagonist atropine (Trzepacz et al. 1992). The behavioral results resemble the EEG and cognitive-behavior changes found in patients with delirium. In autoradiographic studies of the effects of atropine, dose-dependent reductions in glucose metabolism were found in cortex (Gibson et al. 1991). In drug-induced delirium in the elderly, where anticholinergic medications are additive with age-related decreases in cholinergic neurotransmission, the relationship is stronger (see Chapter 4 in this volume). Anticholinergic medications have been shown to impair memory, especially in the elderly (Miller et al. 1988).

Several investigations have found correlations between elevated anticholinergic levels, as measured by serum radioreceptor assay, and the presence of delirium in elderly patients. Mach et al. (1995) found that delirious inpatients have 1) higher serum anticholinergic levels, 2) greater impairments in activities of daily living that correlated with anticholinergic levels, and 3) lower serum anticholinergic levels as the delirium resolved. In a separate study, Flacker et al. (1998) found that elevated serum anticholinergic levels were independently associated with delirium. Self-care capacity in the nursing home is negatively associated with elevated serum anticholinergic levels (Rover et al. 1988). Tollefson et al. (1991) conducted a blinded intervention study of nursing home patients who received more than one anticholinergic medication for more than 2 weeks. Patients were randomly assigned to an intervention (where an attempt was made to reduce anticholinergics by 25%) or nonintervention group. At the conclusion of the study, baseline and end-of-study anticholinergic levels were compared. Patients in the intervention group showed significant improvements in measures of delirium and cognition.

Epidemiology of Delirium

Epidemiological research has been difficult because of differences in study populations and the absence of clear, operationalized criteria for delirium. DSM-IV has provided suitable criteria so that cross-study comparisons are more likely to yield meaningful results. Other methodological issues include 1) absence of reliable and valid research instruments, 2) differences in case-finding methods, and 3) comorbidity, especially with dementing illnesses. For these reasons, it is not surprising that prevalence estimates for medical inpatient units vary from 10% to 30% and incidence estimates range from 4% to 53%. Levkoff et al. (1992) reviewed five previously published studies and applied DSM-III diagnostic criteria. Using these criteria, instead of widely fluctuating incidence and prevalence estimates, the prevalence of delirium was 11%–16%, with an incidence of 4%–10% for five separate groups of medical inpatients. The Commonwealth-Harvard Study (Levkoff et al. 1992) assessed all patients over the age of 65 who were admitted over a 1-year period to the Beth Israel Hospital. Patients came either from a long-term rehabilitation center for the elderly or from a local community catchment area (East Boston). Of the 211 community-based elderly patients who were admitted, 24% satisfied criteria for delirium. Of the 114 patients admitted from the long-term care facility, 65% were delirious on admission. Data from the Epidemiological Catchment Area survey of East Baltimore found that 0.4%–1.1% of the community-based population over the age of 55 were delirious (Folstein et al. 1991).

Etiology and Risk Factors

The commonest identifiable "etiologies" include 1) intoxication syndromes, including drug toxicity resulting from polypharmacy, benzodiazepines, anticholinergics, or alcohol; 2) cerebrovascular diseases; 3) systemic metabolic disorders with known effects on brain function, for example, tumors, heart failure, and infections, especially urinary tract infections and pneumonia; and 4) withdrawal from addicting substances. Table 19–3 provides an expanded list of the commonest causes of delirium. The major risk factors for delirium include age (Schor et al. 1992; Michocki and Lamy 1988), prior brain damage (Berggren et al. 1987; Erkinjuntii et al. 1986; Francis et al. 1990; Schor et al. 1992), drug intoxication (Berggren et al. 1987; Michocki and Lamy 1988), and dementia (Erkinjuntii et al. 1986).

Among hospitalized elderly, several immediate risk factors have been identified and included into predictive models for delirium. Francis et al. (1990) found that the risk of delirium in the elderly was 60% when three or more of the following risk factors were present: hypothermia, severity of illness, dementia, fever, azotemia, and psychoactive drug use. In a separate investigation, the risk of delirium among elderly patients admitted to a medical or surgical ward was greatest among those patients who 1) had

TABLE 19–3. Common causes of delirium in the elderly

Metabolic or endocrine
    Electrolyte abnormality (especially Na^+, K^+, Ca^{++}, and Mg^{++})
    Hyperglycemia or hypoglycemia
    Hypoxia or hypercarbia
    Liver or kidney failure
    Thyroid disorder
    Fever

Infection
    Sepsis
    Pneumonia
    Urinary tract infection or upper respiratory infection in elderly patients

Drug toxicity
    Anticholinergics
    Anticholinergic psychoactive medications (e.g., neuroleptics and tricyclic antidepressants)
    Lithium
    Electroconvulsive therapy
    Steroids

Drug or alcohol withdrawal

Central nervous system lesion
    Postictal states
    Raised intracranial pressure
    Head trauma
    Encephalitis or meningitis
    Vasculitis

Multifactorial

prior cognitive impairment, 2) were older than 80 years, 3) had a fracture on admission, 4) had symptomatic infection, 5) were male, and 6) received either antipsychotic or narcotic analgesic medication (Schor et al. 1992).

Inouye et al. (1996, 1998) incorporated five independent risk factors into a predictive model for delirium. These risk factors were 1) use of physical restraints, 2) malnutrition, 3) more than three medications added while in the hospital, 4) use of bladder catheter, and 5) any iatrogenic event. In one cohort of 196 inpatients, the delirium rate was 3% in patients who had none of these risks in the 24-hour period before admission, 20% in patients with one to two risk factors, and 59% in patients with three or more risk factors. For this latter category, the delirium rate per 100 person-days was 21.3%. Table 19–4 provides a list of risk factors for delirium.

Age and Delirium

One of the most consistently identified risk factors for delirium is age. Potential explanations for this relation include structural brain disease, reduced capacity for homeostasis, impairments in vision and hearing, high prevalence of chronic diseases, reduced resistance to acute disease, age-related changes in pharmacokinetics, and pharmacodynamics of drug disposition. Common psychosocial precipitants of delirium in the elderly include sleep loss, sensory deprivation, sensory overload, and severe psychosocial stress (e.g., death of spouse, relocation).

Dementia and Delirium

One important risk factor for delirium is preexisting cognitive impairment or dementia (Erkinjuntii et al. 1986; Inouye 1998). In a study of patients with delirium admitted to a general medical service, dementia was present in 9.1% of all patients over the age of 55 and in 31% of all patients over the age of 85. Of the patients with dementia, 41% were delirious on admission. Of the delirious patients, 25% were found, on subsequent examination, to have some evidence of prior cognitive impairment. Patients with delirium have more evidence of preexisting cerebrovascular disease (e.g., lacunar infarcts, periventricular white matter disease) on brain imaging than do control subjects.

The relationship between delirium and dementia is less clear, when considering the transition from delirium to dementia. Recovery from delirium in elderly patients with dementia is much less common than that in patients with delirium without dementia. Levkoff et al. (1996) found that only 17.7% of patients with both dementia and delirium had complete resolution of symptoms of delirium at 6-month follow-up.

Drug Toxicity: Focus on Anticholinergic Effects

Drugs are a common cause of delirium. Possible reasons for this relation include 1) age-related changes in drug metabolism and disposition (see Chapters 33 and 34 in this volume), 2) polypharmacy, 3) lack of knowledge regarding drug-drug interactions of multiple medications, 4) medication errors arising from complex regimens that patients who are cognitively impaired are unable to follow, and 5) age-related decreases in neurotransmitter production and turnover. Drug toxicity is one of the commonest causes of delirium in the hospitalized elderly and one of the commonest "treatable dementias" (Larsen et al. 1985; Report of Royal College of Physicians 1984).

The cumulative effect of anticholinergic medications is one likely mechanism of drug-induced delirium in the elderly. Cholinergic neurotransmission declines with age. Many neurodegenerative diseases of brain, especially de-

TABLE 19–4. Risk factors for delirium

Study	Patient sample	Age range	Source	Percent delirious	Risk factors
Schor et al. 1992	291 patients not delirious on first evaluation	> 65	Medical and surgical wards	Incidence in hospital = 31.3%	Prior cognitive impairment Age > 80 Fracture on admission Symptomatic infection Male gender Neuroleptic or narcotic use
Michocki and Lamy 1988	46 orthopedic patients	Mean age = 67.5	Orthopedic inpatient unit	26%	Primary aging factors: slower thought and metabolic factors Secondary aging factors: hypoxia, ischemia, sepsis, uremia, fluid electrolyte imbalance, and anemia Tertiary aging factors: psychosocial stress Drug factors: alcohol, antidepressants, sedatives, and anticholinergics
Rogers et al. 1989	46 orthopedic patients	Mean age = 67.5	Orthopedic inpatient unit	26%	Drugs: propranolol, flurazepam, scopolamine
Berggren et al. 1987	57 patients with femoral neck fracture	> 64 years	Orthopedic inpatients	44%	History of mental confusion History of anticholinergic drug use
Erkinjuntii et al. 1986	2,000 consecutive patients	≥ 55 years	Medical inpatients	41.4% of patients with dementia 12.4% of patients without dementia	Early postoperative hypoxemia and dementia
Francis et al. 1990	229 elderly patients	≥ 70 years	Medical inpatients	22% overall	Predictors include abnormal sodium level, severe illness, chronic cognitive impairment; fever or hypothermia; psychoactive drug use; azotemia

mentia (most notably Alzheimer's disease), have a central cholinergic lesion that further diminishes cholinergic neurotransmission (see Chapter 24 in this volume). These cholinergic impairments are then compounded by medications. More than 600 medications have known anticholinergic effects, and these medications are disproportionately administered to elderly patients (Blazer et al. 1983; Report of Royal College of Physicians 1984; Tollefson 1991). Many commonly prescribed medications have modest anticholinergic effects. In one study, 11.60% of patients with suspected dementia had drug-related cognitive impairments. The risk of drug-induced cognitive toxicity was greatly increased in those patients receiving four to five prescription medications. This study did not include nonprescription medications (Lamy 1986).

Many commonly prescribed medications not typically associated with anticholinergic effects have modest antimuscarinic effects when measured by radioreceptor assay. Table 19–5 shows that 14 of the 25 medications most frequently prescribed for the elderly (Tune et al. 1992) have modest anticholinergic effects. Although many of these medications cannot be avoided, and by themselves usually do not pose a significant challenge to the cholinergic system, physicians must be aware of the potential cumulative effects of these medications. This problem may well be compounded when known potent anticholinergic psychotropic medications (e.g., amitriptyline, clomipramine, imipramine, and doxepin) are added.

TABLE 19–5. Anticholinergic drug levels in 25 medications ranked by the frequency of their prescription for elderly patients

Medication[a]	Anticholinergic drug level (ng/mL of atropine equivalents)
Furosemide	0.22
Digoxin	0.25
Dyazide (hydro-chlorothiazide and triamterene)	0.08
Lanoxin[b]	0.25
Hydrochlorothiazide	0.00
Propranolol	0.00
Salicylic acid	0.00
Dipyridamole	0.11
Theophylline, anhydrous	0.44
Nitroglycerine	0.00
Insulin	0.00
Warfarin	0.12
Prednisolone	0.55
Methyldopa	0.00
Nifedipine	0.22
Isosorbide dinitrate	0.15
Ibuprofen	0.00
Codeine	0.11
Cimetidine	0.86
Diltiazem hydrochloride	0.00
Captopril	0.02
Atenolol	0.00
Metoprolol	0.00
Timolol	0.00
Ranitidine	0.22

[a]Drug concentration = 10^{-8} M.
[b]A digoxin compound.

Detection

The Mini-Mental State Examination (MMSE) (Figure 19–1) is useful in detecting the presence and global severity of cognitive impairments. Although not specifically created to distinguish delirium from dementia, the full MMSE contains a clinical assessment of the patient's level of consciousness. Although this measure may seem a bit simplistic, it serves to identify alterations in level of consciousness. The MMSE is sensitive (87%) and specific (82%) com-

pared with a clinical diagnosis of delirium (Anthony et al. 1982). Thus, the MMSE can be of considerable value in primary care in both the inpatient and outpatient setting. The major caveats are the false-positive ratio for detection of significant cognitive impairment—39%—largely a result of patient-related variables (e.g., low educational status, impaired vision, impaired hearing).

MMSE items most likely to be missed by the patient with delirium are calculation, orientation (especially to time), and three-item recall at 5 minutes. Naming and registration are relatively preserved, even in patients with delirium who are severely impaired. This preservation of naming and registration may partially explain why delirium is often undetected in a routine clinician examination.

Numerous other screening methods are available for detecting delirium. One of the simplest instruments is the Confusion Assessment Method (CAM) (Inouye et al. 1990) (Table 19–6). This scale incorporates the nine operationalized criteria from DSM-III-R into a reliable rating instrument that can be quickly administered by incorporating the elements of the CAM into a routine clinical examination. The CAM has a sensitivity of 94%–100%, a specificity of 90%–95%, and a positive predictive accuracy of 91%–94% for the clinical diagnosis of delirium.

Management

Few systematic studies of the management of delirium have been undertaken. The following recommendations are based largely on collective clinical experience. The first step is the identification of underlying medical condition(s). At times, the etiology is unclear either because it cannot be identified or, more commonly, because multiple etiologies have been identified. It is important to provide an appropriate, supportive environment (Table 19–7).

Because the patient with delirium has a primary disturbance in attention and concentration, professional and family visits should usually be short but frequent. Reassurance and reorientation are often helpful and will likely be required on a frequent basis throughout the day. One goal is to not tax the patient needlessly. Care should be taken to avoid approaches that distress the patient. For example, some patients are comforted by the explanation that they are encountering side effects from their medications or are confused because of their infection. Others are distressed by this news. It is important to observe the patient's response to this type of conversation. If the patient is visibly distressed, then further discussion should be avoided.

Moving the patient out of stressful environments (e.g., the intensive care unit) as soon as medically safe may prove

Patient _____

Examiner _____

Date _____

Maximum score	Score	
		Orientation
5	( )	What is the (year) (date) (day) (month) (season)?
5	( )	Where are we (state) (county) (town) (hospital) (floor)?
		Registration
3	( )	Name 3 objects: 1 second to say each. Then ask the patient all 3 after you have said them. Give 1 point for each correct answer. Then repeat them until he or she learns all 3. Count trial and record.
		Trials
		Attention and calculation
5	( )	Serial 7s: 1 point for each correct. Stop after 5 answers. Alternately spell "world" backwards.
		Recall
5	( )	Ask for 3 objects repeated above. Give 1 point for each correct answer.
		Language
2	( )	Name a pencil and watch (2 points)
1	( )	Repeat the following: "no ifs, ands, or buts" (1 point)
3	( )	Follow a 3-stage command: "Take a paper in your right hand, fold it in half, and put it on the floor."
1	( )	Read and obey the following: "Close your eyes." (1 point)
1	( )	Write a sentence. Must contain subject and verb and be sensible. (1 point)
		Visual-motor integrity
1	( )	Copy design (2 intersecting pentagons. All 10 angles must be present and 2 must intersect.) (1 point)
		Total score _____
30	( )	Assess level of consciousness along a continuum.
		Alert _____ Drowsy _____ Stupor _____ Coma _____

FIGURE 19–1. Mini-Mental State Exam.
Source. Reprinted with permission from Folstein MF, Folstein SE, McHugh PR: "Mini-Mental State: a practical method for grading the cognitive state of patients for the clinician." *J Psychiatr Res* 12:189–198, 1975.

helpful. Having a limited number of family or friends (who have been properly appraised of the circumstances) at hand to reassure and reorient the patient may prove beneficial. Psychiatric consultation is often helpful to provide behavioral management recommendations and to serve as a liaison to staff and family. Many patients with delirium do better in psychiatric environments rather than in a typical medical unit. The general medical management of the patient with delirium includes prevention and/or management of fluid and electrolyte disturbances, aspiration, decubitus ulcers, nutritional status, and other less common medical complications of delirium.

Agitation is a serious problem in patients with delirium (see Chapter 22 in this volume). These patients are at greater risk of falls and of injury to both themselves and their caregivers (Berggren et al. 1987). Because agitation often occurs in response to psychotic symptoms (hallucinations, delusions), short-term pharmacotherapy is often necessary. Although few controlled trials of medications for management of delirium have been performed, haloperidol is the most widely used and accepted medication. Typical well-tolerated doses of haloperidol are 0.5–2.0 mg intramuscularly or intravenously, repeated every 30 minutes to 1 hour as needed to suppress the agitated

TABLE 19–6. Confusion Assessment Method

(1) Acute onset and fluctuating course

Is there evidence of an acute change in mental status from the patient's baseline?

AND

Did this behavior fluctuate during the past day, that is, tend to come and go or increase and decrease in severity?

(2) Inattention

Does the patient have difficulty focusing attention, for example being easily distractible, or having difficulty keeping track of what was being said?

(3) Disorganized thinking

Is the patient's speech disorganized or incoherent, such as rambling or irrelevant conversation, unclear or illogical flow of ideas, or unpredictable switching from subject to subject?

(4) Altered level of consciousness

Overall, how would you rate this patient's level of consciousness?

    Alert (normal)

    Vigilant (hyperalert)

    Lethargic (drowsy, easily aroused)

    Stuporous (difficult to arouse)

    Comatose (unarousable)

The diagnosis of delirium requires the presence/abnormal rating for criteria: (1), (2), and either (3) or (4).

Source.   Reprinted with permission from Inouye SK, van Dyck CH, Alessi C, et al.: "Clarifying Confusion: The Confusion Assessment Method." *Ann Intern Med* 113:941–948, 1990.

behavior. Side effects include drug-induced parkinsonian symptoms. Of concern is akathisia and motor restlessness, which can easily be confused with agitation. A few recent investigations have used atypical antipsychotic medications, such as risperidone, successfully (Sipahimalani et al. 1997). One advantage to these antipsychotics is their favorable side-effect profile. An alternative to antipsychotics is the addition of a short- or intermediate- acting benzodiazepine. Lorazepam 0.5–1.0 mg intravenously, repeated hourly as necessary, has been shown to be effective in the management of agitated delirium.

Summary

Delirium is a common, often unrecognized clinical syndrome characterized by potentially reversible disturbances in attention and other aspects of cognition. The clinical examination is the mainstay of diagnosis, though several screening instruments (e.g., MMSE, CAM) have made the

TABLE 19–7. Management of delirium

A. Pharmacological interventions and physical restraints

  1. Avoid physical restraints if possible. Evaluate their need daily. Consider alternatives, including the use of sitters and family members to calm the patient.

  2. Use lowest possible doses of neuroleptics and/or benzodiazepines.

  3. Reassess need for these interventions *at least* daily. The goal is to discontinue neuroleptics as soon as possible.

  4. When patients are administered neuroleptics, carefully monitor and document the patient's neurological status for presence of extrapyramidal side effects.

B. Psychosocial aspects (providing a predictable, orienting environment)

  1. The room should be adequately lit, including the use of night lights in the evening, to decrease illusions.

  2. Avoid excessive stimulation. Keep exposure to chaotic environments (e.g., intensive care units) to a minimum because many delirious patients are hyperresponsive to stimuli.

  3. The room should have a large calendar and clock.

  4. The staff and family should make an effort to remind the patient of the day and date *frequently*.

  5. If possible, familiar items from home should be brought in.

  6. If clinical state allows, provide eyeglasses and hearing aids to patients who had them before the illness.

  7. Encourage *frequent* interactions with staff and family.

  8. Consider telling the patient he or she is confused and disoriented.

process easier. The neurobiology of delirium may include specific alterations in ascending pathways as well as diffuse disturbances in glucose metabolism. The most consistent risk factors for delirium include age, prior cognitive impairment, increasing number of comorbid medical conditions, and drug toxicity.

References

American Psychiatric Association: Diagnostic and Statistical Manual: Mental Disorders. Washington, DC, American Psychiatric Association, 1952

American Psychiatric Association: Diagnostic and Statistical Manual of Mental Disorders, 4th Edition. Washington, DC, American Psychiatric Association, 1994

Anthony JC, Niaz LU, von Korff M, et al: Limits of the Mini-Mental State as a screening for dementia and delirium among hospital patients. Psychol Med 12:397–408, 1982

Bansky G, Meier PJ, Zeigler WH, et al: Reversal of hepatic coma by benzodiazepine antagonist (RO15-1788). Lancet 1:1324–1325, 1985

Baraldi M, Zeneroli M, Ventura E, et al: Supersensitivity of benzodiazepine receptors in hepatic encephalopathy due to fulminant hepatic failure in the rat: reversal by a benzodiazepine antagonist. Clin Sci (Colch) 67:167–175, 1984

Basile AS, Hughes RD, Harrison PM, et al: Elevated brain concentrations of 1,4-benzodiazepines in fulminant hepatic failure. N Engl J Med 325:473–478, 1991

Bassett ML, Mullen KD, Skolnick P, et al: Amelioration of hepatic encephalopathy by pharmacologic antagonism of the GABA-benzodiazepine receptor complex in a rabbit model of fulminant hepatic failure. Gastroenterology 93:1069–1077, 1987

Beresin EV: Delirium in the elderly. J Geriatr Psychiatry Neurol 1:127–143, 1988

Berggren D, Gustafson Y, Erikssen B, et al: Postoperative confusion after anesthesia in elderly patients with femoral neck fractures. Anesth Analg 66:497–504, 1987

Blazer DG II, Federspiel CF, Ray WA, et al: The risk of anticholinergic toxicity in the elderly: a study of prescribing practices in two populations. J Gerontol A Biol Sci Med Sci 38:31–35, 1983

Chedru F, Geschwind N: Disorders of higher cortical functions in acute confusional states. Cortex 8:395–411, 1972

Erkinjuntii T, Wikstrom J, Palo J, et al: Dementia among medical inpatients. Arch Intern Med 146:1923–1926, 1986

Flacker J, Lipsitz LA: Serum anticholinergic activity changes with acute illness in elderly medical patients. Am J Geriatr Psychiatry 6:47–54, 1998

Flacker JK, Cummings V, Mach JR, et al: The association of serum anticholinergic activity with delirium in elderly medical patients. Am J Geriatr Psychiatry 6:31–41, 1998

Folstein MF, Folstein SE, McHugh PR: Mini-Mental State: a practical method for grading the cognitive state of patients for the clinician. J Psychiatr Res 12:189–198, 1975

Folstein M, Bassett SS, Romanoski A, et al: The epidemiology of delirium in the community: the eastern Baltimore mental health survey. Int Psychogeriatr 3:169–176, 1991

Foote SL, Anton-Jones G, Bloom FE: Impulse activity of locus ceruleus neurons in awake rats and monkeys as a function of sensory stimulation and arousal. Proc Natl Acad Sci U S A 77:3033–3037, 1980

Francis J, Martin D, Kapoor WN: A prospective study of delirium in hospitalized elderly. JAMA 263:1097–1101, 1990

Fries BE, Mehr DR, Schneider D, et al: Mental dysfunction and resource utilization in the nursing home. Medical Care 31:898–920, 1993

Gibson G, Blass JP, Huang H-M, et al: The cellular basis of delirium and its relevance to age related disorders including Alzheimer's disease. Int Psychogeriatr 3:373–395, 1991

Gjedde A, Lockwood AH, Duffy TE, et al: Cerebral blood flow and metabolism in chronically hyperammonemic rats: effect of an acute ammonia challenge. Ann Neurol 3:325–330, 1978

Glennon RA, Titeler M, McKenney JD: Evidence for 5-HT2 involvement in the mechanism of action of hallucinogenic agents. Life Sci 35:2502–2511, 1984

Gottlieb GL, Johnson J, Wanich C, et al: Delirium in the medically ill elderly: operationalizing the DSM-III criteria. Int Psychogeriatr 3:181–196, 1991

Herkenham M: Laminar organization of thalamic projections to the rat neocortex. Science 207:532–534, 1980

Inouye SK, Charpentier PA: Precipitating factors for delirium in hospitalized elderly persons: predictive model and interrelationship with baseline vulnerability. JAMA 275:852–857, 1996

Inouye SK, van Dyck CH, Alessi C, et al: Clarifying confusion: the Confusion Assessment Method. Ann Intern Med 113:941–948, 1990

Jouvet M: The regulation of paradoxical sleep by the hypothalamo-hypophysis. Arch Ital Biol 126:259–274, 1988

Kievet J, Kuypers MGJM: Subcortical afferents to the frontal lobe in the rhesus monkey studied by means of retrograde horseradish peroxidase transport. Brain Res 85:261–266, 1975

Lamy P: The elderly and drug interactions. J Am Geriatric Soc 34:586–592, 1986

Larsen EB, Reifler BV, Sumi S, et al: Diagnostic evaluation of 200 elderly outpatients with suspected dementia. J Gerontol 40:536–543, 1985

Levkoff SE, Besdine RW, Wetle T: Acute confusional states (delirium) in the hospitalized elderly. Annual Review of Gerontology and Geriatrics 6:1–26, 1986

Levkoff SE, Evans D, Liptzin B, et al: Delirium. The occurrence and persistence of symptoms among elderly hospitalized patients. Arch Intern Med 152:334–340, 1992

Lindsley DB, Schreiner LH, Knowles WB, et al: Behavioral and EEG changes following chronic brain stem lesions in the cat. Electroencephalogr Clin Neurophysiol 2:483–498, 1950

Lipowski ZJ: Delirium: Acute Brain Failure in Man, 2nd Edition. Springfield, IL, Charles C Thomas, 1987

Lugaresi E, Medori R, Montagna P, et al: Fatal familial insomnia and dysautonomia with selective degeneration of thalamic nuclei. N Engl J Med 315:997–1003, 1986

Mach JR, Dysken MW, Kuskowski K, et al: Serum anticholinergic activity in hospitalized older persons with delirium: a preliminary study. J Am Geriatric Soc 43:491–445, 1995

Michocki RJ, Lamy PP: A "risk" approach to adverse drug reactions. J Am Geriatr Soc 36:79–81, 1988

Moruzzi G, Magoun HW: Brain stem reticular formation and activation of the EEG. Electroencephalogr Clin Neurophysiol 1:455–473, 1949

Mullen KD, Szauter KK, Kaminsky-Russ K: "Endogenous" benzodiazepine activity in body fluids of patients with hepatic encephalopathy. Lancet 336(8707):81–83, 1990

Nauta WJH: Hypothalamic regulation of sleep in rats: an experimental study. J Neurophysiol 9:285–316, 1946

Pfeiffer E: A short portable mental status questionnaire for the assessment of organic brain deficit in elderly patients. J Am Geriatric 23:433–441, 1975

Posner JB, Plum F: The toxic effects of carbon dioxide and acetazolamide in hepatic encephalopathy. J Clin Invest 39:1246–1258, 1960

Rabins PV, Folstein MF: Delirium and dementia: diagnostic criteria and fatality rates. Br J Psychiatry 140:149–153, 1982

Ranson SW: Somnolence caused by hypothalamic lesions in the monkey. Archives of Neurology and Psychiatry 41:1–23, 1939

Report of Royal College of Physicians: Medication for the elderly. J R Coll Physicians Lond 18:7–17, 1984

Rogers MP, Liang MH, Daltry LH, et al: Delirium after elective orthopedic surgery: risk factors and natural history. Int J Psychiatry Med 19:109–121, 1989

Romano J, Engel GL: Delirium, I: electroencephalographic data. Archives of Neurology and Psychiatry 51:356–377, 1944

Ross CA: CNS arousal systems: possible role in delirium. Int Psychogeriatr 3:353–371, 1991

Rovner B, David A, Blaustein MJ, et al: Self care capacity and anticholinergic drug levels in nursing home patients. Am J Psychiatry 145:378–390, 1988

Saper CB: Organization of cerebral cortical afferent systems in the rat: I; magnocellular basal nucleus. J Comp Neurology 222:313–342, 1984

Saper CB: Organization of cerebral cortical afferent systems in the rat, II: hypothalamocortical projections. J Comp Neurol 237:21–46, 1985

Saper CB: Diffuse cortical projection systems: anatomical organization and role in clinical function, in Handbook of Physiology, Vol 5: The Nervous System. New York, Oxford University Press, 1986, pp 169–210

Schor JD, Levkoff SE, Lipsitz LA, et al: Risk factors for delirium in hospitalized elderly. JAMA 267:827–831, 1992

Shute CCD, Lewis PR: The ascending cholinergic reticular system: neocortical, olfactory, and subcortical projections. Brain Res 90:497–520, 1974

Sipahimalani A, Sime RM, Masand PS: Treatment of delirium with risperadone. International Journal of Geriatric Psychopharmacology 1:24–26, 1997

Thomas R, Cameron DJ, Fahs MC: A prospective study of delirium and prolonged hospital stay. Arch Gen Psychiatry 45:937–940, 1986

Tollefson GD, Montague-Clouse J, Lancaster SP: The relationship of serum anticholinergic activity to mental status performance in an elderly nursing home population. J Neuropsychiatry Clin Neurosci 3:314–319, 1991

Trzepacz PT, Leavitt M, Ciongoli K: An animal model for delirium. Psychosomatics 33:404–415, 1992

Tune L, Bylsma F: Benzodiazepine-induced and anticholinergic induced delirium in the elderly. Int Psychogeriatr 3:397–408, 1991

Tune L, Carr S, Hoag E, et al: Anticholinergic effects of drugs commonly prescribed for the elderly: potential means of assessing risk of delirium. Am J Psychiatry 149:1393–1394, 1992

Tune L, Carr S, Cooper TC, et al: Association of anticholinergic activity of prescribed medications with postoperative delirium. J Neuropsychiatry Clin Neurosci 5:208–210, 1993

Vincent SR, Hokfelt T, Shirboll LR, et al: Hypothalamic gamma aminobutyric acid neurons project to the neocortex. Science 220:1309–1311, 1983

Wada H, Inagaki N, Yamatodani A, et al: Is the histaminergic neuron system a regulatory center for whole-brain activity? Trends Neurosci 14:415–418, 1991

Wolff HG, Curran D: Nature of delirium and allied states: the dysergastic reaction. Archives of Neurology and Psychiatry 33:1175–1215, 1935

20

Contemporary Personality Psychology

Paul T. Costa, Jr., Ph.D.

Robert R. McCrae, Ph.D.

Personality may seem to be too vague and metaphysical a topic to belong in a modern textbook of neuropsychiatry, but in fact it connects squarely with that discipline on two levels. First, it has become increasingly clear in the past decade that personality traits have a biological basis. Although convincing theories of the specific neurological or neurohormonal mechanisms involved are still lacking, strong collateral evidence indicates that such mechanisms must exist. Second, personality is directly relevant to the thoughts, feelings, and behaviors of patients, caregivers, and physicians. Forms of psychopathology, medical compliance, symptom reporting, caregiver burden (Hooker et al. 1998), and the physician's bedside manner are all influenced to a substantial degree by the pervasive and enduring characteristics that define personality.

The personality of patients with neuropsychiatric disorders is often ignored in the belief that neuropsychological assessment is sufficient to understand the patient (Cahn and Gould 1996). When personality is considered, it is typically construed either in terms of personality disorders—as when the premorbid personality of an individual with late-life–onset psychosis is described as paranoid or schizoid (Pearlson and Petty 1994)—or as a catalog of traits discerned by clinical judgment (Todes and Lees 1985). In this chapter, we present a contemporary model of normal personality and discuss its relevance to geriatric neuropsychiatry.

Definition and Measurement of Personality

Although a textbook of personality theories can offer a bewildering array of definitions of its subject matter, two

The authors thank Jamie Berry and Jeffrey Herbst for assistance in the preparation of this chapter.

common and complementary approaches are in use. The first sees personality as a system that organizes and directs the behavior of the individual in ways that allow the satisfaction of needs and the expression of the self. Figure 20–1 provides a contemporary example of this type of model. In this view of the personality system, biologically based basic tendencies interact over time with external influences to create a repertoire of characteristic adaptations (skills, habits, attitudes, preferences, roles, relationships, and so on). These adaptations in turn interact with the immediate situation to determine what the individual does and experiences at a particular moment (McCrae and Costa 1996).

Some such model of the personality system is required to understand how human beings function. For example, Figure 20–1 calls attention to the biological bases of personality dispositions, consistent with a wealth of literature on the heritability of most personality traits (Loehlin 1992; Riemann et al. 1997). But the system approach is limited as a definition of personality because—with the possible exception of patients with severe psychosis or dementia—it applies equally to everyone. The second approach commonly used to define personality calls attention to individual differences.

From the perspective of individual differences, personality refers to the psychological features that confer both individuality and identity. Among the most important of these features are *personality traits*, defined as pervasive and enduring styles of thinking, feeling, and acting. Because they reflect something intrinsic to the person, these traits are manifested in a wide range of situations; because they form a core part of one's identity (McCrae and Costa 1988), they must endure over substantial periods of time. Personality traits are thus to be distinguished from situationally bound habits and relationships and from transient moods and motives, and they are located in Figure 20–1 in the category of basic tendencies.

Personality traits are ubiquitous in laypersons' descriptions of themselves and others, and traitlike constructs have been measured by psychologists for decades. Needs, temperaments, characters, folk concepts, cognitive styles, and a variety of personality disorders have all been proposed as the basic units of personality psychology. For many years, one of the central problems in the field was that so many individual difference variables had been identified that little progress could be made in understanding any of them.

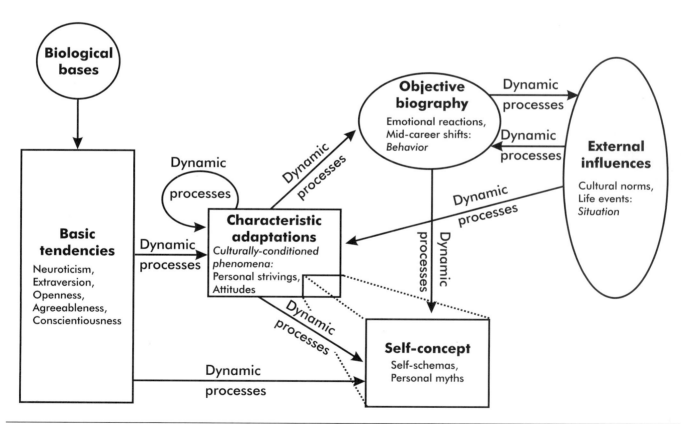

FIGURE 20–1.   A model of the personality system, showing the major components of the system and the principal paths by which they are related.
Source.   Adapted from McCrae and Costa 1996.

It was clear, however, that all these different constructs were heavily redundant: poor ego strength was akin to low psychological resiliency and to general anxiety and negative affectivity (Watson and Clark 1984). Factor analysts such as Cattell (1973) and Eysenck (1960) attempted to summarize the redundancy in terms of a few broad personality factors or dimensions. After years of research and debate, a general (if not universal) consensus has emerged that most specific traits can be understood in terms of five broad factors, usually labeled neuroticism, extraversion, openness to experience, agreeableness, and conscientiousness (Digman 1990; McCrae 1992).

These five factors were initially identified in studies based on English-language trait adjectives, but they were soon replicated in a variety of theoretically based personality questionnaires. One of the first inventories designed specifically to measure the Five-Factor Model was the NEO Personality Inventory (NEO-PI) (Costa and McCrae 1985); Table 20–1 lists the 30 facets that define the five factors and gives some indication of their scope and nature. For example, the table shows that individuals high in openness to experience have an active fantasy life, appreciate art and beauty, are keenly aware of their feelings and emotions, prefer variety and novelty, are intellectually curious, and have liberal value systems.

The Five-Factor Model has proven to be generalizable not only over a wide range of personality instruments but over many different populations. Similar factor structures are found in young and old adults, men and women, and

white and nonwhite subsamples (Costa et al. 1991). Perhaps more importantly, the structure has also been replicated in studies using translations of the revised NEO-PI (NEO-PI-R) into such languages as Portuguese, Korean, and Filipino (McCrae and Costa 1997; McCrae et al. 1998). These cross-cultural replications suggest that personality traits are a specieswide characteristic. Finally, recent studies (Bagby et al., in press; Yang et al., in press) have reported the same structure in psychiatric samples as that found in psychiatrically healthy samples.

Personality trait assessment has been the topic of extensive research for decades. Because traits are abstract constructs that must be inferred from patterns of behavior and experience, no single method or instrument is perfect, but several approaches yield reasonably accurate assessments. Most common are self-report questionnaires or checklists (e.g., Costa and McCrae 1992; Trapnell and Wiggins 1990) that ask respondents to describe their own interests, behaviors, and feelings. More familiar to psychiatrists are structured interviews (Trull and Widiger 1997), in which self-reports are elicited and evaluated by a trained professional. Informant ratings have also been shown to be valid alternatives to self-reports, especially valuable in situations in which self-reports may not be trustworthy. For example, considerable research has been done on personality in patients with dementia by using ratings from spouses or caregivers (Glosser et al. 1995; Siegler et al. 1991).

Personality and Aging

Personality development from infancy through adolescence has been a major focus of personality theory and research for most of this century. From the time of Freud on, however, most psychologists assumed that personality development had ended by adulthood. Until Erikson's (1950) influential epigenetic model extended psychosocial development into old age, little attention was paid to adult personality. Erikson's stage model has received only partial support (e.g., Van de Water and McAdams 1989), but it stimulated cross-sectional and longitudinal research that has led to a clear and consistent picture of what happens to personality in the normal course of aging.

Two important and distinct questions need to be asked about personality and aging. The first concerns the preservation of individual differences; the second, stability or change in mean levels. The first question requires assessment at different points in time and is usually addressed by longitudinal studies that measure the same group of individuals on multiple occasions separated by intervals of years or decades. Questions about mean levels can also be

TABLE 20–1. Revised NEO Personality Inventory Facet scales defining the five basic personality factors

Neuroticism	Actions
Anxiety	Ideas
Angry hostility	Values
Depression	**Agreeableness**
Self-consciousness	Trust
Impulsiveness	Straightforwardness
Vulnerability	Altruism
Extraversion	Compliance
Warmth	Modesty
Gregariousness	Tender-mindedness
Assertiveness	**Conscientiousness**
Activity	Competence
Excitement seeking	Order
Positive emotions	Dutifulness
Openness to experience	Achievement striving
Fantasy	Self-discipline
Aesthetics	Deliberation
Feelings	

addressed by longitudinal data, but they are often approached through cross-sectional comparisons of different age groups.

By definition, traits are enduring dispositions, so if they exist at all, they must show some stability of rank order over a period of months or years. But traits might well change across longer portions of the life span, and most researchers anticipated that life events, changes in physical health, and changing roles and responsibilities would each have profound impact on personality traits. That view is tenable during the first part of adulthood (Siegler et al. 1990); personality scores at age 30 are only moderately predictable from scores at age 18. After age 30, however, evidence shows impressive predictability and thus stability. Longitudinal studies covering periods of up to 30 years (Costa and McCrae 1992; Finn 1986) find substantial stability in rank order for traits from all five factors. Costa and McCrae (1992), for example, reported retest correlations ranging from .61 to .71 over a 24-year interval for a set of 10 traits. In the normal course of aging, extraverts at age 40 are still likely to be relatively extraverted at age 70; conscientious people remain conscientious across the adult life span.

Retest correlations, however, reflect only relative standing; they do not reflect developmental trends that may be common to an entire age group. It is entirely possible to show high retest correlations even when there are dramatic changes in mean level, and reasons have been suggested to hypothesize a number of changes in personality that might accompany aging. Popular stereotypes suggest that old age brings depression, withdrawal, rigidity, and crankiness—although popular stereotypes also suggest that it brings mellowness and wisdom. If predictable age changes in personality do exist, that fact is of considerable importance. Rival disengagement (Cumming and Henry 1961) and activity (Maddox 1963) theories of aging lead to public policy debates on how society should deal with the elderly (Neugarten 1982): should they be allowed to fade away with dignity or should they be surrounded with opportunities and incentives for social interaction?

The major finding from subsequent research is one of stability: most cross-sectional studies of adults over age 30 reported only a small age difference across long portions of the life span (Costa et al. 1986), and many longitudinal studies found no consistent evidence of change at all (Costa and McCrae 1988). Stereotypes about depression, withdrawal, and rigidity are myths, applicable, if at all, only to a small percentage of the elderly.

Coupled with the findings of stability in rank order, mean level stability implies that personality traits are essentially constant across the adult life span. The same range of individual differences is thus found in older men and women as in younger men and women. Social planners—and geriatric physicians—cannot prepare for the "typical" old person; they must learn to appreciate and respond to the full range of individual differences.

Although the major lesson from studies of adult personality development is that personality changes little, more recent research has confirmed that the little it changes is predictable. Between age 18 and age 30, moderately large changes—on the order of one-half standard deviation—are found in the mean levels of all five traits. The pattern, seen in both men and women, makes considerable sense: neuroticism, extraversion, and openness decline and agreeableness and conscientiousness increase—changes that collectively might be described as an increase in psychological maturity. Further, these same trends continue, at a slow rate, after age 30.

So small are these changes that they can be detected usually only by very large samples observed across very long intervals. For example, the correlation of age with neuroticism in a national sample of individuals ages 32 to 88 was −.12 (Costa et al. 1986). It would be easy to dismiss such small effects as meaningless were it not for the fact that similar trends are found in Germany, Croatia, South Korea, Portugal, and Italy (McCrae et al. 1999). Despite differences in language, culture, and recent history, the same developmental pattern appears everywhere. One interpretation of this phenomenon is that personality development is not so much the result of life experience as it is an intrinsic maturational process common to the species.

■ Normal and Abnormal Personality

Neuropsychiatrists are likely to be most familiar with personality in the form of DSM-IV Axis II personality disorders (American Psychiatric Association 1994). Personality disorders—including borderline, paranoid, and antisocial disorders—are marked by extreme and inflexible styles of behaving and experiencing and cause personal distress or social impairment. Ten specific disorders are currently cataloged in DSM-IV, along with a category for disorders "not otherwise specified."

Personality disorders clearly represent significant clinical conditions to which neuropsychiatrists ought to attend. But for many reasons, Axis II is not an optimal system for describing personality (McCrae 1994). The selection of disorders is based on no clear rationale—indeed, several disorders have come and gone in successive editions of the DSM. Many individuals meet criteria for several personality disorder diagnoses—the problem of comorbidity—whereas most people receive no Axis II diagnosis at all and can be characterized only as "normal." Little empirical evidence exists to indicate that the defining symptoms cohere as syndromes (Livesley et al. 1989) or to substantiate the postulated categorical breaks between normal and abnormal personalities (Trull et al. 1990).

In 1989, Wiggins and Pincus proposed a radical alternative to Axis II: they hypothesized that the characteristic maladaptive styles described by personality disorders were in fact variants of the normal personality traits assessed by the Five-Factor Model. Borderline personality disorder, for example, is associated with high neuroticism; histrionic disorder with extraversion; antisocial and paranoid disorders with (low) agreeableness. That hypothesis has subsequently been supported by a number of studies using different samples and measures of the personality disorders (Ball et al. 1997; Costa and Widiger 1994).

From this perspective, personality disorders can be viewed as personality-related problems, the kinds of affective, cognitive, and interpersonal difficulties toward which different personality traits predispose people. Most people have problems and all people have personalities, so the limited applicability of Axis II diagnoses is avoided in this approach. Instead, the clinician can obtain useful insight into the strengths and weaknesses of all patients.

Normal personality traits are also relevant to a number of Axis I disorders (Widiger and Trull 1992). For example, low extraversion is associated with major depression (Bagby et al. 1995); low conscientiousness with substance abuse (Brooner et al. 1993); and high neuroticism with posttraumatic stress disorder (Hyer et al. 1994). Personality traits may predispose individuals to the development of certain forms of psychopathology or they may themselves result from neuropsychiatric disorders. In a later section, we review a body of literature on the effects of Alzheimer's disease on personality traits.

Biological Basis of Personality

Figure 20–1 presented a model of the personality system in which both biology and the environment play prominent shaping roles, reflecting the truism that personality is the result of both nature and nurture. But Figure 20–1 differs fundamentally from most earlier conceptualizations of personality by presuming that personality traits themselves are endogenous and that the environment affects only their expression in acquired habits, tastes, attitudes, and so on. Doubtless the model oversimplifies, but it rests on a rapidly growing body of information on the biological basis of personality.

A long tradition links personality traits directly to neurophysiology. Perhaps most influential is the work of Hans Eysenck (1967), whose theories of the biological basis of neuroticism and extraversion have stimulated many programs of research. More recently, Cloninger (1988) has proposed that personality traits (or at least those related to temperament) reflect activity of the serotonergic, dopaminergic, and noradrenergic systems. Some evidence supports these claims. For example, Cloninger links dopamine to a set of traits he calls novelty seeking, and both novelty seeking (Cloninger et al. 1994) and D_2 dopamine receptors (Roth and Joseph 1994) decline with age.

But the human brain is extraordinarily complex, and personality/brain associations are not readily amenable to experimental study, so it is perhaps not surprising that, at the present time, overall support for Eysenck's and Cloninger's theories is weak (Amelang and Ullwer 1991; Ebstein et al. 1997; Vandenbergh et al. 1997). However, a wealth of evidence shows that personality is firmly rooted in biology and thus that the neurophysiological mechanisms are there to be discovered eventually.

Perhaps the most persuasive evidence comes from adoption and twin studies that have conclusively demonstrated the importance of genetic influences on all five personality factors (Bouchard 1994; Riemann et al. 1997) and on the specific traits that define them (Jang et al. 1998). By contrast, shared environmental influences (such as social class, parental role models, and religious training) appear to have little or no influence on adult personality traits, although they clearly have major effects on characteristic adaptations. In recent years, attempts have been made to identify specific genes associated with personality traits (Benjamin et al. 1996); so far, these findings have not proven to be replicable (Malhotra et al. 1996; Vandenbergh et al. 1997). It seems likely that a large number of genes influence each trait, so the effects of any single gene are small and difficult to detect.

A second line of evidence for the biological basis of personality comes from cross-cultural studies. Both personality structure (McCrae and Costa 1997) and personality development (McCrae et al. 1999) appear to follow universal patterns that transcend language, culture, and history. Although such universal patterns might be attributable to shared experiences—for example, humans everywhere are aware of their own mortality—it is more plausible to see these as results of a common biology.

That argument is even stronger when comparisons are made not across cultures but across species. Research on both primates (King and Figueredo 1997) and nonprimates (Gosling and John 1998) shows that personality characteristics resembling those found in humans can be reliably observed in other animal species. Some personality factors— notably conscientiousness—are absent or difficult to detect, but stable individual differences in aggressiveness, activity level, and shyness are easily demonstrated. Whatever their evolutionary function (if any; see Tooby and Cosmides 1990), personality traits appear to be a part of human beings' mammalian heritage.

A final source of evidence on the neurological basis of personality comes from studies of neuropsychiatric disorders. It has long been recognized that both dementia and traumatic brain injury could affect such characteristics as motivation, mood, and impulse control. However, adequate descriptions of personality changes associated with these conditions was impeded by the lack of a comprehensive model of personality to guide systematic study and by difficulties in personality assessment among impaired patients. Recent advances associated with the Five-Factor Model have resolved both these problems.

Self-report questionnaires are the mainstay of personality assessment in both normal and psychiatric samples, but the validity of such instruments in cognitively impaired individuals is questionable. Instead, most personality assessments of individuals with dementia or those who are otherwise incapacitated have relied on clinician ratings. Although these are of considerable value in describing the current functioning of the patient, they are of limited use in assessing personality changes because clinicians rarely know the premorbid status of the individual. Instead of a consequence, personality traits might be long-term predictors of the neuropsychiatric condition in question.

In the first of a series of papers, Siegler and colleagues (Siegler et al. 1991) asked caregiver informants (spouses and children) to provide personality ratings of 35 patients with memory impairment. Informants described both premorbid and current personality characteristics using the observer rating version of the original NEO-PI (a version that measured all five factors but identified specific facets for only the first three). Premorbid personality profiles showed slightly lower than average levels of openness, but otherwise, mean scores were in the normal range. By contrast, current ratings depicted patients as being high in neuroticism, especially vulnerability to stress, low in extraversion, and very low in conscientiousness. These results were clearly replicated in three other studies (Chatterjee et al. 1992; Siegler et al. 1994; Welleford et al. 1995). Results (expressed as difference between premorbid and current ratings) from all four studies are plotted in Figure 20–2.

These dramatic and remarkably consistent findings are the basis for a number of conclusions. First, they clearly demonstrate that neuropsychiatric status can have profound effects on rated personality—in clear contrast to the

general absence of effects from such physical conditions as heart disease and cancer (Costa et al. 1994). The widespread clinical belief that personality changes are among the more important signs of dementing disorders is apparently well-founded.

Next, these data point to specific traits and factors that are likely to change. At the facet level, the greatest change for patients with Alzheimer's disease is in vulnerability, an inability to deal effectively with stress. At the factor level, these patients became higher in neuroticism and lower in extraversion, but changed relatively little in openness or agreeableness. The largest changes are in conscientiousness, a factor defined by such traits as competence, order, achievement striving, and self-discipline. It is impairment in purposeful, goal-directed striving that most characterizes these individuals.

In hindsight, that finding seems intuitively reasonable because even individuals with mild dementia have difficulty in organizing and directing their lives. But the importance of conscientiousness could not have been predicted from the prior literature. Most attention has been paid to memory loss and other forms of cognitive decline, but conscientiousness is not related to cognitive ability (McCrae and Costa 1985), and neuropsychiatrists should not assume that they can infer levels of conscientiousness from cognitive tests such as measures of executive function. Closer to personality, in the PsycLIT database, of more than 4,000 articles involving Alzheimer's disease that were published between 1991 and 1997, 464 included the word "depression," but only 4 included "conscientiousness"—all from studies informed by the Five-Factor Model. One of the chief advantages of a comprehensive model of personality is that it allows systematic exploration of personality correlates, including traits that might otherwise have been overlooked.

These studies suggest that informant ratings may be useful in the assessment of personality in many neuropsychiatric conditions. Additional studies by Strauss and colleagues (Strauss and Pasupathi 1994; Strauss et al. 1993) show that retrospective ratings are consensually valid and temporally stable and that current ratings are sensitive to progression of the disease. Standardized questionnaires provide an effective way to enlist the aid of caregivers in the comprehensive assessment of the patient.

Personality in Geriatric Neuropsychiatry

The methods and findings of contemporary personality psychology are potentially useful at two levels: in research

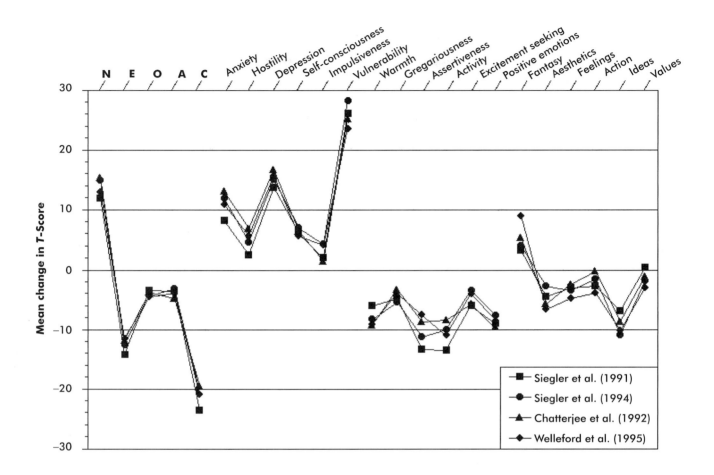

FIGURE 20–2.   Mean changes from premorbid to current personality ratings in four studies of patients with Alzheimer's disease.

on the causes and consequences of neuropsychiatric disorders and in understanding and helping patients and their families. Research on personality correlates of disease is valuable for several reasons. Patterns such as those shown in Figure 20–2 may offer insights into brain/behavior relationships; for example, something about the neurohormonal and neuroanatomical changes that accompany the progression of Alzheimer's disease profoundly affects planning and goal-directed behavior, while leaving intact the quality of interpersonal orientation (agreeableness versus antagonism) (see Chapter 24 in this volume). A comparison of patterns across many different disorders would be particularly illuminating.

Some of that research has already been conducted. Two studies (Glosser et al. 1995; Mendelsohn et al. 1995) have used similar designs to investigate Parkinson's disease and found increased neuroticism and decreased extraversion, openness, and conscientiousness—a pattern very similar to that seen in Alzheimer's disease. Two unpublished studies of patients with traumatic brain injury

(Costa 1996) also showed similar patterns of personality changes. It appears that diffuse brain damage, with or without cognitive impairment, leads to predictable patterns of personality change.

That information has important clinical implications as well. These changes in personality can be detected by lay observers and can provide early signs of dementing disorders. Because these changes are progressive in Alzheimer's disease (Strauss and Pasupathi 1994), their recognition can help caregivers anticipate how the patient is likely to change over the course of the disease. Memory loss is not the only, or even necessarily the most troubling, effect of Alzheimer's disease; loss of purposefulness and vulnerability to stress also present problems with which the caregiver may have to deal.

But information on personality can be valuable to geriatric neuropsychiatrists at a broader level because all patients have personality traits that influence their interactions with physicians (McCrae and Stone 1997). Individuals high in neuroticism are prone to exaggerate medical complaints, whereas those who are low may minimize them. Extraverts are talkative and may more readily volunteer information about their medical condition or ask questions about treatment. Open individuals are unconventional and willing to experiment; they may prefer innovative or nontraditional medical therapies. Disagreeable people are suspicious, demanding, and frequently dissatisfied with the medical treatment they receive (Roter and Hall 1992). Conscientious people have better health habits to begin with and comply more diligently with prescribed medical regimens. Those persons who are chronically low in conscientiousness, such as those whose initial levels of conscientiousness are decreased by dementing disorders, may require extra assistance from family caregivers. For all these reasons, physicians are better equipped to understand, diagnose, and treat their patients if they appreciate the role of enduring individual differences.

References

Amelang M, Ullwer U: Correlations between psychometric measures and psychophysiological as well as experimental variables in studies on extraversion and neuroticism, in Explorations in Temperament: International Perspectives on Theory and Measurement. Edited by Strelau J, Angleitner A. New York, Plenum, 1991, pp 287–316

American Psychiatric Association: Diagnostic and Statistical Manual of Mental Disorders, 4th Edition. Washington, DC, American Psychiatric Association, 1994

Bagby RM, Joffe RT, Parker JDA, et al: Major depression and the Five-Factor Model of personality. J Personal Disord 9: 224–234, 1995

Bagby RM, Costa PT Jr, McCrae RR, et al: Replicating the Five-Factor Model of personality in a psychiatric sample. Personality and Individual Differences (in press)

Ball SA, Tennen H, Poling JC, et al: Personality, temperament, and character dimensions and the DSM-IV personality disorders in substance abusers. J Abnorm Psychol 106: 545–553, 1997

Benjamin J, Li L, Patterson C, et al: Population and familial association between the D_4 dopamine receptor gene and measures of novelty seeking. Nat Genet 12:81–84, 1996

Bouchard TJ: Genes, environment, and personality. Science 264:1700–1701, 1994

Brooner RK, Herbst JH, Schmidt CW, et al: Antisocial personality disorder among drug abusers: relations to other personality diagnoses and the Five-Factor Model of personality. J Nerv Ment Dis 181:313–319, 1993

Cahn G, Gould RE: Understanding head injury and intellectual recovery from brain damage: is IQ an adequate measure? Bulletin of the American Academy of Psychiatry and the Law 24:135–142, 1996

Cattell RB: Personality and Mood by Questionnaire. San Francisco, CA, Jossey-Bass, 1973

Chatterjee A, Strauss ME, Smyth KA, et al: Personality changes in Alzheimer's disease. Arch Neurol 49:486–491, 1992

Cloninger CR: A unified biosocial theory of personality and its role in the development of anxiety states: a reply to commentaries. Psychiatric Developments 2:83–120, 1988

Cloninger CR, Przybeck TR, Svrakic DM, et al: The Temperament and Character Inventory (TCI): A Guide to Its Development and Use. St. Louis, MO, Washington University, 1994

Costa PT Jr: Personality assessment of neurologically impaired patients using Form R of the Revised NEO Personality Inventory (NEO-PI-R). Paper presented at the midwinter meeting of the Society for Personality Assessment, Denver, CO, March 1996

Costa PT Jr, McCrae RR: The NEO Personality Inventory Manual. Odessa, FL, Psychological Assessment Resources, 1985

Costa PT Jr, McCrae RR: Personality in adulthood: a six-year longitudinal study of self-reports and spouse ratings on the NEO Personality Inventory. J Pers Soc Psychol 54: 853–863, 1988

Costa PT Jr, McCrae RR: Trait psychology comes of age, in Nebraska Symposium on Motivation: Psychology and Aging. Edited by Sonderegger T. Lincoln, NE, University of Nebraska Press, 1992, pp 169–204

Costa PT Jr, Widiger TA (eds): Personality Disorders and the Five-Factor Model of Personality. Washington, DC, American Psychological Association, 1994

Costa PT Jr, McCrae RR, Zonderman AB, et al: Cross-sectional studies of personality in a national sample, 2: stability in neuroticism, extraversion, and openness. Psychol Aging 1: 144–149, 1986

Costa PT Jr, McCrae RR, Dye DA: Facet scales for agreeableness and conscientiousness: a revision of the NEO Personality Inventory. Personality and Individual Differences 12:887–898, 1991

Costa PT Jr, Metter EJ, McCrae RR: Personality stability and its contribution to successful aging. Journal of Geriatric Psychiatry 27:41–59, 1994

Cumming E, Henry W: Growing Old. New York, Basic Books, 1961

Digman JM: Personality structure: emergence of the Five-Factor Model. Annu Rev Psychol 41:417–440, 1990

Ebstein RP, Gritsenko I, Nemanov L, et al: No association between the serotonin transporter gene regulatory region polymorphism and the tridimensional personality questionnaire (TPQ) temperament of harm avoidance. Mol Psychiatry 2:224–226, 1997

Erikson EH: Childhood and Society. New York, WW Norton, 1950

Eysenck HJ: The Structure of Human Personality. London, Methuen, 1960

Eysenck HJ: The Biological Basis of Personality. Springfield, IL, Charles C Thomas, 1967

Finn SE: Stability of personality self-ratings over 30 years: evidence for an age/cohort interaction. J Pers Soc Psychol 50:813–818, 1986

Glosser G, Clark C, Freundlich B, et al: A controlled investigation of current and premorbid personality: characteristics of Parkinson's disease patients. Mov Disord 10:201–206, 1995

Gosling SD, John OP: Personality dimensions in dogs, cats, and hyenas. Paper presented at the 10th annual convention of the American Psychological Society, Washington, DC, May 1998

Hooker K, Monahan DJ, Bowman SR, et al: Personality counts for a lot: predictors of mental and physical health of spouse caregivers in two disease groups. J Gerontol B Psychol Sci Soc Sci 53B:P73–P85, 1998

Hyer L, Braswell L, Albrecht B, et al: Relationship of NEO-PI to personality styles and severity of trauma in chronic PTSD victims. J Clin Psychol 50:699–707, 1994

Jang KL, McCrae RR, Angleitner A, et al: Heritability of facet-level traits in a cross-cultural twin study: support for a hierarchical model of personality. J Pers Soc Psychol 74:1556–1565, 1998

King JE, Figueredo AJ: The Five-Factor Model plus dominance in chimpanzee personality. Journal of Research in Personality 31:257–271, 1997

Livesley WJ, Jackson DN, Schroeder ML: A study of the factorial structure of personality pathology. J Personal Disord 3:292–306, 1989

Loehlin JC: Genes and Environment in Personality Development. Newbury Park, CA, Sage, 1992

Maddox GL: Activity and morale: a longitudinal study of selected elderly subjects. Social Forces 42:195–204, 1963

Malhotra AK, Virkkunen M, Rooney W, et al: The association between the dopamine D_4 receptor (D4DR) 16 amino acid repeat polymorphism and novelty seeking. Mol Psychiatry 1:388–391, 1996

McCrae RR: The Five-Factor Model: issues and applications (special issue). J Pers 60(2), 1992

McCrae RR: A reformulation of Axis II: personality and personality-related problems, in Personality Disorders and the Five-Factor Model of Personality. Edited by Costa PT Jr, Widiger TA. Washington, DC, American Psychological Association, 1994, pp 303–310

McCrae RR, Costa PT Jr: Updating Norman's "adequate taxonomy": intelligence and personality dimensions in natural language and in questionnaires. J Pers Soc Psychol 49:710–721, 1985

McCrae RR, Costa PT Jr: Age, personality, and the spontaneous self-concept. J Gerontol B Psychol Sci Soc Sci 43: S177–S185, 1988

McCrae RR, Costa PT Jr: Toward a new generation of personality theories: theoretical contexts for the Five-Factor Model, in The Five-Factor Model of Personality: Theoretical Perspectives. Edited by Wiggins JS. New York, Guilford, 1996, pp 51–87

McCrae RR, Costa PT Jr: Personality trait structure as a human universal. Am Psychol 52:509–516, 1997

McCrae RR, Stone SV: Personality, in Cambridge Handbook of Psychology, Health, and Medicine. Edited by Baum A, Newman S, Weinman J, et al. Cambridge, England, Cambridge University Press, 1997, pp 29–34

McCrae RR, Costa PT Jr, del Pilar GH, et al: Cross-cultural assessment of the Five-Factor Model: the revised NEO Personality Inventory. Journal of Cross-Cultural Psychology 29:171–188, 1998

McCrae RR, Costa PT Jr, Lima MP, et al: Age differences in personality across the adult lifespan: parallels in five cultures. Dev Psychol 35:466–477, 1999

Mendelsohn GA, Dakof GA, Skaff M: Personality change in Parkinson's disease patients: chronic disease and aging. J Pers 63:233–257, 1995

Neugarten BL (ed): Age or Need? Public Policies for Older People. Beverly Hills, CA, Sage, 1982

Pearlson GD, Petty RG: Late-life–onset psychoses, in Textbook of Geriatric Neuropsychiatry. Edited by Coffey CE, Cummings JL. Washington, DC, American Psychiatric Press, 1994, pp 261–277

Riemann R, Angleitner A, Strelau J: Genetic and environmental influences on personality: a study of twins reared together using the self- and peer report NEO-FFI scales. J Pers 65:449–475, 1997

Roter DL, Hall JA: Doctors Talking With Patients/Patients Talking With Doctors: Improving Communication in Medical Visits. Westport, CT, Auburn House, 1992

Roth GS, Joseph JA: Age-related changes in transcriptional and posttranscriptional regulation of the dopaminergic system. Life Sci 55:2031–2035, 1994

Siegler IC, Zonderman AB, Barefoot JC, et al: Predicting personality in adulthood from college MMPI scores: implications for follow-up studies in psychosomatic medicine. Psychosom Med 52:644–652, 1990

Siegler IC, Welsh KA, Dawson DV, et al: Ratings of personality change in patients being evaluated for memory disorders. Alzheimer Dis Assoc Disord 5:240–250, 1991

Siegler IC, Dawson DV, Welsh KA: Caregiver ratings of personality change in Alzheimer's disease patients: a replication. Psychol Aging 9:464–466, 1994

Strauss ME, Pasupathi M: Primary caregivers' descriptions of Alzheimer patients' personality traits: temporal stability and sensitivity to change. Alzheimer Dis Assoc Disord 8: 166–176, 1994

Strauss ME, Pasupathi M, Chatterjee A: Concordance between observers in descriptions of personality change in Alzheimer's disease. Psychol Aging 8:475–480, 1993

Todes CJ, Lees AJ: The premorbid personality of patients with Parkinson's disease. J Neurol Neurosurg Psychiatry 48: 97–100, 1985

Tooby J, Cosmides L: On the universality of human nature and the uniqueness of the individual: the role of genetics and adaptation. J Pers 58:17–68, 1990

Trapnell PD, Wiggins JS: Extension of the Interpersonal Adjective Scales to include the Big Five dimensions of personality. J Pers Soc Psychol 59:781–790, 1990

Trull TJ, Widiger TA: Structured Interview for the Five-Factor Model of Personality (SIFFM) Professional Manual. Odessa, FL, Psychological Assessment Resources, 1997

Trull TJ, Widiger TA, Guthrie P: The categorical versus dimensional status of borderline personality disorder. J Abnorm Psychol 99:40–48, 1990

Van de Water D, McAdams DP: Generativity and Erikson's "belief in the species." Journal of Research in Personality 23: 435–449, 1989

Vandenbergh DJ, Zonderman AB, Wang J, et al: No association between novelty seeking and dopamine D_4 receptor (D4DR) exon III seven repeat alleles in Baltimore Longitudinal Study of Aging participants. Mol Psychiatry 2: 417–419, 1997

Watson D, Clark LA: Negative affectivity: the disposition to experience aversive emotional states. Psychol Bull 96: 465–490, 1984

Welleford EA, Harkins SW, Taylor JR: Personality change in dementia of the Alzheimer's type: relation to caregiver personality and burden. Exp Aging Res 21:295–314, 1995

Widiger TA, Trull TJ: Personality and psychopathology: an application of the Five-Factor Model. J Pers 60:363–393, 1992

Wiggins JS, Pincus AL: Conceptions of personality disorders and dimensions of personality. Psychological Assessment 1:305–316, 1989

Yang J, McCrae RR, Costa PT Jr, et al: Cross-cultural personality assessment in psychiatric populations: the NEO-PI-R in the People's Republic of China. Psychological Assessment (in press)

Mental Retardation

James D. Duffy, M.B., Ch.B.

Eleanore Hobbs, M.D.

Although 1%–3% of the population meet diagnostic criteria for mental retardation (MR), the physical and mental health needs of this large segment of society have remained largely unexplored. In addition, little rigorous research on the assessment and treatment of behavioral disorders in people with MR has been undertaken. Bearing these caveats in mind, and with the understanding that considerable research still needs to be done, in this chapter we attempt to provide a broad overview of the current scientific data available on the neuropsychiatry of MR, with a particular emphasis on the elderly.

Definition of Mental Retardation

Reaching a consensus on the most appropriate definition of MR remains elusive. The diagnostic approach subsumed under DSM-IV provides clear criteria based on the patient's measurable IQ (American Psychiatric Association 1994). Although this approach is concrete and therefore easy to operationalize, it fails to identify many individuals with MR who, through an enriched environmental experi-

ence or because of intellectual competence, are able to score above the cutoff IQ scores. In recognition of these limitations of the DSM-IV's "uni-dimensional" IQ-driven approach, the American Association on Mental Retardation (1992) has proposed a broader definition that is based on an assessment of functional capacity:

> Mental retardation refers to substantial limitations in present functioning. It is characterized by significantly subaverage intellectual functioning, existing concurrently with related limitations in two or more of the following applicable adaptive skills areas: communication, self-care, home living, social skills, community use, self-direction, health and safety, functional academics, leisure and work. Mental retardation manifests before age 18. (American Association on Mental Retardation 1992)

The American Association on Mental Retardation approach also includes a multidimensional classification system that contains a description of the individual's status within the domains of intellectual, psychological, physical, and environmental functioning. This approach provides a broader perspective of the individual's clinical status and assists with treatment planning.

Demographics

Because of the "graying" of the postwar baby boomers and of their increasing life expectancy, the number of elderly persons with MR in the United States is growing rapidly. Current estimates suggest that 6.1%–15.7% of the population with MR in the United States is over age 55, with the greatest proportion of these older individuals residing in state institutions (Jacobson et al. 1985). Current demographic trends indicate that this rate can be expected to double in the next 30 years (National Institute on Aging 1987). The remarkable increase of individuals with MR is reflected in the statistic that between 1932 and 1976 the number of 10-year-old children who were mentally retarded who could expect to survive to age 60 increased from 28% to 46% (Balakrishnan and Wolf 1976; Dayton et al. 1932). This upward trend is most evident in people with Down's syndrome (DS), whose life expectancy has increased from 9 years in 1929 to at least 70% surviving beyond age 30 in 1987 (Penrose 1949). As would be expected, people with mild MR are most likely to live longer than those with severe MR, a fact that dictates that the elderly population with MR is overrepresented by individuals with mild compared with those with severe MR.

Deinstitutionalization programs have resulted in an elderly person with MR being more likely to reside in the community and therefore seek services from community-based health care professionals. Unfortunately, the health care system has failed to anticipate or respond to this demographic trend, with the result that few clinicians possess the skills necessary to provide adequate medical or mental health care for patients with MR. Indeed, in most regions, including urban and suburban areas, the person with MR has difficulty even finding health care professionals willing to provide medical services. This situation is even more dire in the elderly patient with MR whose particular needs demand a composite of skills not currently taught in any professional training programs.

Normal Aging in Mental Retardation

The neurobiology of normal aging is described elsewhere in this text (see Chapter 3 in this volume). People with MR are particularly vulnerable to age-related changes in sensory and cognitive functioning. Hearing loss has been found to be common in people with DS. More than half of patients with DS develop hypothyroidism that is frequently associated with cognitive deficits that may be misinterpreted as indicating Alzheimer's disease (AD). Although little is known about the sleep pattern of persons

with DS, they are predisposed to developing sleep apnea, which, in turn, produces cognitive and behavioral deficits that may become disabling. The association between DS and AD is discussed below.

Social Aspects

Although little is known about the social functioning of the elderly population with MR, the research studies that have been undertaken have reported similar findings. Anderson et al. (1984) examined the living arrangements of adults age 63 and older in four settings: state institutions, private facilities, foster homes, and group homes. Their major finding was that across all settings the subjects with MR had a very low level of social integration. This finding was supported by several other studies that have reported that, regardless of their community placement, elderly patients with MR are likely to be socially withdrawn (Legault 1992; Markova et al. 1992). Interestingly, the most comprehensive study of social integration by elderly patients with MR has reported that those individuals exhibiting mild "anti-social" behavior are more likely to become involved in community activities, probably because of their more assertive and socially aggressive behavior (Moss et al. 1992). The social isolation of the elderly patient with MR is likely to be compounded by the fact that almost three-quarters are physically limited and require mobility aids (e.g., wheelchairs, crutches, canes) (Parette and Vanbiervliet 1992). These findings indicate that community placement programs for elderly patients who are mentally retarded require adequate staffing and support services to ensure that these individuals are able to take advantage of social opportunities.

Although most group homes are willing and able to continue caring for their aging residents with MR, an increasing number of elderly people with MR are residing in nursing homes. Unfortunately, few of these facilities have the resources necessary to provide the most appropriate care environment for their residents with MR (also see Chapter 37 in this volume).

Clinical Assessment of the Elderly Patient With Mental Retardation

The neuropsychiatric assessment of the elderly patient with MR requires a wide range of clinical diagnostic skills. Indeed, probably no other patient population challenges the clinician with such a complex interplay of neuropsychiatric, psychological, and social factors. The clinician repeatedly faces the challenge of diagnosing a specific DSM-IV or ICD-10 disorder in which clinical manifestations are obscured or modified by a premorbid developmental disability. Bearing in mind the complexity of achieving a valid neuropsychiatric diagnosis, a few guiding principles are helpful when evaluating any behaviorally disturbed patient with MR:

- *Individuals with MR have the same psychiatric disorders as those found in the general population.* As many as 40%–70% of individuals with MR have a diagnosable psychiatric disorder, yet their behavioral disturbances are frequently dismissed by clinicians as simply being a manifestation of the patient's premorbid developmental disability. This failure to identify a specific psychiatric disorder inevitably results in a downward spiral of ineffective behavioral strategies or inappropriate psychopharmacological interventions.
- *Wherever possible, psychiatric diagnoses should be made using DSM-IV behavioral checklists and behavioral questionnaires developed specifically for individuals with MR.* DSM checklists have been demonstrated to be more sensitive and specific than either case record reviews or clinical interviews in making a definitive psychiatric diagnosis. These behavioral checklists do, however, have the disadvantage of being skewed toward current or recent behaviors. In addition, the pathological significance of a behavior may be unclear in the case of a person with a developmental disability (Sturmey 1993). Two behavioral questionnaires, the Psychopathology Instrument for Mentally Retarded Adults (PIMRA) (Mattson et al. 1984) and the Diagnostic Assessment for the Severely Handicapped (Mattson et al. 1991), are specifically designed to identify behavioral disorders in the mentally retarded and have demonstrated adequate reliability and inter-

nal consistency. Ideally, the clinical assessment of behaviorally disturbed individuals with MR should employ one of these behavioral checklists in conjunction with a thorough clinical evaluation.
- *The clinical presentation of psychiatric disorders in the patient with MR are modified by his or her comorbid neurodevelopmental disorder.* Most people with MR possess an extremely limited repertoire of behavioral responses. Different subjective states and environmental stressors are therefore likely to produce overtly similar behavioral responses, thereby making it difficult to identify the underlying primary psychiatric disorder or the person's subjective behavioral state. The pathoplastic effects of MR and their impact on the phenomenology of psychiatric disorders have been elegantly distilled by Sovner (1986) (Table 21–1).
- *Patients with MR frequently manifest behavioral symptoms as the herald sign of an underlying physical complaint.* The limited behavioral repertoire of patients with MR dictates that they often have difficulty in localizing the source of their subjective discomfort (e.g., an ear infection can manifest as aggressive irritability). Therefore, it is important that any neuropsychiatric evaluation should include a thorough physical assessment (see Chapter 5 in this volume).
- *Individuals with MR are exquisitely sensitive to their social milieu.* When taking a psychosocial history, the clinician should carefully note all recent changes in the patient's history. Social changes that might normally be considered of little importance (e.g., change of bus route or group home routine) can have an enormous impact upon the patient with MR, who is likely to respond poorly to any change in routine. It is important that the clinician obtain a detailed psychosocial history and be cognizant of the potential significance of apparently minor stressors.

TABLE 21–1. Pathoplastic effects of mental retardation and their clinical impact

Factor	Definition	Clinical impact
Intellectual distortion	Concrete thinking and impaired communication skills	Inability to name and label subjective feeling state
Psychosocial masking	Impoverished social skills and life experience	Inappropriate social behavior can inhibit or modify typical behavior markers for psychopathology.
Cognitive disintegration	Stress-induced disruption of information processing	Cognitive disorganization can be difficult to distinguish from psychopathology.
Baseline exaggeration	Increase in severity of preexisting cognitive deficits and maladaptive behaviors	Atypical clinical features can dominate (increase in incontinence).

Source. Adapted from Sovner 1986.

■ *The etiology of the patient's developmental disability is often an important predictor of behavioral patterns and a predictor of treatment responses.* Although few neurodevelopmental syndromes have a specific behavioral phenotype (e.g., Williams syndrome), an understanding of the patient's neurodevelopmental disorder is often helpful in developing a diagnostic formulation and treatment plan. In particular, the clinician should be alert to the consequences of seizure disorders (see below).

■ *Neurodiagnostic studies have only a limited role to play in the clinical assessment of patients with MR.* Patients with MR, particularly those with more severe disability, are usually unable to tolerate the claustrophobia or inertia necessary to complete a neurodiagnostic study such as a magnetic resonance imaging study or electroencephalogram. This intolerance necessitates that these studies are usually performed under general anesthesia or conscious sedation.

■ *The groups of individuals or community agencies responsible for the care of patients with MR each have their own group dynamics.* The professionals and volunteers who work with people who are mentally retarded have developed a remarkable network of competent agencies that provide outstanding care, sometimes in extremely difficult circumstances. However, each of these groups or agencies has its particular group dynamics. It is important that the clinician understand the dynamics of each patient's living situation, regarding staff and other residents. Changes in group home membership or staffing will usually result in significant stress and consequent behavioral change among other group home residents. In some circumstances, it may be appropriate for the clinician to work with several group home members or staff to identify and treat maladaptive transactional patterns.

■ *Treatment decisions should be driven by a specific diagnostic hypothesis, and treatment response should be monitored with quantified behavioral outcome data.* All too often, clinicians attempt to treat behavioral disorders in patients with MR by simply targeting the most prominent symptom (e.g., aggression) rather than developing a DSM-IV–based diagnosis. This symptom-driven approach inevitably results in a series of medication trials that has only a modest chance of success. In addition to developing a solid testable diagnostic hypothesis, it is important that the clinician and community caregivers work together to develop measurable behavioral data that can be used to assess treatment response. These data are necessary if the clinician is to avoid the trap of reacting to each "cri-

sis." For example, a single destructive act by an aggressive patient may overshadow the fact that a treatment has produced a 50% reduction in the frequency of aggressive acts.

■ Medical Evaluation in the Elderly Patient With Mental Retardation

It has been estimated that 20%–40% of patients with MR who are diagnosed as having a chronic mental illness actually have one or more physical disorders that cause or exacerbate their neuropsychiatric symptoms (Ryan and Sunanda 1997) (see Chapter 31 in this volume). A recent community survey reported that people with MR who are residing in the community have no more medical problems than the general population (McDermott et al. 1997). In stark contradiction to this finding, a survey of New Jersey Medicare health care expenditures for acute care admissions for alternate years between 1983 and 1991 found that, although expenditures for the general population had actually dropped during this period, the number of admissions and length of stay for individuals with MR had increased by 56% and 42%, respectively (Walsh et al. 1997). The total hospital charges for people with MR during the period 1983–1991 rose 206%, almost twice that of the general population (Walsh et al. 1997). These statistics suggest that current health services for persons with MR are inefficient and ineffective—a situation that is likely to increase with the aging of the MR community. The increased utilization of health care services by people with MR in this study was found to be attributable to an increased number of psychiatric admissions and a significant number of "outliers" for whom appropriate community placements could not be found. In addition, elderly patients with MR were found to have unusually long medical and surgical hospitalizations. The authors concluded that these expenditure burdens could have been reduced through coordinated case management and subsequent effective discharge planning (Walsh et al. 1997). Fortunately, the fiscal inefficiencies highlighted in the New Jersey study are likely to focus increasing attention upon the needs of the MR community.

When evaluating the patient with MR, it should be borne in mind that certain syndromes predispose the individual to specific disorders (e.g., hypothyroidism with DS). Ryan et al. (1997) recently reported the results of their survey of the medical problems of 1,135 adults with MR who underwent an extensive medical evaluation (Ryan and Sunanda 1997) (Table 21–2). Conditions that were most likely to produce a behavioral disorder included epilepsy, chronic arthritic pain, hypothyroidism, and lupus. This study highlights the importance of obtaining a thorough medical evaluation of all patients with MR and also suggests that the neuropsychiatrist may be the most appropriate physician to assume the role of primary care provider.

The neuropsychiatrist may frequently encounter elderly patients with MR in whom the etiology of their neurodevelopmental disability has not been previously ascertained. Although certain phenotypic characteristics make the identification of the disability clear (e.g., DS, Angelman syndrome), in the large majority of patients no specific syndrome can be identified. It is important, however, that the clinician be alert for those conditions that have predictable neurobehavioral sequelae (e.g., tuberous sclerosis, Angelman syndrome). The appropriate diagnostic work-up to identify the etiology of MR in a particular elderly patient is open to debate. It is our experience that a thorough history and physical examination provide an adequate screen for those conditions that may warrant specific therapeutic or diagnostic interventions (e.g., hydrocephalus). Although genotyping may provide information regarding inheritability, it is unlikely to provide any helpful clinical data.

Neuropsychiatric Disorders in the Elderly Patient With Mental Retardation

The research literature on the prevalence of neuropsychiatric disorders in the elderly with MR remains extremely

TABLE 21–2. Most common medical conditions seen in a cohort of adults with mental retardation referred for psychiatric evaluation

Condition	Percentage of cases
Epilepsy	45.8%
Hypothyroidism	12.7%
Gastroesophageal reflux	9.7%
Chronic pain	6.3%
Abnormal electroencephalogram	5.4%
Autoimmune arthritis	5.0%
Hypertension	4.7%
Scoliosis	4.1%
Peptic ulcer disease	4.0%
Insulin-dependent diabetes mellitus	3.5%
Asthma	3.0%

Source. Adapted from Ryan and Sunanda 1997.

sparse. In addition, what data are available are confounded by the fact that researchers have studied different patient samples (e.g., community dwellers versus institutionalized subjects) and employed varying and usually imprecise diagnostic methods (e.g., retrospective chart reviews versus diagnostic interviews) and outcome measures. Using a clinical diagnostic interview, Day (1987) reported that approximately one-fifth of 99 patients with MR over age 55 were experiencing a psychiatric disorder. Based on an interview of patient caretakers, Lund (1985) reported that 30% of a random sample of 302 adults with MR met DSM-III criteria (American Psychiatric Association 1980) for a psychiatric disorder. A more recent report (Crews 1994), based on a diagnostic interview of 124 institutionalized patients with MR between the ages of 60 and 94, reported that 12.9% had a dementing illness, 8.9% an affective disorder, and 6.5% schizophrenia (all according to DSM-III-R criteria [American Psychiatric Association 1987]). As might be expected, the prevalence of neuropsychiatric disorders is higher in the elderly population with MR. Cooper (1997a, 1997b) has reported that the psychiatric morbidity among elderly patients with MR is 68.7% compared with 47.9% in younger control subjects with MR. In particular, the prevalence rate for depression (6% versus 4.1%), anxiety disorders (9.0% versus 5.5%), and dementia (21.6% versus 2.7%) is higher in the elderly population with MR (Cooper 1997b).

Myriad factors appear to be responsible for the increase in psychiatric disorders among the elderly with MR. The limited cognitive reserve of the patient with MR makes him or her particularly vulnerable to manifesting the clinical sequelae of dementia, which in turn is more likely to manifest itself in behavioral rather than cognitive symptoms (see discussion below). Furthermore, underlying neurological dysfunction linked to the patient's developmental delay can also produce progressive functional decline; for example, the consequences of repeated seizures and anticonvulsant medication. Unfortunately, as a consequence of self-injurious behavior (SIB) or assault, many patients with MR experience repeated minor neurotrauma throughout their lives—producing a cumulative decline in cognitive capacity (see Chapter 28 in this volume). In addition to physical burden, factors such as social stigmatization, isolation, loss of loved ones and unstable support systems are all likely to place an increasing psychosocial burden upon the elderly person with MR and increase his or her vulnerability to psychiatric illness.

Depression

Adults with DS appear to be more susceptible to depression and dementia, but less susceptible to other psychiatric disorders, compared with the general population of individuals with MR (Collacott et al. 1992). Although depression may be causally related to hypothyroidism, this association has not been established in patients with DS (Collacott et al. 1992). In addition, although the stereotypic characterization of people with DS as happy, loving, and outgoing may be exaggerated, they do appear to manifest a lower incidence of conduct disorders, psychosis, and aggression than other people with MR (Collacott 1992).

Research on the prevalence and clinical characteristics of depression in adults with MR has been largely neglected, and what studies have been undertaken have produced conflicting results. Factors that have led to this confusion include 1) the belief that individuals with impaired intelligence and an immature ego-defense are incapable of becoming depressed, 2) the inability of many patients with MR to provide a subjective report of their depression, and 3) the unusual clinical features of depression in individuals who are severely retarded.

The symptoms of depression in adults with MR are likely to differ from those of the general population. In particular, the person with MR who is depressed is less likely to report subjective feelings of sadness, hopelessness, and guilt and is more likely to manifest external behavioral manifestations such as irritability, aggression, SIB, and declining function (Charlot 1997). This differential in clinical symptomatology is further emphasized in people with more severe degrees of intellectual handicap who are statistically more likely (than those who are mildly retarded) to exhibit SIB, screaming, stereotypy, incontinence, and vomiting. Although no data are available, patients with MR who are experiencing the additional burden of age-related cognitive deficits or a neurodegenerative disorder are also more likely to exhibit these atypical features of depression.

Sovner (1986) has recommended behavioral criteria for the diagnosis of depression in subjects with MR. Under these criteria, a diagnosis of depression is made if there is a disturbance of mood characterized by sadness, withdrawal, or agitation and any four of the following eight symptoms: 1) change in appetite or weight, 2) onset or increase in severity of SIB, 3) apathy, 4) psychomotor retardation, 5) loss of activity of daily living skills (e.g., onset of incontinence), 6) catatonic stupor or rigidity, 7) spontaneous crying, and 8) fearfulness. (In patients with a family history of depression, only three symptoms are required). Although these criteria have not been validated empirically, they do provide a useful reference point for assessing the presence of depression in the person with MR.

Contrary to commonly held beliefs, the depressed person with MR is at risk for suicidal ideation and behavior. The only systematic study in this regard reported that 30%

of the patients with depression who were mildly retarded and 8% of patients with depression who were severely retarded experienced suicidal ideation or attempts (Meins et al. 1995).

As discussed above, the atypical clinical features associated with depression in the patient with MR have made research in this area fraught with difficulties. These methodological difficulties are reflected in the conflicting results of epidemiological studies. Community studies have reported that the population with MR experiences a reduced prevalence of depression compared with that of the general population, that is, 1.7% (Lund 1985) compared with 5.4% (Corbett 1979), respectively. In the only study of the prevalence of depression in the elderly population with MR residing in the community, Cooper (1997a) has reported that they are more likely to be diagnosed as having depression than their younger counterparts (6% versus 4.1%, respectively).

Within institutions, the frequency of affective disorders has been reported as between 1.2% (Heaton-Ward et al. 1977) and 24.4% (Duncan et al. 1936). The study with the soundest methodological design (i.e., employing a psychiatric interview and DSM-III-R criteria) reported a prevalence of 8.4% for affective disorders in adults with MR who were residing in institutions (Sansom et al. 1994).

Although a number of case reports have described the efficacy of antidepressants in treating depression in individuals with MR, no controlled studies have addressed this question (Davis et al. 1997; Rummans et al. 1999). In a recent review of the research literature, Mikkelson et al. (1997) reached the following generalizations about the use of antidepressants in patients with MR: 1) patients with MR experience a positive response and adverse side effects at lower doses than are typically demonstrated in the general population, 2) adverse behavioral responses to antidepressants occur in 5%–20% of subjects, 3) hallucinations and delusional thought content are related to either an adverse response or no response to antidepressant medication, and 4) serotonergic agents appear to be better tolerated and more effective antidepressants than noradrenergic medication (Mikkelson et al. 1997).

The phenomenology and demographic characteristics of bipolar affective disorder in the elderly with MR remain unexplored. The limited data available suggest only that patients with MR and bipolar disorder are less likely to respond to lithium than to anticonvulsant mood stabilizers.

A small literature of uncontrolled clinical reports (and our clinical experience) also suggest that electroconvulsive therapy may be an effective and well-tolerated treatment for mood disorders in patients with MR (Krystal and Coffey 1997). Electroconvulsive therapy may also be effective for self-injurious and other aggressive behaviors (see below) when they occur secondary to a mood disorder in patients with MR.

Anxiety Disorders

Estimates of the prevalence of anxiety disorders within the population with MR vary between 1% and 25% (Benson et al. 1985; Eaton and Menolascino 1982). This wide variance in estimated prevalence reflects the difficulty in assessing both the subjective and objective clinical features of anxiety disorders in patients with MR.

Generalized anxiety disorder in persons with MR typically presents as an increase in maladaptive and oppositional behaviors, increased somatization, nausea, shortness of breath, and fatigue and can become the impetus for a downward spiral in social functioning (Khreim and Mikkelson 1997). Clinically, it is helpful to remember that the person with MR is likely to experience fears similar to those of children at a similar developmental stage (Duff et al. 1981; Vandenberg 1993). Behavioral therapy remains the mainstay of treatment for generalized anxiety disorder, and although several psychotropic agents including buspirone and clonazepam have received anecdotal support (Khreim and Mikkelson 1997; Ratey et al. 1989), no controlled studies have addressed the issue of drug therapy for general anxiety disorders in people with MR (see Chapter 15 in this volume).

Because in most cases it is not possible to assess the presence of cognitive obsessions, the diagnosis of obsessive-compulsive disorder in the patient with MR relies primarily upon the observation of compulsive ritualistic behavior. Distinguishing compulsive rituals from stereotypic motor behaviors, perseveration, and stimulus-bound responses presents the clinician with a formidable challenge. Furthermore, virtually every person with MR feels most comfortable in a well-structured routine, and the anxiety they experience when their schedule is disrupted may be misinterpreted as indicating compulsive behavior. Case studies have reported that clomipramine and sertraline are effective treatments for obsessive-compulsive disorder in patients with MR (Barak et al. 1995).

Although specific phobias are thought to occur more commonly among individuals with MR, the incidence of this disorder in this population remains unknown (Vitiello and Behar 1992). The authors' experience suggests that school and workplace phobias, social phobia, and specific phobias produce significant psychiatric morbidity in the patient with MR and result in a downward spiral of oppositional behavior, somatization, and diminishing functional status. Specific phobias, agoraphobia in particu-

lar, are likely to be prevalent among the elderly population with MR who tend to have limited social interactions or are likely to be intimidated by younger, more aggressive residents in institutional settings. Panic disorder should of course be considered as an historical antecedent to the development of any specific phobia.

The physical and emotional vulnerability and limited cognitive coping capacity of the person with MR, as well as the difficult and sometimes abusive environments they have encountered in institutional and community settings, would suggest that they are at extreme risk for developing posttraumatic stress disorder (PTSD). The prevalence of PTSD within the MR community remains unknown, despite the predictable susceptibility to PTSD of persons with MR. As with other psychiatric disorders, the pathoplastic effects of MR upon the clinical manifestations of PTSD render the diagnosis extremely difficult to make. However, a close review of the clinical cornerstones of the disorder, that is, hyperarousal, intrusive memories, flashbacks, reenactments, and interpersonal irritability, will assist in distinguishing the disorder from other causes of aggression (Ryan 1994, 1996).

Dementia

The identification of dementing illness in individuals with MR presents the clinician and researcher with major challenges. Although attempts are under way to establish standard assessment and diagnostic criteria, currently no gold standard exists for the diagnosis of dementia in the person with MR (Aylward et al., in press).

The increasing life span of people with MR dictates that they will experience an increasing incidence of dementia. A recent study (Holland et al. 1998) of all elderly (i.e., > 65 years) residents of Leicestershire, United Kingdom, who were mentally retarded reported a dementia prevalence of 21.6% (against an expected prevalence of 5.7% in the general population). The prevalence of dementia was found to increase with advancing age. Because this cohort contained few patients with DS, other reasons for the increased prevalence of dementia need to be identified, that is, decreased cognitive reserve, progressive neurological disorders (e.g., hydrocephalus, seizures), acquired neurotrauma, and medication effects.

Patients with MR who have a comorbid dementing process are likely to present to clinicians with a decline in functional capacity or with behavioral symptoms (Cooper 1997a). Psychotic symptoms with persecutory content are the most common neuropsychiatric symptoms in dementia associated with MR and occur in 27.6% of patients (Cooper 1997a). In addition, the patient with MR and dementia is likely to exhibit or experience disrupted sleep, irritability, social withdrawal, aggression, and weight loss (Ballard and Oyebode 1995; Moss and Patel 1995).

The linkage between DS and AD is well established. Several studies have reported that AD-like neuropathological changes occur in virtually all subjects with DS over age 30. The earliest changes of AD (i.e., cerebral amyloid deposition) appear to begin as early as age 10 (Mann and Esiri 1989). The prevalence of AD in patients with DS has been reported at 3.4%, 10.3%, and 40% in the 30–39, 40–49, and 50–59 age groups, respectively (Holland et al. 1998). The association between AD and DS is further strengthened by the finding of an increased risk of AD among the relatives of individuals with DS (Heston et al. 1981). These findings suggested that chromosome 21 might be a possible locus for a candidate gene for familial AD—an association further supported by the identification of the gene responsible for B-amyloid production on chromosome 21 (q11-q22). Royston et al. (1994) have reported a correlation between the presence of dementia and the presence of diffuse and classic amyloid plaque formation in the temporal cortex of 21 patients with DS. These findings have led to the hypothesis that excess amyloid production or abnormalities in the processing of amyloid protein and its subsequent deposition are the critical pathology underlying the pathophysiology of AD. Abnormalities in the distribution of paired helical filament tau protein have also been postulated as an etiological factor in AD, as evidenced by one study that reported a significant reduction in tau protein in patients with DS and dementia, but not those without dementia (Mukaetova-Ladinska, in press). The connection between the apolipoprotein E genotype and AD in DS remains unclear. A recent review of published studies indicates that the risk of the individual with DS of developing AD is probably not influenced by her or his E genotype (Cooper 1998). The possible therapeutic benefits of cholinesterase inhibitors in subjects with MR with depression remains to be explored. (Also see Chapter 24 in this volume.)

Self-Injurious Behavior and Stereotypic Movement Disorder

SIB in the patient with MR has a number of possible etiologies, including depression, psychosis, stereotypic movement disorder, and hyperarousal states including PTSD. In its broadest sense, SIB could be used to cover a wide range of behaviors including self-destructive acts such as smoking or risk-taking behavior. However, in the context of MR, the term SIB is most commonly used to describe the repetitive, sometimes rhythmic acts that are characteristic of ste-

reotypic movement disorder (SMD) and produce concomitant self-injury. Head banging, head hitting, eye gouging, biting, and scratching are the most common stereotypic (and self-injuring) behaviors encountered in individuals with MR. SMD occurs in more than 50% of the population with MR, and the incidence of SMD is inversely related to the subjects' degree of MR (Stein et al. 1998). The incidence of SIB and SMD appears significantly lower in older compared with younger subjects with MR (Stein et al. 1998). Several neurodevelopmental disorders, including autism, pervasive developmental disability, Lesch-Nyhan syndrome, Cornelia de Lange syndrome, and Prader-Willi syndrome, are characterized by SMD.

A number of theories have been developed to understand the functional utility of SMD. Psychological constructs posit that the rhythmic movements represent the individual's attempt to reenact an idealized nurturing relationship with the mother. One behavioral model of SMD suggests that, through their ability to modulate arousal, the behaviors are reinforcing and therefore self-propagating. Another behavioral model suggests that SMD represents a form of displacement behavior that the subject uses to reduce the anxiety produced in situations that engender helplessness.

Although the biochemical basis of SMD still remains to be elucidated, the abnormalities in striate dopaminergic innervation found in rhesus monkeys who have been separated from their mothers early in life have supported the hypothesis that SMD is a consequence of dopaminergic supersensitivity within these striatal systems. In support of this hypothesis, high doses of methylxanthines produce SMD in animals through an effect thought to be mediated through striatal D_2 receptors. Haloperidol has been shown to be effective in reducing stereotypic behaviors in cats and pigs (Willemse 1992; von Burrell and Hurnik, 1991). The efficacy of selective serotonin reuptake inhibitors (SSRIs) and the association of SMD with conditions believed to involve dysregulation of serotonergic systems (e.g., autism, Cornelia de Lange syndrome) have provided indirect evidence that serotonergic dysregulation plays an important role in the genesis of SMD.

Two primary hypotheses have been posited to suggest a pivotal role for endogenous opiates in the genesis of SMD. The *excessive opioid hypothesis* suggests that SMD occurs as a consequence of excessive endogenous opiate release that raises the subject's pain threshold (Hermann et al. 1989). The alternate hypothesis, *opiate addiction hypothesis*, suggests that SMD elicits self-reinforcing opiate release and subsequent dependence upon the reinforcing motor trigger (Cataldo and Harris 1982). In support of these opiate hypotheses, increased plasma enkephalin levels have been found in subjects with MR (Sandman 1988). The results of studies on the clinical efficacy of opiate antagonists remain inconclusive, with various studies on naltrexone reporting that the drug is effective in 0%–50% of subjects with SIB (Bauermeister et al. 1993; Sandman et al. 1993). Those studies that have documented that naltrexone is effective have noted, however, that the opiate antagonist is effective in reducing the subject's SIB but not any associated SMD (Sandman et al. 1993). In addition, it is important to appreciate that many patients receiving opiate antagonists will exhibit an increase in SIB (i.e., preextinction burst) before administration of the medication reducing these behaviors.

The pharmacological management of SMD remains poorly studied and consequently somewhat controversial. Several studies have reported that typical antipsychotics exert a selective effect in inhibiting SMD without producing any significant sedation or deterioration in general function (Aman et al. 1989; Cohen et al. 1980; Heistad et al. 1979). Several other studies have reported that, although neuroleptics are effective in reducing SMD, their efficacy comes at the price of reducing the patient's overall functional capacity (Anderson et al. 1982; Campbell et al. 1982). A recent open-label study reported that risperidone was effective in reducing SIB and aggressive behavior in a small case series of 13 patients (Khan 1997). Although the clinical efficacy of other currently available atypical neuroleptics (i.e., olanzapine and quetiapine) in SMD has not been formally studied, our clinical experience indicates that olanzapine, in particular, may have significant efficacy in this regard. In our experience, the potent sedating and anticholinergic side effects of clozapine limit its use in many patients with MR.

Several studies have confirmed that the SSRIs are effective in reducing self-injurious stereotypic behaviors such as trichotillomania and nail biting (Gordon et al. 1993; Sovner 1993; Swedo et al. 1993) in patients with SIB who are autistic (McDougle et al. 1996). The serotonergic tricyclic clomipramine has been shown to be superior to desipramine (a predominantly noradrenergic reuptake inhibitor) and placebo for the treatment of SMD (Castellanos et al. 1996; Garber 1992; Lewis 1996).

One study has reported the efficacy of valproic acid in reducing SIB in 12 of 18 patients (Kastner et al. 1993). Clinical response in this study was associated with a history of seizure disorder and affective symptoms. Two small studies have reported that the β-blockers propranolol (dose range 90–410 mg/day) and pindolol (40 mg/day) were effective in reducing SIB in small samples of patients with MR (Luchins and Dojka 1989; Ratey and Lindem 1991).

In summary, although SMD and SIB are extremely common and disabling symptoms in patients with MR, their pharmacological treatment remains in its infancy. The development of animal models of stereotypy promise to provide new insights into the neurobiology and treatment of these disorders (Stein and Simeon 1998).

Behavioral modification techniques provide a safe and effective treatment of SMD and SIB that is unfortunately increasingly overlooked (Ammerman 1998; Keuthen and O'Sullivan 1998). Unfortunately, these behavioral approaches are often construed to involve aversive techniques that have been "outlawed" within the MR community. Research data indicate that behavioral modification techniques are effective in reducing SMD, provided the intervention is developed by a skilled behavioral analyst who is able to perform a detailed functional assessment of the particular behaviors and select appropriate behavioral interventions (Keuthen and O'Sullivan 1998). These programs are expensive to implement, however, and require the cooperation of the patient's entire social milieu.

Aggression

Aggression toward others and destruction of property is extremely common among people with MR and has been reported to occur in 30% of the residents of public facilities and in 16% of community facilities (Hill and Bruinicks 1984). Aggression is the most frequent reason why persons with MR are admitted to psychiatric facilities or are prescribed psychotropic medications. Despite the magnitude of the problem and its devastating impact on individuals and public health resources, little is known about its etiology and treatment in persons with MR. It is our clinical experience that these behaviors frequently persist or increase in late life and are the genesis of significant social morbidity among this group.

A number of studies have addressed the efficacy of psychotropic medications in reducing aggression in persons with MR. Unfortunately all of these studies share the same methodological pitfall, that is, they fail to appreciate that, rather than representing a unitary disorder, aggressive behavior in the person with MR may be the manifestation of distinct psychopathological processes. Given the heterogeneity of aggression within the population with MR, any attempt to undertake a clinical trial of any single psychotropic agent in a sample of patients with MR who are aggressive is likely to produce conflicting results.

Numerous studies have reported that neuroleptics (including thioridazine, trifluoperazine, haloperidol, chlorpromazine, and clopenthixol) are effective in reducing aggressive behavior (Bauermeister et al. 1993; Kiernan

1995; Rubin 1997). However, in virtually all studies, in addition to reducing aggressive behaviors, neuroleptics have been reported to produce a decline in the patient's functional status (Bauermeister et al. 1993). Limited case series have reported that clozapine is helpful in reducing the aggression of patients with MR who have any of a wide range of psychiatric disorders (Cohen and Underwood 1994).

Although at least 10 published studies have addressed the efficacy of lithium in aggression in MR, only two of these were methodologically sound (Bauermeister et al. 1993). All these studies have reported that lithium is effective in reducing aggressive behavior with particular susceptibility to the drug's side effects (Bauermeister et al. 1993).

Several recent reports have indicated that SSRIs may be effective for aggressive behavior—most particularly in patients with autism (Markowitz 1992; McDougle et al. 1997). Other medications that have been reported (in poorly controlled studies) to be beneficial in treating aggression in MR include propranolol, reserpine, and diazepam (Bauermeister et al. 1993).

The association between depression and aggression has been described above. Reiss et al. (1993) reported an incidence of depression of 8.9% among 528 individuals with MR who were receiving community-based services. Of particular note, 40% of subjects with depression exhibited aggressive behavior compared with 10% of nondepressed subjects. Charlot et al. (1993) reported that, within a cohort of 16 subjects with MR with depression, 75% displayed aggressive behavior and 50% displayed SIB. The aggression exhibited by these subjects with MR with depression was characterized by interpersonal irritability, dysphoria, and frequent remorse. It is interesting to note that "irritable" mood is an acceptable alternative for the DSM-IV diagnostic criteria for depression in children. Although the issue has not been scientifically assessed, one can reasonably assume that the aggression associated with depression should respond to effective antidepressant treatments.

Sociopathic behavior represents an important cause of aggressive behavior in MR. As in any other social group, people with MR who live together will develop hierarchical patterns of dominance and subordination. Changes in the social milieu, challenges to the social hierarchy, or the arrival of new members into the community will result in power struggles that frequently manifest as aggression. This predatory aggression is typically directed toward a particular individual or individuals and is purposeful, sustained, nonstereotypic, not associated with remorse, and is "cold-blooded" (i.e., there are no associated autonomic symptoms). It is important that predatory aggression be distinguished from other forms of aggression so that behavioral, rather than pharmacological, interventions can

be established. In our experience, elderly patients with MR are typically the victims, rather than the perpetrators, of predatory aggression.

Because some patients with MR may have sustained neurotrauma, they are likely to exhibit the intermittent, stimulus-bound, short-lived, explosive aggression stemming from damage to the orbitofrontal cortex. In addition to behavioral interventions, SSRIs appear to be the treatment of choice for reducing disinhibited violence (Ranen et al. 1996). (Also see Chapter 22 in this volume.)

Seizure Disorders

The epidemiology of seizure disorders in the elderly population with MR has not been studied. However, an extrapolation of data available in the younger population with MR suggests that seizure disorders are a significant problem that produces major behavioral and physical morbidity. Although the data remain contradictory, the overall prevalence of epilepsy in mild MR is approximately 15% and increases to at least 30% in patients with severe MR (Sillanpaa 1996). As one would expect, the prevalence of epilepsy is higher in institutionalized patients and in those with cerebral palsy or specific congenital disorders associated with seizures (e.g., Angelman syndrome, West's syndrome, tuberous sclerosis). As many as 75% of patients with DS and comorbid AD experience seizures (Collacott 1993). Recurrent partial and generalized seizures occur in 25% of patients with fragile X syndrome, many of whom live into old age (Forsgren et al. 1990).

Attempts to classify seizures in the patient with MR according to the classification system of the International League Against Epilepsy are fraught with difficulties. Mariani et al. (1993) reported that they were able to specifically classify the seizure type of only 28% of their sample of patients with MR. Convulsive status epilepticus appears to be more common in this patient population, with one study reporting an incidence of 18.7%. The differential diagnosis of paroxysmal alteration in consciousness is outlined in Table 21–3.

Pseudoseizures appear to be more common in patients with MR with or without epilepsy, and making the diagnosis presents the clinician with a formidable challenge. Although some clinical characteristics aid in distinguishing pseudoseizures from epilepsy (e.g., duration > 3 minutes, gradual termination, absence of cyanosis, whole-body rigidity, pelvic thrusting, absence of a postictal confusion), a definitive diagnosis of pseudoseizures is usually difficult to reach. In particular, temporolimbic or frontal partial seizures can mimic pseudoseizures and can be difficult to diagnose even with videotelemetry, prolactin assays, and depth electrode studies.

TABLE 21–3. Differential diagnosis of nonepileptic "spells" in mental retardation

Cerebral hypoxia
Reflex and mechanical syncope
Transient global cerebral ischemia
Cardiogenic
Migraine

Involuntary paroxysmal movement disorders
Dyskinesias
Stereotypic movement disorders
Exaggerated startle response

Sleep disorders
Night terrors
Pavor nocturnus
Head banging
Rapid-eye-movement sleep disorder
Somnambulism
Benign nocturnal myoclonus
Sleep apnea

Psychogenic episodes
Hyperventilation syndromes
Panic attacks
Dissociative episodes
Breath-holding spells
Pseudoseizures
Posttraumatic stress disorder

Metabolic derangements
Hypoglycemia
Hypokalemia

Patients with MR who experience seizures are more likely to demonstrate behavioral problems such as aggression, emotional lability, and SIB compared with matched control subjects (Hermann 1982). The largest study in this regard reported that, of patients with MR who had seizures, "behavior disorders" occurred in 40%; "temper tantrums" in 38%; hyperkinesis in 30%; and "autism" in 15% (Corbett et al. 1975). The relationship of seizures to secondary thought, mood, and personality disorders in persons with MR has not been investigated.

The effective treatment of epilepsy in patients with MR demands a team approach that takes into account the physical and psychological antecedents and sequelae of the patient's seizures. Caretakers should be educated to identify unusual seizure events such as staring or motor automatisms and are important allies in identifying and avoiding environmental seizure precipitants. The vulnerability of the patient with MR to the adverse effects of anticonvulsants presents the clinician with difficult pharmacological challenges. In particular, agents with sedating side effects (e.g., phenobarbitone, phenytoin) are seldom tolerated and typically produce an unacceptable decline in functional status (Corbett et al. 1985). In addition, the patient with MR and seizures is likely to be sensitive to the ataxic side effects of anticonvulsants. A recent case series described five patients who developed unprovoked aggressive behavior after starting lamotrigine to control their seizures (Beran and Gibson 1998). Wherever possible, the clinician should attempt to employ monotherapy with an anticonvulsant known to exhibit positive psychotropic effects (e.g., carbamazepine, valproic acid, vigabatrin, gabapentin). However, despite the best efforts of the treatment team, epilepsy in the patient with MR is likely to present a formidable therapeutic challenge (also see Chapter 29 in this volume).

Conclusion

In this chapter, we attempt to provide a broad overview of the neuropsychiatric assessment and treatment of elderly patients with MR. Although the scientific foundations of clinical practice remain sparse, by adhering to the basic principles of a thorough clinical assessment and close monitoring, the clinician can provide effective, respectful, and safe care to a population whose needs have been overlooked for too long.

References

Aman MG, Teehan CJ, White AJ, et al: Haloperidol treatment with chronically medicated residents: dose effects on clinical behavior and reinforcement contingencies. Am J Ment Retard 93:452–460, 1989

American Association on Mental Retardation: Mental Retardation: Definition, Classification, and Systems of Support, 9th Edition. Washington, DC, American Association on Mental Retardation, 1992

American Psychiatric Association: Diagnostic and Statistical Manual of Mental Disorders, 3rd Edition. Washington, DC, American Psychiatric Association, 1980

American Psychiatric Association: Diagnostic and Statistical Manual of Mental Disorders, 3rd Edition, Revised. Washington, DC, American Psychiatric Association, 1987

American Psychiatric Association: Diagnostic and Statistical Manual of Mental Disorders, 4th Edition. Washington, DC, American Psychiatric Association, 1994

Ammerman RT: Psychological and behavioral interventions, in Textbook of Pediatric Neuropsychiatry. Edited by Coffey CE, Brumback RA. Washington, DC, American Psychiatric Press, 1998, pp 1429–1448

Anderson LT, Campbell M, Grega DM, et al: Haloperidol in the treatment of infantile autism: effects on learning and behavioral symptoms. Am J Psychiatry 141:1195–1202

Aylward EH, Burt DB, Thorpe LU, et al: Diagnosis of dementia in adults with intellectual disability. J Intellect Disabil Res 41:152–164, 1997

Balakrishnan TR, Wolf LC: Life expectancy of mentally retarded persons in canadaian institutions. Am J Mental Deficiency 80:650–662, 1976

Ballard CG, Oyebode F: Review: psychotic symptoms in patients with dementia. Int J Geriatr Psychiatry 10:743–752, 1995

Barak Y, Ring A, Levy D, et al: Disabling compulsions in 11 mentally retarded adults: an open trial of clomipramine SR. J Clin Psychiatry 56:116–117, 1995

Bauermeister AA, Todd ME, Sevin JA: Efficacy and specificity of pharmacological therapies for behavioral disorders in persons with mental retardation. Clin Neuropharmacol 16:271–294, 1993

Benson BA, Reiss S, Smith DA, et al: Psychosocial correlates of depression in mentally retarded adults, II: poor social skills. American Journal of Mental Deficiency 89:657–659, 1985

Beran RG, Gibson RJ: Aggressive behavior in intellectually challenged patients with epilepsy treated with lamotrigine. Epilepsia 39:280–282, 1988

Campbell M, Anderson LT, Small AM, et al: The effects of haloperidol on learning and behavior in autistic children. J Autism Dev Disord 12:167–175, 1982

Castellanos FX, Ritchie FG, Marsh WI, et al: DSM-IV stereotypic movement disorder: persistence of stereotypies of infancy in intellectually normal adolescents and adults. J Clin Psychiatry 57:116–122, 1996

Cataldo MF, Harris J: The biological basis for self-injury in the mentally retarded. Analysis and Intervention in Developmental Disabilities 2:21–39, 1982

Charlot LR: Irritability, aggression, and depression in adults with mental retardation: a developmental perspective. Psychiatric Annals 27:190–197, 1997

Charlot LR, Doucette AC, Mezzacappa E: Affective symptoms of institutionalized adults with mental retardation. Am J Ment Retard 98:408–416, 1993

Cohen IL, Campbell M, Posner D, et al: Behavioral effects of haloperidol in young autistic children. Journal of the American Academy of Child Psychiatry 19:665–677, 1980

Cohen SA, Underwood MT: The use of clozapine in a mentally retarded and aggressive population. J Clin Psychiatry 55:440–444, 1994

Collacott RA: Epilepsy, dementia and adaptive behavior in Down's syndrome. J Intellect Disabil Res 37:153–160, 1993

Collacott RA, Cooper SA, McGrother C: Differential rates of psychiatric disorders in adults with Down's syndrome compared with other mentally handicapped adults. Br J Psychiatry 161:671–674, 1992

Cooper SA: The psychiatry of elderly people with mental handicaps. Int J Geriatr Psychiatry 7:865–874, 1992

Cooper SA: Epidemiology of psychiatric disorders in elderly compared to younger adults with learning disabilities. Br J Psychiatry 170:375–380, 1997a

Cooper SA: Psychiatric symptoms of dementia among elderly people with learning disabilities. Int J Geriatr Psychiatry 12:662–666, 1997b

Cooper S-A: Ageing in people with learning disabilities: focus on Alzheimer's disease. Current Opinion in Psychiatry 11:535–539, 1998

Corbett JA: Psychiatric morbidity and mental retardation, in Psychiatric Illness and Mental Handicap. Edited by James FE, Snaith RP. London, Gaskell, 1979, pp 11–25

Corbett JA, Harris R, Robinson R: Epilepsy, in Mental Retardation and Developmental Disabilities, Vol VII. Edited by Woprtis J. New York, Raven, 1975, pp 79–111

Corbett JA, Trimble MR, Nichol T: Behavioral and cognitive impairment in children with epilepsy: the long-term effects of anticonvulsant therapy. Journal of the American Academy of Child Psychiatry 23:17–23, 1985

Crews WD, Bonaventura S, Rowe F: Dual diagnosis: prevalence of psychiatric disorders in a large state residential facility for individuals with mental retardation. Am J Mental Retard 98:688–731, 1994

Day KA: The elderly mentally handicapped in hospital: a clinical study. Journal of Mental Deficiency Research 31:131–146, 1987

Davis JP, Judd FK, Herman H: Depression in adults with intellectual disability. Aust N Z J Psychiatry 31:232–242, 1997

Dayton NA, Doering CR, Hilferty MM, et al: Mentality and life expectation in mental deficiency in Massachusetts: analysis of the fourteen year period 1917–1930 206:550–570, 1932

Duff R, LaRocca J, Lizzet A, et al: A comparison of the fears of mildly retarded children with adults of their mental age and chronological age matched controls. J Behav Ther Exp Psychiatry 12:121–124, 1981

Duncan AG, Penrose LC, Turnbull RC: A survey of the patients in a large mental hospital. Journal of Neurology and Psychopathology 16:225–238, 1936

Eaton LF, Menolascino FJ: Psychiatric disorders in the mentally retarded: types, problems and challenges. Am J Psychiatry 139:1297–1303, 1982

Forsgren L, Edvinsson SO, Blomquist HK, et al: Epilepsy in a population of mentally retarded adults. Epilepsy Res 6:234–248, 1990

Garber HJ, McGonigle JJ, Slomka GT, et al: Clomipramine treatment of stereotypic behaviors and self-injury in patients with developmental disabilities. J Am Acad Child Adolesc Psychiatry 31:1157–1160, 1992

Gordon CT, State RC, Nelson JE, et al: A double-blind comparison of clomipramine, desipramine, and placebo in the treatment of autistic disorder. Arch Gen Psychiatry 50:441–447, 1993

Heaton-Ward A: Psychosis in mental handicap. Br J Psychiatry 130:525–533, 1977

Heistad GT, Zimmerman RL: Double-blind assessment of mellaril in a mentally retarded population using detailed evaluations. Psychopharmacol Bull 15:86–88, 1979

Hermann BH, Hammock MK, Egan J: A role for opioid peptides in self-injurious behavior: dissociation from autonomic nervous system functioning. Dev Pharmacol Ther 12:81–89, 1989

Hermann BP: Neuropsychological functioning and psychopathology in children with epilepsy. Epilepsia 23: S45–S54, 1982

Heston LL, Mastri AR, Anderson AR, et al: The genetics of Alzheimer's disease. Association with hematological malignancy and Down's syndrome. Arch Gen Psychiatry 34: 976–981, 1981

Hill BK, Bruinicks RH: Maladaptive behavior of mentally retarded individuals in residential facilities. American Journal of Mental Deficiency 88:380–387, 1984

Holland AJ, Hon J, Hupert FA, et al: Population-based study of the prevalence and presentation of dementia in adults with Down's syndrome. Br J Psychiatry 172:493–498, 1998

Jacobson JW, Sutton MS, Janicki MP: Demography and characteristics of aging and aged mentally retarded persons, in Aging and Developmental Disabilities. Edited by Janicki MP, Wisniewski HM. Baltimore, MD, Brookes, 1985, pp 115–142

Kastner T, Finesmith R, Walsh K: Long-term administration of valproic acid in the treatment of affective symptoms in people with mental retardation. J Clin Psychopharmacol 13:444–451, 1993

Keuthen NJ, O'Sullivan RL: Behavioral treatment of stereotypic movement disorders. Psychiatric Annals 28:335–340, 1998

Khan BU: Brief report: risperidone for severely disturbed behavior and tardive dyskinesia in developmentally disabled adults. J Autism Dev Disord 27:479–489, 1997

Khreim I, Mikkelsen E: Anxiety disorders in adults with mental retardation. Psychiatric Annals 27:175–181

Kiernan C, Reeves D, Alborz A: The use of anti-psychotic drugs with adults with learning disabilities and challenging behavior. J Intellect Disabil Res 39:263–274, 1995

Krystal AD, Coffey CE: Neuropsychiatric considerations in the use of electroconvulsive therapy. J Neuropsychiatry Clin Neurosci 9:283–292, 1997

Legault JR: Study of the relationship of community living situation on independence and satisfaction in the lives of mentally retarded adults. J Intellect Disabil Res 36:129–141, 1992

Leonard HL, Swedo SE, Rapoport JL, et al: Treatment of childhood obsessive compulsive disorder with clomipramine and desipramine: a double-blind crossover comparison. Arch Gen Psychiatry 46:1088–1092, 1989

Lewis MH, Bodfish JW, Powell SB, et al: Clomipramine treatment for self-injurious behavior of individuals with mental retardation: a double-blind comparison with placebo. Am J Ment Retard 100:654–665, 1996

Lowry MA, Sovner R: Severe behavior problems associated with rapid cycling bipolar disorder in two adults with profound mental retardation. J Intellect Disabil Res 36: 269–281, 1992

Luchins DJ, Dojka D: Lithium and propranolol in aggression and self-injurious behavior in the mentally retarded. Psychopharmacol Bull 3:372–375, 1989

Lund J: Epilepsy and psychiatric disorder in the mentally retarded adult. Acta Psychiatr Scand 72:557–562, 1985

Mann DMA, Esiri MM: The pattern of acquisition of plaques and tangles in the brains of patients under age 50 years with Down's syndrome. J Neurol Sci 89:169–179, 1989

Mariani E, Ferini-Strambi L, Sala M, et al: Epilepsy in institutionalized patients with encephalopathy: clinical aspects and nosological considerations. Am J Ment Retard 98 (suppl):27–33, 1993

Markova I, Jahoda A, Catterhole M, et al: Living in hospital and hostel: the pattern of interactions of people with learning disabilities. J Intellect Disabil Res 36:115–127, 1992

Markowitz PI: Effect of fluvoxamine on self-injurious behavior in developmentally disabled: a preliminary study. J Clin Psychopharmacol 12:27–31, 1992

Mattson JL, Kazdin AE, Senatore V: Psychometric properties of the Psychopathology Instrument for Mentally Retarded Adults. Applied Research in Mental Retardation 5: 881–889, 1984

Mattson JL, Coe DA, Ardner WI, et al: A factor analytic study of Diagnostic Assessment for the Severely Handicapped (DASH) scale. Br J Psychiatry 159:404–409, 1991

McDermott S, Breen R, Platt T, et al: Do behavior changes herald physical illness in adults with mental retardation? Community Ment Health J 33:85–97, 1997

McDougle CJ, Naylor ST, Cohen DJ, et al: A double-blind placebo-controlled study of fluvoxamine in adults with autistic disorder. Arch Gen Psychiatry 53:1001–1008, 1996

Meins W: Symptoms of major depression in mentally retarded adults. J Intellect Disabil Res 39:41–45, 1995

Mikkelsen EJ, Albert LG, Emens M, et al: The efficacy of antidepressant medication for individuals with mental retardation. Psychiatric Annals 27: 198–206, 1997

Moss S, Patel P: Psychiatric symptoms associated with dementia in older people with learning disability. Br J Psychiatry 167:663–667, 1995

Moss S, Hogg J, Horne M: Demographic characteristics of a population of people with moderate, severe and profound intellectual disability (mental handicap) over 50 years of age: age structure, IQ and adaptive skills. J Intellect Disabil Res 36:387–401, 1992

Mukaetova-Ladinska EM, Harrington CR, Roth M, et al: Distribution of tau protein in Down's syndrome: quantitative differences from Down's syndrome. Developmental Brain Dysfunction (in press)

National Institute on Aging: Personnel for health needs of the elderly. Washington, DC, Department of Health and Human Services, 1987

Parette HP, Vanbiervliet A: Tentative findings of a study of the technology needs and use patterns of persons with mental retardation. J Intellect Disabil Res 36:7–27, 1992

Penrose LS: The incidence of mongolism in the general population. Journal of Mental Science 9:10, 1949

Ranen NG, Lipsey JR, Treisman G, et al: Sertraline in the treatment of severe aggressiveness in Huntington's disease. J Neuropsychiatry Clin Neurosci 8:338–340, 1996

Ratey JJ, Lindem KJ: β-Blockers as primary treatment for aggression for self-injury in the developmentally disabled, in Mental Retardation: Developing Pharmacotherapies. Edited by Ratey JJ. Washington, DC, American Psychiatric Press, 1991, pp 51–81

Ratey JJ, Sovner R, Mikkelson E, et al: Buspirone therapy for maladaptive behavior and anxiety in developmentally disabled persons. J Clin Psychiatry 50:382–384, 1989

Reiss S, Rojahn J: Joint occurrence of depression and aggression in children and adults with mental retardation. J Intellect Disabil Res 37:287–294, 1993

Royston MC, Kodical NS, Mann DMA: Quantitative analysis of B-amyloid deposition in Down's syndrome using computerised image analysis. Neurodegeneration 3:43–51, 1994

Rubin M: Use of atypical antipsychotics in children with mental retardation, autism, and other developmental disabilities. Psychiatric Annals 27:219–221, 1997

Rummans TA, Lauterbach EC, Coffey CE, et al: Pharmacologic Efficacy in neuropsychiatry: A review of placebo-controlled treatment trials. J Neuropsychiatry and Clinical Neurosciences 11(2):176–179, 1999

Ryan R: Posttraumatic stress disorder in persons with developmental disabilities. Community Ment Health J 30:45–54, 1994

Ryan RM: Post-traumatic stress disorder in persons with developmental disabilities, in Assessment and Treatment of Anxiety Disorders in Persons With Mental Retardation. Edited by Poindexter A. Kingston, NJ, NADD, 1996, pp 41–52

Ryan R, Sunada K: Medical evaluation of persons with mental retardation referred for psychiatric assessment. Gen Hosp Psychiatry 19:274–280, 1997

Sandman CA: β-Endorphin dysregulation in autistic and self-injurious behavior: a neurodevelopmental hypothesis. Synapse 2:193–199, 1988

Sandman CA, Hetrick WP, Taylor DV, et al: Naltrexone reduces self-injury and improves learning. Experimental and Clinical Psychopharmacolgy 1:242–258, 1993

Sansom DT, Singh I, Jawed SH, et al: Elderly people with learning disability in hospital: a psychiatric study. J Intellect Disabil Res 38:45–52, 1994

Sillanpaa M: Epilepsy in the mentally retarded, in Epilepsy in Children. Edited by Wallace S. London, Chapman & Hall, 1996, pp 417–427

Sovner R: Limiting factors in the use of DSM-II criteria in mentally retarded individuals. Psychopharmacol Bull 22: 1055–1059, 1986

Sovner R, Fox CJ, Lowery MJ, et al: Fluoxetine treatment of depression and associated self-injury in two adults with mental retardation. J Intellect Disabil Res 37:307–311, 1993

Stein DJ, Simeon D: Pharmacotherapy of stereotypic movement disorders. Psychiatric Annals 28:327–331, 1998

Stein DJ, Niehaus DJH, Seedat S, et al: Phenomenology of stereotypic movement disorders. Psychiatric Annals 28: 307–312, 1998

Sturmey P: The use of DSM and ICD diagnostic criteria in people with mental retardation. A review of empirical studies. J Nerv Ment Dis 181:38–41, 1993

Swedo SE, Rapoport JL, Leonard H, et al: Obsessive-compulsive disorder in children and adolescents: clinical phenomenology of 70 consecutive cases. Arch Gen Psychiatry 46:335–341, 1989

Vandenberg B: Fears of normal and retarded children. Psychol Rep 72:473–474, 1993

Vitiello B, Behar D: Mental retardation and psychiatric illness. Hosp Community Psychiatry 43:494–499, 1992

Von Burrell E, Hurnik JF: The effect of haloperidol on the performance of stereotyped behavior in sows. Life Sci 49: 309–314, 1991

Walsh KK, Kastner T, Criscione T: Characteristics of hospitalizations for people with developmental disabilities: utilization, costs, and impact of care coordination. Am J Ment Retard 101:505–520, 1997

Willemse T: The effect of dopamine antagonists on psychogenic alopecia in cats. Proceedings of the Second World Congress of Veterinary Dermatology, Montreal, May 13–16, 1992

22

Aggression

Constantine G. Lyketsos, M.D., M.H.S.

Human aggression is a complex topic because of uncertainties in defining the term, because of limited understanding of the underlying neuroscience, and because the environmental contributions to the development of the aggression are also not well delineated. Knowledge regarding aggression among the elderly is further limited by the relative absence of specific research in this age group. Thus, it is necessary to extrapolate knowledge from younger samples to develop a rudimentary understanding of aggression in the elderly. The reader should keep in mind that inferences drawn from the young might not always apply to the old. Nevertheless, from the existing literature, it does appear clear that aggression in the elderly is strongly associated with the presence of neuropsychiatric disorders, particularly dementia.

In this chapter, I focus on physically aggressive behavior (PAB), defined as any observable behavior that threatens to or actually inflicts harm on an individual or on an inanimate object. This definition does not require intent to harm because of the difficulty in ascertaining intent among the elderly, particularly those with dementia. Additionally, this definition excludes other behaviors among the elderly that have been described as "agitated," such as nonthreatening verbal outbursts, wandering, intrusiveness, uncooperativeness, or other aberrant motor behaviors (see Chapter 24 in this volume). In this chapter, I do not discuss aggression directed against the elderly. Although an important public health problem, aggression directed at the elderly is usually perpetrated by younger persons, placing it beyond the scope of this chapter.

The impact of PAB on elderly patients and those around them should immediately be apparent. Physically aggressive elderly patients are at greater risk of harming themselves and others. Additionally, they are much more likely to be restrained, treated with medications, hospitalized, or placed in an institutional setting such as a nursing home (see Chapter 37 in this volume). Similarly, the care of physically aggressive elderly patients is much more labor intensive for direct care providers, whether family or professional, and for clinicians and psychiatrists. Thus, physically aggressive behavior in the elderly represents a serious clinical problem.

Supported in part by National Institute of Mental Health Grant 1R01-MH56511 and by the Copper Ridge Institute. The author is grateful to Cynthia Steele, R.N., M.P.H., for her comments and to Betty Burgeois for preparing this chapter for publication.

In this chapter, I begin with a consideration of the epidemiology of PAB in the elderly as well as its risk factors. A discussion follows of the etiology of PAB by applying the epidemiological causal model of *host, agent, environment*. A segment on the evaluation and differential diagnosis of aggression in the elderly is next, and then I conclude with a review of management approaches for aggression in the elderly. Every effort is made to base the content of this chapter on the empirical literature. Where there are limitations in the available evidence, the discussion is based on the aggression literature in nonelderly populations and on my clinical experience.

Epidemiology

Direct estimates of the prevalence and incidence of PAB among the elderly are not available, and essentially no literature exists on incidence. The general population prevalence is probably approximately 10–20 cases per 1,000 elderly people. This indirect estimate is derived from the prevalence of aggression among a random sample of community-residing elderly persons with dementia in the United Kingdom (Burns et al. 1990). Another indirect estimate comes from the Cabe County Study of Memory in Aging. In that study, 1,002 elderly residents underwent comprehensive neuropsychiatric evaluations and were also rated on the Cummings Neuropsychiatric Inventory. Those without dementia had a prevalence of "agitation-aggression" of 3% (19/672), and those with dementia had a prevalence of 24% (78/330) (Lyketsos et al., unpublished observations, 1999).

Prevalence data from clinical settings are much more widely available. Almost all are from studies of individuals who have cognitive impairment. Most studies reviewed involve small samples ($N < 100$), although a few included a sample size of several hundred.

From community-residing samples, typically of patients who attend geriatric, geropsychiatric, or dementia clinics, it is estimated that 10%–15% of elderly had been physically aggressive in the past month, and that 15%–30% had been physically aggressive in the past year (Aarsland et al. 1996; Deutsch et al. 1991; Eastley et al. 1997; Gibbons et al. 1997; Gilley et al. 1997; Hamel et al. 1990; Malone et al. 1993; Mendez et al. 1990; Paveza et al. 1992; Ryden 1988; Shah 1993; Swearer et al. 1988; Tsai et al. 1996). Some estimates suggest that as many as 50%–60% of elderly patients had been aggressive in the past year (Patel and Hope 1993; Ryden 1988). In our study of community-residing outpatients with dementia, by using a strict definition of physically aggressive behavior we

found that 15% of patients had been aggressive in the past 2 weeks (Lyketsos et al. 1999a).

Samples from nursing homes indicate a somewhat higher prevalence of PAB among elderly patients, with estimates ranging from a low of 23% (Zimmer et al. 1984) to a high of 91% for all types of aggressive behavior (Winger et al. 1987) (see Chapter 37 in this volume). The most consistent estimates suggest that PAB is exhibited by 40%–48% of nursing home residents over a year's time (Chandler and Chandler 1988; Rovner et al. 1986).

Hospital samples from geropsychiatric units indicate that between 20% (Burns et al. 1990) and 47% of elderly are physically aggressive (Rabins et al. 1982). Thus, although physical aggression is uncommon in the community, it is a frequent problem in specific clinical samples.

Studies of the characteristics of PAB among elderly persons have also been reported. In most of these studies, it is unclear what proportion suffered from dementia and what proportion did not. However, it is likely that most elderly in these samples had dementia because these were studies from clinical settings, such as nursing homes or geriatric psychiatry clinics, where the prevalence of dementia is high.

Physical aggression among the elderly usually takes the form of pushing, shoving, kicking, pinching, or hitting (Cohen-Mansfield and Billing 1986; Patel and Hope 1993). Less frequent are biting, scratching, and destroying property (Cohen-Mansfield and Billing 1986; Patel and Hope 1993). Occasionally, elderly patients will trip others, hit themselves, or bang on tables and walls (Cohen-Mansfield and Billing 1986; Patel and Hope 1993). Male elderly patients will also at times exhibit what has been described as "sexually aggressive behaviors," usually meaning grabbing the breasts of women or slapping women on the buttocks (Cohen-Mansfield and Billing 1986; Patel and Hope 1993). These physically aggressive behaviors have been found to be distinct from the other 11 "agitated" behaviors in the elderly in factor analytic and similar studies (Cohen-Mansfield and Billing 1986; Patel and Hope 1992).

Precise estimates of the frequency of individual behaviors (e.g., hitting) are rare and depend on the clinical setting. Ryden (1988) reported that, over a year's time, 27% of elderly persons with dementia in the community exhibited threatening or physical aggression at some point: 26% pushed or shoved, 24% threw an object, 16% damaged property, 14% pinched or squeezed, and another 14% hit. Other aggressive behaviors were much less frequent. In contrast, in a nursing home study (Malone et al. 1993)—with prevalence of dementia uncertain—it was reported that 57% of aggressive behaviors consisted of hitting; 17% of grabbing or throwing; 6% of kicking; 6% of punching; 5% of pushing; 5% of scratching; and 2.1% of biting.

A different study (Bridges-Parlet et al. 1994) investigated to whom the physically aggressive behaviors in a nursing home were directed. Here too, the prevalence of dementia in the sample was unknown. Eighty-two percent of PAB was directed toward nursing staff, and 18% was directed toward other nursing home residents. Fifty-four percent of PAB occurred during personal care, such as bathing, dressing, grooming, etc. Eighteen percent occurred during redirection of the patient. Only 11% had no apparent antecedent.

Evidence indicates two subgroups of elderly patients who exhibit PAB. (This distinction probably applies best to elderly with dementia.) First are the majority who engage in few or infrequent aggressive acts, usually during daily care. Second are a minority who commit repetitive and frequent aggressive acts of a wide variety, who are hard to manage, and who frequently require restraint. For example, in a prospective, 1-year study of aggressive behaviors in a nursing home, Malone et al. (1993) reported that, of a sample of 349 residents (with the proportion with dementia unknown), 47 exhibited PAB at some point during the year. Of these, 6 patients (13%) accounted for 44% of all PAB episodes, whereas the other 41 patients were aggressive fewer than two times.

We had similar findings in routine resident surveillance at Copper Ridge, a specialty residence that includes a nursing home and an assisted-living facility for 126 persons with dementia. At admission to the facility, approximately 28% of residents (of a sample of 116) had been aggressive in the past week. After admission, 9 residents (7 of them men) were responsible for 48% of aggressive acts over a year's time (M. Lavrisha, personal communication, May 1998).

With regard to the temporal characteristics of aggressive episodes among the elderly, reports from nursing home settings provide mixed results. One unreplicated study (Meyer et al. 1991) reported an increased prevalence of aggression in the winter months. Cohen-Mansfield and Billing (1986), in their studies of "agitation" in nursing home elderly, found that aggression was more likely to occur in the late afternoon and evening. In contrast, others suggest that it is more common in the daytime, especially in the morning (Meyer et al. 1991; Patel and Hope 1992). In the surveillance of PAB at Copper Ridge (both in the assisted-living and in the skilled nursing facility), no consistent variation between daytime and evening nursing shifts was found in the frequency of the patients' aggressive behaviors, although they were much less frequent on night

shifts. Also, there was no apparent variation by season or lunar cycle (M. Lavrisha, personal communication, May 1998).

Several risk factors for physical aggression in elderly patients have been described. The most consistent across studies are dementia, delirium, male gender, and the presence of psychotic symptoms (Aarsland et al. 1996; Burns and Levy 1990; Deutsch et al. 1991; Eastley et al. 1997; Gilley et al. 1997; Hamel et al. 1990; Lyketsos et al. 1999a; Malone et al. 1993; Mendez et al. 1990; Mungas 1983; Paveza et al. 1992; Ryden 1988; Shah 1993; Swearer et al. 1988; Tsai et al. 1996). Other risk factors include depression (Lyketsos et al. 1999a), greater severity of dementia (Eastley et al. 1997; Hamel et al. 1990; Ryden 1988; Swearer et al. 1988), earlier age at dementia onset (Tsai et al. 1996), wandering (Tsai et al. 1996), concurrent medical illness (Malone et al. 1993), limited space and living arrangements (Paveza et al. 1992), and sleep disorder (Tsai et al. 1996).

Several environmental risk factors for aggression among the elderly have been described. These factors relate both to the people around the patient, particularly their caregivers, as well as to the ambient environment. Environmental noise, inadequate lighting, and moving to unfamiliar places are risk factors for aggression (Silliman et al. 1988). Also, specific caregiver characteristics are important. Caregivers who are depressed or irritable might precipitate aggression among elderly patients (Tsai et al. 1996). The approach of the caregiver to the patient is also critically important. Caregivers who are demanding, intrusive, confrontational, or who rush patients through tasks that are difficult for them might also precipitate aggression (Minde et al. 1990). One study has found that nursing home caregivers who have "subtly adversarial management styles" may also precipitate aggression from elderly patients (Cooper et al. 1989).

The relationship between physical aggression and psychopathology must be underlined. Several studies have found a relationship between PAB in the elderly, particularly elderly with dementia, and symptoms of psychosis (delusions and hallucinations) or depression (reviewed by Lyketsos et al. 1999a; Patel and Hope 1993). In a study of PAB in outpatients with dementia who were residing in the community, we found that PAB was closely linked to the presence of moderate to severe depressive symptomatology and that this association remained strong after adjusting for severity of dementia, delusions, or hallucinations. Indeed, after adjusting for severity of dementia and depression, the association between aggression and delusions or hallucinations was no longer significant (Lyketsos et al. 1999a).

▮ Etiology of Aggression in the Elderly

The expression of aggressive behavior is phylogenetically quite old. "Adaptive" aggression is present throughout the order Mammalia (Saver et al. 1995). Such adaptive aggression, which is readily observed in animals, has a variety of purposes. These purposes were classified by Moyer (Saver et al. 1995) into seven types of hostile behavior: predatory, territorial, intermale, fear-induced, maternal, irritable, and instrumental. Each of these types of aggression appears to have its own "eliciting stimulus." For example, a natural prey might elicit predatory aggression, whereas frustration, deprivation, or pain might elicit irritable aggression. Each of these aggressive subtypes is probably controlled by a distinct, albeit overlapping, neural system, which in humans is located in the more primitive aspects of the brain (Saver et al. 1995).

As the human species evolved, it developed complex regulatory mechanisms for these more basic aggressive "drives" (Saver et al. 1995). Areas of the brainstem, in particular in the pons and mesencephalon, mediate certain stereotypic movements associated with aggression, including facial expression and the autonomic aspects of aggression (Saver et al. 1995). The hypothalamus appears to be a basic regulator and suppressor of aggression (Saver et al. 1995). Specific cortical structures such as the amygdala, temporolimbic cortex, and prefrontal cortex also appear to be higher level regulators of aggression (Saver et al. 1995). Thus, existing neuroscience proposes that aggression in humans has its origin in basic, phylogenetically old drives, each with a specific purpose and neural structure (Krakowski 1997). These drives are regulated by complex interplay of more primitive and more advanced regulating mechanisms that involve cognitive and affective components.

Several neurotransmitter systems have been found to modulate aggressive behaviors (Saver et al. 1995; Volavka 1997). The systems include serotonin, acetylcholine, dopamine, norepinephrine, and γ-aminobutyric acid (GABA). Serotonin is associated with reduction of aggression; serotonin brain levels are lower in persons who die of violent suicide, and serotonin metabolites in cerebrospinal fluid are decreased in violent criminal offenders (Saver et al. 1995; Volavka 1997). Serotonin agonists, such as buspirone, a relatively selective serotonin subtype 1A agonist, reduce certain types of aggression in mice (Saver et al. 1995; Volavka 1997). The effect of serotonin is most specific in types of aggression that are mediated by testosterone (Saver et al. 1995; Volavka 1997). Also, among patients with Alzheimer's disease who have come to autopsy, absence of aggression has been associated with relative sparing of serotonergic neurons (Proctor et al. 1992).

Acetylcholine is associated with increased aggression, particularly predatory aggression. As well, cholinesterase inhibitors have led to aggressive behavior in humans, as noted in case reports (Volavka 1997).

Catecholamine systems are also associated with aggression (Saver at al. 1995; Volavka 1997). Norepinephrine, particularly when acting on the α_2 receptor, increases aggressive behavior. For example, patients with Alzheimer's disease who were aggressive before death have higher counts of α_2-adrenergic receptors in the cerebellum at autopsy (Russo-Neustadt and Cotman 1997). Norepinephrine antagonists, such as clonidine, reduce such behavior. Adrenergic blocking agents, such as propranolol, reduce aggressive behavior in laboratory animals and in diverse patient groups exhibiting violent behaviors (Saver et al. 1995; Volavka 1997).

Dopamine antagonists also tend to reduce aggression, and dopamine agonists such as apomorphine induce aggressive fighting in rats (Saver et al. 1995; Volavka 1997). In humans with dementia, aggression is associated with relative preservation of the dopaminergic system at autopsy (Victoroff et al. 1996).

GABA is widely known to inhibit aggression in animals and humans (Saver et al. 1995; Volavka 1997). GABA antagonists can induce mouse-killing behavior in mice, and benzodiazepines, which are GABA mediators, can attenuate aggression in animals (Saver et al. 1995; Volavka 1997).

Testosterone and other androgens are important mediators of certain types of aggression in males. Multiple studies suggest that aggression is more common in males across species (Saver et al. 1995). Additionally, androgen antagonists have been associated with reductions of violent behavior across species, including in humans (Saver et al. 1995; Volavka 1997). One small study found that serum testosterone level was correlated with the likelihood of aggression in male elderly patients with dementia (Orengo et al. 1997). Case reports indicate alleviation of aggression in the elderly with dementia by antiandrogen treatment, such as with progesterone and leuprolide (Amadeo 1996; Kyomen et al. 1991; Lyketsos et al. 1998).

Given this rudimentary understanding of the neuroscience and risk factors relating to aggression, and assuming that it applies to the elderly, it is useful to consider an epidemiological model of host, agent, environment as it applies to the development of aggression. Aggressive behaviors among the elderly might be considered the product of one or more perturbations in the host, agent, environment triangle. Different types of aggressive behavior might be the product of different perturbations, and different magnitudes and types of perturbation might give rise to different types of aggressive behavior.

Host factors to consider include direct damage to the

neural substrate regulating aggression (see above). This damage may involve inhibitors of aggression, although it may also involve overactivity of aggressive drives. Damage or dysfunction may come from diseases of the brain, with conditions causing dementia being the most common. Thus, Alzheimer's disease, frontotemporal degeneration (Hooten and Lyketsos 1996), and stroke with damage in amygdala temporolimbic structures, dorsolateral prefrontal cortex, hypothalamus, medulla, or mesencephalon may be most relevant here. Similarly, metabolic disturbances might disrupt brain inhibitory pathways and give rise to aggression. Therefore, elderly people who have brain damage from one of the diseases causing dementia or who have a metabolic disturbance (including delirium) from a general medical condition are more likely to exhibit PAB, as noted by the epidemiological findings.

Brain disease leading to concurrent damage in areas that exercise inhibitory control over aggression might account for the more serious cases of aggression reported in nursing homes and that are chronic and hard to treat. The occurrence of aggression at certain times of day might also be associated with effects of the circadian rhythm on the inhibitory control of aggression.

Other factors that influence a host's ability to modulate aggressive drives include the mood state or the presence of other abnormal mental states, such as delirium, delusions, and hallucinations. A low mood state, such as depression, or an irritable, expansive, or anxious mood state might make an elderly person more likely to exhibit aggression. Delirium, by impairing an elderly person's level of consciousness, might lead to fear, suspiciousness, and irritability and thus be a predisposition to PAB. Similarly, the presence of a delusion or a hallucination might make an elderly person more likely to misinterpret a stimulus or a situation that is otherwise nonthreatening.

As noted, the great majority of aggressive episodes in the elderly are associated with specific antecedent, perhaps provoking, stimuli. The stimulus or provocation plays the role of the agent in the epidemiological triangle. Several features of this stimulus might be considered, including the occurrence of a random stimulus presented to a vulnerable host. For example, hungry elderly persons with dementia might become aggressive if they smell or see food. Agnosia may also increase the likelihood of aggression as frustrated patients attempt to communicate with or assess their surroundings. Patients with aphasia who cannot understand what they are being told might become aggressive in self-defense when someone intrudes in their personal space and attempts to help them bathe or clean. This phenomenon would account for PAB episodes in patients with dementia occurring during daily and physical care. In the same way,

caregivers who approach a vulnerable patient in an inappropriate way might provoke an aggressive behavior.

Environmental features that facilitate the expression of aggressive behaviors may interfere with the host's ability to modulate aggressive behavior, may accentuate certain aspects of the stimulus, or may themselves provide an adverse stimulus to the host. Loud environments might distract a patient's attention and make it harder to inhibit an aggressive drive if the patient is hungry. An unfamiliar environment might provide a stimulus for irritable aggression. The presence of many other people in the environment, such as in a nursing home, might stimulate threat-induced aggression or territorial aggression.

In summary, the etiology of aggression in the elderly is complex and is best understood as an inappropriate display of phylogenetically old, adaptive behavior that is being inappropriately modulated. Damage to modulating systems, specific stimuli that might provoke the expression of aggression, or environments that might interfere with modulation or provide particular stimulation increase the chances of expression of PAB.

Evaluation of Aggression in an Elderly Person

The evaluation of any elderly person with aggression should attempt to *define* the areas outlined in Table 22–1 (Lyketsos et al. 1998). The first goal of evaluation is careful clinical description (define the case). The actual aggressive behavior should be noted in detail as well as its impact, such as injury to the patient and others or damage to property. The temporal characteristics and modifying variables of the behavior (e.g., apparent precipitants) should be described in detail. Other features of the case should also be understood. For example, does the patient show any evidence of cognitive decline or dementia (amnesia, agnosia, aphasia, apraxia, executive disorder)? Does the patient have evident psychiatric symptoms such as depression, anxiety, delusions, or hallucinations? Is there evidence of a medical disorder or symptom (most common are urinary tract infection, pain, constipation)? Exacerbations of preexisting medical conditions should also be considered. What medicines is the patient taking? Are they being consumed properly or could there be a possibility of undermedication or overmedication by accident or on purpose? What is the patient's personal, social, and family history?

The information necessary to describe a PAB should be collected in a standard neuropsychiatric examination as described elsewhere in this textbook (see Chapters 5 and 6 in this volume). A careful history of present illness, sub-

TABLE 22–1. Evaluation of an elderly person with aggression

Define

    Describe the aggressive behaviors in detail

    Ascertain the temporal characteristics of the behavior(s)

        Frequency, duration, time of day

    Specify precipitants, mediators, alleviators of the behavior

    Determine other features of the case

Decode

    Host factors

        Cognitive disorder

        Mental disorder or syndrome

        Medical disorder

        Medications

        Brain damage

    Stimulus/provocation factors

        Caregiver approach

    Environmental factors

        Ambient environment

stance use (especially alcohol), medical status, review of systems, personality, and psychiatric status should all be reviewed and updated. An examination should be conducted including general medical, neurological, cognitive, and general mental status examination directed at describing the behaviors and the associated features of the case.

The evaluation should also include laboratory and other necessary studies as part of determining potential contributing causes of the aggression. Blood tests to investigate abnormalities in electrolyte levels and liver and thyroid function should be considered. Toxicology screens or medication levels to investigate acute intoxication with substances or chronic use of substances should also be conducted. To rule out a urinary tract infection, urinalysis and urine culture with sensitivity should be considered in almost every case of aggressive behavior in an elderly person. If clinically appropriate, electrocardiography and chest X ray should also be ordered. In cases where the aggression is stereotypical and episodic, electroencephalography might be considered to rule out a seizure disorder (see Chapter 29 in this volume). If there is evidence of injury or an acute neurological event, head computed tomography or magnetic resonance imaging should be considered to investigate an intracranial cause of aggression. It is presumed that in patients with dementia who exhibit aggression a complete dementia work-up has already been conducted.

After the evaluation, the psychiatrist should *decode* the case—this is essentially a process of differential diagnosis, looking at host, agent, and environment as they relate to the particular case. Are there important host factors that likely have made the patient vulnerable to expressing aggression by affecting her or his ability to modulate aggression? For example, is the aggressive behavior occurring independently or is it occurring in the context of coexisting brain damage, dementia, psychopathology, delirium, or an active (new or exacerbated) medical condition? Could the aggression be related to one or more medications? Is it linked to specific aspects of dementia, such as aphasia? Physical aggression that occurs in the context of other conditions (e.g., depression, pneumonia) should generally be considered as secondary to these other conditions. The implication is that removal or treatment of the host vulnerability will lead to resolution of the aggression.

Next, stimulus factors should be considered. For example, is the aggression always provoked? What are the features of the provoking stimulus? If there is no apparent stimulus, is additional observation needed to confirm the absence of a provocation? If provoked, is the provocation daily care or some other circumstance? If aggression is occurring during daily care, what exactly is the provocation: caregiver approach, specific activities, other? Does the aggression always occur with a specific caregiver (e.g., a spouse or a nursing aide)? What else in a stimulus may be contributing to the expression of aggression?

Finally, environmental factors should be considered. What is the ambient environment like at the time of the PAB? Is it too cold or hot? Too loud or quiet? Too bright or too dark? Is there inadequate stimulation to the patient by the environment? Does the aggression occur at specific times of day? Are there any other environmental patterns associated with the aggression?

At the conclusion of the decoding process, the clinician should have a good understanding of the aggressive behavior and the contributing causes to its expression from the point of view of host, stimulus, and environment. The neuropsychiatrist should also have a sense of the modifiable and unmodifiable contributors to the aggression. For example, if a contributing factor is believed to be the presence of a depressive illness, this factor may be modifiable through appropriate treatment. The same is true if the contributing factor is a delusion. However, if the contributing factor is advanced dementia, resolution of the underlying disease is more difficult.

Management of Aggressive Behavior in the Elderly

The define and decode process above typically will leave the neuropsychiatrist with an understanding of the causes of aggression in a particular case and with a set of potentially modifiable contributing features. For example, if the patient has a mood disorder, a psychotic disorder, delusions, hallucinations, delirium, or a comorbid medical disorder, primary treatment of those conditions should be initiated first. The principle is that treatment of an underlying primary condition causing aggression should be pursued with the hope that removal of the contributing cause or concurrent removal of several contributing causes will lead to resolution of the aggression.

If the aggression is exacerbated or caused by an environmental circumstance, then steps should be taken to modify the environment. This approach is particularly relevant to patients who have dementing disorders and other brain diseases and for whom modification of brain disease is not always possible. If patients become aggressive in overstimulating, unfamiliar environments, then they should receive one-on-one support in more familiar environments that are less stimulating.

Aggression may also be provoked by factors related to the state of the patient, for example, pain, hunger, and constipation. Attention to these conditions can markedly alleviate aggressive behavior.

If the decode process reveals that the aggression is occurring exclusively in the context of daily care assistance, every effort should be made to modify the approach to the patient during daily care. An experienced clinician should first observe the provision of the care in which the aggression arises in order to study in detail the antecedents of aggression. Is it that the patient strikes out when approached from one particular direction? Does the problem occur when someone makes an effort to take off the patient's pants or to wash particular parts of his or her body? What has the caregiver tried to reduce the behavior? This approach allows the clinician to determine the stimuli and provocations that are immediately followed by aggressive behavior and to find alternative approaches to daily care not involving the aggression-provoking stimuli.

If aggression is provoked by a caregiver who is hostile or otherwise inappropriate with the patient, this caregiver should be provided with education and hands-on modeling of a proper approach to the patient. For example, if a patient with dementia asks a caregiver repetitive questions and the caregiver responds by criticizing the patient for asking these questions, thus leading to aggression, the caregiver should be taught why the patient repeats the questions and given alternative ways to respond other than being critical of the patient.

Caregivers of patients who are at risk for PAB should be instructed in various management techniques. They should be reminded that it is possible to prevent PAB by using structure and routines in the patient's day-to-day life. They should be shown how to approach patients with dementia in a nonconfrontational manner and how to communicate with patients based on what means of communication patients understand best (e.g., to use body language and not words in very aphasic patients). Caregivers should be assisted in learning how to detect when a patient is escalating toward a PAB in order to set limits and attempt a de-escalation before the expression of the PAB.

The success of a variety of nonpharmacological interventions for aggression in the elderly, such those presented above, has been investigated in the literature (Beck et al. 1994; Fritz et al. 1995; Maxfield et al. 1996; Mishima et al. 1994; Satlin et al. 1992). Most studies have supported the use of nonpharmacological interventions in managing aggression or in reducing its impact on the clinical situation. However, the interventions reported have often been unstandardized, expensive, hard to replicate, or assessed in studies without control subjects. The latter issue is important because any intervention, and even no intervention at all, has been associated with a reduction of aggression over time in 40%–50% of aggressive elderly patients, particularly those with dementia. Thus, in the absence of a control condition for intervention studies addressing aggression in the elderly, it is not clear that patients are being helped by anything more than the nonspecific common features of these interventions.

Examples of successful interventions reported from noncontrolled studies include: behavioral analysis, validation, therapy, conditioning, differential reinforcement strategies, and environmental modification (reviewed by Beck et al. 1994). The use of activity programs, stimulus enhancement techniques, relaxation, ambient light manipulation, ambient sound manipulation, and increased social interaction have also been shown in noncontrolled studies to reduce aggression among elderly patients (reviewed by Beck et al. 1994).

Maxfield et al. (1996) provided a detailed behavior analysis approach accompanied by classroom and bedside education for nurses working in a geriatric hospital. The intervention was targeted at preventing and reducing aggressive incidents during bathing and grooming. The intervention was found to impart significant new knowledge to the nursing staff on pretest and posttest assessment. Additionally, the intervention led to a 54% reduction in aggressive incidents during bathing and grooming in the units to which this was applied and a 49% reduction in the use of as-required medications to facilitate the provision of bathing and grooming.

Another study (Fritz et al. 1995) investigated the effect of exposing elderly patients with dementia to companion animals. These patients were residing in the community and being cared for by a family caregiver. Assignment to exposure or nonexposure to animals was not randomly set by the investigators. Over the months after exposure to pets, it was noted that patients exposed to pets had significantly lower rates of aggression, approximately one-third the rates in patients not exposed to pets. Similarly, noncognitive symptoms and other behavior disturbances, including verbal aggression and anxiety, were overall lower in patients exposed to pets.

Noncontrolled studies of bright light therapy (BLT) have indicated some efficacy in reducing aggressive behaviors in patients with dementia (Mishima et al. 1994; Satlin et al. 1992). We recently conducted a study at Copper Ridge assessing the efficacy of BLT versus a control condition (staff attention with dim lights) in reducing aggressive and agitated behavior in patients with dementia (Lyketsos et al. 1999b). Patients in both the control and bright light condition had a 30%–35% reduction in scores on the Behavior Pathology in Alzheimer's Disease Scale (Reisberg et al. 1987). No statistically significant difference was found between the active and control conditions, however, suggesting no specific benefits of BLT in reducing aggression in dementia.

Given that in most cases in the elderly aggression is likely in part the result of a brain dysfunction affecting the patient's ability to modulate aggressive drives, several pharmacological interventions have been attempted and investigated.

It is important to note that, although medications are often efficacious in reducing aggression in elderly patients, this indication has been primarily based on an understanding of the putative neurochemical activity of the medications and of aggression and less so on controlled, randomized clinical trials. The antipsychotic medications (e.g., thiothixene, haloperidol, risperidone, quetiapine, olanzapine) have repeatedly been found superior to placebo in randomized, controlled clinical trials in treating "agitation" in elderly persons or in patients with dementia (Birkett 1997; Katz et al. 1999; Scheider et al. 1990).

A few clinical trials were found that have specifically investigated treatment of aggression in the elderly (reviewed by Rummans et al., in press). One of the notable findings from placebo-controlled trials to treat aggression and agitation in elderly patients, particularly in those with dementia, is that there is a high placebo response, as high as 60% in some cases (Katz et al. 1999). Thus, it is critical that medication treatments for PAB in the elderly be evaluated in rigorously designed and implemented controlled trials, typically with a placebo control.

Placebo-controlled trials of medications for aggression in the elderly have assessed several classes of medications. Most often assessed are the antipsychotic neuro-

leptic agents. Petrie et al. (1982) compared haloperidol and loxapine in the treatment, among other symptoms, of hostility and agitation in 61 elderly persons with dementia. Both antipsychotics were superior to placebo, and similar to each other, in efficacy, although they both produced sedation in study participants. In other studies using similar methods, thioridazine (Barnes et al. 1982), milenperone (DeCuyper et al. 1985), and thiothixene (Finkel et al. 1995) were reported superior to placebo in efficacy for aggression in patients with dementia.

More recent studies have reported efficacy for newer "atypical" antipsychotics for the treatment of aggression in patients with dementia. The latter studies have had several hundred participants and have been well-designed multicenter studies. In one study of the treatment of aggression in institutionalized patients with dementia (Katz et al. 1999), approximately 72% of those on risperidone, as compared with approximately 68% of those on haloperidol and 60% of patients on placebo, had 30% or greater reductions in scores on the Behavioral Pathology in Alzheimer's Disease Scale (Reisberg et al. 1987). Similar data regarding olanzapine have been reported recently as well (Street 1998).

Attention has also been paid to "mood-stabilizing" anticonvulsants as treatments for PAB in the elderly. However, only one randomized placebo-controlled study involving carbamazepine has been reported (Tariot et al. 1998). After 6 weeks of treatment for agitation and aggression, Brief Psychiatric Rating Scale scores (Overall and Gorham 1962) declined from a mean of 53 to a mean of 52 on placebo and from a mean of 55 to 47 in patients treated with carbamazepine. Overt Aggression Scale (Yudofsky et al. 1986) scores in patients treated with placebo were reduced by approximately 15% as compared with approximately 45% in patients treated with carbamazepine.

Serotonin reuptake inhibitors that elevate brain serotonin levels, antipsychotic agents providing dopamine blockade, direct serotonin agonists (buspirone), and β-blockers such as propranolol are useful in reducing PAB in certain elderly patients (Lyketsos et al. 1998; Steinberg and Lyketsos 1997; Yudofsky et al. 1990).

Anecdotal evidence also suggests that other anticonvulsants including divalproex sodium, gabapentin, and lamotrigine have a role to play in the management of episodic aggression in elderly people whether or not seizures are present (Lyketsos et al. 1998; Steinberg and Lyketsos 1997). The anticonvulsants appear to be most effective in patients with advanced dementia, in patients without provoking stimuli, and in patients who have other features of mood instability or evidence of mania and/or hypomania (Lyketsos et al. 1998; Steinberg and Lyketsos 1997).

Medications, such as progesterone and leuprolide, that

interfere with the actions of testosterone are also reported to be effective in reducing PAB in the elderly, particularly if sexual aggression is evident (Amadeo 1996; Kyomen et al. 1991). Combinations of medications have also been useful in this regard. Benzodiazepines, being GABA agonists, also appear effective in reducing aggression (Lyketsos et al. 1998; Steinberg and Lyketsos 1997). However, in some elderly patients, benzodiazepines may have a disinhibiting effect. That effect, coupled with their propensity for addiction, their sedating properties, and their interference with cognitive processing, make benzodiazepines less preferable. Table 22–2 provides a summary of medications useful in treating aggression in the elderly, including reasons why they might be useful and approximate doses.

Carefully designed clinical trials of benzodiazepines, antiandrogens, β-blockers, and other medications, such as stimulants, for PAB in elderly patients have not been conducted. Their use is primarily supported by anecdotal evidence and case reports. However, a substantial literature of noncontrolled studies (e.g., Lyketsos et al. 1998; Steinberg and Lyketsos 1997; Yudofsky et al. 1990) exists on the use of such medications for "agitation" and aggression in dementia, based of the putative ability of these medications to manipulate neurotransmitter systems associated with the modulation of aggression.

No empirical data have been published regarding the reduction of aggression presumed secondary to other psychiatric disorders in an elderly person. For example, if a patient with depression and aggression (or delusions and aggression) is successfully treated for the depression (or the delusions), does the aggression also resolve? Although most clinicians probably would agree that this is the case, no studies substantiating this could be located.

Similarly, clinical belief suggests that detection and treatment of comorbid medical disorders, particularly urinary tract infections, pain, and constipation, will lead to reductions in aggression in the majority of patients. Nevertheless, this belief too has received inadequate research support. In one study, the use of acetaminophen to treat presumed pain in aggressive elderly residents of a nursing home led to significant reductions in aggression and also to reductions in psychotropic drug use (Douzjian et al. 1998).

As reviewed, aggression in elderly persons is often multifactorial in cause and precipitants. Thus, the integration of environmental, educational, caregiver, and pharmacological interventions based on the findings of a solid evaluation as described in this chapter is often the key to effective management of aggression. An example of integrated interventions managing aggression is demonstrated in an important study by Rovner et al. (1996). In this randomized controlled clinical trial, an integrated approach using staff education, activities programming, and careful psychotropic management led to significant reductions in aggression and in use of restraints and psychotropic agents in nursing home patients with dementia.

Currently, recommended treatment for PAB in elderly patients includes the removal of causative or precipitating factors as determined by the evaluation of the patient. Nonpharmacological interventions should be tried next. If pharmacological interventions become necessary, they should be introduced with caution, at low doses, and with slow titration followed by careful side-effect monitoring. The atypical antipsychotics, such as risperidone and olanzapine, are probably the best first-line agents, given their demonstrated efficacy and better tolerability than that of the traditional antipsychotics. These latter should then be considered as second-line treatments, followed by the anticonvulsants, selective serotonin reuptake inhibitors, other antidepressants, β-adrenergic blockers, antiandrogens, and the other medications mentioned in this section.

Conclusion

Physical aggression among the elderly as a whole is relatively uncommon, but it is quite frequent in a variety of geroneuropsychiatric settings. When PAB occurs, it invariably presents a difficult management problem and can be catastrophic. Most instances of PAB in the elderly are associated with a dementing illness or another neuropsychiatric disorder. A basic understanding of the neuroscience underlying human aggression is important to appreciate the complexities of etiology and management. When confronted with elderly patients who are physically aggressive, the neuropsychiatrist must consider host, stimulus, and environmental factors that are underlying the aggression. That evaluation leads to a rational series of interventions whose goal is to modify factors that provoke or contribute to the aggression. In many instances, the aggression is then managed in an empirical fashion by using a variety of integrated behavioral, environmental, and pharmacological approaches. Much research needs to be done in the field of aggression in the elderly, given that most of our understanding of this problem is rudimentary.

References

Aarsland D, Cummings JL, Yenner G, et al: Relationship of aggressive behavior to other neuropsychiatric symptoms in patients with Alzheimer's disease. Am J Psychiatry 153: 243–247, 1996

TABLE 22–2. Medications that may be useful for the treatment of aggression in the elderly

Agent	Starting dose	Weekly titration	Peak effective dose
Antidepressants			
Selective serotonin reuptake inhibitors			
Sertraline	25 mg in A.M.	25 mg/day	175–200 mg/day
Fluoxetine	10 mg in A.M.	10 mg/day	60–80 mg/day
Paroxetine	10 mg at bedtime	10 mg/day	30–50 mg/day
Tricyclics			
Nortriptyline	10 mg at bedtime	10 mg/day	Blood level of 50–150 ng/dL
Desipramine	10 mg at bedtime	10 mg/day	Blood level of 150–200 ng/dL
Clomipramine	25 mg at bedtime	25–50 mg/day	Blood level of 150–200 ng/dL
Other antidepressants			
Venlafaxine	25 mg bid	25 mg bid	400 mg/day
Bupropion	75 mg bid	50 mg bid	40 mg/day
Trazodone	25–50 mg at bedtime	50–100 mg/day	500–600 mg/day
Nefazodone	50 mg at bedtime	50 mg bid	500 mg/day
Neuroleptics			
Haloperidol	0.5 mg at bedtime	0.5 mg/day	500–600 mg/day
Thioridazine	10 mg at bedtime	10 mg/day	60–80 mg/day
Risperidone	0.5 mg at bedtime	0.5 mg/day	4 mg/day
Thiothixene	1 mg at bedtime	1 mg/day	8–10 mg/day
Trifluoperazine	1 mg at bedtime	1 mg/day	8–10 mg/day
Olanzapine	2.5 mg at bedtime	2.5 mg/day	10–15 mg/day
Clozapine	12.5 mg at bedtime	12.5 mg/day	100 mg/day
Other medications			
Anticonvulsants			
Divalproex sodium	125 mg at bedtime or bid	125–250 mg/day	Blood level of 50–100 ng/dL
Carbamazepine	100 mg bid or tid	100–200 mg /day	Blood level of 6–l0 ng/dL
Gabapentin	200–300 mg bid or tid	300–600 mg/day	2–3,000 mg/day
Others			
Lithium	150 mg bid	150 mg/day	Blood level of 0.5–0.8 mEq/dL
Amantadine	50–100 mg bid	50–100 mg bid	300 mg/day
L-dopa (with carbidopa)	100 mg tid	100–200 mg/day	750–1,000 mg/day
Propranolol	10 mg bid	10 mg bid	160 mg/day
Buspirone	10 mg bid	5–10 mg/day	60–80 mg/day
Methylphenidate	2.5 mg bid	2.5–5 mg/day	40–60 mg/day
Progesterone	10 mg/day	10 mg/day	20 mg/day
Leuprolide	2.5–5 mg im q2w	NA	10 mg im q2w

Note.   bid = twice per day; im = intramuscularly; NA = not available; q2w = twice per week; tid = three times per day.

Amadeo M: Antiandrogen treatment of aggressivity in men suffering from dementia. J Geriatr Psychiatry Neurol 9: 142–145, 1996

Barnes R, Veith R, Okimoto J, et al: Efficacy of antipsychotic medications in behaviorally disturbed dementia patients. Am J Psychiatry 139:1170–1174, 1982

Beck CK, Shue VM: Interventions for treating disruptive behavior in demented elderly people. Nurs Clin North Am 29(l):143–155, 1994

Birkett DP: Violence in geropsychiatry. Psychiatric Annals 27(11):752–756, 1997

Bridges-Parlet S, Knopman D, Thompson T: A descriptive study of physically aggressive behavior in dementia by direct observation. J Am Geriatr Soc 42:192–197, 1994

Burns A, Jacoby R, Levy R: Psychiatric phenomena in Alzheimer's disease, IV: disorders of behavior. Br J Psychiatry 157:86–94, 1990

Chandler JD, Chandler JE: The prevalence of neuropsychiatric disorders in a nursing home population. J Geriatr Psychiatry Neurol 1:71–76, 1988

Cohen-Mansfield J, Billing N: Agitated behaviors in the elderly, 1: a conceptual review. J Am Geriatr Soc 34:711–721, 1986

Cooper AJ, Mendonca JD: A prospective study of patient assaults on nursing staff in psychogeriatric unit. Can J Psychiatry 34:399–404, 1989

DeCuyper H, van Praag HM, Verstraeten D: The effect of milenperone on the aggressive behavior of psychogeriatric patients. Biol Psychiatry 13:1–6, 1985

Deutsch LH, Bylsma FW, Rovner BW, et al: Psychosis and physical aggression in probable Alzheimer's disease. Am J Psychiatry 148:1159–1163, 1991

Douzjian M, Wilson C, Shultz M, et al: A program to use pain control medication to reduce psychotropic drug use in residents with difficult behavior. Annals of Long-Term Care 6:174–179, 1998

Eastley R, Wilcock GK: Prevalence and correlates of aggressive behaviours occurring in patients with Alzheimer's disease. Int J Geriatr Psychiatry 12:484–487, 1997

Finkel S, Lyons JS, Anderson RL, et al: A randomized, placebo controlled trial of thiothixene in agitated demented nursing home residents. Int J Geriatr Psychiatry 10:129–136, 1995

Fritz CL, Farver TB, Kass PH, et al: Association with companion animals and the expression of noncognitive symptoms in Alzheimer's patients. J Nerv Ment Dis 183(7):459–463, 1995

Gibbons P, Gannon M, Wrigley M: A study of aggression among referrals to a community-based psychiatry of old age service. Int J Geriatr Psychiatry 12:384–388, 1997

Gilley DW, Wilson RS, Beckett LA, et al: Psychotic symptoms and physically aggressive behavior in Alzheimer's disease. J Am Geriatr Soc 45:1074–1079, 1997

Hamel M, Gold DP, Andres D, et al: Predictors and consequences of aggressive behavior by community-based dementia patients. Gerontologist 30(2):206–211, 1990

Hooten RM, Lyketsos CG: Fronto-temporal dementia: a clinicopathological review of four postmortem studies. J Neuropsychiatry Clin Neurosci 8:10–19, 1996

Katz IR; Jeste DV; Mintzer JE; et al: Comparison of risperidone and placebo for psychosis and behavioral disturbances associated with dementia: a randomized, double-blind trial. J Clin Psychiatry 60:107–115, 1999

Krakowski M: Neurologic and neuropsychologic correlates of violence. Psychiatric Annals 27(10):674–675, 1997

Kyomen HH, Nobel KW, Wei JY: The use of estrogen to decrease aggressive physical behavior in elderly men with dementia. J Am Geriatr Soc 39(11):1110–1112, 1991

Lyketsos CG, Steele CS, Steinberg M: Behavioral disturbances in dementia, in Reichel's Care of the Elderly. Edited by Gallo JJ. Baltimore, MD, Williams & Wilkins, 1998, pp 214–218

Lyketsos CG, Steele C, Galik E, et al: Physical aggression in dementia patients and its relationship to depression. Am J Psychiatry 156:66–71, 1999

Lyketsos CG; Lindell Veiel L; et al: A randomized, controlled trial of bright light therapy for agitated behaviors in dementia patients residing in long-term care. Int J Geriatr Psychiatry 14:520–525, 1999b

Malone ML, Thompson L, Goodwin JS: Aggressive behaviors among the institutionalized elderly. J Am Geriatr Soc 41:853–856, 1993

Maxfield MC, Lewis RE, Cannon S: Training staff to prevent aggressive behavior of cognitively impaired elderly patients during bathing and grooming. Journal of Gerontological Nursing 22:37–43, 1996

Mendez MF, Martin RJ, Smyth KA, et al: Psychiatric symptoms associated with Alzheimer's disease. J Neuropsychiatry Clin Neurosci 2:28–33, 1990

Meyer J, Schalock R, Genaidy H: Aggression in psychiatric hospitalized geriatric patients. Int J Geriatr Psychiatry 6:589–592, 1991

Minde R, Haynes E, Rodenburg M: The ward milieu and its effect on the behaviour of psychogeriatric patients. Can J Psychiatry 35:133–138, 1990

Mishima K, Okawa M, Hishikawa Y, et al: Morning bright light therapy for sleep and behavior disorders in elderly patients with Alzheimer's disease. Acta Psychiatr Scand 89:1–7, 1994

Mungas D: An empirical analysis of specific syndromes of violent behavior. J Nerv Ment Dis 171(6):354–361, 1983

Orengo CA, Kunik ME, Ghusn H, et al: Correlation of testosterone with aggression in demented elderly men. J Nerv Ment Dis 185(5):349–351, 1997

Overall JE, Gorham DR: The Brief Psychiatric Rating Scale. Psychol Rep 10:799–812, 1962

Patel V, Hope T: Aggressive behaviour in elderly psychiatric inpatients. Acta Psychiatr Scand 85:131–135, 1992

Patel V, Hope T: Aggressive behaviour in elderly people with dementia: a review. Int J Geriatr Psychiatry 8:457–472, 1993

Paveza GJ, Cohen D, Eisdorfer C, et al: Severe family violence and Alzheimer's disease: prevalence and risk factors. Gerontologist 12(4):492–497, 1992

Petrie WM, Ban TA, Berney S, et al: Loxapine in psychogeriatrics: a placebo and standard controlled investigation. J Clin Psychopharmacol 2:122–126, 1982

Proctor AW, Francis PT, Stratmann GC, et al: Serotonergic pathology is not widespread in Alzheimer patients without prominent aggressive symptoms. Neurochem Res 17(9):917–922, 1992

Rabins PV, Mace NL, Lucas MJ: The impact of dementia on the family. JAMA 248:333–335, 1982

Reisberg B, Borenstein J, Salob S, et al: Behavioral symptoms in Alzheimer's disease: phenomenology and treatment. J Clin Psychiatry 48 (suppl 5):9–15, 1987

Rovner BW, Kafonek S, Filipp L, et al: Prevalence of mental illness in a community nursing home. Am J Psychiatry 143: 1446–1449, 1986

Rovner BW, Steele CD, Shmuely Y, et al: A randomized trial of dementia care in nursing homes. J Am Geriatr Soc 44(l): 7–13, 1996

Rummans TA, Lauterbach EC, Coffey CE, et al: Pharmacologic efficacy in neuropsychiatry: a review of placebo-controlled treatment trials. J Neuropsychiatry Clin Neurosci 11:176–189, 1999

Russo-Neustadt A; Cotman CW: Adrenergic receptors in Alzheimer's disease brain: selective increases in the cerebella of aggressive patients. J Neurosci 17:5573–5580, 1997

Ryden MB: Aggressive behavior in persons with dementia who live in the community. Alzheimer Dis Assoc Disord 2(4): 342–355, 1988

Satlin A, Volicer L, Ross V, et al: Bright light treatment of behavioral and sleep disturbances in patients with Alzheimer's disease. Am J Psychiatry 149:1028–1032, 1992

Saver JL, Salloway SP, Devinsky O, et al: Neuropsychiatry of aggression, in Neuropsychiatry. Edited by Fogel B, Rao D. Baltimore, MD, Williams & Wilkins, 1995, pp 523–547

Schneider L, Pollack VE, Lyness SA: A meta-analysis of controlled trials of neuroleptic treatment in dementia. J Am Geriatr Soc 38:555–563, 1990

Shah AK: Aggressive behavior among patients referred to a psychogeriatric service. Med Sci Law 32:144–150, 1993

Silliman RA, Sternberg J, Fretwell MD: Disruptive behavior in demented patients living within disturbed families. J Am Geriatr Soc 39:617–618, 1988

Steinberg M, Lyketsos CG: Rational pharmacotherapy for Alzheimer's disease. Medical Update for Psychiatrists 2(l): 5–10, 1997

Street J: Olanzapine versus placebo in the treatment of agitation in patients with dementia. Presentation at the International Conference on Alzheimer's Disease, Amsterdam, July 1998

Swearer JM, Drachman DA, O'Donnell BF, et al: Troublesome and disruptive behaviors in dementia. J Am Geriatr Soc 36:784–790, 1988

Tariot PN, Erb R, Podorski CA, et al: Efficacy and tolerability of carbamazepine for agitation and aggression in dementia. Am J Psychiatry 155:54–61, 1998

Tsai S-J, Hwang J-P, Yang C-H, et al: Physical aggression and associated factors in probable Alzheimer disease. Alzheimer Dis Assoc Disord 10(2):82–85, 1996

Victoroff J, Zarow C, Mack WJ, et al: Physical aggression is associated with preservation of substantia nigra pars compacta in Alzheimer disease. Arch Neurol 53:428–434, 1996

Volavka J: Genetic and neurochemical correlates of violence. Psychiatric Annals 27(10):679–682, 1997

Winger J, Schirm V, Stewart D: Aggressive behavior in long-term care. J Psychosoc Nurs Ment Health Serv 25: 28–33, 1987

Yudofsky SC; Silver JM; Jackson W, et al: The Overt Aggression Scale for the objective rating of verbal and physical aggression. Am J Psychiatry 143:35–39, 1986

Yudofsky SC, Silver JM, Hales RE: Pharmacologic management of aggression in the elderly. J Clin Psychiatry 51 (suppl 10):22–28, 1990

Zimmer JG, Watson N, Treat A: Behavioral problems among patients in skilled nursing facilities. Am J Public Health 74:1118–1121, 1984

Neuropsychiatric Aspects of Neurological Disease in the Elderly

Jeffrey L. Cummings, M.D., Section Editor

CHAPTER 23

Nondegenerative Dementing Disorders

CHAPTER 24

Alzheimer's Disease and Frontotemporal Dementia

CHAPTER 25

Hyperkinetic Movement Disorders

CHAPTER 26

Parkinson's Disease and Parkinsonism

CHAPTER 27

Stroke

CHAPTER 28

Traumatic Brain Injury

CHAPTER 29

Epilepsy

CHAPTER 30

Neoplastic, Demyelinating, Infectious, and
Inflammatory Brain Disorders

CHAPTER 31

Medical Therapies

CHAPTER 32

Neurobehavioral Syndromes

23

Nondegenerative Dementing Disorders

William E. Reichman, M.D.

ementia is a syndrome of acquired persistent decline in several realms of intellectual ability. Individuals display combinations of impaired memory, disturbed language, visuospatial abnormalities, and loss of cognitive abilities such as calculation, abstraction, and problem solving. In concert with these changes, patients may manifest impaired recognition (agnosia) and disturbances in motor planning and sequencing (executive functions deficits).

In addition to the intellectual impairment that characterizes dementia, alteration often occurs in the patient's behavior and mood. Neuropsychiatric symptoms such as hallucinations, delusions, anxiety, aggression, and excessively disinhibited or passive behavior commonly occur. Many patients with dementia develop sleep-wake cycle abnormalities, alterations in sexual behavior, and dietary changes. Performance in the activities of daily living such as grooming, dressing, eating, toileting, and managing household and personal affairs is universally disturbed in dementia. These clinical features of the syndrome, taken together with any concomitant neurological or medical disability, severely impede the patient's ability to fulfill important vocational, social, and familial obligations. The emotional and financial costs associated with the care of patients with dementia have achieved staggering proportions. Dementia has become and will continue to be a major public health concern.

In this chapter, I review the nondegenerative dementing disorders with emphasis on their recognition, underlying pathophysiology, and treatment. Alzheimer's disease and frontotemporal dementia are discussed in Chapter 24 and dementia associated with movement disorders is addressed in Chapters 25 and 26 in this volume.

Nondegenerative Causes of Dementia

The nondegenerative causes of dementia in the elderly population are a heterogeneous group of conditions that include cerebrovascular disease (vascular dementia [VaD]) and other less common states such as hydrocephalus, the dementia syndrome of depression (DOD), infections of the central nervous system, neoplasms, toxic and metabolic encephalopathies, endocrinopathies, and trauma (Table 23–1). Although these individual conditions may alone cause dementia, they may also exacerbate the dementia

TABLE 23–1.   Nondegenerative dementing disorders

Vascular dementia

Hydrocephalus

Dementia syndrome of depression and other psychiatric disorders

Infectious disorders

     Neurosyphilis and other spirochetal illnesses (e.g., Lyme disease)

     Acquired immunodeficiency syndrome (AIDS)

     Other viral and prion encephalitides (e.g., Creutzfeldt-Jakob disease)

     Fungal and bacterial infections

Neoplastic conditions

     Primary and metastatic brain tumors

     Meningeal carcinomatosis

     Paraneoplastic dementia

Metabolic and toxic encephalopathies

     Systemic disorders

         Cardiopulmonary failure

         Chronic hepatic encephalopathy

         Chronic uremic encephalopathy

         Anemia

         Endocrinopathy

         Inflammatory conditions

         Porphyria

         Chronic electrolyte disturbances

     Nutritional deficiency (e.g., vitamin B_{12}, folate, and niacin)

     Toxic disorders

         Medication toxicity

         Alcoholic dementia

         Polysubstance abuse

         Heavy metal intoxication

Posttraumatic dementia

resulting from degenerative diseases such as Alzheimer's disease or Parkinson's disease.

With the exception of VaD, many of the nondegenerative causes of dementia have been described as "reversible" (Cummings et al. 1980; Rabins 1981). In such cases, implementation of a specific therapy, such as thyroid hormone replacement in hypothyroidism or vitamin B_{12} supplementation in pernicious anemia, is expected to result in restoration of intellectual function. The proportion of dementia cases that actually fulfills this criterion is unknown. The reversibility of dementia associated with such conditions has been subjected to increasing scrutiny and

challenge (Barry and Moskowitz 1988; Clarfield 1988; Larson et al. 1986). Across several studies, potentially reversible conditions compose approximately 13% of all cases of dementia (Clarfield 1988). Although substantially more research is needed to explore the validity of "reversibility" of dementia, it appears that many of the so-called reversible conditions may be more accurately referred to as "modifiable." Treatment of the underlying cause of a nondegenerative dementia may halt or slow the progression of intellectual decline but not necessarily result in complete restoration of function.

Vascular Dementia

VaD is a clinical syndrome of acquired intellectual and functional impairment resulting from the effects of cerebrovascular disease. VaD is characterized by a wide range of neurological and neuropsychological signs and symptoms reflecting the heterogeneity of responsible lesions. Different causes of VaD demonstrate variability in onset (abrupt or insidious) and course (static, remitting, or progressive) (Roman et al. 1993). Until recently, the lack of established diagnostic criteria for VaD hampered effective research into its causes, prognosis, and treatment. The application of different terms to describe dementia resulting from cerebrovascular disease such as *multi-infarct* (MID) or *arteriosclerotic dementia* has been imprecise or misleading. For example, it is now clear that neither multiple large infarctions nor arteriosclerosis is a necessary prerequisite for the development of dementia associated with vascular causes. Whereas multiple large cortical infarctions invariably cause VaD, single, strategically placed lesions; small-vessel disease including lacunar infarction; hemorrhage; and hypoperfusion may all independently cause dementia syndromes (Roman et al. 1993).

The risk factors for stroke leading to dementia are still incompletely understood. Factors such as arterial hypertension, cardiac disease, diabetes, hyperlipidemia, and smoking are noted to increase the risk for stroke. Factors that may increase the likelihood that stroke is associated with dementia include the presence of aphasia, a major dominant stroke clinical syndrome, a history of prior cerebrovascular disease, and low educational level (Pohjasvaara et al. 1998).

Importantly, the contribution of stroke to the cause of dementia in an individual patient remains a matter of clinical judgment (Hachinski 1991). In older patients, it is frequently unclear as to whether identified cerebrovascular lesions are the sole cause of dementia, are significantly contributing to the clinical features of an underlying neurodegenerative disease ("mixed dementia"), or are neuropsychologically silent (Erkinjuntti and Sulkava 1991). In recent years, it has been noted that "pure" VaD may actually be uncommon as the sole cause of dementia (Hulette et al. 1997). Many, if not most, cases appearing as VaD may actually represent cerebrovascular disease complicating Alzheimer's disease (mixed dementia). Diagnostic criteria for research in VaD are readily available that attempt to provide improved clarity of diagnosis and standardization of nomenclature (Roman et al. 1993) (Table 23–2).

Epidemiology of Vascular Dementia

Historically, the lack of an accurate definition for dementia of vascular etiology has confounded attempts to reliably establish the epidemiology of the condition (Kase 1991; Mirsen and Hachinski 1988). In studies of the causes of dementia, the diagnosis may have been established by clinical criteria or neuroimaging data such as computed tomography (CT) or magnetic resonance imaging (MRI). Only a few studies have had confirmatory pathological diagnoses. In some studies, the co-occurrence of stroke and Alzheimer's disease is described as "mixed dementia" or is not addressed. As a result, the percentage of all cases of dementia that are secondary to stroke has varied among studies from 4.5% to 39%. The frequency of VaD is generally quoted in the 12%–20% range (Kase 1991). Despite the methodological limitations of epidemiological surveys, it appears that after Alzheimer's disease VaD is the second most common cause of dementia in Western societies (Roman 1991).

Clinical Features of Vascular Dementia

The Ischemia Scale (IS) (Hachinski et al. 1975) and subsequent modifications (Loeb and Gandolfo 1983; Small 1985) have enumerated the clinical features of VaD in an attempt to distinguish it from Alzheimer's disease. These general features include all or some of the following: abrupt onset, prior history of stroke, fluctuating course, focal neurological signs, focal neurological symptoms, stepwise deterioration, nocturnal confusion, relative preservation of personality, depression, somatic complaints, emotional lability, hypertension, and associated atherosclerosis. Despite a sensitivity and specificity of 70%–80% in separating VaD from Alzheimer's disease (Chui et al. 1992), the IS is less able to reliably diagnose the co-occurrence of these two conditions in the same individual and may significantly overdiagnose VaD in patients later found to have Alzheimer's disease (Roman et al. 1993).

Subtypes of Vascular Dementia

As a result of improved recognition of the clinical and pathological variability produced by cerebrovascular disease, subtypes of VaD have been described (Table 23–3). These subtypes present with variable combinations of motor, sensory, and neuropsychological impairment reflecting the anatomical region disrupted. In addition to clinical features such as hemiparesis and hemisensory loss, patients may demonstrate parkinsonism, gait instability, urinary incontinence, visual field defects, hemineglect, and pseudobulbar palsy (dysarthria, dysphagia, exaggerated facial and gag reflexes, and pseudobulbar affect). Along with neuropsychological deficits such as impaired memory, language, cognition, and visuospatial ability, patients may also manifest impairment in frontal systems functions (Wolfe et al. 1990). Disturbances of mood, behavior, and perception (hallucinosis) may complicate the clinical course of VaD. In some patients, delusional thinking develops. In most cases of VaD, many different types of lesions are identified in the brain parenchyma and its vascular supply. The clinical features of VaD reflect the location of the lesions, the volume of infarcted tissue, the number of lesions, and their laterality (Olsson et al. 1996).

Multi-infarct dementia. The cumulative effect of multiple large complete cortical infarctions throughout the distributions of the anterior, middle, or posterior cerebral artery circulations can result in dementia. Generally, occlusion of these arteries is the consequence of atherosclerotic thrombosis or cardiac embolization. Multi-infarct dementia is typically reported as having an abrupt onset with stepwise progression. The resulting clinical picture is characterized by variable impairment across several areas of intellectual function. Patients may demonstrate "patchiness" of deficits such that certain intellectual functions are spared, and others are significantly affected. As the syndrome progresses, most areas of intellectual function become disturbed. Patients typically manifest neurological signs and symptoms such as dysarthria, hemiparesis, hemisensory loss, visual field disturbances, and pathological reflexes or reflex asymmetries. Disturbances of recognition (agnosia) and praxis (apraxia) are occasionally noted. In many patients, multi-infarct dementia results from a combination of cortical and subcortical infarctions (see below).

Strategic single-infarct dementia. A solitary infarction may abruptly cause dementia if it occurs in a cortical or subcortical region critical to intellectual functions. Strategically placed single lesions in the distributions of the

TABLE 23–2.   **Diagnostic criteria for probable, possible, and definite vascular dementia**

I.   The criteria for the clinical diagnosis of *probable* vascular dementia include *all* of the following:

1.   *Dementia*, defined by cognitive decline from a previously higher level of functioning and manifested by impairment of memory and of two or more cognitive domains (orientation, attention, language, visuospatial functions, executive functions, motor control, and praxis), preferably established by clinical examination and documented by neuropsychological testing; deficits should be severe enough to interfere with activities of daily living not due to physical effects of stroke alone.

Exclusion criteria: Cases with disturbance of consciousness, delirium, psychosis, severe aphasia, or major sensorimotor impairment precluding neuropsychological testing. Also excluded are systemic disorders or other brain diseases (e.g., Alzheimer's disease [AD]) that in and of themselves could account for deficits in memory and cognition.

2.   *Cerebrovascular disease* (CVD), defined by the presence of focal signs on neurological examination (e.g., hemiparesis, lower facial weakness, Babinski's sign, sensory deficit, hemianopsia, and dysarthria) consistent with stroke (with or without history of stroke) and evidence of relevant CVD by brain imaging (computed tomography [CT] or magnetic resonance imaging [MRI]) including multiple large-vessel strokes or a single, strategically placed infarct (angular gyrus, thalamus, basal forebrain, posterior cerebral artery, or anterior cerebral artery territories), as well as multiple basal ganglia and white matter lacunes or extensive periventricular white matter lesions or combinations thereof.

3.   A relationship between the above two disorders, manifested or inferred by the presence of one or both of the following:

a.   Onset of dementia within 3 months after a recognized stroke.

b.   Abrupt deterioration in cognitive functions or fluctuating, stepwise progression of cognitive deficits.

II. Clinical features consistent with the diagnosis of *probable* vascular dementia include the following:

1.   Early presence of a gait disturbance (small-step gait or marché a petits-pas, magnetic, apraxic-ataxic, or parkinsonian gait).

2.   History of unsteadiness and frequent unprovoked falls.

3.   Early urinary frequency, urgency, and other urinary symptoms not explained by urological disease.

4.   Personality and mood changes, abulia, depression, emotional incontinence, other subcortical deficits including psychomotor retardation, and abnormal executive function.

III. Features that make the diagnosis of vascular dementia uncertain or unlikely include:

1.   Early onset of memory deficit and progressive worsening of memory and other cognitive functions such as language (transcortical sensory aphasia), motor skills (apraxia), and perception (agnosia), in the absence of corresponding focal lesions on brain imaging.

2.   Absence of focal neurological signs other than cognitive disturbance.

3.   Absence of cerebrovascular lesions on brain CT or MRI.

IV. Clinical diagnosis of *possible* vascular dementia: May be made in the presence of dementia (Section I) with focal neurological signs, but in the absence of brain imaging confirmation of definite CVD; or in the absence of clear temporal relationship between dementia and stroke; or in patients with subtle onset and variable course (plateau or improvement of cognitive deficits and evidence of relevant CVD).

V.   Criteria for diagnosis of *definite* vascular dementia are:

1.   Clinical criteria for probable vascular dementia.

2.   Histopathological evidence of CVD obtained from biopsy or autopsy.

3.   Absence of neurofibrillary tangles and neuritic plaques exceeding those expected for age.

4.   Absence of other clinical or pathological disorder capable of producing dementia.

VI. Classification of vascular dementia for research purposes may be made on the basis of clinical, radiological, and neuropathological features for subcategories or defined conditions such as:

- Cortical vascular dementia
- Subcortical vascular dementia
- Binswanger's disease
- Thalamic dementia

The term *AD with CVD* should be reserved to classify patients fulfilling the clinical criteria for probable AD and who also present clinical or brain imaging evidence of relevant CVD. Traditionally, these patients have been included with vascular dementia in epidemiological studies. The term *mixed dementia* used hitherto should be avoided.

Source.   Adapted from Roman et al. 1993.

TABLE 23–3. Subtypes of vascular dementia

Subtype	Features
Multi-infarct	Abrupt onset, stepwise progression, "patchy" neuropsychological deficits, pyramidal signs, hemiparesis, hemisensory loss, and impaired memory
Strategic single-infarct	Abrupt onset
Carotid artery	Aphasia (left-sided), visuospatial deficits, and contralateral hemiparesis and hemisensory loss
Anterior cerebral artery	Abulia, dyspraxia, transcortical motor aphasia, dysarthria, apraxia, impaired memory; contralateral hemiparesis and hemisensory loss in lower extremities, and incontinence
Middle cerebral artery	Severe aphasia (left-sided)[a], alexia, agraphia, dyscalculia, psychosis, contralateral pyramidal signs, hemiparesis, hemisensory loss, and visual field deficits
Dominant angular gyrus	Aphasia, alexia, agraphia, impaired verbal memory, visuospatial deficits, right-left disorientation, finger agnosia, and dyscalculia
Posterior cerebral artery	Impaired memory, agnosia, alexia without graphia, visual field deficits, brainstem signs
Branches to thalamic region	Aphasia (left-sided), impaired attention and memory, and variable motor and sensory loss
Hypoperfusion of watershed (borderzone)	Transcortical aphasias, impaired memory, apraxia, and visuospatial deficits
Small-vessel disease	
Lenticulostriate arteries (lacunar state)	Memory loss, psychomotor slowing, apathy, depression, multifocal motor symptoms, parkinsonism, and pseudobulbar palsy
Subcortical arterioles	Memory loss, psychomotor slowing, euphoria, psychosis, symmetric hemiparesis, ataxia supranuclear palsy, incontinence, and parkinsonism (often without tremor)

[a]In the setting of severe aphasia, one cannot adequately determine whether, in fact, dementia exists.

carotid, anterior, middle, and posterior cerebral arteries (left angular gyrus, thalamus, caudate nucleus) give rise to well-recognized dementia syndromes with a variety of neurological and neurobehavioral features (Mahler and Cummings 1991) (Table 23–3).

Hypoperfusion of watershed areas (borderzone infarction) producing dementia. The borderzone regions exist at the borders between the vascular territories of the major cerebral arteries. Reduced cerebral perfusion resulting from cardiac arrest, severe hypotension, or loss of blood volume causes stroke in these cortical areas. The most vulnerable border-zone region appears to be the area between the territories of the middle and posterior cerebral arteries.

Small-vessel disease dementia. Occlusion of small vessels most prominently causes lesions of subcortical structures such as the basal ganglia, thalamus, internal capsule, and subhemispheric white matter. Disruption of these structures and their connections to the dorsolateral frontal cortex leads to a syndrome called subcortical dementia. This state is characterized by psychomotor slowing, dilapidation in cognitive functions, memory impairment, frontal systems dysfunction, and behavioral alterations such as depression and apathy (Cummings 1990). Neurologically, such patients frequently manifest parkinsonism, ataxia, and urinary incontinence.

Lacunar state (etat lacunaire) refers to a pattern of infarction in which multiple small lesions in the basal ganglia, thalamus, and internal capsule produce dementia. Neurological signs and symptoms include, but are not limited to, pseudobulbar palsy, gaze abnormalities, psychomotor slowing, and pyramidal and extrapyramidal disorders. Depression, apathy, and emotional lability are frequent accompanying psychiatric features. Dementia often features prominent frontal systems dysfunction (Ishii et al. 1986; Wolfe et al. 1990). Affected patients typically have a history of hypertension.

Ischemic injury of the frontal hemispheric white matter produces a chronic progressive state called *subcortical arteriosclerotic encephalopathy* or *Binswanger's disease* (Babikian and Ropper 1987; Peterson and Summergrad

1989; Summergrad and Peterson 1989). Like lacunar infarction, the signs and symptoms of Binswanger's disease reflect pathology localized to subcortical structures. Disturbances of cortical origin such as agnosia or apraxia are generally absent. Hypertension has been noted in 80% or more of cases (Kinkel et al. 1985). Because the clinical triad of dementia, gait disturbance, and urinary incontinence may be seen in Binswanger's disease, it is occasionally misdiagnosed as normal-pressure hydrocephalus (NPH), in which these features have been considered pathognomonic. As compared with patients with NPH, patients with Binswanger's disease demonstrate an earlier age at onset, less frequent early gait abnormalities, longer illness duration, and more prominent signs of hypertension and cerebrovascular disease (Gallassi et al. 1991).

Evaluation of Vascular Dementia

After review of the patient's history, the evaluation of VaD includes thorough physical, neurological, and mental status examinations. This approach is complemented by CT or MRI of the brain to identify changes consistent with vascular lesions such as gray matter infarctions or ischemic white matter changes.

The frequency of infarctions noted on CT scans of patients given the clinical diagnosis of VaD has varied considerably (from 20% to 86%) (Erkinjuntti and Sulkava 1991). Infarctions appear on CT as regions of lucency. With the advent of MRI, the ability to detect ischemic changes in the subhemispheric white matter has improved, leading to increased speculation regarding their significance. In many intellectually and neurologically intact older patients, MRI may demonstrate patchy and diffuse white matter changes evident as increased signal, especially on T2-weighted images (Almkvist et al. 1992; Boone et al. 1992; Leys et al. 1990). These lesions frequently appear in close proximity to the ventricles and may consist of caps or thickened, irregular rims. These changes have been often referred to as *leukoariosis*. When these lesions are confined to the periventricular region, their clinical significance is unclear (Bondareff et al. 1990). In general, these changes are thought to represent localized areas of demyelination and increased amounts of free water (Zimmerman et al. 1986). In some patients, the periventricular findings are accompanied by single or multiple lesions of the basal ganglia, internal capsule, and thalamus. Large confluent lesions in the subhemispheric white matter may also be noted. Arteriosclerosis may or may not be identified in these subcortical lesions and seems to occur depending on their location (Chimowitz et al. 1992). In general, widespread white matter lesions on neuroimaging are a frequent finding in patients with VaD (Erkinjuntti and Sulkava 1991) (Figure 23–1). However, it remains that these lesions have different pathological correlates and may be of variable clinical significance (Chimowitz et al. 1992).

In VaD, functional neuroimaging techniques such as single photon emission computed tomography (SPECT) and positron-emission tomography (PET) (Figure 23–2) demonstrate focal areas of hypoperfusion and hypometabolism, respectively.

Although most cases of VaD occur on the basis of arteriosclerosis in the setting of prominent vascular risk factors, in some patients, stroke can result from inflammatory vasculitis. In these individuals, the clinician often encounters other prominent signs of collagen-vascular disease such as an elevated sedimentation rate and confirmatory serologic abnormalities. Inflammatory diseases such as systemic lupus erythematosus, temporal arteritis, and sarcoidosis have been associated with VaD. Hematologic disorders such as polycythemia, sickle-cell disease, and thrombotic thrombocytopenic purpura may also cause stroke and should be considered when routine blood work is reviewed. Attention to potential embolic sources such as cardiac valvular disease is an important component of the diagnostic assessment.

Treatment of Vascular Dementia

At present, no medication has demonstrated definitive sustained efficacy in preventing, reversing, or modifying the course of VaD. Smoking cessation and optimal control of hypertension or diabetes mellitus have been found to reduce mortality from stroke but have not yet been sufficiently studied to demonstrate such an effect specifically in VaD (Hier et al. 1989). Some data suggest intellectual improvement with moderately lowered blood pressure in hypertensive patients, but other individuals with VaD may experience further cognitive decline (Meyer et al. 1986). Meyer and colleagues (Meyer et al. 1988, 1989; Wade 1991) have observed therapeutic benefit from cigarette smoking abstinence, aspirin therapy, and surgical interventions such as endarterectomy and/or cardiac bypass surgery. Though stroke prophylaxis has been shown with the antiplatelet agent ticlopidine, its usefulness for the treatment of VaD is unproven (Gent et al. 1989).

Pharmacological approaches to the treatment of VaD have included vasodilating agents such as dihydroergotamine (Hydergine) and pentoxifylline (Trental) and calcium channel blocking agents. Although data analysis is still preliminary, no agent has demonstrated unequivocal efficacy over placebo.

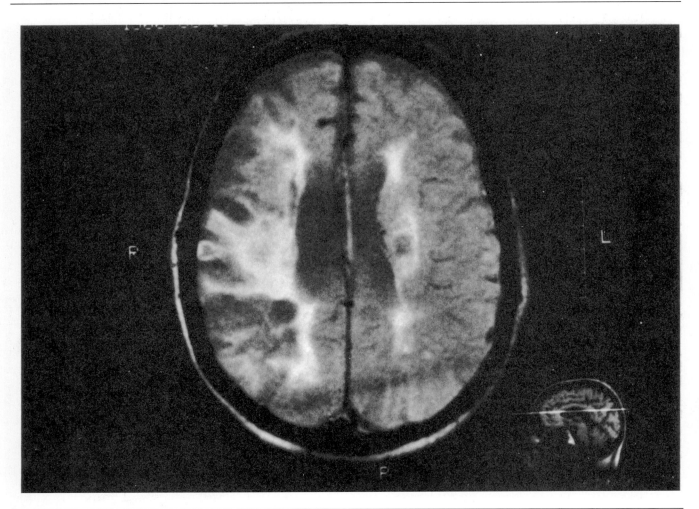

FIGURE 23–1. Magnetic resonance image of a patient with vascular dementia. Large irregular periventricular hyperintensities, as well as large confluent deep white matter hyperintensities, are shown.

Hydrocephalic Dementia

The clinical hallmarks of hydrocephalic dementia include dementia, gait instability, and urinary incontinence. Symptoms usually evolve over several months or years. The dementia syndrome has subcortical features including slowness, bradyphrenia, and inattentiveness. Although memory is invariably impaired, patients also appear apathetic and excessively concrete (Benson 1985).

NPH is associated with normal intracranial pressure (Adams et al. 1965). The disorder results from impaired absorption of cerebrospinal fluid into the venous circulation at the level of the arachnoid granulations. Although NPH can be idiopathic in occurrence, it can follow cerebral trauma, subarachnoid hemorrhage, encephalitis, or meningitis. Despite its frequent consideration in the differential diagnosis of dementia, NPH is a rare cause of dementia, accounting for less than 2% of cases (Clarfield 1988).

In addition to NPH, other forms of hydrocephalus cause dementia in elderly people. Mass lesions or inflammatory conditions such as ependymitis or arachnoiditis can obstruct the normal flow of cerebrospinal fluid (CSF) (obstructive, noncommunicating hydrocephalus). When obstruction due to these causes is relatively acute, the patient demonstrates signs of increased intracranial pressure (headache, papilledema, lethargy, nausea, and emesis) and eventually progresses to somnolence and coma. Bilateral abducens palsies and quadriparesis also can be present. When the obstruction is subacute, however, the onset of symptomatology is more gradual and frequently presents as dementia without other neurological signs (Benson 1985).

Ataxia and urinary incontinence associated with hydrocephalic dementia are thought to result from displacement by the enlarging lateral ventricles of those periventricular corticospinal tracts that control lower-extremity and bladder-motor function. Ataxia with hydrocephalus tends to vary in severity and may be accompanied by

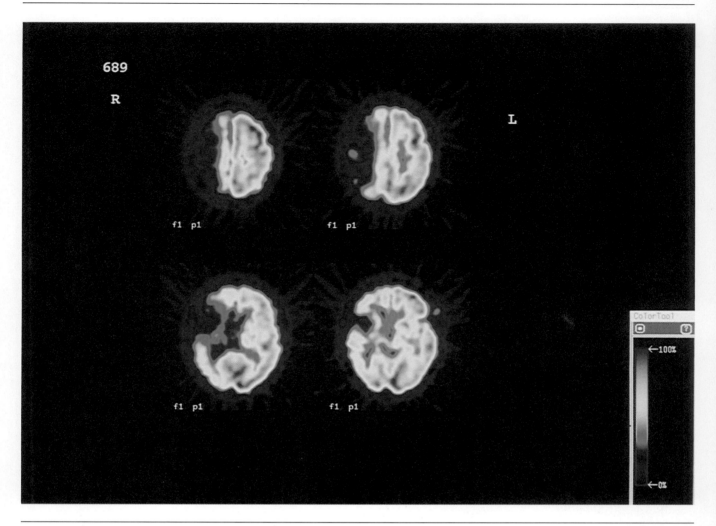

FIGURE 23–2. Positron-emission tomography scan of a patient with vascular dementia. Multiple areas of reduced glucose metabolism are shown.

spasticity of the legs and extensor plantar responses. Difficulty initiating gait is common. Once the patient is ambulatory, however, the patient's strides are noted to improve (Fisher 1982).

Whereas ataxia is often a prominent feature of hydrocephalic dementia, urinary incontinence may be mild or only late occurring (Benson 1985). Although frequently cited as a pathognomonic feature of hydrocephalus, urinary incontinence is a common feature of Alzheimer's disease and other dementing disorders and is of limited diagnostic specificity.

Evaluation of Hydrocephalic Dementia

The accurate diagnosis of NPH is often difficult as the characteristic signs and symptoms of the disorder occur in other progressive causes of dementia (Cox et al. 1988). Classically, the radiological appearance of NPH has been

reported to consist of ventricular dilation in the absence of sulcal widening. Although this finding on CT or MRI strengthens the diagnosis of NPH, it is not invariably present; cortical atrophy can be present in some hydrocephalic patients. In some cases, elderly patients with dementia and with clear radiological evidence of NPH may not have the associated features of incontinence or ataxia (Mulrow et al. 1987). Additional diagnostic techniques including radioisotope or CT cisternography are of limited value in improving diagnostic accuracy (Vanneste et al. 1992). Although most patients with NPH may be expected to decline intellectually over time, some may remain stable without additional intervention (Clarfield 1989).

Treatment of Hydrocephalic Dementia

The treatment of hydrocephalic dementia, particularly NPH, involves surgical shunting procedures. Surgical success rates have been variable, and treatment complications have been common (Graff-Radford et al. 1989). Dementia appears to be the symptom of NPH that is least responsive to treatment. Even when the diagnosis is reasonably certain, accurate, consistent predictive tests for surgical outcome are still lacking. In general, those patients best suited for shunt placement are those who initially present with the full clinical triad, have a readily identified cause for NPH, and have had a relatively short duration of symptoms (Clarfield 1989).

Dementia Syndrome of Depression

Pseudodementia has been the term historically applied to describe memory and other cognitive impairments caused by psychiatric disorders such as depression, mania, and schizophrenia (Kiloh 1961). It has been argued that dementia could be "mimicked" or "caricatured" by functional psychiatric illness, implying a hysterical component to the clinical presentation (Wells 1979). Although still controversial, it is now generally accepted that the intellectual deficits that result from psychiatric illness, in particular depression, constitute a "true dementia" that may be modifiable or perhaps reversed with appropriate therapy.

Four essential criteria have been proposed to diagnostically define dementia resulting from functional psychiatric disorders (Caine 1981). First, there must be evidence of a primary psychiatric disorder accompanied by intellectual impairment. Second, the clinical features of the disorder must resemble those noted in degenerative brain disorders with neuropathological confirmation. Third, the intellectual deficit should reverse with psychiatric treatment. Fourth, there must not be evidence of a primary neurodegenerative process that can cause dementia.

Dementia specifically resulting from depressed mood has been aptly termed the *dementia syndrome of depression* (Folstein and McHugh 1978). The true prevalence of DOD among the elderly population is unknown, reflecting variability in sampled populations and assessment methods. Across studies, from 2% to 32% of patients evaluated for dementia meet criteria for pseudodementia, of whom 50%–100% have DOD (Cummings and Benson 1992). In elderly patients, depression is the psychiatric state most often responsible for dementia. In younger patients, there may be greater variability in the psychiatric causes of intellectual impairment.

The onset of DOD is most typically subacute, occurring in an elderly individual with a personal or family history of depression. As the major depressive episode evolves, intellectual impairment rapidly progresses. Patients appear dysphoric and may complain of poor motivation, anhedonia, and feelings of worthlessness. Heightened levels of anxiety and nihilistic or persecutory delusions also may be present. Neurovegetative features of depression are evident and include disrupted sleep, impaired appetite, anergia, constipation, and impotence. Patients are often hypophonic and appear cognitively and psychomotorically slowed; they may demonstrate diminished affective intensity and range.

The neuropsychological deficits of DOD tend to be variable, and they include some or all of the following: impaired attention and concentration, restricted verbal fluency, memory-retrieval deficits, visuoconstructional disturbances, concreteness, and disrupted calculation ability (Weingartner et al. 1981). Disturbances such as aphasia, apraxia, and agnosia are notably absent. The severity of the patient's underlying depression is highly correlated with the motivation to perform and the level of intellectual impairment (Cohen et al. 1982). The degree of depression is also strongly correlated with the individual's tendency to complain about memory impairment, irrespective of its severity (Kahn et al. 1975; O'Connor et al. 1990). Patients with depression often complain about forgetfulness, as well as indecisiveness, poor concentration, and mental slowing (O'Connor et al. 1990). The degree of awareness and concern verbalized by the typical patient with DOD is far greater than that evidenced by the patient with a degenerative cause of dementia such as Alzheimer's disease.

Several studies have documented reduced complaints of impaired memory (Plotkin et al. 1985) and improved intellectual functioning following successful treatment of depression with pharmacotherapy (tricyclic antidepressants and monoamine oxidase inhibitors) or electroconvulsive therapy (Janowsky 1982; Kral and Emery 1989; McAllister and Price 1982). It remains uncertain whether intellectual improvement is complete or whether some deficits persist despite a fully recovered mood (Ames et al. 1990; Greenwald et al. 1989; Jacoby et al. 1981; Savard et al. 1980).

The long-term prognosis of DOD is also uncertain. Some studies suggest that, over time, many patients with DOD develop a progressive dementia (Ames et al. 1990; Kral 1983; Reding et al. 1985), whereas other studies, using relatively rigorous criteria for the diagnosis of DOD, have concluded that the risk for developing an irreversible progressive dementia is no greater in patients who have had DOD than in nondepressed elderly patients (Pearlson et al. 1989; Rabins et al. 1984).

Preliminary neuroimaging investigations have demonstrated some structural abnormalities in DOD. In one study (Pearlson et al. 1989), CT scans of patients with

DOD had ventricle-to-brain ratios that were smaller than those of patients with Alzheimer's disease, but larger than those recorded in depressed, age-matched control subjects without dementia. However, in another series, no significant differences between control subjects and patients with DOD were detected with CT (Abas et al. 1990). Elderly patients with late-onset depression have significantly more white matter ischemic changes on MRI than do psychiatrically healthy, age-matched control subjects (Coffey et al. 1990). Whether these lesions predispose to the development of DOD is unknown. In patients with left-hemisphere stroke, concurrent major depression further impairs neuropsychological test performance irrespective of lesion size, lesion location, or other clinical variables (Bolla-Wilson et al. 1989; Robinson et al. 1986).

The diagnosis of DOD rests on the demonstration of a major depressive episode in a patient with secondarily acquired intellectual impairment. The patient must not meet diagnostic criteria for another dementing illness that may cause similar clinical features (especially Parkinson's disease or subcortical cerebrovascular disease). It is also crucial to exclude potentially toxic effects of medications. Centrally acting antihypertensive drugs (reserpine, clonidine, and propranolol) or neuroleptics can disrupt intellectual ability and produce depression, confounding diagnostic accuracy. Final certainty in the diagnosis depends on discriminating improvement in intellectual function with resolution of the mood disorder.

Although less common in elderly patients, dementia has also been noted to secondarily arise from mania or schizophrenic psychosis (Wright and Silove 1988). Patients with mania are generally easily distractible and forgetful and exhibit psychomotor agitation. Their mood is grandiose or exceptionally irritable. They may have relatively florid hallucinations or delusions and disturbances of thought processes such as circumstantiality or flight of ideas. Other manic features are variable. Dementia arising solely from the manic phase of bipolar disorder must be distinguished from manic-like behavior encountered in dementia syndromes that disrupt frontal systems. Disorders such as the frontal lobe degenerations, general paresis, alcoholic dementia, cerebral neoplasms, strokes, trauma, and the toxic effects of medications (steroids and levodopa) may cause manic symptoms (secondary mania).

In many patients with schizophrenia, dementia has been noted, especially when "negative symptoms" (withdrawal, emotional blunting, loss of reactivity, and apathy) dominate the clinical picture. These features have been correlated with frontal ventricular prominence and sulcal widening (Andreasen et al. 1982). The neuropsychological profile of dementia in patients with schizophrenia who have prominent negative symptoms has been shown to preferentially, but not exclusively, consist of impaired executive functions (Breier et al. 1991; Perlick 1992). Less frequently, impaired intellectual ability in subjects with schizophrenia can be seen during episodes of psychotic agitation. During such periods, impaired motivation to perform and inattentiveness may underlie the observed deficits. Lastly, a subgroup of elderly subjects with schizophrenia demonstrate chronic neuropsychological deficits.

Treatment of DOD follows the usual approach to treatment of depression in the elderly and is described in elsewhere in this volume.

■ Infectious Disorders

Infectious disorders of the central nervous system are uncommon causes of dementia in the elderly population. Dementia resulting from chronic fungal, helminthic, or protozoan infectious processes most often presents clinically as a chronic confusional state with impaired attention and arousal. Along with features of meningeal irritation, signs of increased intracranial pressure such as papilledema, headache, nausea, and emesis can be present. Seizures and cranial nerve dysfunction can also be evident.

Bacterial infection (meningitis or brain abscess) more often develops as an acute, rapidly progressive clinical state with neuropsychiatric features more reminiscent of delirium than of dementia. Chronic treponemal infections of the nervous system that can cause dementia include neurosyphilis and Lyme disease.

Dementia can be a long-term consequence of viral encephalitis. In herpes simplex encephalitis, severe memory impairment can be a chronic residual feature reflecting the virus's predilection for the anterior medial temporal cortex. Affected patients may demonstrate aphasia and mild cognitive deficits. Apart from herpes simplex infection, other viral encephalitides can also cause enduring intellectual deficits.

Creutzfeldt-Jakob disease is a rare disorder with onset in the sixth or seventh decade. The disorder, arising from a proteinaceous infectious particle (prion), is rapidly progressive, leading to death within several months. Patients manifest progressive dementia with prominent language disturbance, myoclonus, extrapyramidal features, and pyramidal signs. Cerebellar signs, cranial nerve pathology, and choreoathetosis also can occur (Brown et al. 1986; Cummings and Benson 1992).

Patients infected with the human immunodeficiency virus (HIV) can have a variety of neuropsychiatric disorders including depression, anxiety, and dementia

(Faulstich 1987; Hintz et al. 1990; Perry 1990). Dementia is the most frequent neurological complication of acquired immunodeficiency syndrome (AIDS) (Navia and Price 1987). Since early reports of the AIDS epidemic, the tendency of HIV to cause neuropsychological impairment has been well established. Although originally dementia was thought to be the result of opportunistic infection, it has been increasingly recognized that dementia can occur as the direct consequence of HIV infection of the central nervous system (Lunn et al. 1991; Navia et al. 1986). The acquired intellectual impairment directly resulting from HIV infection has been termed the *AIDS dementia complex* (ADC) or *AIDS cognitive-motor complex*. The disorder may be a presenting manifestation of AIDS (Navia and Price 1987) and has been noted in at least two-thirds of patients who die from an AIDS-related illness (Navia et al. 1986).

ADC has clinical features indicative of subcortical dysfunction including impairment in concentration, forgetfulness, and slowed psychomotor speed. Additionally, patients have poor balance, lower-extremity weakness, hyperreflexia, and an action tremor. Headache, impaired handwriting, and loss of motivation have also been noted frequently (Benson 1987). Other associated behavioral features such as depression and hallucinations can be present also. In the end stage of AIDS, patients may be incontinent, strikingly apathetic, and mute (Lunn et al. 1991). Though not having AIDS, people with asymptomatic HIV infection may demonstrate subclinical impairment in verbal memory and psychomotor speed (Lunn et al. 1991; Stern et al. 1991).

It remains unclear how HIV enters the central nervous system to produce ADC. One view is that the retrovirus is initially contained within macrophages that cross the blood-brain barrier. With evolving immunosuppression, the virus replicates within the brain in an uncontrolled fashion (Perry 1990).

Although ADC is most commonly seen in younger age groups, in which risk factors such as homosexuality, intravenous drug use, and prior blood transfusion increase the risk of HIV infection, the disorder may also be seen in the elderly. The diagnosis should be considered in the older patient with any of the above risk factors and a subcortical dementia.

The treatment of ADC involves substantial psychological support for patients and their caregivers, augmented by pharmacotherapy. Antiviral therapy, specifically zidovudine (AZT), has been shown to improve intellectual impairment associated with AIDS (Schmitt et al. 1988; Yarchoan et al. 1987), and many patients with combination ADC receive protease inhibitors and antiviral treatment regimens. Psychotropic, neurological, and analgesic medications are used where indicated for pertinent symptoms. Specifically, psychotropic agents including psychostimulants for withdrawal and apathy and high-potency neuroleptics for associated psychosis have demonstrated consistent efficacy (Ostrow et al. 1988; Perry 1990).

Neoplasia-Associated Dementia

Primary neoplasms that arise from the brain parenchyma, cerebral blood vessels, pituitary, meninges, and cranial nerves may all sufficiently disrupt neural function to produce dementia. Metastatic lesions from extracranial tumors, granulomas, and lymphomas can all invade the central nervous system to exert profound effects on mentation. The wide variety of cerebral neoplasms that can cause dementia accounts for significant variability in the onset and progression of intellectual impairment and the occurrence of associated neurological signs and symptoms (Rowland 1989).

The clinical features associated with intracranial tumors arise from parenchymal invasion, mass effects, hydrocephalus, vascular occlusion, or any combination of these. Most often, signs and symptoms of intracranial mass lesions arise insidiously and are progressive. Symptoms such as depression, lethargy, apathy, impaired concentration, disturbed memory, and headache can slowly evolve over several weeks to months (Anderson et al. 1990). When other symptoms such as unsteady gait, incontinence, and emesis are noted, a cerebral mass lesion must be strongly suspected. Additional features consistent with the presence of a brain tumor include papilledema, vasomotor symptoms, focal motor or sensory signs, diplopia, vertigo, and visual field defects (Bannister 1986). Less frequently, the initial manifestations of a cerebral tumor include the abrupt onset of a seizure, focal motor weakness, or hemisensory loss (Adams and Victor 1989).

The pattern of intellectual impairment noted with a cerebral mass lesion is in part a function of neuroanatomic location. Direct pressure effects can cause relatively focal disturbances in language, praxis, or memory. In certain locations, dementia is particularly likely to occur. For example, global intellectual impairment is found in 70% of patients with frontal tumors, whereas language disturbances are particularly prominent with left-temporal masses (Cummings and Benson 1992). Increased intracranial pressure gives rise to altered arousal, attention, and concentration. Tumors disrupting subcortical structures such as the basal ganglia also cause dementia in which there are prominent attentional disturbances and depression.

Masses affecting the diencephalic structures can cause dementia associated with personality changes, endocrinological abnormalities, dietary disturbances, and sleep alterations (Cummings and Benson 1992).

Widespread metastasis to the meninges with dissemination throughout the ventricles has been termed *meningeal carcinomatosis*. Malignant melanoma and carcinomas of the breast, lung, and gastrointestinal tract have been associated with this condition. Affected patients demonstrate signs of increased intracranial pressure, cranial nerve dysfunction, and dementia typified by prominent attention and concentration difficulties (Theodore and Gendelman 1981).

Distant tumors such as occult neoplasms of the lung (oat-cell carcinoma), ovary, or breast may be associated with limbic encephalitis. This disorder has been considered a paraneoplastic condition of unknown pathogenesis. Intellectual impairment is often accompanied by depression and anxiety. There can be impairment of arousal and hallucinatory phenomena. Signs or symptoms of cerebellar dysfunction such as ataxia, nystagmus, tremor, hyporeflexia, dysarthria, and impairment of rapid alternating movements may be noted. Seizures, myopathy, and myeloradiculoneuropathy have been documented in this condition (Posner 1989). Although the medial temporal lobe appears to be the site most severely affected, neuronal loss and inflammatory changes have been discovered throughout the cortex and subcortical regions. Paraneoplastic dementia is an untreatable condition that typically progresses to death within 2 years of onset (Cummings and Benson 1992).

The diagnosis of an intracranial mass is contingent on confirmation by CT or MRI. The addition of contrast enhancement to these procedures increases their sensitivity to detect cerebral neoplasms. These procedures also help to differentiate other dementing conditions such as stroke, cerebral abscess, subdural hematoma, and NPH from brain tumors. Electroencephalography (EEG) may demonstrate diffuse or excessive focal slow-wave activity. CSF examination often reveals a mild leukocytosis with elevated protein and normal glucose levels. (For a more complete discussion of the neuropsychiatric aspects of neoplastic, demyelinating, infectious, and inflammatory diseases of the brain, see Chapter 30 in this volume.)

■ Metabolic and Toxic Encephalopathies

Elderly people are particularly vulnerable to the neuropsychiatric effects of systemic illness, nutritional deficiency, and toxin exposure. In most cases, metabolic or toxic derangements of the central nervous system produce acute, time-limited disturbances in cognition and behavior (delirium). However, when the effects persist for an extended period of time, dementia results. The most prominent effects of metabolic and toxic disorders on mentation include fluctuating arousal, impaired attention, and disturbances in memory. Depending on the underlying disorder, other associated neuropsychological deficits may appear. However, severe disturbances of language and the other higher cortical functions such as apraxia and agnosia are uncommon. Motor system abnormalities including tremor, asterixis, and myoclonus often accompany the observed confusional state. EEG shows diffuse slow-wave activity, whereas CT and MRI are generally unrevealing.

Systemic Disorders

Disturbances of the cardiopulmonary, hematological, hepatic, renal, and endocrinological systems produce transient or chronic disruptions in intellectual function. Such systemic disorders can cause dementia in the elderly or, more commonly, contribute to the intellectual impairment caused by other conditions such as Alzheimer's disease or stroke. Diseases such as systemic lupus erythematosus, sarcoidosis, temporal arteritis, and rheumatoid arthritis also cause dementia through inflammation of cerebral vessels leading to stroke.

Nutritional Deficiencies

Deficiency of vitamins such as cyanocobalamin (vitamin B_{12}), folic acid, and niacin has been associated with dementia in elderly patients (Bell et al. 1990a, 1990b). Cyanocobalamin and folic acid are biochemically interrelated vitamins that exert both a separate and concomitant influence on cognition and mood (Bell et al. 1990a). Most often, vitamin B_{12} deficiency leads to impaired memory, psychosis, and depression. Additional neuropsychological impairment is an infrequent finding. Clouding of consciousness appears to be a consistent feature of the alteration in mental status associated with this nutritional cause of dementia (Hector and Burton 1988). The neuropsychiatric manifestations of vitamin B_{12} deficiency and associated neurological deficits such as myelopathy, neuropathy, and seizures may occur in subtle or atypical vitamin B_{12} deficiency states in which hematological indices and the Schilling test results are normal (Karnaze and Carmel 1990).

The diagnosis of dementia caused by vitamin B_{12} deficiency rests on demonstration of diminished serum cobalamin levels. Diagnostic accuracy can be improved by measurement of pretreatment and posttreatment serum levels of methylmalonic acid and/or total homocysteine (Lindenbaum et al. 1988).

Replacement therapy of vitamin B_{12} deficiency rarely leads to complete restoration of intellectual function. In some patients, however, supplementation with the deficient vitamin can lead to partial improvement in neuropsychological function (Gross et al. 1986).

It is less clear to what extent isolated folic acid deficiency may cause dementia. Some have speculated that increased levels of folic acid in elderly patients cause a variety of neuropsychiatric symptoms, most importantly depression. In general, disruptions in the delicate balance between cyanocobalamin and folic acid probably underlie the emergence of most neuropsychiatric features. The complex relationship between these two vitamins and neuropsychiatric syndromes is uncertain. However, dysfunction in brain cyanocobalamin and folic acid status does appear to have important consequences for neurotransmitter metabolism, particularly those pathways related to serotonergic function (Bell et al. 1990b).

Toxic Disorders

The neuropsychological impairment of chronic alcoholism has been historically considered to be a severe amnestic disorder related to a nutritional deficiency of thiamine (Korsakoff's psychosis). Contemporary research, however, supports the view that, along with anterograde and retrograde memory impairment, alcoholism is associated with visuoperceptual and problem-solving disability. Impaired performance of verbal fluency tasks and poor abstract concept formation have also been noted (Butters 1985; Cummings and Benson 1992; Tuck et al. 1984). Improvement of dementia may occur with abstinence, but complete restoration of intellectual function is rare.

Alcohol-associated dementia is more common in the elderly population than in younger alcoholic populations; this finding is independent of the duration of excessive intake of alcohol (Cummings and Benson 1992). The dementia associated with alcoholism may be in part a product of thiamine deficiency but is likely also to reflect a direct toxic effect of alcohol. Also largely unexplained is the reversible CT scan finding of enlarged ventricles and widened cortical sulci in the brains of alcoholic patients. The degree of atrophy does not appear to correlate with the severity of intellectual impairment. In elderly alcoholic patients with dementia, the EEG frequently shows abnormal slowing.

Although hemorrhagic lesions of the medial diencephalon have been thought to underlie the memory impairment of alcoholism, evidence has arisen implicating pathology of the nucleus basalis of Meynert and cortical structures (Butters 1985). Postmortem studies of alcoholic patients reveal greater degrees of white matter atrophy than of cortical atrophy, implicating a toxic effect of alcohol on myelin (Cummings and Benson 1992).

With aging of patients, the risk of medication toxicity increases as a consequence of alterations in drug metabolism, distribution, binding, and excretion. Aside from being vulnerable to excessive dosing or polypharmacy, elderly patients can be vulnerable also to pharmacotoxicity because of increased sensitivity to the psychotropic effects of various medications (Mahler et al. 1987). Centrally acting antihypertensive agents, anticholinergic drugs, neuroleptics, benzodiazepines, hypnotics, and antidepressants can all impair intellectual function in the susceptible elderly patient.

Posttraumatic Dementia

Elderly people are especially at risk for suffering closed head injury (see Chapter 28 in this volume). Physical frailty, disturbances of gait secondary to orthopedic disability, and an increased occurrence of orthostatic hypotension in this population increase the risk of falls and traumatic brain injury. Injury to the brain in this fashion includes hemorrhage, contusion, laceration, or shearing effects. With subtle trauma, older patients have an increased tendency for the bridging veins to rupture and hemorrhage as they course from the cortical surface to the dural sinuses. As a result, subdural collections of blood may form (subdural hematoma), giving rise to altered mentation. The onset of dementia may be subacute or chronic. Affected patients manifest a gradually progressive, chronic confusional state with transient, relatively minor, focal neurological signs that can be mistaken for stroke or tumor.

With chronic subdural hematomas, the collection of blood can be isodense on CT scanning of the brain and thus difficult to detect unless there is obvious shift of the midline structures or obscuring of the cortical sulci. For this lesion, MRI provides significantly improved imaging sensitivity and is the diagnostic procedure of choice (Cummings and Benson 1992). When the patient is symptomatic, subdural collections of blood may be surgically evacuated to produce some clinical improvement.

Standard Evaluation of Dementia

The standard evaluation of the nondegenerative causes of dementia includes assimilating a thorough history of the patient's present illness, with comprehensive attention to cognitive, medical, neurological, and psychiatric features. The interview must review the patient's medical, educational, social, vocational, and family histories. Any significant exposure of the individual to alcohol, medications, and other potential toxins must be considered. Because the intellectually impaired individual can only rarely provide such comprehensive data accurately, it is recommended that the caregiver be extensively interviewed with and without the patient present. Physical, neurological, and mental status examinations should be conducted. A quantifiable screening assessment of the patient's intellectual ability, such as the Mini-Mental State Exam (MMSE) (Folstein et al. 1975), allows the physician to establish a baseline of function for the patient and follow disease course. More extensive neuropsychological assessment can help fully elucidate the patient's deficits.

Several laboratory studies should be conducted to augment evaluation of the body's cardiopulmonary, renal, hepatic, endocrinological, and hematological systems. When cardiac or pulmonary dysfunction is clinically apparent, electrocardiography, chest radiography, or arterial blood gas determinations may be indicated. Additionally, an assay for vitamin B_{12} should be accompanied by blood tests to detect the presence of systemic infection or inflammation.

The thorough evaluation of dementia requires a neuroimaging study such as CT or MRI of the brain to document the presence of atrophy, mass lesions, stroke, or hydrocephalus. When diagnostic uncertainty is prominent, functional neuroimaging techniques, such as SPECT or PET, if available, can be useful to detect perfusion or metabolic abnormalities characteristic of dementing disorders such as Alzheimer's disease or the frontal lobe degenerations.

When infection or inflammation of the brain parenchyma or meninges is suspected, lumbar puncture is indicated. EEG is an especially useful study to support the presence of seizures or an infectious, toxic, or metabolic encephalopathy. Additionally, EEG studies can be repeated to monitor disease progression or response to treatment (Table 23–4). A diagnostic brain biopsy is infrequently indicated in the evaluation of dementia. The procedure is associated with substantial morbidity and rarely leads to the diagnosis of a reversible condition (Hulette et al. 1992; Kaufman and Catalano 1979). Brain biopsy can be helpful for the diagnosis of Creutzfeldt-Jakob disease (Gajdusek et al. 1977). However, this technique is being largely supplanted by the recent availability of CSF protein markers for the disease (Zerr et al. 1998). Published practice parameters for the diagnosis and evaluation of dementia are readily available for reference (Quality Standards Subcommittee of the American Academy of Neurology 1994).

TABLE 23–4. **History of illness**

Review of systems
Medical history
Medication review
Family history
Psychiatric interview
Physical examination
Neurological examination
Mental status examination (with rating of dementia severity)
Laboratory evaluation (mandatory)
    Complete blood count with differential
    Liver function tests
    Serum electrolytes, calcium, phosphorus, and glucose
    High-sensitivity thyroid-stimulating hormone
    Syphilis serology
    Erythrocyte sedimentation rate
    Serum creatinine and blood urea nitrogen
    Urinalysis
    Serum B_{12} and folic acid
Laboratory evaluation (selective)
    Lyme disease antibody titer
    Human immunodeficiency virus titer
    Rheumatologic studies (rheumatoid factor, antinuclear antibody titer, and so on)
    Endocrine studies (serum cortisol, parathyroid hormone, and so on)
    Arterial blood gas determination
Neuroimaging (mandatory)
    Computed tomography or magnetic resonance imaging of the head
Neuroimaging (selective)
    Single photon emission computed tomography
    Positron-emission tomography
Ancillary studies
    Chest radiograph
    Electrocardiogram
    Electroencephalogram
    Neuropsychological evaluation

The comprehensive evaluation of dementia must be augmented by careful surveillance for caregiver anxiety or depression. It is necessary to define any potential causes of excessive burden such as disruptive patient behavior, a lack of familial or social supports, or any financial losses, real or imagined. On establishing a diagnosis, the patient and his or her caregiver must be fully informed and apprised of the prognosis and any potential treatment options. Referral should be made for specialized medical evaluation and care as indicated. Additionally, caregivers often need to be referred for legal counseling and ancillary social services such as home health care, day care, and nursing home care.

Treatment of Dementia: General Considerations

For the nondegenerative dementing disorders, improvement in intellectual function following treatment is often incomplete. Therapies such as resection of a mass lesion, ventricular shunting for NPH, or correction of a metabolic disorder such as vitamin B_{12} deficiency or hypothyroidism often lead to symptomatic improvement, but rarely to complete recovery. The essential requirement for therapy is to halt disease progression and minimize disability. In VaD, for example, this generally entails optimal control of risk factors such as hypertension, smoking, and hyperlipidemia.

Although the neuropsychological features of dementia are rarely completely reversible, accompanying neuropsychiatric symptoms such as depression, anxiety, psychosis, sleep disorders, and aggressivity are often successfully treated with a combination of behavioral approaches and pharmacotherapy. The contribution of disruptive behavior to caregiver burden cannot be overemphasized and must receive comprehensive attention.

The nonpharmacological approaches to dysfunctional behavior generally consist of reassurance, distraction, redirection, and structure. Generally, the caregiver should try to respond to the behavior in a calm and direct manner. In the setting of aggressive behavior, caregivers must ensure their own safety before attempting to relax the patient. When patients experience hallucinations or verbalize persecutory thoughts such as delusions of theft or infidelity, caregivers should acknowledge the expressed fears and offer calm reassurance and distraction. Wandering behavior should be accommodated whenever possible by providing an open space that is secure and well lit. Exceptionally restless patients or those who frequently wander must be observed for signs of dehydration and the development of sores on the bottom of the feet.

Disrupted sleep is best treated with improvements in sleep hygiene. This often includes avoiding stimulants and nocturnal fluids, limiting daytime naps, and discouraging all non–sleep-related activities in bed (with the possible exception of sexual relations). A diligent search for coexistent medical conditions that may disturb sleep is also required. (For a fuller discussion of sleep disorders in the elderly, see Chapter 17 in this volume.)

Augmentation with pharmacotherapy is often necessary to effectively treat disruptive behavior in dementia. Tables 23–5 through 23–7 provide guides for the pharmacotherapy of behavioral changes in dementia. (Pharmacotherapy in the elderly is covered more extensively in Chapter 34 in this volume.) In addition to managing disruptive behavior, treatment of dementia must also include astute attention to the other causes of excessive caregiver burden, such as social isolation and inadequate social and familial supports.

Summary

The nondegenerative causes of dementia in the elderly population include cerebrovascular disease, hydrocephalus, psychiatric disorders such as depression, infectious and

TABLE 23–5. Pharmacotherapy of behavioral changes in dementia—antidepressants

Agent	Dosing guidelines	Side effects
Nortriptyline, desipramine	Initiate at 10 mg/day; increase dose by 10 mg/week until treatment response or side effects emerge.	Confusion, sedation, anticholinergic effects, and cardiac conduction delay
Trazodone	Initiate at 50 mg/day; increase dose by 50 mg/week until response or side effects emerge.	Sedation, orthostasis, confusion, and priapism (in males)
Fluoxetine, paroxetine	Initiate at 10 mg/day; increase dose to 20 mg/day after 1 week.	Restlessness, insomnia, anxiety, anorexia, and confusion
Sertraline	Initiate at 25 mg/day; increase dose to 50 mg/day after 1 week (may need to go to 150 mg/day depending on clinical response).	Restlessness, insomnia, anxiety, anorexia, diarrhea
Bupropion	Initiate at 75 mg/day; increase dose after 4 days to 150 mg/day; maintain at 300 mg/day maximum.	Insomnia, anxiety, confusion, seizures

TABLE 23–6. Pharmacotherapy of behavioral changes in dementia—antipsychotics

Agent	Starting daily dose[a]	Relative side effects	
		Parkinsonism	Anticholinergic/sedation
Haloperidol	0.5–1 mg	High	Low/low
Trifluoperazine	1 mg	Moderate	Moderate/moderate
Thiothixene	1 mg	Moderate	Moderate/low
Thioridazine	10 mg	Low	High/high
Risperidone	0.5 mg	Low	None/low
Olanzapine	2.5 mg	Very low	Low/moderate
Quetiapine	12.5 mg	Very low	Low/moderate
Clozapine	12.5 mg	Very low	High/high

[a]Maintain dosage at lowest possible effective dose; increase as needed every 4–7 days.

TABLE 23–7. Pharmacotherapy of behavioral changes in dementia—alternative agents for agitation and aggressivity

Agent	Starting daily dose[a]	Side effects
Carbamazepine[b]	100 mg bid	Sedation, ataxia, dysarthria, bone marrow suppression, and hepatotoxicity
Sodium valproate	125 mg bid	Sedation, ataxia, dysarthria, bone marrow suppression, and hepatotoxicity
Trazodone	50 mg/day	Sedation, orthostasis, and priapism (in males)
Buspirone	5 mg bid	Dizziness, nausea, and sedation
Clonazepam	0.5 mg bid	Sedation, ataxia, and dysarthria
Propranolol[c]	10 mg bid	Sedation, bradycardia, hypotension, depression, and worsening of chronic obstructive pulmonary disease

[a]Dosing will need to be increased for all agents at weekly intervals until response or emergence of side effects.
[b]Monitor serum levels, complete blood count, and liver function tests.
[c]Monitor pulse and blood pressure closely.

of the major organ systems, endocrinopathies, nutritional deficiencies, toxic disorders, and trauma. Although any of these conditions may be the primary cause of acquired intellectual impairment, more characteristically, their presence complicates the clinical course of degenerative disorders such as Alzheimer's disease. The standard evaluation of these disorders must be sufficiently broad in scope to detect their occurrence but should be specifically guided by the data available. Treatment of the nondegenerative dementing disorders is directed at halting progression, restoring intellectual function, managing associated neuropsychiatric features, and relieving caregiver burden.

References

Abas MA, Sahakian BJ, Levy R: Neuropsychological deficits and CT scan changes in elderly depressives. Psychol Med 20: 507–520, 1990

Adams RD, Victor M: Principles of Neurology, 4th Edition. New York, McGraw-Hill, 1989

Adams RD, Fisher CM, Hakim S, et al: Symptomatic occult hydrocephalus with "normal" cerebrospinal fluid pressure: a treatable syndrome. N Engl J Med 273:117–126, 1965

Almkvist O, Wahlund LO, Andersson-Lundman G, et al: White-matter hyperintensity and neuropsychological functions in dementia and healthy aging. Arch Neurol 49: 626–633, 1992

Ames D, Dolan R, Mann A: The distinction between depression and dementia in the very old. Int J Geriatr Psychiatry 5:193–198, 1990

Anderson SW, Damasio H, Tranel D: Neuropsychological impairments associated with lesions caused by tumor or stroke. Arch Neurol 47:397–405, 1990

Andreasen NC, Olsen SA, Dennert JW, et al: Ventricular enlargement in schizophrenia: relationship to positive and negative symptoms. Am J Psychiatry 139:297–301, 1982

Babikian V, Ropper AH: Binswanger's disease: a review. Stroke 18:2–12, 1987

Bannister R: Brain's Clinical Neurology, 6th Edition. New York, Oxford University Press, 1986

Barry PB, Moskowitz MA: The diagnosis of reversible dementia in the elderly: a critical review. Arch Intern Med 148: 1914–1918, 1988

Bell IR, Edman JS, Marby DW, et al: Vitamin B_{12} and folate status in acute geropsychiatric inpatients: affective and cognitive characteristics of a vitamin nondeficient population. Biol Psychiatry 27:125–137, 1990a

Bell IR, Edman JS, Miller J, et al: Relationship of normal serum vitamin B_{12} and folate levels to cognitive test performance in subtypes of geriatric major depression. J Geriatr Psychiatry Neurol 3:98–105, 1990b

Benson DF: Hydrocephalic dementia, in Handbook of Clinical Neurology: Neurobehavioral Disorders, Vol 2. Edited by Frederiks JAM. New York, Elsevier, 1985, pp 323–333

Benson DF: The spectrum of dementia: a comparison of the clinical features of AIDS/dementia and dementia of the Alzheimer type. Alzheimer Dis Assoc Disord 1:217–220, 1987

Bolla-Wilson K, Robinson RG, Starkstein SE, et al: Lateralization of dementia of depression in stroke patients. Am J Psychiatry 146:627–634, 1989

Bondareff W, Raval J, Woo B, et al: Magnetic resonance imaging and the severity of dementia in older adults. Arch Gen Psychiatry 47:47–51, 1990

Boone KB, Miller BL, Lesser IM, et al: Neuropsychological correlates of white-matter lesions in healthy elderly subjects. Arch Neurol 40:549–554, 1992

Breier A, Schreiber JL, Dyer J, et al: National Institute of Mental Health longitudinal study of chronic schizophrenia: prognosis and predictors of outcome. Arch Gen Psychiatry 48:239–246, 1991

Brown P, Cathala F, Castaigne P, et al: Creutzfeldt-Jakob disease: clinical analysis of a consecutive series of 230 neuropathologically verified cases. Ann Neurol 20: 597–602, 1986

Butters N: Alcoholic Korsakoff's syndrome: some unresolved issues concerning etiology, neuropathology, and cognitive deficits. Journal of Clinical Experimental Neurology 7:181–210, 1985

Caine ED: Pseudo-dementia. Arch Gen Psychiatry 38: 1359–1364, 1981

Chimowitz MI, Estes ML, Furlan AJ, et al: Further observations on the pathology of subcortical lesions identified on magnetic resonance imaging. Arch Neurol 49:747–752, 1992

Chui HC, Victoroff JI, Margolin D, et al: Criteria for the diagnosis of ischemic vascular dementia proposed by the State of California Alzheimer's Disease Diagnostic and Treatment Centers. Neurology 42:473–480, 1992

Clarfield AM: The reversible dementias: do they reverse? Ann Intern Med 109:476–486, 1988

Clarfield AM: Normal-pressure hydrocephalus: saga or swamp? JAMA 262:2592–2593, 1989

Coffey CE, Figiel GS, Djang WT, et al: Subcortical hyperintensity on magnetic resonance imaging: a comparison of normal and depressed elderly subjects. Am J Psychiatry 147:187–189, 1990

Cohen RM, Weingartner H, Smallberg SA, et al: Effort and cognition in depression. Arch Gen Psychiatry 39:593–597, 1982

Cox J, Knox J, Brocklehurst G: Normal pressure hydrocephalus (letter). JAMA 36:650, 1988

Cummings JL (ed): Subcortical Dementia. New York, Oxford University Press, 1990

Cummings JL, Benson DF: Dementia: A Clinical Approach, 2nd Edition. Boston, MA, Butterworth-Heinemann, 1992

Cummings JL, Benson DF, LoVerme S Jr: Reversible dementia: illustrative cases, definition, and review. JAMA 243:2434–2439, 1980

Cummings JL, Miller B, Hill MA, et al: Neuropsychiatric aspects of multi-infarct dementia and dementia of the Alzheimer type. Arch Neurol 44:389–393, 1987

Erkinjuntti T, Sulkava R: Diagnosis of multi-infarct dementia. Alzheimer Dis Assoc Disord 5(2):112–121, 1991

Faulstich ME: Psychiatric aspects of AIDS. Am J Psychiatry 144:551–556, 1987

Fisher CM: Hydrocephalus as a cause of disturbances of gait in the elderly. Neurology 32:1358–1363, 1982

Folstein MF, McHugh PR: Dementia syndrome of depression, in Alzheimer's Disease: Senile Dementia and Related Disorders. Edited by Katzman R, Terry RD, Bick KL. New York, Raven, 1978, pp 87–96

Folstein MF, Folstein SE, McHugh PR: Mini-Mental State: a practical method for grading the cognitive state of patients for the clinician. J Psychiatr Res 12:189–198, 1975

Gajdusek DC, Gibbs CS, Asher DM, et al: Precautions in medical care of, and in handling materials from, patients with transmissible virus dementia (Creutzfeldt-Jakob disease). N Engl J Med 297:1253–1258, 1977

Gallassi R, Morreale AN, Montagna P, et al: Binswanger's disease and normal-pressure hydrocephalus. Arch Neurol 48:1156–1159, 1991

Gent M, Blakely JA, Easton JD, et al: The Canadian American Ticlopidine Study (CATS) in thromboembolic stroke. Lancet 1:1215–1220, 1989

Graff-Radford NR, Godersky JC, Jones MP: Variables predicting surgical outcome in symptomatic hydrocephalus in the elderly. Neurology 39:1601–1604, 1989

Greenwald BS, Kramer-Ginsberg E, Marin DB, et al: Dementia with coexistent major depression. Am J Psychiatry 146:1472–1478, 1989

Gross JS, Weintraub NT, Neufeld RR, et al: Pernicious anemia in the demented patient without anemia or macrocytosis: a case for early recognition. J Am Geriatr Soc 34:612–614, 1986

Hachinski VC: Multi-infarct dementia: a reappraisal. Alzheimer Dis Assoc Disord 5(2):64–68, 1991

Hachinski VC, Iliff LD, Zilhka E, et al: Cerebral blood flow in dementia. Arch Neurol 32:632–637, 1975

Hector M, Burton JR: What are the psychiatric manifestations of vitamin B$_{12}$ deficiency? J Am Geriatr Soc 36:1105–1112, 1988

Hier DB, Warach JD, Gorelick PB, et al: Predictors of survival in clinically diagnosed Alzheimer's disease and multi-infarct dementia. Arch Neurol 46:1213–1216, 1989

Hintz S, Kuck J, Peterkin JJ, et al: Depression in the context of human immunodeficiency virus infection: implications for treatment. J Clin Psychiatry 51:497–501, 1990

Hulette CM, Earl NL, Crain BJ: Evaluation of cerebral biopsies for the diagnosis of dementia. Arch Neurol 49:28–31, 1992

Hulette C, Nochlin D, McKeel D, et al: Clinical-neuropathological findings in multi-infarct dementia: a report of six autopsied cases. Neurology 48(3):668–672, 1997

Ishii N, Nishihara Y, Imamura T: Why do frontal lobe symptoms predominate in vascular dementia with lacunes? Neurology 36:340–345, 1986

Jacoby RJ, Levy R, Bird JM: Computed tomography and the outcome of affective disorder: a follow-up study of elderly patients. Br J Psychiatry 139:288–292, 1981

Janowsky DS: Pseudodementia in the elderly: differential diagnosis and treatment. J Clin Psychiatry 49:19–25, 1982

Kahn RL, Zarit SH, Hilbert NM, et al: Memory complaint and impairment in the aged. Arch Gen Psychiatry 32:1569–1573, 1975

Karnaze DS, Carmel R: Neurologic and evoked potential abnormalities in subtle cobalamin deficiency states, including deficiency without anemia and with normal absorption of free cobalamin. Arch Neurol 47:1008–1012, 1990

Kase CS: Epidemiology of multi-infarct dementia. Alzheimer Dis Assoc Disord 5(2):71–76, 1991

Kaufman HK, Catalano LW: Diagnostic brain biopsy: a series of 50 cases and a review. Neurosurgery 4:129–136, 1979

Kiloh LG: Pseudo-dementia. Acta Psychiatr Scand 37:336–351, 1961

Kinkel WR, Jacobs L, Polachini I, et al: Subcortical arteriosclerotic encephalopathy (Binswanger's disease): computed tomographic, nuclear magnetic resonance and clinical correlations. Arch Neurol 42:951–959, 1985

Kral VA: The relationship between senile dementia (Alzheimer type) and depression. Can J Psychiatry 28:304–305, 1983

Kral VA, Emery OB: Long-term follow-up of depressive pseudodementia of the aged. Can J Psychiatry 34:445–446, 1989

Larson EB, Reifler BV, Sumi SM, et al: Diagnostic tests in the evaluation of dementia: a prospective study of 200 elderly outpatients. Arch Intern Med 146:1917–1922, 1986

Leys D, Soetaert G, Petit H, et al: Periventricular and white matter magnetic resonance imaging hyperintensities do not differ between Alzheimer's disease and normal aging. Arch Neurol 47:524–527, 1990

Lindenbaum J, Healton EB, Savage DG, et al: Neuropsychiatric disorders caused by cobalamin deficiency in the absence of anemia or macrocytosis. N Engl J Med 318:1720–1728, 1988

Loeb C, Gandolfo C: Diagnostic evaluation of degenerative and vascular dementia. Stroke 14:399–401, 1983

Lunn S, Skydsbjerg M, Schulsinger H, et al: A preliminary report on the neuropsychologic sequelae of human immunodeficiency virus. Arch Gen Psychiatry 48:139–142, 1991

Mahler ME, Cummings JL: Behavioral neurology of multi-infarct dementia. Alzheimer Dis Assoc Dis 5:122–130, 1991

Mahler ME, Cummings JL, Benson DF: Treatable dementias. West J Med 146:705–712, 1987

McAllister TW, Price TRP: Severe depressive pseudodementia with and without dementia. Am J Psychiatry 137:1449–1450, 1982

Meyer JS, Judd BW, Tawakina T, et al: Improved cognition after control of risk factors for multi-infarct dementia. JAMA 256:2203–2209, 1986

Meyer JS, McClintic K, Sims P, et al: Etiology, prevention, and treatment of vascular and multi-infarct dementia, in Vascular and Multi-infarct Dementia. Edited by Meyer JS, Lechner H, Marshall J, et al. Mount Kisco, NY, Futura, 1988, pp 129–147

Meyer JS, Rogers RL, McClintic K, et al: Randomized clinical trial of daily aspirin therapy in multi-infarct dementia: a pilot study. J Am Geriatr Soc 37:549–555, 1989

Mirsen T, Hachinski V: Epidemiology and classification of vascular and multi-infarct dementia, in Vascular and Multi-infarct Dementia. Edited by Meyer JS, Lechner H, Marshall J, et al. Mount Kisco, NY, Futura, 1988, pp 61–75

Mulrow CD, Feussner JR, Williams BC, et al: The value of clinical findings in the detection of NPH. J Gerontol 42:277–279, 1987

Navia BA, Price RW: The acquired immunodeficiency syndrome dementia complex as the presenting or sole manifestation of human immunodeficiency virus infection. Arch Neurol 44:65–69, 1987

Navia BA, Jordan BD, Price RW: The AIDS dementia complex, I: clinical features. Ann Neurol 19:517–524, 1986

O'Connor DW, Pollitt PA, Roth M, et al: Memory complaints and impairment in normal, depressed, and demented elderly persons identified in a community survey. Arch Gen Psychiatry 47:224–227, 1990

Olsson Y, Brun A, Englund E: Fundamental pathological lesions in vascular dementia. Acta Neurol Scand Suppl 168:31–38, 1996

Ostrow D, Grant I, Atkinson H: Assessment and management of the AIDS patient with neuropsychiatric disturbances. J Clin Psychiatry 49 (suppl):14–22, 1988

Pearlson GD, Rabins PV, Kim WS, et al: Structural brain CT changes and cognitive deficits in elderly depressives with and without reversible dementia ("pseudodementia"). Psychol Med 19:573–584, 1989

Perlick D: Negative symptoms are related to both frontal and nonfrontal neuropsychological measures in chronic schizophrenia. Arch Gen Psychiatry 49:245–246, 1992

Perry SW: Organic mental disorders caused by HIV: update on early diagnosis and treatment. Am J Psychiatry 147: 696–710, 1990

Peterson B, Summergrad P: Binswanger's disease, II: pathogenesis of subcortical arteriosclerotic encephalopathy and its relation to other dementing processes. J Geriatr Psychiatry Neurol 2–4:171–181, 1989

Plotkin DA, Mintz J, Jarvik LF: Subjective memory complaints in geriatric depression. Am J Psychiatry 142:1103–1105, 1985

Pohjasvaara T, Erkinjuntti T, Ylikoski R, et al: Clinical determinants of poststroke dementia. Stroke 29(1):75–81, 1998

Posner TB: Paraneoplastic syndromes involving the nervous system, in Neurology and General Medicine. Edited by Aminoff MT. New York, Churchill Livingstone, 1989, pp 342–364

Quality Standards Subcommittee of the American Academy of Neurology: Practice parameter for diagnosis and evaluation of dementia (summary statement). Neurology 44:2203–2206, 1994

Rabins PV: The prevalence of reversible dementia in a psychiatric hospital. Hosp Community Psychiatry 32:490–492, 1981

Rabins PV, Merchant A, Nestadt G: Criteria for diagnosing reversible dementia caused by depression: validation by 2-year follow-up. Br J Psychiatry 144:488–492, 1984

Reding M, Haycox J, Blass J: Depression in patients referred to a dementia clinic; a three-year prospective study. Arch Neurol 42:894–896, 1985

Robinson RG, Bolla-Wilson K, Kaplan E, et al: Depression influences intellectual impairment in stroke patients. Br J Psychiatry 148:541–547, 1986

Roman GC: The epidemiology of vascular dementia, in Cerebral Ischemia and Dementia. Edited by Hartmann A, Kuschinsky W, Hoyer S. Berlin, Springer-Verlag, 1991, pp 9–15

Roman GC, Tatemichi TK, Erkinjuntti T, et al: Vascular dementia: diagnostic criteria for research studies (report of the NINCDS-AIREN International Work Group). Neurology 43:250–260, 1993

Rowland LP: Merritt's Textbook of Neurology, 8th Edition. Philadelphia, PA, Lea & Febiger, 1989

Savard RJ, Rey A, Post RM: Halstead-Reitan category test in bipolar and unipolar affective disorders: relationship to age and phase of illness. J Nerv Ment Dis 168:297–304, 1980

Schmitt FA, Bigley JW, McKinnis R, et al: Neuropsychological outcome of zidovudine (AZT) treatment of patients with AIDS and AIDS-related complex. N Engl J Med 319: 1573–1578, 1988

Small GW: Revised ischemic score for diagnosing multi-infarct dementia. J Clin Psychiatry 46:514–517, 1985

Stern Y, Marder K, Bell K, et al: Multidisciplinary baseline assessment of homosexual men with and without human immunodeficiency virus infection, III: neurologic and neuropsychological findings. Arch Gen Psychiatry 48: 131–138, 1991

Summergrad P, Peterson B: Binswanger's disease, I: the clinical recognition of subcortical arteriosclerotic encephalopathy in elderly neuropsychiatric patients. J Geriatr Psychiatry Neurol 2–3:123–133, 1989

Theodore WH, Gendelman S: Meningeal carcinomatosis. Arch Neurol 38:696–699, 1981

Tuck RR, Brew BJ, Britton AM, et al: Alcohol and brain damage. British Journal of Addiction 79:251–259, 1984

Vanneste J, Augustijn P, Davies GAG, et al: Normal-pressure hydrocephalus; is cisternography still useful in selecting patients for a shunt? Arch Neurol 49:366–370, 1992

Wade JPH: Multi-infarct dementia: prevention and treatment. Alzheimer Dis Assoc Disord 5(2):144–148, 1991

Weingartner H, Cohen RM, Murphy DL, et al: Cognitive processes in depression. Arch Gen Psychiatry 38:42–47, 1981

Wells CE: Pseudodementia. Am J Psychiatry 136:895–900, 1979

Wolfe N, Linn R, Babikian VL, et al: Frontal systems impairment following multiple lacunar infarcts. Arch Neurol 47: 129–132, 1990

Wright JM, Silove D: Pseudodementia in schizophrenia and mania. New Zealand Journal of Psychiatry 22:109–114, 1988

Yarchoan R, Berg G, Brouwers P, et al: Response of human immunodeficiency–virus-associated neurological disease to 3-azido-3-deoxythymidine. Lancet 1:132–135, 1987

Zerr I, Bodemer M, Gefeller O, et al: Detection of 14-3-3 protein in the cerebrospinal fluid supports the diagnosis of Creutzfeldt-Jakob disease. Ann Neurol 43(1):32–40, 1998

Zimmerman RD, Fleming CA, Lee BCP, et al: Periventricular hyperintensity as seen by magnetic resonance: prevalence and significance. AJR 146:443–450, 1986

Alzheimer's Disease and Frontotemporal Dementia

Bruce L. Miller, M.D.

Andrew Gustavson, M.D.

Recent advances in the diagnosis and treatment of the degenerative disorders have been enormous. Both Alzheimer's disease (AD) and frontotemporal dementia (FTD) have distinct epidemiological, clinical, and pathological profiles, and recent work suggests that the two can be differentiated during life (Miller et al. 1997a). Accurate diagnosis is no longer purely academic because new disease-specific treatments for AD and FTD have emerged. Another exciting advance related to these disorders has been the discovery of a series of different genetic mutations causal for AD or FTD. These findings are beginning to change our understanding of the pathogenesis of these disorders, and ultimately they offer hope for the development of disease-specific therapies that will modify disease progression.

AD is still considered a unitary disorder despite clinical, genetic, and pathological variability. In contrast, with FTD there is marked controversy as to how to classify the clinically and pathologically diverse syndromes associated with progressive frontotemporal degeneration. Some experts lump patients with Pick's disease, FTD without Pick's bodies, progressive subcortical gliosis, primary progressive aphasia, and corticobasal degeneration into the same category (Kertesz 1997), whereas others insist that these are each distinct disease entities (Neary 1997). A problem associated with previous attempts to classify these diseases was that little was known concerning the primary cause of FTD. This led to a taxonomy based largely upon clinical and pathological phenomenology. However, genetic breakthroughs are changing the understanding of both FTD and AD. In this chapter, we discuss AD and FTD separately and address the evolving understanding of their epidemiological, clinical, genetic, imaging, chemical, and pathological features.

Alzheimer's Disease

Epidemiology

During the final stages of AD, the patient is bedridden and unable to swallow or mobilize, so that death often is secondary to dehydration or sepsis. Therefore, many deaths of patients with end-stage AD are coded on death certificates as caused by infection. This problem, along with serious obstacles associated with determining a proper diagnosis, make ascertainment of the exact prevalence of AD difficult (Hay and Ernst 1987). In addition, the clinical and pathological standards regarding what constitutes AD, although improving, continue to be flawed, which also complicates accurate determination of AD prevalence. One community-based study (Evans et al. 1989), estimates the prevalence of AD at four million cases in the United States. Assuming this is correct, AD is the fourth leading cause of death in adults, ranking behind heart disease, cancer, and stroke (Office of Technology Assessment Task Force 1988).

A major risk factor for AD is aging, and AD rises with each decade of life. AD has a prevalence of approximately 6.2% over age 65 (Roth 1978), 20% over 80 (Mortimer 1983), and 45% over 95 (Gottfries 1990). The reason for the increase of AD with age is complex and multifactorial, although the cumulative loss of neuronal synapses is one important factor. Monozygotic twin studies (Gatz et al. 1997; Nee et al. 1987) suggest a strong genetic component to AD; when one twin manifests AD, approximately 40% of the co-twins also develop the disorder. However, often there is a long delay between the onset of AD for the second twin, suggesting both environmental and genetic contributions to AD (Creasey et al. 1989).

Nearly all patients with Down's syndrome who live beyond 40 years develop amyloid plaques in the cortex (Ropper and Williams 1980). Because Down's syndrome is caused by an extra chromosome 21, it was suggested that a gene on this chromosome might be key in the pathogenesis of AD. Subsequent studies of familial AD led to the discovery of a mutation in the amyloid precursor protein (APP) on chromosome 21 (Goate et al. 1991; St. George-Hyslop et al. 1990). Although such patients represent only 3% of all familial AD, they firmly connect amyloid to AD pathogenesis. Transgenic mice with the APP mutation develop a progressive dementing disorder (D'Hooge et al. 1996) with AD-like neuropathology (Hsiao et al. 1995), further implicating amyloid in the pathogenesis of AD. Therefore, overproduction of amyloid as occurs with Down's syndrome or the presence of a mutation on chromosome 21 in the gene coding for amyloid predispose to AD.

Beyond amyloid, a complex picture regarding AD and genetics is emerging. The most common mutation associated with early onset AD is found in the presenilin 1 gene on chromosome 14 (Schellenberg 1995), and it accounts for approximately 50% of all early onset familial AD. With this mutation, AD usually begins in the fifth decade. A mu-

tation in a homologous protein on chromosome 1 (presenilin 2) has been found in a few families (Rogaev et al. 1995). The function of the presenilins is unknown, but this is an area of intense research (Mattson and Guo 1997).

Finally, apolipoprotein E4 greatly increases the risk that the carrier will develop AD. Unlike the presenilin and APP mutations, most cases associated with this allele develop AD after the age of 60. Carrying one apolipoprotein E4 increases the risk for AD by 2.5 times. Two E4 proteins increase the risk by 20-fold, with 90% of carriers developing AD by age 90 (Mayeux et al. 1998; Roses 1995). As with the APP mutations, transgenic mice carrying the apolipoprotein E4 allele also develop a progressive dementing disorder. Some researchers suggest that screening for apolipoprotein E4 will help the clinician to pinpoint cases of dementia that are not a result of AD (Mayeux et al. 1998). However, this concept is still controversial because there are individuals with dementias not the result of AD who carry the apolipoprotein E4 allele, and there are patients with AD in whom the E4 allele is not present.

Environmental risk factors play a role in the pathogenesis of AD. Head injury (Graves et al. 1990) and possibly small head size (Graves et al. 1996) increase the risk for AD. Also, there is a greater prevalence of AD in low socioeconomic groups (Zhang et al. 1990). Diminished idea density in a young group of nuns proved to be a risk factor for developing AD later in life (Snowdon et al. 1996). The association between low education and AD is now accepted, although the exact mechanism for the association is still unknown. Whether it is related to diminished education or represents a genetic factor (Gatz et al. 1997; Pedersen et al. 1996) that influences the likelihood that an individual will obtain a good education is debated. However, an emerging consensus has developed that individuals with diminished synaptic concentration, whether genetic or acquired, are at greater risk for AD.

Various studies have found nongenetic factors offering protection from AD. Women who take estrogen postmenopause appear to be at a lower risk for AD than women who do not (Paganini-Hill and Henderson 1994). Inflammation is an important component of AD pathology (McGeer and McGeer 1997) and nonsteroidal anti-inflammatory compounds may lower the risk for developing AD (Stewart et al. 1997). Currently, larger studies are under way to determine whether or not these purported protective agents will truly benefit those at risk for AD.

Cognitive Features

AD is a progressive dementia characterized by a slow decline in memory, language, visuospatial skills, personality, and cognition (Cummings and Benson 1992). Often, the first symptom of AD is loss of the ability to learn new information—amnesia. Three major types of memory—episodic, semantic, and working—are lost with AD. Episodic memory, or memory for events, is highly dependent on the hippocampus, and loss of episodic memory is a key deficit in AD (Graham and Hodges 1997). Initially, the patient is forgetful and repetitive, losing objects, repeating stories, and missing appointments. Eventually, both storage and retrieval of episodic memory become severely impaired. Unlike the memory problems seen with frontal or subcortical injury, clues do not dramatically help the patient to remember.

Semantic memory, or memory for facts and general information, deteriorates in AD. In the early stages of AD, it is not as severely impaired as episodic memory. The deficit in semantic memory leads to loss of recall for historical facts or names. Work with a subgroup of patients with FTD (Hodges et al. 1992) suggests that semantic memory is highly dependent on the function of the left anterior temporal neocortex, a region that is also vulnerable to AD pathology.

Also abnormal in AD is working memory, the ability to briefly hold and then manipulate small bits of information. This relies upon intact prefrontal cortex and posterior temporoparietal cortex (Waltz et al., in press) and is markedly impaired with AD. The amnesia of AD is the result of the deficiency of brain acetylcholine (Bartus et al. 1982; Whitehouse et al. 1981) and pathological damage in areas involved with learning and memory.

Language decline follows a characteristic course. Diminished list generation is the first deficit, and this is followed by word-finding trouble. Then, a fluent aphasia emerges, associated with diminished comprehension (Cummings et al. 1985). Neuropathology is extensive in brain regions posterior to Wernicke's area, and a transcortical sensory aphasia often develops. Next, AD spreads anteriorly to Wernicke's area, and a Wernicke's aphasia is seen. Finally, patients become mute.

Visuospatial deficits develop early. Navigating, cooking, or manipulating mechanical objects in the home are visuospatial tasks, and the ability to perform them is often lost in the first stages of AD. Drawing becomes abnormal, and one should question the diagnosis of AD if the patient can copy intersecting pentagons or a three-dimensional figure. Eventually, ability to perform overlearned visuospatial tasks such as using household items and dressing are lost. Simultaneously, many patients develop an apraxia and lose the ability to perform organized motor movements. Injury to the right parietal lobe is largely responsible for the visuospatial deficits, whereas left parietal dysfunction accounts for the apraxia.

Deficits occur in cognition, the ability to manipulate new information. Mathematical and business skills, judgments about wills, and driving ability deteriorate. At times, this impairment in cognition can lead to complex legal problems. Driving, in particular, has been an area of intense research (Fitten et al. 1995; Lundberg et al. 1997), and patients with AD are more likely to suffer serious consequences (Friedland et al. 1988) than elderly patients without dementia. Therefore, many states require that patients with a diagnosis of dementia be reported to the department of motor vehicles. Parietal and frontal injury both contribute to this aspect of the disease.

The period from onset to death typically takes from 7 to 11 years. In some patients, AD progresses with extreme rapidity over several years, whereas in others, it advances slowly over many decades. Initially, deficits in higher cortical function predominate, whereas during the middle stages of the disease patients often develop behavioral and motor problems that progressively impair movement. Finally, inability to swallow leads to aspiration pneumonia, often the cause of death.

Neuropsychiatric Features

Subtle personality changes occur in AD, sometimes as an early symptom (Petry et al. 1989; Rubin et al. 1987). Patients may show decreased energy, indifference, egocentricity, impulsivity, or irritability. Sometimes, social withdrawal and selfishness develop. However, in contrast to patients with FTD, many with AD show normal social skills. Also, profound changes in judgment or behavior are unusual in the early stages of AD.

Estimates for the prevalence of depression in AD range from zero to 57% (Cummings et al. 1987). Major depression is uncommon, but many patients with AD have periods of depressed mood associated with a feeling of inadequacy and hopelessness. This depression is often modifiable by environmental manipulations, although pharmacological treatment with the selective serotonin reuptake inhibitors is sometimes necessary and can be highly effective. As AD progresses, delusions, agitation, and even violence are seen. Delusions in AD often relate to theft, infidelity, or Capgras's syndrome (Cummings et al. 1987; Ponton et al. 1995). Hallucinations are unusual until the later stages and can signify a confusional state. The anatomical basis for these psychiatric syndromes is injury to the parietal, frontal, and limbic cortex (Cummings 1992).

Disorders of sleep, eating, sexual behavior, and psychomotor activity are common. Over 50% of caregivers describe sleep disturbances in the AD patient (Swearer et al. 1988). Telemetry with electroencephalography (EEG) shows more awake time in bed, longer latencies to rapid-eye-movement (REM) sleep, and loss of slow-wave sleep (Prinz et al. 1982). Decreased appetite is common, although weight gain is seen. Loss in sexual drive is more common than increased drive. Psychomotor activity is increased, and motor restlessness, wandering, agitation, and aggression occur. These behaviors lead to severe problems for the caregivers and often precipitate institutionalization. Pathological changes in the hypothalamus and ascending catecholaminergic, serotoninergic, and cholinergic cortical projection systems may account for these alterations in behavior.

Differential Diagnosis

Inaccuracy of diagnosis continues to plague AD research and clinical care. In one study (Boller et al. 1989), the diagnosis of two clinicians was compared with findings at pathology. In 63% of cases, both clinicians were correct; in 17% of cases, one was correct; and in 20% of cases, neither was correct. Still, diagnostic accuracy rarely reaches 95%, and studies with this degree of accuracy usually come from the assessment of groups of highly selected patients for whom diagnosis is more certain (Galasko et al. 1994; Read et al. 1995). In many settings, AD is overdiagnosed and patients with FTD, Parkinson's disease, Lewy body disease, and vascular dementia often are diagnosed during life as having AD. In addition, medically treatable dementias continue to be reported in postmortem studies from research centers (Joachim et al. 1988).

Research has helped improve diagnostic accuracy for AD and non-AD dementias. The National Institute of Neurological and Communicative Disorders and Stroke–Alzheimer's Disease and Related Disorders Association (NINCDS-ADRDA) work group established research criteria for probable and possible AD (McKhann et al. 1984). The Mini-Mental State Examination (MMSE) (Folstein et al. 1975) is a simple test that allows quantification of dementia severity. The Ischemia Scale identifies those patients in whom a vascular contribution to dementia is likely (Hachinski et al. 1975). Such tools have helped to refine AD diagnosis.

AD is no longer a "diagnosis of exclusion," that is, diagnosed by excluding other treatable disorders. Rather, an effective approach has been championed by various researchers (Cummings and Benson 1992; Gustafson 1987; Neary et al. 1988) who diagnose AD and other disorders by their clinical phenomenology. Because AD leads to dysfunction in brain regions different from those affected in FTD and most cases of vascular dementia, a clinical (and imaging) evaluation that focuses upon the brain areas that

are not functioning properly can be effective in improving diagnosis (Read et al. 1995).

Many metabolic and toxic illnesses cause cognitive impairment, and elderly patients are particularly vulnerable to developing delirium or dementia from systemic insults. Examples of systemic diseases and conditions that can lead to a dementia are thyroid disease, hyponatremia, B_{12} deficiency, depression, vasculitis, and brain hypoxia from pulmonary disease or arrhythmia (Giombetti and Miller 1990); see also Chapter 26 in this volume. Psychoactive medications can also lead to dementia. Primary brain diseases that may mimic AD include brain tumor, stroke, hydrocephalus, syphilis, Lyme encephalopathy, and Whipple's disease. Some of these conditions are treatable, and the dementia can be reversed.

Neuroimaging

Neuroimaging techniques show promise for further improving diagnosis. Computed tomography (CT) helps to identify focal brain masses or hydrocephalus and detects many, but not all, previous strokes. AD leads to generalized cerebral atrophy, although atrophy also occurs in elderly individuals without AD and in patients with non-AD degenerative dementias. Therefore, atrophy by itself is unreliable as a diagnostic marker for AD.

Magnetic resonance imaging (MRI) is better than CT at defining pathology in the temporal and basofrontal lobes, brainstem, and white matter. However, as with CT, atrophy on MRI cannot be used to make a presumptive diagnosis of AD, although quantitative analyses using MRI distinguish most patients with AD from elderly control subjects without AD by showing reductions in brain size and increases in cerebrospinal fluid in the AD group (DeCarli et al. 1990, 1996). MRI is better than CT for defining vascular disease, particularly white matter disease, a common finding in elderly populations (Boone et al. 1992).

White matter disease has many causes, with hypertension and genetics the strongest known risk factors (Carmelli et al. 1998; Pedersen et al., in press; Salerno et al. 1992). White matter hyperintensities can cause dementia, but large confluent lesions must be present before gross cognitive impairment is seen (Boone et al. 1992; DeCarli et al. 1996; Liu et al. 1992).

Positron-emission tomography (PET) and single photon emission computed tomography (SPECT) help to define dysfunctional brain areas in AD. With both PET (Benson et al. 1983; DeCarli et al. 1996) and SPECT (Jagust et al. 1987), marked deficits in metabolism or perfusion in the temporoparietal cortex and hippocampus, areas where plaques, tangles, and neuronal loss are most intense, can be seen. In contrast, in brain regions where function is better, such as motor, sensory, and visual cortex, these techniques reveal relatively normal metabolic activity or perfusion.

Neither technique has perfect sensitivity nor specificity. Temporoparietal hypoperfusion is not specific to AD and is seen with hypoxia, sleep apnea, and sometimes vascular dementia or Creutzfeldt-Jakob disease (Miller et al. 1990). Many patients with AD show marked asymmetry with SPECT or PET (Grady et al. 1990), and others show normal patterns. However, functional imaging is helpful in the differential diagnosis of degenerative brain disease, particularly in separating AD from FTD (Brun et al. 1994). Several groups (Read et al. 1995; Risberg et al. 1993) report that greater than 90% of patients with FTD can be differentiated from those with AD based upon SPECT. Also, many, but not all, patients with Creutzfeldt-Jakob disease show with PET a mottled multifocal pattern of cerebral metabolism (Benson 1983), which is distinct from that of AD or FTD. With PET (Kuhl et al. 1984) and SPECT (Miller et al. 1996), many patients with parkinsonian dementia show temporoparietal hypometabolism. However, this overlap does not reflect a deficiency of functional imaging because many patients with parkinsonian dementia have AD (Hansen and Samuel 1997).

With PET and SPECT and perfusion MRI (Sandson et al. 1996), temporoparietal changes are shown occurring early. Using SPECT, Johnson and colleagues (1998) found deficits in memory circuitry before the onset of clinical disease. With PET, apolipoprotein E4–positive subjects showed temporoparietal metabolic deficits in preclinical stages (Reiman et al. 1996; Small et al. 1996). Other researchers have used activation paradigms with functional MRI to determine the earliest deficits associated with this illness (Gabrieli 1996).

Finally, magnetic resonance spectroscopy shows promise for AD diagnosis. In AD, decreased n-acetyl-aspartate (a neuronal marker) and increased myoinositol are found (Miller et al. 1993a). More recently, Weiner and colleagues (Schuff et al. 1998) have developed a sophisticated technique for quantifying both hippocampal atrophy and neuronal loss. The combination of these two parameters led to the correct classification of 94% of control subjects and 90% of subjects with AD. Comparisons between spectroscopy and functional imaging have not yet been performed.

Neurochemistry

Many neurochemical deficits occur in AD. The cholinergic deficit was discovered approximately 20 years ago

(Bowen et al. 1976; Davies and Malony 1976; Perry et al. 1977), and this finding was the theoretical basis for the anticholinesterase medications that were developed for the treatment of AD. Other AD-related neurochemical deficits include the loss of somatostatin and serotonin (Bowen and Davison 1986), whereas dopamine loss is more variable. In contrast, patients with FTD have normal levels of cortical acetylcholine, but marked decreases in brain serotonin (Sparks and Markesbery 1991).

Neuropathology

The main features of AD are amyloid plaques, neurofibrillary tangles, and neuronal and synaptic loss. The center of the amyloid plaque consists of a 42–amino acid protein derived from the APP (Glenner and Wong 1984) found on chromosome 21 (St. George-Hyslop et al. 1990). Surrounding the plaque is an area of gliosis and degenerating synapses. Plaque density is greatest in hippocampus and posterior temporoparietal cortex. Although plaques are found in elderly individuals without AD, plaque concentration is far less than that in patients with AD (Blessed et al. 1968). Amyloid accumulates in meningeal vessels (Vinters et al. 1990) and fatal hemorrhages can occur as a result of the effect of amyloid on these vessels (Vinters and Gilbert 1983).

Neurofibrillary tangles are present within neurons and stain positively with antibodies to both tau and ubiquitin (Dickson et al. 1990). Abnormal phosphorylation of the neuronal tau protein is a major factor in the formation of the tangle. Few or no tangles are seen in the neocortex of elderly subjects without AD, but tangles occur with many non-AD dementing conditions including subacute sclerosing panencephalitis, dementia pugilistica, aluminum intoxication, postencephalitic parkinsonism, and the parkinsonian–amyotrophic lateral sclerosis (ALS)–dementia complex of Guam (Wisniewski et al. 1979).

Because elderly individuals without AD have both plaques and tangles, research criteria for AD (Khachaturian 1985) use both the patient age and the concentration of plaques and tangles to determine diagnosis. To meet AD research criteria, patients younger than 50 years must have two to five senile plaques per high-power field in the cortex, whereas subjects between 50 and 65 must have eight plaques per high-power field.

The role of cerebrospinal fluid markers in the diagnosis of AD is still limited. Cerebrospinal fluid tau is elevated in patients with AD compared with that in control subjects without AD (Galasko et al. 1997), but it is also elevated in other dementing disorders such as vascular dementia (Andreasen et al. 1998), FTD, and diffuse Lewy body disease (Arai et al. 1997). Similarly, APP is diminished in AD (Motter et al. 1996), although this may not differentiate subjects with AD from subjects without AD (Southwick et al. 1996). Efforts toward imaging amyloid as a diagnostic test are ongoing (Walker 1991).

Treatment

Both nonpharmacological and pharmacological therapies are beneficial in the treatment of AD. The patient's caregivers will require advice and education regarding the dementia, superimposed psychiatric and medical conditions, and psychosocial problems and resources. The best therapies for psychiatric symptoms associated with dementia often involve manipulation of the environment. For example, the patient who awakens during the night will sleep during the day. Increasing daytime exercise and eliminating naps is often more effective than a sleeping medication. It is difficult to manage aggressive behaviors in the home, and their presence often means that the patient will require long-term care.

Most families need extensive advice regarding psychosocial issues. The physician will need to know when the patient might benefit from day care and when a nursing home is required. Similarly, families will need advice regarding the nursing homes most appropriate for their relative. Families often benefit from consultation with attorneys. The Alzheimer's Association, a lay organization dedicated to helping patients and families of patients with AD, is an excellent community resource for family referrals.

Many medications have been unsuccessful in the treatment of the dementia associated with AD. These include calcium channel blockers, vasodilators, anticoagulants, nootropic agents, and acetylcholine precursors (Mody and Miller 1990). But, recently, a variety of medications have shown efficacy in the treatment of AD. Such treatments can be divided into drugs targeted at acute symptom management, improvement of cognition, slowing progression of the disease, and prevention.

Anticholinesterases such as tacrine and donepezil ameliorate deficits in cognition and activities of daily living. Donepezil has a major benefit over tacrine in that it does not have liver toxicity and has become the treatment of choice for AD. Although the gains seen with these compounds are often modest (Growdon 1992), there are patients in whom these medications can lead to spectacular enhancement of day-to-day functions (Kaufer and Cummings 1996). Memory is not the only component of the dementia that will improve, and some subjects showed striking changes in attention, focus, or neuropsychiatric symptoms. In fact, Kaufer and Cummings (1996) found

that improvement on anticholinesterases was greatest in patients in the middle stages of the illness and in whom psychiatric symptomatology was prominent.

Recent efforts have attempted to predict which patients will respond to therapy. In preliminary neuroimaging studies, pretherapy perfusion deficits of the dorsolateral parietal, orbitofrontal, and anterior cingulate regions predicted anticholinesterase responders (Mega et al. 1998). Similarly, the anticholinesterase inhibitor metrifonate has been shown to improve behavioral symptoms, in addition to the cognitive deficits, of patients with AD (Cummings et al. 1998).

Preventive therapy is directed at increase of neuronal survival, inhibition of amyloid plaque formation, and suppression of abnormal tau protein formation. Nonsteroidal anti-inflammatory compounds, selective COX-2 inhibitors, neurotrophic factors, vitamin E, and other antioxidants are being investigated as possibly increasing neuronal survival. In a large clinical trial (Sano et al. 1996), 2000 IU of vitamin E delayed institutionalization and death. Attempts to replicate a benefit for vitamin E in patients with early AD are under way.

As is noted earlier in this chapter, estrogen replacement therapy in postmenopausal women has been shown to prevent cognitive decline (Paganini-Hill and Henderson 1994). The mechanisms for estrogens are not completely known although they can increase neuronal sprouting and survival. Androgens are also being explored as a potential therapeutic agent for men.

Treating superimposed medical conditions can be difficult, as they are often subtle and hard to diagnose. The patient with advanced AD who has little or no verbal expression cannot communicate, and even small problems such as constipation or a tooth cavity can go unrecognized, leading to serious complications such as bowel obstruction or orofacial abscess. Immobility and aspiration pneumonia are the major causes of mortality in AD. Because patients do not suddenly deteriorate as a result of AD, when sudden deterioration occurs one should suspect an infection, stroke, myocardial infarction, or drug-induced delirium (Giombetti and Miller 1990).

Drug therapies for AD-associated psychiatric symptoms often have substantial side effects. Depression responds to antidepressants, but also to placebo (Teri et al. 1991). Violent psychosis is improved with traditional antipsychotics, but these medications are sedating, and sudden death has been described in patients with AD who exhibit parkinsonian features (McKeith et al. 1992). New atypical antipsychotics such as risperidone and olanzapine may be safer based on clinical experience, though controlled trials have not been conducted. Benzodiazepines rarely help anxiety and may cause a paradoxical increase in agitation.

Dementia With Lewy Bodies

Dementia with Lewy bodies (DLB) is a clinicopathological entity with histological features overlapping with those of AD. The clinical characteristics of DLB include a dementia syndrome and two of the three following features: fluctuating cognition, visual hallucinations, and parkinsonism. The typical dementia syndrome of DLB resembles that of AD, but the patients typically have less severe memory impairments early in their clinical course and may have more evidence of executive dysfunction. Fluctuating cognition refers to relatively dramatic day-to-day fluctuations in patient cognitive function. In some cases, periods of loss of consciousness or syncope can occur. The typical visual hallucinations of DLB are silent, well-formed images of people, objects, or animals that the patient endorses as real. Parkinsonism in DLB is usually mild and features rigidity and bradykinesia with little tremor. Supportive features of the diagnosis of DLB include delusions, hallucinations in other sensory modalities, hypersensitivity to neuroleptic medication, falls, syncope, and episodic loss of consciousness (McKeith et al. 1996). The course of DLB from recognition of symptoms to death is 6–8 years, shorter than the natural history of AD. Death may be hastened by the use of conventional neuroleptic medication.

Neuropathologically, patients with DLB are found at autopsy to have extensive neurotic plaque similar to that found in patients with AD. Patients with DLB have few neurofibrillary tangles, and they have extensive Lewy body formation, particularly in paralimbic cortical areas such as anterior cingulate gyrus, insular cortex, and medial temporal regions. Lewy bodies also are found in neocortex. Patients with DLB have brainstem pathology, with Lewy bodies in the substantia nigra. The pathological changes in the brainstem are typically less extensive than those found in Parkinson's disease.

Patients with DLB have a marked deficit in choline acetyltransferase and a consequent deficiency in acetylcholine synthesis in the cortex (Perry et al. 1990). The cholinergic deficiency is more marked in patients with prominent visual hallucinations than those without. Also, a modest loss of dopamine in the striatum is seen, corresponding to the reduction of cells in the substantia nigra (Perry et al. 1990).

The approach to treatment of DLB is similar to that for AD. Cholinesterase inhibitors may ameliorate the cognitive deficit and often produce a beneficial behavioral response. Conventional neuroleptic medications must be avoided because of excessive neuroleptic sensitivity, but delusions and hallucinations may respond well to novel antipsychotics including risperidone, olanzapine, or quetiapine. Depressive symptoms are common in DLB and should be treated with selective serotonin reuptake inhibitors.

Frontotemporal Dementia

Nosology

The second group of dementing disorders, the FTDs, are associated with degeneration of the anterior frontal and temporal lobes. The taxonomy connected with FTD is both confusing and controversial, related in large part to our fundamental lack of knowledge concerning the pathogenesis of these conditions. Compounding this problem, many researchers have described new disease entities (or resurrected diagnoses from prior decades) to describe patients in whom clinical or pathological findings are slightly different from those found in classical Pick's disease.

Some terms used to describe diverse syndromes with similar pathology include progressive subcortical gliosis (Neumann and Cohn 1967), dementia of frontal lobe type (Neary et al. 1988), frontal lobe dementia of non-Alzheimer type (Brun 1987), dementia lacking distinctive histological features (Knopman et al. 1990), primary progressive aphasia (Mesulam 1982), semantic dementia (Snowden et al. 1992), and the temporal lobe variant of FTD (Edwards-Lee et al. 1997). Further complicating this nomenclature dilemma is the discovery that some patients with ALS develop FTD and, in these patients, the pathological findings in cortex suggest Pick's disease (Sam et al. 1991) or FTD without Pick's bodies (Mitsuyama 1984). Recently, some have suggested that corticobasal degeneration is a subtype of FTD due to the clinical and pathological overlap of the two conditions (Jackson and Lowe 1996; Kertesz 1997).

The Lund and Manchester research groups established guidelines for diagnosis and suggested the term frontotemporal dementia (Brun et al. 1994); this term is used in this chapter. As described below, new genetic findings related to FTD may help to clarify whether or not these entities should be split or lumped together.

Epidemiology

The prevalence of FTD is hard to estimate, in part, because many patients with FTD are either not recognized during life or are misdiagnosed as having AD (Mendez et al. 1993). The best data on prevalence come from studies in Lund, Sweden, and Manchester, England. In the Swedish study (Gustafson et al. 1990), 20 of 150 (13.3%) patients with presenile dementia had the characteristic pathological findings of FTD including frontal and usually anterior temporal lobe gliosis, spongiosis, and neuronal dropout. Only four patients (2.7% of total) had classical Pick's disease, whereas 16 (10.6% of total) had FTD without Pick's bodies. In the Manchester study (Neary et al. 1987), 21.9% of 41 patients with a presenile dementia had FTD.

The typical age at onset for FTD is the sixth to seventh decade, with duration of illness being approximately 7 years. Between 38% and 60% of patients with FTD have a family history of dementia; often the history suggests a dominantly inherited illness (Gustafson 1993; Miller et al. 1998; Stevens et al. 1998). In the University of California–Los Angeles (UCLA) cohort, approximately one-half of the patients had at least one first-degree relative with FTD or a related disorder such as ALS. Of this group, 86% appeared to have a dominant pattern of inheritance (Chow et al. 1999).

The genetic basis for FTD is being aggressively studied. Some suggest that the E4 allele is slightly overrepresented in FTD (Stevens et al. 1997), whereas others disagree with this (Geschwind et al. 1998; Mesulam et al. 1997). Wilhelmsen and colleagues (1994) showed linkage of FTD to chromosome 17 in a large family with "disinhibition-dementia-Parkinsonism and amyotrophy." Later, linkage to this region was also found in patients with progressive subcortical gliosis, multiple tauopathy, hereditary dysphasic dementia, pallidopontonigral degeneration, and bilateral amygdala degeneration (Foster et al. 1997). In some families with 17-linkage there are mutations in the tau gene (Clark et al., in press; Hutton et al. 1998; Poorkaj et al., in press). In contrast to the rapid advances in FTD genetics, epidemiological studies have yielded little fruit because clinical cohorts used to study FTD have been too small for study results to make meaningful statements about other risk factors.

Clinical Features and Differential Diagnosis

Although the varied syndromes associated with FTD have slightly different clinical features, similarities among the different entities are far outweighed by differences. Usually, changes in personality precede gross dementia by several years (Miller et al. 1991). Many patients are socially withdrawn and apathetic (Cummings and Duchen 1981; Gustafson 1987; Neary et al. 1987). Also, behavioral

disinhibition and loss of judgment and insight are common. This can lead to legal difficulties; in one study, nearly 50% of patients with FTD committed an antisocial act that either led to or could have led to arrest (Miller et al. 1997a). Insight or concern into these legal problems is usually diminished or absent.

The symptoms of apathy and disinhibition can be explained by dysfunction of the frontal lobes. Blumer and Benson (1975) called these the pseudodepressed and pseudopsychopathic personality disorders of frontal lobe dysfunction. Apathy occurs as a result of medial frontal injury, whereas disinhibition is the result of basofrontal dysfunction (Cummings 1993). Both areas are usually involved in FTD.

Peculiar behaviors develop that are in part a result of involvement of the anterotemporal lobes. Klüver-Bucy syndrome was described in macaque monkeys after the anterotemporal lobes and amygdala were removed (Klüver and Bucy 1939). These monkeys developed hyperorality, hypersexuality, visual hypermetamorphosis, placidity, and sensory agnosia. In addition, anterotemporal lobectomized primates lose socially affiliative behavior (Kling and Steklis 1976). Common behavioral findings that can be attributed to anterotemporal lobe dysfunction include hyperorality, placidity, compulsive motor behaviors, bizarre and remote affect, hyperreligiosity, and development of eccentric ideas.

Another possible explanation for the hyperorality, carbohydrate craving, and compulsions found in FTD is the loss of brain serotonin associated with this condition (Sparks and Markesbery 1991). Approximately two-thirds of subjects with FTD show hyperorality, carbohydrate craving, and compulsions (Miller et al. 1995). These symptoms are manifested by compulsive gum chewing or smoking, massive weight gain, and an intense craving for sweets. Compulsive collecting and ritualistic obsessions related to urination or bowel movements are common.

Once cognitive symptoms develop, a characteristic pattern of decline ensues. Initially, language output is economical, and, as the disease progresses, verbal stereotypes, such as "let's go, let's go," are seen. Some patients become mute while other cognitive skills are still relatively intact. As in AD, an early change in language is difficulty in generating a word list, but, unlike in AD, semantic anomia is common, particularly in those patients with left anterotemporal lobe dysfunction. With this anomia, the patient is not helped by clues, and, when told that an object is a key, the patient might say, "Key, key, I don't know what a key is." Hodges and colleagues (1992) and Snowden and colleagues (1992) have named this *semantic dementia*. Patients with predominantly frontal lobe pathology do not typically show this type of language disorder.

Parietal and posterior language functions such as reading, writing, and calculation are spared in the early and even middle stages of FTD (Neary et al. 1988). Unlike in AD, visuospatial skills are usually normal or near normal, and many patients can draw in three dimensions without difficulty. Some patients can draw complex designs and multiply three-number integers at a time when they are mute and behaviorally impaired.

Neuropsychological testing shows selective impairment of executive skills in the early stages. This includes perseveration and difficulties in set shifting, impairments in verbal and design fluency, poor attention, and impaired response inhibition. Word retrieval, memory, calculation, and pencil-and-paper constructional skills are generally spared relative to executive abilities (Miller et al. 1991). However, it is difficult to use neuropsychological testing alone to differentiate patients with FTD from those with AD (Pachana et al. 1996).

Motor systems are initially normal. However, as FTD advances, parkinsonian symptoms including diminished eye movements, tremor, and bradykinesia develop in some patients. Some patients develop ALS months to years after the onset of their dementia, whereas in others manifestations of ALS precede dementia. In the end stages, FTD is difficult to distinguish from AD.

The EEG shows frontal slowing over a normal background in the early phases (Yener et al. 1996). CT and MRI can be normal at first, although often both show anterior atrophy at the time of presentation (Gustafson et al. 1990; Miller et al. 1991). SPECT and PET detect cerebral dysfunction in the frontal and temporal regions even in patients without major cognitive deficits. SPECT shows frontal and sometimes temporal hypoperfusion in early FTD (Brun et al. 1994; Jagust et al. 1989; Neary et al. 1988) (Figure 24–1). In some patients, the temporal lobes are more severely involved than the frontal regions. Unlike in AD, posterior temporal areas show relatively normal perfusion. PET demonstrates frontotemporal hypometabolism (Kamo et al. 1987). Using careful clinical parameters and SPECT, several groups (Read et al. 1995; Risberg et al. 1993) achieved diagnostic accuracy of greater than 90%. SPECT and PET show promise for improving clinical diagnosis; with these modalities, patients with FTD can usually be distinguished from those with AD (see SPECT images in Figure 24–2).

The Lund and Manchester research groups have suggested a series of items that help to diagnose FTD. They listed 26 items, all graded as "yes" or "no." The items are divided into the following categories: behavior, speech, affect, spatial orientation/praxis, physical signs, investiga-

tions, and supportive findings. Also, there are 14 exclusion items. We studied the sensitivity and specificity of these items in separating patients with FTD from those with AD. We scored every patient on each item and compared the two groups. A discriminant function showed that loss of personal awareness, hyperorality, stereotyped and perseverative behavior, progressive reduction of speech, and preserved spatial orientation differentiated 100% of FTD and AD subjects (Miller et al. 1997b). Items relating to affect and physical findings were not different in FTD versus AD. Loss of personal awareness, eating, perseverative behavior, and reduction of speech are the Lund-Manchester Research Criteria items that most clearly differentiate FTD from AD. Tables 24–1 and 24–2 compare and contrast the neuropsychiatric and neuropsychological differences of AD and FTD.

Neuropathological Findings

All of the clinical entities described show neuropathological similarities. Brain weight is slightly to moderately reduced. Grossly, the brain has mild-to-severe frontal and/or frontal and anterotemporal atrophy. Neuronal loss, gliosis, and mild-to-moderate spongiform changes are found, primarily in the first three layers of the cortex. Gliosis is visualized with stains for glial acid fibrillary protein. Neuronal loss can be subtle, but disruption of neuronal cytoskeleton is seen, and there is dying back of neurons, which stain as periodic acid–Schiff (PAS)-positive spheroids (Zhou et al., in press). Plaques and tangles do not occur beyond what is seen in elderly individuals without FTD. Subcortical structures, such as the substantia nigra, are often abnormal. Severe degeneration of the substantia nigra was observed in 79% of patients with dementia lacking distinctive histology (Knopman et al. 1990), in 78% of patients with Pick's disease (Kosaka et al. 1991), and in three patients with dementia with motor neuron disease (Horoupian et al. 1984). Table 24–3 contrasts the pathology of AD versus FTD.

Clinical and Pathological Features of Frontotemporal Dementia Subtypes

As is noted in the section on nosology, a variety of disorders can be considered clinical and pathological subtypes of FTD. These entities are described below.

Pick's disease.   Pick first described the clinical and gross morphological features of his patients in 1892, but it took almost 20 years before Alzheimer noted the presence of cellular inclusions in Pick's original cases. Pick's disease

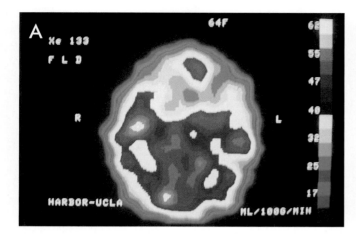
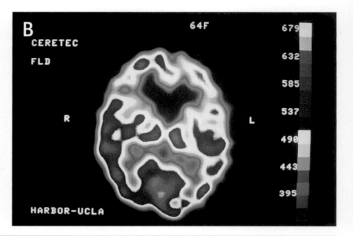

FIGURE 24–1. *Panel A:* Xenon-133 scan from a patient with early frontal lobe dementia (FLD). Note marked decreases in frontal perfusion. *Panel B:* A technetium–99m-labeled hexamethylpropyleneamine oxime (HMPAO) study from the same subject, showing marked frontal hypoperfusion with normal temporoparietal perfusion.

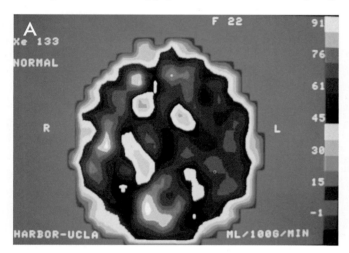
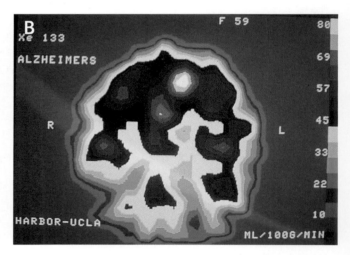

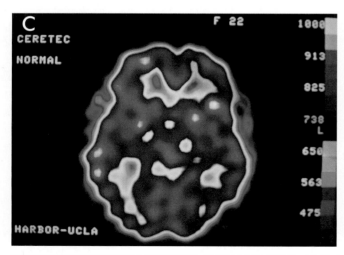
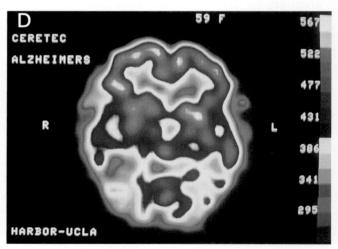

FIGURE 24–2. *Panel A:* Cerebral blood flow with xenon-133 in an elderly control subject. Cerebral blood flow is color coded to mL/100 g tissue per minute. Parietotemporal flow is normal. *Panel B:* Xenon-133 scan in a patient with Alzheimer's disease. Note markedly decreased perfusion to the temporoparietal cortex. *Panel C:* High-resolution scan of cerebral blood flow in an elderly control subject using technetium–99m-labeled hexamethylpropyleneamine oxime (HMPAO). The scan is color coded, and areas of yellow are 50%–62% of maximal cortical perfusion; areas of green are 40%–50%. Perfusion is symmetrical throughout the cortex. *Panel D:* HMPAO scan showing cerebral blood flow in a patient with Alzheimer's disease. Temporoparietal perfusion is approximately 50%–60% of normal (yellow color).

TABLE 24–1. Psychiatric distinctions

Diagnosis	Behavior	Affect	Apathy	Delusions	Compulsions	Eating
Alzheimer's disease	Socially correct	Normal	Mild	Simple	Mild	Weight loss
Frontotemporal dementia	Early disinhibition	Remote, bizarre	Severe	Bizarre	Severe	Weight gain

TABLE 24–2. Neuropsychological features

Diagnosis	Drawing	Memory	Executive	Generation	Anomia
Alzheimer's disease	Impaired	Impaired	Impaired	Impaired	Lexical
Frontotemporal dementia	Spared	Variable	Severely impaired	Severely impaired	Semantic (often)

TABLE 24–3. Neuropathology features

Diagnosis	Plaques	Neurofibrillary tangles	Gliosis	Abnormal genes	Neurochemistry
Alzheimer's disease	Yes	Yes	Proportional to neuronal loss	Amyloid precursor protein, presenilin 1 and 2 Apolipoprotein E4 Tau mutations	Presynaptic cholinergic and serotonergic
Frontotemporal dementia	No	No (except for familial tauopathy)	Out of proportion to neuronal loss		Postsynaptic cholinergic, presynaptic and postsynaptic serotonergic

accounts for 2%–3% of all degenerative dementias (Gustafson et al. 1990), but it is not possible to clinically distinguish patients with Pick's disease from patients with FTD without Pick's bodies. In the early stages, patients develop the Klüver-Bucy syndrome (Cummings and Duchen 1981), whereas in patients with AD this tends to occur in the later stages (Cummings and Benson 1992). As with the other FTDs, deterioration in personality in Pick's disease contrasts with relatively preserved visuospatial skills (Gustafson 1987). Also, language disturbances are common and may consist of semantic anomia, circumlocution, and verbal stereotypies with echolalia (Cummings and Duchen 1981; Miller et al. 1993a). Pick's disease can present as a highly selective language disturbance rather than as a dementia (Pick 1892; Wechsler et al. 1982), though this is more characteristic of the focal atrophies (Malamud and Boyd 1940; Mesulam 1982; Snowden et al. 1992). Neuropsychological tests show mainly frontal lobe dysfunction. These clinical, neuropsychological, and pathological findings are reflected in metabolic alterations revealed by PET (Kamo et al. 1987).

At autopsy, the brains of patients with Pick's disease show circumscribed atrophy of the frontal and/or temporal lobes. Microscopically there is neuronal loss, gliosis, and Pick's bodies, which are argentophilic cytoplasmic inclusions that fill inflated neurons (Pick's cells) (Corsellis 1976). These cells may be rare, and an extensive search may be necessary to achieve diagnosis. Asymmetric involvement of the frontotemporal lobes is seen in 70% of patients; 50% have more left-sided atrophy (Corsellis 1976; Cummings and Benson 1992). PET identifies reduced perfusion and metabolism in the frontal and temporal lobes (Kamo et al. 1987). However, tissue confirmation of Pick's bodies is needed for diagnosis, and functional imaging cannot distinguish patients with Pick's disease from those with FTD without Pick's bodies.

Frontal lobe dementia of the non-Alzheimer type and dementia of the frontal type. During the 1980s, studies performed by the Lund, Sweden, and Manchester, England, groups brought FTD into the modern era. In Lund, Brun, Gustafson, and Risberg carefully characterized the clinical, perfusion, and pathological features of a large population with dementia. Of their first 150 patients, 20 showed non-AD pathology that affected the frontal and temporal regions. Hence the name "frontal lobe dementia of the non-Alzheimer type." Four patients showed classical Pick's disease whereas 16 showed frontal and temporally predominant gliosis, spongiosus, and neuronal loss without Pick's bodies. Brun emphasized that the gliosis selectively involved the first three layers of cortex (Brun 1987).

Similarly, the Manchester group, led by Neary and Bowen, performed a biopsy study of patients with presenile dementia. Histology was performed immediately following biopsy so that a diagnosis was quickly obtained. Neary and colleagues (1988) noted the distinctive frontal clinical and imaging features of a subtype in whom biopsy showed gliosis, neuronal loss, and spongiosus. They chose the term "dementia of the frontal lobe type" to describe this population who shared the clinical and pathological features of the patients seen in Lund. In 1994, the Lund and Manchester groups (Brun et al. 1994) established research criteria for these conditions and replaced previous nomenclature with the term FTD.

Dementia lacking distinctive histological features.

The categories "dementia of the frontal lobe type" (Neary et al. 1988), "frontal lobe dementia of the non-Alzheimer type" (Brun 1987), and "dementia lacking distinctive histological features" (Knopman et al. 1990) seem to be describing the same disorders. In the study by Knopman et al. (1990), the authors emphasized memory loss, prominent personality changes, and prominent dysphagia and dysarthria in later stages. Death of patients occurred within 7 years of onset of dementia. Fifty percent of patients had a positive family history of dementia, and cases of ALS were seen rarely in these families. It was difficult to distinguish these patients from those with classical Pick's disease at autopsy.

Progressive subcortical gliosis.

Neumann and Cohn (1967) described a "new disease entity" for which they coined the term *progressive subcortical gliosis*. Clinically, their patients showed personality changes including social impropriety, poor judgment, and perseveration. Memory impairment was common. One patient was unable to recognize family members and had paraphasias; another had childish behavior and paranoid delusions. Some developed muscle atrophy before death. Functional imaging studies were not performed, but clinically and pathologically these patients seemed similar to patients with FTD.

Pathologically, frontotemporal atrophy was seen. Also, neuronal loss with reactive astrocytosis occurred in cortex, whereas rich gliosis was found in the subcortical areas. Ventral horns and substantia nigra showed abnormal gliosis. The presence of muscle atrophy and ventral horn gliosis in patients with progressive subcortical gliosis suggested a possible relationship between this disease and ALS. Our own most recent patient with this syndrome had a fulminant ALS associated with a progressive frontal syndrome. He resembled many of our patients with FTD on clinical and imaging features. A familial incidence has been found with progressive subcortical gliosis and linkage to chromosome 17 (Petersen et al. 1995). The prominent pathological feature of these patients is intense gliosis at the junction of six-layer cortex and white matter. However, because of the overlap between this entity and Pick's disease, the original authors called it "Pick's disease, type II" (Neumann 1949).

Focal lobar atrophies.

Although awareness of an entity associated with focal degeneration of language areas dates back at least to Alajouanine's description of the composer Ravel (Alajouanine 1948), it was Mesulam (1982) who first defined the entity of primary progressive aphasia. Mesulam described six patients with a progressive aphasia without signs of global dementia. Symptoms in five patients began with anomic aphasia, whereas symptoms in the sixth started with pure word deafness. Most progressed for years with language disturbance, while right-hemisphere functions and memory remained intact. Studies with both SPECT (Mesulam 1982; Snowden et al. 1992) and PET (Chawluk et al. 1986) demonstrated focal hypoperfusion in the left anterior hemisphere, whereas the right hemisphere showed mild or no hypoperfusion. Focal degeneration of the left anterior hemisphere can be genetically programmed, and Morris and colleagues (Lendon et al. 1998; Morris et al. 1984) have described a large family with this syndrome in whom linkage to chromosome 17 is present.

Although there are many reports on left frontotemporal lobar atrophies, only isolated reports exist concerning the behavioral and neuropsychological changes associated with right frontotemporal degeneration (Tyrrell et al. 1990). We described five patients with progressive right frontotemporal dysfunction, all of whom differed clinically and neuropsychologically from patients previously studied with left frontotemporal degeneration (Miller et al. 1993b). Our five patients exhibited dramatic changes in personality characterized by remote affect, severe behavioral disinhibition, agitation, hyperreligiosity, and impaired judgment. They showed profound disruption of social conduct. Also, they had difficulty recognizing familiar faces and voices, and, surprisingly, some had a semantic anomia. They had less language difficulty and slightly more visuoconstructive problems than patients with left frontotemporal involvement.

Patients with progressive aphasia have been examined neuropathologically. In this population, the anatomical abnormalities typically are neuronal loss, gliosis, and atrophy localized primarily to the left temporal region, particularly the left-inferior and middle-temporal gyri. These findings mimic what is seen with FTD. We have seen similar changes in patients with right temporal atrophy.

Amyotrophic lateral sclerosis.

Classically, lesions in ALS are localized to the upper and lower motor neurons. However, studies show that other areas of the cortex are often involved (Hudson 1991). Clinically, up to 15% of patients with ALS develop mental symptoms (Hudson 1981), and the cognitive changes often suggest frontal involvement (Hudson 1991; Mitsuyama 1984; Morita et al. 1987). Also, Klüver-Bucy syndrome has been described.

Patients with ALS show deficits in neuropsychological testing (Peavy et al. 1992). Although many patients are neuropsychologically normal, others show serious deficits in frontal systems tasks and memory. In vivo studies with PET, using $[^{18}F]$fluoro-2-deoxyglucose, have shown generalized hypometabolism, most severe in the sensorimotor cortex and putamen (Dalakas et al. 1987; Hatazawa et al. 1988). Focal frontal and temporal hypometabolism was not reported. Similar patterns have been observed in ALS using SPECT (Figure 24–3). At autopsy, patients with ALS show nonspecific neuronal degeneration and gliosis (particularly in the upper cortical layers) and sponginess of the neuropil, most severely in the frontal and medial temporal regions (Horoupian et al. 1984).

Secondary frontotemporal dementias.

Finally, there are diseases that cause frontal lobe dysfunction where the main pathology is not at the level of the frontal lobes. Several different mechanisms lead to secondary FTDs. One occurs in patients in whom the primary pathology occurs at the level of the basal ganglia, as in patients with Parkinson's disease, Huntington's disease, and Wilson's disease (Benson 1993). Because there are extensive connections between the basal ganglia and the frontal lobes, injury to the substantia nigra and neostriatum can cause frontal lobe–type dysfunction (Cummings 1993). These illnesses can usually be differentiated from primary FTD because a movement disorder is prominent. Also, the dementia with these diseases is characterized by marked awareness and concern and mental slowing, in marked contrast to the dementia associated with FTD.

A similar mechanism is associated with diseases of subfrontal white matter, which can disconnect the frontal lobes from their subcortical connections. This occurs in some types of vascular dementia such as Binswanger's disease, a few inherited metabolic diseases such as metachromatic leukodystrophy, and a variety of demyelinating illnesses such as multiple sclerosis. These patients can appear clinically similar to those with FTD, although MRI shows extensive white matter lesions not typically present with primary FTD.

With alcoholism, general paresis of the insane, some cases of Creutzfeldt-Jakob disease, and acquired immunodeficiency syndrome (AIDS) dementia, there is a primary attack on the frontal lobes. History, serological testing, and lumbar puncture should differentiate these patients from those with primary FTD. With some diseases, such as

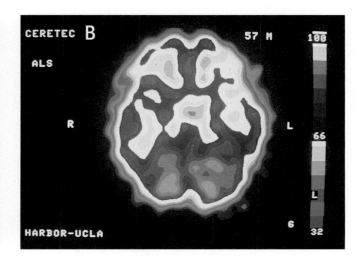

FIGURE 24–3. *Panel A:* Xenon-133 scan of a patient with amyotrophic lateral sclerosis (ALS). Note mild frontal and temporal hypoperfusion. *Panel B:* Hexamethylpropyleneamine oxime (HMPAO) scan of the same patient, showing frontal and temporal hypoperfusion.

corticobasal degeneration, parkinsonian-ALS-dementia complex of Guam, Lewy body dementia, many cases of Creutzfeldt-Jakob disease, and AIDS dementia, both the frontal and the subcortical systems are involved. Patients with these diseases can be hard to differentiate from patients with advanced FTD in whom both the subcortical and the frontal lobes are dysfunctional.

Treatment

There has been little effort to systematically assess treatment associated with FTD. However, we have had some success using selective serotonin reuptake inhibitors. Swartz and colleagues (1997) found that in more than one-half of subjects with FTD the eating disorder, compulsions, irritability, and depressed mood improved with these compounds. Anecdotally, we have found that some patients with FTD show greater irritability when given anticholinesterase compounds, although this has not been formally studied. To date, no therapy has been found that will slow progression or improve cognition.

▌ Summary

In this chapter, we outlined the clinical, genetic, imaging, and neuropathological characteristics of the two major cortical dementias: AD and FTD. As our knowledge of these conditions advances and as diagnostic tools are refined, improved diagnosis and a better understanding of pathogenesis will become possible. With this, better treatments will emerge.

▌ References

Alajouanine T: Aphasia and artistic realization. Brain 17:229–241, 1948

Andreasen N, Vanmechelen E, Van de Voorde A, et al: Cerebrospinal fluid tau protein as a biochemical marker for Alzheimer's disease: a community-based follow-up study. J Neurol Neurosurg Psychiatry 64:298–305, 1998

Arai H, Morikawa Y, Higuchi M: Cerebrospinal fluid tau levels in neurodegenerative diseases with distinct tau-related pathology. Biochem Biophys Res Commun 236:262–264, 1997

Bartus RT, Dean RL, Beer B, et al: The cholinergic hypothesis of geriatric memory dysfunction. Science 217:408–414, 1982

Benson DF: Progressive frontal dysfunction. Dementia 4:149–153, 1993

Benson DF, Kuhl DE, Hawkins DR, et al: The fluorodeoxyglucose ^{18}F scan in Alzheimer's disease and multi-infarct dementia. Arch Neurol 40:711–714, 1983

Blessed G, Tomlinson BE, Roth M: The association between quantitative measures of dementia and of senile change in the cerebral grey matter of elderly subjects. Br J Psychiatry 117:797–811, 1968

Blumer D, Benson DF: Personality changes with frontal and temporal lobe lesions, in Psychiatric Aspects of Neurological Disease. Edited by Benson DF, Blumer D. New York, Grune & Stratton, 1975, pp 151–170

Boller F, Lopez OL, Moossy J: Diagnosis of dementia: clinicopathologic correlations. Neurology 39:76–79, 1989

Boone KB, Miller BL, Lesser IM, et al: Neuropsychological correlates of white matter lesions in healthy elderly subjects: a threshold effect. Arch Neurol 49:549–554, 1992

Bowen DM, Davison AN: Biochemical studies of nerve cells and energy metabolism in Alzheimer's disease. Br Med Bull 42:75–80, 1986

Bowen DM, Smith CB, White P, et al: Neurotransmitter-related enzymes and indices of hypoxia in senile dementia and other abiotrophies. Brain 99:459–496, 1976

Brun A: Frontal lobe degeneration of non-Alzheimer type, I: neuropathology. Archives of Gerontology and Geriatrics 6:193–208, 1987

Brun A, Englund B, Gustafson L, et al: Clinical and neuropathological criteria for frontotemporal dementia. J Neurol Neurosurg Psychiatry 57:416–418, 1994

Carmelli D, Swan GE, Reed T, et al: Midlife cardiovascular risk factors ApoE, and cognitive decline in elderly male twins. Neurology 50:1580–1585, 1998

Chawluk JB, Mesulam MM, Hurtig H, et al: Slowly progressive aphasia without generalized dementia: studies with positron emission tomography. Ann Neurol 19:68–74, 1986

Chow TW; Miller BL; Hayashi VN, et al: Inheritance of frontotemporal dementia. Arch Neurol 56:817–822, 1999

Clark LN, Poorkaj P, Wszolek Z, et al: Pathogenic implications of mutations in the tau gene in pallido-ponto-nigral degeneration and related chromosome 17–linked neurodegenerative disorders. Proc Natl Acad Sci U S A 95:13103–13107, 1998

Corsellis JAN: Aging and the dementias, in Greenfield's Neuropathology. Edited by Blackwood W, Corsellis JAN. Chicago, IL, Year Book Medical, 1976, pp 796–848

Creasey H, Jorm A, Longley W, et al: Monozygotic twins discordant for Alzheimer's disease. Neurology 39:1474–1476, 1989

Cummings JL: Psychosis in neurologic disease: neurobiology and pathogenesis. Neuropsychiatry Neuropsychol Behav Neurol 5:144–150, 1992

Cummings JL: Frontal-subcortical circuits and human behavior. Arch Neurol 50:873–880, 1993

Cummings JL, Benson DF: Dementia: A Clinical Approach, 2nd Edition. Boston, MA, Butterworth, 1992

Cummings JL, Duchen LW: Kluver-Bucy syndrome in Pick's disease: clinical and pathological correlations. Neurology 31:1415–1422, 1981

Cummings JL, Benson F, Hill MA, et al: Aphasia in dementia of Alzheimer's type. Neurology 35:394–397, 1985

Cummings JL, Miller BL, Hill MA, et al: Neuropsychiatric aspects of multi-infarct dementia and dementia of the Alzheimer type. Arch Neurol 44:389–393, 1987

Cummings JL, Cyrus PA, Ruzicka B, et al: The efficacy of metrifonate in improving the behavioral disturbances of Alzheimer's disease patients. Neurology 50:A252, 1998

Dalakas MC, Hatazawa J, Brooks RA, et al: Lowered cerebral glucose utilization in amyotrophic lateral sclerosis. Ann Neurol 22:580–586, 1987

Davies P, Malony AJF: Selective loss of central cholinergic neurons in Alzheimer's disease (letter). Lancet ii:1403, 1976

DeCarli C, Kaye JA, Rapoport SI: Critical analysis of the use of computer assisted transverse axial tomography to study human brain in aging and dementia of the Alzheimer type. Neurology 40:884–886, 1990

DeCarli C, Grady CL, Clark CM, et al: Comparison of positron emission tomography, cognition, and brain volume in Alzheimer's disease with and without severe abnormalities of white matter. J Neurol Neurosurg Psychiatry 60:158–167, 1996

D'Hooge R, Nagels G, Westland CE, et al: Spatial learning deficit in mice expressing human 751–amino acid beta–amyloid precursor protein. Neuroreport 7:2807–2811, 1996

Dickson DW, Wertkin A, Mattiace LA, et al: Ubiquitin immunoelectron microscopy of dystrophic neurites in cerebellar senile plaques of Alzheimer's disease. Acta Neuropathol (Berl) 79:486–493, 1990

Edwards-Lee T, Miller BL, Benson DF, et al: The temporal lobe variant of frontotemporal dementia. Brain 120:1027–1040, 1997

Evans DA, Funkenstein HH, Albert M, et al: Prevalence of Alzheimer's disease in a community population of older persons: higher than previously reported. JAMA 262:2551–2556, 1989

Fitten LJ, Perryman K, Wilkinson CJ: Alzheimer and vascular dementias and driving: a prospective road and laboratory study. JAMA 273:1360–1365, 1995

Folstein MF, Folstein SE, McHugh PR: Mini-Mental State: a practical method for grading the cognitive state of patients for the clinician. J Psychiatr Res 12:189–198, 1975

Foster NL, Wilhelmsen K, Sima AF, et al: Frontotemporal dementia and parkinsonism linked to chromosome 17: a consensus conference. Ann Neurol 41:706–715, 1997

Friedland RP, Koss E, Kumar V, et al: Motor vehicle crashes in dementia of the Alzheimer type. Ann Neurol 24:782–786, 1988

Gabrieli JD: Memory systems analyses of mnemonic disorders in aging and age-related diseases. Proc Natl Acad Sci U S A 93(24):13534–13540, 1996

Galasko D, Hansen LA, Katzman R, et al: Clinical-neuropathological correlations in Alzheimer's disease and related dementias. Arch Neurol 51:888–895, 1994

Galasko D, Clark C, Chang L: Assessment of CSF levels of tau protein in mildly demented patients with Alzheimer's disease. Neurology 48:632–635, 1997

Gatz M, Pedersen NL, Berg S: Heritability for Alzheimer's disease: the study of dementia in Swedish twins. J Gerontol 52:M117–125, 1997

Geschwind D, Karrim J, Nelson S, et al: The apo E4 allele is not a significant risk factor for frontotemporal dementia. Ann Neurol 44:134–138, 1998

Giombetti RJ, Miller BL: Recognition and management of superimposed medical conditions, in Alzheimer's Disease Treatment and Long Term Management. Edited by Cummings JL, Miller BL. New York, Marcel Dekker, 1990, pp 253–261

Glenner GG, Wong CW: Alzheimer's disease: initial report of the purification and characterization of a novel cerebrovascular amyloid protein. Biochem Biophys Res Commun 120:885–890, 1984

Goate A, Chartier-Harlin MC, Mullan M, et al: Segregation of a missense mutation in the amyloid precursor protein gene with familial Alzheimer's disease. Nature 349:704–706, 1991

Gottfries CG: Neurochemical aspects of dementia disorders. Dementia 1:56–64, 1990

Grady CL, Haxby JV, Schapiro MB, et al: Subgroups in dementia of the Alzheimer type identified using positron emission tomography. J Neuropsychiatry Clin Neurosci 2:373–384, 1990

Graham KS, Hodges JR: Differentiating the roles of the hippocampal complex and the neocortex in long-term memory storage: evidence from the study of semantic dementia and Alzheimer's disease. Neuropsychology 11:77–89, 1997

Graves AB, White E, Koepsell TD, et al: The association between head trauma and Alzheimer's disease. Am J Epidemiol 131:491–501, 1990

Graves AB, Mortimer JA, Larson EB, et al: Head circumference as a measure of cognitive reserve. Association with severity of impairment in Alzheimer's disease. Br J Psychiatry 169:86–92, 1996

Growdon JH: Treatment for Alzheimer's disease? N Engl J Med 327:1306–1308, 1992

Gustafson L: Frontal lobe degeneration of non-Alzheimer type, II: clinical picture and differential diagnosis. Archives of Gerontology and Geriatrics 6:209–223, 1987

Gustafson L: Clinical picture of frontal lobe degeneration of non-Alzheimer type. Dementia 4:143–148, 1993

Gustafson L, Brun A, Risberg J: Frontal lobe dementia of non-Alzheimer type, in Advances in Neurology: Alzheimer's Disease, Vol 51. Edited by Wurtman RJ, Corkin S, Growdon J, et al. New York, Raven, 1990, pp 65–71

Hachinski VC, Iliff LD, Zilhka E, et al: Cerebral blood flow in dementia. Arch Neurol 32:632–637, 1975

Hansen LA, Samuel W: Criteria for Alzheimer's disease and the nosology of dementia with Lewy bodies. Neurology 48:126–132, 1997

Hatazawa J, Brooks RA, Dalakas MC, et al: Cortical motor-sensory hypometabolism in amyotrophic lateral sclerosis: a PET study. J Comput Assist Tomogr 12:630–636, 1988

Hay JJ, Ernst RL: The economic costs of Alzheimer's disease. Am J Public Health 77:1169–1175, 1987

Hodges JR, Patterson K, Oxbury S, et al: Semantic dementia. Progressive fluent aphasia with temporal lobe atrophy. Brain 115:1783–1806, 1992

Horoupian DS, Thal L, Katzman R, et al: Dementia and motor neuron disease: morphometric, biochemical, and Golgi studies. Ann Neurol 16:305–313, 1984

Hsiao KK, Borchlet DR, Olson K, et al: Age-related CNS disorder and early death in transgenic FVB mice overexpressing Alzheimer amyloid precursor proteins. Neuron 15:1203–1218, 1995

Hudson AJ: Amyotrophic lateral sclerosis and its association with dementia, parkinsonism and other neurological disorders: a review. Brain 1041:217–247, 1981

Hudson AJ: Dementia and parkinsonism in amyotrophic lateral sclerosis, in Handbook of Clinical Neurology: Diseases of Motor System, Vol 15 (59). Edited by de Jong JMBV. New York, Elsevier, 1991, pp 231–240

Hutton M, Lendon CL, Rizzu P, et al: Association of missense and 5'-splice-site mutations in tau with the inherited dementia FTDP-17. Nature 393:702–705, 1998

Jackson M, Lowe J: The new neuropathology of degenerative frontotemporal dementias. Acta Neuropathol (Berl) 91:127–134, 1996

Jagust WJ, Budinger TF, Reed BR: The diagnosis of dementia with single photon emission computed tomography. Arch Neurol 44:258–262, 1987

Jagust WJ, Reed BR, Seab JP, et al: Clinical-physiological correlates of Alzheimer's disease and frontal lobe dementia. American Journal of Physiological Imaging 4:89–96, 1989

Joachim CL, Morris JH, Selkoe DJ: Clinically diagnosed Alzheimer's disease: autopsy results in 150 cases. Ann Neurol 24:50–56, 1988

Johnson K, Jones K, Holman BL, et al: Preclinical prediction of Alzheimer's disease using SPECT. Neurology 50:1563–1572, 1998

Kamo H, McGeer PL, Harrop R, et al: Positron emission tomography and histopathology in Pick's disease. Neurology 37:439–445, 1987

Kaufer D, Cummings JL: Neuropsychiatric aspects of Alzheimer's disease: the cholinergic hypothesis revisited. Neurology 47:871–875, 1996

Kertesz A: Frontotemporal dementia, Pick disease and corticobasal degeneration. One entity or 3? 1. Arch Neurol 54:1427–1429, 1997

Khachaturian ZS: Diagnosis of Alzheimer's disease. Arch Neurol 42:1097–1105, 1985

Kling A, Steklis HD: A neural substrate for affiliative behavior in nonhuman primates. Brain Behav Evol 13:216–238, 1976

Klüver H, Bucy PC: Preliminary analysis of functions of the temporal lobes in monkeys. Arch Neurol Psychiatry 42:547–554, 1939

Knopman DS, Mastri AR, Frey WH, et al: Dementia lacking distinctive histologic features: a common non-Alzheimer degenerative dementia. Neurology 40:251–256, 1990

Kosaka K, Ikeda KK, Kobayashi K, et al: Striato-pallidonigral degeneration in Pick's disease: a clinico-pathological study of 41 cases. J Neurol 238:151–160, 1991

Kuhl DE, Metter EJ, Riege WH: Patterns of local cerebral glucose utilization determined in Parkinson's disease by [^{18}F]fluorodeoxyglucose method. Ann Neurol 15:419–424, 1984

Lendon CL, Lynch T, Norton J, et al: Hereditary dysphasic disinhibition dementia: a frontotemporal dementia linked to 17q21-22. Neurology 50:1546–1555, 1998

Liu CK, Miller BL, Cummings JL, et al: A quantitative MRI study of vascular dementia. Neurology 42:138–143, 1992

Lundberg C, Johansson K, Ball K, et al: Dementia and driving: an attempt at consensus. Alzheimer Dis Assoc Disord 11:28–37, 1997

Malamud N, Boyd DA: Pick's disease with atrophy of the temporal lobes. Archives of Neurology and Psychiatry 43:210–222, 1940

Mattson MP, Guo Q: Cell and molecular neurobiology of presenilins: a role for the endoplasmic reticulum in the pathogenesis of Alzheimer's disease. J Neurochem 66:259–265, 1997

Mayeux R, Saunders AM, Shea S, et al: Utility of the apolipoprotein E genotype in the diagnosis of Alzheimer's disease. Alzheimer's disease centers consortium on apolipoprotein E and Alzheimer's disease. N Engl J Med 338:506–511, 1998

McGeer EG, McGeer PL: The role of the immune system in neurodegenerative disorders. Mov Disord 12:855–858, 1997

McKeith I, Fairbairn A, Perry R, et al: Neuroleptic sensitivity in patients with senile dementia of Lewy body type. BMJ 305:673–678, 1992

McKeith IG, Galasko D, Kosaka K, et al, for the Consortium on Dementia with Lewy Bodies: Consensus guidelines for the clinical and pathologic diagnosis of dementia with Lewy bodies (DLB): Report of the consortium on DLB international workshop. Neurology 47:1113–1124, 1996

McKhann G, Drachman D, Folstein MF, et al: Clinical diagnosis of Alzheimer's disease: report of the NINCDS-ADRDA Work Group under the auspices of the Department of Health and Human Services Task Force on Alzheimer's Disease. Neurology 34:939–944, 1984

Mega MS, O'Connor SM, Lee L, et al: Orbital frontal and anterior cingulate pretreatment perfusion defects on 99m-Tc-HMPAO-SPECT are associated with behavioral response to cholinesterase inhibitor therapy in Alzheimer's disease. Neurology 50:A250, 1998

Mendez MF, Selwood A, Mastri AF, et al: Pick's disease versus Alzheimer's disease: a comparison of clinical characteristics. Neurology 43:289–292, 1993

Mesulam MM: Slowly progressive aphasia without generalized dementia. Ann Neurol 11:592–598, 1982

Mesulam MM, Johnson N, Grujic Z, et al: Apolipoprotein E genotypes in primary progressive aphasia. Neurology 49:51–55, 1997

Miller BL, Mena I, Daly J, et al: Temporal-parietal hypoperfusion with single photon electron computer tomography in conditions other than Alzheimer's disease. Dementia 1:41–45, 1990

Miller BL, Cummings JL, Villanueva-Meyer J, et al: Frontal lobe degeneration: clinical, neuropsychological and SPECT characteristics. Neurology 41:1374–1382, 1991

Miller BL, Moats R, Shonk T, et al: Abnormalities of cerebral *myo*-inositol in patients with early Alzheimer disease. Radiology 187(2):334–339, 1993a

Miller BL, Chang L, Mena I, et al: Clinical and imaging features of right focal frontal lobe degenerations. Dementia 4:204–213, 1993b

Miller BL, Darby AL, Swartz JR, et al: Dietary changes, compulsions and sexual behavior in fronto-temporal degeneration. Dementia 6:195–199, 1995

Miller BL, Urrutia L, Cornford M, et al: The clinical and functional imaging characteristics of parkinsonian-dementia, in Lewy Body Dementia. Edited by Perry E, McKeith I, Perry R. Cambridge, England, Cambridge University Press, 1996, pp 132–144

Miller BL, Darby A, Benson DF, et al: Aggressive, socially disruptive and antisocial behavior in frontotemporal dementia. Br J Psychiatry 170:150–156, 1997a

Miller BL, Ikonte C, Ponton MP, et al: A study of the Lund-Manchester research criteria for frontotemporal dementia. Neurology 48:937–942, 1997b

Miller BL, Boone K, Mishkin F, et al: Frontotemporal dementias, in Pick's Complex Disorders. Edited by Kertesz A. New York, Wiley, 1998, pp 23–33

Mitsuyama Y: Presenile dementia with motor neuron disease in Japan: clinico-pathological review of 26 cases. J Neurol Neurosurg Psychiatry 47:953–959, 1984

Mody CK, Miller BL: Unsuccessful treatments, in Alzheimer's Disease Treatment and Long Term Management. Edited by Cummings JL, Miller BL. New York, Marcel Dekker, 1990, pp 69–85

Morita K, Kaiya HK, Ikeda T, et al: Presenile dementia combined with amyotrophy: a review of 34 Japanese cases. Archives of Gerontology and Geriatrics 6:263–277, 1987

Morris JC, Cole M, Banker BQ, et al: Hereditary dysphasic dementia and the Pick-Alzheimer spectrum. Ann Neurol 16:455–466, 1984

Mortimer JA: Alzheimer's disease and senile dementia: prevalence and incidence, in Alzheimer's Disease. Edited by Reisberg B. New York, Free Press, 1983, pp 144–148

Motter R, Vigo-Pelfrey C, Kholodenko D, et al: Reduction of amyloid beta peptide 42 in the CSF of Alzheimer's patients. Ann Neurol 38:263–267, 1996

Neary D: Frontotemporal degeneration, Pick disease and corticobasal degeneration. One entity or 3? 3. Arch Neurol 54:1425–1427, 1997

Neary D, Snowden JS, Shields RA: Single photon emission tomography using 99mTc-HMPAO in the investigation of dementia. J Neurol Neurosurg Psychiatry 50:1101–1109, 1987

Neary D, Snowden JS, Northen B, et al: Dementia of frontal lobe type. J Neurol Neurosurg Psychiatry 51:353–361, 1988

Nee LE, Eldridge R, Sunderland T, et al: Dementia of the Alzheimer type: clinical and family study of 22 twin pairs. Neurology 37:359–363, 1987

Neumann MA: Pick's disease. J Neuropathol Exp Neurol 8:255–282, 1949

Neumann MA, Cohn R: Progressive subcortical gliosis; a rare form of presenile dementia. Brain 90:405–418, 1967

Office of Technology Assessment Task Force: Confronting Alzheimer's Disease and Other Dementias. Philadelphia, PA, JB Lippincott, 1988

Pachana N, Boone KB, Miller BL, et al: Comparison of neuropsychological functioning in Alzheimer's disease and frontotemporal dementia. J Int Neuropsychol Soc 2:505–510, 1996

Paganini-Hill A, Henderson V: Estrogen deficiency and risk of Alzheimer's disease in women. Am J Epidemiol 140(3):256–261, 1994

Peavy GM, Herzog AG, Rubin NP, et al: Neuropsychological aspects of dementia of motor neuron disease: a report of two cases. Neurology 42:1004–1008, 1992

Pedersen NL, Reynolds CA, Gatz M: Sources of covariation among Mini-Mental State Examination scores, educational and cognitive abilities. J Gerontol B Psychol Sci Soc Sci 51:55–63, 1996

Pedersen NL, Miller BL, Wetherell JL, et al: Neuroimaging findings in twins discordant for dementia. Dement Geriatr Cogn Disord 10:51–58, 1999

Perry EK, Perry RH, Blessed G, et al: Necropsy evidence of central cholinergic deficits in senile dementia (letter). Lancet i:189, 1977

Perry EK, Marshall E, Perry RH, et al: Cholinergic and dopaminergic activities in senile dementia of Lewy body type. Alzheimer Dis Assoc Disord 4:87–95, 1990

Petersen RB, Tabaton M, Chen SG, et al: Familial progressive subcortical gliosis: presence of prions and linkage to chromosome 17. Neurology 45(6):1062–1067, 1995

Petry S, Cummings JL, Hill MA, et al: Personality alterations in dementia of the Alzheimer type: a three-year follow up study. J Geriatr Psychiatry Neurol 2:203–207, 1989

Pick A: On the relation between senile atrophy of the brain, in Neurological Classics in Modern Translation. Translated by Schoene WS; edited by Rottenberg DA, Hochberg FH. New York, Hafner Press, 1892, pp 35–40

Ponton M, Darcourt J, Miller BL, et al: Psychometric and SPECT studies in Alzheimer's disease with and without delusions. Neuropsychiatry Neuropsychol Behav Neurol 8:264–270, 1995

Poorkaj P, Bird TD, Wijsman E, et al: Tau is a candidate gene for chromosome 17 frontotemporal dementia. Ann Neurol 1998 43:815–825, 1998

Prinz PN, Vitiliano PP, Vitiello MV, et al: Sleep, EEG, and mental function changes in dementia of the Alzheimer type. Neurobiol Aging 3:361–370, 1982

Read SL, Miller BL, Mena I, et al: SPECT in dementia: clinical and pathological correlation. J Am Geriatr Soc 43:1243–1247, 1995

Reiman EM, Caselli RJ, Yun LS, et al: Preclinical evidence of a genetic risk factor for Alzheimer's disease in apolipoprotein E type 4 homozygotes using positron emission tomography. N Engl J Med 334:752–758, 1996

Risberg J, Passant U, Warkentin S, et al: Regional cerebral blood flow in frontal lobe dementia of non-Alzheimer type. Dementia 4:186–187, 1993

Rogaev E, Sherrington R, Liang Y, et al: Familial Alzheimer's disease in kindreds with missense mutations in a gene on chromosome 1 related to the Alzheimer's disease type 3 gene. Nature 376:600–602, 1995

Ropper AH, Williams RS: Relationship between plaques, tangles, and dementia in Down syndrome. Neurology 30:639–644, 1980

Roses AD: Apolipoprotein E genotyping in the differential diagnosis, not prediction, of Alzheimer's disease. Ann Neurol 38:6–14, 1995

Roth M: The diagnosis of senile and related forms of dementia, in Alzheimer's Disease: Senile Dementia and Related Disorders. Edited by Katzman R, Terry RD, Bick KL. New York, Raven, 1978, pp 337–339

Rubin EH, Morris JC, Berg L: The progression of personality changes in senile dementia of the Alzheimer type. J Am Geriatr Soc 37:721–725, 1987

Salerno JA, Murphy DGM, Horwitz B, et al: Brain atrophy in hypertension: a volumetric magnetic resonance imaging study. Hypertension 20:340–348, 1992

Sam M, Gutmann L, Scohchet S, et al: Pick's disease: a case clinically resembling amyotrophic lateral sclerosis. Neurology 41:1831–1833, 1991

Sandson TA, O'Connor M, Sperling RA, et al: Perfusion MRI with EPISTAR in Alzheimer's disease: preliminary results. Neurology 47:1339–1342, 1996

Sano M, Ernesto C, Thomas RG, et al: A controlled trial of selegiline, alpha-tocopherol, or both as treatment for Alzheimer's disease. N Engl J Med 336:1216–1222, 1996

Schellenberg GD: Genetic dissection of Alzheimer disease, a heterogeneous disorder. Proc Natl Acad Sci U S A 92:8552–8559, 1995

Schuff N, Amend DL, Meyerhoff DJ, et al: Alzheimer disease: quantitative H-1 MR spectroscopic imaging of frontoparietal brain. Radiology 207:91–102, 1998

Small GW, Komo S, LaRue A, et al: Early detection of Alzheimer's disease by combining apolipoprotein E and neuroimaging. Ann N Y Acad Sci 802:70–78, 1996

Snowden JS, Neary D, Mann DMA, et al: Progressive language disorder due to lobar atrophy. Ann Neurol 31:174–183, 1992

Snowdon DA, Kemper SJ, Mortimer JA, et al: Linguistic ability in early life and cognitive function and Alzheimer's disease in late life. Findings from the Nun study. JAMA 275:528–532, 1996

Southwick PC, Yamagata SK, Echols CL, et al: Assessment of amyloid beta protein in cerebrospinal fluid as an aid in the diagnosis of Alzheimer's disease. J Neurochem 66:259–265, 1996

Sparks DL, Markesbery WR: Altered serotonergic and cholinergic synaptic markers in Pick's disease. Arch Neurol 48:796–799, 1991

St. George-Hyslop PH, Haines JL, Farer LA, et al: Genetic linkage studies suggest that Alzheimer's disease is not a single homogeneous disorder. Nature 347:194–197, 1990

Stevens M, van Duijn CM, de Kniff P, et al: Apolipoprotein E gene and sporadic frontal lobe dementia. Neurology 48:1526–1529, 1997

Stevens M; van Duijn CM; Kamphorst W; et al: Familial aggregation in frontotemporal dementia. Neurology 50:1541–1545, 1998

Stewart WF, Kawas C, Corrado M, et al: Risk of Alzheimer's disease and duration of NSAID use. Neurology 48:626–632, 1997

Swartz R, Miller BL, Darby A, et al: Frontotemporal dementia: treatment response to serotonin selective reuptake inhibitors. J Clin Psychiatry 58:212–216, 1997

Swearer JM, Drachman DA, O'Donnell BF, et al: Troublesome and disruptive behaviors in dementia. J Am Geriatr Soc 36:784–790, 1988

Teri L, Reifler BV, Veith RC, et al: Imipramine in the treatment of depressed Alzheimer's patients: impact on cognition. J Gerontol 46:P372–P377, 1991

Tyrrell PJ, Warrington EK, Frackowiak RSJ, et al: Progressive degeneration of the right temporal lobe studied with positron-emission tomography. J Neurol Neurosurg Psychiatry 53:1046–1050, 1990

Vinters HV, Gilbert JJ: Cerebral amyloid angiopathy: incidence and complications in the aging brain, II: the distribution of amyloid vascular changes. Stroke 14:924–928, 1983

Vinters HV, Nishimura GS, Secor DL, et al: Immunoreactive A4 and gamma-trace peptide co-localization in amyloidotic arteriolar lesions in the brains of patients with Alzheimer's disease. Am J Pathol 137:233–240, 1990

Walker L: Animal models of cerebral amyloidosis. Bulletin of Clinical Neuroscience 56:86–96, 1991

Waltz J, Knowlton B, Holyoak K, et al: A system for relational reasoning in human prefrontal cortex. Psychol Sci 10: 119–125, 1999

Wechsler AF, Verity A, Rosenschein S, et al: Pick's disease: a clinical, computed tomographic and histological study. Arch Neurol 39:287–290, 1982

Whitehouse PJ, Price DL, Clark AW, et al: Alzheimer disease: evidence for selective loss of cholinergic neurons in the nucleus basalis. Ann Neurol 10:122–126, 1981

Wilhelmsen K, Lynch T, Pavlou E, et al: Localization of disinhibition-dementia-parkinsonism-amyotrophy complex to 17q21-22. Am J Hum Genet 55:1150–1165, 1994

Wisniewski K, Jervis GA, Moretz RC, et al: Alzheimer neurofibrillary tangles in disease other than senile and presenile dementia. Ann Neurol 5:288–294, 1979

Yener GG, Leuchter A, Jenden D, et al: Quantitative EEG in fronto-temporal dementias and Alzheimer disease. Clin Electroencephalogr 27:1–8, 1996

Zhang M, Katzman R, Salmon D, et al: The prevalence of dementia and Alzheimer's disease in Shanghai, China: impact of age, gender, and education. Ann Neurol 27:428–437, 1990

Zhou L, Miller BL, McDaniel CH, et al: Fronto-temporal dementia: neuropil spheroids contain modified tau. Ann Neurol 44:99–109, 1998

Hyperkinetic Movement Disorders

George R. Jackson, M.D., Ph.D.

Anthony E. Lang, M.D., F.R.C.P.

Movement disorders constitute a spectrum of abnormalities that in broadest terms can be classified as either hypokinetic or hyperkinetic (Weiner and Lang 1989). *Hypokinetic* disorders are characterized by significant impairment in the initiation of movement (akinesia) and reduction in the amplitude and speed of movement (bradykinesia), as well as increased muscle tone (rigidity). Idiopathic Parkinson's disease is a prototypic akinetic-rigid syndrome (see Chapter 26 in this volume). In contrast, *hyperkinetic* disorders are characterized by excessive motor activity manifesting as involuntary movements (or dyskinesias). Common types of dyskinesias include tremor, chorea, dystonia, myoclonus, and tics.

Abnormal movements in elderly patients may occur in a wide variety of primary central nervous system disorders (e.g., neurodegenerative diseases). Alternatively, movement disorders in the elderly may be secondary to systemic processes, such as drug exposure, metabolic disturbances, vascular disease, or hypoxic-ischemic injury. A systematic approach to a patient presenting with abnormal movements must include a careful history of the onset and course of illness as well as a detailed physical examination. Evaluation should include a remote and current drug history and documentation of family history. It is often necessary to review this information repeatedly or to seek additional details from other sources (e.g., other family members or physicians). When assessing a hyperkinetic movement disorder, the physician must first attempt to classify the nature of the dyskinesia. This "what is the dyskinesia?" step is a critical first component of the diagnostic approach to patients with movement disorders. It precedes the classic neurological questions of "where is the lesion?" and "what is the lesion?" Once the dyskinesia has been classified accurately using the definitions provided in the following sections, knowledge of the differential diagnosis of a particular dyskinesia guides the diagnostic evaluation and approach to treatment. Investigations will vary depending on clinical suspicion.

Many hyperkinetic movement disorders arise from dysfunction of the basal ganglia. Although the pathophysiology of hyperkinetic movement disorders, such as

Huntington's disease, often may be understood by examining the effects of known anatomical and neurochemical alterations on basal ganglia circuitry, in other instances, such as tics, examination of basal ganglia pathways sheds little light on pathophysiology. Moreover, in many cases, theories of basal ganglia dysfunction in movement disorders do not guide therapeutic interventions. For these reasons, this chapter does not summarize current theories of basal ganglia function and dysfunction in movement disorders. Interested readers are referred to several excellent reviews on this subject (Albin et al. 1989; Weiner and Lang 1989; Wichmann 1997). In the remainder of this chapter, we review the hyperkinetic movement disorders seen in older patients. The behavioral changes that commonly occur in these patients, either as a primary component of the disorder or secondary to the resulting disability, are highlighted.

Tremor

Tremor is defined as involuntary rhythmic oscillatory movement resulting from alternating or synchronous contraction of antagonist muscles. Tremor can be an exaggerated normal physiological process, an isolated monosymptomatic illness, or a component of a variety of neurological disorders. Usually, tremor is classified according to the circumstances in which it occurs. A rest tremor is seen with the body part in complete repose. Maintenance of a posture, such as extending the arms parallel to the floor, elicits a postural tremor. Kinetic tremor (or intention tremor) is seen during volitional movement. Other important descriptive qualities include the frequency, amplitude, and topographic distribution of the tremor (e.g., face or lower extremities).

Rest tremor is most commonly a sign of idiopathic Parkinson's disease or its drug-induced counterpart, but it sometimes may be seen in other conditions. Approximately 75% of patients with Parkinson's disease exhibit a 4- to 6-Hz rest tremor, which usually begins unilaterally in the upper or lower extremity. The well-recognized appearance of a "pill-rolling" tremor of the arm is characteristic of Parkinson's disease and results from rhythmic extension-flexion of the wrist, pronation-supination of the forearm, and grasping movements of the fingers. Many patients with Parkinson's disease also have an 8- to 12-Hz postural tremor of the arms that is clinically indistinguishable from essential tremor. (For further discussion of Parkinson's disease, see Chapter 26 in this volume.)

Unlike the close association between rest tremor and Parkinson's disease, postural and kinetic tremors occur in a wide range of disorders. In the elderly, pathological postural and kinetic tremors usually represent essential tremor or side effects of medications. Table 25–1 provides a summary of the various causes of tremor in elderly people.

In normal individuals, a low-amplitude, 10- to 12-Hz

TABLE 25–1. Classification and differential diagnosis of tremor in elderly patients

Rest tremor

Parkinson's disease

Other parkinsonian syndromes (less commonly)

Midbrain ("rubral") tremor: the rest tremor is less prominent than the postural tremor, which is less prominent than the kinetic tremor

Essential tremor—only if severe: rest tremor is much less severe than the postural and kinetic tremors

Postural tremor (typically with terminal accentuation)

Physiological tremor

Exaggerated physiological tremor

Stress, fatigue, and emotion

Endocrine: hypoglycemia, thyrotoxicosis, pheochromocytoma, and steroids

Drugs and toxins: β agonists, dopamine agonists, lithium, tricyclic antidepressants, neuroleptics, theophylline, caffeine, valproic acid, amphetamines, alcohol withdrawal, mercury, lead, arsenic, and others

Essential tremor

Primary writing tremor

With other central nervous system disorders

Parkinson's disease and other akinetic-rigid syndromes

Idiopathic dystonia, including focal dystonias

With peripheral neuropathy

Cerebellar tremor

Kinetic tremor

Disease of cerebellar "outflow" (dentate nucleus and superior cerebellar peduncle): vascular, tumor, acquired hepatocerebral degeneration, drugs, toxins (e.g., mercury), multiple sclerosis, and others

Miscellaneous rhythmical movement disorders

Psychogenic tremor

Orthostatic tremor

Rhythmical myoclonus (segmental myoclonus, such as palatal myoclonus and spinal myoclonus)

Asterixis

Clonus

Epilepsia partialis continua

Source. Adapted from Weiner and Lang 1989.

physiological tremor may be seen in the fingers when the arms are extended. This physiological tremor may be accentuated by a variety of emotional and metabolic factors such as stress, fatigue, thyrotoxicosis, or hypoglycemia. Accentuated physiological tremor may also be a result of treatment with a number of drugs, including caffeine, sympathomimetics, tricyclic antidepressants, and corticosteroids.

Essential Tremor

Essential tremor is arguably the most common movement disorder. Its prevalence increases with advancing age. Essential tremor is thought to follow an autosomal dominant pattern of inheritance with variable expression. When a positive family history is elicited, the disorder is referred to as *familial tremor*. When it appears for the first time after age 65, it has been called *senile tremor*. Essential tremor is a slowly progressive disorder that usually begins as an 8- to 10-Hz postural tremor of the hands. The tongue, head, voice, trunk, and (less commonly) legs are involved. Typically, the tremor persists during action and worsens at the end point of movement (terminal accentuation). In more severe cases, tremor may also be present at rest. More severe forms of tremor with wider amplitude tend to be of lower frequency (4–6 Hz) and are more common in older individuals.

In many patients, the functional impact of essential tremor is minimal; hence, it is believed that only a small percentage of persons with the disorder seek medical attention. In others, however, the tremor interferes substantially with handwriting, eating, drinking, and fine manipulations and is a source of social embarrassment. As the disease progresses, increased tremor amplitude further compromises the performance of discrete movements. The prefix "benign" is often a misnomer, as essential tremor can be disabling (Koller et al. 1986). In some patients, notably those with prominent head tremor, embarrassment plays a major role in disability. Typically, stress and anxiety accentuate tremor and thus aggravate the problem, resulting in reactive depression in some individuals.

A clinical feature having both diagnostic and therapeutic significance is that most patients with essential tremor note dramatic reduction in tremor after ingesting alcohol. The judicious use of small amounts of alcohol before meals and important events is not contraindicated. Surprisingly, the risk of alcohol abuse among these patients is low (Koller 1983a).

For patients who require treatment, the two most effective drugs for essential tremor are primidone and propranolol or other β-adrenergic blockers (mainly those with relatively selective peripheral β-adrenergic antagonist properties; e.g., metoprolol, nadolol, atenolol, or timolol). Acute vestibulocerebellar side effects—such as vertigo, ataxia, and nausea—are common in response to primidone, even when given in low doses (50–62.5 mg/day). These side effects may be more common in elderly patients and can be both disabling and protracted. A useful approach in elderly patients is to administer small doses of primidone elixir using a tuberculin syringe and incrementally adjust the dosage before beginning therapy with tablets. Many elderly patients cannot tolerate β-blockers because of cardiac or pulmonary disease. In patients with asthma, metoprolol may be preferable to propranolol because of relative cardiac selectivity (Koller and Biary 1984). A single daily dose of nadolol may be useful if patient compliance is a problem (Koller 1983c). Like β-blockers, alternative treatments such as alprazolam and phenobarbital also may not be well tolerated in the elderly (Huber and Paulson 1988). Other second-line drugs include clonazepam and carbonic anhydrase inhibitors (Busenbark et al. 1993; C. Thompson et al. 1984). Because of drug contraindications, intolerance, and poor efficacy, a significant number of elderly patients with essential tremor are left with persistent disability.

Patients with medically refractory, disabling tremor have been effectively treated with stereotactic thalamotomy (Goldman and Kelly 1992). More recently, high-frequency deep brain stimulation (DBS) of the ventral intermediate thalamic nucleus has proved to be effective in patients with severe essential and other types of tremor (Benabid et al. 1996; Hubble et al. 1996). This procedure is now widely available in major medical centers.

The physiological basis for essential tremor is incompletely understood, but the disorder is thought to be caused by an abnormal oscillation of a central nervous system "pacemaker" (the location of which is uncertain) that is influenced by peripheral reflex pathways. No neurotransmitter or structural abnormalities have yet been identified. Although linkage analysis of several kindreds has identified potential loci for essential tremor-related genes, none has yet been cloned (Gulcher et al. 1997; Higgins et al. 1997).

Other Tremors

Primary writing tremor is induced almost exclusively by writing. It is characterized predominantly by pronation-supination movements of the forearm at 5–7 Hz. Because many such patients have an associated mild postural tremor, primary writing tremor may be related to essential tremor. However, the task specificity suggests that it may be a form of focal dystonia akin to dystonic "writer's cramp." Botulinum toxin injection probably affords the best relief in this disorder (Wissel et al. 1996).

Patients with orthostatic tremor develop rapid rhythmic contractions of the legs and sometimes the buttocks within a few minutes of assuming a standing position (T. C. Britton et al. 1992; FitzGerald and Jankovic 1991; P. D. Thompson et al. 1986). Walking, sitting, or lying will cause the tremor to cease. Most patients respond to clonazepam, primidone, or propranolol.

Cerebellar disease most commonly causes slow, irregular tremor of the head and trunk (titubation) when the patient is upright. Cerebellar tremor of the limbs is typically absent at rest and during the initial stages of motion but becomes manifest through the course of and at the end of a trajectory. The term *intention tremor* has been used to describe the increase in tremor as the limb approaches a precise destination; this is not specific to cerebellar tremor, however, but is common to most forms of postural tremor.

Lesions in the midbrain involving the superior cerebellar peduncle and possibly the substantia nigra near the red nucleus result in midbrain or "rubral" tremor. This type of tremor is present at rest, increases with maintenance of posture, and increases still further with action. It is believed to result from interruption of the connections between cerebellar dentate nuclei and the thalamus. A lesion anywhere in this outflow pathway may cause such a tremor (thus the term *cerebellar outflow tremor*). Additional involvement of the dopaminergic nigrostriatal pathway may contribute to the tremor. Demyelinating lesions in multiple sclerosis are the most common cause of midbrain tremor overall, whereas posterior circulation stroke accounts for most cases in elderly patients. Other features of midbrain or diencephalic dysfunction typically accompany the tremor in this setting. Sometimes the onset of tremor may be delayed for weeks after a brain stem event (e.g., stroke or head injury). Often, medications are ineffective for this tremor type. Stereotactic thalamotomy or DBS may be useful in patients with severe debility; however, the disabling proximal component of the tremor is often resistant to this approach.

Numerous drugs can produce tremor (Table 25–1). As indicated above, often this is an accentuation of normal physiological tremor. Any patient who develops tremor acutely or subacutely after initiation of a new medication should be suspected of having a drug-induced tremor regardless of whether tremor is a recognized side effect. Some individuals may have a further predisposition to develop tremor from medications by virtue of underlying disorders such as essential tremor or subclinical Parkinson's disease. Pronounced mixed postural and resting tremor may develop in patients with preexisting essential tremor

who are treated with neuroleptic drugs. A number of medications used in psychiatric practice are capable of causing tremor. Tricyclic antidepressants may accentuate physiological tremor; however, this rarely poses a management problem. Tremor is an extremely common side effect of lithium therapy, which occasionally requires treatment with β-blockers or primidone.

Neuroleptic agents may cause a either a postural or a parkinsonian resting tremor. One variant of the latter is a tremor of the perinasal and oral region known as the *rabbit syndrome*. Neuroleptic-induced parkinsonian tremor typically subsides after drug withdrawal. Patients who require ongoing neuroleptic therapy and who have sufficiently bothersome or disabling tremor may be treated with anticholinergics or amantadine. However, because of the frequency of cognitive and psychiatric side effects, anticholinergics should be avoided in patients over age 65 and are contraindicated in patients with known cognitive disturbance. Other considerations include a change to a less potent neuroleptic or to an atypical agent such as clozapine.

Chorea

The term *chorea* is derived from the Greek word for dance. Choreic movements are brief, jerky, purposeless involuntary movements that occur in random sequence. They can involve the distal or proximal limbs, face, or trunk. The movements may be brisk and abrupt as in Sydenham's chorea or more slow and flowing as in Huntington's disease. Various causes of chorea in elderly patients are listed in Table 25–2. Because the types of chorea most frequently encountered in psychiatric practice include Huntington's disease and tardive dyskinesia, these topics are emphasized in the following discussion.

Huntington's Disease

Huntington's disease is a progressive, autosomal dominant disorder characterized by chorea, personality changes, and dementia. The prevalence of Huntington's disease in North America ranges from 4 to 7 per 100,000 (Harper 1991). Symptoms usually appear insidiously in the fourth decade, although symptom onset as late as the tenth decade has been reported. Typically, the movement disorder and the cognitive and personality changes are present at the onset of the disease, although one may precede the other by a matter of years.

Movement disorders.   Initially, involuntary movements most often involve the upper limbs and face with

TABLE 25–2.   Causes of chorea in elderly patients

Hereditary causes

    Huntington's disease

    Benign hereditary chorea (typically childhood onset)

    Neuroacanthocytosis

Other central nervous system degenerations

    Olivopontocerebellar atrophy

    Machado-Joseph disease

    Kufs disease

    Dentatorubropallidoluysian atrophy

Aging-related causes

    Spontaneous orofacial dyskinesias

    "Edentulous orodyskinesia"

    "Senile chorea" (probably several etiologies)

Drug-induced causes

    Neuroleptics, metoclopramide, flunarizine, cinnarizine, antiparkinsonian drugs, amphetamines, methylphenidate, tricyclic antidepressants, monoamine oxidase inhibitors, lithium, estrogens (including estrogen creams for atrophic vaginitis), steroids, antihistamines, α-methyldopa, anticonvulsants (phenytoin, ethosuximide, carbamazepine, and phenobarbital), benzodiazepines, digoxin, methadone, and toluene

Metabolic causes

    Hyperthyroidism

    Hypoparathyroidism

    Hypo- and hypernatremia, hypomagnesemia, hypocalcemia

    Hypo- and hyperglycemia (latter may cause hemichorea or hemiballism)

    Acquired hepatocerebral degeneration, Wilson's disease

Infectious causes

    Encephalitides

    Subacute bacterial endocarditis

    Creutzfeldt-Jakob disease

Toxins

    Alcohol intoxication and withdrawal, anoxia, carbon monoxide, manganese, mercury, toluene, and thallium

Immunological causes

    Systemic lupus erythematosus

    Recurrence of Sydenham's chorea

    Primary anticardiolipin antibody syndrome

Vascular causes

    Infarctions usually involving striatum, subthalamic nucleus region

    Hemorrhage

    Arteriovenous malformation

    Polycythemia rubra vera

    Migraine

Tumors

Trauma: subdural hematoma

Miscellaneous: including paroxysmal choreoathetosis

Source.   Adapted from Lang 1992a.

"fidgeting" of the hands, shrugging of the shoulders, grimacing of the face, or pursing of the lips. With time, more obvious and generalized choreic movements develop. Patients often try to incorporate these movements into normal purposeful acts, such as raising the hand to the head as if to smooth the hair; this incorporation of involuntary into seemingly voluntary movement is referred to as parakinesia. Chorea may be aggravated by mental concentration, emotional stimuli, performance of complex motor tasks, or walking.

There is early impersistence of motor tasks such as the inability to sustain tongue protrusion or hand grip ("milk-maid grip"). Oculomotor disturbances are invariably present and include slowed pursuit and saccadic eye movements (Lasker and Zee 1997). Initially, patients may be unable to rapidly direct their gaze in a given direction (i.e., generate a saccade) without blinking the eyes or thrusting the head. Later, gaze palsies may be pronounced. Other prominent findings include decreased fine motor coordination, dysarthria, dysphagia, orolingual apraxia (inability to perform complex motor tasks such as licking the lips or sucking an imaginary straw), and ideomotor apraxia. The gait takes on a dancing, stuttering character, which may be associated with lateral swaying or decreased arm swing. As the disease progresses, postural stability becomes impaired and axial chorea may throw the patient off balance. Later, dystonia and rigidity often become superimposed on chorea. Involuntary movements may become so severe that routine activities of daily living are impossible. Importantly, apraxia and bradykinesia also contribute greatly to later motor disability.

Neuropsychological and psychiatric features.

Early mental disturbances in patients with Huntington's disease include personality and behavioral changes such as irritability, apathy, depression, decreased work performance, violence, impulsivity, and emotional lability (Morris 1995). Intellectual decline usually follows the personality changes. The neuropsychological profile characteristically includes a memory disturbance suggesting selective impairment of information retrieval with retention of the ability to register new information. Patients often have difficulty recalling information on command but are able to give the correct answer if provided categorical cues or a multiple-choice format. Other deficits in memory include loss of detailed recollections (equally severe across all decades of the patient's life). There is difficulty with organization, planning, and sequencing even when all the necessary information is available (Caine et al. 1978). Additional prominent abnormalities include visuospatial deficits, dyscalculia, impaired judgment, and ideomotor apraxia (the inability to perform previously learned tasks in the context of intact elementary motor function) (Brouwers et al. 1984; Cummings 1995). As the disease advances, there are more global intellectual deficits.

A wide range of psychiatric disturbances is seen in Huntington's disease. Thirty-eight percent of patients have an affective disorder. Depression is the most common psychiatric symptom and does not appear to be simply a reaction to fatal illness. Evidence for this is the fact that mood disorders are not randomly distributed but occur in subsets of families with Huntington's disease (Peyser and Folstein 1990). Impaired motivation and reinforcement of rewarding behavior may be caused by interruption of the anterior cingulate circuit by striatal dysfunction (Cummings 1993). Apathy and loss of spontaneity may result from impairment of the medial frontal–anterior cingulate subcortical circuit (Cummings 1993). Ten percent of patients develop mania. Psychosis is less common. Suicide accounts for 5.7% of deaths in patients with Huntington's disease, and 25% of all patients attempt suicide at least once (Farrer 1986). This tendency to suicide may be due to impulsivity related to dysfunction of the orbitofrontal circuit. Obsessive-compulsive symptoms such as handwashing may also be seen in patients with Huntington's disease (Cummings and Cunningham 1992).

Course. The duration of Huntington's disease from onset to death is typically 15–20 years. Death is often caused by pneumonia, trauma, or suicide. In 10% of patients, the disease begins before age 20. Juvenile-onset Huntington's disease (the so-called Westphal variant) usually presents as an akinetic-rigid disorder, occasionally with seizures. The predominant signs are bradykinesia, rigidity, dementia, and cerebellar disturbance, often with little or no chorea. This form of Huntington's disease may be more rapidly progressive and the duration of illness shorter than the adult-onset type. Occasionally the akinetic-rigid variant is seen in adults either de novo or developing after a choreic presentation.

Twenty-five percent of patients have late-onset Huntington's disease, which is usually defined as the onset of motor manifestations after age 50. One study of this population of patients (Myers et al. 1985) revealed that the average age at onset of chorea was 57.5 years and the average age at the time of diagnosis was 63 years. The clinical features are similar to those of the typical adult-onset variety, but the progression of motor signs is slower and the cognitive changes are less severe.

Genetics. Huntington's disease is inherited as an autosomal dominant trait with complete penetrance. Thus, all people who inherit the gene will develop symptoms of the disease if they do not die prematurely. The Huntington gene has been localized to the short arm of chromosome 4 (Gusella et al. 1983). It has been found to contain an expanded and unstable CAG trinucleotide repeat within exon 1 of a large gene, the protein product of which is called Huntington's disease (Huntington's Disease Collaborative Research Group 1993). The genetic "stutter" of trinucleotide repeats gives rise to elongated polyglutamine tracts within huntingtin. Normal alleles contain 34 or fewer CAG repeats, whereas repeats of 37–150 or more occur in affected individuals (Gusella et al. 1997). Patients with juvenile-onset disease show predominantly paternal inheritance of the expanded allele (Gusella and MacDonald 1995). A younger age at onset is associated with longer trinucleotide repeat lengths. Age at onset is correlated with repeat length; however, for any given repeat length, the age at onset may vary by 15 or more years, suggesting that factors other than repeat length alone determine the onset of symptoms (Gusella et al. 1997). It is not known whether such factors are genetic, environmental, or stochastic.

Diagnosis. A diagnosis of Huntington's disease can be made with confidence when a patient has dominantly inherited chorea and dementia with onset in adult life. Before the characterization of the genetic defect, the diagnosis was always clinical. There are no definite biochemical or radiological markers for Huntington's disease. Routine imaging demonstrates atrophy of the striatum (caudate nucleus and putamen), most easily appreciated as enlargement of the frontal horns of the lateral ventricles (Figure 25–1). In elderly patients this may be a less useful diagnostic feature unless it is very pronounced, given the normal reduction in brain mass with age and the occurrence of atrophy in other disorders that might be confused with Huntington's disease. [18F]fluorodeoxyglucose positron-emission tomography (PET) demonstrates striatal hypometabolism even before atrophy is seen on computed tomography (CT) or magnetic resonance imaging (MRI). However, this is a

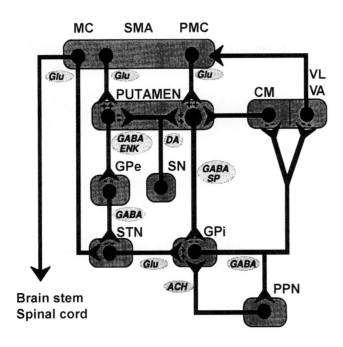

FIGURE 25–1. Current concept of neuronal connections and neurotransmitters of the basal ganglia, thalamus, and motor cortex. MC = motor cortex; SMA = supplementary motor cortex; PMC = premotor cortex; GPe = globus pallidus externa; GPi = globus pallidus interna (which is functionally similar to the substantia nigra pars reticulata); STN = subthalamic nucleus; SN = substantia nigra; CM = centromedian nucleus of the thalamus; VL = ventrolateral nucleus of the thalamus; VA = ventral anterior nucleus of the thalamus; PPN = pedunculopontine nucleus. The circled letters represent neurotransmitters. ACH = acetylcholine; GABA = γ-aminobutyric acid; DA = dopamine; ENK = enkephalin; Glu = glutamic acid; SP = substance P. *Source.* Reprinted with permission from Nutt JG: "Dyskinesia Induced by Levodopa and Dopamine Agonists in Patients With Parkinson's Disease," in Drug-Induced Movement Disorders. Edited by Lang AE, Weiner WJ. Mount Kisco, NY, Futura, 1992, p. 296.

nonspecific finding and may be seen in other disorders combining striatal degeneration and chorea (e.g., neuroacanthocytosis). The onset of symptoms may occur soon after the development of PET abnormalities in Huntington's disease; thus, this technique is of limited value in the evaluation of persons at risk for Huntington's disease.

Until 1993, the most sensitive method for detecting gene carriers had been genetic linkage analysis. It is now possible to evaluate the CAG repeat length in an individual patient. Repeat lengths of 40 or more are diagnostic of the disorder. There is a "gray area" of repeat lengths in the 36–39 unit range; that is, some but not all individuals with intermediate repeat lengths will live long enough to manifest symptoms of disease (Gusella et al. 1997). Predictive

testing is a problematic issue, because no effective treatment is currently available. A carefully designed counseling service is a necessary component of any presymptomatic or diagnostic testing program (International Huntington Association and the World Federation of Neurology Research Group on Huntington's Chorea 1994).

Difficulties in diagnosis often arise when the family history is negative. It may be necessary to interview several relatives on more than one occasion to be certain of the family history. Some families deny the presence of cognitive or psychiatric disease in other family members. Patients should be asked about extramarital conception. If the affected parent had late-onset Huntington's disease, the diagnosis may have been missed because the symptoms may have been so mild as to go unnoticed, or the parent may have died before clinically apparent symptoms developed. Furthermore, physicians may fail to consider the possibility of Huntington's disease in elderly patients, preferring to label the problem as "senile chorea." Spontaneous mutations have been described, in some instances in children of fathers with an "intermediate" repeat length. The true incidence of new mutations is not known. The availability of CAG repeat length analysis will now allow a definitive diagnosis in many patients with Huntington's disease who lack a clear family history.

The differential diagnosis of Huntington's disease in the elderly patient includes various degenerative, systemic, and drug-related conditions, including tardive dyskinesia (Table 25–2). One important source of confusion is the patient treated with neuroleptics for a psychiatric presentation of Huntington's disease. The subsequent development of a movement disorder may then be mistaken for a complication of the drug therapy rather than an important clue to the underlying neurological diagnosis. Knowledge of the clinical differences between the movement disorders of Huntington's disease and the abnormal movements typically seen in tardive dyskinesia may help to avoid this confusion (Table 25–3).

Treatment. Management of Huntington's disease requires a team approach involving a wide variety of medical, paramedical, and social services. Education of patients and their families about the implications of the disease is extremely important. Genetic, psychological, and social counseling is regularly required, and lay organizations such as the Huntington's Disease Society of America often assist greatly in these tasks.

Medical treatment is symptomatic. Drugs that block postsynaptic dopamine receptors (neuroleptics) or deplete presynaptic dopamine terminals (reserpine and tetra-

TABLE 25–3. Clinical features that help distinguish tardive dyskinesia (TD), oromandibular dystonia (OMD), and Huntington's disease (HD)

Feature	TD	OMD	HD
Forehead chorea	0	+	+++
Blepharospasm	+	++++	+/–
Movements of mouth	++++	++++	+
Platysma	+/–	++++	+/–
Nuchal muscles	+	+++	+/–
Trunk, arms, and legs	+++	0	+++
Stereotyped nature of movements	++++	++	0
Flowing movements	0	0	+++
Akathisia	+++	0	0
Marching in place	+++	0	0
Truncal rocking	+++	0	+
Dysarthria	+/–	+++	++++
Facial apraxia	0	0	+++
Impersistence of tongue protrusion	0	0	+++
Oculomotor defects	0	0	+++
Respiratory dyskinesia	++	+/–	+
Gait disorder	+	0	+++
Postural instability	0	0	+++
Dementia	+	0	+++
Effect of			
Talking or chewing	Decrease	Increase	+/–
Tongue protrusion to command	Decrease	+/–	+/–
Antidopaminergics	Decrease	Decrease	Decrease
Anticholinergics	Increase	Decrease	+/–
Effect on			
Talking or chewing	+	++++	+
Swallowing	0	++	++++

Note. ++++ = Extremely common or marked; +++ = common or frequent; ++ = often; + = occasional; +/– = rarely present or variable; 0 = usually absent.
Source. From S. Fahn, personal communication, July 1992.

benazine) are the most useful in reducing chorea. The mechanism whereby antidopaminergic drugs decrease chorea is unknown. Neuroleptics may also help control emotional outbursts, paranoia, psychosis, and irritability sometimes seen in Huntington's disease. With respect to the movement disorder, these medications should be reserved for disabling dyskinesias because of the high incidence of serious side effects. Newer atypical agents such as clozapine may be of some use in selected patients, although the necessity of performing weekly complete blood counts (because of a risk of agranulocytosis) may limit its utility (Factor and Friedman 1997). Other atypical agents such as risperidone and olanzapine have been useful anecdotally; the risk of tardive side effects with these agents, though less than with older neuroleptics, is not negligible. In younger patients, concern about the superimposition of tardive dyskinesia on the underlying choreic disorder encourages the use of dopamine-depleting agents rather than neuroleptics (Jankovic and Beach 1997; van Vugt et al. 1997). Reserpine is associated with problematic hypotension, which may limit its utility. Tetrabenazine, although not approved for use in the United States, can be obtained from England or Canada and may be of considerable utility. Sedation is common, however, and use of the medication does carry a long-term risk of parkinsonism. In elderly patients one might turn to neuroleptics more readily, because there may be less concern regarding long-term side effects. Despite the ability of dopamine antagonists to reduce chorea, motor disability may not be altered given other deficits, such as bradykinesia and apraxia, which may be worsened by these drugs.

Depression may be treated with conventional antidepressant agents, such as fluoxetine (Como et al. 1997). Sertraline may also be helpful in aggressive patients (Ranen et al. 1996b). Benzodiazepines are often helpful with anxiety. (See Chapter 34 in this volume for discussion of psychopharmacological agents in geriatric neuropsychiatric disorders.)

Akinetic-rigid patients occasionally benefit from antiparkinsonian medications such as carbidopa/levodopa or dopamine agonists; however, increasing chorea and psychiatric disturbances may ensue. Although clinical trials are under way of agents (such as antioxidants and coenzyme Q) that are intended to modify the course of the disease rather than treat it symptomatically, none of these agents has been demonstrated to be effective (Huntington Study Group 1998; Koroshetz et al. 1997; Ranen et al. 1996a). Recently, anecdotal reports have suggested a beneficial effect of fetal striatal transplants (Kopyov et al. 1998; Philpott et al. 1997). The efficacy and long-term outcome of this approach, however, remain to be proved. At present, it cannot be recommended.

Other Choreas

Spontaneous orofacial dyskinesia. Spontaneous abnormal movements in the lingual-facial-buccal region occur in a variety of populations and are not exclusive to patients treated with neuroleptics. The prevalence of this disorder has been estimated as being 0.8% between the ages of 50 and 59, increasing to 7.8% between the ages of 70 and 79 (Klawans and Barr 1982). Spontaneous orodyskinesia may be more likely to develop in the context of underlying brain dysfunction such as in patients with schizophrenia or Down's syndrome (Dinan and Golden 1990; Waddington and Youssef 1990). The true incidence of the disorder, however, is difficult to ascertain because of difficulties in obtaining complete drug histories (Ticehurst 1990). Many patients described as having spontaneous orofacial dyskinesia actually have cranial dystonia or Meige's syndrome (discussed below) (Table 25–3).

"Edentulous orodyskinesia" in elderly patients. Elderly patients may develop orofacial dyskinesias following tooth extraction (Koller 1983b). This occurs in about 16% of patients, but only after a long period of edentulousness (average of 12 years). The movements are similar to those seen in tardive dyskinesia with stereotyped smacking and pursing of the lips and lateral deviation of the tongue or jaw. However, the absence of vermicular movements of the tongue when inside the mouth and the lack of involuntary movements of the limbs or trunk help distinguish edentulous orodyskinesia from tardive dyskinesia. Most often, patients are unaware of these movements, and they never cause disability. Wearing dentures often diminishes or dampens the movements.

"Senile chorea." The uncommon condition called senile chorea is best considered a "syndrome" of late-onset generalized chorea (beginning after age 65) for which no underlying cause can be determined. There is no cognitive deterioration, nor is there a family history of psychiatric disturbance or chorea. Few cases with pathological documentation are available. The findings are not uniform, but they may resemble less severe degrees of the changes seen in Huntington's disease with degeneration of the caudate nucleus and putamen (Alcock 1936) or the putamen alone (J. H. Friedman and Ambler 1990). Senile chorea probably represents a heterogeneous group of disorders, which may inadvertently include late-onset Huntington's disease (J. W. Britton et al. 1995; Garcia Ruiz et al. 1997). Genotyping for CAG repeat length should aid in distinguishing late-onset, sporadic Huntington's disease from true senile chorea. Symptomatic treatment with dopamine-depleting agents or low-dose neuroleptics may be tried if necessary, as discussed above for Huntington's disease.

Vascular chorea. An important consideration when assessing chorea presenting in elderly patients is the potential role of multiple infarctions involving the basal ganglia, particularly the caudate nucleus, putamen, and subthalamic nucleus. This syndrome usually occurs in the setting of lacunar disease as a result of chronic hypertension. A wide range of other causes of cerebral infarction must also be considered. Vascular malformations also may give rise to chorea. Typically, vascular chorea is of abrupt onset and spares the face. The majority of patients recover within a few weeks of the vascular insult. Treatment with neuroleptics or dopamine-depleting agents may be tried. Although chorea due to systemic lupus erythematosus is usually a disorder of the young, it may also occur in older individuals, as may chorea due to the primary anticardiolipin syndrome (Asherson et al. 1987; Cervera et al. 1997; Lang et al. 1991). Here, the chorea is probably the result of vascular or immunologic processes. Treatment is directed toward control of the underlying disease.

Polycythemia rubra vera has been known to cause generalized chorea of acute, subacute, or gradual onset; indeed, chorea may be the presenting sign of polycythemia in up to two-thirds of cases (Bruyn and Padberg 1984).

Haloperidol or other antidopaminergic agents may diminish the chorea; however, the abnormal movements often improve after treatment of the underlying disorder by phlebotomy or treatment with phosphorus 32.

Hemiballismus

The term *hemiballismus* describes involuntary, proximal, large-amplitude flailing or throwing movements that can be violent and potentially dangerous in severe cases. Hemiballismus is often classified as one extreme in the spectrum of chorea because of the clinical and pathological overlap between the two conditions. Many patients with hemiballismus have concomitant distal choreic movements. As patients with hemiballismus improve, they often go through a hemichoreic phase.

Most patients with hemiballismus have a lesion in the contralateral subthalamic nucleus, although lesions of the caudate nucleus, putamen, thalamus, and possibly even the cortex are able to induce similar movements (Dewey and Jankovic 1989; Ghika-Schmid et al. 1997; Lee and Marsden 1994; Shannon 1990; Vidakovic et al. 1994). Most hemiballism is secondary to vascular insult in the form of either lacunar infarction or hemorrhage, typically presenting with sudden onset of the involuntary movements. Given the common causes, hemiballism is most often a disorder of elderly individuals, particularly those with predisposing factors such as hypertension and diabetes. The diagnostic study of choice is brain MRI. Other possible causes include metastatic tumor, basilar meningitis, vascular malformations, infections (e.g., toxoplasmosis), drugs, and metabolic derangement (e.g., hyperglycemic nonketotic states) (Glass et al. 1984; Lin and Chang 1994; Tamaoka et al. 1987).

Vascular hemiballism usually resolves spontaneously after weeks or months, but it may occasionally be persistent. Given the severe disability caused by the pronounced abnormal movements, most patients require treatment with either neuroleptics or dopamine-depleting agents. Clozapine may be helpful in refractory cases (Stojanovic et al. 1997). Drug-resistant or persistent hemiballism sometimes requires stereotactic thalamotomy.

Tardive Dyskinesia

Tardive dyskinesia refers to a variety of persistent, involuntary movements caused by drugs that are dopamine receptor blocking agents (DRBAs). Neuroleptic antipsychotic drugs are the most common responsible agents. Medications less commonly recognized as DRBAs such as metoclopramide, promethazine, amoxapine, and per-

phenazine-amitriptyline (Etrafon) can also cause tardive dyskinesia. Other drugs such as antidepressants, antihistamines, and phenytoin may induce movements similar to those seen in tardive dyskinesia; however, such movements are not classified as tardive dyskinesia. Dopamine-depleting drugs such as reserpine, tetrabenazine, and α-methylparatyrosine have not been shown to cause tardive dyskinesia.

Tardive dyskinesia usually begins insidiously after several years of therapy with a DRBA but can occur after only 3 months of exposure. Often, tardive dyskinesia also appears after a decrease in dosage or drug withdrawal. There is no definite period of time between stopping a DRBA and the onset of involuntary movements that excludes a diagnosis of tardive dyskinesia. However, it is widely accepted that the movement disorder must begin within 3 months of stopping the DRBA (Fahn 1992) for a diagnosis of tardive dyskinesia to be applied. In contrast to other neuroleptic-induced movement disorders—such as acute dystonic reactions, parkinsonism, and acute akathisia—the movements of tardive dyskinesia usually worsen when the offending agent is withdrawn and improve when the dose of the DRBA is increased.

Tardive dyskinesia is now considered a syndrome that includes several categories of abnormal involuntary movements (Table 25–4). The typical movements of tardive dyskinesia are choreic in speed and amplitude, but their stereotypical and almost rhythmic pattern distinguish them from the classic random, flowing choreic movements seen in Huntington's disease. Occasionally, a more typical choreic picture is seen. The involuntary movements usually reach maximal severity quickly after onset and then tend to stabilize.

The oral-buccal-lingual muscles tend to be involved earliest and most frequently in tardive dyskinesia. One early sign is a fine, vermicular movement of the tongue when inside the mouth. This may progress to horizontal tongue movements and later to rolling, twisting, or curling with pressing of the tongue against the cheek ("bon bon sign"). There may be brief or prolonged involuntary tongue protrusion ("fly catcher's tongue"). Jaw movements

TABLE 25–4. Tardive dyskinesia subtypes

"Classic" tardive dyskinesia
Tardive dystonia
Tardive akathisia
Withdrawal-emergent syndrome
Tardive myoclonus
Tardive tics

include chewing, biting, teeth clenching, and lateral side-to-side movements. There may be pouting, pursing, smacking, or sucking movements of the lips, which sometimes have an audible component. The corners of the mouth may retract ("bridling"), or the cheeks may puff out intermittently. Despite these movements, speech and eating are often unaffected, as volitional activity of the affected muscles often dampens or alleviates the dyskinesia. The hands, feet, neck, and trunk may also be affected. Movements of the fingers may have a "piano-playing" appearance. There may be tapping motions of the feet, side-to-side oscillations of the foot at the ankle, or marching in place without the report of restlessness. Respiratory dyskinesia due to diaphragm and intercostal muscle involvement may produce an irregular respiratory pattern, periodic tachypnea, or grunting. The term *copulatory dyskinesia* colorfully describes a rocking, undulating movement of the pelvis sometimes encountered as a manifestation of tardive dyskinesia. Surprisingly, the gait is usually little affected.

Many patients seem unaware of even pronounced involuntary movements. However, a significant minority of patients are embarrassed and/or disabled by the dyskinesias because of interference with speech and swallowing, oral ulceration, or life-threatening respiratory involvement. Patients with both schizophrenia and tardive dyskinesia may have twice the mortality rate of patients with schizophrenia and no tardive dyskinesia, but the reasons for this are uncertain (Yagi et al. 1989; Youssef and Waddington 1987).

The movements described above refer to "classic" tardive dyskinesia, which should be distinguished from other subtypes of tardive dyskinesia such as tardive dystonia, tardive akathisia, and the withdrawal-emergent syndrome. Often, tardive dyskinesias represent combinations of different movement disorders, such as dystonia and chorea or dystonia and myoclonus (Cardoso and Jankovic 1997).

Unlike classic tardive dyskinesia, which occurs more frequently in elderly individuals, tardive dystonia is seen equally in all age groups. The prevalence of this condition among chronic psychiatric patients is approximately 2% (Yassa et al. 1986). Younger patients tend to have more generalized involvement, whereas older patients usually have a focal or segmental distribution. Retrocollis may be especially common in tardive dystonia, with more severe forms demonstrating opisthotonic posturing, often with the arms extended and pronated. A history of exposure to DRBAs, early facial and neck involvement, and concomitant signs of other tardive syndromes (e.g., classic tardive dyskinesia and tardive akathisia) can support a diagnosis of tardive

dystonia. Tardive dystonia is usually more disabling and more difficult to treat than classic tardive dyskinesia.

Patients taking neuroleptics often complain of inner restlessness or akathisia, usually involving the legs. Most often this is an early, dose-related complication referred to as *acute akathisia*, which occurs after initiating or increasing the dosage of a neuroleptic agent and resolves when the offending drug is stopped. In contrast, tardive akathisia is a persistent problem that results from long-term exposure to DRBAs and occurs in the context of a constant or decreasing drug dosage. Patients demonstrate a variety of "akathitic" movements, including rubbing the scalp, marching in place, crossing and uncrossing the legs, or rocking at the trunk. Moaning and shouting also may occur. As is true of the other tardive syndromes, tardive akathisia usually worsens on withdrawal of the DRBA and improves if the dose is increased. Like tardive dystonia, tardive akathisia can result in profound disability.

The withdrawal-emergent syndrome involves involuntary movements (usually choreic) that typically appear in children following the abrupt discontinuation of DRBAs. This is a self-limited disorder that usually disappears within 6–12 weeks of onset. Other tardive syndromes include myoclonus, tics, and possibly tremor, but they are much less common than those described above.

Differential diagnosis. The differential diagnosis of tardive dyskinesia is extensive, given the spectrum of movements seen in this condition (Table 25–5), and includes a variety of abnormal movements seen in elderly psychiatric populations. Manneristic movements such as rubbing, picking, or grimacing may also improve with administration of neuroleptic agents and may be mistaken for tardive dyskinesia. Patients with Huntington's disease who have been receiving chronic neuroleptic therapy may develop superimposed tardive dyskinesia. Clinical points of distinction between Huntington's disease and tardive dyskinesia are listed in Table 25–3.

Epidemiology. Estimates of the prevalence of tardive dyskinesia among patients receiving long-term neuroleptic therapy have ranged between 17% and 30% (Cardoso and Jankovic 1997; Kane and Smith 1982). Proven risk factors for the development of tardive dyskinesia include advanced age, female sex, and extended duration of treatment. The incidence of tardive dyskinesia in elderly patients may be four times higher than that in young adults. The incidence is higher in women. The risk of developing tardive dyskinesia increases with duration of DRBA treatment: the cumulative incidence is estimated to

TABLE 25–5. Differential diagnosis of tardive dyskinesia in elderly patients

Schizophrenic stereotyped movements

Spontaneous orofacial dyskinesia

"Edentulous orodyskinesia"

Infarcts of the basal ganglia

Huntington's disease or other choreiform disorders (see Table 25–2)

Dyskinesias induced by other drugs (see Table 25–2)

Idiopathic dystonias: Meige's syndrome or oromandibular dystonia (see Table 25–3)

Hemifacial spasm

Mouthing movements said to be associated with cerebellar vermis lesions

be 5% after 1 year, 10% after 2 years, and 19% after 4 years (Khot et al. 1992). Other proposed but controversial risk factors include preexisting "organic brain dysfunction," "negative features of schizophrenia," and affective disorders (said to be a greater risk than schizophrenia).

Pathophysiology. Although tardive dyskinesia has been recognized for more than 30 years, its pathogenesis remains poorly understood. The most commonly proposed mechanism is supersensitivity of postsynaptic striatal dopamine receptors as a consequence of chemical denervation caused by long-term use of DRBAs (Egan et al. 1997). Supersensitive striatal neurons may then respond abnormally to the presence of dopamine and produce the movements of tardive dyskinesia. The discontinuation of DRBAs would be expected to facilitate more interaction between dopamine and supersensitive receptors, leading to worsening of symptoms. Increasing the dosage of the offending drug would increase receptor blockade and improve (or mask) symptoms. The appearance of tardive dyskinesia during ongoing neuroleptic therapy suggests that competitive receptor blockade can sometimes be overcome by endogenous dopamine; the latter may be increased through enhanced activity of presynaptic nigrostriatal neurons responding to blockade of the postsynaptic receptors. Most neuroleptic agents are antagonists of the D_2 receptor. The atypical neuroleptic clozapine is a D_4 agonist, which is believed to explain its lack of association with tardive dyskinesias. Other newer atypical DRBAs show varying degrees of selectivity for other dopamine receptors (Baldessarini and Frankenburg 1991). The postsynaptic receptor hypersensitivity hypothesis has a number of limitations but is still useful in attempting to rationalize therapy for tardive dyskinesia.

Prevention. Given the iatrogenic nature of tardive dyskinesia, prevention should be emphasized. The indications for long-term antipsychotic medication should be delineated clearly and reevaluated regularly. Patients requiring ongoing neuroleptic therapy should be maintained on the minimal dose needed for a therapeutic effect. Patients should be evaluated regularly for signs of tardive dyskinesia. Neuroleptics should be avoided in psychiatric conditions for which other categories of drugs may be effective. Antiemetics such as metoclopramide should not be given for maintenance therapy unless other drugs have failed. The use of anticholinergic agents in addition to neuroleptics should be minimized because they may aggravate movements of tardive dyskinesia and are thought to increase the likelihood of its developing, although this remains to be proved. The former practice of using intermittent neuroleptic therapy, or "drug holidays," in hopes of determining whether early tardive dyskinesia has developed but is being masked by ongoing treatment is no longer recommended, given the clinical impression that drug holidays may be associated with an increased risk of tardive dyskinesia (Jeste et al. 1979).

Treatment. Once the diagnosis of tardive dyskinesia is established, the offending agent should be gradually withdrawn if the psychiatric state allows (Figure 25–2). Anticholinergic and other antiparkinsonian medications should be discontinued. In patients who must continue receiving neuroleptic therapy, the movements of tardive dyskinesia usually remain static but may gradually improve or even remit (Casey et al. 1986; Jeste et al. 1983; Koshino et al. 1991). During the drug-withdrawal phase, involuntary movements will often worsen transiently over weeks, and it may be necessary to add a benzodiazepine or phenobarbital to ease the patient's discomfort and anxiety. Between one-quarter and one-half of patients will improve within 1 year of drug withdrawal, but others may require up to 5 years (Klawans et al. 1984). Sometimes tardive dyskinesia may be permanent. The severity of the movements does not predict outcome after drug withdrawal. The chance of remission may be greater if DRBAs are discontinued soon after the onset of symptoms. Elderly patients have less chance for spontaneous remission once drugs are discontinued.

Patients requiring long-term neuroleptic treatment should be considered for conversion to a novel antipsychotic such as clozapine, olanzapine, quetiapine, or risperidone (Casey 1998; Factor and Friedman 1997; Peacock et al. 1996; Silberbauer 1998; Tollefson et al. 1997). The risk of developing tardive dyskinesia with other atypical agents such as risperidone and olanzapine is lower than

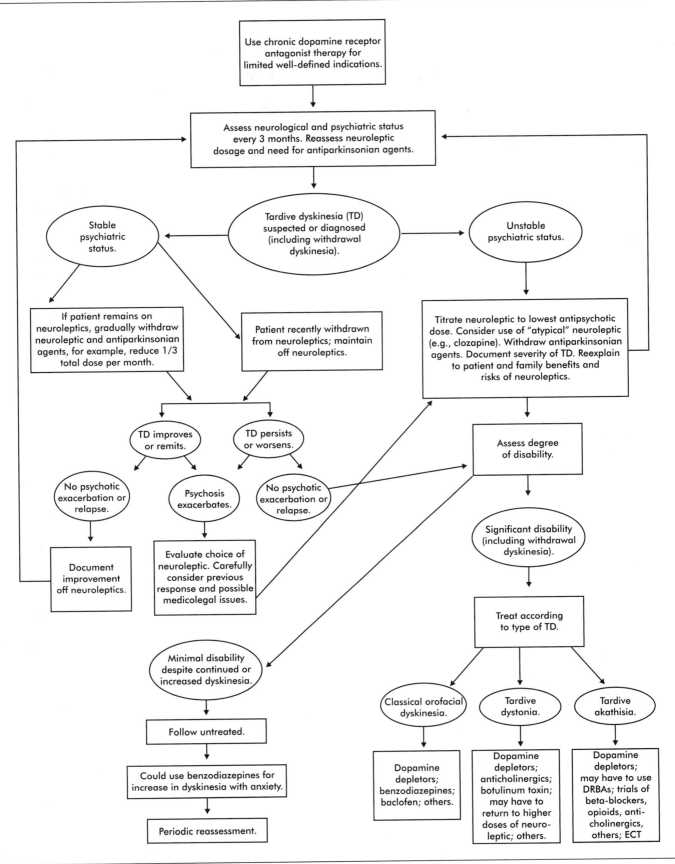

FIGURE 25–2.   Approach to the management of tardive dyskinesia. DRBAs = dopamine receptor blocking agents; ECT = electroconvulsive therapy.
Source.   Adapted from Weiner and Lang 1989.

with older agents but is not negligible.

For patients with disabling classic tardive dyskinesia, dopamine antagonists offer the most effective therapy for suppressing abnormal movements. Treatment with DRBAs, however, significantly decreases the chance of remission. Presynaptic depleting agents such as reserpine and tetrabenazine may be very effective in suppressing tardive dyskinesia, but these agents may not be well tolerated because of secondary parkinsonism, akathisia, and depression. Therapeutic trials of GABA agonists (clonazepam, valproic acid, diazepam, and baclofen), noradrenergic antagonists (propranolol and clonidine), and cholinergic agonists (lecithin and choline chloride) may also be helpful, but these drugs are rarely as effective as treatment with dopamine antagonists. Second-line agents include vitamin E, buspirone, and calcium channel blockers.

Whereas younger patients with tardive dystonia may benefit from anticholinergic agents such as trihexyphenidyl and ethopropazine, older patients are more likely to develop memory loss and confusion, and thus these drugs are relatively contraindicated in elderly patients. Dopamine antagonists—especially dopamine-depleting drugs, but sometimes even DRBAs—have the greatest likelihood of therapeutic success in disabling tardive dystonia, and some patients have been helped by anticholinergic therapy. Dopamine-depleting drugs alone or in combination with other agents are helpful in more than 50% of patients (Kang et al. 1986). Atypical neuroleptics have been effective in some cases (Yoshida et al. 1998). Botulinum toxin injection may be extremely effective in selected patients with prominent focal involvement of cranial and cervical musculature.

In contrast to acute akathisia, tardive akathisia usually does not respond to β-blockers, antiparkinsonian agents (e.g., anticholinergics and amantadine), or benzodiazepines. Management of this disabling tardive variant is difficult and usually involves dopamine-depleting agents or receptor blockers. Opioids may be helpful in some cases.

Dystonia

Dystonia is characterized by abnormal involuntary twisting movements that tend to be sustained and can result in abnormal postures. Some dystonic movements are slow and writhing and, when they occur distally, may be referred to as *athetosis*. Dystonic movements also may be quite rapid and resemble the lightning-like jerks of myoclonus. There may be superimposed rhythmic movements that are especially prominent when the patient tries to actively resist the dystonia (sometimes referred to as *dystonic tremor*). Dystonic movements frequently occur only during specific actions (e.g., writer's cramp). The movements are often increased by stress and improve with relaxation. Patients often use a variety of sensory tricks or antagonistic gestures to decrease the severity of the movements. Spontaneous remissions may occur in some forms of idiopathic dystonia, especially torticollis. Failure to recognize these unusual features has commonly resulted in dystonia being misdiagnosed as hysteria.

Dystonia is often classified by distribution, age at onset, and etiology. When a single body part is affected it is called *focal dystonia*. Involvement of two or more contiguous parts is called *segmental dystonia*, whereas it is called *multifocal dystonia* when distribution is not contiguous. The term *generalized dystonia* indicates involvement of one or both legs, the trunk, and some other body part. *Hemidystonia* is the involvement of one side of the body.

Dystonia beginning in adulthood typically affects the neck, face, or arm. Involuntary movements tend to remain limited to one or a small number of contiguous regions (e.g., face and neck). This is unlike dystonia of childhood onset, in which signs usually begin in the legs and frequently generalize.

With respect to etiology, dystonia may be idiopathic or secondary to other disorders (Table 25–6). The age at onset and the distribution of the dystonia are often helpful in determining the cause. For example, in adulthood, generalized involvement or onset in the legs suggests that the dystonia is secondary to some underlying condition, whereas isolated focal or segmental dystonia is usually idiopathic. Involvement of one side of the body (hemidystonia) is often associated with a contralateral basal ganglia lesion. The nature of the dystonic movements also may assist in diagnosis. For example, as mentioned above, early in the course of dystonia, patients may exhibit the abnormal movements only when performing specific actions. This feature is particularly common in idiopathic dystonia. When a patient demonstrates constant abnormal posturing of a limb early in the disease (i.e., dystonia at rest), this is suggestive of secondary cause.

Idiopathic Dystonia

Idiopathic torsion dystonia typically begins in childhood and often leads to severe disability by age 20. Occasional members of families with idiopathic torsion dystonia have onset delayed until later adulthood. The inheritance of idiopathic torsion dystonia seen in Ashkenazi Jewish and non-Jewish populations is autosomal dominant with variable penetrance. Linkage studies have localized the genes

TABLE 25–6. Causes of late-onset dystonia

Idiopathic dystonia

    Generalized dystonia (rare)

    Segmental/multifocal dystonia

    Focal dystonias

        Spasmodic torticollis

        Cranial dystonia

            Blepharospasm

            Oromandibular dystonia

            Spasmodic dysphonia

    Writer's cramp

Secondary dystonia

    Drugs: including neuroleptics, dopamine agonists, anticonvulsants, and antimalarial drugs

    Stroke: hemorrhage or infarction[a]

    Other focal lesions: vascular malformation, tumor, abscess, and demyelination

    Trauma: head injury or peripheral injury[a] and subdural hematoma

    Encephalitis

    Toxins: manganese, carbon monoxide poisoning, methanol, and carbon disulfide

    Paraneoplastic

    Hypoparathyroidism

    Central pontine myelinolysis

    Degenerative diseases

        Parkinson's disease

        Progressive supranuclear palsy

        Cortical-basal ganglionic degeneration

        Multiple system atrophy (Shy-Drager syndrome, olivopontocerebellar atrophy, and striatonigral degeneration)

Disorders that may simulate dystonia

    Psychogenic dystonia

    Orthopedic: atlantoaxial subluxation[b]

    Neurological: seizures, posterior fossa tumor, and oculomotor disturbance

[a]Dystonia is often delayed.
[b]Typically a disorder of childhood.

for idiopathic torsion dystonia in Jewish and some non-Jewish families to chromosome 9 (Ozelius et al. 1989). More recently, the DYT1 gene has been cloned and has been shown to encode an ATP-binding protein (Ozelius et al. 1997).

Focal dystonias. Idiopathic adult-onset focal dystonia is much more common than idiopathic torsion dystonia (Dauer et al. 1998). Marsden (1976) provided compelling arguments in favor of classifying these disorders as variants of idiopathic torsion dystonia. However, efforts to link focal dystonia to the DYT1 mutation have been unproductive to this point (Dauer et al. 1998).

The most common forms of idiopathic adult-onset focal dystonia are spasmodic torticollis (cervical dystonia), cranial dystonia, including blepharospasm and oromandibular dystonia, spasmodic dysphonia (laryngeal dystonia), and dystonia of the upper limb most often manifested as writer's cramp.

Spasmodic torticollis is the most common type of adult-onset focal dystonia (Dauer et al. 1998). It usually begins in the fourth or fifth decade and is more common in women. Involuntary activity of neck muscles causes abnormal postures and movements of the head. The movements may be sustained or may appear as twisting, shaking, or turning of the head. Commonly the head is turned to one side (torticollis) or is tilted with the ear toward the shoulder (laterocollis). Less often there is excessive head flexion (anterocollis) or extension (retrocollis). The continuous muscle contraction may lead to muscle hypertrophy, frequently evident in the sternocleidomastoid muscle, and there may be associated shoulder elevation. Neck discomfort and pain are common (Chan et al. 1991). Although many patients initially report an involuntary pulling of the head in one direction, some are unaware of the abnormal head posture until a family member draws it to their attention. Up to 50% of patients will have additional dystonic features, usually in the face or arm. Associated postural tremor of the hands is common (Dauer et al. 1998).

Many patients use sensory tricks (*geste antagoniste*) to decrease the severity of the dystonic movements. Resting the head against a high-back chair, holding the back of the neck, or lightly touching the cheek may return the head to the normal position. Activities such as walking, writing, and combing the hair often aggravate the symptoms.

Symptoms usually increase during the first 5 years. Partial or full remission occurs in up to one-fifth of patients, but this is almost always transient (A. Friedman and Fahn 1986; Jahanshahi et al. 1990). Symptoms may be mild, but most patients experience some degree of disability related to pain, abnormal head posture, and embarrassment. Patients with long-standing symptoms occasionally develop cervical root or cord compression. This complication may be more likely in elderly patients, who have a higher incidence of underlying cervical spondylosis.

Focal or segmental dystonia involving cranial muscles is called *cranial dystonia*. The usual age at onset is the sixth decade, and women are more commonly affected than are men. The most common component of cranial dystonia is blepharospasm, characterized by involuntary, forced eye closure caused by excessive contraction of the orbicularis oculi muscles (Grandas et al. 1988). The disorder usually begins with an increase in blink rate, which gradually progresses to more forceful closure of both eyelids. Aggravating factors include talking, watching television, reading, and exposure to bright lights. Tricks such as rubbing or lightly touching the eye, yawning or opening the mouth, or extending the neck may interrupt the eyelid closure. Blepharospasm may eventually result in functional blindness despite normal visual acuity.

Another component of cranial dystonia is oromandibular dystonia, featuring involuntary spasms of lower cranial muscles that cause mouth opening, jaw clenching, platysma contraction, tongue muscle contractions and protrusion, and contractions of the soft palate. There may be associated grunting, throat clearing, and inspiratory noises. This type of dystonia is usually seen in combination with blepharospasm as Meige's syndrome, or as spasmodic dysphonia (see below), but it may occur in isolation (Tolosa and Marti 1988). In contrast to classic tardive dyskinesia (for which oromandibular dystonia is commonly mistaken), the movements of oromandibular dystonia are typically brought out or aggravated by use of the involved muscles, such as in talking or chewing (Table 25–3). Injuries of the tongue, lips, and teeth are common. Touching the finger to the lips or teeth may lessen the spasms.

Involvement of laryngeal muscles is known as *spasmodic dysphonia*. Most patients have a voice disturbance due to hyperadduction of the vocal cords (adductor spasmodic dysphonia) (Blitzer et al. 1988). The voice is strained, tight, hoarse, and often tremulous. The less common hyperabduction variety (abductor spasmodic dysphonia) results in breathy phonation and sudden drops in pitch.

Writer's cramp is the most common form of task-specific focal limb dystonia (P. D. Thompson 1993). Typically, the fingers and wrist flex excessively, causing the hand to tightly grasp the pen and press unnecessarily hard on the paper. Alternatively, the fingers may involuntarily extend or splay, making it difficult to hold the pen. Tremor or myoclonic jerks also may occur while writing. Initially, only writing may be affected (simple writer's cramp). Later, other manual tasks also may be impaired (dystonic writer's cramp). There are a wide variety of other "occupational palsies" or task-specific dystonias (Rosenbaum and Jankovic 1988). As in the case of writer's cramp, these typically begin in mid-adult life and subsequently persist or progress. Like all other forms of dystonia, these disorders are commonly misdiagnosed as being due to anxiety or "nerves." Both the chronic disability caused by the focal dystonia and the frequent mislabeling as a psychological disorder often result in emotional upset and reactive depression.

Pathophysiology.   Little is known of the etiology or pathophysiology of idiopathic dystonia. Electrophysiological studies suggest disturbances of inhibitory mechanisms in the brainstem and spinal cord (Hallett 1998; Marsden and Quinn 1990). These changes may be secondary to aberrant suprasegmental influences, for example, originating from the basal ganglia. Routine histopathology studies have failed to demonstrate consistent abnormalities. Study of secondary dystonias may provide further clues to the origin and nature of the abnormalities in idiopathic dystonia.

Secondary Dystonia

Drug-induced dystonia.   Levodopa-induced dystonia in Parkinson's disease is probably the most common form of drug-induced dystonia. Other important agents that can cause dystonia include DRBAs and, less commonly, anticonvulsants, selective serotonin reuptake inhibitors, antimalarial agents, and other miscellaneous drugs (Lang 1992b; Leo 1996). With respect to neuroleptics (antipsychotics and antiemetics such as metoclopramide), these drugs may cause short-lived dystonia very early in their course (acute dystonic reactions) or prolonged dystonia usually after long-term use (tardive dystonia). Unlike tardive dystonia, which has no age preference, and tardive dyskinesia and drug-induced parkinsonism, which are more common in elderly patients, neuroleptic-induced acute dystonia is more common in younger patients and indeed rarely develops in elderly patients. It may be more common in men and is more likely to occur with higher-potency neuroleptics. Although it is rare, acute dystonia has been reported with clozapine (Kastrup et al. 1994; Thomas et al. 1994). Dystonic reactions usually develop within the first 5 days of starting a neuroleptic, most often occurring on day 2 (Casey 1992). Patients may develop a sensation of thickness of the tongue, involuntary opening or closing of the mouth, facial grimacing, tongue protrusion, tightness in the throat, torticollis, retrocollis, oculogyric crisis (rolling of the eyes upward or off to the side), or laryngopharyngeal spasms. Limb or truncal spasm may result in bizarre posturing.

The pathophysiology of acute dystonia may involve an idiosyncratic response to D_2 receptor antagonists, although this is controversial (Casey 1994). Treatment consists of parenteral administration of anticholinergic or antihistaminic agents followed by oral anticholinergics for 1–2 days.

Miscellaneous secondary dystonias.

In childhood a wide variety of storage diseases and neurometabolic disorders can cause dystonia. All children presenting with dystonia require a trial of levodopa to exclude the diagnosis of dopa-responsive dystonia. This disorder is caused in many instances by mutations in the gene encoding GTP cyclohydrolase, which is necessary for synthesis of tetrahydrobiopterin, a cofactor for tyrosine hydroxylase (Ichinose et al. 1994; Tamaru et al. 1998). Adults presenting with this disorder typically demonstrate features of Parkinson's disease rather than dystonia. Wilson's disease is an extremely important consideration; however, it rarely if ever presents de novo after age 45.

Dystonia can be seen after various acute brain insults such as stroke (Lee and Marsden 1994; Marsden et al. 1985) or head trauma (Krauss et al. 1996; Lee et al. 1994). The dystonia secondary to stroke usually occurs weeks or even years after the initial insult. The involuntary movements often develop as hemiparesis resolves. Lesions resulting in hemidystonia occur most often in the contralateral putamen, thalamus, caudate nucleus, and globus pallidus. Occasionally, blepharospasm has been associated with lesions in the brainstem, thalamus, or basal ganglia (Jankovic 1986).

Many of the secondary dystonias due to environmental causes, such as encephalitis and exposure to toxins, have stabilization of symptoms once the destructive process is completed. However, for reasons that are not clearly known, the symptoms of a static encephalopathy, including dystonia, choreoathetosis, myoclonus, and even pyramidal tract deficits, may progress in later adult life (Scott and Jankovic 1996).

There is increasing evidence that peripheral trauma may be associated with various forms of dystonia (Fletcher et al. 1991; Jankovic 1994). Post-traumatic dystonia tends to have a rapid onset after the inciting injury. In some instances, there may be a genetic predisposition to idiopathic dystonia, although to date this has not been proved. Sometimes a seemingly inconsequential injury can result in severe, fixed dystonic postures with features of reflex sympathetic dystrophy.

Dystonia is common to a variety of neurodegenerative diseases. It is common in Parkinson's disease both as a manifestation of the disorder and as a complication of therapy with dopamine agonists (e.g., levodopa, bromocriptine, pergolide, and newer agents such as pramipexole and ropinirole). Patients often develop transient dystonia as their medications are "wearing off," in the fully developed "off" period, on awakening in the morning, or as a peak-of-dose effect (Poewe et al. 1988). Patients with progressive supranuclear palsy usually have pronounced neck and trunk rigidity, sometimes with nuchal extension, which has been referred to as *axial dystonia*. There may be associated dystonic posturing of the limbs, sometimes in a hemidystonic pattern (Barclay and Lang 1997). Cortical-basal ganglionic degeneration causes an akinetic-rigid syndrome with apraxia, cortical sensory deficit, action tremor, myoclonus, and frequent limb dystonia (Rinne et al. 1994). Multiple system atrophy, which includes striatonigral degeneration, Shy-Drager syndrome, and olivopontocerebellar atrophy, may also manifest various forms of dystonia, including excessive neck flexion (or anterocollis) (Wenning et al. 1994). An occasional feature of multiple system atrophy is laryngeal stridor, possibly secondary to vocal cord paralysis (Isozaki et al. 1996) or even laryngeal dystonia (Marion et al. 1992). Dystonia may be a prominent feature of Machado-Joseph disease, a dominant spinocerebellar ataxia, which, like Huntington's disease, is associated with expansion of unstable CAG repeats (Schols et al. 1996).

Psychogenic dystonia is uncommon, but when it does occur it can be severe enough to cause permanent contractures. Clinical clues that suggest psychogenic dystonia include "giving way" weakness, nondermatomal sensory loss, fixed postures, absence of sensory tricks, multiple somatizations, and especially inconsistency and incongruity of the abnormal movements (Fahn and Williams 1988; Lang 1995).

Treatment

Dystonia has traditionally been one of the most difficult movement disorders to manage. Drug therapy is often unrewarding. The most effective drugs have a high incidence of side effects, especially in elderly patients. High doses of anticholinergic drugs (e.g., trihexyphenidyl, ethopropazine, and benztropine) may be at least partially effective in up to 50% of patients. Adults frequently experience intolerable side effects secondary to both peripheral and central anticholinergic effects. Peripheral side effects such as blurred vision and constipation may be lessened by the use of concomitant pilocarpine eye drops and oral bethanechol or pyridostigmine. However, central side effects including memory loss and confusion remain a major limiting factor, especially in older patients. Tricyclic antidepressants, benzodiazepines, carbamazepine, and baclofen may also be helpful. Dopamine antagonists, particularly clozapine, may be of some benefit. Tetrabenazine may also be useful, particularly in tardive dystonia.

Botulinum toxin injection has revolutionized the therapy of focal dystonia, particularly blepharospasm, spasmodic torticollis, spasmodic dysphonia, and oromandibular dystonia (Jankovic and Brin 1991). The toxin acts presynaptically at nerve terminals to decrease the amount of acetylcholine released into the neuromuscular junction. Chemical denervation of the muscle results in weakness and wasting. The duration of benefit is usually 3–4 months. Side effects are mainly related to excessive weakness of injected muscles and to spread of the toxin locally to other areas (e.g., causing dysphagia in patients treated for cervical dystonia).

Myoclonus

Myoclonus refers to sudden, brief, shock-like involuntary movements that are usually caused by active muscle contraction (positive myoclonus) but can also be caused by inhibition of ongoing muscle activity (negative myoclonus, including asterixis) (Caviness 1996). Myoclonus may be focal, multifocal, segmental (involving two or more contiguous regions), or generalized. There is a wide clinical spectrum of myoclonic movements (Obeso et al. 1993). They may be single, rare jerks or constant repetitive contractions. The amplitude may vary from a mild twitch that fails to move a joint to a gross jerk that moves the entire body. The pattern is usually irregular but sometimes may be rhythmic, giving a superficial appearance of tremor. Myoclonus may occur spontaneously at rest or on attempting movement (action myoclonus). Myoclonus is frequently triggered (stimulus sensitive) by a variety of stimuli such as sudden noise, light, visual threat, soft touch, pinprick, or muscle stretch.

Myoclonus can originate from a variety of locations in the central nervous system (Shibasaki 1995). Electrophysiological studies, including back-average recording of electroencephalographic (EEG) potentials, evoked potentials, long-latency reflex recordings, and multichannel electromyographic (EMG) assessment, are capable of separating myoclonus of cortical and subcortical (reticular) origin. Less often, myoclonus originates at a segmental (brainstem or spinal) level, in which case the movements are often rhythmical. Rarely, myoclonic movements are caused by lesions in the peripheral nervous system. Clinically, it is sometimes difficult to distinguish myoclonus from tics. Unlike tics, myoclonus cannot be willfully controlled nor is it associated with a conscious urge to move or with relief once the movement has been completed. Myoclonic movements are usually of shorter duration and less patterned than tics and are typically increased rather than diminished when the patient performs a motor act.

Causes of myoclonus in the elderly may include idio-

pathic disorders such as physiological myoclonus, nocturnal myoclonus, essential myoclonus, and startle syndromes. More commonly, however, myoclonus in elderly patients is secondary to metabolic disorders, infections, drug administration, hypoxia, and degenerative diseases (Table 25–7). In earlier life, myoclonus is a common feature of idiopathic seizure disorders (epileptic myoclonus), and it may be a feature of progressive encephalopathies associated with seizures such as Lafora's disease (i.e., progressive myoclonic epilepsies).

Idiopathic Myoclonus

Physiological myoclonus.   Physiological myoclonus occurs in healthy individuals and is often worsened by fatigue or stress. Hiccups and the jerking that most people experience on falling asleep (sleep starts or hypnic jerks) are other forms of myoclonus seen in healthy individuals.

Nocturnal myoclonus.   Periodic movements in sleep are stereotyped, repetitive movements of the legs that appear during stages 1 and 2 of sleep (Silber 1997; Wetter and Pollmacher 1997). Typically, there is myoclonic jerking of one or both legs followed by tonic flexion at the knee and hip, dorsiflexion at the ankle, and extension of the big toe. The duration of the movements may be as long as 5 seconds, implying that they are not truly myoclonic in nature; they occur at regular intervals, usually every 20–40 seconds. The prevalence of periodic movements in sleep appears to increase with age, being present in 29% of patients over age 50 (Lugaresi 1986).

Restless legs syndrome consists of nighttime unpleasant paresthesia and restlessness of the legs. These symptoms are relieved or lessened by activity, and patients may demonstrate a variety of secondary purposeful movements such as stretching, rubbing the legs, wiggling the ankles, or arising and pacing. Some patients also have myoclonic or dystonic involuntary movements in the legs while awake, and periodic movements in sleep are almost universal (Walters and Hening 1987). The symptoms interfere with sleep and, in fact, restless legs syndrome is the fourth leading cause of insomnia after psychiatric disorders, drug abuse, and sleep apneas (Coleman 1982). Restless legs syndrome can develop at any age, but symptoms may become more severe in old age. Most cases are idiopathic, although strong associations exist with iron deficiency anemia, rheumatoid arthritis, and uremia. When no cause is apparent, restless legs syndrome may be inherited as an autosomal dominant trait. Neuroleptic treatment can exacerbate the symptoms of restless legs syndrome. Peripheral neuropathies may cause similar symptoms. Both periodic

TABLE 25–7. Causes of myoclonus in elderly patients

Physiological myoclonus
- Hiccup
- Sleep starts
- Exercise induced
- Anxiety induced

Essential myoclonus

Secondary myoclonus
- Metabolic causes
  - Hepatic failure
  - Renal failure
  - Dialysis syndrome
  - Hyponatremia
  - Hypoglycemia
  - Nonketotic hyperglycemia
- Viral encephalopathies
  - Herpes simplex encephalitis
  - Arbovirus encephalitis
  - Encephalitis lethargica
  - Postinfectious encephalomyelitis
- Drugs and toxins
  - Bismuth
  - Heavy metal poisons
  - Methyl bromide, DDT
  - Drugs: tricyclic antidepressants, levodopa, monoamine oxidase inhibitors, antibiotics, and lithium
- Physical encephalopathies
  - Postanoxic (Lance-Adams syndrome)
  - Posttraumatic
  - Heat stroke
  - Electric shock
  - Decompression injury
- Dementing and degenerative diseases
  - Creutzfeldt-Jakob disease
  - Alzheimer's disease
  - Cortical-basal ganglionic degeneration
  - Parkinson's disease
  - Huntington's disease
  - Multiple system atrophy
  - Pallidal degenerations
- Focal central nervous system damage
  - Poststroke
  - Olivodentate lesions (palatal myoclonus)
  - Spinal cord lesions (segmental/spinal myoclonus)
  - Tumor
  - Trauma
  - Following thalamotomy (often unilateral asterixis)

Source. Adapted from Fahn et al. 1986.

movements in sleep and restless legs syndrome respond to benzodiazepines, including clonazepam and nitrazepam; dopamine agonists such as levodopa, pergolide, and pramipexole; or μ-receptor opiate agonists such as codeine or propoxyphene (Kaplan et al. 1993; Winkelmann et al. 1998).

Essential myoclonus. Essential myoclonus is an idiopathic disorder that is often inherited in an autosomal dominant pattern (Quinn 1996). Symptoms typically begin in childhood or early adult years and persist with a variable course over the remainder of the patient's life. Disability may be pronounced. Some patients also demonstrate a postural tremor, and others have features of focal or segmental dystonia. Whether these features are all manifestations of the same genotype or whether "essential myoclonus" represents several different genetic diseases remains to be determined (Bressman and Fahn 1986). Some patients experience a pronounced beneficial response with alcohol, and this has led to problematic alcohol abuse (Quinn 1996).

Startle syndromes. The startle syndromes represent exaggerations of the normal human alerting reaction (startle). There is excessive motor response to unexpected auditory or visual stimuli. Typically, this consists of a blink, contortion of the face, and flexion of the neck, trunk, and arms. Sometimes the condition is inherited in autosomal dominant fashion (hyperexplexia) and may be associated with a mutation in the α_1-glycine receptor subunit (Shiang et al. 1993), but in rare cases it may result from acquired brain stem pathology such as anoxia, hemorrhage, or sarcoidosis (Brown et al. 1991b). Clonazepam is currently the treatment of choice.

Secondary Myoclonus

Myoclonus secondary to metabolic disturbances. Myoclonus may result from a wide range of metabolic disturbances, including severe hepatic failure, hyponatremia, hypoglycemia, and nonketotic hyperglycemia. The myoclonus commonly seen in uremia involves the face and upper extremities and is often aggravated by auditory or tactile stimuli. A significant number of patients with metabolic derangements will demonstrate asterixis. These brief lapses in postural tone (negative myoclonus) can be demonstrated by attempting to hold the wrist actively extended or the foot dorsiflexed. Toxic levels of anticonvulsants, especially phenytoin, may cause asterixis as well as typical myoclonus. Unilateral asterixis may be caused by focal central nervous system lesions, which often involve the thalamus (Young and Shahani 1986).

Myoclonus secondary to infections or tumors. Multifocal or generalized myoclonus may be seen in patients with systemic infections, acute encephalitides, or postinfectious encephalomyelitis. Myoclonus may be accompanied by opsoclonus (dancing eye movements) as a paraneoplastic syndrome. In adults, this may accompany gynecological tumors and has been associated with the Ri antineuronal antibody (Dropcho 1998).

Myoclonus secondary to drug administration. A wide variety of medications may cause myoclonus. Most often this occurs in the context of an acute toxic encephalopathy. For example, antibiotics, especially the penicillins and cephalosporins, can cause isolated myoclonus or more severe toxic encephalopathy with seizures, especially if given to patients with compromised renal function. A number of other drugs may cause myoclonus even in the absence of other features of toxicity; these include tricyclic antidepressants, levodopa, dopamine agonists, monoamine oxidase inhibitors, and lithium. In psychiatric practice, myoclonus occurs in up to 40% of patients taking tricyclic antidepressants (Garvey and Tollefson 1987).

Postanoxic myoclonus. Postanoxic myoclonus usually results from cardiac arrest, respiratory failure, or an anesthetic accident. Pronounced myoclonus in a patient with one of these conditions usually indicates a severe anoxic encephalopathy with poor prognosis. A unique syndrome of action myoclonus (Lance-Adams syndrome) occurs in a minority of patients surviving severe cerebral anoxia. As the patient awakens from coma, action-induced myoclonic jerks emerge, as do lapses in posture (negative myoclonus), which frequently result in falling. In more severely affected individuals, myoclonus interferes with all voluntary movement, including speech and swallowing. Additional cognitive and behavioral disturbances may accompany the myoclonus depending on the extent of anoxic cerebral damage.

The pathophysiology of postanoxic action myoclonus is strongly associated with dysfunction of brainstem serotonin pathways. The major metabolite of serotonin, 5-hydroxyindoleacetic acid, is typically reduced in the cerebrospinal fluid of these patients. Agents that increase serotonin activity, such as the serotonin precursor L-5-hydroxytryptophan (L5HTP) given with carbidopa are often markedly effective in reducing myoclonus. However, L-5HTP may cause a variety of side effects and is not readily available. For these reasons, the treatments of choice are valproic acid and/or clonazepam, agents that can also result in a striking reduction in the severity of the myoclonus.

Myoclonus related to dementing and neurodegenerative diseases. Myoclonus is a prominent feature of Creutzfeldt-Jakob disease (see Chapter 23 in this volume), a disorder that causes subacute onset of dementia and personality change. Myoclonus may begin in the face or limbs, but it later becomes more generalized as the disease progresses. Although present at rest, the myoclonus can often be triggered by loud noise. The EEG often shows periodic sharp discharges, occurring approximately once per second. The myoclonic jerks are sometimes time locked to these abnormal EEG discharges.

Myoclonus is present in 10% or more of patients with Alzheimer's disease. It can occur at any time in the course of the illness but is often a late manifestation (Hauser et al. 1986). Focal, stimulus-sensitive myoclonus is a common feature of cortical-basal ganglionic degeneration and multiple system atrophy, including striatonigral degeneration, Shy-Drager syndrome, and olivopontocerebellar degeneration. In Parkinson's disease, myoclonus rarely occurs as an early feature. Most often it develops as a late-stage side effect of levodopa, especially in patients with psychiatric complications and concomitant dementia.

Segmental Myoclonus

Palatal myoclonus is characterized by unilateral or bilateral 1.5- to 3-Hz rhythmic (thus the more appropriate designation as a "tremor") movements of the soft palate (Deuschl et al. 1994). Synchronous movements of adjacent muscles of the face and neck frequently accompany the palatal activity. In most patients, a definitive cause can be identified, and these patients are said to have symptomatic palatal tremor. The most common cause of symptomatic palatal tremor is stroke affecting the brainstem and cerebellum (Deuschl et al. 1990). The palatal tremor usually develops after a delay of up to 10 months after the initial stroke and persists as a permanent sequela.

Patients do not typically complain of the involuntary palatal movements, but rather they are more bothered by limb, gait, and oculomotor disturbances from the underlying infarction. MRI often shows a hyperintense signal in the inferior olive (Pierot et al. 1992). Pathological examination shows vacuolar hypertrophic transsynaptic degeneration of the inferior olive with a lesion involving the connection between the cerebellar dentate nucleus (via the superior cerebellar peduncle) and the central tegmental tract to the contralateral inferior olive. When the lesion is unilateral, the olivary hypertrophy is on the side opposite the myoclonus.

One-quarter of patients with palatal tremor (myoclonus) have no underlying cause identified (Deuschl et al.

1990). These patients are considered to have essential palatal tremor, which typically occurs in young adulthood and presents with a clicking sound in the ear that can often also be heard by the examiner. The cause of the ear click is probably the sudden opening and closing of the eustachian tube as a result of intermittent contraction of the tensor veli palatini muscle.

Palatal myoclonus is typically resistant to pharmacological therapy, although occasional patients will respond to drugs such as clonazepam or anticholinergics. Bothersome ear click may be reduced by focal injections of botulinum toxin into the tensor veli palatini muscle (Deuschl et al. 1991).

Spinal myoclonus is also usually slow and rhythmic, involving the muscles of several spinal segments and resulting in movements of one or more limbs and/or trunk. Lesions in the spinal cord that may give rise to myoclonus include infection, demyelination, tumor, degenerative disease, and cervical myelopathy (Jankovic and Pardo 1986). Another rare form of spinal myoclonus is thought to originate in slowly conducting propriospinal pathways. Propriospinal myoclonus includes spontaneous and stimulus-sensitive nonrhythmic axial jerks causing symmetric flexion of the neck, trunk, hips, and knees (Brown et al. 1991a).

Hemifacial Spasm

Hemifacial spasm typically begins in adulthood and is more common in women. It begins as brief twitches around the eye that gradually increase in severity and may evolve to sustained contractions lasting many seconds to minutes. The movements may remain isolated to the orbicularis oculi or may spread to other ipsilateral facial muscles. The movements cannot be voluntarily suppressed and tend to persist in sleep. In most instances it is thought that hemifacial spasm is caused by mechanical compression of the facial nerve at the nerve root exit zone by an aberrant blood vessel (less commonly by a tumor, aneurysm, or other compressive lesion). Although surgical decompression of the facial nerve can be curative (Jannetta et al. 1977), botulinum toxin injection is extremely effective in reducing the involuntary movements and is the treatment of choice (Jankovic and Brin 1991).

▮ Tics

Tics are intermittent, repetitive, stereotyped abnormal movements (motor tics) or sounds (vocal tics) that vary in intensity and are repeated at irregular intervals. Tics encompass an extremely broad range of movements and sounds. Although most tics are abrupt and brief, some tics may be slower in onset and prolonged (dystonic tics). Motor and vocal tics may be further classified as simple or complex. Simple motor tics involve one group of muscles and include eye blinking, shoulder shrugging, or facial grimacing. Complex motor tics are coordinated sequences of movement such as touching, hitting, jumping, or copropraxia (obscene gestures). Simple vocal tics are inarticulate noises or sounds, including throat clearing, sniffing, and grunting. Complex phonic tics involve saying words and include echolalia (repetition of others), palilalia (repetition of self), and coprolalia (swearing). Patients usually experience an inner urge to perform the movement that is temporarily relieved by the execution of the movement. More than most other movement disorders, tics can be suppressed for prolonged periods of time and are decreased by distraction or concentration on complex mental or motor tasks.

Tics are most commonly idiopathic but may result from a variety of other conditions such as encephalitis, head injury, stroke, and drug administration (Table 25–8). Tics usually begin in childhood either as a simple transient motor tic or as part of the spectrum of manifestations of Gilles de la Tourette syndrome (Tourette syndrome). Many patients with Tourette syndrome remit in adolescence, but for the remainder the syndrome is a lifelong disorder. Tourette syndrome is probably inherited in an autosomal dominant pattern, with incomplete penetrance and sex-related expression. A close association exists with obsessive-compulsive disorder; indeed, behavioral mani-

TABLE 25–8. **Causes of tics in elderly patients**

Idiopathic

  Persistent childhood-onset tic disorder

  Simple tic

    Multiple motor tics

    Multiple motor and vocal tics (Tourette syndrome)

  Adult-onset tic disorder

Secondary

  Postencephalitic

  Head injury

  Carbon monoxide poisoning

  Poststroke

  Drugs: stimulants, levodopa, neuroleptics ("tardive Tourette"), carbamazepine, phenytoin, and phenobarbital

  Mental retardation syndromes: including chromosomal abnormalities

  Postrheumatic chorea (probably not seen in the elderly)

festations in the absence of motor tics may be a variant.

Unfortunately, there is limited information regarding the course of Tourette syndrome as patients reach the geriatric age period. Interestingly, the first well-described patient with Tourette syndrome reported by Itard in 1825 (included in Gilles de la Tourette's first paper) was 85 years old (Bruun 1988). The results of studies including elderly patients with Tourette syndrome indicate that most patients improve with maturity (except for occasional worsening in the fourth decade) and that when symptoms persist beyond age 50 they are typically mild (Bruun 1988; Burd et al. 1986). On the other hand, we have seen one patient with lifelong multiple simple motor tics who at the age of 72 developed the complex vocal tic of shouting the names of friends and 2 years later developed echolalia and coprolalia (Lang et al. 1983). Additional studies are required to understand the effects of aging on the course of tics. Further complicating this issue is the rare occurrence of idiopathic adult-onset tics. Epidemiological and clinical aspects of tics beginning in mid to late adult life have yet to be formally studied. The relationship between adult-onset tics and the more common childhood-onset tics, including Tourette syndrome, is unknown at present.

In the treatment of tics, the goal should be satisfactory alleviation rather than complete elimination of motor manifestations. In mild cases, treatment with clonidine may suffice. Neuroleptics (most commonly haloperidol) may then be tried if this is unsuccessful. Other medications that have been reported in tic treatment include tetrabenazine and clonazepam. Botulinum toxin injection may be helpful in cases of painful dystonic tics. Compulsive symptoms that accompany tics may be treated with serotonin selective reuptake inhibitors such as fluoxetine.

◼ Summary

The hyperkinetic movement disorders include tremor, chorea, dystonia, myoclonus, and tics. A wide variety of these dyskinesias begin in late life or have a course affected in some manner by the aging process. The idiopathic focal dystonias, including spasmodic torticollis, cranial dystonia, and writer's cramp, begin in mid to late life and can result in significant disability. Neurodegenerative disorders such as multiple system atrophy, progressive supranuclear palsy, cortical basal ganglionic degeneration, Alzheimer's disease, and Creutzfeldt-Jakob disease all may be associated with variable degrees of dystonia, myoclonus, or tremor. Patients with Parkinson's disease who have been receiving long-term levodopa therapy often develop prominent choreiform and dystonic movements.

Aging is associated with an increased risk of cerebrovascular disease, which can sometimes result in "cerebellar outflow tremor," chorea (including hemiballismus), delayed dystonia, palatal myoclonus, and occasionally asterixis. Elderly patients have a greater chance of developing tardive dyskinesia when exposed to neuroleptics and appear to have less potential for improvement after discontinuation of these drugs than do younger patients. The incidence of periodic movements in sleep and "spontaneous orofacial dyskinesia" also increases with advancing age. Some disorders, such as essential tremor, may worsen with age. Conversely, there are examples in which advanced age appears to be an attenuating factor in the expression of hyperkinetic disorders. The incidence of neuroleptic-induced acute dystonic reactions decreases with age, and these reactions rarely occur in the elderly. Tics appear to lessen in severity after the third decade.

Treatment of hyperkinetic movements in older patients is often limited by medical contraindications or poor drug tolerance. An informed trial-and-error sequential use of several different medications may be necessary in disabled patients. Botulinum toxin has revolutionized the treatment of dystonia. Neuroleptics might be used more readily in elderly patients for the management of choreiform disorders, as there is less concern about long-term sequelae such as tardive dyskinesia; however, this possibility should remain a concern, as should the greater risk of disabling drug-induced parkinsonism.

In summary, an elderly patient with a movement disorder may pose a diagnostic and therapeutic challenge for the clinician. The important first step is the classification of the dyskinesia, which then focuses the diagnostic considerations and guides the approach to treatment.

◼ References

Albin RL, Young AB, Penney JB: The functional anatomy of basal ganglia disorders. Trends Neurosci 12:366–375, 1989

Alcock NS: A note on the pathology of senile chorea (non-hereditary). Brain 59:376–387, 1936

Asherson RA, Derksen RH, Harris EN, et al: Chorea in systemic lupus erythematosus and "lupus-like" disease: association with antiphospholipid antibodies. Semin Arthritis Rheum 16:253–259, 1987

Baldessarini RJ, Frankenburg FR: Clozapine. A novel antipsychotic agent. N Engl J Med 324:746–754, 1991

Barclay CL, Lang AE: Dystonia in progressive supranuclear palsy. J Neurol Neurosurg Psychiatry 62:352–356, 1997

Benabid AL, Pollak P, Gao D, et al: Chronic electrical stimulation of the ventralis intermedius nucleus of the thalamus as a treatment of movement disorders. J Neurosurg 84: 203–214, 1996

Blitzer A, Brin MF, Fahn S, et al: Clinical and laboratory characteristics of focal laryngeal dystonia: study of 110 cases. Laryngoscope 98:636–640, 1988

Bressman S, Fahn S: Essential myoclonus, in Myoclonus (Advances in Neurology Series, Vol 43). Edited by Fahn S, Marsden CD, Van Woert M. New York, Raven, 1986, pp 287–294

Britton JW, Uitti RJ, Ahlskog JE, et al: Hereditary late-onset chorea without significant dementia: genetic evidence for substantial phenotypic variation in Huntington's disease. Neurology 45:443–447, 1995

Britton TC, Thompson PD, van der Kamp W, et al: Primary orthostatic tremor: further observations in six cases. J Neurol 239:209–217, 1992

Brouwers P, Cox C, Martin A, et al: Differential perceptual-spatial impairment in Huntington's and Alzheimer's dementias. Arch Neurol 41:1073–1076, 1984

Brown P, Thompson PD, Rothwell JC, et al: Axial myoclonus of propriospinal origin. Brain 114:197–214, 1991a

Brown P, Rothwell JC, Thompson PD, et al: The hyperekplexias and their relationship to the normal startle reflex. Brain 114:1903–1928, 1991b

Bruun RD: The natural history of Tourette's syndrome, in Tourette's Syndrome and Tic Disorders. Edited by Cohen DJ, Bruun RD, Leckman JF. New York, Wiley, 1988, pp 21–40

Bruyn GW, Padberg G: Chorea and polycythaemia. Eur Neurol 23:26–33, 1984

Burd L, Kerbeshian J, Wikenheiser M, et al: Prevalence of Gilles de la Tourette's syndrome in North Dakota adults. Am J Psychiatry 143:787–788, 1986

Busenbark K, Pahwa R, Hubble J, et al: Double-blind controlled study of methazolamide in the treatment of essential tremor. Neurology 43:1045–1047, 1993

Caine ED, Hunt RD, Weingartner H, et al: Huntington's dementia. Clinical and neuropsychological features. Arch Gen Psychiatry 35:377–384, 1978

Cardoso F, Jankovic J: Dystonia and dyskinesia. Psychiatr Clin North Am 20:821–838, 1997

Casey DE: Neuroleptic-induced acute dystonia, in Drug-Induced Movement Disorders. Edited by Lang AE, Weiner WJ. Mount Kisco, NY, Futura, 1992, pp 21–40

Casey DE: Motor and mental aspects of acute extrapyramidal syndromes. Acta Psychiatr Scand Suppl 380:14–20, 1994

Casey DE: Effects of clozapine therapy in schizophrenic individuals at risk for tardive dyskinesia. J Clin Psychiatry 59 (suppl 3):31–37, 1998

Casey DE, Povlsen UJ, Meidahl B, et al: Neuroleptic-induced tardive dyskinesia and parkinsonism: changes during several years of continuing treatment. Psychopharmacol Bull 22:250–253, 1986

Caviness JN: Myoclonus. Mayo Clin Proc 71:679–688, 1996

Cervera R, Asherson RA, Font J, et al: Chorea in the antiphospholipid syndrome. Clinical, radiologic, and immunologic characteristics of 50 patients from our clinics and the recent literature. Medicine 76:203–212, 1997

Chan J, Brin MF, Fahn S: Idiopathic cervical dystonia: clinical characteristics. Mov Disord 6:119–126, 1991

Coleman RM: Periodic movements in sleep (nocturnal myoclonus) and restless legs syndrome, in Sleeping and Waking Disorders: Indications and Techniques. Edited by Guilleminault C. Palo Alto, CA, Addison-Wesley, 1982, pp 265–295

Como PG, Rubin AJ, O'Brien CF, et al: A controlled trial of fluoxetine in nondepressed patients with Huntington's disease. Mov Disord 12:397–401, 1997

Cummings JL: Frontal-subcortical circuits and human behavior. Arch Neurol 50:873–880, 1993

Cummings JL: Behavioral and psychiatric symptoms associated with Huntington's disease. Adv Neurol 65:179–186, 1995

Cummings JL, Cunningham K: Obsessive-compulsive disorder in Huntington's disease. Biol Psychiatry 31:263–270, 1992

Dauer WT, Burke RE, Greene P, et al: Current concepts on the clinical features, aetiology and management of idiopathic cervical dystonia. Brain 121:547–560, 1998

Deuschl G, Mischke G, Schenck E, et al: Symptomatic and essential rhythmic palatal myoclonus. Brain 113:1645–1672, 1990

Deuschl G, Lohle E, Heinen F, et al: Ear click in palatal tremor: its origin and treatment with botulinum toxin. Neurology 41:1677–1679, 1991

Deuschl G, Toro C, Valls-Sole J, et al: Symptomatic and essential palatal tremor. 1. Clinical, physiological and MRI analysis. Brain 117:775–788, 1994

Dewey RB Jr, Jankovic J: Hemiballism-hemichorea. Clinical and pharmacologic findings in 21 patients. Arch Neurol 46:862–867, 1989

Dinan TG, Golden T: Orofacial dyskinesia in Down's syndrome. Br J Psychiatry 157:131–132, 1990

Dropcho EJ: Neurologic paraneoplastic syndromes. J Neurol Sci 153:264–278, 1998

Egan MF, Apud J, Wyatt RJ: Treatment of tardive dyskinesia. Schizophr Bull 23:583–609, 1997

Factor SA, Friedman JH: The emerging role of clozapine in the treatment of movement disorders. Mov Disord 12:483–496, 1997

Fahn S: The tardive syndromes: phenomenology, concepts on pathophysiology, and treatment. Mov Disord 7 (suppl 1):7, 1992

Fahn S, Williams DT: Psychogenic dystonia. Adv Neurol 50:431–455, 1988

Fahn S, Marsden CD, Van Woert MH: Definition and classification of myoclonus, in Myoclonus (Advances in Neurology Series, Vol 43). Edited by Fahn S, Marsden CD, Van Woert M. New York, Raven, 1986, pp 1–5

Farrer LA: Suicide and attempted suicide in Huntington disease: implications for preclinical testing of persons at risk. Am J Med Genet 24:305–311, 1986

FitzGerald PM, Jankovic J: Orthostatic tremor: an association with essential tremor. Mov Disord 6:60–64, 1991

Fletcher NA, Harding AE, Marsden CD: The relationship between trauma and idiopathic torsion dystonia. J Neurol Neurosurg Psychiatry 54:713–717, 1991

Friedman A, Fahn S: Spontaneous remissions in spasmodic torticollis. Neurology 36:398–400, 1986

Friedman JH, Ambler M: A case of senile chorea. Mov Disord 5:251–253, 1990

Garcia Ruiz PJ, Gomez-Tortosa E, del Barrio A, et al: Senile chorea: a multicenter prospective study. Acta Neurol Scand 95:180–183, 1997

Garvey MJ, Tollefson GD: Occurrence of myoclonus in patients treated with cyclic antidepressants. Arch Gen Psychiatry 44:269–272, 1987

Ghika-Schmid F, Ghika J, Regli F, et al: Hyperkinetic movement disorders during and after acute stroke: the Lausanne Stroke Registry. J Neurol Sci 146:109–116, 1997

Glass JP, Jankovic J, Borit A: Hemiballism and metastatic brain tumor. Neurology 34:204–207, 1984

Goldman MS, Kelly PJ: Stereotactic thalamotomy for medically intractable essential tremor. Stereotact Funct Neurosurg 58:22–25, 1992

Grandas F, Elston J, Quinn N, et al: Blepharospasm: a review of 264 patients. J Neurol Neurosurg Psychiatry 51:767–772, 1988

Gulcher JR, Jonsson P, Kong A, et al: Mapping of a familial essential tremor gene, FET1, to chromosome 3q13. Nat Genet 17:84–87, 1997

Gusella JF, MacDonald ME: Huntington's disease: CAG genetics expands neurobiology. Curr Opin Neurobiol 5:656–662, 1995

Gusella JF, Wexler NS, Conneally PM, et al: A polymorphic DNA marker genetically linked to Huntington's disease. Nature 306:234–238, 1983

Gusella JF, Persichetti F, MacDonald ME: The genetic defect causing Huntington's disease: repeated in other contexts? Mol Med 3:238–246, 1997

Hallett M: The neurophysiology of dystonia. Arch Neurol 55:601–603, 1998

Harper PS: The epidemiology of Huntington's disease, in Huntington's Disease. Edited by Harper PS. London, WB Saunders, 1991, pp 251–280

Hauser WA, Morris ML, Heston LL, et al: Seizures and myoclonus in patients with Alzheimer's disease. Neurology 36:1226–1230, 1986

Higgins JJ, Pho LT, Nee LE: A gene (ETM) for essential tremor maps to chromosome 2p22-p25. Mov Disord 12:859–864, 1997

Hubble JP, Busenbark KL, Wilkinson S, et al: Deep brain stimulation for essential tremor. Neurology 46:1150–1153, 1996

Huber SJ, Paulson GW: Efficacy of alprazolam for essential tremor. Neurology 38:241–243, 1988

Huntington Study Group: Safety and tolerability of the free radical scavenger OPC-14117 in Huntington's disease. Neurology 50:1366–1373, 1998

Huntington's Disease Collaborative Research Group: A novel gene containing a trinucleotide repeat that is expanded and unstable on Huntington's disease chromosomes. Cell 72:971–983, 1993

Ichinose H, Ohye T, Takahashi E, et al: Hereditary progressive dystonia with marked diurnal fluctuation caused by mutations in the GTP cyclohydrolase I gene. Nat Genet 8:236–242, 1994

International Huntington Association (IHA) and the World Federation of Neurology (WFN) Research Group on Huntington's Chorea: Guidelines for the molecular genetics predictive test in Huntington's disease. Neurology 44:1533–1536, 1994

Isozaki E, Naito A, Horiguchi S, et al: Early diagnosis and stage classification of vocal cord abductor paralysis in patients with multiple system atrophy. J Neurol Neurosurg Psychiatry 60:399–402, 1996

Jahanshahi M, Marion MH, Marsden CD: Natural history of adult-onset idiopathic torticollis. Arch Neurol 47:548–552, 1990

Jankovic J: Blepharospasm with basal ganglia lesions. Arch Neurol 43:866–868, 1986

Jankovic J: Post-traumatic movement disorders: central and peripheral mechanisms. Neurology 44:2006–2014, 1994

Jankovic J, Beach J: Long-term effects of tetrabenazine in hyperkinetic movement disorders. Neurology 48:358–362, 1997

Jankovic J, Brin MF: Therapeutic uses of botulinum toxin. N Engl J Med 324:1186–1194, 1991

Jankovic J, Pardo R: Segmental myoclonus. Clinical and pharmacologic study. Arch Neurol 43:1025–1031, 1986

Jannetta PJ, Abbasy M, Maroon JC, et al: Etiology and definitive microsurgical treatment of hemifacial spasm. Operative techniques and results in 47 patients. J Neurosurg 47:321–328, 1977

Jeste DV, Potkin SG, Sinha S, et al: Tardive dyskinesia—reversible and persistent. Arch Gen Psychiatry 36:585–590, 1979

Jeste DV, Jeste SD, Wyatt RJ: Reversible tardive dyskinesia: implications for therapeutic strategy and prevention of tardive dyskinesia. Mod Probl Pharmacopsychiatry 21:34–48, 1983

Kane JM, Smith JM: Tardive dyskinesia: prevalence and risk factors, 1959 to 1979. Arch Gen Psychiatry 39:473–481, 1982

Kang UJ, Burke RE, Fahn S: Natural history and treatment of tardive dystonia. Mov Disord 1:193–208, 1986

Kaplan PW, Allen RP, Buchholz DW, et al: A double-blind, placebo-controlled study of the treatment of periodic limb movements in sleep using carbidopa/levodopa and propoxyphene. Sleep 16:717–723, 1993

Kastrup O, Gastpar M, Schwarz M: Acute dystonia due to clozapine. J Neurol Neurosurg Psychiatry 57:119, 1994

Khot V, Egan MF, Hyde TM, et al: Neuroleptics and classic tardive dyskinesia, in Drug-Induced Movement Disorders. Edited by Lang AE, Weiner WJ. Mount Kisco, NY, Futura, 1992, pp 121–166

Klawans HL, Barr A: Prevalence of spontaneous lingual-facial-buccal dyskinesias in the elderly. Neurology 32:558–559, 1982

Klawans HL, Tanner CM, Barr A: The reversibility of "permanent" tardive dyskinesia. Clin Neuropharmacol 7:153–159, 1984

Koller WC: Alcoholism in essential tremor. Neurology 33:1074–1076, 1983a

Koller WC: Edentulous orodyskinesia. Ann Neurol 13:97–99, 1983b

Koller WC: Nadolol in essential tremor. Neurology 33:1076–1077, 1983c

Koller WC, Biary N: Metoprolol compared with propranolol in the treatment of essential tremor. Arch Neurol 41:171–172, 1984

Koller W, Biary N, Cone S: Disability in essential tremor: effect of treatment. Neurology 36:1001–1004, 1986

Kopyov OV, Jacques S, Lieberman A, et al: Safety of intrastriatal neurotransplantation for Huntington's disease patients. Exp Neurol 149:97–108, 1998

Koroshetz WJ, Jenkins BG, Rosen BR, et al: Energy metabolism defects in Huntington's disease and effects of coenzyme Q10. Ann Neurol 41:160–165, 1997

Koshino Y, Wada Y, Isaki K, et al: A long-term outcome study of tardive dyskinesia in patients on antipsychotic medication. Clin Neuropharmacol 14:537–546, 1991

Krauss JK, Trankle R, Kopp KH: Post-traumatic movement disorders in survivors of severe head injury. Neurology 47:1488–1492, 1996

Lang AE: Movement disorders: approach, definitions, and differential diagnosis, in Drug-Induced Movement Disorders. Edited by Lang AE, Weiner WJ. Mount Kisco, NY, Futura, 1992a, pp 1–20

Lang AE: Miscellaneous drug-induced movement disorders, in Drug-Induced Movement Disorders. Edited by Lang AE, Weiner WJ. Mount Kisco, NY, Futura, 1992b, pp 339–381

Lang AE: Psychogenic dystonia: a review of 18 cases. Can J Neurol Sci 22:136–143, 1995

Lang AE, Moldofsky H, Awad AG: Long latency between the onset of motor and vocal tics in Tourette's syndrome. Ann Neurol 14:693–694, 1983

Lang AE, Sethi KD, Provias JP, et al: What is it? Case 1, 1991: a severe and fatal systemic illness first presenting with a movement disorder. Mov Disord 6:362–370, 1991

Lasker AG, Zee DS: Ocular motor abnormalities in Huntington's disease. Vision Res 37:3639–3645, 1997

Lee MS, Marsden CD: Movement disorders following lesions of the thalamus or subthalamic region. Mov Disord 9:493–507, 1994

Lee MS, Rinne JO, Ceballos-Baumann A, et al: Dystonia after head trauma. Neurology 44:1374–1378, 1994

Leo RJ: Movement disorders associated with the serotonin selective reuptake inhibitors. J Clin Psychiatry 57:449–454, 1996

Lin JJ, Chang MK: Hemiballism-hemichorea and non-ketotic hyperglycaemia. J Neurol Neurosurg Psychiatry 57:748–750, 1994

Lugaresi E, Cirignotta F, Coccagna G, et al: Nocturnal myoclonus and restless legs syndrome, in Myoclonus (Advances in Neurology Series, Vol 43). Edited by Fahn S, Marsden CD, Van Woert MH. New York, Raven, 1986, pp 295–307

Marion MH, Klap P, Perrin A, et al: Stridor and focal laryngeal dystonia. Lancet 339:457–458, 1992

Marsden CD: Dystonia: the spectrum of the disease, in The Basal Ganglia. Edited by Yahr MD. New York, Raven, 1976, pp 351–367

Marsden CD, Quinn NP: The dystonias. BMJ 300:139–144, 1990

Marsden CD, Obeso JA, Zarranz JJ, et al: The anatomical basis of symptomatic hemidystonia. Brain 108:463–483, 1985

Morris M: Dementia and cognitive changes in Huntington's disease. Adv Neurol 65:187–200, 1995

Myers RH, Sax DS, Schoenfeld M, et al: Late onset of Huntington's disease. J Neurol Neurosurg Psychiatry 48:530–534, 1985

Obeso JA, Arteida J, Marsden CD: Different clinical presentations of myoclonus, in Parkinson's Disease and Movement Disorders. Edited by Jankovic J, Tolosa E. Baltimore, MD, Williams & Wilkins, 1993, pp 315–328

Ozelius L, Kramer PL, Moskowitz CB, et al: Human gene for torsion dystonia located on chromosome 9q32-q34. Neuron 2:1427–1434, 1989

Ozelius LJ, Hewett JW, Page CE, et al: The early onset torsion dystonia gene (DYT1) encodes an ATP-binding protein. Nat Genet 17:40–48, 1997

Peacock L, Solgaard T, Lublin H, et al: Clozapine versus typical antipsychotics. A retro- and prospective study of extrapyramidal side effects. Psychopharmacology (Berl) 124:188–196, 1996

Peyser CE, Folstein SE: Huntington's disease as a model for mood disorders. Clues from neuropathology and neurochemistry. Mol Chem Neuropathol 12:99–119, 1990

Philpott LM, Kopyov OV, Lee AJ, et al: Neuropsychological functioning following fetal striatal transplantation in Huntington's chorea: three case presentations. Cell Transplant 6:203–212, 1997

Pierot L, Cervera-Pierot P, Delattre JY, et al: Palatal myoclonus and inferior olivary lesions: MRI-pathologic correlation. J Comput Assist Tomogr 16:160–163, 1992

Poewe WH, Lees AJ, Stern GM: Dystonia in Parkinson's disease: clinical and pharmacological features. Ann Neurol 23:73–78, 1988

Quinn NP: Essential myoclonus and myoclonic dystonia. Mov Disord 11:119–124, 1996

Ranen NG, Peyser CE, Coyle JT, et al: A controlled trial of idebenone in Huntington's disease. Mov Disord 11: 549–554, 1996a

Ranen NG, Lipsey JR, Treisman G, et al: Sertraline in the treatment of severe aggressiveness in Huntington's disease. J Neuropsychiatry Clin Neurosci 8:338–340, 1996b

Rinne JO, Lee MS, Thompson PD, et al: Corticobasal degeneration. A clinical study of 36 cases. Brain 117:1183–1196, 1994

Rosenbaum F, Jankovic J: Focal task-specific tremor and dystonia: categorization of occupational movement disorders. Neurology 38:522–527, 1988

Schols L, Amoiridis G, Epplen JT, et al: Relations between genotype and phenotype in German patients with the Machado-Joseph disease mutation. J Neurol Neurosurg Psychiatry 61:466–470, 1996

Scott BL, Jankovic J: Delayed-onset progressive movement disorders after static brain lesions. Neurology 46:68–74, 1996

Shannon KM: Hemiballismus. Clin Neuropharmacol 13: 413–425, 1990

Shiang R, Ryan SG, Zhu YZ, et al: Mutations in the alpha 1 subunit of the inhibitory glycine receptor cause the dominant neurologic disorder, hyperekplexia. Nat Genet 5:351–358, 1993

Shibasaki H: Myoclonus. Curr Opin Neurol 8:331–334, 1995

Silber MH: Restless legs syndrome. Mayo Clin Proc 72: 261–264, 1997

Silberbauer C: Risperidone-induced tardive dyskinesia. Pharmacopsychiatry 31:68–69, 1998

Stojanovic M, Sternic N, Kostic VS: Clozapine in hemiballismus: report of two cases. Clin Neuropharmacol 20:171–174, 1997

Tamaoka A, Sakuta M, Yamada H: Hemichorea-hemiballism caused by arteriovenous malformations in the putamen. J Neurol 234:124–125, 1987

Tamaru Y, Hirano M, Ito H, et al: Clinical similarities of hereditary progressive/dopa responsive dystonia caused by different types of mutations in the GTP cyclohydrolase I gene. J Neurol Neurosurg Psychiatry 64:469–473, 1998

Thomas P, Lalaux N, Vaiva G, et al: Dose-dependent stuttering and dystonia in a patient taking clozapine. Am J Psychiatry 151:1096, 1994

Thompson C, Lang A, Parkes JD, et al: A double-blind trial of clonazepam in benign essential tremor. Clin Neuropharmacol 7:83–88, 1984

Thompson PD: Writers' cramp. British Journal of Hospital Medicine 50:91–94, 1993

Thompson PD, Rothwell JC, Day BL, et al: The physiology of orthostatic tremor. Arch Neurol 43:584–587, 1986

Ticehurst SB: Is spontaneous orofacial dyskinesia an artefact due to incomplete drug history? J Geriatr Psychiatry Neurol 3:208–211, 1990

Tollefson GD, Beasley CM Jr, Tamura RN, et al: Blind, controlled, long-term study of the comparative incidence of treatment-emergent tardive dyskinesia with olanzapine or haloperidol. Am J Psychiatry 154:1248–1254, 1997

Tolosa E, Marti MJ: Blepharospasm-oromandibular dystonia syndrome (Meige's syndrome): clinical aspects. Adv Neurol 49:73–84, 1988

van Vugt JP, Siesling S, Vergeer M, et al: Clozapine versus placebo in Huntington's disease: a double blind randomised comparative study. J Neurol Neurosurg Psychiatry 63: 35–39, 1997

Vidakovic A, Dragasevic N, Kostic VS: Hemiballism: report of 25 cases. J Neurol Neurosurg Psychiatry 57:945–949, 1994

Waddington JL, Youssef HA: The lifetime outcome and involuntary movements of schizophrenia never treated with neuroleptic drugs. Br J Psychiatry 156:106–108, 1990

Walters AS, Hening W: Clinical presentation and neuropharmacology of restless legs syndrome. Clin Neuropharmacol 10:225–237, 1987

Weiner WJ, Lang AE: An introduction to movement disorders and the basal ganglia, in Movement Disorders: A Comprehensive Survey. Edited by Weiner WJ, Lang AE. Mount Kisco, NY, Futura, 1989, pp 1–22

Wenning GK, Ben Shlomo Y, Magalhaes M, et al: Clinical features and natural history of multiple system atrophy. An analysis of 100 cases. Brain 117:835–845, 1994

Wetter TC, Pollmacher T: Restless legs and periodic leg movements in sleep syndromes. J Neurol 244 (suppl 1):37–45, 1997

Wichmann T: Physiology of the basal ganglia and pathophysiology of movement disorders of basal ganglia origin, in Movement Disorders: Neurologic Principles and Practice. Edited by Koller W, Watts RL. New York, McGraw-Hill, 1997, pp 87–97

Winkelmann J, Wetter TC, Stiasny K, et al: Treatment of restless leg syndrome with pergolide—an open clinical trial. Mov Disord 13:566–569, 1998

Wissel J, Kabus C, Wenzel R, et al: Botulinum toxin in writer's cramp: objective response evaluation in 31 patients. J Neurol Neurosurg Psychiatry 61:172–175, 1996

Yagi G, Takamuja, M, Kauba, S, et al: Mortality rates of schizophrenic patients with tardive dyskinesia during 10 years: a controlled study. Keio J Med 38:70–72, 1989

Yassa R, Nair V, Dimitry R: Prevalence of tardive dystonia. Acta Psychiatr Scand 73:629–633, 1986

Yoshida K, Higuchi H, Hishikawa Y: Marked improvement of tardive dystonia after replacing haloperidol with risperidone in a schizophrenic patient. Clin Neuropharmacol 21:68–69, 1998

Young RR, Shahani BT: Asterixis: one type of negative myoclonus, in Myoclonus (Advances in Neurology Series, Vol 43). Edited by Fahn S, Marsden CD, Van Woert M. New York, Raven, 1986, pp 137–156

Youssef HA, Waddington JL: Morbidity and mortality in tardive dyskinesia: associations in chronic schizophrenia. Acta Psychiatr Scand 75:74–77, 1987

Parkinson's Disease and Parkinsonism

Alexander I. Tröster, Ph.D.

Julie A. Fields

William C. Koller, M.D., Ph.D.

James Parkinson (1817), in his treatise of the disease now bearing his name, considered the senses and intellect to be spared in Parkinson's disease (PD), but alterations of mental function have been recognized since the late 1800s (Charcot 1878). These alterations may take the form of cognitive dysfunction, clinical psychiatric illness, sleep disturbance, or any combination thereof. The alterations are commonly encountered by clinicians who manage this illness or provide general medical care. In PD, the diagnosis of cognitive and behavioral disturbances, such as dementia and depression, is usually based on *Diagnostic and Statistical Manual of Mental Disorders* (American Psychiatric Association 1994) criteria. The appropriateness of these criteria to PD remains debated, and the criteria provide no guidance in the diagnosis of circumscribed cognitive impairments in PD without dementia. The establishment of specific diagnostic guidelines would facilitate recognition of, and reinforce the cause-and-effect relationship be-

tween, these abnormalities of mental function and PD.

In this chapter, our goal is to provide a description of the various neurobehavioral changes encountered in PD. In doing so, we emphasize the clinical features and discuss the proposed pathogenetic mechanisms and treatment options currently available.

Clinical Features

The four cardinal signs of parkinsonism are tremor, bradykinesia, rigidity, and postural abnormalities (including disturbance of balance). However, the clinical onset may be heralded by nonspecific symptoms such as generalized fatigue; muscle tightness, aching, or cramping; focal dystonias; decreased manual dexterity; restlessness; sensory symptoms (e.g., extremity pain or paresthesias); and psychiatric complaints (e.g., anxiety and/or depression). Complaints may also be related to autonomic nervous system dysfunction such as postural hypotension, constipation, and/or paroxysmal sweating.

Epidemiology

Two measures are used to express the frequency with which a given disease occurs. Prevalence refers to the total number of cases present within a population at a given time. Incidence refers to the number of new cases that occur within a given time, usually per year, in a given population. Prevalence rates are sensitive to factors related to disease survival. For example, a slowly progressive disease such as PD will have a much higher prevalence than another disease with comparable incidence but a short survival time. Consequently, incidence is considered a more accurate measure of disease frequency. Unfortunately, incidence rates are more difficult to establish, and the majority of epidemiological studies of PD have examined its prevalence.

The first comprehensive study (Kurland 1958), a community-based study in Rochester, Minnesota, recognized persons receiving medical attention for PD and found a 187/100,000 prevalence and a 20/100,000 annual incidence. Prevalences found by community-based studies worldwide have varied from 31 to 347 per 100,000 (Table 26–1).

A number of risk factors for the development of PD have been investigated. Among demographic factors, increasing age has been the most consistently identified risk factor. Onset of PD before the fifth decade is rare, and age-specific prevalence is highest for the seventh and eighth decades (Tanner et al. 1997). Gender and race may be other risk factors: PD is almost twice as common in men as in women; its prevalence may be higher among whites than among blacks (Schoenberg et al. 1985), but this finding remains controversial.

Several putative environmental risk factors (e.g., toxins) have also been identified. The most striking example of toxins causing parkinsonism (Table 26–2) is 1-methyl-4-phenyl-1,2,3,6- tetrahydropyridine (MPTP), which produces clinical and cognitive changes closely resembling those of idiopathic PD (Langston et al. 1983; Stern and Langston 1985). Other neurotoxins cause more widespread injury resulting in parkinsonism and a constellation of other clinical findings (Goetz 1985). Several other factors, probably by virtue of involving toxicant exposure, have been linked to a heightened prevalence of PD: residence in industrialized nations (Aquilonius and Hartvig 1986); farming (Gorell et al. 1998) and residence in rural areas with exposure to well water, herbicides, or pesticides (Hubble et al. 1993; Koller et al. 1990; Tanner et al. 1987); and employment in chemical, wood pulp, and steel-manufacturing industries (Tanner 1989).

Genetic factors do not appear to play a primary role in the pathogenesis of PD. Studies of several large family kindreds suggested an autosomal-dominant inheritance mechanism in atypical PD (e.g., Golbe et al. 1990a, 1993; Waters and Miller 1994), but only rarely in typical PD (Wszolek et al. 1995). Interpretation of some of these studies is complicated by possible intermarriage in preceding generations (which may result in a spurious autosomal-dominant inheritance pattern) and by disease ascertainment methods (Wszolek et al. 1996). A significantly greater concordance of PD in monozygotic than dizygotic twins, which would support a genetic basis for the disease, also has not been found (e.g., Marsden 1987; Ward et al. 1983).

Genetic factors may, however, predispose to PD. Such a genetic predisposition, together with environmental fac-

TABLE 26–1. Estimated prevalence of Parkinson's disease in community-based studies

Study	Location	Patient acquisition setting	Prevalence per 100,000
Kurland 1958	Rochester, MN	Clinical	187
Gudmundsson 1967	Iceland	Clinical	162
Kessler 1972	Baltimore, MD	Clinical	128
Marttila and Rinne 1967	Finland	Clinical	120
Li et al. 1982	China	Door-to-door	44
Schoenberg et al. 1985	Copian County, MS	Door-to-door	347
Mutch et al. 1986	Scotland	Clinical	164
Ashok et al. 1986	Libya	Clinical	31
Schoenberg et al. 1988	Nigeria	Door-to-door	59
Okada et al. 1990	Japan	Clinical	82
Rocca and Morgante 1990	Sicily, Italy	Door-to-door	243

TABLE 26–2. Classification of parkinsonism

Infectious and postinfectious causes of parkinsonism
Encephalitis lethargica
Encephalitides
Syphilis
Toxic causes of parkinsonism
Manganese
Carbon monoxide
Carbon disulfide
Cyanide
Methanol
1-methyl-4-phenyl-1,2,3,6-tetrahydropyridine (MPTP)
Pharmacological causes of parkinsonism
Neuroleptics
Phenothiazines
Butyrophenones (e.g., haloperidol)
Thioxanthenes (e.g., thiothixene)
Benzamides (e.g., metoclopramide)
Reserpine, tetrabenazine
Miscellaneous agents
α-Methyldopa
Lithium
Multiple system atrophies with parkinsonian features
Striatonigral degeneration
Progressive supranuclear palsy
Olivopontocerebellar degeneration
Shy-Drager syndrome
Other degenerative diseases of the nervous system with parkinsonian features
Primary pallidal atrophy
Idiopathic dystonia-parkinsonism
Corticobasal ganglionic degeneration

Hemiatrophy-hemiparkinsonism
Parkinsonism–amyotrophic lateral sclerosis (ALS)–dementia complex of Guam
"Atherosclerotic" or "senile" parkinsonism
Alzheimer's and Pick's diseases
Creutzfeldt-Jakob disease
Gerstmann–Sträussler–Schneider disease
Rett's disease
Central nervous system disorders that may cause parkinsonism
Normal pressure hydrocephalus
Stroke
Tumor
Trauma
Subdural hematoma
Syringomesencephalia
Metabolic causes of parkinsonism
Hypoparathyroidism and basal ganglia calcification
Chronic hepatocerebral degeneration
Hereditary diseases of the nervous system associated with parkinsonism
Wilson's disease
Huntington's disease
Disorder with diffuse pathology
Spinocerebellonigral degeneration
Parkinsonism with ataxia and neuropathy
Parkinsonism with alveolar hypoventilation
Psychogenic disorders
Factitious disorder
Somatoform disorder
Malingering

---

tors, may lead to the appearance of the clinical syndrome (Barbeau and Pourcher 1982). For instance, individuals with defective xenobiotic-metabolizing enzymes (e.g., CYP2D6, a subfamily of the cytochrome P450 enzymes) may be at greater risk for PD when exposed to toxins usually broken down by these enzymes, but the relationship between CYP2D6 alleles and PD remains unclear (Tanner et al. 1997).

Several factors have been suggested to protect against PD, including smoking (e.g., Grandinetti et al. 1994) and ingesting of foods rich in antioxidant vitamins (Golbe et al. 1990b; Li et al. 1982).

Differential Diagnosis

The differential diagnosis includes any disorder manifesting parkinsonism (Table 26–2), a syndrome that may result from a variety of etiologies. PD is thought to have a long prodromal phase (Koller and Montgomery 1997), and no set of universally accepted diagnostic criteria for early PD exists. Research criteria (Table 26–3) and probabilistic criteria (Table 26–4) are commonly employed, and various exclusionary criteria (Table 26–5) have been proposed to enhance diagnostic accuracy. Probability criteria based on inclusionary and exclusionary features were recently proposed by Gelb et al. (1999), but, like other criteria, their utility remains to be evaluated. Clinical diagnostic accuracy defined on the basis of postmortem neuropathological examination is approximately 75% (Hughes et al. 1992; Rajput et al. 1991).

The group of disorders designated multiple system atrophies (also known as parkinsonism-plus syndromes) share parkinsonian features with PD, but manifest additional findings (e.g., supranuclear ophthalmoplegia in progressive supranuclear palsy and dysautonomia in

TABLE 26–3. Research criteria for probable Parkinson's disease

1. Evidence of disease progression
2. Presence of at least two of the three cardinal features of parkinsonism:
   a. Tremor
   b. Rigidity
   c. Bradykinesia
3. Presence of at least two of the following:
   a. Marked response to levodopa (functional improvement or dyskinesia)
   b. Asymmetry of signs
   c. Asymmetry at onset
4. Absence of clinical features of alternative diagnosis
5. Absence of etiology known to cause similar features

Source. Reprinted with permission from Koller WC, Montgomery EB: "Issues in the Early Diagnosis of Parkinson's Disease." *Neurology* 49 (suppl 1): S10–S25, 1997. Copyright 1997 Lippincott Williams & Wilkins.

TABLE 26–4. Probabilistic classification scheme for the diagnosis of Parkinson's disease

Clinically possible

The presence of any one of the salient features:

Tremor

Rigidity

Bradykinesia

Impairment of postural reflexes is not included because it is too nonspecific. The tremor must be of recent onset but may be postural or resting.

Clinically probable

A combination of any two of the cardinal features:

Resting tremor

Rigidity

Bradykinesia

Impaired postural reflexes

Alternatively, asymmetrical resting tremor, asymmetrical rigidity, or asymmetrical bradykinesia is sufficient.

Clinically definite

Any combination of three of the cardinal features (above).

Alternatively sufficient are two of these features, with one of the first three displaying asymmetry.

Source. Reprinted with permission from Koller WC, Montgomery EB: "Issues in the Early Diagnosis of Parkinson's Disease." *Neurology* 49 (suppl 1): S10–S25, 1997. Copyright 1997 Lippincott Williams & Wilkins.

Shy-Drager syndrome). Early in their courses, these disorders may be difficult to distinguish from PD. One useful characteristic in this regard is their poor responsiveness to levodopa or dopamine agonists. Parkinsonian signs and symptoms may also be of psychogenic origin. In these instances, it becomes important to determine whether the signs are a manifestation of malingering, a somatoform disorder, or a factitious disorder (Koller et al. 1998a).

Treatment

Treatment goals should be individualized for each patient. A treatment algorithm for PD is presented in Figure 26–1. Patient and family education is important for the patient newly diagnosed with PD (Figure 26–2), and patients should be encouraged to contact a PD support group.

Pharmacotherapy

Levodopa. Levodopa has been the mainstay of drug therapy for the motor manifestations of the disease. Its absorption is highly variable in the proximal small intestine, with competition for transport from amino acid components of ingested protein (Riley and Lang 1988). It is decarboxylated to dopamine in the gut and liver and, after crossing the blood-brain barrier, in the brain by the surviving dopaminergic neurons and by decarboxylase-containing serotonergic and adrenergic neurons (Melamed et al. 1980).

The initiation of levodopa therapy, most often when PD has begun to interfere with activities of daily living, usually results in dramatic improvement in motor symptoms. The absence of a therapeutic effect at high doses necessitates reappraisal of the diagnosis. Bradykinesia and rigidity respond best. Tremor may improve somewhat, but usually there is no improvement in postural stability, mental state, or autonomic nervous system dysfunction.

Levodopa is combined with a peripheral dopa decarboxylase inhibitor (carbidopa in the United States, benserazide in Europe) to counteract the adverse effects of peripherally produced dopamine (e.g., nausea, vomiting, and postural hypotension). Domperidone, a peripheral dopamine antagonist not yet available in the United States, may also be used to treat levodopa-associated nausea (Olanow and Koller 1998). Most patients are started at a dose of one tablet of Sinemet 25/100 (25 mg carbidopa and 100 mg levodopa) thrice daily, 30 minutes before or 1 hour after meals. The subsequent dosage is adjusted to obtain an optimal motor response.

A long-acting preparation, Sinemet CR (controlled-release) 50/200, is a slowly eroding tablet that is absorbed

TABLE 26–5. Proposed exclusion criteria for the diagnosis of Parkinson's disease

Suggested exclusion criteria	Author		
	Gibb 1988	Koller 1992	Quinn 1994
More than one affected relative	X		
Remitting course	X	X	
History of definite encephalitis lethargica	X	X	
Oculogyric crises	X	X	
Neuroleptic therapy within the previous year	X	X	
Supranuclear down or lateral gaze palsy	X	X	
Cerebellar signs	X	X	
Autonomic neuropathy	X		
Alzheimer-type dementia from onset of symptoms	X	X	
Pyramidal signs not explained by discrete strokes	X	X	
Cerebrovascular disease[a]	X		
Abrupt onset of symptoms		X	
Stepwise progression		X	
Lower motor neuron signs		X	
Severe autonomic failure causing repeated syncope		X	
Postural instability, with falling, early in disease course		X	
Rapid disease progression			X
Permanently wheelchair-bound despite therapy			X
Irregular jerk tremor			X
Marked dysarthria			X
Marked dysphagia			X
Disproportionate antecollis			X
Cold, dusky hands (Raynaud's phenomenon)			X

[a]Implied by ataxic gait, stroke at onset, incontinence in first year, or early severe dementia; or two of the following: hypertension, emotional incontinence, spastic gait.
Source.   Reprinted with permission from Koller WC, Montgomery EB: "Issues in the Early Diagnosis of Parkinson's Disease." *Neurology* 49 (suppl 1): S10–S25, 1997. Copyright 1997 Lippincott Williams & Wilkins.

over a more protracted period of time. Its onset of effect is slower than that of standard Sinemet, but it has been shown to decrease "off" time (return of symptoms as a result of subtherapeutic drug effects), early morning dystonia, and nocturnal disturbances. Sinemet and Sinemet CR may be given separately or in combination based on the desired clinical effect.

Dyskinesias are prominent among the adverse effects caused by levodopa. Choreic movements are most common, and dyskinesias may interfere with speech, swallowing, respiration, and balance (Tanner 1986). Dyskinesias are dose-related and may improve by lowering the dose, although this may exacerbate the parkinsonism. In addition, motor fluctuations (e.g., early morning akinesia), "wearing-off," and "on-off" phenomena are more severe in patients treated with levodopa. Smaller and multiple doses may improve this end-of-dose deterioration. The neurobehavioral complications of levodopa therapy are discussed later in this chapter.

The natural history of PD includes gradual deterioration of speech and posture and gait abnormalities. Levodopa does little to affect progression to disability in this regard. However, its efficacy may continue for rigidity, bradykinesia, tremor, and micrographia after many years of levodopa therapy (Klawans 1986), and levodopa has reduced premature mortality in patients with PD (Curtis et al. 1984).

Selegiline and neuroprotection.   Because oxidant stress might play a role in the pathogenesis of PD, selegiline (L-deprenyl, Eldepryl), a monoamine oxidase-B (MAO-B) inhibitor, might exert a neuroprotective effect by reducing stress associated with MAO-B oxidation of dopamine. Selegiline has been shown to delay evolution of

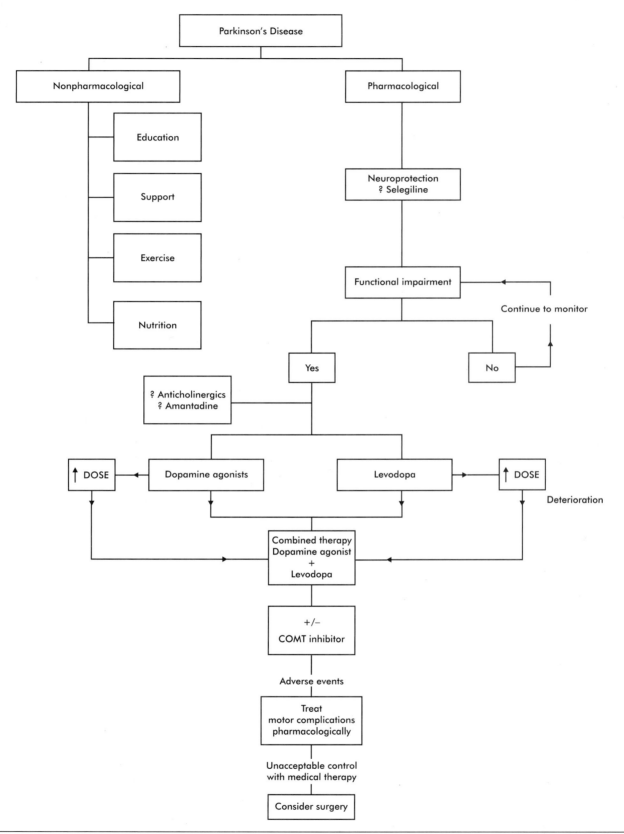

FIGURE 26–1.   Algorithm outlining treatment strategies for Parkinson's disease. COMT = catechol-*O*-methyltransferase.
Source.   Reprinted with permission from Olanow CW, Koller WC: "An Algorithm (Decision Tree) for the Management of Parkinson's Disease: Treatment Guidelines." *Neurology* 50 (suppl 3):S1–S57, 1998. Copyright 1998 Lippincott Williams & Wilkins.

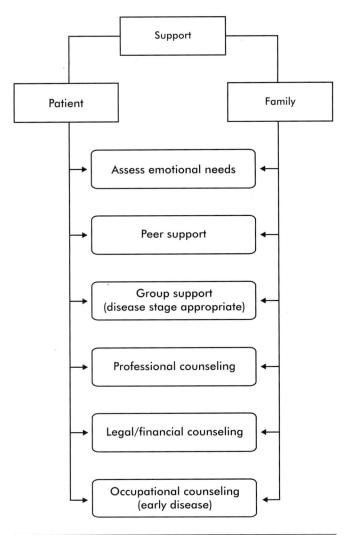

FIGURE 26–2. Algorithm outlining types of supports for patients and caregivers.
Source. Reprinted with permission from Olanow CW, Koller WC: "An Algorithm (Decision Tree) for the Management of Parkinson's Disease: Treatment Guidelines." *Neurology* 50 (suppl 3):S1–S57, 1998. Copyright 1998 Lippincott Williams & Wilkins.

disability requiring symptomatic therapy and to slow disease progression (Parkinson Study Group 1989, 1993). A report that selegiline plus levodopa treatment was associated with significantly higher mortality than was levodopa treatment alone (Parkinson's Disease Research Group in the United Kingdom 1995) has eluded replication and been criticized on methodological grounds (Olanow et al. 1996). Lazabemide, another selective and reversible MAO-B inhibitor, may affect PD progression in a manner similar to selegiline (Parkinson Study Group 1996).

Anticholinergic drugs and tremor. Anticholinergics (e.g., benztropine and trihexyphenidyl) and

amantadine (which acts as an anticholinergic and stimulates dopamine release) may be beneficial when tremor is a major problem. Because of their adverse effects (especially cognitive changes), they are best avoided in patients older than 70 years.

Dopamine agonists. The action of these agonists on various receptors is shown in Table 26–6. Bromocriptine and pergolide, both ergot derivatives, have traditionally been used in combination with levodopa once motor fluctuations emerge. They are started in small, once-daily (bedtime) doses to minimize the occurrence of orthostatic hypotension. The dosage may be gradually increased until the desired therapeutic benefit is realized. Dopamine agonists are also being evaluated as an initial monotherapy for PD. Used in this fashion, they are less likely than levodopa to lead to motor fluctuations and dyskinesias, but such monotherapy conveys adequate benefit for more than 3 years in only approximately 30% of patients (Poewe 1998).

Two relatively new, non-ergoline dopamine agonists (pramipexole and ropinirole) are anticipated to have fewer side effects than the ergot-derived dopamine agonists, but there is limited clinical experience with these agents. Ropinirole monotherapy was well tolerated and improved motor function in early PD (Adler et al. 1997) and effectiveness persisted at least 3 years in one study (Korczyn et al. 1999). As an adjunct to levodopa, ropinirole permitted reductions in levodopa dosage without loss of function (Brooks et al. 1995). Pramipexole also improved motor function in early PD, and, when given with levodopa or other antiparkinsonian medications in advanced PD, it reduced motor fluctuations, yielded further motor improvements, and permitted a decrease in levodopa dosage (Lieberman et al. 1997; Parkinson Study Group 1997; Pinter et al. 1999). It is hypothesized that early use of dopamine agonist may also exert a neuroprotective effect (Olanow 1997).

Catechol-*O*-methyltransferase inhibitors. Because peripheral degradation of levodopa by catechol-*O*-methyltransferase (COMT) is linked to motor fluctuations and dyskinesias, COMT inhibition is thought to be one means of extending the therapeutic effect of levodopa. Entacapone (a new, peripheral COMT inhibitor) and tolcapone (a peripheral and central COMT inhibitor), when used as an adjunct to levodopa, reduce motor fluctuations and "off" time (Martínez-Martín and O'Brien 1998; Rinne et al. 1998). Improvements in activities of daily living, motor function, and quality of life were observed in a randomized, double-blind, placebo-controlled study of stable patients with PD, taking 100 mg or 200 mg

TABLE 26–6.   Dopamine agonist receptor activity

Agonist	D_1	D_2	D_3	D_4	D_5	$5\text{-}HT_{1/2}$	$\alpha_{1/2}$
Bromocriptine	–	++	++	+	+	++	++
Cabergoline	0	+++	?	?	?	0	0
Lisuride	+	++	?	?	?	0	0
Pergolide	+	+++	++++	+	+	++	++
Pramipexole	0	++	++++	++	?	0	+
Ropinirole	0	++	++++	+	0	0	0

5-HT = 5-hydroxytryptamine; ? = not known; 0 = no effect; – = inhibitory effect; + = minimal effect; ++ = mild effect; +++ = moderate effect; ++++ = marked effect.
Source.   Reprinted with permission from Olanow CW, Koller WC: "An Algorithm (Decision Tree) for the Management of Parkinson's Disease: Treatment Guidelines." *Neurology* 50 (suppl 3):S1–S57, 1998. Copyright 1998 Lippincott Williams & Wilkins.

tolcapone three times per day, and these improvements were maintained at 12-month follow-up (Waters et al. 1997). In patients with "wearing-off" phenomena, treatment with 100 mg or 200 mg tolcapone three times daily was associated with significant reductions in "off" time and increases in "on" time (Baas et al. 1997; Rajput et al. 1997). In both studies the development or worsening of dyskinesias, often within the first 30 days of treatment, was the most frequent complication (in up to 62% of patients). Although peripheral COMT inhibitors are a promising adjunct to levodopa therapy, the effects of both their early and long-term use remain to be documented.

Stereotactic and Functional Neurosurgery

Stereotactic surgery for PD (particularly thalamotomy) reached its height in the 1950s and 1960s but declined rapidly after the introduction of levodopa in 1968 (Wilkinson and Tröster 1998). Acknowledgment of the limitations of pharmacotherapy, together with advances in neurophysiology, radiology, and stereotaxy, led to a resurgence of the surgical treatment of movement disorders (Goetz and Diederich 1996; Koller et al. 1998b). Laitinen and colleagues' (1992) rediscovery of Leksell's pallidotomy brought about a renaissance in ablative surgery. Alternative treatments, such as chronic deep brain stimulation and neural transplantation, were also further developed and refined. Surgical intervention may be considered in patients who no longer derive significant benefit from levodopa and/or dopamine agonists or who develop intolerable side effects from these medications. Patients with dementia or major affective disorder are typically not considered surgical candidates.

Ablative surgery.   Unilateral thalamotomy is effective for severe tremor, especially if there is an action component. Burchiel (1995) estimated that significant changes

in memory and language functions may occur in up to 31% of cases (in 60% of bilateral and in 31% of unilateral thalamotomy cases). Outcomes in early and more recent thalamotomy series are difficult to compare, but, in the largest, most recently reported series, no significant neurobehavioral morbidity was observed (Lund-Johansen et al. 1996).

Modern unilateral pallidotomy has been reported to alleviate all parkinsonian motor signs, predominantly on the side contralateral to surgery, and dyskinesias bilaterally (Kishore et al. 1997; Lang et al. 1997; Laitinen 1995). Long-term effects of pallidotomy remain to be adequately evaluated. In one study, contralateral parkinsonian signs remained improved at 2-year follow-up, but improvements in gait, balance, and ipsilateral dyskinesia were more short lived (Lang et al. 1997). Another study reported that overall motor function and dyskinesias remained improved for up to 4 years (Fazzini et al. 1997). Significant improvements in quality of life have been observed after pallidotomy, at least in the short term (Baron et al. 1996; Scott et al. 1998; Tröster et al. 1998b). Some patients experience typically mild and transient cognitive morbidity, most often affecting verbal fluency, learning and memory, and executive functions (Baron et al. 1996; Cahn et al. 1998; Scott et al. 1998; Trépanier et al. 1998; Uitti et al. 1997). Patients with mild or incipient dementia before surgery appear at greater risk for more severe and permanent cognitive declines (Alterman et al. 1997; Lang et al. 1997). Depression (Lang et al. 1997; Sutton et al. 1995), psychosis (Friedman et al. 1996; Johansson et al. 1997), euphoria (Narabayashi et al. 1997), a "reduction in motivation" (Samuel et al. 1998), and perseveration, impulsivity, lability, unawareness of deficits, and poor social judgment (Trépanier et al. 1998) have been observed after unilateral pallidotomy, but the frequency, persistence, and etiology of these disturbances remain to be established. Bilateral pallidotomy has been associated with marked cognitive impairment (Gálvez-Jiménez et al. 1996), but Scott et al. (1998) reported generalized cognitive impairment in only one of eight cases.

Deep brain stimulation. Deep brain stimulation (DBS) involves stereotactic placement of a typically quadripolar electrode within the ventral intermediate nucleus of the thalamus, the internal globus pallidus, or the subthalamic nuclei. The electrode is connected subcutaneously to a programmable pulse generator, implanted in the subclavicular region, via an extension lead. In cases of bilateral DBS, two independently programmable stimulators are implanted. At this time, only unilateral thalamic DBS is an approved treatment in the United States.

Relative to ablative procedures, DBS has both advantages and disadvantages (Pollak et al. 1998). Potential disadvantages include cost, need for replacement of the battery, need for additional visits to adjust the stimulator settings, infection, discomfort, and device failure. Advantages include the adaptability over time and reversibility of DBS, and consequently the minimization of morbidity. DBS is less likely than a permanent lesion to compromise potential benefit from future medical therapies. Adaptability of thalamic DBS may obviate the need for reoperation as is occasionally necessary after unsatisfactory thalamotomy (Tasker 1997).

DSS of the various targets differentially affects parkinsonian signs and symptoms (Table 26–7). Thalamic DBS has been shown effective in controlling tremor and improving disability (Benabid et al. 1996; Koller et al.

TABLE 26–7. **Estimated effects of stimulating subthalamic nucleus (STN), globus pallidus internus (Gpi), and ventral intermediate nucleus (Vim) on the main symptoms of PD**

	STN	Gpi	Vim
Tremor	+++	++	+++
Akinesia	+++	+(+)	0
Rigidity	+++	++	+
Dyskinesia	0/– (short-term) ++ (long-term)	+++	+(++VL)
Off-period dystonia	+++	++	0/–

+ = mildly effective; ++ = moderately effective; +++ = greatly effective; 0/– = may be deleterious; VL = ventrolateral thalamus.

Source. Reprinted with permission from Pollak P, Benabid A-L, Krack P, et al: "Deep Brain Stimulation," in *Parkinson's Disease and Movement Disorders*, 3rd Edition. Edited by Jankovic J, Tolosa E. Baltimore, MD, Williams & Wilkins, 1998, pp. 1085–1101. Copyright 1998 Williams & Wilkins.

1997; Tasker 1997). Pallidal DBS appears to alleviate akinesia, rigidity, and dyskinesia, but the effect on tremor and gait appears less reliable (Gross et al. 1997; Siegfried and Wellis 1997). Subthalamic DBS reportedly alleviates akinesia, rigidity, tremor, dyskinesias, and gait and balance disturbances (Pollak et al. 1998).

Unilateral thalamic (Caparros-Lefebvre et al. 1992; Tröster et al. 1997a) and pallidal DBS (Tröster et al. 1997b) appear relatively safe from the standpoint of cognitive morbidity, although decrements in verbal fluency are occasionally observed (see Fields and Tröster, in press). It has been anecdotally reported that subthalamic DBS entails no neuropsychological morbidity except "for those with poor presurgical neuropsychological performance" (Pollak et al. 1998), although another study (Kumar et al. 1999) reported mild memory and/or personality changes in some patients after subthalamic DBS. Given concerns about cognitive morbidity after bilateral ablative procedures, the safety of bilateral pallidal DBS (Fields et al., in press; Ghika et al. 1998) is noteworthy. The cognitive effects of stimulation, rather than of the combined effects of electrode implantation and stimulation, have been evaluated in only one case (Tröster et al. 1998c). DBS in PD tends to be associated with improvements in quality of life and mood state (Straits-Tröster et al., in press; Vingerhoets et al. 1999). Psychiatric morbidity has not been formally studied in DBS.

Transplantation. The intrastriatal implantation of autologous adrenal medullary tissue, despite its early promise (Goetz et al. 1989), has been virtually abandoned given the lack of lasting benefit and considerable morbidity and mortality. Psychiatric morbidity was considerable in a multicenter study (22% by 2-year follow-up) (Goetz et al. 1991), and complications such as confusion, hallucinations, delusions, depression, hypomania, and somnolence were reported in several other studies (Stebbins and Tanner 1992), especially after open as opposed to stereotactic procedures (Rehncrona 1997). The few studies formally evaluating cognition after adrenal tissue implantation did not find significant morbidity (Goetz et al. 1990; Ostrosky-Solis et al. 1988).

More recently, intrastriatal grafting of fetal mesencephalic tissue has been attempted. Although studies' variable outcomes are difficult to compare given methodological differences (e.g., surgical approach, number and site of grafts), a recent report indicated continued clinical benefit in 7 of 10 patients 5 years after unilateral grafting (López-Lozano et al. 1997). Graft viability, as indexed by positron–emission tomography (PET)-imaged increases in fluorine–18-labeled dopa uptake, appears a robust predictor of clinical benefit (Hagell et al. 1999; Rehncrona 1997).

Neurobehavioral outcomes after fetal tissue grafting are inadequately documented. Transient, perioperative psychiatric disturbances such as depression, paranoia, and hallucinations have been reported after open operations (Madrazo et al. 1990; Molina et al. 1991), but not after stereotactic procedures (Price et al. 1995). Sass et al. (1995) reported improvements in verbal memory in three patients 12 and 24 months after grafting, but these improvements were not maintained 36 months after surgery. Among five patients evaluated neuropsychologically before and 12 months after unilateral grafting, one patient demonstrated significant cognitive decline whereas two patients improved (Leroy et al. 1996).

Several other treatment approaches—for example, xenografts, intraventricular delivery of neurotrophic factors, and gene therapy—are currently under study (see Lang and Lozano 1998).

Cognitive Impairment in Early Parkinson's Disease

Parkinson's disease, even early in its course, is often accompanied by mild cognitive disturbances and affective disorders such as depression. Although the prevalence of cognitive impairment without dementia is difficult to ascertain given the lack of specific criteria, a review of 20 studies of treated and untreated patients with PD without dementia estimated the prevalence at 19% (range 17%–53%) (Lieberman 1998). Dementia is almost never evident in the earliest disease stage. A dementia preceding or accompanying the evolution of the motor signs of PD raises the suspicion that the dementia is related to another condition, for example, Alzheimer's disease (AD) or depression.

When cognitive impairment is present in early PD, it is typically mild and circumscribed, most often affecting executive functions (e.g., planning, reasoning, abstraction, conceptualization, cognitive flexibility), visuoperceptual functions, and memory (Bondi and Tröster 1997). Bradyphrenia, a slowing of thought and information processing speed, is also observable early in the disease and has been linked to noradrenergic changes (Mayeux et al. 1987).

Executive deficits have been ascribed to frontal lobe dysfunction secondary to cortical-striatal-thalamic-cortical circuit pathophysiology and are most apparent on tasks requiring spontaneous, self-directed strategy formulation and deployment (Taylor and Saint-Cyr 1995).

The existence of a pure, primary impairment of visuoperceptual processes remains controversial. Although visuoperceptual impairments have been frequently observed in early PD, even when tasks' motor demands are minimized (Huber et al. 1986; Taylor et al. 1986), it has been argued that some instances of visuospatial impairment may reflect deficient motor speed and dexterity, spatial memory, and shift of mental set from one orientation to another and/or executive dysfunction (e.g., Bondi et al. 1993; Brown and Marsden 1986).

The memory impairment of PD is characterized predominantly by retrieval deficits, as evident from patients' disproportionately better performance on recognition than recall tests (Beatty et al. 1989; Pillon et al. 1993). The memory deficits in early PD have also been ascribed to frontal lobe dysfunction (Taylor et al. 1986, 1990a, 1990b), although it is unlikely that frontal lobe dysfunction is the sole determinant of memory impairment (Tröster and Fields 1995). Unlike the ability to learn new information, remote memory content is typically spared in early PD (Freedman et al. 1984; Leplow et al. 1997; Sagar et al. 1988; but see Venneri et al. 1997).

Performance on simple attention tasks such as digit span is often preserved. Impairments are readily observed on more complex tasks involving working memory (Gabrieli et al. 1996).

Language functions such as repetition, comprehension, and word knowledge are typically preserved (Cummings et al. 1988; Lewis et al. 1998; Tröster et al. 1996a). Patients with early PD may demonstrate subtle reductions in the syntactic complexity of spontaneous speech (Illes 1989; Lieberman et al. 1990) and difficulty in comprehension of syntax (Grossman et al. 1992; Lieberman et al. 1992). Visual confrontation naming, typically preserved, may be impaired (Globus et al. 1985; Levin et al. 1989). Some studies have observed mild impairments on verbal fluency tasks requiring oral generation of words belonging to a given semantic category or beginning with a given letter of the alphabet (Lewis et al. 1998; Troyer et al. 1998). These verbal fluency impairments probably reflect difficulties with the initiation and maintenance of systematic word retrieval strategies and are attributed to frontostriatal dysfunction. The presence of verbal fluency impairments in the earliest stages of PD may be a strong predictor of the subsequent development of dementia (Jacobs et al. 1995; Mahieux et al. 1998).

Dementia in Parkinson's Disease

Epidemiology

Reported prevalence rates range from 8% (Taylor et al. 1985) to 81% (Martin et al. 1973). Sampling and case definition and ascertainment methods differ across studies. As Cummings (1988a) pointed out, studies employing nonstandardized clinical examinations report the lowest prevalence rates of dementia, whereas studies employing formal neuropsychological evaluation report the highest rates. Commonly accepted prevalence estimates range from 20% to 40% (Mohr et al. 1995). Incidence of dementia in PD has rarely been reported. Mayeux et al. (1990) reported an incidence of 69 per 1,000 person-years, whereas Biggins et al. (1992) reported one of 48 per 1,000.

A genetic predisposition to the dementia of PD has been proposed. The risk of dementia among the first-degree relatives of patients with PD with dementia is sixfold greater than that in relatives of patients with PD without dementia (Marder et al. 1990). A familial association between PD and AD has been reported; first-degree relatives with AD had a threefold risk of PD, suggesting a common genetic etiology (Hofman et al. 1989). However, the risk factors most often associated with AD are not found in patients with PD with dementia. For example, the apolipoprotein E e4 allele is associated with an increased risk of AD, but dementia in PD appears not to be related to apolipoprotein E genotype (Koller et al. 1995; Marder et al. 1994).

Putative risk factors for the development of dementia in PD include increasing age (Stern et al. 1993a), older age at disease onset (Glatt et al. 1996; Lieberman et al. 1979), low socioeconomic status and education (Glatt et al. 1996; Salganik and Korczyn 1990), greater severity of extrapyramidal signs (Marder et al. 1995) (although the specific extrapyramidal signs associated with dementia remain to be specified), susceptibility to psychosis or confusion in response to levodopa (Stern et al. 1993a), and depression (Marder et al. 1995; Stern et al. 1993a).

Diagnostic Criteria and Definitions of Dementia in Parkinson's Disease

Diagnostic criteria for dementia have been defined in the DSMs. In DSM-IV, the most recent edition of this work, dementia as a result of PD is classified under Dementia Due to Other General Medical Conditions (Table 26–8). These criteria remain subject to the concerns and criticisms leveled against earlier versions of DSM. One criterion for the diagnosis of dementia in PD is that the required decline in occupational or social functioning is *caused* by cognitive deficits. A modification of this criterion has been recommended (Brown and Marsden 1984; McCarthy et al. 1985) because it is difficult to determine the extent to which functional impairment in PD reflects motor disability as opposed to cognitive decline. It has also been sug-

gested that because of performance expectations, especially in the workplace, dementia in men may be recognized sooner than that in women homemakers (Rajput et al. 1990).

DSM criteria for dementia require the presence of a memory impairment. Because bradyphrenia and impairments in executive and visuoperceptual functions may precede significant memory impairment, it is possible that a patient without memory impairment, but functional impairment comparable to that of a patient with dementia, would not meet DSM criteria for dementia. Another unresolved issue is whether the required memory impairment must be a *primary* memory impairment. As noted earlier, subtle encoding and retrieval strategy deficiencies, attributed to frontal or executive dysfunction, are observed in early PD. It is unclear whether such changes in memory *processes* should be classified as memory or executive dysfunction when the diagnostic possibility of dementia arises.

Cummings and Benson (1992) proposed alternate criteria for dementia. These criteria define dementia as an acquired, persistent impairment in at least three of five domains: 1) language, 2) memory, 3) complex cognition (executive functions), 4) visuospatial functions, and 5) personality or emotion. Occupational and social functioning

TABLE 26–8. DSM-IV criteria for dementia as a result of Parkinson's disease

A. The development of multiple cognitive deficits manifested by both

  1. Memory impairment (impaired ability to learn new information or to recall previously learned information)

  2. One (or more) of the following cognitive disturbances:

    a. Aphasia (language disturbance)

    b. Apraxia (impaired ability to carry out motor activities despite intact motor function)

    c. Agnosia (failure to recognize or identify objects despite intact sensory function)

    d. Disturbance in executive functioning (e.g., planning, organizing, sequencing, abstracting)

B. The cognitive deficits in criteria A1 and A2 both cause significant impairment in social or occupational functioning and represent a significant decline from a previous level of functioning.

C. There is evidence from the history, physical examination, or laboratory findings that the disturbance is the direct physiological consequence of Parkinson's disease.

D. The deficits do not occur exclusively during the course of a delirium.

need *not* be affected. These criteria are more liberal than those in DSM, and it is possible that a patient with relatively mild cognitive impairments would meet the Cummings and Benson but not the DSM criteria for dementia (McPherson and Cummings 1996). The possibly differential validity of DSM and Cummings and Benson criteria remains to be addressed.

Neuropathology

PD is characterized by the loss of pigmented neurons from the pars compacta of the substantia nigra, reactive gliosis at sites of cell loss, and the appearance of Lewy bodies in the substantia nigra, locus ceruleus, ventral tegmental area, nucleus basalis of Meynert, thalamus, dorsal raphe nuclei, cerebral cortex, and autonomic nervous system. The mechanism of Lewy body formation is unknown but is thought to be related to a disruption of neurofilament metabolism, perhaps in reaction to cell stress (Esiri and McShane 1997).

Neuronal loss in the substantia nigra pars compacta is associated with decreased levels of dopamine and its metabolites in the substantia nigra, caudate, putamen, globus pallidus, and nucleus accumbens. This neuronal loss, together with that in the ventral tegmental area, is also associated with reductions in dopamine in mesocortical projection sites such as entorhinal, hippocampal, cingulate, and frontal cortices. Ventral tegmental neuronal degeneration is associated with reduction of dopamine in mesolimbic projection areas (e.g., nucleus accumbens, hypothalamus, amygdaloid nucleus). Reductions in norepinephrine and serotonin concentrations are linked to neuronal loss in the locus ceruleus and dorsal raphe nuclei, respectively.

It is likely that there are several dementia syndromes in PD (Cummings 1988b). From a neurochemical perspective, dementia may be related to either dopaminergic or combined dopaminergic and cholinergic deficits (McPherson and Cummings, 1996). Alternatively, dementia might occur when damage of both the basal ganglia and several mutually interactive ascending neuronal pathways (including serotonergic, cholinergic, dopaminergic, and noradrenergic) reaches the threshold for expression of severe cognitive impairment (Dubois and Pillon 1998).

The most common cause of dementia in PD appears to be coexistent AD (Esiri and McShane 1997). Up to 35% of patients with PD with dementia have been found at autopsy to have the neuropathological hallmarks (neuritic plaques, neurofibrillary tangles, and granulovacuolar degeneration) of AD (Boller et al. 1980; Gaspar and Gray 1984; Hughes et al. 1993). However, AD does not account for all, or even the majority of, cases of dementia in PD. Some in-

vestigators (e.g., Ball 1984; Perry et al. 1983) have reported only an infrequent association between PD and AD, and dementia has been present in patients without cortical pathology (Xuereb et al. 1990). The observations that frontal cognitive deficits (Dubois et al. 1990) and severity of dementia (Nakano and Hirano 1984; Perry et al. 1985) are related to cholinergic abnormalities and that neuronal loss in the nucleus basalis of patients with PD with dementia is usually more severe than in those without dementia (Whitehouse et al. 1983) are mitigated by the observation that dementia in PD may occur in the absence of both Alzheimer-type changes and atrophy of the nucleus basalis (Helig et al. 1985). The role of AD in the dementia of PD is further clouded by the description of another neuropathological entity, namely dementia with Lewy bodies, and the recent observation that severity of dementia in patients with PD without AD changes was related to density of Lewy neurites in the hippocampal CA2 cell field (Churchyard and Lees 1997).

Dementia With Lewy Bodies

Kosaka et al. (1980) introduced the notion of a spectrum of Lewy body diseases, and they described a new clinicopathological entity characterized by Lewy bodies present not only in brainstem neurons but distributed throughout the cerebral cortex. The spectrum of Lewy body diseases includes several variants (Lennox and Lowe 1997): a cortical Lewy body variant characterized by cortical and brainstem Lewy bodies in the absence of plaques or tangles (most closely resembling what has been termed "pure" Lewy body disease); variants of cortical Lewy body disease with plaques and tangles (resembling cortical Lewy body disease with AD) or with only plaques; and a brainstem Lewy body disease variant (in which very few cortical Lewy bodies are seen), corresponding closely with the clinical correlate of PD. Lennox and Lowe (1997) define "Alzheimer's disease and Parkinson's disease" as an entity meeting pathological criteria for AD with the additional feature of brainstem but not cortical Lewy bodies. It remains debated whether dementia with Lewy bodies (DLB) is a distinct disease entity, a form of AD, or a form of PD. Proposed clinical criteria and neuropathological features of DLB (Table 26–9) will likely facilitate research to clarify this issue.

The clinical picture of DLB is heterogeneous. Kosaka (1990) noted that a dementia, often with cortical features (e.g., aphasia, apraxia), was the presenting syndrome in more than half the cases. Other cases may present initially with psychiatric disorders or extrapyramidal signs. Psychosis is estimated to occur in 60% of cases (Morris et al. 1998). Hallucinations (visual more often than auditory)

TABLE 26–9. Consensus criteria for the clinical diagnosis of probable and possible dementia with Lewy bodies (DLB) and pathological features associated with disease of DLB

Diagnostic criteria

1. The central feature required for a diagnosis of DLB is progressive cognitive decline of sufficient magnitude to interfere with normal social or occupational function. Prominent or persistent memory impairment may not necessarily occur in the early stages, but is usually evident with progression. Deficits on tests of attention and of frontosubcortical skills and visuospatial ability may be especially prominent.

2. Two of the following core features are essential for a diagnosis of probable DLB, and one is essential for possible DLB:

   a. Fluctuating cognition with pronounced variations in attention and alertness

   b. Recurrent visual hallucinations that are typically well formed and detailed

   c. Spontaneous motor features of parkinsonism

3. Features supportive of the diagnosis are

   a. Repeated falls

   b. Syncope

   c. Transient loss of consciousness

   d. Neuroleptic sensitivity

   e. Systematized delusions

   f. Hallucinations in nonvisual modalities

4. A diagnosis of DLB is less likely in the presence of

   a. Stroke disease, evident as focal neurological signs or on brain imaging

   b. Evidence on physical examination and investigation of any physical illness or other brain disorder sufficient to account for the clinical picture

Pathological features

Essential for diagnosis of DLB

Lewy bodies

Associated but not essential

   a. Lewy-related neurites

   b. Plaques (all morphological types)

   c. Neurofibrillary tangles

   d. Regional neuronal loss, especially brainstem (substantia nigra and locus ceruleus) and nucleus basalis of Meynert

   e. Microvacuolation (spongiform change) and synapse loss

   f. Neurochemical abnormalities and neurotransmitter deficits

Source. Adapted from McKeith et al. 1996.

have been estimated to occur in 20%–80% of cases (Morris et al. 1998), and more often in DLB than AD, but as frequently as in PD (Klatka et al. 1996). The estimated prevalence of delusions (often persecutory in nature) in DLB ranges between 20% and 80%. Delusions in DLB were found in one study to be as common as those found in AD, but more common than those found in PD (Klatka et al. 1996). Morris et al. (1998) recommended that nonpharmacological approaches to treating psychosis be used first, given the potential increased morbidity and mortality associated with use of conventional antipsychotics in DLB. When pharmacological intervention is necessary, the newer atypical antipsychotics (e.g., clozapine or risperidone) were recommended, although these are prescribed in lower than typical doses. Affective disturbances are common in DLB, and prevalence of depression has been estimated to be about 40% (Klatka et al. 1996; Weiner et al. 1996).

The dementia of DLB is characterized by pronounced impairments in attention, visuospatial and visuoconstructive functions, psychomotor speed, and memory retrieval (Salmon and Galasko 1996). When compared with AD, DLB involves more marked impairments in visuospatial, visuoconstructive, and attentional functions, and in lexical verbal fluency (Hansen et al. 1990; Salmon et al. 1996). When DLB is characterized by additional AD pathology, the dementia resembles a superimposition of the cognitive deficits of AD and PD (Salmon and Galasko 1996), although the memory deficit may be more pronounced in AD than DLB with AD pathology (Connor et al. 1998).

Clinical Features of Dementia in Parkinson's Disease: Cortical Versus Subcortical

Dementia is an acquired clinical syndrome, not a single entity or outcome. It may result from a number of etiologies and present in various forms depending on underlying neuropathology and which cognitive functions are most affected. Neuropsychological deficits have not been found to develop in a uniform manner during the progression of PD (Huber et al. 1989c).

Dementia syndromes have been subdivided on the basis of neurobehavioral deficits into two categories: cortical and subcortical (Cummings 1986). The prototypical cortical dementia is AD. Examples of subcortical dementia occur in PD, Huntington's disease, and progressive supranuclear palsy. Criticized because cortical and subcortical pathology eventually becomes evident in all dementias and because the features of dementias within a given class vary, the cortical-subcortical classification nonetheless serves as a useful clinical shorthand for describing cognitive and behavioral deficits early in the course of dementias. A comparison of the features of cortical and subcortical dementias is presented in Table 26–10. Such differences in the features between cortical and subcortical dementias are observable even on cognitive screening examinations such as the Dementia Rating Scale (Paolo et al. 1995).

Attention.   Performance on digit span is generally preserved in patients with PD with dementia (Huber et al. 1986, 1989b; Pillon et al. 1986). Performance on tasks requiring the self-allocation of attentional resources is impaired (Brown and Marsden 1988; Wright et al. 1990), and, as the disease progresses, patients may have difficulty performing tasks even when external cues are provided (Yamada et al. 1990).

Memory.   The memory deficits of PD, although variable in quality (Filoteo et al. 1997), are not as pervasive as those in AD. The diminished ability to learn and remember new information is characterized by predominantly a retrieval deficit, as evident from relatively preserved recogni-

tion, as opposed to free recall, and the ability to benefit from cuing. There may also be an increased reliance on serial encoding (remembering words in the order presented) and diminished semantic encoding (remembering words in clusters according to the semantic category to which they belong) (Buytenhuijs et al. 1994).

Spared early in the disease, remote memory becomes affected in PD with dementia (Freedman et al. 1984; Huber et al. 1986). However, the impairment is milder in PD than in AD. Furthermore, unlike in AD, in which the retrograde amnesia is characterized by a temporal gradient with relative preservation of memories of more distant than recent events, the remote memory impairment in PD with dementia is equally severe across previous decades of life.

Nondeclarative memory refers to "knowing how" and a form of remembering that can be expressed only through the performance of task operations. Performance on nondeclarative memory tasks appears task dependent. Early in PD, patients show intact priming (facilitation in processing a previously presented stimulus). Impairments in the learning of new motor, perceptual, and cognitive skills may or may not be evident (Ferraro et al. 1993; Heindel et al. 1989; Huberman et al. 1994; Knowlton et al.

TABLE 26–10.   **Comparison of cortical and subcortical types of dementia**

Feature	Cortical dementia	Subcortical dementia
Language	Aphasia	Relatively preserved
Memory functions		
Recall	Impaired	Impaired
Recognition cues	Ineffective	Effective
Encoding	Ineffective	Effective or mildly impaired
Priming	Absent	Present
Procedural	Intact	Impaired
Visuoperception	Severe impairment	Mild impairment
Calculation	Acalculia	Relatively preserved
Executive/frontal systems function	Proportionate to overall intellectual impairment	Affected greater than overall impairment
Speed of information processing	Normal	Slowed
Personality and mood	No insight; unconcerned; depression infrequent	Insight; apathetic; depression frequent
Motor functions		
Speech	Normal articulation until late	Dysarthria early
Motor speed	Normal until late	Slowed
Posture	Normal until late	Stooped, rigid
Gait	Normal until late	Abnormal
Coordination	Normal until late	Abnormal
Adventitious movements	Absent except for myoclonus late in course	Chorea, tremor, dystonia, and tics

Source.   Adapted from Ross et al. 1992.

1996). In contrast, patients with dementia typically perform poorly on nondeclarative memory tasks (Heindel et al. 1989).

Language. AD involves early difficulties with word finding as evident from poor performance on tests of lexical and semantic verbal fluency and visual confrontation naming. Spontaneous speech is characterized by circumlocutions and occasional paraphasias. The language impairments in AD progress to resemble a transcortical sensory aphasia (dysnomia, paraphasias, impaired written and auditory comprehension, and aphasic dysgraphia). Speech remains fluent, with relatively intact repetition and ability to read aloud (Cummings and Benson 1983).

Speech in PD is marked by hypophonia and dysarthria, with rare paraphasic errors. Mild impairments of word generation and retrieval early in PD are believed to be consistent with frontal lobe dysfunction (Matison et al. 1982). In PD with dementia, performance on lexical and semantic verbal fluency tasks is as poor as in AD (Tröster et al. 1998a), or even worse (Stern et al. 1993b). The visual confrontation naming impairment is less pronounced than that in AD (Tröster et al. 1996b, 1998a). Comprehension and writing (limited by motor impairments) are relatively preserved in PD.

Visuospatial functions. Impaired visuospatial and visuoconstructive abilities are characteristic of AD. Similar deficits have been found consistently in patients with PD with dementia relative to patients with PD without dementia and psychiatrically healthy control subjects, even when tasks minimize or eliminate motor demands (Globus et al. 1985; Huber et al. 1989b; Pillon et al. 1986). The results of studies comparing the abilities of groups with PD and AD are not conclusive. Huber et al. (1986) found that patients with AD outperformed patients with PD with dementia on Raven's Progressive Matrices (a test of spatial reasoning) (Raven 1958). In contrast, patients with PD performed better at Block Design than did the group with AD, suggesting more severe involvement of frontal systems in PD and more severe posterior hemispheric changes in AD. Visuospatial impairments do not improve with dopamine replacement and do not vary during "on" and "off" periods. If the dopamine deficit plays a role in these abnormalities, it must be in conjunction with other neurochemical or pathological processes (Pillon and Dubois 1989).

Executive functions. Executive functions depend critically on the integrity of the frontal lobes and their thalamostriatal connections, especially the dorsolateral circuit (Mega and Cummings 1994). Frontal lobe dysfunc-

tion in PD most likely results from the deficit of dopamine within the basal ganglia (Taylor et al. 1990b), although cholinergic dysfunction secondary to neuronal loss in the septal and basal nuclei has also been implicated (Dubois et al. 1990).

Executive deficits are especially notable on tasks requiring the self-initiated or internally guided planning and execution of information processing strategies. Poor performance of tasks that require coordination of mental and motor functions (e.g., resulting in frequent falling or poor operation of an automobile) has also been attributed to the disturbance of frontal-subcortical pathways. The loss of these abilities may be conditioned by visuospatial deficits leading to the defective planning and execution of strategies to accomplish a task (e.g., turning a corner while walking or driving) (Marsden 1982). This gives rise to the hypothesis that the basal ganglia serve as a subcognitive, internal navigational system that places limits on the options available to efficiently solve a problem (Robertson and Flowers 1990; Taylor et al. 1990b).

Affect. Disorders of mood are more extensively discussed below. In contrast to AD, depression is much more frequently seen in PD dementia. It is considered an important feature that distinguishes subcortical from cortical syndromes.

Neuroimaging

Structural neuroimaging. Brain-imaging studies often accompany the workup of the patient manifesting a dementia syndrome. These studies are most useful in eliminating the possibility of dementia secondary to a structural brain abnormality, such as a space-occupying lesion (tumor or vascular malformation) or hydrocephalus. The contribution of these studies to the evaluation of dementia secondary to other types of brain disease is less clear.

Cerebral atrophy is the most frequent finding of brain-imaging studies in neurodegenerative disorders. Computed tomography (CT) studies attempting to relate nonspecific measures of atrophy (e.g., ventricular enlargement or size of the sulci) with the severity of dementia, determined by less than rigorous neuropsychological criteria, have yielded conflicting results (deLeon and Ferris 1980; Wilson et al. 1982). Even when it was demonstrated that greater atrophy was present in patients with dementia, significant overlap was shown with the control groups.

Subsequent studies relating specific neuropsychological test results to measures of structural brain changes (from CT) (Inzelberg et al. 1987; Lichter et al. 1988) also failed to demonstrate strong relationships between measures of cortical atrophy and dementia. However, findings suggesting subcortical atrophy (e.g., increase in inter-caudate distance or ventricular enlargement) or frontal atrophy (e.g., increased width of the anterior interhemispheric fissure) were associated with the presence of cognitive dysfunction (Inzelberg et al. 1987; Starkstein and Leiguarda 1993).

Magnetic resonance imaging (MRI) provides more precise visualization of brain abnormalities including cerebral cortical loss, ventricular enlargement, and changes in the periventricular white matter. Despite this enhanced sensitivity, the correlation of MRI abnormalities and dementia in patients with PD parallels that of the CT studies (Huber et al. 1989a). Cerebral cortical atrophy correlates poorly with dementia. Findings consistent with subcortical atrophy (e.g., ventricular enlargement and increase in intercaudate width) were associated with cognitive impairment (Inzelberg et al. 1987; Korczyn et al. 1986; Lichter et al. 1988). Laakso et al. (1996) observed hippocampal atrophy in patients with PD both with and without dementia, and this atrophy might relate to memory impairment.

Functional neuroimaging. Functional neuroimaging studies in PD have utilized both single photon emission computed tomography (SPECT) and PET. SPECT studies of resting cerebral blood flow in PD with dementia have revealed frontotemporoparietal decreases (Sawada et al. 1992). Estimates of oxygen and glucose metabolism via the utilization of oxygen-15 ($^{15}O_2$) or ^{18}F-2-fluoro-2-deoxyglucose (^{18}FDG) are measurable by PET. Cerebral metabolism in patients with PD (without dementia) is decreased globally (especially in the frontal lobes) (Brooks and Frackowiak 1989) and related to psychometric test performance (Kuhl et al. 1984; Peppard et al. 1988). These findings would be consistent with the current concept that cognitive deficits in early PD are most likely symptomatic of frontal lobe dysfunction. However, ^{18}FDG PET studies in PD with dementia have generally revealed changes closely paralleling those in AD, that is, decreased glucose utilization in the posterior parietal and temporal areas (Otsuka et al. 1991; Wolfson et al. 1985). It is thus unclear whether metabolic changes in PD dementia reflect AD, DLB, or some other degenerative process (Brooks 1997).

In addition to providing measures of blood flow and metabolism during the resting state, PET has been used to demonstrate changes in cerebral blood flow and metabolism in response to activation with motor and cognitive tasks. Owen et al. (1998) recently demonstrated the importance of neostriatal outflow to frontal cortex in working memory and planning tasks, observing diminished internal

globus pallidus activation in PD during performance of these cognitive tasks. Motor activation studies have shown reduced lentiform nucleus (putamen and globus pallidus), anterior cingulate, supplementary motor area, and dorsolateral prefrontal cortex activation in PD when the patient is operating a joystick or extending the index finger (Brooks 1997). Activation studies in PD with dementia have not been carried out, but cognitive activation PET provides one avenue for exploring cerebral correlates of specific cognitive impairments.

PET also provides images that measure the binding of positron-emitting radiopharmaceuticals to specific neurochemical receptors. Numerous tracers are now available to study dopamine transport, storage, uptake, and binding. Initial studies suggest that such functional imaging is useful in detecting disease early, tracking PD progression, and evaluating graft survival (Brooks 1997). Studies have yet to take advantage of these techniques to demonstrate the role of dopaminergic abnormalities in neurobehavioral changes in PD.

Treatment of Dementia

The drugs piracetam and phosphatidylserine (both nootropics) have been the subjects of controlled clinical trials in the treatment of dementia in PD. Neither resulted in improvement of cognition (Fünfgeld et al. 1989; Sano et al. 1990). Selegiline appears to have no effect on cognition in early PD (Kieburtz et al. 1994). Other studies of the effects of selegiline on cognition are difficult to interpret, given the small numbers of patients studied and study differences in patient characteristics and assessment. One study reported that a dose of 5 mg selegiline twice per day was associated with modest improvements on the Mini-Mental State Exam (Folstein et al. 1975) in PD with dementia (Tarczy and Szirmai 1995). Cholinomimetics such as tacrine, which may be beneficial in AD, have not been used in controlled clinical trials, perhaps because they might exacerbate parkinsonism (Ott and Lannon 1992). Lieberman (1998) indicated that trials of donepezil (5 to 10 mg/day) or exelon (6–12 mg/day) may be useful in some patients but that such treatment can be accompanied by agitation and worsening of tremor.

■ Disease-Related Psychiatric Conditions

The psychiatric manifestations of PD may be as, or more, disabling than the motor dysfunction and may occur as a result of the disease itself or as a complication of pharmacotherapy for the motor symptoms of the disease. The specific disease-related syndromes are discussed below. Treatment-related syndromes are discussed in a subsequent section.

Depression

General considerations.

Parkinson's original description characterized his patients as manifesting melancholy and appearing dejected. Subsequent studies found a wide ranging prevalence of depression (7%–90%) in PD, with the most commonly accepted prevalence being about 40% (Cummings 1992). Approximately 50% of patients become depressed at some time during the disease (Dooneief et al. 1992; Mayeux 1982), and depression is present in up to one-third of patients at the time of their diagnosis (Santamaria et al. 1986). Recent studies (Hantz et al. 1994; Tandberg et al. 1996) suggest that minor depression, or dysthymia, might be more common than major depression in PD, but other studies indicate that approximately half the patients have a dysthymia and the other half have a major depression (Davous et al. 1995; Starkstein et al. 1990).

Both dysthymia and major depression deemed to be a feature of PD itself are defined in DSM-IV under the criteria for mood disorders due to a general medical condition (Table 26–11). These criteria make it clear that a mood disorder due to PD must be differentiated from an adjustment reaction. Although some patients develop depression in reaction to having PD and limitations in activities of daily living (e.g., Gotham et al. 1986), the diagnosis of an adjustment reaction in PD is rare. Numerous findings can be cited to support both a "reactive" and an "endogenous" basis for the depression in PD, but, as Brown and Jahanshahi (1995) pointed out, the debate about reactive versus endogenous depression in PD has become a sterile issue. They view the distinction as overly simplistic, and one that needs to be replaced by an interactionistic perspective.

Depression and cognitive impairment.

Depression in patients without PD is associated with cognitive deficits, particularly in the encoding and retrieval of information from memory (Zakzanis et al. 1998). Not surprisingly, depression also affects cognition and memory in PD. Given that depression is a risk factor for dementia in PD (Stern et al. 1993a), that depression exacerbates cognitive impairment in PD (Kuzis et al. 1997; Tröster et al. 1995a, 1995b) when the depression is sufficiently severe (Boller et al. 1998), and that depression is associated with more rapid declines over time in cognition and ability to successfully perform activities of daily living (Starkstein et al. 1992), it is

TABLE 26–11. DSM-IV diagnostic criteria for mood disorder as a result of Parkinson's disease

A. A prominent and persistent disturbance in mood predominates in the clinical picture and is characterized by either (or both) of the following:
　1. Depressed mood or markedly diminished interest or pleasure in all, or almost all, activities
　2. Elevated, expansive, or irritable mood

B. Evidence from the history, physical examination, or laboratory findings suggests that the disturbance is the direct physiological consequence of Parkinson's disease.

C. The disturbance is not better accounted for by another mental disorder (e.g., adjustment disorder with depressed mood in response to the stress of having Parkinson's disease).

D. The disturbance does not occur exclusively during the course of a delirium.

E. The symptoms cause clinically significant distress or impairment in social, occupational, or other important areas of functioning.

Specify types:

With depressive features: if the predominant mood is depressed, but the full criteria are not met for a major depressive episode

With major depressive-like episode: if the full criteria are met (except for criterion D) for a major depressive episode

With manic features: if the predominant mood is elevated, euphoric, or irritable

With mixed features: if the symptoms of both mania and depression are present but neither predominates

---

important to determine whether a dementia in PD is related to depression. Prompt treatment of depression is essential to enhance the patient's quality of life (Valldeoriola et al. 1997): treatment of depression may retard the rate of cognitive decline (Starkstein et al. 1992) and ameliorate depression-related functional decline (Cole et al. 1996). Unfortunately, no studies have examined the extent to which cognition and function improve with treatment of depression and whether such gains would be observed in patients with a depressive dementia or a depression overlaid on another dementia.

Pathophysiology.

Serotonergic pathophysiology has been more consistently linked to depression in PD than have dopaminergic and noradrenergic abnormalities. Several findings implicate serotonergic abnormalities in depression in PD. Studies of the cerebrospinal fluid of patients with PD with depression have shown decreased concentrations of the serotonin metabolite 5-hydroxy-indoleacetic acid (5-HIAA) (Kostic et al. 1987; Mayeux et al. 1984). Furthermore, depression improves following administration of 5-hydroxytryptophan (5-HTP), the precursor of serotonin, and concomitant increases in cerebrospinal fluid 5-HIAA (Mayeux et al. 1988; McCance-Katz et al. 1992). The brain content of serotonin at autopsy in patients with PD is reduced, and the raphe nuclei have a reduced ability to decarboxylate amino acids in PD.

A dopaminergic role in depression in PD is suggested by the finding of pronounced dopaminergic cell loss in the ventral tegmentum of patients with PD who are depressed (Torack and Morris 1988). Dose-related elevations in mood and reductions in anxiety were found in a placebo-controlled study of acute levodopa infusion in patients with motor fluctuations (Maricle et al. 1995), and this response is less pronounced in early PD (Maricle et al. 1998), presumably when dopaminergic depletion is not as pronounced as that in patients with motor fluctuations. The observation that chronic treatment with dopaminergic agents does not alleviate depression (but see Miyoshi et al. 1996) does not entirely discount a dopaminergic role in depression. Dopaminergic drugs may have a greater impact on the nigrostriatal than the mesolimbic system, which is more likely to be involved in depression. Indeed, in response to methylphenidate infusion, thought to activate the mesolimbic system, patients with PD who are depressed showed a much lesser euphoric response than patients with PD who are not depressed (Cantello et al. 1989). Evidence linking noradrenergic changes to depression in PD is generally based on the response of depression to tricyclics (Fields et al. 1998).

Functional neuroimaging studies have highlighted the involvement of frontosubcortical systems, and especially the paralimbic pathways linking frontal and temporal cortices and striatum, in depression in PD. Depression in PD has been associated with hypometabolism in the inferior orbital and anterior temporal cortex (Mayberg et al. 1990) and in the medial frontal and anterior cingulate cortex (Ring et al. 1994). Medial prefrontal blood flow abnormalities are also seen in patients without PD who are depressed, and they are more strongly related to cognitive dysfunction than to mood (Bench et al. 1993; Dolan et al. 1994). Dorsolateral and medial prefrontal regional cerebral blood flow (rCBF) normalization occurs with remission of depression (Bench et al. 1995), but it is unknown if cognitive dysfunction improves and if similar changes would be seen in patients with PD with depression. It is of interest that frontal dysfunction indexed by cognitive screening and

psychophysiological methods may be a harbinger of poor or delayed response to antidepressant treatment in the elderly (Kalayam and Alexopoulos 1999). Whether frontal dysfunction in PD might be related to treatment response remains to be investigated.

Clinical features. Among patients with PD and depression, approximately half have a major affective disorder and the other half have a dysthymia. Major depression and dysthymia differ in that the former is characterized by periods of depression separated by intervals with normal affect; the latter is a chronic condition with more mild mood changes. The depression is usually mild to moderate; very infrequently is it severe. Several features of depression in PD distinguish it from idiopathic depression (Meyerson et al. 1997): comorbid anxiety and panic, a relative lack of self-reproach and guilt, and a low suicide rate.

Clinical features of PD have been only inconsistently related to depression. Tentative evidence suggests that patients with an early disease onset age, with rapid disease progression, and in the early and advanced stages of the disease are more likely to be depressed (Brown and Jahanshahi 1995). There does not appear to be a linear or parallel relationship between depression and disease severity or between depression and disability. Cummings (1992) proposed that membership in patient groups with or without depression remains relatively stable over time, suggesting the possibility that there are two distinct disease types.

Treatment: pharmacotherapy. Before discussing specific drug therapy for depression in PD, we consider the effects of antiparkinsonian medication on mood. Levodopa therapy has been found to transiently improve mood, but this effect is rarely sustained (Shaw et al. 1980), and levodopa is not effective as an antidepressant (Mindham et al. 1976; Taylor and Saint-Cyr 1990). In addition, because of its effects on serotonin metabolism, levodopa may predispose to depression (Anderson and Aabro 1980). Pergolide does not ameliorate depression (Factor et al. 1995). Several other antiparkinsonian agents do, however, appear to improve mood in some cases. Bromocriptine (Jouvent et al. 1983; Sitland-Marken et al. 1990), anticholinergic drugs (e.g., trihexyphenidyl) (Kaspar et al. 1981), amantadine (Bavazzano and Guarducci 1980), and selegiline (Allain et al. 1993; Baronti et al. 1992; Eisler et al. 1981; Parkinson Study Group 1989) had beneficial effects on mood in some studies. It remains unknown if these agents are also useful in treating major depression. Should levodopa exacerbate the symptoms of depression, either lowering the dosage or combining it with one of the above agents may be effective in treating motor and depressive symptoms (Silver and Yudofsky 1992). The effects on mood of the newer dopamine agonists and COMT inhibitors remain to be documented.

Tom and Cummings (1998) provided an algorithm (Figure 26–3) for the treatment of depression in PD. A listing of some commonly used antidepressants and their neurotransmitter actions appears in Table 26–12. Few methodologically rigorous, controlled clinical trials of antidepressants in PD (Klaasen et al. 1995) have been performed. Among the 12 trials these authors defined as methodologically adequate, positive outcomes were reported for selegiline (10 mg/day), nortriptyline (100 mg/day), desipramine (100 mg/day), imipramine (30–75 mg in patients older than 55 years; 50–100 mg in patients younger than 55), and bupropion (maximum 450 mg).

The side-effect profiles of some commonly used antidepressants are detailed in Table 26–13. Because of the side effects, these medications require caution in their administration. Patients with PD are particularly sensitive to certain of these effects. Many experience orthostatic hypotension that may be exacerbated by drugs, resulting in syncope with injury (e.g., fractures and lacerations). Nortriptyline is less likely to cause postural hypotension than is imipramine (Roose and Glassman 1981). The anticholinergic effects of some agents may cause confusion and worsen preexisting cognitive problems. Among the heterocyclic antidepressants, desipramine and nortriptyline are less likely than amitriptyline to cause these effects. Trazodone and selective serotonin reuptake inhibitors (e.g., fluoxetine and sertraline) have no significant anticholinergic effects.

Several antidepressant agents, via different actions, are known to cause parkinsonian symptoms. These agents include amoxapine (which is metabolized to loxapine) (Thornton and Stahl 1984), fluoxetine (Bouchard et al. 1989), and phenelzine (Gillman and Sandy 1986; Waldmeier and Delini-Stula 1979). Fluoxetine has a known dopamine-antagonistic activity (Brod 1989). Steur (1993) reported a transient increase in parkinsonian signs and symptoms in four patients with PD taking fluoxetine (20 mg/day). On the other hand, Caley and Friedman (1982) reported no exacerbation of parkinsonian symptoms in 20 patients with PD with depression receiving up to 40 mg/day of fluoxetine. An additional three patients experienced mild worsening of symptoms. This antidepressant should be administered with caution to patients with PD. Bupropion is mildly dopaminergic and may induce dyskinesias or hallucinations.

Drugs that may offer specific advantages include selegiline, which, when given at dosages selective for MAO-B receptor activity, may improve mood (Parkinson Study Group 1989). Caution has been advised in using selegiline together with tricyclic antidepressants or selective serotonin reuptake inhibitors. Such combinations may give rise to "serotonin syndrome," the symptoms of which overlap with those of malignant neuroleptic syndrome and include tremor, agitation, restlessness, reduced consciousness, and hyperpyrexia. Nonetheless, Richard et al. (1997), based on a survey of investigators, concluded that adverse reactions to combinations of selegiline and antidepressants were rare. They concluded that, among 4,568 patients treated with selegiline and an antidepressant, 0.24% experienced symptoms consistent with a possible serotonin syndrome, and only 0.04% had serious adverse events. Trazodone and fluoxetine, by virtue of negligible anticholinergic properties, have little adverse effect on cognition. Sertraline and fluvoxamine have not been adequately evaluated in PD. An open-label pilot study found depression in PD to respond to sertraline (25 mg/day for 1 week, then 50 mg/day) (Hauser and Zesiewicz 1997). One case report supports the efficacy of fluvoxamine in treating depression in PD (McCance-Katz et al. 1992).

No long-term studies of antidepressant therapy in patients with PD have been conducted, although one study of 21 patients found that depression remitted in only four of these cases after a 2.5-year follow-up (Mayeux et al. 1988). Given the absence of long-term treatment studies, general principles of antidepressant drug therapy are applicable. Tom and Cummings (1998) suggest that an adequate trial should last at least 6 weeks. The drug should be titrated to the dose necessary (within the recommended guidelines) to achieve a satisfactory antidepressant effect in the absence of intolerable side effects. Once an adequate effect is achieved, therapy should be continued for at least 6 months before the medication is gradually tapered.

Plasma levels are not required for the management of patients receiving antidepressant therapy. Guidelines were developed by the American Psychiatric Association Task Force on the Use of Laboratory Tests in Psychiatry (1985) to determine optimal plasma levels in patients with major depression (excluding patients with neurodegenerative disorders, such as PD). An optimal trial of the medication is assumed when plasma levels fall within the guidelines. It is not known if the results of these determinations are applicable to more complicated clinical settings (i.e., in the setting of a documented brain disorder). Levels of imipramine and its desmethyl metabolite, desipramine, should be greater than 200–250 ng/mL; levels of desipramine, greater than 125 ng/mL; and a level of nortriptyline, between 50 and 150 ng/mL. Levels should be drawn 10–14 hours after the last dose.

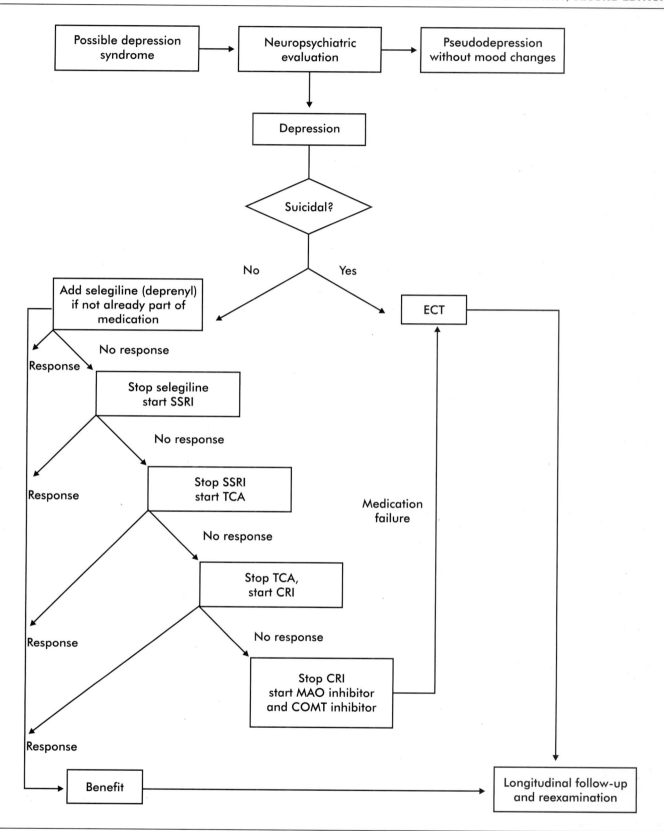

FIGURE 26–3. Algorithm for treatment of depression in Parkinson's disease (PD). COMT = catechol-*O*-methyltransferase; CRI = combined reuptake inhibitor; ECT = electroconvulsive therapy; MAO = monoamine oxidase; SSRI = selective serotonin (5-hydroxytryptamine; 5-HT) reuptake inhibitor; TCA = tricyclic antidepressant.
Source. Reprinted with permission from Tom T, Cummings JL: "Depression in Parkinson's Disease: Pharmacological Characteristics and Treatment." *Drugs Aging* 12:55–74, 1998. Copyright 1998 Adis International.

TABLE 26–12. Neurotransmitter effects of selected antidepressants

Agent (trade name)	Serotonin	Norepinephrine	Dopamine
Amitriptyline (Elavil)	++	+	0
Bupropion (Wellbutrin)	0	+	+[a]
Desipramine (Norpramin)	+	+++	+/−
Fluoxetine (Prozac)	+++	0	+/−[b]
Nefazodone (Serzone)	++[c]	+/−	0
Nortriptyline (Pamelor)	+	++	0
Sertraline (Zoloft)	+++	0	+/−[b]
Venlafaxine (Effexor)	+++	++	+[a]

Note. Values are approximations, derived from in vivo, in vitro, and clinical studies. +++ = marked effects; ++ = moderate effects; + = modest effects; +/− = minimal effects; 0 = virtually no effects.
[a]Dopaminergic effects probably significant only at higher doses.
[b]Selective serotonin reuptake inhibitors (SSRIs) have variable effects on dopamine, perhaps decreasing dopamine in some brain regions. However, sertraline has substantial dopamine reuptake inhibition compared with the other SSRIs, and this may have implications for its apparently beneficial effects on cognitive function in some patients.
[c]Nefazodone antagonizes the 5-HT$_2$ receptor but shows modest blockade of 5-HT reuptake.
Source. Adapted from Pies 1998.

Treatment: electroconvulsive therapy. Electroconvulsive therapy (ECT) has been shown to be effective in the treatment of psychiatric disorders, especially depression (Brandon et al. 1984; Faber and Trimble 1991; Gregory et al. 1985). In controlled comparisons with antidepressant medications, ECT has been demonstrated to be superior (Abrams 1988). Dating back to the 1950s (Lebensohn and Jenkins 1975; Savitsky and Karliner 1953; Shapiro and Goldberg 1957), ECT has been observed to also benefit the tremor and motor symptoms of patients with PD who are undergoing the procedure for depression, as well as to improve parkinsonism secondary to neuroleptic medications (Goswami et al. 1989). Furthermore, ECT improved the motor symptoms of patients with PD without psychiatric illness in five of six reports (in 22 of 34 patients) (Faber and Trimble 1991).

Several studies (Andersen et al. 1987; Douyon et al. 1989; Zervas and Fink 1991) have reported ECT to be effective in relieving depression and transiently improving the motor symptoms of PD. The total number of patients studied is, however, small: Faber and Trimble (1991) noted that between 1975 and 1991 there had been a total of 21 reports detailing ECT in 44 patients with PD and psychiatric morbidity. A recent retrospective study of 25 patients with PD and one or more of major depression with psychosis (4), major depression without psychosis (15), unspecified anxiety disorder (2), dementia (6), or unspecified other disorders (12) found improvements in mental state, depression, and anxiety (Moellentine et al. 1998). Transient improvement in 14 of the 25 patients' parkinsonian symptoms was found.

The primary indication for ECT in PD is in the treatment of depression, especially when antidepressant medications are ineffective or when side effects make them intolerable. The latter may include impairment of cognition, glaucoma, ileus, heart conduction block, or urinary retention. In addition, ECT may be preferable in life-threatening situations requiring a more rapid response (e.g., suicidal depression or malnutrition secondary to apathy and psychomotor retardation).

Other psychiatric uses of ECT include the treatment of mania (Small and Millstein 1986), which is uncommon in patients with PD. Roth et al. (1988) reported improvement in both motor and affective signs in a patient with PD with mania treated with ECT. ECT has been used effectively in the treatment of psychosis induced by dopaminergic therapy (see section on Drug-Related Psychiatric Conditions below).

TABLE 26–13. Side-effect profiles of selected antidepressants

Drug (trade name)	Anticholinergic (blurry vision, dry mouth, constipation)	Sedation/ drowsiness	Insomnia/ agitation	Orthostatic hypotension	Cardiac arrhythmia	Gastrointestinal distress/diarrhea	Weight gain
Amitriptyline (Elavil)	4	4	½	4	3	½	4
Bupropion (Wellbutrin)	0	½	2	0	½	1	0
Desipramine (Norpramin)	1	1	1	2	3	½	1
Doxepin (Sinequan)	3	4	½	3	2	½	3
Fluoxetine (Prozac)	0	½	2	0	½	3	0[a]
Imipramine (Tofranil)	3	3	1	4	3	1	3
Nefazodone (Serzone)	½	½	0	2	½	2	½
Nortriptyline (Pamelor)	1	2	½	1	2	½	2
Paroxetine (Paxil)	½	½	1	0	½	3	0[a]
Sertraline (Zoloft)	0	½	1	0	½	3	0[a]
Venlafaxine (Effexor)	½	½	2	0	½	3	0

Note. All values are rough guidelines and may vary according to dose, duration of treatment, and age of patient. 4 = high; 3 = moderately high; 2 = significant; 1 = modest; ½ = minimal; 0 = virtually none.

[a]Despite published data showing little or no weight gain with the selective serotonin reuptake inhibitors (SSRIs), clinical experience has shown that some patients, often after an initial period of weight loss, may gain substantial weight with fluoxetine, paroxetine, and perhaps other SSRIs.

Source. Adapted from Pies 1998.

Included with the risks of ECT are those attendant with the induction of and recovery from anesthesia. Psychotropic drugs are discontinued before ECT, and levodopa dosage should be reduced. The latter is required to minimize the occurrence of dyskinesias and post-treatment delirium, which may result from increased dopamine sensitivity. The cardiovascular risks of ECT are small (Kramer 1985), with a mortality of one death per 50,000 treatments. Neither permanent electroencephalographic changes nor subsequent spontaneous seizures follow ECT. Postictal confusion is common for up to 30 minutes after the procedure. In comparison to a control group of patients without PD undergoing ECT, patients with PD had a higher rate of complications (56% vs. 12% in the control group) (Moellentine et al. 1998). The most common complication was an intertreatment delirium (52%). Indeed, two other studies suggested that patients with PD may be at greater risk for prolonged delirium than other patients receiving ECT (Douyon et al. 1989; Figiel et al. 1991), suggesting that pathological changes in the basal ganglia may play a role in the pathogenesis of this mental status abnormality. Moellentine et al. (1998) also found that length of hospitalization was longer for the PD than the control group. Bilateral electrode placement results in some degree of memory impairment for at least 6 months (Weiner et al. 1986). However, unilateral electrode placement with brief pulse stimulation produces a memory disturbance no greater in ECT-treated patients than in antidepressant-treated control subjects.

ECT is safe and effective in patients with dementia in general (Tsuang et al. 1979). Moellentine et al. (1998) observed no relationship between dementia and the occurrence of prolonged delirium in PD and an increase in Mini-Mental State Exam scores after ECT in both the patient and control groups.

Mania

Manic behavior (occurring in 1%–5% of patients with PD) is rarely a manifestation of bipolar illness in PD; it is associated with levodopa therapy (Celesia and Barr 1970) and dementia. Hyperactivity may also occur as a manifestation of a schizophrenic-like disorder that has been described rarely in PD (Crow et al. 1976). Management is difficult because of the likelihood of the exacerbation of manic symptoms by levodopa and the risk of increasing extrapyramidal symptoms (e.g., tardive dyskinesia) by lithium.

Anxiety Disorders

Anxiety disorders such as generalized anxiety, panic, and social phobia occur in up to 40% of patients with PD, frequently with comorbid depression (Richard et al. 1996). Optimal treatments have not been established, but some guidelines are provided below and by Lieberman's (1998) algorithm (Figure 26–4).

Generalized anxiety disorder. Generalized anxiety is a frequent finding in patients with PD. Stein et al. (1990) found the disorder in 38% of patients with PD and with no relationship to their degree of motor disability or treatment with levodopa. Symptoms of anxiety or panic may also coexist with depression (Henderson et al. 1992; Schiffer et al. 1988; Starkstein et al. 1993).

Benzodiazepines are effective in the treatment of anxiety. In addition, they may be used in conjunction with antidepressants and are effective in counteracting the not infrequent occurrence of stimulant effects by small, initial doses of antidepressants (e.g., in the treatment of panic disorder). Buspirone, a nonbenzodiazepine with both anxiolytic and antidepressant properties, may be administered in conjunction with antidepressant drugs to treat coexistent anxiety (Fabre 1990). However, in a double-blind placebo-controlled crossover study of 16 patients with PD, buspirone in doses of 10–100 mg/day had no effect on anxiety, depression scales, or extrapyramidal symptoms (Ludwig et al. 1986).

Panic. Among 131 levodopa-treated patients with PD, Vázquez et al. (1993) found 24% to have recurrent panic attacks, with 90% of the attacks occurring during the "off" state. In cases with panic related to the "off" state, management of motor fluctuations is indicated. Panic disorder may be effectively treated with the heterocyclic antidepressants nortriptyline, desipramine, and imipramine or with fluoxetine (Silver and Yudofsky 1988).

Phobic disorder. Phobic disorders are characterized by irrational fear (fully defined by DSM-IV), such as fear of crowded places. Initially, fear manifested by patients with PD may be justified (e.g., fear of falling because of impaired postural reflexes), but later it may be exaggerated to include situations in which it is not reasonable. This disorder rarely begins before the onset of PD.

Obsessive-compulsive disorder. Obsessive-compulsive symptomatology (OCS) has been linked to dysfunction of the basal ganglia. OCS is sometimes present in disorders involving the basal ganglia (e.g., Gilles de la Tourette's syndrome, Huntington's disease, and Sydenham's chorea) and has been observed in postencephalitic parkinsonism. It has also been associated with lateralized brain abnormalities in both left and right hemispheres.

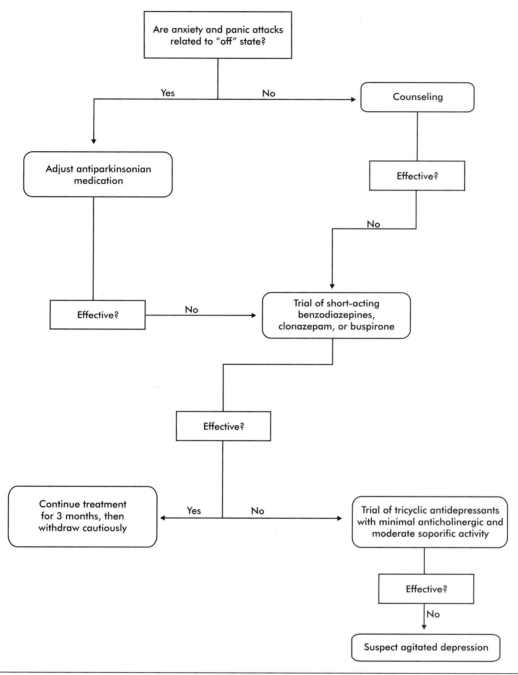

FIGURE 26–4.   Algorithm for treatment of anxiety in Parkinson's disease. Reprinted with permission from Lieberman A: "Managing the Neuropsychiatric Symptoms of Parkinson's Disease." *Neurology* 50 (suppl 6):S33–S38, 1998. Copyright 1998 Lippincott Williams & Wilkins.

Tomer et al. (1993), using the Leyton Obsessional Inventory (Cooper 1970), studied the relationship between OCS and the lateralization of motor symptoms in 30 patients with idiopathic PD. The severity of left-sided motor dysfunction was found to be a reliable predictor of the overall severity of OCS. The variables that most significantly correlated with left-sided motor impairment were overconscientiousness, repetition, disturbing thoughts, and obsessions with cleanliness. This may reflect a relatively greater deficiency of dopamine in the right basal ganglia of patients with PD manifesting OCS.

Psychosis

Symptoms of psychosis occur in up to 40% of patients with PD (Peyser et al. 1998). Based on their literature review,

Peyser et al. (1998) identified six types of psychotic disorders in PD: 1) hallucinations with preserved insight (usually in the context of dopaminergic treatment); 2) medication-induced psychoses (delusions, hallucinations, and/or thought disorder) without clouding of consciousness but partial or total loss of insight; 3) delirium (usually provoked by dopaminergic treatment or another medical condition); 4) schizophrenia-like psychoses not related to medications; 5) schizophrenia predating PD; and 6) other psychoses (including psychotic depression and mania). Many of the psychoses in PD not related to medical treatment have been the subject of case reports, and it is evident that most of the studies reveal psychotic disorders to usually occur with dopaminergic treatments or in the context of dementia. Recent studies indicate psychotic symptoms to be common in DLB, even in the absence of medications (Morris et al. 1998). No convincing association has been found between PD and psychosis (i.e., schizophrenia).

Drug-Related Psychiatric Conditions

Virtually every drug used in the treatment of PD can produce clinically significant psychiatric symptoms (for review, see Young et al. 1997). Included are the anticholinergics, amantadine, selegiline, levodopa, MAO-B inhibitors, and dopamine receptor agonists. These adverse effects significantly limit the efficacy of antiparkinsonian medication in some patients. Data reported in some studies regarding the incidence of certain effects (e.g., hallucinations, delusions, and delirium) may be inaccurate (i.e., underestimates) because of imprecise psychiatric interviewing techniques, the reluctance of patients and families to relate these disturbing events, and failure to distinguish the exact nature of the adverse effect.

Hallucinations

Visual hallucinations are the most common medication-induced side effect (tactile and auditory hallucinations are rare) and may occur with the use of any antiparkinsonian medication. The overall incidence is estimated to be about 20% and is greatest with the use of dopaminergic agents (Goetz et al. 1982). It is thought that bromocriptine has a greater potential to cause psychiatric side effects than levodopa.

Hallucinations most frequently occur in the absence of delirium, at night, and most often they involve seeing formed objects (e.g., people or animals) (Sanchez-Ramos et al. 1996). Sleep disturbances may also be present. Increasing age, a history of multiple-drug therapy, a premorbid history of psychiatric illness, and the use of

anticholinergic medications have been found to be predictors for the occurrence of hallucinations (Glantz et al. 1986; Tanner et al. 1983).

Hallucinatory syndromes differ depending on the offending agent. Anticholinergic drugs are more likely to produce hallucinations that are threatening, be combined with tactile or auditory components, and be accompanied by delirium (Goetz et al. 1982). Patients usually respond to decreasing the dosage of the causative agent(s). A few patients with PD experience benign hallucinations: vivid, nonthreatening visual hallucinations in the absence of delirium or other cognitive impairment, with insight remaining intact. Dosage reduction, if possible, is usually effective in lessening or eliminating hallucinations. An algorithm for the treatment of hallucinations and delirium (Olanow and Koller 1998) is presented in Figure 26–5.

Delusions

Delusions (false beliefs based on faulty inference, held despite evidence to the contrary, and ordinarily not accepted by members of a person's culture or subculture) have been reported with all types of antiparkinsonian medication. The reported incidence ranges from 3% to 30% (but may be higher if more scrupulously sought), and it is greater at higher doses.

If caused by levodopa, delusions may often be predicted by the occurrence of dreams and/or visual hallucinations (Klawans 1978). Delusions may occur in the setting of a clear or clouded sensorium (Moskovitz et al. 1978) and are typically of the paranoid type but may be self-persecutory. A case of amantadine-induced Othello syndrome (pathological jealousy) has also been described (McNamara and Durso 1991). Older patients with dementia are particularly susceptible (Fischer et al. 1990), and delusions are rarely associated with a schizophrenic-like thought disorder (Beardsley and Puletti 1971).

Management of delusions includes withdrawal of anticholinergic agents and amantadine and reduction of the dosage of levodopa or other dopaminergic drugs.

Treatment of Drug-Induced Psychoses

Drug-induced psychoses resulting from antiparkinsonian medications have been successfully treated using neuroleptic medications. They are limited by their tendencies to produce extrapyramidal symptoms and, thus, worsen the parkinsonism. Low dosages of molindone, thioridazine, perphenazine, and haloperidol may be administered with caution to alleviate symptoms (Hale and Bellizzi 1980). However, in our experience, a successful

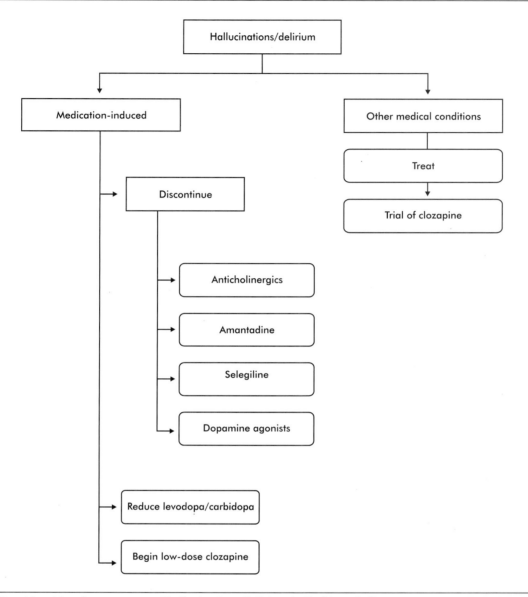

FIGURE 26–5. Algorithm for treatment of hallucinations/delirium in Parkinson's disease.
Source. Reprinted with permission from Olanow CW, Koller WC: "An Algorithm (Decision Tree) for the Management of Parkinson's Disease: Treatment Guidelines." *Neurology* 50 (suppl 3):S1–S57, 1998. Copyright 1998 Lippincott Williams & Wilkins.

result is rarely achieved because of exacerbation of the parkinsonian features with these drugs. In addition, L-tryptophan has been reported to reduce paranoid delusions in a few patients (Miller and Nieburg 1974).

Several newer, atypical antipsychotics, thought to produce fewer extrapyramidal side effects, have been evaluated in the treatment of psychotic symptoms (including delusions) in PD. The neurotransmitter receptor antagonism profile and the side-effect profile of some of these agents are presented in Tables 26–14 and 26–15, respectively.

Clozapine has been used successfully in the treatment of drug-induced psychosis. Auzou et al. (1996), in their review of studies detailing clozapine treatment in more than 200 patients, concluded that good results were obtained in 90% of patients without worsening of extrapyramidal symptoms. Indeed, some researchers have observed improvements in one or more of tremor, gait disorder, rigidity, bradykinesia, and dyskinesia with clozapine treatment (Bennett et al. 1994; Durif et al. 1997; Friedman and Lannon 1989, 1990; Friedman et al. 1997; Parkinson Study Group 1999). Clozapine may cause bone marrow suppression, and hematological monitoring (i.e., weekly complete blood counts) is required. However, one study (Ruggieri et al. 1997) reported no cases of agranulocytosis in 36 patients with PD who were treated for 12 months with a mean dosage of 10.59 ± 6.48 mg/day. In the Parkinson Study Group

TABLE 26–14. Relative receptor antagonism of atypical antipsychotic agents (trade names in parentheses)

Receptor	Risperidone (Risperdal)	Clozapine (Clozaril)	Olanzapine (Zyprexa)	Quetiapine (Seroquel)	Sertindole (SerLect)
D_2	1	+/–	½	+/–	4
$5\text{-}HT_{2A}$	3	2	1	+/–	4
M_1 (muscarinic cholinergic)	+/–	3	4	1	+/–
H_1 (histaminic)	½	4	2	1	+/–
α_1- adrenergic	2	1	½	½	4

Note. Data are semiquantitative comparisons of in vitro affinities for a given receptor. Values should not be compared "vertically"; for example, a "4" on D_2 antagonism may not be quantitatively equivalent to a "4" on α_2 antagonism in the same column. In vitro affinities do not always correspond with clinical effects. 4 = marked; 3 = substantial; 2 = moderate; 1 to ½ = slight; +/– = minimal; 5-HT = 5-hydroxytryptamine.
Source. Adapted from Pies 1998.

TABLE 26–15. Side effects of selected atypical antipsychotic agents (trade names in parentheses)

Side-effect profile[a]	Risperidone (Risperdal)	Clozapine[b] (Clozaril)	Olanzapine[b] (Zyprexa)	Quetiapine (Seroquel)	Sertindole (SerLect)
Extrapyramidal symptoms[c]	+	+/–	+/–	+/–	+/–
Tardive dyskinesia	?	+/–	?	?	?
Seizures	+/–	+++	+/–	+/–	+/–
Agranulocytosis	+/–	+++	+/–	+/–	+/–
Drowsiness	+	+++	++	+/+	+/–
Hypotension	+	++	+	+	+
Dizziness	+	++	+	+	+
Dry mouth	+/–	+	+	+	+/–
Constipation	+	++	+	+	+/–
Weight gain[d]	+	+++	+	+	+

Note. +++ = high incidence; ++ = moderate incidence; + = low incidence; +/– = negligible incidence; ? = data too preliminary.
[a]Based on various dosages of agents, with *no direct drug-to-drug comparisons available.*
[b]Values for clozapine and olanzapine not directly comparable with those in other tables because data may be derived from different sources.
[c]Sum of dystonia, parkinsonism, akathisia.
[d]Reports of weight gain are often underestimated during early experience with atypical antipsychotics; thus, weight gain with olanzapine, for example, may well prove to exceed the 5%–7% rates reported thus far.
Source. Adapted from Pies 1998.

(1999) study, only one patient treated with clozapine developed leukopenia. Clozapine has been associated with an increased risk of seizures, but the risk in patients with PD appears to be less than 1% (Factor et al. 1995).

Given its anticholinergic properties, clozapine must be used with caution in patients with dementia, who may be at increased risk for confusion (Factor et al. 1994). Indeed, lower dosages of clozapine are used in patients with PD than in patients with schizophrenia (Musser and Akil 1996). Factor et al. (1995) recommended a starting dose of 6.25–12.5 mg/day or every other day, which is increased by 12.5 mg every 4–7 days until symptoms are controlled.

Other new atypical antipsychotics have been studied in too few patients with PD to permit compelling conclusions about these agents' efficacy and safety in this disease. Nonetheless, some of these agents do show promise. Risperidone has been found to be effective and safe in some patients with PD (Ford et al. 1994; Meco et al. 1997; Rich et al. 1995), although motor symptoms may be exacerbated at higher doses. A recent study of 9 patients with PD and dementia found the drug to be effective and well tolerated without exacerbating motor symptoms or cognitive impairment (Workman et al. 1997). An initial study indicated that olanzapine (1–15 mg/day) was effective and well tolerated in 15 patients with PD without dementia with drug-induced psychoses (Wolters et al. 1996). Olanzapine may also be effective in PD patients with dementia (Aarsland et al. 1999). Quetiapine has been evaluated in only two cases with PD (Parsa and Bastani 1998). Remoxipride may be effective in controlling psychosis in PD (Lang et al. 1995; Mendis et al. 1994), but higher doses (mean 161 mg/day) may worsen parkinsonism in a significant percentage of patients. Zotepine (not available in the United States) failed to improve psychosis without worsening motor symptoms in two studies (Arnold et al. 1994; Spieker et al. 1995). New serotonin antagonists such as ondansetron (Zoldan et al. 1995) and mianserin (Ikeguchi and Kuroda 1995) have also had inadequate evaluation in PD. Although efficacy data are encouraging, the cost of ondansetron may be prohibitive.

Confusion/Delirium/Cognitive Impairment

The terms confusion and delirium are often used interchangeably and refer to a syndrome consisting of an altered state of consciousness, incoherent speech, altered psychomotor activity, memory impairment, and sudden onset and rapid fluctuation. Mild forms may go unrecognized. This syndrome has been noted to complicate all forms of antiparkinsonian therapy with a prevalence of 5%–25% and seems to be more frequent among

higher-potency ergot derivatives (e.g., bromocriptine and pergolide). Confusional states are likely to be induced by anticholinergic agents, especially in those patients with preexisting cognitive impairment (Saint-Cyr et al. 1993). One algorithm for treatment of cognitive impairment is presented in Figure 26–6. Agitation may occur with or without delirium. An algorithm for treatment of agitation is presented in Figure 26–7.

Depression

Table 26–16 lists DSM-IV criteria for substance-induced mood disorders. Despite its mood-elevating effects in some patients with PD, levodopa has also been implicated in causing depression. Huber et al. (1988) found that patients with PD and depression had taken the drug for longer periods and were receiving significantly higher dosages than were patients with PD without depression. However, the prevalence range of depressive symptoms in patients with PD treated with levodopa compared with those untreated is approximately the same, ranging from 2% to 50%. Levodopa may affect the appearance of depressive symptoms but not make them more prevalent. Treatment of depression in the setting of levodopa therapy is by the conventional use of antidepressants and ECT.

Mania

Levodopa has the capability of mood elevation along a spectrum from a simple feeling of well-being to full-blown episodes of mania (elation, grandiosity, pressured speech, racing thoughts, hyperactivity, reduced requirement for sleep, increased libido, and risk-taking behavior) (Celesia and Barr 1970; Ryback and Schwab 1971). Pergolide has also been reported to cause mania (Lang and Quinn 1982). In patients with PD with a *premorbid* history of mania, hypomania has resulted from levodopa and bromocriptine therapy (Goodwin 1971; Jouvent et al. 1983). It usually subsides with dosage reduction.

Anxiety

Symptoms of anxiety and panic (e.g., apprehension, irritability, nervousness, feelings of impending doom, palpitations, and hyperventilation) have been attributed to levodopa therapy, especially when occurring in patients not so predisposed before the onset of PD (Celesia and Barr 1970). Those with similar prior symptomatology have reported worsening of their anxiety syndromes (Rondot et al. 1984). Pergolide and selegiline (in combination with levodopa) therapies have also been associated with a significant incidence of anxiety (Lang and Quinn 1982; Yahr et al. 1983). Anxiety occurs in approximately two-thirds of

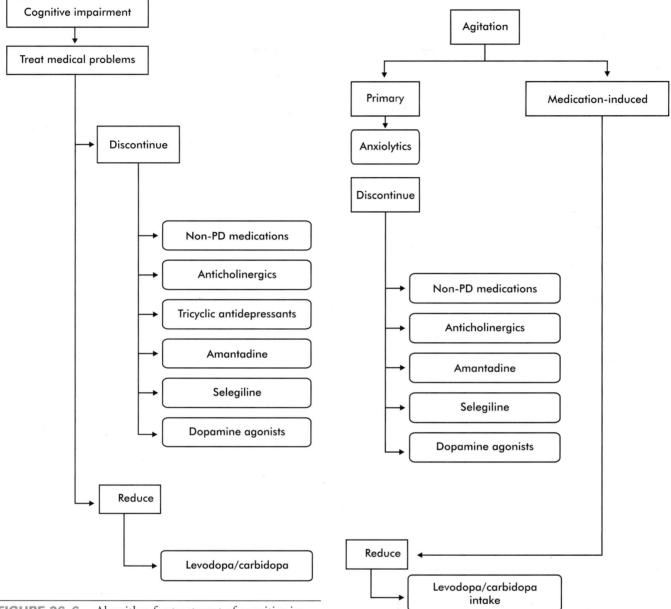

FIGURE 26–6. Algorithm for treatment of cognitive impairment in Parkinson's disease (PD).
Source. Reprinted with permission from Olanow CW, Koller WC: "An Algorithm (Decision Tree) for the Management of Parkinson's Disease: Treatment Guidelines." *Neurology* 50 (suppl 3):S1–S57, 1998. Copyright 1998 Lippincott Williams & Wilkins.

FIGURE 26–7. Algorithm for treatment of agitation in Parkinson's disease (PD).
Source. Reprinted with permission from Olanow CW, Koller WC: "An Algorithm (Decision Tree) for the Management of Parkinson's Disease: Treatment Guidelines." *Neurology* 50 (suppl 3):S1–S57, 1998. Copyright 1998 Lippincott Williams & Wilkins.

patients with motor fluctuations, especially in the "off" state (Nissenbaum et al. 1987). Treatment is by adjustment (usually reduction) of the agent and use of anxiolytic agents (e.g., benzodiazepines).

Altered Sexual Behavior

Increased libido, resulting from antiparkinsonian therapy, may occur in conjunction with or in the absence of a manic syndrome. Its expression may range from a renewed sexual interest with increased potency to a pathological state (i.e., hypersexuality). Increases in libido in case series reports range from 1% to 10% but may be more frequent. Hypersexuality may be manifested by increased masturbation or sexual intercourse. Males are predominantly

TABLE 26–16. DSM-IV diagnostic criteria for substance-induced mood disorder

A. A prominent and persistent disturbance in mood predominates in the clinical picture and is characterized by either (or both) of the following:

   1. Depressed mood or markedly diminished interest or pleasure in all, or almost all, activities

   2. Elevated, expansive, or irritable mood

B. There is evidence from the history, physical examination, or laboratory findings of either items 1 or 2:

   1. The symptoms in criterion A developed during, or within a month of, substance intoxication or withdrawal

   2. Medication use is etiologically related to the disturbance

C. The disturbance is not better accounted for by a mood disorder that is not substance-induced. Evidence that the symptoms are better accounted for by a mood disorder that is not substance-induced might include the following: the symptoms precede the onset of the substance use (or medication use); the symptoms persist for a substantial period of time (e.g., about a month) after the cessation of acute withdrawal or severe intoxication or are substantially in excess of what would be expected, given the type or amount of the substance used or the duration of use; or other evidence suggests the existence of an independent non–substance-induced mood disorder (e.g., a history of recurrent major depressive episodes).

D. The disturbance does not occur exclusively during the course of a delirium.

E. The symptoms cause clinically significant distress or impairment in social, occupational, or other important areas of functioning.

Specify types:

With depressive features: if the predominant mood is depressed

With manic features: if the predominant mood is elevated, euphoric, or irritable

With mixed features: if symptoms of both mania and depression are present and neither predominates

---

affected, and levodopa is the most common causative agent (Harvey 1988; Vogel and Schifter 1983). The behavior has also been reported with pergolide (Quinn et al. 1984). Sexually deviant behavior has been reported in patients with PD both with and without a history but is more likely in those with a predisposition. Paraphiliac disorders that have been reported include sexual masochism, pedophilia, voyeurism, sadomasochistic fantasies, and exhibitionism.

Sleep Disturbances

Sleep disturbances are more likely in patients with PD with drug-related psychiatric conditions, although sleep disturbance can be a manifestation of PD itself, depression, pain, nightmares, and dyskinesias (Olanow and Koller 1998). Vivid dreams and nightmares complicate both levodopa and pergolide treatment (Lang and Quinn 1982). Sleep studies in patients with PD have found diminished stage III and IV sleep, with multiple arousals and awakenings (Emser et al. 1988). Hypnotic agents (e.g., chloral hydrate or benzodiazepines) and antidepressants (if the sleep disorder is related to depression) may be effective.

Summary

Cognitive and psychiatric disorders are important aspects of the clinical syndrome resulting from PD. Although the motor symptoms often receive the majority of attention, deterioration of the mental state is not uncommon and virtually inevitable if the disease is long-standing. Behavioral disturbances may result from the disease itself and from medical and surgical treatments used to improve motor function.

Following recognition of changes in the mental state, it is necessary to distinguish those who may be more likely to respond to treatment (e.g., patients with depression and drug-induced psychosis) from those who will not (e.g., patients with dementia and bradyphrenia). This determination will be facilitated when specific diagnostic guidelines are formulated that take into account both the behavioral and the motor manifestations of PD. For the neuropsychiatric manifestations, effective therapies (e.g., drug and ECT) are available and may significantly improve the quality of life of the patient with PD.

References

Aarslandd, Larsen JP, Lim NG, et al: Olanzapine for psychosis in patients with Parkinson's disease with and without dementia. J Neuropsychiatry Clin Neurosci 11:392–394, 1999

Abrams R: Electroconvulsive Therapy. New York, Oxford University Press, 1988

Adler CH, Sethi KD, Hauser RA, et al: Ropinirole for the treatment of early Parkinson's disease. Neurology 49:393–399, 1997

Allain H, Pollak P, Neukirch HC: Symptomatic effect of selegiline in *de novo* parkinsonian patients: the French Selegiline Multicenter Trial. Mov Disord 8 (suppl 1): S36–S40, 1993

Alterman RL, Kelly P, Sterio D, et al: Selection criteria for unilateral posteroventral pallidotomy. Acta Neurochir Suppl (Wien) 68:18–23, 1997

American Psychiatric Association: Diagnostic and Statistical Manual of Mental Disorders, 4th Edition. Washington, DC, American Psychiatric Association, 1994

American Psychiatric Association Task Force on the Use of Laboratory Tests in Psychiatry: Blood level measurements and clinical outcome: an APA Task Force report. Am J Psychiatry 142:155–162, 1985

Andersen K, Balldin J, Gottfries CG, et al: A double-blind evaluation of electroconvulsive therapy in Parkinson's disease with "on-off" phenomena. Acta Neurol Scand 76:191–199, 1987

Anderson J, Aabro E: Antidepressant treatment in Parkinson's disease: a controlled trial of the effect of nortriptyline in patients with Parkinson's disease treated with L-dopa. Acta Neurol Scand 62:210–219, 1980

Aquilonius SM, Hartvig P: A Swedish country with unexpected high utilization of antiparkinsonian drugs. Acta Neurol Scand 74:379–382, 1986

Arnold G, Trenkwalder C, Schwartz J, et al: Zotepine reversibly induces akinesia and rigidity in Parkinson's disease patients with resting tremor or drug induced psychosis. Mov Disord 9:238–240, 1994

Ashok PP, Radhakrishan K, Sridharan R, et al: Parkinsonism in Benghazi, East Libya. Clin Neurol Neurosurg 88:109–113, 1986

Auzou P, Ozsancak C, Hannequin D, et al: Clozapine for the treatment of psychosis in Parkinson's disease: a review. Acta Neurol Scand 94:329–336, 1996

Baas H, Beiske AG, Ghika J, et al: Catechol-*O*-methyltransferase inhibition with tolcapone reduces the "wearing off" phenomenon and levodopa requirements in fluctuating parkinsonian patients. J Neurol Neurosurg Psychiatry 63:421–428, 1997

Ball M: The morphological basis of dementia in Parkinson's disease. Can J Neurol Sci 11:180–184, 1984

Barbeau A, Pourcher E: New data on the genetics of Parkinson's disease. Can J Neurol Sci 9:53–60, 1982

Baron MS, Vitek JL, Bakay RAE, et al: Treatment of advanced Parkinson's disease by posterior Gpi pallidotomy: 1-year results of a pilot study. Ann Neurol 40:355–366, 1996

Baronti F, Davis TL, Boldry RC, et al: Deprenyl effects on levodopa pharmacodynamics, mood, and free radical scavenging. Neurology 42:541–544, 1992

Bavazzano A, Guarducci R: Clinical trial with amantadine and hydergine in elderly patients. Journal of Clinical Neuropsychology 2:289–299, 1980

Beardsley JV, Puletti F: Personality (MMPI) and cognitive (WAIS) changes after levodopa treatment. Arch Neurol 25:145–150, 1971

Beatty WW, Staton RD, Weir WS, et al: Cognitive disturbances in Parkinson's disease. J Geriatr Psychiatry Neurol 2:22–33, 1989

Benabid AL, Pollak P, Gao D, et al: Chronic electrical stimulation of the ventralis intermedius nucleus of the thalamus as a treatment of movement disorders. J Neurosurg 84:203–214, 1996

Bench CJ, Friston KJ, Brown RG, et al: Regional cerebral blood flow in depression measured by positron emission tomography: the relationship with clinical dimensions. Psychol Med 23:579–590, 1993

Bench CJ, Frackowiak RS, Dolan RJ: Changes in regional blood flow on recovery from depression. Psychol Med 25:247–261, 1995

Bennett JP, Landow ER, Dietrich S, et al: Suppression of dyskinesias in advanced Parkinson's disease: moderate daily clozapine doses provide long-term dyskinesia reduction. Mov Disord 9:409–414, 1994

Biggins CA, Boyd JL, Harrop FM, et al: A controlled, longitudinal study of dementia in Parkinson's disease. J Neurol Neurosurg Psychiatry 55:566–571, 1992

Boller F, Mizutani R, Roessmann U, et al: Parkinson's disease, dementia and Alzheimer's disease: clinicopathologic correlations. Ann Neurol 7:329–335, 1980

Boller F, Marcie P, Starkstein S, et al: Memory and depression in Parkinson's disease. European Journal of Neurology 5:291–295, 1998

Bondi MW, Tröster AI: Parkinson's disease: neurobehavioral consequences of basal ganglia dysfunction, in Handbook of Neuropsychology and Aging. Edited by Nussbaum PD. New York, Plenum, 1997, pp 216–245

Bondi MW, Kaszniak AW, Bayles KA, et al: Contributions of frontal system dysfunction to memory and perceptual abilities in Parkinson's disease. Neuropsychology 7:89–102, 1993

Bouchard RH, Bourcher E, Vincent P: Fluoxetine and extrapyramidal side effects. Am J Psychiatry 146:1352–1353, 1989

Brandon S, Cowley P, McDonald C, et al: Electroconvulsive therapy: results in depressive illness from the Leicestershire trial. BMJ 288:22–25, 1984

Brod TM: Fluoxetine and extrapyramidal side effects. Am J Psychiatry 146:1352–1353, 1989

Brooks DJ: PET and SPECT studies in Parkinson's disease. Baillieres Clin Neurol 6:69–87, 1997

Brooks DJ, Frackowiak R: PET and movement disorder. J Neurol Neurosurg Psychiatry 52 (suppl):68–77, 1989

Brooks DJ, Torjanski N, Burn DJ: Ropinirole in the symptomatic treatment of Parkinson's disease. J Neural Transm Suppl 45:231–238, 1995

Brown R, Jahanshahi M: Depression in Parkinson's disease: a psychosocial viewpoint, in Advances in Neurology Series, Vol 65. Edited by Weiner JA, Lang AE. New York, Raven, 1995, pp 61–84

Brown RG, Marsden CD: How common is dementia in Parkinson's disease? Lancet 2:1262–1265, 1984

Brown RG, Marsden CD: Visuospatial function in Parkinson's disease. Brain 109:987–1002, 1986

Brown RG, Marsden CD: Internal versus external cues and the control of attention in Parkinson's disease. Brain 111: 323–345, 1988

Burchiel KJ: Thalamotomy for movement disorders. Neurosurg Clin N Am 6:55–71, 1995

Buytenhuijs EL, Berger HJC, Van Spaendonck KPM, et al: Memory and learning strategies in patients with Parkinson's disease. Neuropsychologia 32:335–342, 1994

Cahn DA, Sullivan EV, Shear PK, et al: Neuropsychological and motor functioning after unilateral anatomically guided posterior ventral pallidotomy: pre-operative performance and three-month follow-up. Neuropsychiatry Neuropsychol Behav Neurol 11:136–145, 1998

Caley CF, Friedman JH: Does fluoxetine exacerbate Parkinson's disease? J Clin Psychiatry 53:278–282, 1982

Cantello R, Maguggia M, Gilli M, et al: Major depression in Parkinson's disease and the mood response to intravenous methylphenidate: possible role of the "hedonic" dopamine synapse. J Neurol Neurosurg Psychiatry 52:724–731, 1989

Caparros-Lefebvre D, Blond S, Pécheux N, et al: Évaluation neuropsychologique avant et après stimulation thalamique chez 9 parkinsoniens. Rev Neurol (Paris) 148:117–122, 1992

Celesia GG, Barr AN: Psychosis and other psychiatric manifestations of levodopa therapy. Arch Neurol 23:193–200, 1970

Charcot JM: Lectures on Diseases of the Nervous System, Vol 1. English translation by Sigerson G. London, New London Society, 1878

Churchyard A, Lees AJ: The relationship between dementia and direct involvement of the hippocampus and amygdala in Parkinson's disease. Neurology 49:1570–1576, 1997

Cole SA, Woodard JL, Juncos JL, et al: Depression and disability in Parkinson's disease. J Neuropsychiatry Clin Neurosci 8:20–25, 1996

Connor DJ, Salmon DP, Sandy TJ, et al: Cognitive profiles of autopsy-confirmed Lewy body variant vs pure Alzheimer's disease. Arch Neurol 55:994–1000, 1998

Cooper J: The Leyton Obsessional Inventory. Psychol Med 1:48–64, 1970

Crow TJ, Johnstone EC, McClelland HA: The coincidence of schizophrenia and parkinsonism: some neurochemical implications. Psychol Med 6:227–233, 1976

Cummings JL: Subcortical dementia: neuropsychology, neuropsychiatry and pathophysiology. Br J Psychiatry 149: 682–687, 1986

Cummings JL: The dementias of Parkinson's disease: prevalence, characteristics, neurobiology, and comparison with dementia of the Alzheimer type. Eur Neurol 28 (suppl 1):15–23, 1988a

Cummings JL: Intellectual impairment in Parkinson's disease: clinical, pathologic, and biochemical correlates. J Geriatr Psychiatry Neurol 1:24–36, 1988b

Cummings JL: Depression and Parkinson's disease: a review. Am J Psychiatry 149:443–454, 1992

Cummings JL, Benson DF: Dementia: A Clinical Approach. Boston, MA, Butterworths, 1983

Cummings JL, Benson DF: Dementia: A Clinical Approach, 2nd Edition. Boston, MA, Butterworth-Heinemann, 1992

Cummings JL, Darkins A, Mendez M, et al: Alzheimer's disease and Parkinson's disease: comparison of speech and language alterations. Neurology 38:680–684, 1988

Curtis L, Lees AJ, Stern GM, et al: Effect of L-dopa on the course of Parkinson's disease. Lancet 2:211–212, 1984

Davous P, Auquier P, Grignon S, et al: A prospective study of depression in French patients with Parkinson's disease: the Depar study. European Journal of Neurology 2:455–461, 1995

deLeon MJ, Ferris SH: Computed tomography evaluation of brain-behavior relationships in senile dementia of the Alzheimer's type. Neurobiol Aging 1:59–79, 1980

Dolan RJ, Bench CJ, Brown RG, et al: Neuropsychological dysfunction in depression: the relationship to regional cerebral blood flow. Psychol Med 24:849–857, 1994

Dooneief G, Mirabello E, Bell K, et al: An estimate of the incidence of depression in idiopathic Parkinson's disease. Arch Neurol 49:305–307, 1992

Douyon R, Serby M, Klutchko B, et al: ECT and Parkinson's disease revisited: a "naturalistic" study. Am J Psychiatry 146:1451–1455, 1989

Dubois B, Pillon B: Cognitive and behavioral aspects of movement disorders, in Parkinson's Disease and Movement Disorders, 3rd Edition. Edited by Jankovic J, Tolosa E. Baltimore, MD, Williams & Wilkins, 1998, pp 837–858

Dubois B, Pillon B, Lhermitte F, et al: Cholinergic deficiency and frontal dysfunction in Parkinson's disease. Ann Neurol 28:117–121, 1990

Durif F, Vidailhet M, Assal F, et al: Low-dose clozapine improves dyskinesias in Parkinson's disease. Neurology 48: 658–662, 1997

Eisler T, Teravainen H, Nelson R, et al: Deprenyl in Parkinson's disease. Neurology 31:19–23, 1981

Emser W, Brenner M, Stober T, et al: Changes in nocturnal sleep in Huntington's and Parkinson's diseases. J Neurol 235:177–179, 1988

Esiri MM, McShane RH: Parkinson's disease and dementia, in The Neuropathology of Dementia. Edited by Esiri MM, Morris JH. Cambridge, Cambridge University Press, 1997, pp 174–193

Faber R, Trimble MR: Electroconvulsive therapy in Parkinson's disease and other movement disorders. Mov Disord 6:293–303, 1991

Fabre LF: Buspirone in the management of major depression: a placebo-controlled comparison. J Clin Psychiatry 51 (suppl):55–61, 1990

Factor SA, Brown D, Molho ES, et al: Clozapine: a two year open trial in Parkinson's disease patients with psychosis. Neurology 44:544–546, 1994

Factor SA, Molho ES, Podskalny GD, et al: Parkinson's disease: drug-induced psychiatric states, in Advances in Neurology Series, Vol 65. Edited by Weiner JA, Lang AE. New York, Raven, 1995, pp 115–138

Fazzini E, Dogali M, Sterio D, et al: Stereotactic pallidotomy for Parkinson's disease: a long-term follow-up of unilateral pallidotomy. Neurology 48:1273–1277, 1997

Ferraro FR, Balota DA, Connor LT: Implicit memory and the formation of new associations in nondemented Parkinson's disease individuals and individuals with senile dementia of the Alzheimer type: a serial reaction time (SRT) investigation. Brain Cogn 21:163–180, 1993

Fields JA, Tröster AI: Cognitive outcomes after deep brain stimulation for Parkinson's disease: a review of initial studies and recommendations for future research. Brain Cogn (in press)

Fields JA, Norman S, Straits-Tröster KA, et al: The impact of depression on memory in neurodegenerative disease, in Memory in Neurodegenerative Disease: Biological, Cognitive and Clinical Perspectives. Edited by Tröster AI. Cambridge, Cambridge University Press, 1998, pp 314–337

Fields JA, Tröster AI, Wilkinson SB, et al: Cognitive outcome following staged bilateral pallidal stimulation for the treatment of Parkinson's disease. Clin Neurol Neurosurg (in press)

Figiel GS, Hassen MA, Zorumski C, et al: ECT-induced delirium in depressed patients with Parkinson's disease. J Neuropsychiatry Clin Neurosci 3:405–411, 1991

Filoteo JV, Rilling LM, Cole B, et al: Variable memory profiles in Parkinson's disease. J Clin Exp Neuropsychol 19:878–888, 1997

Fischer P, Danielczyk W, Simyani M, et al: Dopaminergic psychosis in advanced Parkinson's disease, in Advances in Neurology Series, Vol 53. Edited by Streifter MB, Korczyn AD, Melamed E, et al. New York, Raven, 1990, pp 391–397

Folstein MF, Folstein SE, McHugh PR: Mini-Mental State: a practical method for grading the cognitive state of patients for the clinician. J Psychiatr Res 12:189–198, 1975

Ford B, Lynch T, Greene P: Risperidone in Parkinson's disease (letter). Lancet 344:681, 1994

Freedman M, Rivoira P, Butters N, et al: Retrograde amnesia in Parkinson's disease. Can J Neurol Sci 11:297–301, 1984

Friedman JH, Lannon MC: Clozapine in the treatment of psychosis in Parkinson's disease. Neurology 39:1219–1221, 1989

Friedman JH, Lannon MC: Clozapine-responsive tremor in Parkinson's disease. Mov Disord 5:225–229, 1990

Friedman JH, Epstein M, Sanes JN, et al: Gamma knife pallidotomy in advanced Parkinson's disease. Ann Neurol 39:535–538, 1996

Friedman JH, Koller WC, Lannon MC, et al: Benztropine versus clozapine in the treatment of tremor in Parkinson's disease. Neurology 48:1077–1081, 1997

Fünfgeld EW, Baggen M, Nedwidek P, et al: Double-blind study with phosphatidylserine in parkinsonian patients with senile dementia of the Alzheimer's type. Prog Clin Biol Res 317:1235–1246, 1989

Gabrieli JDE, Singh J, Stebbins G, et al: Reduced working memory span in Parkinson's disease: evidence for the role of a frontostriatal system in working and strategic memory. Neuropsychology 10:322–332, 1996

Gálvez-Jiménez N, Lozano AM, Duff J, et al: Bilateral pallidotomy: amelioration of incapacitating levodopa-induced dyskinesias but accompanying cognitive decline (abstract). Mov Disord 11 (suppl 1):242, 1996

Gaspar P, Gray F: Dementia in idiopathic Parkinson's disease. Acta Neuropathol 64:43–52, 1984

Gelb DJ, Oliver E, Gilman S: Diagnostic criteria for Parkinson's disease. Arch Neurol 56:33–39, 1999

Ghika J, Villemure J-G, Frankhauser H, et al: Efficiency and safety of bilateral contemporaneous pallidal stimulation (deep brain stimulation) in levodopa-responsive patients with Parkinson's disease with sever motor fluctuations: a 2-year follow-up review. J Neurosurg 89:713–718, 1998

Gibb WR: The neuropathology of Parkinson's disease, in Parkinson's Disease and Movement Disorders. Edited by Jankovic J, Tolosa E. Baltimore, MD, Urban & Schwarzenberg, 1988, pp 205–223

Gillman MA, Sandy KR: Parkinsonism induced by a monoamine oxidase inhibitor. Postgrad Med J 62:235–236, 1986

Glantz RH, Bieliauskuas L, Paleogos N: Behavioral indicators of hallucinosis in levodopa-treated Parkinson's disease, in Advances in Neurology Series, Vol 45. Edited by Yahr MD, Bergmann KJ. New York, Raven, 1986, pp 417–420

Glatt SL, Hubble JP, Lyons K, et al: Risk factors for dementia in Parkinson's disease: effect of education. Neuroepidemiology 15:20–25, 1996

Globus M, Mildworf B, Melamed E: Cerebral blood flow and cognitive impairment in Parkinson's disease. Neurology 35:1135–1139, 1985

Goetz CG: Neurotoxins in Clinical Practice. New York, SP Medical & Scientific Books, 1985

Goetz CG, Diederich NJ: There is a renaissance of interest in pallidotomy for Parkinson's disease. Nat Med 2:510–514, 1996

Goetz CG, Tanner CM, Klawans HL: Pharmacology of hallucinations induced by long-term drug therapy. Am J Psychiatry 139:494–497, 1982

Goetz CG, Olanow C, Koller WC, et al: Multicenter study of autologous adrenal medullary transplantation to the corpus striatum in patients with advanced Parkinson's disease. N Engl J Med 320:337–341, 1989

Goetz CG, Tanner CM, Penn RD, et al: Adrenal medullary transplant to the striatum of patients with advanced Parkinson's disease: 1-year motor and psychomotor data. Neurology 40:273–276, 1990

Goetz CG, Stebbins GT, Klawans HL, et al: United Parkinson Foundation Neurotransplantation registry on adrenal medullary transplants: presurgical, and 1- and 2-year follow-up. Neurology 41:1719–1722, 1991

Golbe LI, DiIorio G, Bonavita V, et al: A large kindred with autosomal dominant Parkinson's disease. Ann Neurol 27:276–282, 1990a

Golbe LI, Farrell TM, Davis PH: Follow-up study of early life protective and risk factors in Parkinson's disease. Mov Disord 5:66–70, 1990b

Golbe LI, Lazzarini AM, Schwarz KO, et al: Autosomal dominant parkinsonism with benign course and typical Lewy-body pathology. Neurology 43:2222–2227, 1993

Goodwin FK: Psychiatric side effects of levodopa in man. JAMA 218:1915–1920, 1971

Gorell JM, Johnson CC, Rybicki BA, et al: The risk of Parkinson's disease with exposure to pesticides, farming, well water, and rural living. Neurology 50:1346–1350, 1998

Goswami U, Dutta S, Kuruvilla K, et al: Electroconvulsive therapy in neuroleptic-induced parkinsonism. Biol Psychiatry 26:234–238, 1989

Gotham A-M, Brown RG, Marsden CD: Depression in Parkinson's disease: a quantitative and qualitative analysis. J Neurol Neurosurg Psychiatry 49:381–389, 1986

Grandinetti A, Morens DM, Reed D, et al: Prospective study of cigarette smoking and the risk of developing idiopathic Parkinson's disease. Am J Epidemiol 139:1129–1138, 1994

Gregory S, Schawcross CR, Gill D: The Nottingham ECT study: a double-blind comparison of bilateral, unilateral and simulated ECT in depressive illness. Br J Psychiatry 146:520–524, 1985

Gross C, Rougier A, Guehl D, et al: High-frequency stimulation of the globus pallidus internalis in Parkinson's disease: a study of seven cases. J Neurosurg 87:491–498, 1997

Grossman M, Carvell S, Stern MB, et al: Sentence comprehension in Parkinson's disease: the role of attention and memory. Brain Lang 42:347–384, 1992

Gudmundsson KR: A clinical survey of parkinsonism in Iceland. Acta Neurol Scand 33:9–61, 1967

Hagell P, Schrag A, Piccini P, et al: Sequential bilateral transplantation in Parkinson's disease: effects of the second graft. Brain 122:1121–1132, 1999

Hale MS, Bellizzi J: Low-dose perphenazine and levodopa/carbidopa therapy in a patient with parkinsonism and a psychotic illness. J Nerv Ment Dis 168:312–314, 1980

Hansen LA, Salmon DP, Galasko D, et al: The Lewy body variant of Alzheimer's disease: a clinical and pathological entity. Neurology 40:1–8, 1990

Hantz P, Caradoc-Davies G, Caradoc-Davies T, et al: Depression in Parkinson's disease. Am J Psychiatry 151:1010–1014, 1994

Harvey NS: Serial cognitive profiles in levodopa-induced hypersexuality. Br J Psychiatry 153:833–836, 1988

Hauser RA, Zesiewicz TA: Sertraline for the treatment of depression in Parkinson's disease. Mov Disord 12:756–759, 1997

Heindel WC, Salmon D, Shults C, et al: Neuropsychological evidence for multiple implicit memory systems: a comparison of Alzheimer's, Huntington's and Parkinson's disease patients. J Neurosci 9:582–587, 1989

Helig CW, Knopman DS, Mastri AR, et al: Dementia without Alzheimer pathology. Neurology 35:762–765, 1985

Henderson R, Kurlan R, Kersun JM, et al: Preliminary examination of the comorbidity of anxiety and depression in Parkinson's disease. J Neuropsychiatry Clin Neurosci 4:257–264, 1992

Hofman A, Schulte W, Tanja TA, et al: History of dementia and Parkinson's disease in first-degree relative of patients with Alzheimer's disease. Neurology 39:1589–1592, 1989

Hubble JP, Cao T, Hassanein RES, et al: Risk factors for Parkinson's disease. Neurology 43:1693–1697, 1993

Huber SJ, Shuttleworth EC, Paulson GW: Dementia in Parkinson's disease. Arch Neurol 43:987–990, 1986

Huber SJ, Paulson GW, Shuttleworth EC: Depression in Parkinson's disease. Neuropsychiatry Neuropsychol Behav Neurol 1:47–51, 1988

Huber SJ, Shuttleworth EC, Christy JA, et al: Magnetic resonance imaging in dementia of Parkinson's disease. J Neurol Neurosurg Psychiatry 52:1221–1227, 1989a

Huber SJ, Shuttleworth EC, Freidenberg DL: Neuropsychological differences between the dementias of Alzheimer's and Parkinson's diseases. Arch Neurol 46:1287–1291, 1989b

Huber SJ, Freidenberg DL, Shuttleworth EC, et al: Neuropsychological impairments associated with the severity of Parkinson's disease. J Neuropsychiatry Clin Neurosci 1:154–158, 1989c

Huberman M, Moscovitch M, Freedman M: Comparison of patients with Alzheimer's and Parkinson's disease on different explicit and implicit tests of memory. Neuropsychiatry Neuropsychol Behav Neurol 7:185–193, 1994

Hughes AJ, Daniel SE, Kilford L, et al: Accuracy of the clinical diagnosis of idiopathic Parkinson's disease: a clinico-pathological study of 100 cases. J Neurol Neurosurg Psychiatry 55:181–184, 1992

Hughes AJ, Daniel SE, Blankson S, et al: A clinicopathologic study of 100 cases of Parkinson's disease. Arch Neurol 50:140–148, 1993

Ikeguchi K, Kuroda A: Mianserin treatment of patients with psychosis induced by antiparkinsonian drugs. Eur Arch Psychiatry Clin Neurosci 244:320–324, 1995

Illes J: Neurolinguistic features of spontaneous language production dissociate three forms of neurodegenerative disease: Alzheimer's, Huntington's, and Parkinson's. Brain Lang 37:628–642, 1989

Inzelberg R, Treves T, Reider I, et al: Computed tomography brain changes in Parkinson's disease. Neuroradiology 29:535–539, 1987

Jacobs DM, Marder K, Côté LJ, et al: Neuropsychological characteristics of preclinical dementia in Parkinson's disease. Neurology 45:1691–1696, 1995

Johansson F, Malm J, Nordh E, et al: Usefulness of pallidotomy in advanced Parkinson's disease. J Neurol Neurosurg Psychiatry 62:125–132, 1997

Jouvent R, Abensour P, Bonnet AM, et al: Antiparkinsonian and antidepressant effects of high doses of bromocriptine. J Affect Disord 5:141–145, 1983

Kalayam B, Alexopoulos GS: Prefrontal dysfunction and treatment response in geriatric depression. Arch Gen Psychiatry 56:713–718, 1999

Kaspar S, Moises HW, Beckman H: The anticholinergic biperiden in depressive disorders. Pharmacopsychiatry 14:195–198, 1981

Kessler II: Epidemiologic studies of Parkinson's disease, III: a community-based survey. Am J Epidemiol 96:242–254, 1972

Kieburtz K, McDermott M, Como P, et al: The effect of deprenyl and tocopherol on cognitive performance in early untreated Parkinson's disease. Neurology 44:1756–1759, 1994

Kishore A, Turnbull IM, Snow BJ, et al: Efficacy, stability and predictors of outcome of pallidotomy for Parkinson's disease: six-month follow-up with additional 1-year observations. Brain 120:729–737, 1997

Klaasen T, Verhey FRJ, Sneijders GHJM, et al: Treatment of depression in Parkinson's disease: a meta-analysis. J Neuropsychiatry Clin Neurosci 7:281–286, 1995

Klatka LA, Louis ED, Schiffer RB: Psychiatric features in diffuse Lewy body disease: a clinicopathologic study using Alzheimer's disease and Parkinson's disease comparison groups. Neurology 47:1148–1152, 1996

Klawans HL: Levodopa-induced psychosis. Am J Psychiatry 8:447–451, 1978

Klawans HL: Individual manifestations of Parkinson's disease after ten or more years of levodopa. Mov Disord 1: 187–192, 1986

Knowlton BJ, Mangels JA, Squire LR: A neostriatal habit learning system in humans. Science 273:1399–1402, 1996

Koller WC: How accurately can Parkinson's disease be diagnosed? Neurology 42 (suppl 1):6–16, 1992

Koller WC, Montgomery EB: Issues in the early diagnosis of Parkinson's disease. Neurology 49 (suppl 1):S10–S25, 1997

Koller WC, Vetere-Overfield B, Gray C, et al: Environmental risk factors in Parkinson's disease. Neurology 40: 1218–1221, 1990

Koller WC, Glatt SL, Hubble JP, et al: Apolipoprotein E genotypes in Parkinson's disease with and without dementia. Ann Neurol 37:242–245, 1995

Koller WC, Pahwa R, Busenbark K, et al: High-frequency unilateral thalamic stimulation in the treatment of essential and parkinsonian tremor. Ann Neurol 42:292–299, 1997

Koller WC, Marjama J, Tröster AI: Psychogenic movement disorders, in Parkinson's Disease and Movement Disorders, 3rd Edition. Edited by Jankovic J, Tolosa E. Baltimore, MD, Williams & Wilkins, 1998a, pp 859–868

Koller WC, Wilkinson S, Pahwa R, et al: Surgical treatment options in Parkinson's disease. Neurosurg Clin N Am 9: 295–306, 1998b

Korczyn AD, Inzelberg R, Treves T, et al: Dementia of Parkinson's disease, in Advances in Neurology Series, Vol 45. Edited by Yahr MD, Bergmann KJ. New York, Raven, 1986, pp 399–403

Korczyn AD, Brunt ER, Larsen JP, et al: A 3-year randomized trial of ropinirole and bromocriptine in early Parkinson's disease. Neurology 53:364–370, 1999

Kosaka K: Diffuse Lewy body disease in Japan. J Neurol 237:197–204, 1990

Kosaka K, Matsushita M, Oyanagi S, et al: A clinicopathological study of the "Lewy body disease." Seishin Shinkeigaku Zasshi (Psychiatria et Neurologia Japonica) 82:292–311, 1980

Kostic VS, Djuricic BM, Covickovic-Sternic N, et al: Depression and Parkinson's disease: possible role of serotonergic mechanisms. J Neurol 12:94–96, 1987

Kramer BA: The use of ECT in California, 1977–1983. Am J Psychiatry 142:1190–1192, 1985

Kuhl DE, Metter EJ, Riege WH, et al: Patterns of cerebral glucose utilization in Parkinson's disease and Huntington's disease. Ann Neurol 15 (suppl):S119–S125, 1984

Kumar R, Lozano AM, Sime E, et al: Comparative effects of unilateral and bilateral subthalamic nucleus deep brain stimulation. Neurology 53:561–566, 1999

Kurland LT: Epidemiology: incidence, geographic distribution and genetic consideration, in Pathogenesis and Treatment of Parkinsonism. Edited by Field W. Springfield, IL, Charles C Thomas, 1958, pp 5–43

Kuzis G, Sabe L, Tiberti C, et al: Cognitive functions in major depression and Parkinson's disease. Arch Neurol 54: 982–986, 1997

Laakso MP, Partanen K, Riekkinen P, et al: Hippocampal volumes in Alzheimer's disease, Parkinson's disease with and without dementia and in vascular dementia: an MRI study. Neurology 46:678–681, 1996

Laitinen LV: Pallidotomy in Parkinson's disease. Neurosurg Clin N Am 6:105–112, 1995

Laitinen LV, Bergenheim AT, Hariz MI: Leksell's posteroventral pallidotomy in the treatment of Parkinson's disease. J Neurosurg 76:53–61, 1992

Lang AE, Lozano AM: Parkinson's disease: second of two parts. N Engl J Med 339:1130–1143, 1998

Lang AE, Quinn N: Pergolide in late-stage Parkinson's disease. Ann Neurol 12:243–247, 1982

Lang AE, Sandor P, Duff J: Remoxipride in Parkinson's disease: differential response in patients with dyskinesia fluctuations versus psychosis. Clin Neuropharmacol 18:39–44, 1995

Lang AE, Lozano AM, Montgomery E, et al: Posteroventral medial pallidotomy in advanced Parkinson's disease. N Engl J Med 337:1036–1042, 1997

Langston JW, Ballard PA, Tetrud JW, et al: Chronic parkinsonism in humans due to a product of meperidine-analog synthesis. Science 219:979–980, 1983

Lebensohn ZM, Jenkins RB: Improvement of parkinsonism in depressed patients treated with ETC. Am J Psychiatry 132: 283–285, 1975

Lennox GG, Lowe JS: Dementia with Lewy bodies. Baillieres Clin Neurol 6:147–166, 1997

Leplow B, Dierks C, Herrmann P, et al: Remote memory in Parkinson's disease and senile dementia. Neuropsychologia 35:547–557, 1997

Leroy A, Michelet D, Mahieux F, et al: Examen neuropsychologique de 5 patients parkinsoniens avant et après greffe neuronale. Rev Neurol (Paris) 152:158–164, 1996

Levin BE, Llabre BM, Weiner WJ: Cognitive impairments associated with early Parkinson's disease. Neurology 39:557–561, 1989

Lewis FM, Lapointe LL, Murdoch BE, et al: Language impairment in Parkinson's disease. Aphasiology 12:193–206, 1998

Li SC, Schoenberg BS, Wang CC, et al: A prevalence study of Parkinson's disease and other movement disorders in the People's Republic of China. Arch Neurol 42:655–657, 1982

Lichter DG, Corbett AJ, Fitzgibbon GM, et al: Cognitive and motor dysfunction in Parkinson's disease. Arch Neurol 45:854–860, 1988

Lieberman A: Managing the neuropsychiatric symptoms of Parkinson's disease. Neurology 50 (suppl 6):S33–S38, 1998

Lieberman A, Dziatolowski M, Kupersmith M, et al: Dementia in Parkinson's disease. Ann Neurol 6:335–359, 1979

Lieberman A, Ranhosky A, Korts D, et al: Clinical evaluation of pramipexole in advanced Parkinson's disease. Neurology 49:162–168, 1997

Lieberman P, Friedman J, Feldman LS: Syntax comprehension deficits in Parkinson's disease. J Nerv Ment Dis 178: 360–365, 1990

Lieberman P, Kako E, Friedman J, et al: Speech production, syntax comprehension, and cognitive deficits in Parkinson's disease. Brain Lang 43:169–189, 1992

López-Lozano JJ, Bravo G, Brera B, et al: Long-term improvement in patients with severe Parkinson's disease after implantation of fetal ventral mesencephalic tissue in a cavity of the caudate nucleus: 5-year follow up in 10 patients. J Neurosurg 86:931–942, 1997

Ludwig CL, Weinberger DR, Bruno G, et al: Buspirone, Parkinson's disease and the locus ceruleus. Clin Neuropharmacol 9:373–378, 1986

Lund-Johansen M, Hugdahl K, Wester K: Cognitive function in patients with Parkinson's disease undergoing stereotaxic thalamotomy. J Neurol Neurosurg Psychiatry 60:564–571, 1996

Madrazo I, Franco-Bourland R, Ostrosky-Solis F, et al: Fetal homotransplants (ventral mesencephalon and adrenal tissue) to the striatum of parkinsonian subjects. Arch Neurol 47:1281–1285, 1990

Mahieux F, Fenelon G, Flahault A, et al: Neuropsychological prediction of dementia in Parkinson's disease. J Neurol Neurosurg Psychiatry 64:178–183, 1998

Marder K, Mirabello E, Chen J, et al: Death rates among demented and nondemented patients with Parkinson's disease (abstract). Ann Neurol 28:295, 1990

Marder K, Maestre G, Côté L, et al: The apolipoprotein e4 allele in Parkinson's disease with and without dementia. Neurology 44:1330–1331, 1994

Marder K, Tang M, Côté L, et al: The frequency and associated risk factors for dementia in patients with Parkinson's disease. Arch Neurol 52:695–701, 1995

Maricle RA, Nutt JG, Valentine RJ, et al: Dose-response relationship of levodopa with mood and anxiety in fluctuating Parkinson's disease: a double-blind, placebo-controlled study. Neurology 45:1757–1760, 1995

Maricle RA, Valentine RJ, Carter J, et al: Mood response to levodopa infusion in early Parkinson's disease. Neurology 50:1890–1892, 1998

Marsden CD: The mysterious motor function of the basal ganglia: the Robert Wartenberg lecture. Neurology 32: 514–539, 1982

Marsden CD: Parkinson's disease in twins. J Neurol Neurosurg Psychiatry 50:105–106, 1987

Martin WE, Loewenson RB, Resch JA, et al: Parkinson's disease: analysis of 100 patients. Neurology 23:783–790, 1973

Martínez-Martín P, O'Brien CF: Extending levodopa action: COMT inhibition. Neurology 50 (suppl 6):S27–S32, 1998

Marttila RJ, Rinne UK: Epidemiology of Parkinson's disease in Finland. Acta Neurol Scand 43 (suppl 33):9–61, 1967

Matison R, Mayeux R, Rosen J, et al: "Tip-of-the-tongue" phenomenon in Parkinson's disease. Neurology 32:567–570, 1982

Mayberg HS, Starkstein SE, Sadzot B, et al: Selective hypometabolism in the inferior frontal lobe of depressed patients with Parkinson's disease. Ann Neurol 26:57–64, 1990

Mayeux R: Depression and dementia in Parkinson's disease, in Movement Disorders. Edited by Marsden CD, Fahn S. London, Butterworth, 1982, pp 75–95

Mayeux R, Stern Y, Cote L, et al: Altered serotonin metabolism in depressed patients with Parkinson's disease. Neurology 34:642–646, 1984

Mayeux R, Stern Y, Sano M, et al: Clinical and biochemical correlates of bradyphrenia in Parkinson's disease. Neurology 37:1130–1134, 1987

Mayeux R, Stern Y, Sano M, et al: The relationship of serotonin to depression in Parkinson's disease. Mov Disord 3: 237–244, 1988

Mayeux R, Chen J, Mirabello E, et al: An estimate of the incidence and prevalence of dementia in idiopathic Parkinson's disease. Neurology 40:1513–1516, 1990

McCance-Katz EF, Marek KL, Price LH: Serotonergic dysfunction in depression associated with Parkinson's disease. Neurology 42:1813–1814, 1992

McCarthy R, Gresty M, Findley LJ: Parkinson's disease and dementia. Lancet 1:407–408, 1985

McKeith IG, Galasko D, Kosaka K, et al: Consensus guidelines for the clinical and pathological diagnosis of dementia with Lewy bodies (DLB): report of the consortium on DLB international workshop. Neurology 47:1113–1124, 1996

McNamara P, Durso R: Reversible pathologic jealousy (Othello syndrome) associated with amantadine. J Geriatr Psychiatry Neurol 4:157–159, 1991

McPherson S, Cummings JL: Neuropsychological aspects of Parkinson's disease and parkinsonism, in Neuropsychological Assessment of Neuropsychiatric Disorders, 2nd Edition. Edited by Grant I, Adams KM. New York, Oxford University Press, 1996, pp 288–311

Meco G, Alessandri A, Giustini P, et al: Risperidone in levodopa-induced psychosis in advanced Parkinson's disease: an open-label, long-term study. Mov Disord 12: 610–612, 1997

Mega MS, Cummings JL: Frontal-subcortical circuits and neuropsychiatric disorders. J Neuropsychiatry Clin Neurosci 6:358–370, 1994

Melamed E, Hefti F, Wurtman RJ: Nonaminergic striatal neurons convert exogenous L-dopa to dopamine in parkinsonism. Ann Neurol 8:558–563, 1980

Mendis T, Mohr E, George A, et al: Symptomatic relief from treatment-induced psychosis in Parkinson's disease: an open label pilot study with remoxipride. Mov Disord 9:197–200, 1994

Meyerson RA, Richard IH, Schiffer RB: Mood disorders secondary to demyelinating and movement disorders. Seminars in Clinical Neuropsychiatry 2:252–264, 1997

Miller EM, Nieburg HA: L-Tryptophan in the treatment of levodopa-induced psychiatric disorders. Diseases of the Nervous System 35:20–23, 1974

Mindham RHS, Marsden CD, Parkes JD: Psychiatric symptoms during L-dopa therapy for Parkinson's disease and their relationship to physical disability. Psychol Med 6:23–33, 1976

Miyoshi K, Ueki A, Nagano O: Management of psychiatric symptoms of Parkinson's disease. Eur Neurol 36 (suppl 1):49–54, 1996

Moellentine C, Rummans T, Ahlskog JE, et al: Effectiveness of ECT in patients with parkinsonism. J Neuropsychiatry Clin Neurosci 10:187–193, 1998

Mohr E, Mendis T, Grimes JD: Late cognitive changes in Parkinson's disease with an emphasis on dementia, in Advances in Neurology Series, Vol 65. Edited by Weiner JA, Lang AE. New York, Raven, 1995, pp 97–113

Molina H, Quinones R, Alvarez L, et al: Transplantation of human fetal mesencephalic tissue in caudate nucleus as treatment for Parkinson's disease: the Cuban experience, in Intracerebral Transplantation in Movement Disorders: Experimental Basis and Clinical Experiences. Edited by Lindvall O, Björklund A, Widner H. Amsterdam, Elsevier, 1991, pp 99–110

Morris SK, Olichney JM, Corey-Bloom J: Psychosis in dementia with Lewy bodies. Seminars in Clinical Neuropsychiatry 3:51–60, 1998

Moskovitz C, Moses H III, Klawans HL: Levodopa-induced psychosis: a kindling phenomenon. Am J Psychiatry 135: 669–675, 1978

Musser WS, Akil M: Clozapine as a treatment for psychosis in Parkinson's disease: a review. J Neuropsychiatry Clin Neurosci 8:1–9, 1996

Mutch WJ, Dingwall-Fordyce I, Downie AW, et al: Parkinson's disease in a Scottish city. BMJ 292:534–536, 1986

Nakano I, Hirano A: Parkinson's disease: neuron loss in the nucleus basalis without concomitant Alzheimer's disease. Ann Neurol 15:415–418, 1984

Narabayashi H, Miyashita N, Hattori Y, et al: Posteroventral pallidotomy: its effect on motor symptoms and scores of MMPI test in patients with Parkinson's disease. Parkinsonism and Related Disorders 3:7–20, 1997

Nissenbaum H, Quinn NP, Brown RG, et al: Mood swings associated with the "on-off" phenomenon in Parkinson's disease. Psychol Med 17:899–904, 1987

Okada K, Kobayashi S, Tsunematso T: Prevalence of Parkinson's disease in Izumo City, Japan. Gerontology 36: 340–344, 1990

Olanow CW: Attempts to obtain neuroprotection in Parkinson's disease. Neurology 49 (suppl 1):S26–S33, 1997

Olanow CW, Koller WC: An algorithm (decision tree) for the management of Parkinson's disease: treatment guidelines. Neurology 50 (suppl 3):S1–S57, 1998

Olanow CW, Fahn S, Langston JW, et al: Selegiline and mortality in Parkinson's disease. Ann Neurol 40:841–845, 1996

Ostrosky-Solis F, Quintanar L, Madrazo I, et al: Neuropsychological effects of brain autograft of adrenal medullary tissue for the treatment of Parkinson's disease. Neurology 38:1442–1450, 1988

Otsuka M, Ichiya Y, Hosokawa S, et al: Striatal blood flow, glucose metabolism, and ^{18}F-dopa uptake: difference in Parkinson's disease and atypical parkinsonism. J Neurol Neurosurg Psychiatry 54:898–904, 1991

Ott BR, Lannon MC: Exacerbation of parkinsonism by tacrine. Clin Neuropharmacol 15:322–325, 1992

Owen AM, Doyon J, Dagher A, et al: Abnormal basal ganglia outflow in Parkinson's disease identified with PET: implications for higher cortical functions. Brain 121:949–965, 1998

Paolo AM, Tröster AI, Glatt SL, et al: Differentiation of the dementias of Alzheimer's and Parkinson's disease with the Dementia Rating Scale. J Geriatr Psychiatry Neurol 8:184–188, 1995

Parkinson J: An Essay on the Shaking Palsy. London, Sherwood, Neely & Jones, 1817

Parkinson's Disease Research Group in the United Kingdom: Comparison of therapeutic effects and mortality data of levodopa and levodopa combined with selegiline in patients with early, mild Parkinson's disease. BMJ 311: 1602–1606, 1995

Parkinson Study Group: Effect of deprenyl on the progression of disability in early Parkinson's disease. N Engl J Med 321:1364–1371, 1989

Parkinson Study Group: Effects of tocopherol and deprenyl on the progression of disability in early Parkinson's disease. N Engl J Med 328:176–183, 1993

Parkinson Study Group: Effect of lazabemide on the progression of disability in early Parkinson's disease. Ann Neurol 40:99–107, 1996

Parkinson Study Group: Safety and efficacy of pramipexole in early Parkinson disease. JAMA 278:125–130, 1997

Parkinson Study Group: Low-dose clozapine for the treatment of drug-induced psychosis in Parkinson's disease. N Engl J Med 340:757–763, 1999

Parsa MA, Bastani B: Quetiapine (Seroquel) in the treatment of psychosis in patients with Parkinson's disease. J Neuropsychiatry Clin Neurosci 10:216–219, 1998

Peppard RF, Martin WRW, Guttman M, et al: The relationship of cerebral glucose metabolism to cognitive deficits in Parkinson's disease. Neurology 38 (suppl 1):364, 1988

Perry EK, Curtis M, Dick DJ, et al: Cholinergic correlates of cognitive impairment in Parkinson's disease: comparison with Alzheimer's disease. J Neurol Neurosurg Psychiatry 48:413–421, 1985

Perry RH, Tomlinson BE, Candy JM, et al: Cholinergic deficit in mentally impaired parkinsonian patients. Lancet 2: 789–790, 1983

Peyser CE, Naimark D, Zuniga R, et al: Psychoses in Parkinson's disease. Seminars in Clinical Neuropsychiatry 3: 41–50, 1998

Pies RW: Handbook of Essential Psychopharmacology. Washington, DC, American Psychiatric Press, 1998

Pillon B, Dubois B: Cognitive slowing in Parkinson's disease fails to respond to levodopa treatment: the 15-objects test. Neurology 39:762–768, 1989

Pillon B, Dubois B, Lhermitte F, et al: Heterogeneity of cognitive impairment in progressive supranuclear palsy, Parkinson's disease and Alzheimer's disease. Neurology 36: 1179–1185, 1986

Pillon B, Deweer B, Agid Y, et al: Explicit memory in Alzheimer's, Huntington's, and Parkinson's diseases. Arch Neurol 50:374–379, 1993

Pinter MM, Pogarell O, Oertel WH: Efficacy, safety, and tolerance of the non-ergoline dopamine agonist pramipexole in the treatment of advanced Parkinson's disease: a double blind, placebo controlled, randomised, multicentre study. J Neurol Neurosurg Psychiatry 66:436–441, 1999

Poewe W: Adjuncts to levodopa therapy: dopamine agonists. Neurology 50 (suppl 6):S23–S26, 1998

Pollak P, Benabid A-L, Krack P, et al: Deep brain stimulation, in Parkinson's Disease and Movement Disorders, 3rd Edition. Edited by Jankovic J, Tolosa E. Baltimore, MD, Williams & Wilkins, 1998, pp 1085–1101

Price LH, Spencer DD, Marek KL, et al: Psychiatric status after human fetal mesencephalic tissue transplantation in Parkinson's disease. Biol Psychiatry 38:498–505, 1995

Quinn NP: Multiple system atrophy, in Movement Disorders, Vol 3. Edited by Marsden CD, Fahn S. London, Butterworth-Heinemann, 1994, pp 262–281

Quinn NP, Lang AE, Thompson C, et al: Pergolide in the treatment of Parkinson's disease, in Advances in Neurology Series, Vol 40. Edited by Hassler RG, Christ JF. New York, Raven, 1984, pp 509–513

Rajput AH, Rozdilsky B, Rajput A: Alzheimer's disease with idiopathic Parkinson's disease: clinical, pharmacological and pathological observations (abstract). Neurology 40:339, 1990

Rajput AH, Rozdilsky B, Rajput A: Accuracy of clinical diagnosis in parkinsonism: a prospective study. Can J Neurol Sci 18:275–278, 1991

Rajput AH, Martin W, Saint-Hilaire MH, et al: Tolcapone improves motor function in parkinsonian patients with the "wearing off" phenomenon: a double-blind, placebo-controlled, multicenter trial. Neurology 49: 1066–1071, 1997

Raven JC: Standard Progressive Matrices. New York, The Psychological Corporation, 1958

Rehncrona S: A critical review of the current status and possible developments in brain transplantation, in Advances and Technical Standards in Neurosurgery, Vol 23. Edited by Cohadon F, Dolenc VV, Lobo Atunes J, et al. Vienna, Springer-Verlag, 1997, pp 3–46

Rich SS, Friedman JH, Ott BR: Risperidone versus clozapine in the treatment of psychosis in six patients with Parkinson's disease and other akinetic-rigid syndromes. J Clin Psychiatry 56:556–559, 1995

Richard IH, Schiffer RB, Kurlan R: Anxiety and Parkinson's disease. J Neuropsychiatry Clin Neurosci 8:383–392, 1996

Richard IH, Kurlan R, Tanner C, et al: Serotonin syndrome and the combined use of deprenyl and an antidepressant in Parkinson's disease. Neurology 48:1070–1077, 1997

Riley D, Lang AE: Practical application of a low-protein diet for Parkinson's disease. Neurology 38:1026–1031, 1988

Ring HA, Bench CJ, Trimble MR, et al: Depression in Parkinson's disease: a positron emission study. Br J Psychiatry 165:333–339, 1994

Rinne UK, Larsen JP, Siden A, et al: Entacapone enhances response to levodopa in parkinsonian patients with motor fluctuations: Nomecomt Study Group. Neurology 51:1309–1314, 1998

Robertson C, Flowers KA: Motor set in Parkinson's disease. J Neurol Neurosurg Psychiatry 59:583–592, 1990

Rocca WA, Morgante M: Prevalence of Parkinson's disease and other parkinsonisms: a door-to-door survey in two Sicilian communities. Neurology 40 (suppl 1):422, 1990

Rondot P, de Recondo J, Coignet A, et al: Mental disorders in Parkinson's disease after treatment with L-dopa, in Advances in Neurology Series, Vol 40. Edited by Hassler RG, Christ JF. New York, Raven, 1984, pp 259–269

Roose SP, Glassman AH: Comparison of imipramine- and nortriptyline-induced orthostatic hypotension: a meaningful difference. J Clin Psychopharmacol 1:316–319, 1981

Ross GW, Mahler ME, Cummings JL: The dementia syndromes of Parkinson's disease: cortical and subcortical features, in Parkinson's Disease: Neurobehavioral Aspects. Edited by Huber SJ, Cummings JL. New York, Oxford University Press, 1992, pp 132–148

Roth SD, Mukherjee S, Sackeim HA: Electroconvulsive therapy in a patient with mania, parkinsonism and tardive dyskinesia. Convulsive Therapy 4:92–97, 1988

Ruggieri S, De Pandis MF, Bonamartini A, et al: Low dose of clozapine in the treatment of dopaminergic psychosis in Parkinson's disease. Clin Neuropharmacol 20:204–209, 1997

Ryback RS, Schwab RS: Manic response to levodopa therapy: report of a case. N Engl J Med 285:788–789, 1971

Saint-Cyr JA, Taylor AE, Lang AE: Neuropsychological and psychiatric side effects in the treatment of Parkinson's disease. Neurology 43 (suppl 6):S47–S52, 1993

Sagar HJ, Cohen NJ, Sullivan EV, et al: Remote memory function in Alzheimer's disease and Parkinson's disease. Brain 111:185–206, 1988

Salganik I, Korczyn A: Risk factors for dementia in Parkinson's disease, in Advances in Neurology Series, Vol 53. Edited by Streifler MB, Korczyn AD, Melamed E, et al. New York, Raven, 1990, pp 343–347

Salmon DP, Galasko D: Neuropsychological aspects of Lewy body dementia, in Lewy Body Dementia. Edited by Perry EK, Perry RH, McKeith IG. Cambridge, Cambridge University Press, 1996, pp 99–113

Salmon DP, Galasko D, Hansen LA, et al: Neuropsychological deficits associated with diffuse Lewy body disease. Brain Cogn 31:148–165, 1996

Samuel M, Caputo E, Brooks DJ, et al: A study of medial pallidotomy for Parkinson's disease: clinical outcome, MRI location and complications. Brain 121:59–75, 1998

Sanchez-Ramos JR, Ortoll R, Paulson GW: Visual hallucinations associated with Parkinson's disease. Arch Neurol 53:1265–1268, 1996

Sano M, Stern Y, Marder K, et al: A controlled trial of piracetam in intellectually impaired patients with Parkinson's disease. Mov Disord 5:230–234, 1990

Santamaria J, Tolosa E, Valles A: Parkinson's disease with depression: a possible subgroup of idiopathic parkinsonism. Neurology 36:1130–1133, 1986

Sass KJ, Buchanan CP, Westerveld M, et al: General cognitive ability following unilateral and bilateral fetal ventral mesencephalic tissue transplantation for treatment of Parkinson's disease, Arch Neurol 52:680–686, 1995

Savitsky N, Karliner W: Electroshock in the presence of organic disease of the central nervous system. Journal of the Hillside Hospital 2:3–22, 1953

Sawada H, Udaka F, Kameyama M, et al: SPECT findings in Parkinson's disease associated with dementia. J Neurol Neurosurg Psychiatry 55:960–963, 1992

Schiffer RB, Kurlan R, Rubin A, et al: Evidence for atypical depression in Parkinson's disease. Am J Psychiatry 145:1020–1022, 1988

Schoenberg BS, Anderson DW, Haerer AF, et al: Prevalence of Parkinson's disease in the biracial population of Copiah County, Mississippi. Neurology 35:841–845, 1985

Schoenberg BS, Osuntokun BO, Adeuja AO, et al: Comparison of the prevalence of Parkinson's disease in black populations in the rural US and Nigeria: door-to-door community studies. Neurology 38:645–646, 1988

Scott R, Gregory R, Hines N, et al: Neuropsychological, neurological and functional outcome following pallidotomy for Parkinson's disease: a consecutive series of eight simultaneous bilateral and twelve unilateral procedures. Brain 121:659–675, 1998

Shapiro MF, Goldberg HH: Electroconvulsive therapy in patients with structural disease of the nervous system. Am J Med Sci 233:186–195, 1957

Shaw KM, Lees AJ, Stern GM: The impact of treatment with levodopa on Parkinson's disease. Quarterly Journal of Medicine 49:283–293, 1980

Siegfried J, Wellis G: Chronic electrostimulation of ventroposterolateral pallidum: follow-up. Acta Neurochir (Wien) 68 (suppl):11–13, 1997

Silver JM, Yudofsky SC: Psychopharmacology and electroconvulsive therapy, in The American Psychiatric Press Textbook of Psychiatry. Edited by Talbott JA, Hales RE, Yudofsky SC. Washington, DC, American Psychiatric Press, 1988, pp 767–853

Silver JM, Yudofsky SC: Drug treatment of depression in Parkinson's disease, in Parkinson's Disease: Neurobehavioral Aspects. Edited by Huber SJ, Cummings JL. New York, Oxford University Press, 1992, pp 240–254

Sitland-Marken PA, Wells BG, Froemming JH, et al: Psychiatric applications of bromocriptine therapy. J Clin Psychiatry 51:68–82, 1990

Small JG, Millstein V: Electroconvulsive therapy in the treatment of manic episodes, in Electroconvulsive Therapy: Clinical and Basic Research Issues. Edited by Malitz S, Sackeim HA. New York, New York Academy of Sciences, 1986, pp 37–49

Spieker S, Stetter F, Klockgether T: Zotepine in levodopa-induced psychosis (editorial). Mov Disord 10: 795–796, 1995

Starkstein SE, Leiguarda R: Neuropsychological correlates of brain atrophy in Parkinson's disease: a CT-scan study. Mov Disord 1:51–55, 1993

Starkstein SE, Preziosi TJ, Bolduc PL, et al: Depression in Parkinson's disease. J Nerv Ment Dis 178:27–31, 1990

Starkstein SE, Mayberg HS, Leiguarda R, et al: A longitudinal prospective study of depression, cognitive decline and physical impairments in patients with Parkinson's disease. J Neurol Neurosurg Psychiatry 55:377–382, 1992

Starkstein SE, Robinson RG, Leiguarda R, et al: Anxiety and depression in Parkinson's disease. Behavioural Neurology 6:151–154, 1993

Stebbins GT, Tanner CM: Behavioral effects of intrastriatal adrenal medullary surgery in Parkinson's disease, in Parkinson's Disease: Neurobehavioral Aspects. Edited by Huber SJ, Cummings JL. New York, Oxford University Press, 1992, pp 328–345

Stein MB, Heuser IJ, Juncos JL, et al: Anxiety disorders in patients with Parkinson's disease. Am J Psychiatry 147: 217–220, 1990

Stern Y, Langston JW: Intellectual changes in patients with MPTP-induced parkinsonism. Neurology 35:1506–1507, 1985

Stern Y, Marder K, Tang MX, et al: Antecedent clinical features associated with dementia in Parkinson's disease. Neurology 43:1690–1692, 1993a

Stern Y, Richards M, Sano M, et al: Comparison of cognitive changes in patients with Alzheimer's and Parkinson's disease. Arch Neurol 50:1040–1045, 1993b

Steur ENHJ: Increase of Parkinson disability after fluoxetine medication. Neurology 43:211–213, 1993

Straits-Tröster K, Fields JA, Wilkinson SB, et al: Health-related quality of life in Parkinson's disease after pallidotomy and deep brain stimulation. Brain Cogn (in press)

Sutton JP, Couldwell W, Lew MF, et al: Ventroposterior medial pallidotomy in patients with advanced Parkinson's disease. Neurosurgery 36:1112–1117, 1995

Tandberg E, Larsen JP, Aarsland D, et al: The occurrence of depression in Parkinson's disease: a community-based study. Arch Neurol 53:175–179, 1996

Tanner CM: Drug-induced movement disorders, in Extrapyramidal Disorders: Handbook of Clinical Neurology, Vol 5. Edited by Vinken PJ, Bruyn GW, Klawans HL. Amsterdam, Elsevier Science, 1986, pp 185–204

Tanner CM: The role of environmental toxins in the etiology of Parkinson's disease. Trends Neurosci 12:49–54, 1989

Tanner CM, Vogel C, Goetz CG, et al: Hallucinations in Parkinson's disease: a population study (abstract). Ann Neurol 14:136, 1983

Tanner CM, Chen B, Wang WZ, et al: Environmental factors in the etiology of Parkinson's disease. Can J Neurol Sci 14:419–423, 1987

Tanner CM, Hubble JP, Chan P: Epidemiology and genetics of Parkinson's disease, in Movement Disorders: Neurologic Principles and Practice. Edited by Watts RL, Koller WC. New York, McGraw-Hill, 1997, pp 137–152

Tarczy M, Szirmai I: Failure of dopamine metabolism: borderline of parkinsonism and dementia. Acta Biomed Ateneo Parmense 66:93–97, 1995

Tasker RR: Deep brain stimulation is preferable to thalamotomy for tremor suppression. Surg Neurol 49: 145–154, 1997

Taylor AE, Saint-Cyr JA: Depression in Parkinson's disease: reconciling physiological and psychological perspectives. J Neuropsychiatry Clin Neurosci 2:92–98, 1990

Taylor AE, Saint-Cyr JA: The neuropsychology of Parkinson's disease. Brain Cogn 28:281–296, 1995

Taylor AE, Saint-Cyr JA, Lang AE: Dementia prevalence in Parkinson's disease. Lancet 1(8436):1037, 1985

Taylor AE, Saint-Cyr JA, Lang AE: Frontal lobe dysfunction in Parkinson's disease: the cortical focus of neostriatal outflow. Brain 109:845–883, 1986

Taylor AE, Saint-Cyr JA, Lang AE: Memory and learning in early Parkinson's disease: evidence for a "frontal lobe syndrome." Brain Cogn 13:211–232, 1990a

Taylor AE, Saint-Cyr JA, Lang AE: Sub-cognitive processing in the frontocaudate "complex loop." Alzheimer Dis Assoc Disord 4:150–160, 1990b

Thornton JE, Stahl SM: Case report of tardive dyskinesia associated with amoxapine therapy. Am J Psychiatry 141: 704–705, 1984

Tom T, Cummings JL: Depression in Parkinson's disease: pharmacological characteristics and treatment. Drugs Aging 12:55–74, 1998

Tomer R, Levin BE, Weiner WJ: Obsessive-compulsive symptoms and motor asymmetries in Parkinson's disease. Neuropsychiatry Neuropsychol Behav Neurol 6:26–30, 1993

Torack RM, Morris JC: The association of ventral tegmental area histopathology with adult dementia. Arch Neurol 45:211–218, 1988

Trépanier LL, Saint-Cyr JA, Lozano AM, et al: Neuropsychological consequences of posteroventral pallidotomy for the treatment of Parkinson's disease. Neurology 51:207–215, 1998

Tröster AI, Fields JA: Frontal cognitive function and memory in Parkinson's disease: toward a distinction between prospective and declarative memory impairments? Behavioural Neurology 8:59–74, 1995

Tröster AI, Paolo AM, Lyons KE, et al: The influence of depression on cognition in Parkinson's disease: a pattern of impairment distinguishable from Alzheimer's disease. Neurology 45:672–676, 1995a

Tröster AI, Stalp LD, Paolo AM, et al: Neuropsychological impairment in Parkinson's disease with and without depression. Arch Neurol 52:1164–1169, 1995b

Tröster AI, Fields JA, Paolo AM, et al: Performance of individuals with Parkinson's disease on the Vocabulary and Information subtests of the WAIS-R as a Neuropsychological Instrument. Journal of Clinical Geropsychology 2:215–223, 1996a

Tröster AI, Fields JA, Paolo AM, et al: Visual confrontation naming in Alzheimer's disease and Parkinson's disease with dementia (abstract). Neurology 46 (suppl):A292–A293, 1996b

Tröster AI, Fields JA, Wilkinson SB, et al: Neuropsychological functioning before and after unilateral thalamic stimulating electrode implantation in Parkinson's disease (electronic manuscript). Neurosurgical Focus 2(3):1–6, 1997a

Tröster AI, Fields JA, Wilkinson SB, et al: Unilateral pallidal stimulation for Parkinson's disease: neurobehavioral functioning before and 3 months after electrode implantation. Neurology 49:1078–1083, 1997b

Tröster AI, Fields JA, Testa JA, et al: Cortical and subcortical influences on clustering and switching in the performance of verbal fluency tasks. Neuropsychologia 36:295–304, 1998a

Tröster AI, Fields JA, Straits-Tröster KA, et al: Motoric and psychosocial correlates of quality of life in Parkinson's disease four months after unilateral pallidotomy (abstract). Neurology 50 (suppl 4):A299, 1998b

Tröster AI, Wilkinson SB, Fields JA, et al: Chronic electrical stimulation of the left ventrointermediate (Vim) thalamic nucleus for the treatment of pharmacotherapy-resistant Parkinson's disease: a differential impact on access to semantic and episodic memory? Brain Cogn 38:125–149, 1998c

Troyer AK, Moscovitch M, Winocur G, et al: Clustering and switching on verbal fluency tests in Alzheimer's and Parkinson's disease. J Int Neuropsychol Soc 4:137–143, 1998

Tsuang MT, Tidball JS, Geller D: ECT in a depressed patient with shunt in place for normal pressure hydrocephalus. Am J Psychiatry 136:1205–1206, 1979

Uitti RJ, Wharen RE, Turk MF, et al: Unilateral pallidotomy for Parkinson's disease: comparison of outcome in younger versus elderly patients. Neurology 49:1072–1077, 1997

Valldeoriola F, Nobbe FA, Tolosa E: Treatment of behavioural disturbances in Parkinson's disease. J Neural Transm Suppl 51:175–204, 1997

Vázquez A, Jiménez-Jiménez FJ, García-Ruiz P, et al: "Panic attacks" in Parkinson's disease: a long-term complication of levodopa therapy. Acta Neurol Scand 87:14–18, 1993

Venneri A, Nichelli P, Modonesi G, et al: Impairment in dating and retrieving remote events in patients with early Parkinson's disease. J Neurol Neurosurg Psychiatry 62:410–413, 1997

Vingerhoets G, Lannoo E, van der Linden C, et al: Changes in quality of life following unilateral pallidal stimulation in Parkinson's disease. J Psychosom Res 46:247–255, 1999

Vogel HP, Schifter R: Hypersexuality: a complication of dopaminergic therapy in Parkinson's disease. Pharmacopsychiatry 16:107–110, 1983

Waldmeier PC, Delini-Stula AA: Serotonin-dopamine interactions in the nigrostriatal system. Eur J Pharmacol 55: 363–373, 1979

Ward CD, Duvoisin RC, Ince SE, et al: Parkinson's disease in 65 pairs of twins and in a set of quadruplets. Neurology 33: 815–824, 1983

Waters CH, Miller CA: Autosomal dominant transmission of Parkinson's disease in a four generation family. Ann Neurol 35:59–64, 1994

Waters CH, Kurth M, Bailey P, et al: Tolcapone in stable Parkinson's disease: efficacy and safety of long-term treatment. Neurology 49:665–671, 1997

Weiner MF, Risser RC, Cullum CM, et al: Alzheimer's disease and its Lewy body variant: a clinical analysis of postmortem verified cases. Am J Psychiatry 153:1269–1273, 1996

Weiner RD, Rogers HJ, Davidson JR, et al: Effects of stimulus parameters on cognitive side effects, in Electroconvulsive Therapy: Clinical and Basic Research Issues. Edited by Malitz S, Sackeim HA. New York, New York Academy of Sciences, 1986, pp 315–325

Whitehouse PJ, Hedreen JC, White CL III, et al: Basal forebrain neurons in the dementia of Parkinson's disease. Ann Neurol 13:243–248, 1983

Wilkinson SB, Tröster AI: Surgical interventions in neurodegenerative disease: impact on memory and cognition, in Memory Disorders in Neurodegenerative Disease: Biological, Cognitive and Clinical Perspectives. Edited by Tröster AI. Cambridge, Cambridge University Press, 1998, pp 362–376

Wilson RS, Fox JH, Huckman MS, et al: Computed tomography in dementia. Neurology 32:1054–1057, 1982

Wolfson LI, Leenders KL, Brown LL, et al: Alterations of regional cerebral blood flow and oxygen metabolism in Parkinson's disease. Neurology 35:1399–1405, 1985

Wolters EC, Jansen EN, Tuynman-Qua HG, et al: Olanzapine in the treatment of dopaminomimetic psychosis in patients with Parkinson's disease. Neurology 47:1085–1087, 1996

Workman RH, Orengo CA, Bakey AA, et al: The use of risperidone for psychosis and agitation in demented patients with Parkinson's disease. J Neuropsychiatry Clin Neurosci 9:594–597, 1997

Wright MJ, Burns GM, Geffen GM, et al: Covert orientation of visual attention in Parkinson's disease: an impairment in the maintenance of attention. Neuropsychologia 28:151–159, 1990

Wszolek ZK, Pfeiffer B, Fulgham JR, et al: Western Nebraska family (family D) with autosomal dominant parkinsonism. Neurology 45:502–505, 1995

Wszolek ZK, Pfeiffer RF, Denson MA, et al: Danish-American family (family E) with "Parkinson's disease": pitfalls of genetic studies. Parkinsonism and Related Disorders 2:47–49, 1996

Xuereb JH, Tomlinson BE, Irving D, et al: Cortical and subcortical pathology in Parkinson's disease: relationship to parkinsonian dementia. Adv Neurol 53:35–40, 1990

Yahr MD, Mendoza MR, Moros D, et al: Treatment of Parkinson's disease in early and late phases: use of pharmacological agents with special reference to deprenyl (selegiline). Acta Neurol Scand 95 (suppl):95–102, 1983

Yamada T, Izyuuinn M, Schulzer M, et al: Covert orientation in Parkinson's disease. J Neurol Neurosurg Psychiatry 53:593–596, 1990

Young BK, Camicioli R, Ganzini L: Neuropsychiatric adverse effects of antiparkinsonian drugs: characteristics, evaluation and treatment. Drugs Aging 10:367–383, 1997

Zakzanis KK, Leach L, Kaplan E: On the nature and pattern of neurocognitive function in major depressive disorder. Neuropsychiatry Neuropsychol Behav Neurol 11:111–119, 1998

Zervas IM, Fink M: ECT for refractory Parkinson's disease (letter). Convulsive Therapy 7:222–223, 1991

Zoldan J, Friedberg G, Livneh M, et al: Psychosis in advanced Parkinson's disease: treatment with ondansetron, a 5-HT$_3$ receptor antagonist. Neurology 45:1305–1308, 1995

27

Stroke

Sergio E. Starkstein, M.D., Ph.D.

Robert G. Robinson, M.D.

Cerebrovascular disease is one of the most common life-threatening problems among the elderly population in the United States, and it ranks as the third leading cause of death (behind only heart disease and cancer) in patients over age 50. The prevalence of stroke increases steadily with age, rising from 10/100,000 for those under age 35 to 5,970/100,000 for those over age 75 (Wolf et al. 1984). The National Survey of Stroke estimated that there will be 500,000 new cases of stroke each year (Walker et al. 1981). During the past 10 years, however, there has been a steady decline in the incidence of stroke, which most investigators have attributed to the improved control of hypertension (Hachinski and Norris 1985; Wolf et al. 1984). Nevertheless, 75% of stroke survivors are left with physical or intellectual impairments of sufficient severity to limit their vocational capacity (Hachinski and Norris 1985).

The psychiatric complications of stroke lesions, although recognized for more than 100 years (Kraepelin 1921), have never received the attention that has been devoted to poststroke motor deficits, language problems, or intellectual disturbances. This relative neglect of emo-

tional impairments following stroke is difficult to understand for several reasons. First, psychiatric complications of stroke, such as depression or apathy, have a high prevalence (Robinson et al. 1983; Starkstein et al. 1993a). Second, these behavioral disorders have been shown to significantly impair the physical recovery (Parikh et al. 1990) and to increase the long-term mortality (Morris et al. 1993) of stroke patients. Everson et al. (1998) examined the association between depression symptoms and stroke mortality in a prospective study of behavioral, social, and psychological factors related to health and mortality in a community sample. They confirmed a significant relationship between depressive symptoms and stroke mortality. Third, clinicopathological correlations derived from the study of stroke lesions may constitute a valuable model for illuminating the mechanisms of psychiatric disorders in patients without known neuropathological disorders (i.e., functional disorders).

In this chapter, we briefly review the classification and nature of cerebrovascular disease and then discuss the most frequent emotional-behavioral sequelae of stroke lesions. Some of these psychiatric complications of stroke, such as depression, have been the focus of intense research, whereas other complications, such as anxiety or emotional lability, have not been characterized as well.

Cerebrovascular Disease

Classification

One obvious way of classifying cerebrovascular disease is based on the cause of the anatomic-pathological process within the blood vessels that perfuse the central nervous system. Such a classification would include infectious, connective tissue, neoplastic, hematologic, pharmacological, and traumatic causes. Alternatively, the classification of cerebrovascular disease may be based on the mechanisms of these different pathological processes, such as the interactive effects of systemic hypertension and atherosclerosis on the resilience of large arteries, the integrity of vessel lumens, and the production of end-organ ischemia; developmental abnormalities leading to the formation of aneurysmal dilations or weakness of the arterial wall; or the effect of cardiac arrhythmias on the propagation of emboli.

The most pragmatic way of classifying cerebrovascular disease, however, is categorizing disorders based on the way in which parenchymal changes in the brain do or do not occur (Starkstein and Robinson 1992). The first of these, ischemia, may occur with or without parenchymal infarction. Ischemic disorders include transient ischemic attacks, which may not produce parenchymal changes, and infarctions, which do produce parenchymal lesions. The causes of infarctions include atherosclerotic thrombosis, cerebral embolism, lacunae, and others, such as arteritis and fibromuscular dysplasia. The other cause of parenchymal changes is hemorrhage. Hemorrhages may cause direct parenchymal damage by extravasation of blood into the surrounding brain tissue, as in intracerebral hematoma, or indirect parenchymal damage by hemorrhage into the ventricles, subarachnoid space, extradural space, or subdural regions.

There are five major categories of cerebrovascular disease that produce focal parenchymal lesions: atherosclerotic thrombosis, cerebral embolism, lacunae, intracranial hemorrhage, and vascular malformations, such as aneurysms and arteriovenous malformations. Ischemic infarcts constitute the most prevalent type of stroke, and the ratio of infarcts to hemorrhages is about 5:1; atherosclerotic thrombosis and cerebral embolism account for about one-third of all strokes (Caplan and Stein 1986).

Atherosclerotic Thrombosis

Atherosclerotic thrombosis is often a result of a dynamic interaction between hypertension and atherosclerotic deposition of hyaline-lipid material in the walls of peripheral, coronary, and cerebral arteries. Hypertension is the most important risk factor for thrombotic stroke; other factors such as hyperlipidemia, diabetes mellitus, smoking, and obesity are of less importance. Atheromatous plaques tend to propagate at the bifurcation of the internal carotid artery or the carotid sinus, the "top" of the basilar artery, the posterior cerebral arteries at the midbrain level, and the anterior cerebral arteries as they curve over the corpus callosum. These plaques may lead to stenosis of one or more of these cerebral arteries or to complete occlusion.

Transient ischemic attacks, defined as periods of transient focal ischemia associated with reversible neurological deficits within a few hours, are usually produced by a thrombotic process. Most commonly, transient ischemic attacks have a duration of 2–15 minutes, with a range from a few seconds to up to 12–24 hours. Whereas the neurological examination between episodes of transient ischemic attacks is entirely normal, permanent neurological deficits (i.e., those lasting more than 24 hours) indicate that infarction has occurred.

Cerebral Embolism

Cerebral embolism, which accounts for approximately one-third of all strokes, is usually caused by a fragment breaking away from a thrombus within the heart and traveling up the carotid artery. The embolism may also originate from an atheromatous plaque within the lumen of the carotid sinus or from the distal end of a thrombus within the internal carotid artery, or less frequently it may represent a fat, tumor, or air embolus within the internal carotid artery. The causes of thrombus formation within the heart include cardiac arrhythmias, congenital heart disease, infectious processes, valve prostheses, postsurgical complications, and myocardial infarction with mural thrombus. Of all strokes, those caused by cerebral embolism develop most rapidly. A large embolus may occlude the internal carotid artery or the stem of the middle cerebral artery, producing a severe hemiplegia. More often, however, the embolus is smaller and passes into one of the branches of the middle cerebral artery, producing infarction distal to the site of the arterial occlusion. This is characterized by a pattern of neurological deficits consistent with that specific vascular distribution, which may be transient if the embolus fragments and travels into more distal arteries.

Lacunae

Lacunae, which account for nearly one-fifth of strokes, are the result of occlusion of small penetrating cerebral arteries. These small infarcts may produce no recognizable deficits, or (depending on their location) they may be associated with pure motor or sensory deficits. There is a strong association between lacunae and both atherosclerosis and hypertension, suggesting that lacunar infarction is the result of the effect of arteriosclerosis on small-diameter vessels.

Intracranial Hemorrhage

Intracranial hemorrhage is the fourth most frequent cause of stroke. The main causes of intracranial hemorrhage are hypertension, rupture of saccular aneurysms or arteriovenous malformations, hemorrhagic disorder, and trauma. Primary (hypertensive) intracranial hemorrhage occurs in deep parenchymal brain areas. The extravasation of blood forms a roughly circular or oval-shaped mass that disrupts and displaces the parenchyma. Adjacent tissue is compressed, and seepage into the ventricular system may occur. Intracranial hemorrhages can range in size from massive bleeds of several centimeters in diameter to petechial hemorrhages of a millimeter or less. They most commonly occur within the putamen and the adjacent internal capsule, thalamus, cerebellum, lobar white matter, and brainstem. Severe headache is a common accompaniment of intracranial hemorrhage and occurs in about 50% of cases. The prognosis is grave, with 70%–75% of patients dying within 1–30 days (Adams and Victor 1985).

Aneurysms and Arteriovenous Malformations

Ruptured aneurysms and arteriovenous malformations are the most common type of cerebrovascular disease after thrombosis, embolism, lacunae, and intracranial hemorrhage. Aneurysms are usually located at arterial bifurcations and are presumed to result from developmental defects in the formation of the arterial wall; rupture occurs when the intima bulges outward and eventually breaks through the adventitia. Arteriovenous malformations consist of a tangle of dilated vessels that form an abnormal communication between arterial and venous systems. They are developmental abnormalities consisting of persistent embryonic blood vessels. Hemorrhage from aneurysms or arteriovenous malformations may occur within the subarachnoid space or the brain parenchyma.

■ Neuropsychiatric Syndromes

Poststroke Depression

Frequency. Depression is one of the most common psychiatric sequelae to occur after a cerebrovascular lesion. Cross-sectional studies have demonstrated that 20%–50% of consecutive samples of stroke patients have depression, regardless of whether these patients are in specialized stroke units, general clinical units, rehabilitation hospitals, or the community (Eastwood et al. 1989; Robinson et al. 1983; Wade et al. 1987). In our studies of patients admitted to the hospital with an acute stroke, 25% met DSM-III (American Psychiatric Association 1980) criteria for major depression, whereas another 20% met criteria for dysthymic (minor) depression (Robinson et al. 1983). This high prevalence of poststroke depression was observed in both short-term and long-term stroke patients (Morris et al. 1990; Robinson et al. 1987) and was also replicated in incidence studies (Kotila et al. 1998). In a rural Chinese community, as many as 62.2% (28 of 45) of stroke survivors met criteria for depression. The mood disorder correlated with loss of daily living activities (Fuh et al. 1997). A recent Finish study (Pohjasvaara et al. 1998) found major depression in 26% and minor depression in 14% of a consecutive series of 486 patients with ischemic stroke.

Phenomenology of poststroke depression. We have identified two types of poststroke depressive disorders: the diagnosis of major depression is based on DSM-IV (American Psychiatric Association 1994) criteria for major depressive episode (excluding the time constraint), and the diagnosis of minor (dysthymic) depression is based on patients meeting DSM-IV criteria for dysthymic disorder (also excluding the time constraint) (Table 27–1). Lipsey et al. (1986) compared the frequency and type of depressive symptoms in a group of 43 patients with major poststroke depression and a group of 43 age-matched patients with "functional" major depression. Both groups showed the same frequency and types of depressive symptoms (Figure 27–1). The only exception was that the major poststroke depression group had a greater frequency of "slowness" than did the other group. This study, however, demonstrated that major poststroke depression is not an atypical form of depression and that these patients present with symptoms identical to elderly patients with major depression. Paradiso et al. (1997) demonstrated that only 2%–3% of stroke patients have depressive symptoms without a depressed mood and suggested that DSM-IV criteria do not overdiagnose major depression

TABLE 27–1.   DSM-IV criteria for major depressive episode and dysthymic disorder

Major depressive episode

A.   Five (or more) of the following symptoms have been present during the same 2-week period and represent a change from previous functioning; at least one of the symptoms is either (1) depressed mood or (2) loss of interest or pleasure.

Note: Do not include symptoms that are clearly due to a general medical condition, or mood-incongruent delusions or hallucinations.

   (1)   Depressed mood most of the day, nearly every day, as indicated by either subjective report (e.g., feels sad or empty) or observation made by others (e.g., appears tearful).   **Note:** In children and adolescents, can be irritable mood.

   (2)   Markedly diminished interest or pleasure in all, or almost all, activities most of the day, nearly every day (as indicated by either subjective account or observation made by others)

   (3)   Significant weight loss when not dieting or weight gain (e.g., a change of more than 5% of body weight in a month), or decrease or increase in appetite nearly every day.   **Note:** In children, consider failure to make expected weight gains.

   (4)   Insomnia or hypersomnia nearly every day

   (5)   Psychomotor agitation or retardation nearly every day (observable by others, not merely subjective feelings of restlessness or being slowed down)

   (6)   Fatigue or loss of energy nearly every day

   (7)   Feelings of worthlessness or excessive or inappropriate guilt (which may be delusional) nearly every day (not merely self-reproach or guilt about being sick)

   (8)   Diminished ability to think or concentrate, or indecisiveness, nearly every day (either by subjective account or as observed by others)

   (9)   Recurrent thoughts of death (not just fear of dying), recurrent suicidal ideation without a specific plan, or a suicide attempt or a specific plan for committing suicide

B.   The symptoms do not meet criteria for a mixed episode.

C.   The symptoms cause clinically significant distress or impairment in social, occupational, or other important areas of functioning.

D.   The symptoms are not due to the direct physiological effects of a substance (e.g., a drug of abuse, a medication) or a general medical condition (e.g., hypothyroidism).

E.   The symptoms are not better accounted for by bereavement, i.e., after the loss of a loved one, the symptoms persist for longer than 2 months or are characterized by marked functional impairment, morbid preoccupation with worthlessness, suicidal ideation, psychotic symptoms, or psychomotor retardation.

Dysthymic disorder

A.   Depressed mood for most of the day, for more days than not, as indicated either by subjective account or observation by others, for at least 2 years.   **Note:** In children and adolescents, mood can be irritable and duration must be at least 1 year.

B.   Presence, while depressed, of two (or more) of the following:

   (1)   Poor appetite or overeating

   (2)   Insomnia or hypersomnia

   (3)   Low energy or fatigue

   (4)   Low self-esteem

   (5)   Poor concentration or difficulty making decisions

   (6)   Feelings of hopelessness

C.   During the 2-year period (1 year for children or adolescents) of the disturbance, the person has never been without the symptoms in Criteria A and B for more than 2 months at a time.

D.   No major depressive episode has been present during the first 2 years of the disturbance (1 year for children and adolescents); i.e., the disturbance is not better accounted for by chronic major depressive disorder, or major depressive disorder, in partial remission.

Note: There may have been a previous major depressive episode provided there was a full remission (no significant signs or symptoms for 2 months) before development of the dysthymic disorder. In addition, after the initial 2 years (1 year in children or adolescents) of dysthymic disorder, there may be superimposed episodes of major depressive disorder, in which case both diagnoses may be given when the criteria are met for a major depressive episode.

E.   There has never been a manic episode, a mixed episode, or a hypomanic episode, and criteria have never been met for cyclothymic disorder.

F.   The disturbance does not occur exclusively during the course of a chronic psychotic disorder, such as schizophrenia or delusional disorder.

G.   The symptoms are not due to the direct physiological effects of a substance (e.g., a drug of abuse, a medication) or a general medical condition (e.g., hypothyroidism).

H.   The symptoms cause clinically significant distress or impairment in social, occupational, or other important areas of functioning.

Specify if:

Early onset: if onset is before age 21 years
Late onset: if onset is age 21 years or older
Specify (for most recent 2 years of dysthymic disorder):
With atypical features

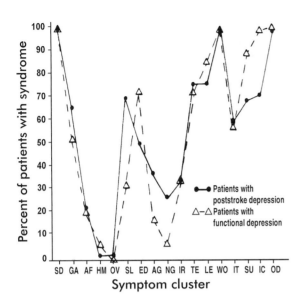

FIGURE 27–1. Symptom clusters from the present state examination in 43 patients with major poststroke depression and 43 patients with functional depression. SD = simple depression; GA = general anxiety; AF = affective flattening; HM = hypomania; OV = overactivity; SL = slowness; ED = special features of depression; AG = agitation; NG = self-neglect; IR = ideas of reference; TE = tension; LE = lack of energy; WO = worrying; IT = irritability; SU = social unease; IC = loss of interest and concentration; OD = other symptoms of depression.
Source. Reprinted with permission from Lipsey JR, Spencer WC, Rabins PV, et al: "Phenomenological Comparison of Functional and Post-stroke Depression." *American Journal of Psychiatry* 143:527–529, 1986.

among stroke patients. Several studies have validated the distinction between major and minor poststroke depression and have demonstrated these two types of depression to have different courses of longitudinal evolution (Morris et al. 1990; Robinson et al. 1987), biological markers (Barry and Dinan 1990; Lipsey et al. 1985), effects on cognitive function (Robinson et al. 1986), and correlation with brain lesion location (Robinson et al. 1984; Starkstein et al. 1988b). Kishi et al. (1996) reported that 7% of short-term stroke patients and 11% of long-term (i.e., > 3 months) stroke patients had suicidal ideation. Whereas early suicidal ideation was related to premorbid alcohol abuse, delayed suicidal ideation was related to greater physical impairment and poorer social support during the immediate poststroke period.

Clinical correlates. Gender differences in the prevalence of poststroke depression have recently been reported by Paradiso and Robinson (1998). These research-

ers found that the prevalence of major depression in women was double that found in men. Among women, greater severity of depression was associated with prior diagnosis of psychiatric disorder and cognitive impairment, whereas among men depression was significantly associated with greater impairment in daily activities and social functioning.

Poststroke depression has a significant influence on both the recovery in activities of daily living (ADLs) and the intellectual impairment of stroke patients. In a recent study, Ramasubbu et al. (1998) examined the independent association of depression following acute stroke with impairment in ADLs in a cross-sectional epidemiological study. They found that depressed stroke patients had significantly greater impairments in ADLs than nondepressed patients, independent of all other factors that influenced poststroke physical disabilities. Parikh et al. (1990) compared the 2-year recovery from impairments in ADLs between 25 patients with poststroke depression (either major or minor depression) and 38 stroke patients with no mood disorders who were matched for their in-hospital severity of ADL impairments. After controlling for all the variables that have been shown to influence stroke outcome (e.g., short-term treatment on a stroke unit; size, nature and location of brain injury; age; education; and duration of rehabilitation services), patients with in-hospital poststroke depression had significantly poorer recovery than did nondepressed stroke patients even after their depressions had subsided (Figure 27–2).

In another study, we (Robinson et al. 1986) compared patients with major poststroke depression and nondepressed stroke patients for the presence of cognitive impairments. We found that patients with major poststroke depression after left-hemisphere lesions had significantly more cognitive deficits than did nondepressed patients with a similar size and location of brain lesion. These deficits were observed in a wide range of cognitive tasks, including orientation, language, visuoconstructional ability, executive motor functions, and frontal lobe tasks (Figure 27–3) (Bolla-Wilson et al. 1989). In contrast, among patients with right-hemisphere lesions, patients with major depression did not differ from nondepressed patients on any of the measures of cognitive impairment. This finding suggests that left-hemisphere lesions that lead to major depression may produce a different kind of depression than do right-hemisphere lesions. Left-hemisphere lesions can produce a dementia of depression, which does not occur with major depressions following right-hemisphere lesions. It remains to be determined whether these dementias of depression will improve with treatment of depression.

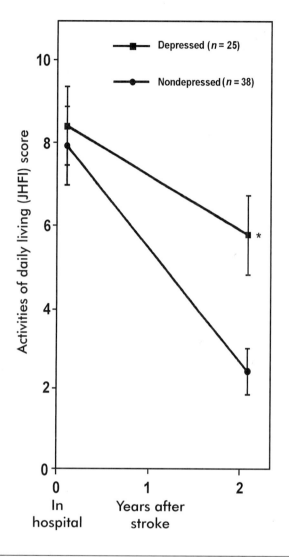

FIGURE 27–2. Johns Hopkins Functioning Inventory (JHFI) scores in the hospital and at 2-year follow-up in patients who were depressed or nondepressed. Higher scores on the JHFI indicate greater impairment in activities of daily living. There was a significant group-by-time interaction, with the nondepressed patients having significantly lower (i.e., less impaired) scores than the depressed patients at 2-year follow-up.

* $P < .05$.

Source. Reprinted with permission from Parikh RM, Robinson RG, Lipsey JR, et al: "The Impact of Post-Stroke Depression on Recovery in Activities of Daily Living Over Two-Year Follow-Up." *Archives of Neurology* 47:785–789, 1990.

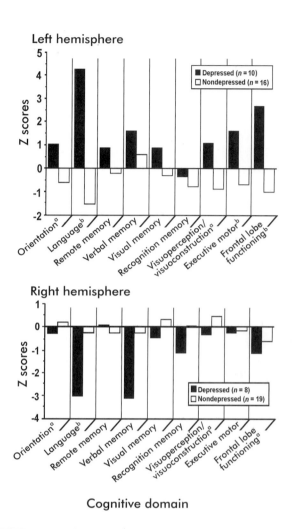

FIGURE 27–3. Performance on the nine cognitive domains by depressed and nondepressed patients with left- or right-hemisphere stroke.

[a]$P < .05$ comparing depressed and nondepressed groups using one-way analysis of variance (ANOVA).

[b]$P < .01$ comparing depressed and nondepressed groups using one-way ANOVA.

Source. Reprinted with permission from Bolla-Wilson K, Robinson RG, Starkstein SE, et al: "Lateralization of Dementia of Depression in Stroke Patients." *American Journal of Psychiatry* 146:627–634, 1989.

Clinical-pathological correlates and mechanism. In several prospective studies using different samples of stroke patients, we have consistently found a significant association between poststroke depression and lesion location: patients with major poststroke depression showed a significantly higher frequency of lesions in anterior areas of the left hemisphere, namely the left frontal dorsolateral cortex and the head of the caudate nucleus (Robinson et al. 1984; Starkstein et al. 1987). Among patients with right-hemisphere stroke lesions, those with frontal or parietal damage showed the highest frequency of depression (Starkstein et al. 1989). Although some, but not all, of these findings have been replicated by other investigators (Eastwood et al. 1989; House et al. 1991; Morris et al. 1992), a consensus has emerged that there is a significant correlation between the proximity of the lesion to the frontal pole and the severity of depression.

In 1981, we first reported that in a group of 29 patients with left-hemisphere lesions produced by trauma or stroke there was an inverse correlation between severity of depression and distance of the anterior border of the lesion from the frontal pole ($r = -.76$, $P < .001$) (Figure 27–4) (Robinson and Szetela 1981). Since then, using computed tomographic (CT) imaging, we found the same phenomenon in another group of 10 right-handed patients with single stroke lesions of the anterior left hemisphere ($r = -.92$, $P < .001$) (Robinson et al. 1984). When patients with lesions in the left posterior hemisphere were added ($n = 18$), the correlation decreased ($r = -.54$, $P < .05$) (Table 27–2). This inverse correlation was also found in other groups of patients with purely cortical lesions of the left hemisphere ($n = 16$; $r = -.52$, $P < .05$) (Starkstein et al. 1987), purely left-sided subcortical lesions ($n = 13$) ($r = -.68$, $P < .01$) (Starkstein et al. 1987), and single left-hemisphere lesions in left-handed patients ($n = 13$; $r = -.78$, $P < .01$) (Robinson et al. 1985). This phenomenon has now been replicated by four different groups of investigators using patients from Canada, England, and Australia (Table 27–2).

Some investigators have found a correlation between severity of depression and proximity of the lesion to the frontal pole in combined right- and left-hemisphere lesion groups, whereas others found it only with left-sided lesions

(Table 27–2). Although there is some difference in the strength of this correlation (and therefore the amount of variance in severity of depression explained by lesion location), this phenomenon has emerged as one of the most consistent and robust clinical-pathological correlations ever described in neuropsychiatry. Future experiments aimed at elucidating the mechanism of poststroke depression must provide an explanation for this remarkably consistent phenomenon.

The mechanism by which left anterior lesions produce depression is not known. One possibility is that both the frontal dorsolateral cortex and the dorsal caudate nucleus play an important role in mediating locomotor, intellectual, and instinctive behavior through their connection with the supplementary motor area, temporoparietal association cortex, and limbic system. A lesion of these anterior brain areas may result in low activation of locomotor, sensory, or limbic areas and produce the autonomic and affective symptoms of depression. We (Robinson et al. 1984) have suggested that biogenic amines may also play an important role in poststroke depression. The anatomy of these pathways (i.e., they begin in brainstem nuclei and ascend through subcortical regions, around the corpus callosum to the posterior cortex) may explain the correlations with lesion location, as anterior lesions close to the frontal pole would interrupt more "downstream" pathways than posterior lesions (Robinson et al. 1984).

Treatment. In a randomized, double-blind, and placebo-controlled study of the efficacy of treatment of poststroke depression, we demonstrated the utility of the tricyclic antidepressant nortriptyline in the treatment of poststroke depression (Lipsey et al. 1984). Patients received 25 mg for 1 week, 50 mg for 2 weeks, 75 mg for 1 week, and 100 mg for 2 weeks. The group receiving the active drug (11 completed the study) showed a significant decrease in depression scores compared with the placebo group (15 completed) (Figure 27–5). Side effects were observed in 6 of 17 patients: 3 developed delirium, 1 had syncope, 1 complained of oversedation, and 1 complained of dizziness.

Andersen et al. (1994a) demonstrated the efficacy of the selective serotonin reuptake inhibitor citalopram in a 6-week double-blind, placebo-controlled trial that included 66 patients with poststroke depression. Significantly greater mood improvement was demonstrated in patients treated with 10 to 40 mg/day of citalopram compared with the placebo group. The only significant side effects of citalopram were nausea and vomiting during the first week of treatment.

One other controlled study demonstrated the useful-

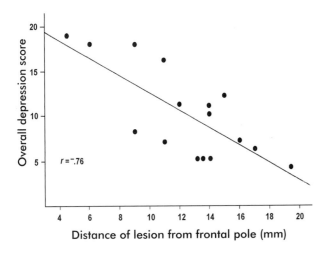

FIGURE 27–4. Relationship between severity of depression as measured by overall depression score and mean distance of the lesion from the frontal pole for patients with lesions that extended into the frontal lobe. The closer the lesion was to the frontal pole, the greater the depression was ($r = -.76$, $P < .001$).

Source. Reprinted with permission from Robinson RG, Szetela B: "Mood Change Following Left Hemispheric Brain Injury." *Annals of Neurology* 9:447–453, 1981.

TABLE 27–2. Depression severity and proximity of lesion to frontal pole

Study	N patients	Patient population	Lesion hemisphere	Correlation	P
Robinson and Szetela 1981	29	Stroke or trauma	Left	−.76	< .001
Robinson et al. 1984	10	Single stroke, right handed	Left anterior	−.92	< .001
	18	Single stroke, right handed	Left anterior and posterior	−.54	< .05
Lipsey et al. 1983	15	Bilateral stroke lesions	Left only	−.65	< .01
Robinson et al. 1985	13	Left handed, single stroke	Left	−.78	< .01
Starkstein et al. 1987	16	Cortical lesions only	Left	−.52	< .05
	13	Subcortical lesion only	Left	−.68	< .01
Sinyor et al. 1986	27	Single stroke	Left and right	−.47	< .05
Eastwood et al. 1989	11	Single stroke	Left	−.74	< .01
House et al. 1991	63	Single stroke	Left and right	−.28	< .01
	33	6 months	Left	−.38	< .05
Morris et al. 1992	14	Single stroke remove prior depression	Left	−.87	< .001

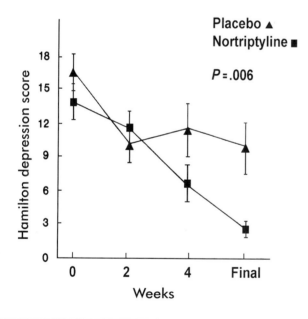

FIGURE 27–5. Hamilton depression scores during 6 weeks of treatment for poststroke depression.
Source. Reprinted with permission from Lipsey JR, Robinson RG, Pearlson GD, et al: "Nortriptyline Treatment of Post-Stroke Depression: A Double-Blind Treatment Trial." *Lancet* 1:297–300, 1984.

ness of another antidepressant drug (trazodone) for poststroke depression (Reding et al. 1986). Depressed patients taking trazodone were found to have greater improvements in ADL scores than were patients treated with placebo. This trend became statistically significant when the treatment groups were restricted to patients with abnormal dexamethasone tests. Although antidepressants are effective in the treatment of poststroke depression, the high rate of complications such as delirium dictate that tricyclic drugs should be used cautiously in elderly stroke patients.

Poststroke Anxiety

Although anxiety is one of the most frequent complaints in the general population, it has rarely been the focus of empirical research among stroke patients.

Phenomenology and frequency. In a study on the prevalence of anxiety disorders in stroke patients, we examined 309 patients admitted to the hospital with acute stroke using DSM-III criteria for generalized anxiety disorders (Castillo et al. 1993). We found that 78 patients (26.9%) met criteria for generalized anxiety disorder, whereas the prevalence of anxiety in the chronic stage was 23% (Castillo et al. 1995). In a 3-year longitudinal study, Aström (1996) found a prevalence of anxiety in the acute poststroke period of 28%, and there was no significant decrease through the 3 years of follow-up. However, the presence of the disorder was strongly associated with the presence of depression, as 58 of 78 stroke patients meeting criteria for generalized anxiety disorder in the study by Castillo et al. (1993) were also depressed. Thus, although generalized anxiety disorder is a common finding among stroke patients, it frequently coexists with depression. A recent study by Shimoda and Robinson (1998) demonstrated a significant interaction of depression and anxiety in stroke. In this study, patients with both anxiety and depression had greater impairment in ADLs at long-term follow-up and worse recovery in social functioning than nondepressed patients.

Clinical correlates and mechanism. We examined the clinical and lesion correlates of anxiety and depression in the study of 309 patients with acute stroke (Castillo et al. 1993). The anxious and nonanxious groups were not significantly different in their demographic backgrounds or neurological findings. The nondepressed anxious patients, however, had a significantly higher frequency of alcoholism than did the nonanxious patients (26% generalized anxiety disorder versus 8% nonanxious, $P < .05$). When patients with both generalized anxiety disorder and depression were compared to patients with depression only, patients with anxiety and depression had a significantly higher frequency of cortical lesions (mainly left frontal), whereas the patients with depression only had a significantly higher frequency of subcortical lesions (mainly left basal ganglia) (Starkstein et al. 1990b). Among the anxious patients without depression, 67% had right-hemisphere lesions compared with 43% of the anxious depressed patients ($P = .04$) (Castillo et al. 1993). Finally, among patients with right-hemisphere lesions, the anxious patients had lesions that were significantly more posterior than those of the nonanxious patients ($P = .038$) (Castillo et al. 1993). Aström (1996) found that at the acute

stage after stroke, anxiety plus depression was associated with left-hemisphere lesions, whereas anxiety alone was associated with right-hemisphere lesions.

Although the mechanism of anxiety is still unknown, several studies have reported a significant decrease in cortical metabolic activity with increased anxiety, as well as a lack of correlation between the severity of anxiety and subcortical metabolic rate (Bartlett et al. 1988; Gur et al. 1987). This is in agreement with our finding of significantly more severe anxiety after cortical lesions than after subcortical lesions and suggests a critical role for cortical-subcortical interaction in the modulation of anxious states.

Poststroke Apathy

Apathy is the absence or lack of feeling, emotion, interest, or concern and has been reported frequently among stroke patients. We examined a consecutive series of 80 patients with single stroke lesions and no significant impairment in comprehension using the Apathy Scale (Figure 27–6). We demonstrated both the validity and reliability of this scale in the assessment of apathy in patients with cerebrovascular lesions (Starkstein et al. 1993a). A score of 14 on this scale separated apathetic from nonapathetic patients with high sensitivity and specificity.

Prevalence and clinical correlates. In a study of poststroke apathy (Starkstein et al. 1993a), we found that

Questions	Not at all	Slightly	Some	A lot
1. Are you interested in learning new things?	❑	❑	❑	❑
2. Does anything interest you?	❑	❑	❑	❑
3. Are you concerned about your condition?	❑	❑	❑	❑
4. Do you put much effort into things?	❑	❑	❑	❑
5. Are you always looking for something to do?	❑	❑	❑	❑
6. Do you have plans and goals for the future?	❑	❑	❑	❑
7. Do you have motivation?	❑	❑	❑	❑
8. Do you have the energy for daily activities?	❑	❑	❑	❑
9. Does someone have to tell you what to do each day?	❑	❑	❑	❑
10. Are you indifferent to things?	❑	❑	❑	❑
11. Are you unconcerned with many things?	❑	❑	❑	❑
12. Do you need a push to get started on things?	❑	❑	❑	❑
13. Are you neither happy nor sad, just in between?	❑	❑	❑	❑
14. Would you consider yourself apathetic?	❑	❑	❑	❑

Note. For questions 1–8, the scoring system is the following: *not at all* = 3 points; *slightly* = 2 points; *some* = 1 point; *a lot* = 0 points. For questions 9–14, the scoring system is the following: *not at all* = 0 points; *slightly* = 1 point; *some* = 2 points; *a lot* = 3 points.

FIGURE 27–6. Apathy scale.

9 of 80 patients (11%) showed apathy as their only psychiatric disorder, whereas another 11% had both apathy and depression. The only demographic correlate of apathy was age, as apathetic patients (with or without depression) were significantly older than were nonapathetic patients. Also, apathetic patients showed significantly more severe deficits in ADLs, and there was a significant interaction between depression and apathy (i.e., Johns Hopkins Functioning Inventory [JHFI] scores were 4.8 ± 4.0 for patients with no disorder, 6.21 ± 3.9 for depressed patients, 7.6 ± 5.8 for apathetic patients, and 13.7 ± 5.5 for depressed and apathetic patients; effect of apathy $P < .001$, effect of depression $P < .002$, and interaction $P = .05$).

Clinical-pathological correlates and mechanism of poststroke apathy.

Patients with apathy (without depression) showed a significantly higher frequency of lesions involving the posterior limb of the internal capsule compared with patients with no apathy (Starkstein et al. 1993a). Lesions in the internal globus pallidus and the posterior limb of the internal capsule have been reported to produce important behavioral changes, such as motor neglect, psychic akinesia, and akinetic mutism (Helgason et al. 1988). The ansa lenticularis is one of the main internal pallidal outputs, and it ends in the pedunculopontine nucleus after going through the posterior limb of the internal capsule (Nauta 1989). In rodents, this pathway has a prominent role in goal-oriented behavior (Bechara and van der Kooy 1989), and dysfunction of this system may explain the presence of apathy in stroke patients.

Poststroke Psychosis

The phenomenon of hallucinations and delusions in stroke patients has been called *agitated delirium, acute atypical psychosis, peduncular hallucinosis, release hallucinations,* or *acute organic psychosis.* We consider *secondary hallucinations* to be sensory perceptions in the absence of appropriate stimuli, with the important qualifications that, first, the patient believes the (nonexistent) sensory perception is real, and, second, this disorder started after a lesion. We use the term *secondary hallucinosis* to refer to a perception without a stimulus, when the patient does not believe the (nonexistent) sensory perception is real and the disorder occurs after a stroke lesion. Finally, we use the term *secondary psychosis* to refer to patients who develop either secondary hallucinations or secondary hallucinosis after stroke lesions. Patients with secondary psychosis, hallucination type, are delusional (i.e., they do not recognize the perception as false), whereas those with secondary psychosis,

hallucinosis type, are usually not delusional unless there is some other independent delusional idea.

Prevalence and clinical-pathological correlates.

In a study of secondary psychosis after stroke lesions, we (Rabins et al. 1991) found a very low prevalence of this phenomenon among stroke patients (only five in more than 300 consecutive admissions). All five patients had right-hemisphere lesions, primarily involving frontoparietal regions. When compared with five age-matched patients with cerebrovascular lesions in similar locations but no psychosis, patients with secondary psychosis had significantly greater subcortical atrophy, as manifested by significantly larger areas of both the frontal horn of the lateral ventricle and the body of the lateral ventricle (measured on the side contralateral to the brain lesion). Several other investigators have reported a high frequency of seizures among patients with secondary psychosis (e.g., Levine and Finklestein 1982). These seizures usually started after the brain lesion but before the onset of psychosis. We also found seizures in three of our five patients with poststroke psychosis, compared with none of the five poststroke nonpsychotic control subjects.

Mechanism.

We conclude from these observations that three factors may be important in the mechanism of secondary psychosis, hallucination type: a right-hemisphere lesion involving the temporoparietal cortex, seizures, and subcortical brain atrophy. The mechanism of secondary hallucinosis is even less clear than secondary hallucinations. Although in the literature most patients with secondary hallucinosis had peduncular lesions, patients with lesions in other brain areas, such as the diencephalon, also showed the phenomenon (Cascino and Adams 1986; Geller and Bellur 1987). These lesions have frequently been found to involve primary sensory pathways, mainly visual and auditory. Thus, secondary hallucinosis may be a "release phenomenon" secondary to damage to reticular activating brainstem pathways, and the presence of primary sensory deficits in these patients may be a necessary predisposing factor.

In conclusion, secondary psychosis is a rare finding in stroke patients. We believe that there are at least two types of secondary psychosis. The first is the hallucination type, which is characterized by hallucinations perceived by the patient as real and may result from right temporoparietal lesions in the presence of preexisting subcortical brain atrophy and poststroke seizures. The second is the hallucinosis type, which is characterized by hallucinations perceived by the patient as unreal and may be secondary to lesions in primary sensory or reticular activating pathways.

Anosognosia

The term *anosognosia* was coined by Babinski (1914) to describe the lack of awareness of hemiplegia, but it was later used to refer to the unawareness of other poststroke deficits, such as cortical blindness, hemianopia, and amnesia (Heilman 1991).

Prevalence and clinical correlates. We examined the prevalence of anosognosia in a consecutive series of 80 patients with single acute stroke lesions (Starkstein et al. 1992). We developed an anosognosia questionnaire (Figure 27–7), which we used to determine the existence of anosognosia. To rate the severity of this phenomenon, we also developed the Denial of Illness Scale (Figure 27–8), which allows the classification of patients into those with mild, moderate, or severe anosognosia. Patients with aphasia were included only if they had intact verbal comprehension as measured by their ability to complete Part 1 of the Token Test (De Renzi and Vignolo 1962). The assessment of anosognosia, however, examined only motor, sensory, and visual field disturbances and did not evaluate anosognosia for aphasia.

1. Why are you here?
2. What is the matter with you?
3. Is there anything wrong with your arm or leg?
4. Is there anything wrong with your eyesight?
5. Is your arm or leg weak, paralyzed, or numb?
6. How does your arm or leg feel?

If denial is elicited ask the following:

    a. (*pick up the patient's arm*) What is this?

    b. Can you lift it?

    c. Do you have some problem with this?

    d. (*ask the patient to lift both arms*) Can you see that your two arms are not at the same level?

    e. (*ask the patient to identify finger movements in and out of the abnormal visual field*) Can't you see that you have a problem with your eyesight?

Scoring

0, The disorder is spontaneously reported or mentioned following a general question about the patient's complaints.

1, The disorder is reported only after a specific question about the strength of the patient's limb, or visual problems.

2, The disorder is acknowledged only after its demonstration through routine techniques of neurological examination.

3, The disorder is not acknowledged.

FIGURE 27–7. Anosognosia questionnaire.

The first important finding from this study was that about one-third of this consecutive series of patients had anosognosia (19% mild, 11% moderate, and 13% severe) (Starkstein et al. 1992). We also examined potential correlates of anosognosia and found this phenomenon to be significantly associated with the presence of a neglect syndrome (i.e., failure to respond to or orient to stimuli contralateral to the lesion), as well as deficits in recognizing facial emotions and the emotional content of speech (prosody). There also was a significant association between anosognosia and right-hemisphere lesions involving the temporal and parietal lobes, thalamus, and basal ganglia.

Two important negative findings should be noted. First, the frequency of depression was similar among patients with and without anosognosia. Thus the existence of anosognosia does not preclude stroke patients from experiencing or reporting depressive feelings. Second, anosognosic patients did not show more severe sensory deficits than did nonanosognosic patients (i.e., anosognosia is not related to the presence of sensory deficits) (Starkstein et al. 1992).

Mechanism. In our study (Starkstein et al. 1992), we found that brain atrophy, probably preexisting the brain lesion, may have been an important predisposing factor for anosognosia, as anosognosic patients had significantly more frontal subcortical and diencephalic atrophy (but not cortical atrophy) than did patients with no anosognosia. Moreover, patients with anosognosia had significantly more deficits in frontal lobe–related cognitive tasks than did patients with no anosognosia but with lesions in similar brain areas.

These findings suggest that lesions in specific cortical and subcortical areas of the right hemisphere, although necessary, may not be sufficient to produce anosognosia; concomitant frontal lobe dysfunction (as expressed by frontal subcortical atrophy and deficits in frontal lobe–related cognitive tasks) may be necessary to produce the syndrome.

Heilman (1991) proposed that anosognosia may result from a dysfunction of a system that monitors the intention to move as well as the actual performance of movements. This mismatch between the intention to move and the (lack of) movement may convey the impression that the movement was actually performed and that the limb is normal. The systems monitoring single sensory and motor modalities may be located in the right parietal lobe, whereas the frontal lobe may constitute a supramodal monitoring structure.

In conclusion, anosognosia is present in one-third of acute stroke patients and is significantly associated with

Items	Scoring		
1. Patient minimizes present symptoms (at interview).	0 (no)	1 (once or twice)	2 (more than twice)
2. Patient alludes to there being nothing really wrong with her or him and that she or he is ready to go home.	0 (no)	1 (once or twice)	2 (more than twice)
3. Patient (past or present) displaces source of symptoms to organs other than brain or complains of symptoms unrelated to the central nervous system.	0 (no)	1 (once or twice)	2 (more than twice)
4. Patient at any time admits to fear of death.	0 (yes)	1 (no)	
5. Patient at any time admits to fear of invalidism.	0 (yes)	1 (no)	
6. Patient verbally denies being in the hospital.	0 (not at all)	1 (sometimes)	2 (every time)
7. Patient displays, at least on the surface, a carefree, cheerful, jovial approach to life.	0 (no)	1 (once or twice)	2 (more than twice)
8. Patient's behavior during interview is characterized by nonchalance, coolness, imperturbability.	0 (no)	1 (once or twice)	2 (more than twice)
9. Patient displaces fear for his or her own illness to family, older patients, weaker patients, and so on.	0 (no)	1 (at least 1 time during the interview)	
10. Patient projects illness or weakness to family, spouse, and so on.	0 (no)	1 (at least 1 time during the interview)	

FIGURE 27–8.   Denial of Illness Scale.

right-hemisphere lesions in the temporoparietal cortex, basal ganglia, or thalamus. The presence of neglect and frontal lobe dysfunction may constitute important predisposing factors.

Catastrophic Reaction

Catastrophic reaction is a term coined by Goldstein (1939) to describe the "inability of the organism to cope when faced with physical or cognitive deficits." It is expressed by anxiety, tears, aggressive behavior, swearing, displacement, refusal, renouncement, and, sometimes, compensatory boasting.

Prevalence and clinical correlates.   The catastrophic reaction has been reported to be a frequent finding among aphasic patients (Gainotti 1972) and has been given the status of a separate neuropsychiatric syndrome. There are no empirical studies regarding the construct validity of the catastrophic reaction, however, and it is possible that the catastrophic reaction may represent a symptom of a major depressive syndrome or anxiety disorder in stroke patients. To empirically examine this issue, we evaluated a consecutive series of 62 patients by using the Catastrophic Reaction Scale (CRS), which we developed to assess the existence and severity of the catastrophic reaction (Figure 27–9). We have demonstrated the CRS to be a reliable instrument in the measurement of catastrophic reaction symptoms (Starkstein et al. 1993b).

We identified the catastrophic reaction in 12 of 62 consecutive patients (19%) with acute stroke lesions (Starkstein et al. 1993b). Three major findings emerged from this study. First, patients with catastrophic reaction were found to have a significantly higher frequency of familial and personal history of psychiatric disorders (mostly depression) than were patients without the catastrophic reaction. Second, catastrophic reaction was not significantly more frequent among aphasic than with nonaphasic patients, which does not support the suggestion that catastrophic reaction is more frequent among "frustrated" aphasic patients (Gainotti 1972). Third, 9 (75%) of the 12 patients with catastrophic reaction also had major depression, 2 (17%) had minor depression, and only 1 (8%) was not depressed. On the other hand, among patients without catastrophic reaction (i.e., 50 patients), 7 (14%) had major depression, 6 (12%) had minor depression, and 37 (74%) were not depressed. Thus catastrophic reaction was significantly associated with major depression ($\chi^2 = 20.9$, df = 2, $P = .0001$). Moreover, patients with a catastrophic reaction had significantly higher scores on the Hamilton Anxiety and Depression Scales compared with patients with no catastrophic reaction.

Mechanism.   Patients with a catastrophic reaction had a significantly higher frequency of lesions involving the

1. Patient appeared to be anxious (i.e., patient showed an apprehensive attitude or expressed fears).

2. Patient complained of feeling anxious or afraid (i.e., patient referred to feeling tense or having psychological concomitants of anxiety).

3. Patient became tearful (i.e., patient cried at some point during the evaluation).

4. Patient complained of feeling sad or depressed (i.e., patient spontaneously reported sad feelings during the evaluation).

5. Patient behaved in angry manner (i.e., patient shouted, contradicted the examiner, or performed tasks in a careless way).

6. Patient complained of feeling angry (i.e., patient reported being upset with the evaluation and/or the examiner).

7. Patient swore (i.e., patient swore at some point during the evaluation).

8. Patient expressed displaced anger (i.e., patient complained about the hospital, doctors, and fellow patients).

9. Patient refused to do something (i.e., patient stopped doing a task or refused to answer some questions).

10. Patient described a feeling of suddenly becoming depressed or hopeless (i.e., patient reported feeling worthless and sad and had a lack of confidence).

11. Patient boasted about self (i.e., patient reported being able to perform the tasks flawlessly; he or she explained failures as due to lack of concentration and tiredness).

Note. Scoring key: 0 = none; 1 = slight (once during the interview); 2 = moderate (several times during the interview); 3 = extreme (most of the interview).

FIGURE 27–9. Catastrophic Reaction Scale.

basal ganglia (Starkstein et al. 1993b). When 10 depressed patients with a catastrophic reaction were compared to 10 depressed patients without a catastrophic reaction, the catastrophic reaction group showed significantly more anterior lesions, which were located mostly in subcortical regions (8 of 9 depressed patients with catastrophic reaction had subcortical lesions; 3 of 9 depressed patients without catastrophic reaction had subcortical lesions) (χ^2 = 5.84, df = 1, P = .01).

We may conclude from the above evidence that the catastrophic reaction is not just a behavioral response of patients confronted with their limitations, as patients with and without a catastrophic reaction showed a similar frequency of aphasia and physical impairments. On the contrary, the catastrophic reaction seems to characterize a specific type of poststroke major depression (i.e., major depressions associated with anterior subcortical lesions). An-

terior brain lesions (both cortical and subcortical) have been consistently associated with poststroke depression. Subcortical damage, however, has usually been hypothesized to underlie the "release" of emotional display by removing inhibitory input to the limbic areas of the cortex (Ross and Stewart 1987).

In conclusion, the catastrophic reaction occurs in about 20% of stroke patients (Starkstein et al. 1993b), mainly among those with a positive familial or personal history of psychiatric disorders. The catastrophic reaction is significantly associated with major depression and may be mediated by a release of emotional display produced by anterior subcortical lesions. Thus the catastrophic reaction may not represent an independent clinical syndrome but may be a behavioral and emotional expression of depressed patients with anterior subcortical damage.

Emotional Lability

Emotional lability is a common complication of stroke lesions. It is characterized by sudden, easily provoked episodes of crying, which, although occurring frequently, generally occur in appropriate situations and are accompanied by a congruent mood change. Pathological laughing and crying is a more severe form of emotional lability and is characterized by episodes of laughing and/or crying that are not appropriate to the context. They may appear spontaneously or may be elicited by nonemotional events and do not correspond to underlying emotional feelings. Other terms that have been applied to these disorders are *emotional incontinence* and *pseudobulbar affect*.

Prevalence and clinical correlates. We examined the clinical correlates and treatment of emotional lability (including pathological laughter and crying) in 28 patients with either acute or chronic stroke (Robinson et al. 1993). We developed a Pathological Laughter and Crying Scale (PLACS) (Appendix 27–1) to assess the existence and severity of emotional lability. We demonstrated in 18 treatment patients and 54 acute stroke patients the reliability and validity of this instrument in the assessment of emotional lability (Robinson et al. 1993). We also found that PLACS scores did not correlate with either Hamilton Depression Scale scores, Mini-Mental State Exam scores, ADL scores, or Social Ties scores, indicating that the PLACS was assessing a factor other than the ones being measured by these instruments.

A double-blind drug trial of nortriptyline was conducted in 31 patients with emotional lability (Robinson et al. 1993). After randomization, patients were given active drug or placebo in a single bedtime dose. Patients were first given 25 mg of nortriptyline for 1 week, then 50 mg for 2 weeks, 70 mg for 1 week, and 100 mg for the last 2 weeks of the study. One patient dropped out during the study, and two patients withdrew before initiation of the study; there were 28 who completed the 6-week protocol. Patients receiving nortriptyline showed significant improvements in PLACS scores compared with the placebo-treated patients; these differences became statistically significant at weeks 4 and 6 (Figure 27–10). Although a significant improvement in depression scores also was observed, improvements in PLACS scores were significant for both depressed and nondepressed patients with pathological laughing and crying, indicating that treatment response was not related simply to an improvement in depression.

Mechanism. Pseudobulbar affect has classically been explained as being secondary to the bilateral interruption of neocortical upper motor neuron innervation of bulbar motor nuclei (Poeck 1969). The finding that emotional lability can be successfully treated with tricyclic drugs suggests that biogenic amine systems may also play a role in the pathogenesis of this disorder. Andersen et al. (1994b) reported that stroke patients with relatively large bilateral pontine lesions had more severe pathological crying than did patients with cortical or subcortical hemisphere le-

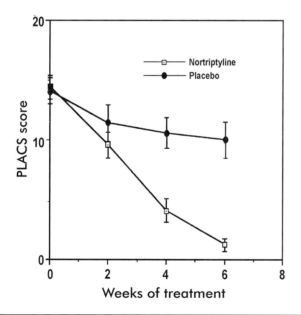

FIGURE 27–10. Mean Pathological Laughter and Crying Scale (PLACS) scores during 6 weeks of double-blind treatment. The nortriptyline-treated group had significantly lower (more improved) PLACS scores at 4 ($t = 3.9$, df = 26, $P = .0005$) and 6 ($t = 5.1$, df = 26, $P = .0001$) weeks of treatment compared with the placebo-treated group.
Source. Adapted from Robinson et al. 1993.

sions; the researchers speculated that pathological crying may result from partial destruction of the serotonergic raphe nuclei or their ascending projections to the hemispheres.

In conclusion, our study (Robinson et al. 1993) suggests that poststroke depression and emotional lability are independent phenomena, although they may coexist. Moreover, we also found that both depressed and nondepressed patients with emotional lability showed significant improvements in the severity of their emotional lability after treatment with nortriptyline.

Mania

Prevalence and clinical correlates. Mania, or disinhibited behavior, is a relatively rare consequence of acute stroke lesions. Using DSM-III criteria for affective disorder, manic type, we found only three cases of secondary mania among a consecutive series of 309 acute stroke patients in an unpublished study. On the other hand, secondary mania is more frequent among patients with traumatic brain injury. In a study of 66 patients with acute traumatic brain injury (Jorge et al. 1993), we found six cases (9%) of secondary mania. Patients with traumatic brain injury frequently sustain damage to orbitofrontal and basotemporal cortical areas, which may be related to the mechanism of mania. These brain areas are rarely damaged in stroke patients, and this difference in the frequency of frontal and temporal cortical injury between traumatic and ischemic brain injury may explain the different prevalence of mania in these two populations. Cummings and Mendez (1984) found right thalamic stroke lesions in two cases of secondary mania.

In a series of 17 patients with post–brain-injury mania, we (Robinson et al. 1988) reported a high frequency of lesions involving the basal and polar areas of the right temporal lobe and subcortical areas of the right hemisphere, such as the head of the caudate nucleus and right thalamus. Similar lesion location was recently reported in patients with bipolar affective disorder (Berthier et al. 1996). In a study using positron-emission tomography (PET) with [^{18}F]fluorodeoxyglucose, we (Starkstein et al. 1990a) examined metabolic abnormalities in three patients with mania following right basal ganglia strokes. The patients had focal hypometabolic deficits in the right basotemporal cortex. This finding suggested that lesions leading to secondary mania may do so through their distant effects on the right basotemporal cortex. This phenomenon of lesions producing distant effects is a well-recognized consequence of some brain lesions and has been termed *diaschisis*.

Because not every patient with a right orbitofrontal or basotemporal lesion develops a manic syndrome, we have also looked for potential predisposing factors for secondary mania (Robinson et al. 1988; Starkstein et al. 1987). In these studies, we found that patients with secondary mania had a significantly higher frequency of familial history of psychiatric disorders, as well as significantly more subcortical brain atrophy (as determined by increased ventricular-to-brain ratios), than did patients with similar brain lesions but no mania. Interestingly, those patients without a genetic predisposition had significantly more subcortical atrophy than did secondary mania patients with a genetic burden, suggesting that subcortical atrophy and genetic predisposition may be independent risk factors for mania following brain injury.

Mechanism. To postulate a mechanism for secondary mania, two clinical-pathological correlations need to be explained. First, most lesions associated with secondary mania involve, directly or indirectly, limbic or limbic-related areas of the brain. Second, virtually all of these lesions are localized to the right hemisphere.

The basotemporal cortex appears to be a crucial area in the production of mania. This paralimbic area receives projections from secondary sensory and multimodal association regions (e.g., the frontal, temporal, and parietal association areas), limbic regions, and paralimbic areas (e.g., the insula and the parahippocampal gyrus) (Moran et al. 1987). The basotemporal cortex is strongly connected to the orbitofrontal cortex through the uncinate fasciculus, and both may exert a tonic inhibitory control over limbic and dorsal cortical regions. Thus, lesions or dysfunction of these areas may result in motor disinhibition (i.e., hyperactivity and pressured speech), intellectual disinhibition (i.e., flight of ideas and grandiose delusions), and instinctive disinhibition (i.e., hyperphagia and hypersexuality).

The second finding, which needs to be incorporated into any explanation of poststroke mania, is that the manias almost always occur following right-hemisphere lesions. In our laboratory studies of the neurochemical and behavioral effects of brain lesions in rats (Robinson 1979), we found that small suction lesions in the right (but not left) frontal cortex of rats produced a significant increase in locomotor activity. Similar abnormal behavior was also found after electrolytic lesions of the right (but not left) nucleus accumbens (which is considered part of the ventral striatum) (Kubos et al. 1987). Moreover, right frontocortical suction lesions also produced a significant increment in dopaminergic turnover in the nucleus accumbens that was not seen with left-hemisphere lesions (Starkstein et al. 1988a). Thus it is possible that, in the presence of pre-disposing factors such as a genetic burden or subcortical atrophy, significant increments in biogenic amine turnover in the nucleus accumbens produced by specific right-hemisphere lesions may be part of the mechanism that results in a manic syndrome.

In conclusion, secondary mania is a rare complication of stroke lesions. We have identified two risk factors: a genetic burden for psychiatric disorders and increased subcortical atrophy. Most patients with secondary mania have right-hemisphere lesions that involve the orbitofrontal or basotemporal cortex or subcortical structures, such as the thalamus or head of the caudate nucleus. Secondary mania may result from disinhibition of dorsal cortical and limbic areas and/or dysfunction of asymmetric biogenic amine pathways.

Conclusions

We have discussed several of the emotional and behavioral disorders that occur following cerebrovascular lesions (Table 27–3). Depression occurs in about 40% of stroke patients, with approximately equal distributions of major depression and minor depression. Patients with poststroke depression often have a greater degree of cognitive impairment (i.e., dementia of depression) and significantly less recovery in ADLs than do patients who never develop depression. Poststroke depression is significantly associated with left frontal and left basal ganglia lesions and may be successfully treated with tricyclic antidepressants. Anxiety, which is present in about 27% of stroke patients, is associated with depression in the vast majority of cases. Among the few patients with poststroke anxiety and no depression, there was a high frequency of alcoholism and lesions of the right hemisphere. Apathy is present in about 20% of stroke patients. It is associated with older age, more severe deficits in ADLs, and a significantly higher frequency of lesions involving the posterior limb of the internal capsule.

Hallucinations and hallucinosis are rare complications of stroke lesions. Poststroke hallucinations are associated with right-hemisphere temporoparietal lesions, subcortical brain atrophy, and seizures. Poststroke hallucinosis is associated with damage to reticular activating and primary sensory pathways. Anosognosia is present in about 30% of patients with acute stroke lesions. It is associated with right-hemisphere temporoparietal, basal ganglia, and thalamic lesions; neglect; and subcortical brain atrophy.

Catastrophic reactions occur in about 20% of stroke patients; they are not related to the severity of impairment or the presence of aphasia but may represent a defining symptom for one clinical type of poststroke major depres-

TABLE 27–3. Poststroke neuropsychiatric syndromes

Neuropsychiatric syndrome	Prevalence	Neuropathological correlates
Depression		
Major	10.25%	Left frontal cortex and basal ganglia; enlarged ventricles
Minor	10%–40%	Not established
Generalized anxiety		
With depression	20%	Left frontal cortex
Without depression	7%	Right parietal cortex
Apathy		
With depression	11%	Left frontal cortex and basal ganglia
Without depression	11%	Posterior internal capsule
Psychosis	Unknown, rare	Right parietal-temporal-occipital junction
Anosognosia	24%–43%	Right hemisphere and enlarged ventricles; frontal dysfunction
Catastrophic reaction	19%	Anterior cortical lesion
Emotional lability	20%	Bilateral injury
Mania	Unknown, rare	Right hemisphere, or bifrontal, basotemporal, basal ganglia, and thalamus

sion. Catastrophic reactions are associated with anterior subcortical lesions and may result from a "release" of emotional display in depressed patients. Emotional lability is another common complication of stroke lesions that sometimes coexists with depression and may be successfully treated with tricyclic antidepressants. Finally, mania is a rare complication of stroke lesions. It is strongly associated with right-hemisphere damage involving the orbitofrontal cortex, basal temporal cortex, thalamus, or basal ganglia. Risk factors for mania include a family history of psychiatric disorders and subcortical atrophy.

References

Adams RD, Victor M: Principles of Neurology. New York, McGraw-Hill, 1985

American Psychiatric Association: Diagnostic and Statistical Manual of Mental Disorders, 3rd Edition. Washington, DC, American Psychiatric Association, 1980

American Psychiatric Association: Diagnostic and Statistical Manual of Mental Disorders, 4th Edition. Washington, DC, American Psychiatric Association, 1994

Andersen G, Vestergaard K, Lauritzen L: Effective treatment of poststroke depression with the selective serotonin reuptake inhibitor citalopram. Stroke 25:1099–1104, 1994a

Andersen G, Ingeman-Nielsen M, Vestergaard K, Riis JO: Pathoanatomic correlation between poststroke pathological crying and damage to brain areas involved in serotonergic neurotransmission. Stroke 25:1050–1052, 1994b

Aström M: Generalized anxiety disorder in stroke patients: a 3 year longitudinal study. Stroke 27:270–275, 1996

Babinski J: Contribution a l'etude des troubles mentaux dans l'hemiplegie organique cerebrale (anosognosie). Rev Neurol (Paris) 27:845–848, 1914

Barry S, Dinan TG: Alpha-2 adrenergic receptor function in post-stroke depression. Psychol Med 10:305–309, 1990

Bartlett EJ, Brodie JD, Wolf AP, et al: Reproducibility of cerebral glucose metabolic measurements in resting human subjects. J Cereb Blood Flow Metab 8:502–512, 1988

Bechara A, van der Kooy D: The tegmental pedunculopontine nucleus: a brainstem output of the limbic system critical for the conditioned place preferences produced by morphine and amphetamine. J Neurosci 9:3400–3409, 1989

Berthier ML, Kulisevsky J, Gironell A, Fernandez Benitez JA: Poststroke bipolar affective disorder: subtypes, concurrent movement disorders, and anatomical correlates. J Neuropsychiatry Clin Neurosci 8:160–167, 1996

Bolla-Wilson K, Robinson RG, Starkstein SE, et al: Lateralization of dementia of depression in stroke patients. Am J Psychiatry 146:627–634, 1989

Caplan LR, Stein RW: Stroke: A Clinical Approach. Boston, MA, Butterworth, 1986

Cascino GD, Adams RD: Brainstem auditory hallucinosis. Neurology 36:1042–1047, 1986

Castillo CS, Starkstein SE, Fedoroff JP, et al: Generalized anxiety disorder following stroke. J Nerv Ment Dis 181:100–106, 1993

Castillo CS, Schultz SK, Robinson RG: Clinical correlates of early onset and late-onset poststroke generalized anxiety. Am J Psychiatry 152:1174–1179, 1995

Cummings JL, Mendez MF: Secondary mania with focal cerebrovascular lesions. Am J Psychiatry 141:1084–1087, 1984

De Renzi E, Vignolo LA: The Token Test: a sensitive test to detect disturbances in aphasics. Brain 85:665–678, 1962

Eastwood MR, Rifat SL, Nobbs H, et al: Mood disorder following cerebrovascular accident. Br J Psychiatry 154:195–200, 1989

Everson SA, Roberts RE, Goldberg DE, et al: Depressive symptoms and increased risk of stroke mortality over a 29-year period. Arch Intern Med 158:1133–1138, 1998

Fuh JL, Liu HC, Wang SJ, et al: Poststroke depression among the Chinese elderly in a rural community. Stroke 28:1126–1129, 1997

Gainotti G: Emotional behavior and hemispheric side of the brain. Cortex 8:41–55, 1972

Geller TJ, Bellur SW: Peduncular hallucinosis: magnetic confirmation of mesencephalic infarction during life. Ann Neurol 21:602–604, 1987

Goldstein K: The Organism: A Holistic Approach to Biology Derived From Pathological Data in Man. New York, American Books, 1939

Gur RC, Gur RE, Resnick SM, et al: The effect of anxiety on cortical cerebral blood flow and metabolism. J Cereb Blood Flow Metab 7:173–177, 1987

Hachinski V, Norris JW: The Acute Stroke. Philadelphia, PA, FA Davis, 1985

Heilman KM: Anosognosia: possible neuropsychological mechanisms, in Awareness of Deficit After Brain Injury. Edited by Prigatano GP, Schacter DL. New York, Oxford University Press, 1991, pp 53–62

Helgason C, Wilbur A, Weiss A, et al: Acute pseudobulbar mutism due to discrete bilateral capsular infarction in the territory of the anterior choroidal artery. Brain 111:507–519, 1988

House A, Dennis M, Mogridge L, et al: Mood disorders in the year after stroke. Br J Psychiatry 158:83–92, 1991

Jorge RE, Robinson RG, Starkstein SE, et al: Secondary mania following traumatic brain injury. Am J Psychiatry 150:916–921, 1993

Kishi Y, Robinson RG, Kosier JT: Suicidal plans in patients with stroke: comparison between acute-onset and delayed-onset suicidal plans. Int Psychogeriatr 8:623–634, 1996

Kotila M, Numminen H, Waltimo O, Kaste M: Depression after stroke: results of the FINNSTROKE study. Stroke 29:368–372, 1998

Kraepelin E: Manic Depressive Insanity and Paranoia. Edinburgh, Livingstone, 1921

Kubos KL, Moran TH, Robinson RG: Mania after brain injury: a controlled study of etiological factors. Arch Neurol 44:1069–1073, 1987

Levine DN, Finklestein S: Delayed psychosis after right temporoparietal stroke or trauma: relation to epilepsy. Neurology 32:267–273, 1982

Lipsey JR, Robinson RG, Peralson GD, et al: Mood change following bilateral hemisphere brain injury. Br J Psychiatry 143:266–273, 1983

Lipsey JR, Robinson RG, Pearlson GD, et al: Nortriptyline treatment of post-stroke depression: a double-blind treatment trial. Lancet 1:297–300, 1984

Lipsey JR, Robinson RG, Pearlson GD, et al: Dexamethasone suppression test and mood following stroke. Am J Psychiatry 142:318–323, 1985

Lipsey JR, Spencer WC, Rabins PV, et al: Phenomenological comparison of functional and post-stroke depression. Am J Psychiatry 143:527–529, 1986

Moran MA, Mufson EJ, Mesulam MM: Neural inputs into the temporopolar cortex of the rhesus monkey. J Comp Neurol 256:88–103, 1987

Morris PLP, Robinson RG, Ralphael B: Prevalence and course of depressive disorders in hospitalized stroke patients. Int J Psychiatry Med 20:349–364, 1990

Morris PLP, Robinson RG, Ralphael B: Lesion location and depression in hospitalized stroke patients: evidence supporting a specific relationship in the left hemisphere. Neuropsychiatry Neuropsychol Behav Neurol 3:75–82, 1992

Morris PLP, Robinson RG, Andrezejewski P, et al: Association of depression with 10-year post-stroke mortality. Am J Psychiatry 150:124–129, 1993

Nauta WJH: Reciprocal links of the corpus striatum with the cerebral cortex and the limbic system: a common substrate for movement and thought? in Neurology and Psychiatry: A Meeting of Minds. Edited by Muller J. Basel, Karger, 1989, pp 43–63

Paradiso S, Robinson RG: Gender differences in poststroke depression. J Neuropsychiatry Clin Neurosci 10:41–47, 1998

Paradiso S, Ohkubo T, Robinson RG: Vegetative and psychological symptoms associated with depressed mood over the first two years after stroke. Int J Psychiatry Med 27:137–157, 1997

Parikh RM, Robinson RG, Lipsey JR, et al: The impact of post-stroke depression on recovery in activities of daily living over two-year follow-up. Arch Neurol 47:785–789, 1990

Poeck K: Pathophysiology of emotional disorders associated with brain damage, in Handbook of Clinical Neurology. Edited by Vinken PJ, Bruyn GW. Amsterdam, North-Holland, 1969

Pohjasvaara T, Lepptlavuori, Siira I, et al: Frequencey and clinical determinants of poststroke depression 29:2311–2317, 1998

Rabins PV, Starkstein SE, Robinson RG: Risk factors for developing atypical (schizophreniform) psychosis following stroke. J Neuropsychiatry Clin Neurosci 3:6–9, 1991

Ramasubbu R, Robinson RG, Flint AJ, et al: Functional impairment associated with acute post-stroke depression: the stroke data bank study. J Neuropsychiatry Clin Neurosci 10:26–33, 1998

Reding MJ, Orto LA, Winter SW, et al: Antidepressant therapy after stroke: a double-blind trial. Arch Neurol 43:763–765, 1986

Robinson RG: Differential behavioral and biochemical effects of right and left hemispheric cerebral infarction in the rat. Science 105:707–710, 1979

Robinson RG, Szetela B: Mood change following left hemispheric brain injury. Ann Neurol 9:447–453, 1981

Robinson RG, Starr LB, Kubos KL, et al: A two-year longitudinal study of post-stroke mood disorders: findings during the initial evaluation. Stroke 14:736–744, 1983

Robinson RG, Kubos KL, Starr LB, et al: Mood disorders in stroke patients: importance of location of lesion. Brain 107:81–93, 1984

Robinson RG, Lipsey JR, Bolla-Wilson K, et al: Mood disorders in left-handed stroke patients. Am J Psychiatry 142:1424–1429, 1985

Robinson RG, Bolla-Wilson K, Kaplan E, et al: Depression influences intellectual impairment in stroke patients. Br J Psychiatry 148:541–547, 1986

Robinson RG, Bolduc P, Price TR: A two-year longitudinal study of post-stroke depression: diagnosis and outcome at one- and two-year follow-up. Stroke 18:837–843, 1987

Robinson RG, Boston JD, Starkstein SE, et al: Comparison of mania with depression following brain injury: causal factors. Am J Psychiatry 145:172–178, 1988

Robinson RG, Parikh RM, Lipsey JR, et al: Pathological laughing and crying following stroke: validation of measurement scale and double blind treatment study. Am J Psychiatry 150:286–293, 1993

Ross ED, Stewart RS: Pathological display of affect in patients with depression and right frontal brain damage. J Nerv Ment Dis 175:165–172, 1987

Shimoda K, Robinson RG: Effect of anxiety disorder on impairment and recovery from stroke. J Neuropsychiatry Clin Neurosci 10:34–40, 1998

Sinyor D, Jacques P, Kaloupek DG, et al: Post-stroke depression and lesion location: an attempted replication. Brain 109:537–546, 1986

Starkstein SE, Robinson RG: Neuropsychiatric aspects of cerebral vascular disorders, in The American Psychiatric Press Textbook of Neuropsychiatry, 2nd Edition. Edited by Yudofsky SC, Hales RE. Washington DC, American Psychiatric Press, 1992, pp 449–472

Starkstein SE, Pearlson GD, Robinson RG: Mania after brain injury: a controlled study of etiological factors. Arch Neurol 44:1069–1073, 1987

Starkstein SE, Moran TH, Bowersox JA, et al: Behavioral abnormalities induced by frontal cortical and nucleus accumbens lesions. Brain Res 473:74–80, 1988a

Starkstein SE, Robinson RG, Berthier ML, et al: Differential mood changes following basal ganglia versus thalamic lesions. Arch Neurol 45:725–730, 1988b

Starkstein SE, Robinson RG, Honig MA, et al: Mood changes after right hemisphere lesion. Br J Psychiatry 155:79–85, 1989

Starkstein SE, Mayberg HS, Berthier ML, et al: Mania after brain injury: neuroradiological and metabolic findings. Ann Neurol 27:652–659, 1990a

Starkstein SE, Cohen BS, Fedoroff P, et al: Relationship between anxiety disorders and depressive disorders in patients with cerebrovascular injury. Arch Gen Psychiatry 47:246–251, 1990b

Starkstein SE, Fedoroff JP, Price TR, et al: Anosognosia in patients with cerebrovascular lesions: a study of causative factors. Stroke 23:1446–1453, 1992

Starkstein SE, Fedoroff JP, Price TR, et al: Apathy following cerebrovascular lesions. J Neurol Neurosurg Psychiatry 24:1625–1630, 1993a

Starkstein SE, Fedoroff JP, Price TR, et al: Catastrophic reaction after cerebrovascular lesions: frequency, correlates, and validation of a scale. J Neuropsychiatry Clin Neurosci 5:189–194, 1993b

Wade DT, Legh-Smith J, Hewer RA: Depressed mood after stroke: a community study of its frequency. Br J Psychiatry 151:200–205, 1987

Walker AE, Robins M, Weinfeld FD: Clinical findings in the National Survey of Stroke. Stroke 12(suppl 1):I13–I31, 1981

Wolf PA, Kannel WB, Verter J: Cerebrovascular disease in the elderly: epidemiology, in Clinical Neurology of Aging. Edited by Albert ML. New York, Oxford University Press, 1984, pp 458–477

APPENDIX 27–1. Pathological Laughter and Crying Scale (PLACS)

Ratings are based on clinical assessment. Initial probe questions are given for each item. However, further questions may be used for clarification. Write the number in the spaces provided that most accurately reflects clinical symptoms.

Part I: Patient Interview

1. Have you recently experienced sudden episodes of laughter?
___ Rate the frequency of the episodes during the past two weeks.
   0. Rarely or not at all
   1. Occasionally
   2. Quite often
   3. Frequently

2. Have you recently experienced sudden episodes of crying?
___ Rate the frequency of the episodes during the past two weeks.
   0. Rarely or not at all
   1. Occasionally
   2. Quite often
   3. Frequently

*If you have experienced sudden **episodes of laughter**, please answer the following (questions 3–10), otherwise skip to question 11.*

3. Have these episodes occurred without any cause in your surroundings?
___ Rate the frequency with which the episodes have occurred without external stimuli in the past 2 weeks.
   0. Rarely or not at all
   1. Occasionally
   2. Quite often
   3. Frequently

4. Have these episodes lasted for a long period of time?
___ Rate the average duration of the episodes during the past two weeks.
   0. Very brief
   1. Few seconds
   2. Moderate (less than 30 seconds)
   3. Prolonged (more than 30 seconds)

5. Have these episodes been uncontrollable by you?
___ Rate the ability to control the episodes during the past two weeks.
   0. Rarely or not at all
   1. Occasionally
   2. Quite often
   3. Frequently

6. Have these episodes occurred as a result of feelings of happiness?
___ Rate the frequency with which the episodes have occurred as a result of happiness in the past two weeks.
   0. Rarely or not at all
   1. Occasionally
   2. Quite often
   3. Frequently

7. Have these episodes occurred in excess of feelings of happiness?
___ Rate the frequency with which the episodes have been disproportionate to the emotional state in the past two weeks.
   0. Rarely or not at all
   1. Occasionally
   2. Quite often
   3. Frequently

8. Have these episodes of laughter occurred with feelings of sadness?
___ Rate the frequency of association between the episode and the paradoxical emotion in the past two weeks. The sadness must precede or accompany the episode and not be a reaction to it.
   0. Rarely or not at all
   1. Occasionally
   2. Quite often
   3. Frequently

9. Have these episodes occurred with any emotions other than happiness or sadness, such as, nervousness, anger, fear, etc.?
___ Rate the frequency of association between the episodes and emotions in the past two weeks. The emotions must precede or accompany the episode and not be a reaction to it.
   0. Rarely or not at all
   1. Occasionally
   2. Quite often
   3. Frequently

10. Have these episodes caused you any distress or social embarrassment?
___ Rate the degree of distress or embarrassment caused by the episodes in the past two weeks.
   0. Rarely or not at all
   1. Occasionally
   2. Quite often
   3. Frequently

(continued)

APPENDIX 27–1. Pathological Laughter and Crying Scale (PLACS) *(continued)*

If you have experienced sudden **episodes of crying,** *please answer the following (questions 11–18).*

11. Have these episodes occurred without any cause in your surroundings?

___ Rate the frequency with which the episodes have occurred without an external stimuli in the past two weeks.

    0. Rarely or not at all

    1. Occasionally

    2. Quite often

    3. Frequently

12. Have these episodes lasted for a long period of time?

___ Rate the average duration of the episodes during the past two weeks.

    0. Very brief

    1. Short (few seconds)

    2. Moderate (less than 30 seconds)

    3. Prolonged (more than 30 seconds)

13. Have these episodes been uncontrollable by you?

___ Rate the ability to control the episodes during the past two weeks.

    0. Rarely or not at all

    1. Occasionally

    2. Quite often

    3. Frequently

14. Have these episodes occurred as a result of feelings of sadness?

___ Rate the frequency with which the episodes have occurred as a result of sadness in the past two weeks. The sadness must proceed or accompany the crying and not be a reaction to it.

    0. Rarely or not at all

    1. Occasionally

    2. Quite often

    3. Frequently

15. Have these episodes occurred in excess of feelings of sadness?

___ Rate the frequency with which the episodes have been disproportionate to the emotional state in the past two weeks.

    0. Rarely or not at all

    1. Occasionally

    2. Quite often

    3. Frequently

16. Have these episodes of crying occurred with feelings of happiness?

___ Rate the frequency of association between the episode and the paradoxical emotion in the past two weeks. The happiness must precede or accompany the crying.

    0. Rarely or not at all

    1. Occasionally

    2. Quite often

    3. Frequently

17. Have these episodes occurred with any emotions other than sadness or happiness, such as nervousness, anger, fear, etc.?

___ Rate the frequency of association between the episodes and emotions in the past two weeks. The emotions must precede or accompany the episode and not be a reaction to it.

    0. Rarely or not at all

    1. Occasionally

    2. Quite often

    3. Frequently

18. Have these episodes caused you any distress or social embarrassment?

___ Rate the degree of distress or embarrassment caused by the episodes in the past two weeks.

    0. Rarely or not at all

    1. Occasionally

    2. Quite often

    3. Frequently

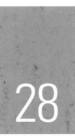

28

Traumatic Brain Injury

Robert B. Fields, Ph.D.

Dawn Cisewski

C. Edward Coffey, M.D.

More than 2 million people in the United States sustain traumatic brain injuries (TBIs) each year (Kraus et al. 1994). Among individuals under the age of 50, TBI is the leading cause of death and neuropsychiatric dysfunction (Sosin et al. 1989). After young adults and children, older adults compose a third at-risk group for TBI. Although the pathophysiology and neurobehavioral consequences of TBI among young adults are becoming better understood, the corresponding literature on TBI among older adults is relatively sparse. Age is a well-established general risk factor for negative outcome following TBI. However, the specific role that age plays in contributing to outcome is less clear. For example, we do not yet know whether all elderly are at risk for negative outcome following TBI or whether the risk of negative outcome is limited to a subset of vulnerable elderly. Similarly, the specific mechanisms by which aging may make the brain more susceptible to a TBI or through which a TBI may provoke, or exacerbate, a neurodegenerative process in an aging brain are not well understood.

Interest in the topic of TBI in older adults has been increasing for at least three reasons. First, because the population is aging, cases of geriatric TBI now account for a greater percentage of all patients with TBI treated in emergency rooms and on trauma services, making findings such as the age-related increase in mortality rates and lengths of hospital stay following geriatric TBI more relevant to clinicians, hospital administrators, and insurance companies. Second, the increased referral of patients for neuropsychiatric and neuropsychological evaluation following geriatric TBI has increased the need for practical guidelines for the differentiation of the syndrome of geriatric TBI from other conditions, such as dementia. A third reason for increased interest in geriatric TBI is the growing body of literature on the apparent epidemiological and pathogenetic association between TBI in adulthood and risk for Alzheimer's disease (AD) in later life (see Chapter 24 in this volume).

This chapter begins with an overview of the general literature on TBI. In subsequent sections, we review the unique characteristics of geriatric TBI, the neurobehavioral consequences of TBI and geriatric TBI, and the diagnosis and treatment of geriatric TBI. Finally, we also include a review of the proposed relationship between TBI and AD within the context of current conceptualizations about the pathogenesis of AD.

Overview of Traumatic Brain Injury

Terminology

Definition of traumatic brain injury. Universal agreement on the definition of a TBI has been difficult to establish, in part because of differences of opinion about where to place the theoretical threshold between non-injury and mild TBI. For example, some definitions of TBI require loss of consciousness, whereas others take into account the finding that loss of consciousness is not necessary for subsequent brain dysfunction to occur. Most definitions of TBI require that the known or suspected injury to the brain was sufficiently severe to cause at least one of the following: 1) alterations in consciousness, 2) posttraumatic amnesia, or 3) physical, radiological, or objective evidence of injury-related abnormalities.

Utility of the term "traumatic brain injury." The use of terms such as *traumatic brain injury*, *head injury*, or *brain injury* can be both informative and problematic. The utility of these terms stems from the implied causal connection between an acquired lesion and abnormal behavior. For patients who have sustained a TBI, there is an assumption that subsequent alterations in thinking, mood, and behavior are the results of the specific neurological damage associated with the traumatic event. The well-known case of Phineas Gage in the 1860s is an example of a TBI (i.e., penetration by a railroad spike through the left frontal lobe) that produced specific and dramatic changes in personality and comportment (Harlow 1868).

However, the use of these terms can also be misleading. In younger adults, for example, the term brain injury typically connotes a traumatic injury, whereas in older adults, the term brain injury is often used to describe a variety of etiologies (e.g., stroke, aneurysm, and tumor), as well as traumatic injury. The terms also imply a misleading homogeneity of patients across studies. Just as strokes of different types, sizes, and locations can produce a wide range of neurological and neurobehavioral dysfunctions, so too can traumatic brain injuries of different types and severities cause different symptoms. Comparing studies of outcome following "TBI," therefore, will likely produce different conclusions if this anatomic heterogeneity is not

taken into account. A third problem with these terms is the risk of assuming a direct correspondence between the brain injury and subsequent behavior and of minimizing other factors that have been shown to contribute to outcome. These factors include, but are not limited to, premorbid personality, previous brain injury or dysfunction, substance abuse, vocational history, social support network, involvement in treatment, involvement in litigation, and the experience of being in a traumatic event (Parker 1990; Richardson 1990; Wood 1990).

Types of traumatic brain injury. TBIs are categorized as *open* or *closed*, depending on whether or not the skull has been penetrated (and the brain exposed). The manner in which an injury is sustained has important implications for the neuroanatomical, neurochemical, metabolic, and neurobehavioral disruption that follows. Dysfunction following open head injuries such as a gunshot wound is dependent on factors such as the path of the bullet, tissue disruption by associated force waves, the spread of bone chips, and the development of cerebral edema (Bigler 1991; Kirkpatrick and DiMaio 1978). In contrast, the dysfunction that follows a closed head injury may be the result of *focal* damage caused by impact at the site of the injury (e.g., from a fall or an assault) or *diffuse* damage caused by rapid acceleration/deceleration or twisting movements of the brain within the cranial vault (e.g., from a high-speed motor vehicle collision). *Primary* brain injuries are those that occur at the moment the TBI takes place (e.g., cerebral contusion from impact). *Secondary* brain injuries are those that develop following the initial trauma (e.g., edema, increased intracranial pressure, delayed hemorrhage).

Severity of traumatic brain injury. TBIs are typically characterized as being either mild, moderate, or severe, based on criteria such as degree of initial neurological dysfunction, duration of unconsciousness, and duration of memory loss for events following the injury (i.e., posttraumatic amnesia [PTA]). TBIs are considered to be mild when there is no, or brief, loss of consciousness and less than 60 minutes of PTA. In contrast, TBIs are considered severe when unconsciousness lasts hours to days and PTA lasts more than 24 hours. While specific estimates vary, the majority (i.e., 70%–90%) of TBIs are classified as mild (Lezak 1995). Because severity of injury is a good predictor of outcome, the use of additional categories of severity has been suggested (e.g., very mild, no loss of consciousness, less than 5 minutes of PTA; very severe, 1–4 weeks of unconsciousness or PTA; extremely severe, more than 4 weeks of unconsciousness or PTA) (Bigler 1990b).

Several objective measures of severity of TBI have

been developed. Of these instruments, the Glasgow Coma Scale (GCS) (Teasdale and Jennett 1974) remains the "gold standard" because of its quick and convenient numerical quantification of level of consciousness and its widespread use in trauma data banks (Diringer and Edwards 1997; Juarez and Lyons 1995; Menegazzi et al. 1993). The GCS is a 15-point global index of consciousness that assesses functioning in three domains (eye opening, verbal response, and motor response) (Teasdale and Jennett 1974) (Table 28–1). GCS scores are generally interpreted as follows: 13–15, mild; 9–12, moderate; and 3–8, severe. Although the GCS has been found to have high interrater reliability and to be a reasonable predictor of poor outcome in TBI (i.e., death or vegetative state), it appears to have limited predictive power in terms of functional and cognitive outcome (Diringer and Edwards 1997; Zafonte et al. 1996) and is also limited when used with selected populations (e.g., children, patients with chronic disabilities, elderly patients with hearing loss, and patients whose injuries affect the eyes and mouth) (Menegazzi et al. 1993; Sorenson and Kraus 1991). These limitations are becoming more pronounced as prehospital treatment (i.e., pharmacological paralysis, sedation, and intubation) increases (Marion and Carlier 1994), thereby limiting the ability to obtain accurate GCS scores for many individuals (Marion and Carlier 1994; Prasad 1996).

As a result of these limitations, several other scales of

injury severity have been developed. Examples include 1) the Abbreviated Injury Scale (AIS) (American Association for Automotive Medicine 1985), which incorporates the Injury Severity Scale (ISS) (Baker et al. 1976) and which was designed to rate overall injury by measuring the cumulative damage across six body regions, including the head; 2) the revised APACHE (Acute Physiology, Age, and Chronic Health Evaluation, II and III) (Knaus et al. 1985; Wagner et al. 1989) system, which also measures more physiological variables than the GCS, including underlying diseases and comorbidity; and 3) the Reaction Level Scale (RLS85) (Starmark et al. 1988), which allows the assessment of TBIs among individuals who are intubated or have severe preorbital swelling. Although these measures overcome some of the problems with the GCS, many of them have significant limitations (e.g., limited information on reliability and validity, increased time and difficulty of administration). Thus, the GCS remains the most widely used tool to measure severity of TBI.

Pathophysiology of Traumatic Brain Injury

Excellent reviews of the biomechanics and pathophysiology of TBI can be found elsewhere (e.g., Alexander 1995; Bigler 1991; Gennarelli 1993; Gualtieri 1995; McIntosh et al. 1996; Parker 1990; Richardson 1990). The following is a brief overview of the pathophysiology of primary and secondary brain injuries.

Primary brain injury. Among patients who experience closed TBIs, primary brain injuries usually occur as a result of impact/contact forces or inertial/acceleration motions (Katz 1992; McIntosh et al. 1996). Impact/contact injuries can cause local skull distortion as well as stress waves through the brain from the point of impact. The consequences of contact injuries include distorted or fractured skulls (with or without extradural hematomas) and contusions or lacerations of the brain. Contrecoup injuries are also common, although the term contrecoup may be somewhat misleading because the location of these injuries may not be exactly opposite the point of initial impact (McIntosh et al. 1996; Richardson 1990).

Many TBIs also involve linear or rotational movements of the brain within the skull. The accelerating and decelerating or twisting movements of the brain produce lacerations or contusions when the moving brain comes into contact with the more stationary bony protuberances of the base of the skull. Within the cranial vault, the orbital, frontal, and temporal areas are most vulnerable to this type of injury (Adams et al. 1977; Bigler 1990a, 1991; Gennarelli

TABLE 28–1. Glasgow Coma Scale

Eye opening response	Spontaneous	4
	To voice	3
	To pain	2
	None	1
Best verbal response	Oriented	5
	Confused	4
	Inappropriate words	3
	Incomprehensible sounds	2
	None	1
Best motor response	Obeys commands	6
	Localizes pain	5
	Withdraws (pain)	4
	Flexion (pain)	3
	Extension (pain)	2
	None	1

Source. Reprinted with permission from Teasdale G, Jennett B: "Assessment of Coma and Impaired Consciousness: A Practical Scale." *Lancet* 2:81–84, 1974.

1993; McIntosh et al. 1996; Ommaya et al. 1971; Richardson 1990). An important by-product of these movements is diffuse axonal injury (Adams 1988; Adams et al. 1982; Alexander 1995; Gualtieri 1995; McIntosh et al. 1996). Straining, shearing, and rupture of axonal fibers are common following TBI of all severities and are generally associated with more significant neuropsychiatric disorders (Alexander 1995; Bigler 1990a; Jennett and Teasdale 1981; McIntosh et al. 1996; Parker 1990; Richardson 1990). In severe cases, dramatic rotation of the brain around the brainstem may lead to coma (Parker 1990).

Secondary brain injury.   Some damage to brain structure and function may be initiated at the time of the TBI but may not be clinically present for minutes, hours, or even days following the injury. Examples of secondary brain injuries include: hematoma, edema, ischemia, increased intracranial pressure, infection, ventricular enlargement, seizures, and alterations in neurochemical functioning (Bachman 1992; Katz 1992; McIntosh et al. 1996; Parker 1990; Richardson 1990).

Intracranial hematomas and cerebral edema are considered to be two of the most frequent types of acute secondary brain injury (Richardson 1990). In his review of this literature, Richardson (1990) reported that intracranial hemorrhage occurs in approximately 50% of patients with severe injuries and often is responsible for the development of delayed coma or other types of neurological deterioration. The presence of a skull fracture dramatically increases the risk of intracranial hematomas (Jennett and Teasdale 1981). Diffuse brain swelling develops in approximately 10% of patients who have sustained severe brain injuries (Adams et al. 1989; Richardson 1990). Brain edema may lead to herniation, occlusion of intracranial vessels with secondary strokes (e.g., subfacial herniation may occlude the anterior cerebral artery, and transtentorial herniation may occlude the posterior cerebral artery), or to strain effects on axonal fibers (Bigler 1990a; Cummings and Benson 1992). The occurrence of subdural hematomas secondary to the tearing of veins is particularly problematic in elderly patients in whom brain atrophy increases the distance from the brain surface to the venous sinuses, thus increasing the vulnerability of bridging veins to rupture with even minor trauma (Bachman 1992; Cummings and Benson 1992; Levy et al. 1993; McIntosh et al. 1996).

Regarding other secondary brain injuries that may complicate the postinjury course, ventricular enlargement is common following moderate-to-severe TBI (Levin et al. 1981) and has been associated with greater neuropsychological impairment (Cullum and Bigler 1986) and worse prognosis (Gudeman et al. 1981; Kishore et al.

1978). Changes in ventricular size may not be fully apparent (via computed tomography [CT] scan analysis) until 1–3 months after the injury (Cope et al. 1988; Gudeman et al. 1981).

Posttraumatic epilepsy is another delayed consequence of brain injury that can affect eventual outcome. Approximately 5% of patients develop seizures within the first week after a TBI (Bachman 1992; Teasdale 1995). Risk factors for early posttraumatic epilepsy include prolonged posttraumatic amnesia, depressed skull fracture, intracranial hematoma, and a history of childhood seizures (Bachman 1992; Hendrick and Harris 1968; Jennett and Teasdale 1981). Late seizures (i.e., beyond the first week) have also been reported in approximately 5% of patients following TBI but may not develop until more than a year after the injury. Risk factors for late epilepsy include severity of injury, early epilepsy, and depressed skull fracture (Annegers et al. 1980b; Bachman 1992; Jennett and Teasdale 1981). Mathematical models exist to predict the likelihood of seizures for individual patients (Feeney and Walker 1990). Among patients who have already had one late seizure, 75% continue to have seizures (Bachman 1992). The use of prophylactic anticonvulsant medication following brain injury reduces the risk of early seizures, but not late seizures (Malec and Basford 1996; Schierhout and Roberts 1998; Temkin et al. 1990). Because anticonvulsants often produce sedation, their use among elderly patients may be problematic (e.g., increased risk of subsequent head injuries as a result of falls) (see Chapter 34 in this volume).

In addition to the structural damage caused by primary and secondary brain injuries, changes in brain neurochemistry also occur following a TBI (Bohnen and Jolles 1992; Gennarelli 1993; Gualtieri 1995; McIntosh et al. 1996). These changes appear to be related to the nature and extent of the structural damage and can be seen as "neuroprotective" or "autodestructive" (McIntosh et al. 1996). For example, it has been suggested that because of their location, size, and widespread projections from the lower brainstem to subcortical and cortical areas, the monoaminergic pathways are particularly vulnerable for disruption as a result of diffuse axonal injury (Gualtieri 1995). Alterations in acetylcholine, norepinephrine, and dopamine have been reported following experimentally induced TBI in animals (McIntosh et al. 1996). Such changes have been postulated to be linked to the changes in intracranial pressure and blood pressure that sometimes follow TBI. Similarly, postinjury changes in arousal, attention, and information processing have been attributed to disruption of dopaminergic and noradrenergic pathways, whereas postinjury changes in mood, appetite, sleep, sexual function, motor activity, anxiety, and aggression have been associated with disruption of serotonergic neurons (Gualtieri 1995) (see Chapter 2 in this volume).

Changes in neurochemistry can result from primary or secondary brain injuries. For example, the immediate disruption of neural pathways and vasculature following diffuse brain injuries may cause a defect in the axonal membrane that results in changes in intracellular ions (particularly calcium). The sudden loading of calcium ultimately leads to a depolarization of axons that then disrupts neural transmission. Secondary brain injuries such as ischemia can also lead to disruptions in cerebral metabolism, which can, in turn, lead to the release of excitatory amino acids (EAAs) such as glutamate and aspartate. EAAs have been called "excitotoxic" because of their destructive effect on cells in vitro. EAAs can excessively stimulate neurons, leading to cellular exhaustion or the formation of free radicals that are toxic to cells. Choi (1987) has postulated that two sequential mechanisms mediate cell death resulting from excitotoxin exposure: 1) acute neuronal swelling resulting from an influx of chloride and sodium and 2) delayed damage resulting from an influx of calcium. Other neurochemical changes that have been reported following TBI include the release of: 1) oxygen free radicals, which can cause perioxidative damage to membrane phospholipids, and 2) neurotrophic substances (e.g., nerve growth factor), which may play a role in reducing damage and promoting recovery from brain injury (McIntosh et al. 1996). The possibility that increased deposition of β-amyloid protein (βAP) following brain injury may increase the risk of AD is reviewed below.

Outcome Following Traumatic Brain Injury

For patients who experience TBIs, and their families, the most pressing injury-related concerns pertain to survival, rate of recovery, and quality of life following the injury.

Measurement strategies. Assessment of global progress through the initial stages of recovery can be accomplished with several instruments. The most frequently used outcome measure is the Glasgow Outcome Scale (GOS) (Clifton et al. 1993; Jennett and Bond 1975). The GOS uses a 5-point scale to classify outcome: 1) good recovery, 2) moderate disability, 3) severe disability, 4) persistent vegetative state, and 5) death (Clifton et al. 1993; Hofer 1993; Zafonte et al. 1996). Although widely used, the GOS has several significant limitations. These include 1) lack of sensitivity to change during recovery because the categories of outcome are too broad (Clifton et al. 1993),

2) reduced sensitivity to the multidimensional nature of patients' deficits with an overemphasis on physical disability and an underemphasis on cognitive and neurobehavioral problems (Anderson et al. 1993), and 3) few or no guidelines regarding the incorporation of problems such as epilepsy, preexisting personality disorders, chronic illness, and preexisting substance abuse, which are common among patients with TBIs.

Other outcome measures exist, some of which address the limitations of the GOS. These measures include 1) the Rancho Los Amigos Levels of Cognitive Function Scale, which uses an 8-level categorical scoring system to evaluate level of awareness, interaction with the environment, cognition, and behavior; 2) the Disability Rating Scale (DRS), which measures arousal, awareness, cognitive ability for self-care, physical dependence, and psychosocial abilities; and 3) the Functional Independence Measure (FIM), which assesses the amount of assistance an individual needs in performing daily activities.

In addition to the aforementioned instruments, global indices have also been used in assessing outcome. These include survival rates, length of hospital stay, discharge destination, and ability to return to preinjury activities. Although these indices can provide important information about functional status, the determination of more subtle or specific neurobehavioral deficits requires comprehensive neuropsychiatric assessment and neuropsychological testing.

General predictors of outcome. Severity of the injury is the best general predictor of outcome following TBI. Regarding outcome in the first few weeks following the injury, patients whose injuries are more severe are at greater risk for death, longer hospital stays, and placement in supervised care settings following hospitalization (Combes et al. 1996; Cowen et al. 1995; Jennett and Teasdale 1981; Katz 1992; Marshall et al. 1983; Richardson 1990; Russell and Smith 1961). For example, in one sample of adults (ages 25–54 [$N = 1,487$]) hospitalized for TBI (Fields 1991), the rate of in-hospital mortality following a severe injury was 23 times greater than the mortality rate following a mild injury. Similarly, in this sample, length of hospital stay was 3.8 times longer and likelihood of transfer to a rehabilitation or skilled nursing facility (rather than home) was 9.6 times greater following severe TBI than following mild TBI.

Other specific variables that have been associated with poor initial outcome include 1) alterations in pupillary response, systolic blood pressure, and intracranial pressure; 2) duration of posttraumatic amnesia; and 3) presence of CT scan abnormalities such as skull fractures and hematomas. For example, Cowen et al. (1995) found an inverse relationship between CT abnormalities and good prognosis. Specifically, 81% of patients in their study who had normal CT scans, but only 45% of patients with one CT scan abnormality, were classified as having a good recovery. Furthermore, among patients with a skull fracture, 67% were classified as having a poor outcome.

Severity of injury is also the most important predictor of longer-term outcome. Severe injuries are associated with greater generalized impairment than are mild injuries (Cifu et al. 1997; Ip et al. 1995; Masson et al. 1996; Mazaux et al. 1997). Vollmer et al. (1991) found the following outcome statistics (based on GOS) for a sample of adults (ages 26–55 [N = 279]) 6 months after a severe brain injury: good recovery, 22%; moderate-to-severe disability, 35%; and vegetative survival or death, 43%. Other studies have also documented that more severe TBIs are associated with greater difficulty in areas such as ability to return to work, drive, initiate participation in social and recreational activities, use public transportation, and perform administrative tasks such as banking, writing letters, and making a weekly schedule (Mazaux et al. 1997; Ponsford et al. 1995; Tennant et al. 1995).

Summary

Much has been learned during the past few decades about the pathophysiology of, and outcome following, TBI. Rather than considering TBI a unitary phenomenon, it is probably more appropriate, and more useful, to conceptualize TBI as an ongoing process during which numerous events take place, many of which have implications for subsequent neurobehavioral functioning. In addition to considering noninjury factors, an understanding of postinjury outcome can be enhanced greatly by knowledge of factors such as mechanism of primary injury, types of secondary injuries, and disruption of neurochemical functioning. Much of our current understanding about the pathophysiology of TBI comes from animal models of TBI and from studies of adults who did not survive their TBI. Although severity of injury is clearly the most important factor in predicting outcome following TBI, it appears that age also plays an important, but less well-understood, role in mediating the consequences of TBI.

▮ Unique Characteristics of Geriatric Traumatic Brain Injury

The available literature suggests that there are age-related differences in both occurrence and outcome of TBI.

Occurrence

Epidemiology. Several factors make it difficult to determine the exact prevalence of TBI and geriatric TBI. These factors include variability in diagnostic criteria used in different countries and different hospitals, double counting of patients transferred between acute hospitals, variation in hospital documentation policies, and the estimate that 20%–40% of individuals who sustain mild TBIs do not seek medical treatment (Bohnen and Jolles 1992; Gualtieri 1995; Jennett 1996).

Despite these limitations, most epidemiological studies have estimated the incidence of TBI as approximating 200–300 cases per 100,000 individuals (Bigler 1990b; Bohnen and Jolles 1992; Gualtieri 1995; Jennett 1996; Kraus et al. 1984; Naugle 1990; Sorenson and Kraus 1991). These injuries do not, however, occur randomly, with the risk for TBI being clearly age-related. TBIs are most common among young adult males (ages 16–25), for whom the incidence is approximately 400 per 100,000. Typically, these injuries occur in motor vehicle accidents where alcohol is often involved (Bigler 1990b; Goldstein and Levin 1990; Goldstein et al. 1994; Jennett 1996; Naugle 1990). Children, between the ages of 1 and 5, are a second risk group, with the incidence rate approximating 150 per 100,000 individuals (Goldstein and Levin 1990; Rosenthal et al. 1990). The elderly population comprises a third at-risk group. As can be seen in Figure 28–1, following a period of relative low risk in middle adulthood, the risk for TBI steadily increases after age 65, to a rate of 200 per 100,000 (Goldstein and Levin 1990; Goldstein et al. 1994; Roy et al. 1986). In addition, the large gender difference in incidence rates that exists in young adults is not present in elderly adults. Whereas young adult men are approximately three times more likely than young adult women to sustain a TBI, in the elderly population, men and women are at equal risk (Jennett 1996; Kraus and Nourjah 1989; Naugle 1990).

Mechanism of injury. Differences also exist across age groups in how injuries are sustained. Among the general population, motor vehicle collisions are the leading cause of TBI, and falls are the second leading cause. Among the elderly, this order is reversed (Jennett 1996; Levy et al. 1993; Parker 1990; Rakier et al. 1995; Sorenson and Kraus 1991). Although geographic differences exist for other types of injuries (e.g., more assaults with firearms in larger cities), a consistent finding across studies is that with advancing age there is an increased risk of TBI as a result of falls and pedestrian accidents and a corresponding decreased risk of TBI as a result of motor vehicle collisions (Figure 28–2).

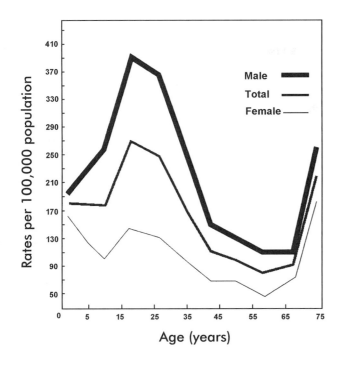

FIGURE 28–1. Incidence rates of traumatic brain injury by age and sex.
Source. Adapted from Kraus et al. 1984.

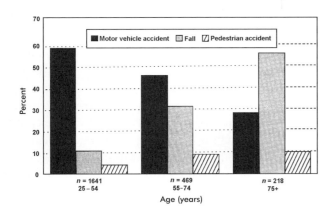

FIGURE 28–2. Causes of traumatic brain injury by age.
P < .0001
Source. Reprinted from Fields RB: "The Effects of Head Injuries on Older Adults" (abstract). *Clinical Neuropsychologist* 5:252, 1991.

Prior traumatic brain injury. Among young adults, previous TBI is a known risk factor for future head injury (Annegers et al. 1980a; Edna 1987; Naugle 1990; Sims 1985). Documentation of prior TBIs is somewhat difficult because it is typically based on self-report, memory, and

subjective interpretation. With these limitations in mind, preliminary data collected in one large trauma database (M. Lovell and S. Smith, personal communication, September 1994) suggest that the frequency of patients hospitalized following a TBI reporting a previous TBI is higher among younger adults than older adults. Specifically, in this sample, prior TBI was reported by 32% of a young to middle-aged sample (ages 20–50, *n* = 535), but only 20% of an older adult sample (ages 60–90, *n* = 97).

Role of alcohol. Alcohol is another factor that is significantly related to etiology and outcome following TBI in young adults (Desai et al. 1983; Edna 1987; Frankowski 1986; Parkinson et al. 1985; Ruff et al. 1990). It is also another factor that has not been adequately addressed in the literature on geriatric TBI and one for which our data suggest that the assumptions based on young adults may not apply to older adults. As expected, among a sample of more than 3,500 patients hospitalized following a TBI at Allegheny General Hospital in Pittsburgh, the frequency of young adults with blood alcohol levels at or above the legal definition of intoxication when brought to the emergency room was relatively high (e.g., ages 15–24, 44%; ages 35–54, 39%). Alcohol was associated with the TBI much less often among the older sample (e.g., ages 65–95, with legally intoxicated blood alcohol levels, 11%).

Another unique characteristic of the geriatric population is the age difference in the circumstances in which alcohol is involved in the TBI. In our database, legally intoxicated blood alcohol levels were found among young and middle-aged adults whose TBIs occurred in motor vehicle accidents (39%) at approximately the same rate as among those whose TBI occurred because of a fall (35%). In contrast, in the older adult group, among whom alcohol use was less prevalent overall, a legally intoxicated blood alcohol level was significantly more likely when the injury occurred during a fall (17.3%) than when the injury occurred during a motor vehicle accident (6.1%). These data suggest that drinking and driving is less of a problem for the elderly than for younger adults and that our understanding of outcome following TBIs that occur as the result of a fall in the elderly must take into account the role of alcohol.

Outcome

Older adults are usually thought to have less favorable outcomes than younger adults following TBI. In 1932, for example, Russell (Russell and Smith 1961) reported an increase in mortality associated with TBI beginning in the fifth decade of life. In their influential work, Jennett and Teasdale (1981) described a "continuous" and essentially linear relationship between age and negative outcome across the life span. Other studies have also documented increased mortality rates, increased length of hospital stay, increased likelihood of nursing home placement, increased long-term disability, and other signs of poor prognosis among older adults following brain injury (Annegers et al. 1980a; Carlsson et al. 1968; Cartlidge and Shaw 1981; Cifu et al. 1996; Edna 1983; Fife et al. 1986; Jennett and Teasdale 1981; Kilaru et al. 1996; Kotwica and Jakubowski 1992; Levy et al. 1993; Luerssen et al. 1988; Marshall et al. 1991; Pentland et al. 1986; Ross et al. 1992). In addition, the literature on general trauma in humans (Dries and Gamelli 1992) and the limited experimental literature on brain injury in animals (Hamm et al. 1991) also suggest that advanced age is a risk factor for adverse outcome.

Although the weight of evidence is impressive, studies comparing the effects of TBI on older versus younger adult humans have been problematic for a number of reasons. First is the influence of preexisting conditions on subsequent outcome. Preexisting neurological impairment may affect the cause of injury (e.g., a patient with dementia who falls), initial presentation (e.g., inaccurate history or delay in seeking treatment), postinjury course (e.g., exaggeration of preinjury neuropsychological deficits), and diagnosis (e.g., attribution of dementia-related cognitive impairment to the brain injury). Whether a TBI is the cause or the result of brain dysfunction is more likely to be a question among older adults in whom, for example, degenerative brain changes or medication sensitivity is more common than in younger adults. In a study of brain injury among the "old old" (ages 80–96), for example, a factor that contributed to the injury (e.g., previous stroke, postural dizziness, and medication) could be identified for 75% of the patients whose injury was the result of a fall (Amacher and Bybee 1987). Assessing outcome in this sample, therefore, might underestimate the potential recovery of "normal" elderly individuals who fall for other reasons.

A second problem has been controlling for severity of brain injury, as well as for total body injuries, when comparing samples of different age groups. If older adults have more severe injuries (as Sorenson and Kraus [1991] contend), increased negative outcome among the elderly may be simply a reflection of severity of injury rather than of age. A third problem is that even when severity of injury is controlled, comparisons of different age groups generally do not control for differences in the type of injury sustained. Finally, the definition of "old" varies considerably from study to study. Many reports of change in outcome with "age" involve a comparison between young adults (usually ages 20–40) and middle-aged adults (ages 40–65), with very little representation of geriatric patients including the "old old." With these cautions in mind, the following is a review of specific outcome measures.

Postinjury neurological sequelae. Advanced age is a risk factor for subdural hematomas, intracranial hemorrhages, and posttraumatic infections following TBI (Amacher and Bybee 1987; Dries and Gamelli 1992; Fogel and Duffy 1994; Miller and Pentland 1989). Postinjury bleeds are more common and more problematic in the elderly for a number of reasons. First, the incidence of nontraumatic intracerebral hemorrhage in the general population increases exponentially with age, making the elderly an at-risk population in general (Broderick et al. 1993). Second, as noted above, older adults are also at greater risk for subdural hematomas because age-related brain atrophy increases the distance from the brain surface to the venous sinuses (Cummings and Benson 1992). Third, because falls are the most common cause of geriatric TBI and because subdural hematomas are common consequences of falls, the elderly are particularly vulnerable for subdural bleeds. Finally, these types of injuries may develop in a delayed fashion over time and may go unrecognized in the presence of other injuries (Fogel and Duffy 1994). For example, in one study of older patients admitted to a hospital because of a fractured bone, 10% were found to have a subdural hematoma as well (Oster 1977).

The age-related increased risk of posttraumatic intracranial hematomas is particularly problematic after injuries that are classified as being in the mild-to-moderate range of severity. For example, in their comparison of older (i.e., > 65 years, $n = 449$) and younger (i.e., < 65 years, $n = 1,571$) patients following TBI of all severities, Pentland et al. (1986) reported a threefold increase in intracranial hematomas among the older sample. However, there was no age difference in the patients whose injuries were severe, among whom intracranial bleeds were common at all ages. In contrast, following TBIs of mild-to-moderate severity, the frequency of intracranial hematoma was six times greater in the older group. In our study (Fields and Ackerman 1991) of patients who sustained a mild TBI as the result of a fall or a motor vehicle accident, the incidence of intracranial bleeds was related to age and type of injury. Specifically, intracranial bleeds were significantly more common in the elderly sample in general but were also more common among those whose injury was sustained in a fall than among those whose injury occurred during a motor vehicle accident.

For other neurological sequelae, there are no age differences or the effects of age are not well known. Despite the logical prediction that an older skull might be more vulnerable to fracture than a younger skull during a TBI, no consistent evidence indicates that this is the case. For example, in one large study of patients with TBI of all severities (Pentland et al. 1986), no age differences were found in the frequency of skull fracture; in another study of patients with severe TBIs (Vollmer et al. 1991), only a slight increase in frequency of fracture with age was found. In our study of the effects of mild TBI across the life span, the developing skulls of children were found to be more vulnerable to fracture than the aging skulls of the adult and elderly samples, and no significant increase in the frequency of skull fracture was found with advancing age (Fields 1997).

Older adults do not appear to be at increased risk of developing brain swelling or a posttraumatic seizure disorder following a TBI (Richardson 1990). Similar to the data on skull fractures, posttraumatic seizures are in fact more common following TBI in children than TBI in adults (Dalmady-Israel and Zasler 1993; Fields 1997) (Table 28–2). Although it has been postulated that axonal shearing and damage from the release of excitotoxic neurotransmitters are greater among the elderly (Hamm et al. 1991, 1992), this prediction has not yet been definitively proven.

Indices of general outcome.

Following TBIs that are classified as severe, death, permanent disability, and inability to return to work are more common at all ages. However, age appears to play an independent and significant role in increasing the risk of negative outcome. In the most comprehensive study of age differences in outcome following severe TBI to date, Vollmer et al. (1991) found dramatic age-related differences in outcome at 6 months. The mortality rate at 6 months was 28% for the 26- to 35-year-old group and 80% for the over 55-year-old group. In addition, 28% of the younger group were rated as having made a good recovery (based on the GOS) after 6 months, whereas among the older group, 0% had made a good recovery. One of the advantages of this study was that the role of age in influencing outcome was assessed by systematically ruling out the effect of other variables. The authors concluded that the variable of age clearly made an independent contribution to outcome in their sample. Other studies have also documented the independent contributions of age to slower recovery and more negative eventual outcome (as measured by GOS) following TBI, particularly following moderate-to-severe injuries (e.g., Cifu et al. 1996; Katz et al. 1990; Kilaru et al. 1996; Pentland et al. 1986; Ross et al. 1992; Ruff et al. 1990).

Mortality.

With regard to the specific question of survival rate following TBI, in keeping with the Vollmer et al. (1991) study, a fairly robust finding in the literature is that older adults are at greater risk for death following head injury than are young adults or children (e.g., Amacher and Bybee 1987; Annegers et al. 1980a; Edna 1983; Fields 1991; Fife et al. 1986; Kilaru et al. 1996; Pentland et al. 1986; Rakier et al. 1995; Ross et al. 1992). However, as noted above, most studies of this outcome measure did not control for factors such as severity of brain injury or severity of other nonbrain injuries. In our attempts to do so (Table 28–3), an age by severity of injury interaction was found. As can be seen in Figure 28–3, when all patients were included regardless of severity of injury, mortality rate was relatively stable through middle adulthood, but it increased significantly beginning at age 55 and continued to increase with advancing age. In follow-up analyses (Table 28–3), among patients whose injuries were severe, mor-

TABLE 28–2. Based on age and type of injury, differences in neurological sequelae following mild traumatic brain injury

| Age group | Type of injury | n | Percentage of patients with | | |
			Skull fracture	Intracranial bleed	Seizures
0–10	Fall	63	29	6	6
	MVA	42	12	9	0
15–24	Fall	82	15	18	5
	MVA	795	10	4	1
35–54	Fall	169	17	19	5
	MVA	545	11	2	2
65–95	Fall	248	16	40	1
	MVA	229	13	15	0

Note. MVA = motor vehicle accident.
Source. Reprinted from Fields RB: "Geriatric Head Injury," in *Handbook of Neuropsychology and Aging.* Edited by Nussbaum PD. New York, Plenum, 1997, pp. 280–297.

TABLE 28–3. Age differences in mortality rates following traumatic brain injuries of different severity

Severity of injury	Age			
	0–10	15–24	35–54	65–95
Severe TBI	24%	19%	21%	54%
(GCS = 3–8)	(*n* = 42)	(*n* = 289)	(*n* = 196)	(*n* = 162)
Mild TBI	0%	0.3%	1%	8%
(GCS = 13–15)	(*n* = 189)	(*n* = 1,139)	(*n* = 952)	(*n* = 545)
Mild overall	0%	0%	0%	0.5%
(GCS = 13–15)	(*n* = 125)	(*n* = 628)	(*n* = 458)	(*n* = 187)
(ISS < 10)				

Note. GCS = Glasgow Coma Scale; ISS = Injury Severity Scale.; TBI = traumatic brain injury
Source. Reprinted from Fields RB: "Traumatic Brain Injury in the Elderly." Paper presented at the annual meeting of the National Academy of Neuropsychology, Orlando, FL, November 1994; Fields RB: "Geriatric Head Injury," in *Handbook of Neuropsychology and Aging.* Edited by Nussbaum PD. New York, Plenum, 1997, pp. 280–297.

tality was greater for patients at all ages but again was highest among the oldest group.

Among patients whose TBIs were considered to be mild, but whose total injuries were not accounted for in the analysis, the mortality rate among the oldest group was approximately 8 times greater than the middle-aged group and 24 times greater than the young adult group. However, when severity of head injury (e.g., mild, GCS = 13–15) and severity of total body injury (e.g., mild, ISS < 10) were controlled, mortality was extremely low for all age groups (Table 28–3). These data suggest that although age increases the risk for in-hospital mortality following a TBI at any level of severity, other factors (e.g., severity of other injuries) play a role in the apparent age difference in outcome.

Length of hospital stay and discharge destination. Several outcome studies have documented that, following TBIs of similar severity, older adults stay in hospital longer and are more likely to be discharged to a nursing home and less likely to be discharged to their home (e.g., Edna 1987; Fields 1991; Fife et al. 1986; Katz et al. 1990; Roy et al. 1986). Given changes in reimbursement for health-care services, these age-related differences have enormous practical and economic significance. Although length of hospital stay increases with age, this increase appears to be a reflection of the interaction between length of stay and discharge destination. In our sample, the mean length of stay for patients discharged to home or to a nursing home did not differ significantly by age (Fields 1991). That is, patients of any age who are discharged to nursing homes had stayed in hospital much longer than patients who return home. Because more older adults are discharged to nursing homes and fewer older adults are discharged home, the overall increase in hospital length of

stay for the elderly actually reflects that a larger percentage of elderly are discharged to nursing homes, rather than the implied impression that it takes all older adults longer to recover from their injuries.

Return to preinjury functioning. Finally, the literature on young and middle-aged adults suggests that advanced age is a relevant factor in the prediction of return to previous level of functioning. One frequently used index of outcome among young adults is return to school or work. Although this indicator is not meaningful for many older adults (who are retired), and despite the fact that the majority of the studies in this area do not include patients above age 65, it is worth noting that conclusions about the effect of age are, nevertheless, often made. For example, in three studies (Ip et al. 1995; Ponsford et al. 1995; Ruff et al. 1993), age was found to be a small but significant predictor of eventual outcome following severe TBI (among young and middle-aged adults). In the few studies that have assessed this variable among older adults (Alberico et al. 1987; Davis and Acton 1988; Pentland et al. 1986), advanced age has also been found to predict increased difficulty with activities of daily living, increased general disability, and decreased likelihood of returning to work (among those who were working prior to their injury).

Summary

There are several unique characteristics of geriatric TBI. First, TBI occurs more frequently among older adults than among middle-aged adults. Second, in contrast to TBI among young adults, no gender difference exists in the occurrence of TBI among older adults. Third, with advancing age there is an increase in the likelihood that TBIs

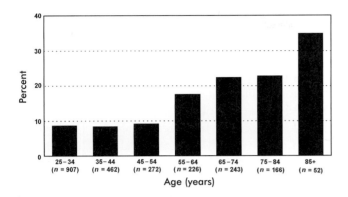

FIGURE 28–3. Age differences in mortality rate following traumatic brain injury—all levels of severity. $\chi^2 = 87.8$; $P < 10^{-8}$.

occur as the result of a fall or pedestrian accident and a decrease in the likelihood that the TBI occurred as the result of a motor vehicle collision. Fourth, a history of TBI is more common in younger adults than it is in older adults who are treated for TBIs. Fifth, alcohol is involved less often in the TBI among older adults, but when it is a factor, the TBI is more likely to be caused by a fall than by a motor vehicle collision. Finally, as a group, older adults are at greater risk for negative outcome (e.g., mortality, disability) following TBI than are younger adults. Elderly are at risk for some (e.g., subdural bleeds), but not all (e.g., skull fractures), postinjury sequelae. Furthermore, not all elderly are at greater risk for negative outcome, and some preliminary evidence suggests that factors such as preexisting impairment and the severity of other injuries contribute to the findings of worse outcome with advancing age.

Neuropsychiatric Consequences of Traumatic Brain Injury

As with other consequences of TBI, severity of injury is the best predictor of the type and severity of neuropsychiatric problems. Sufficient differences exist between groups of patients with mild TBIs and patients with severe TBIs to consider them separately.

Mild Traumatic Brain Injury

Cognitive and postconcussive symptoms. Following mild TBI, patients frequently display time-limited neuropsychological impairment and report a constellation of symptoms known at the *postconcussive syndrome*

(PCS). Neuropsychological deficits are typically seen in the areas of attention/concentration, speed and efficiency of information processing, and short-term memory (Alexander 1995; Barth et al. 1983; Bigler 1990a; Bohnen and Jolles 1992; Fann et al. 1995; Gentilini et al. 1989; Gronwall 1989; Gualtieri 1995; Klonoff and Lamb 1998; Kutner and Barth 1998; Masson et al. 1996; Mazaux et al. 1997; Ruff et al. 1989b). In addition to problems with cognitive processing (e.g., concentration), the PCS includes physical symptoms (e.g., headache, dizziness, blurred vision, tinnitus, fatigue, and increased sensitivity to light and noise) and mood/behavioral symptoms (e.g., anxiety, depression, and irritability) (Alexander 1995; Barth et al. 1983; Bigler 1990a; Binder 1986; Bohnen and Jolles 1992; Gronwall 1991; Gualtieri 1995; Masson et al. 1996; Mazaux et al. 1997). Symptoms of posttraumatic stress disorder (e.g., intrusive recollections, nightmares, avoidance, increased startle response) are also common following mild TBI because the traumatic event is more likely to be remembered than following severe TBI.

The majority of patients who sustain a mild TBI experience a relatively complete recovery of neuropsychiatric symptoms within 1–3 months of their injury. However, a minority of patients report that these symptoms persist for months, or in some cases years, after the injury (Alexander 1995; Bigler 1990a; Gronwall 1991; Gualtieri 1995; Kutner and Barth 1998; Masson et al. 1996; Mazaux et al. 1997; Raskin et al. 1998). For example, in studies by Masson et al. (1996) and Mazaux et al. (1997), a subgroup of patients reported ongoing problems in areas such as headache, dizziness, mood, memory, energy, sleep, and initiative/motivation 5 years following a mild TBI.

The etiology of persistent neuropsychiatric deficits remains controversial. The role that psychological factors including "secondary gain" play in mediating response to a traumatic event has not been clearly defined. In addition, factors such as premorbid psychiatric problems, previous head injury, chronic pain, little education, and litigation have been correlated with persistent neurobehavioral complaints (Dikmen et al. 1989). Some studies, for example, have found that patients involved in litigation following a mild TBI performed more poorly on neuropsychological tests than did patients with documented severe TBI (Youngjohn et al. 1995). However, other studies suggest that, for at least some patients, the persistence of neuropsychiatric symptoms may be caused by unknown or undetected neurological damage. For example, in one study of patients evaluated 6 months following a TBI, Bohnen et al. (1992) found that those who reported postconcussive symptoms also performed less well on tests of divided and selective attention than did patients without postconcussive symptoms or healthy control subjects. Prigatano (1992) has suggested that symptoms that remain relatively stable over time, such as emotional lability, irritability, and restlessness, may be primary effects resulting from neurological damage, whereas symptoms that worsen over time, such as fatigue, sensitivity to distress, and apathy, may be secondary effects resulting from having to cope with the neurological deficits. Although the development of postconcussive symptoms occurs independent of litigation status (Merskey and Woodforde 1972; Steadman and Graham 1970), several factors including pending litigation, preinjury personality, length of posttraumatic amnesia, alcohol use, fault for injury, and social network all must be evaluated when assessing the relationship between a TBI and late postconcussive symptomatology (Alexander 1992; Rutherford 1989).

Depression.   Reports of depressive symptomatology are common following mild TBI, with studies identifying approximately 22%–36% of individuals with mild TBI meeting criteria for a major depressive episode (Busch and Alpern 1998). Although it can be difficult to distinguish between depression and PCS, such a distinction is important for accurate and effective treatment. Complicating the issue is that many individuals who report depressive symptoms have significant premorbid conditions (e.g., psychiatric/psychological histories, substance abuse, neurological disorders) that can contribute to depressive symptomatology following a TBI. In addition, the psychological reaction to the consequences of the accident (e.g., death of friends/family) and to the subsequent cognitive and physical deficits may influence the development or exacerbation of depressive symptomatology.

When trying to isolate the cause of depression following mild TBI, several conflicting findings have emerged. Pharmacological studies indicate little or no improvement with antidepressants for depression in persons with mild TBI cases (Busch and Alpern 1998). Other studies examining relationships between lesion location and depression following mild TBIs have found significant associations (Busch and Alpern 1998). For example, Federoff et al. (1992) found a significant association between a major depressive episode and left dorsolateral frontal, left basal ganglia, and, to a lesser extent, right parieto-occipital lesions. Although this study did not exclusively use mild TBI cases, 35% of the group with depression were identified as having a mild TBI. In another study by Gasparrini et al. (1978), a significant difference was found between left and right hemisphere damage and depressive symptomatology in mild TBI cases. Using the Minnesota Multiphasic Personality Inventory (Hathaway and McKinley 1970), their

results indicated that left hemispheric damage produced significantly higher scores on the depression scale.

Neuroimaging studies also support the relationship between neurological impairment following mild TBI and depression. In several studies, abnormal CT scans and magnetic resonance imaging (MRI) results indicate a possible relationship between depression and lesions in the frontal, temporal, or frontotemporal areas (Jenkins et al. 1986; Levin et al. 1987a; Sekino et al. 1981). Thus, there appears to be increasing evidence suggesting an interactional relationship between the location of brain injury following a mild TBI and the development of depressive symptomatology. However, further research in this area is needed to help differentiate secondary psychological reactions from primary neurological factors.

Severe Traumatic Brain Injury

Cognitive deficits.   Following severe TBI, patients often display significant deficits in the areas of attention/concentration, speed of information processing, memory, and executive functioning (Cullum et al. 1990; Levin et al. 1982; Mazaux et al. 1997; Olver et al. 1996; Ponsford et al. 1995; Tennant et al. 1995). Specifically, impairments have been reported on measures of divided attention; the ability to tune out distractions; speed of processing, learning, and retaining new information; initiation; planning; organization; and awareness/insight. As a result, even without deficits in basic language, perceptual, or motor capacities, patients who have had severe TBIs often have difficulty following conversations, sustaining attention, sustaining efficiency at work, learning without repeated exposure, initiating activity, making plans, correcting errors, shifting cognitive sets, and having insight into their changes in behavior.

In contrast to the majority of patients with mild TBI, neuropsychological dysfunction following severe TBI is more significant and more long lasting (Parker 1990). Persistent deficits in intellectual functioning have been found in most patients following severe TBI (Levin et al. 1979) although the pattern of impairment is not always uniform. For example, Levin et al. (1990) found that although basic language and visuospatial skills had returned to normal 1 year after a severe TBI, young adult patients continued to demonstrate memory impairment and slowed information processing. Other studies documented deficits 5–7 years postinjury. For example, Tennant et al. (1995) found that 56% of their sample were continuing to report memory problems 7 years after a severe TBI. Similarly, Mazaux et al. (1997) found that mental fatigability, memory difficulties, lack of initiative and motivation, conceptual disorganization, difficulties in mental flexibility, and poor planning were common complaints 5 years following severe TBI.

Mood. With regard to affective symptoms following severe TBI, consistent findings are lacking in the literature. This inconsistency is probably the result of the considerable variability in methodologies used to assess severity of injury, time since injury, definition of mood symptoms, and approach to assessment. For example, studies of depressive symptoms following severe brain injury have found prevalence rates varying from 10% to 70% (Silver et al. 1991, 1992). Depressive symptoms are apparently not related to factors such as length of unconsciousness, length of posttraumatic amnesia, or presence of skull fracture (Silver et al. 1992) but may be related to neuropsychological status (Bornstein et al. 1989) and, as described above, lesion location (Federoff et al. 1992).

Other causes of mood or behavioral change following TBI include grief or other adjustment-related mood disturbances and neuropsychiatric syndromes such as apathy, amotivation, slowed cognitive processing, and affective lability (Mazaux et al. 1997; Ponsford et al. 1995; Prigatano 1992; Raskin 1998; Silver et al. 1991; Tennant et al. 1995). In addition, whether depressive symptoms predated or caused the head injury (e.g., suicidal car crash) must be taken into account when assessing the role of brain injury in "causing" depression (Silver et al. 1991).

The use of comprehensive assessment procedures and an agreed-on classification system to diagnose mood disturbance (and other neuropsychiatric disorders) following TBI has been rare. Even when structured interviews and specific diagnostic criteria are used, reported prevalence rates vary and depend, in part, on the point at which patients are assessed. For example, in a sample of patients who were assessed during the first year after a TBI (Jorge et al. 1993b), the frequency of major depression diagnosed according to DSM-III (American Psychiatric Association 1980) was 42%, whereas the frequency of major depression among a sample assessed 2–8 years after their injury was 77% (Varney et al. 1987). In both studies, a substantial portion of these patients reported that their depressive symptoms developed at least 3–6 months after the injury (39% in the Jorge et al. [1993b] study and 46% in the Varney et al. [1987] study).

One series of studies took an important step toward clarifying the causes and course of depressive symptoms following TBI (Federoff et al. 1992; Jorge et al. 1993a, 1993b). The presence of neuropsychiatric disturbance was assessed among 66 young adults on an inpatient trauma service with a structured psychiatric interview (i.e., modified Present State Examination [Wing et al. 1974]) and scales of depression, cognitive capacity, activities of daily living, and social functioning. Patients were initially evaluated during the acute postinjury period and then reassessed 3, 6, and 12 months later. During the 1-year follow-up period, 42.4% of the patients met DSM-III criteria for major depression (25.7% during the acute period and 16.7% during one of the follow-up examinations). Patients with the "acute-" and the "delayed-"onset depression had a higher frequency of previous psychiatric problems and impaired social functioning than did the patients without depression, but these groups also differed on a number of other dimensions. Lesions in the left frontal region (particularly left dorsolateral frontal or left basal ganglia) were associated with major depression among only the patients with the acute-onset depression. In contrast, patients with delayed-onset depression had significantly poorer social functioning, but less severe depression and less impairment in activities of daily living, than did the group with acute-onset depression. In addition, no specific relationship between location of brain lesion and the occurrence of delayed-onset depression has been found (Fann et al. 1995). Based on these findings, Jorge et al. (1993b) suggested that acute-onset depression may be more related to biological changes in an injured brain, whereas delayed-onset depression may be more psychologically based.

Behavior and personality. Long-term alterations in behavior and personality are also common following severe TBI. For example, Jennett and Teasdale (1981) found personality changes in approximately two-thirds of patients who sustained severe brain injuries. Changes that are commonly associated with TBI include impulsivity, irritability, diminished drive, altered frustration tolerance, agitation, aggression, and impaired social judgment (Bigler 1991; Jennett and Teasdale 1981; Mazaux et al. 1997; Olver et al. 1996; Ponsford et al. 1995; Prigatano 1992; Silver et al. 1987; Tennant et al. 1995).

Prigatano (1986) described three types of personality and behavioral disturbances that occur following severe TBI: organic disturbances, emotional reactions to injury or attempts to cope with injury, and preinjury personality characteristics that influence the expression of neurological damage. "Organic" personality changes, such as reduced tolerance for stimulation, mental fatigue, irritability, and difficulty with impulse control, are presumed to be linked to the site of the injury. For example, specific lesions in the orbitofrontal area have been linked to a behavioral dyscontrol syndrome that includes disinhibition, impulsivity, emotional lability, hyperactivity, and diminished awareness or concern for the implications of one's behavior (Cummings 1985; Gualtieri 1991; Mattson and Levin 1990) (see Chapter 32 in this volume). Generalized frontal lobe lesions have also been associated with perseveration, apathy, indifference, amotivation, abulia, loss of empathy, poor social judgment, and a loss of the capacity for accurate self-monitoring (Lewis et al. 1992). Temporal lobe injuries have been associated with irritability and aggression. Frontotemporal lesions have been associated with mood lability, inappropriate laughing and crying, and hypersexuality or hyposexuality. Temporoparietal injuries have been associated with suspiciousness, paranoia, and a tendency to misinterpret the intentions of others (Gualtieri 1991).

Summary

While significant gaps in our knowledge remain, the neuropsychiatric sequelae of TBI are becoming better understood. Following mild TBI, time-limited deficits in areas of higher level cognitive processing such as complex attention and working memory are common, as are mild symptoms of mood and behavioral disturbance. For the majority of patients, symptom resolution occurs within 3 months of the injury. For a minority of patients, symptoms of cognitive and behavioral disturbance persist. The persistence of symptoms in these patients appears to be related to multiple factors, ranging from "secondary gain" in some to documented brain dysfunction in others. Among patients whose TBIs are severe, more long-standing changes in cognitive processing and behavior are likely. Although more research is needed, preliminary evidence suggests that some types of mood and behavioral disturbances do correlate with TBI lesion location.

▌ Neuropsychiatric Consequences of Geriatric Traumatic Brain Injury

Animal Studies

Most of the experimental literature has focused on the neuropathological changes that are associated with TBIs and the course of these injuries over time. Experimentally induced TBIs via methods such as fluid percussion, weight drop, rigid indentation, and angular acceleration have been helpful in elucidating the type and extent of injuries that occur following TBIs at different levels of severity (McIntosh et al. 1996; Povlishock and Coburn 1989). Studies have demonstrated that the greater plasticity of an immature central nervous system enhances the ability of very young animals to recover from experimental brain in-

juries (Finger 1978). To date, however, the effect of advanced age on head injury in animals has received only limited attention (Hamm et al. 1992).

In one study, Hamm et al. (1991) reported that the mortality rate for older rats (20 months) was approximately three times greater than that for younger rats (3 months) following experimentally produced (fluid percussion) "mild" brain injury. Following a more severe fluid percussion brain injury (i.e., "moderate injury") mortality was five times greater among the older rats. Using a similar model, Hamm et al. (1992) also found age-related motoric and cognitive deficits following a lower level (i.e., "mild") fluid percussion brain injury. In this study, weight was used as an index of general health, balance beam performance as an index of motor skill, and the Morris Water Maze Task as an index of cognitive capacity. Older rats (20 months) had no general health changes following the injury but did demonstrate significant motoric and cognitive deficits. In contrast, the younger rats (3 months) did not display any postinjury motor deficits and had less severe cognitive deficits than did the older rats. Other investigators have demonstrated slower and more deficient neuronotropic response following experimentally induced TBI in older rats relative to that in younger rats (Needles et al. 1985; Whittemore et al. 1985). Finally, as reviewed in the last section of this chapter, specific genetic factors also appear to mediate neuronal repair and neurobehavioral recovery following TBI in animals (Chen et al. 1997).

Human Studies

Although limited, the available data on the neuropsychiatric consequences of geriatric TBI have begun to shed light on some of the central questions that must be addressed to define the syndrome of geriatric TBI. These questions include 1) Can the effects of geriatric TBI be differentiated from the effects of normal aging? 2) Do the neuropsychological effects of TBI differ with age? 3) Can the syndrome of geriatric TBI be differentiated from the syndrome of dementia on the basis of neuropsychological test performance? and 4) Do the neuropsychiatric and psychosocial consequences of TBI differ with age?

Can geriatric traumatic brain injury be differentiated from normal aging? Indirect support for the hypothesis that the neuropsychological effects of TBI in the elderly can be differentiated from the effects of normal aging comes from the extensive literature on the effects of TBI among young adults (e.g., Levin et al. 1982, 1990) as well as one study (Mazzucchi et al. 1992) that found a high rate of generalized cognitive impairment (e.g., approximately 50%) among a sample of older adults (e.g., 50–75 years of age) who had recently sustained a TBI.

Two studies have directly tested and supported this hypothesis. In the first, Goldstein et al. (1994) compared the performance of older (50 years and older) patients who had sustained a TBI of mild (*n* = 6) or moderate severity (*n* = 16) with the performance of an older adult control group (*n* = 16) on selected measures in four cognitive domains: attention (e.g., reciting alphabet, reciting serial 3s, reciting months forward and backward), language (e.g., visual naming, controlled oral word associating), memory (e.g., California Verbal Learning Test [CVLT] [Delis et al. 1986], Continuous Visual Recognition Test [Hannay and Levin 1998]), and executive functioning (Wechsler Adult Intelligence Scale—Revised [WAIS-R] [Wechsler 1981], similarities, modified card sorting). Nineteen of the 22 patients with geriatric TBI were tested within 3 months of their injury. Consistent with the literature on TBI among young adults, significant between-group differences were found in three of the four domains (language, memory, and executive functioning). The authors concluded that their "findings indicate that mild to moderate closed head injury in older adults produces cognitive deficits involving the same neurobehavioral areas affected in young survivors" (Goldstein et al. 1994, p. 964).

In a second study (Goldstein et al. 1996), the performance of 15 geriatric patients with TBI was compared with the performance of 15 normal elderly control subjects (and 15 patients with AD; see below) on measures of memory (dementia version of the CVLT) and language processing (naming and verbal fluency). Consistent with the findings of their previous study (Goldstein et al. 1994), the geriatric TBI group in this study performed significantly worse than the elderly control group on measures of memory and language.

An important methodological issue was raised by a third recent study in this area. Aharon-Peretz et al. (1997) also found that older patients (i.e., 60 years or older) with TBI performed more poorly on neuropsychological tests than did psychiatrically normal elderly control subjects. However, in this study, the patients with TBI did not perform more poorly than orthopedic patients, suggesting that the postinjury deficits in both patient groups may have been partly the result of preexisting cognitive impairments, which may have contributed to the etiology of the injuries.

Do the neuropsychological effects of traumatic brain injury differ with age? To provide conclusive support for the contention that TBI produces similar deficits among young and older survivors, a large-scale study of young and older adult patients with TBI is needed that takes into account factors such as premorbid level of functioning, role of substance abuse, history of prior head injury, type of injury, severity of injury, type and severity of other nonbrain injuries, and availability of rehabilitation and psychosocial support resources. No such study exists. The assumption that older age is associated with greater impairment comes from studies such as the one by Raskin et al. (1998) in which it was reported that older adults performed more poorly than younger adults following TBI on a memory test. However, in this study, the mean age of the sample was 38.1, "old" was defined as over 40, and raw scores were used rather than age-corrected scores.

In an attempt to address one aspect of this question, Fields (1994) compared the neuropsychological test performance of young (*n* = 472) and older (*n* = 96) adults who 1) sustained a mild TBI (GCS = 13–15) and 2) recovered sufficiently within the first week following their injury to complete a neuropsychological evaluation. A limitation of this study was that it did not address the issue of whether more elderly than young adults were too impaired to be tested (i.e., had more severe initial outcome). However, this design did ensure the comparability of the two groups by requiring that all patients met the same inclusion criteria.

As can be seen in Table 28–4, while the raw scores of the older adults were significantly worse on seven of the eight measures chosen, when the effects of age were controlled by converting raw scores to age-based percentile scores, the groups differed on only one of the eight measures (Digit Span Backward) (Table 28–4). These preliminary data support the conclusion of Goldstein et al. (1994) and suggest that the *acute* neuropsychological effects of mild TBI among patients whose initial recovery is relatively uncomplicated are not significantly different with age. However, whether there are age differences in the *long-term* neuropsychological effects of TBI or the course of neuropsychological recovery over time is not yet known.

Can geriatric traumatic brain injury be differentiated from dementia? The ability to differentiate the syndrome of geriatric TBI from dementia is important for clinical, as well as legal, reasons. Two studies have provided preliminary guidelines in this area. Goldstein et al. (1996) compared the performance of 15 geriatric patients following mild-to-moderate TBI (GCS = 9–15) with the performance of 15 patients with probable AD (all of whom were considered to be in the early stages of the disease) and 15 elderly control subjects. Geriatric patients with TBI were tested approximately 6 weeks postinjury.

TABLE 28–4.   Comparison of neuropsychological test performance of geriatric patients (*n* = 96) versus that of young adult patients (*n* = 472) following mild traumatic brain injury

	Results	
	Raw	Percentile
Test	score	score
Digit span forward	NS	NS
Digit span backward	$P < .01$	$P < .05$
Trails A	$P < .001$	NS
Trails B	$P < .001$	NS
Wechsler Memory Scale–Revised		
Logical Memory–I	$P < .05$	NS
Logical Memory–II	$P < .01$	NS
Visual Reproduction–I	$P < .001$	NS
Visual Reproduction–II	$P < .001$	NS

Note.   NS = not significant.
Source.   Reprinted from Fields RB: "Traumatic Brain Injury in the Elderly." Paper presented at the annual meeting of the National Academy of Neuropsychology, Orlando, FL, November 1994.

The test battery chosen for this study specifically included two areas that are impaired in early AD, that is, memory (via the dementia version of the CVLT) and language processing (via tests of object naming and verbal fluency). Not surprisingly, the elderly control subjects performed better on the language and memory tasks than did both of the patient groups. Of relevance to the current discussion, compared to the patients with TBI, the patients with AD 1) displayed poorer recall on the dementia version of the CVLT, and 2) did not show the normal facilitation of verbal fluency when asked to generate words in specific semantic catego-

ries (fruits/vegetables), as opposed to the generation of word lists in more specific phonemic categories (words beginning with specific letters).

In a second study, Young et al. (1995) compared the test performance of 33 geriatric patients who had sustained a recent TBI (in the previous week) with 35 elderly patients who met criteria for mild dementia on measures of attention (Digit Span [Wechsler 1987], Trails A [Army Individual Test Battery 1944]), memory (Hopkins Verbal Learning Test [HVLT] [Brandt 1991]), and executive functioning (Trails B [Army Individual Test Battery 1944]). In keeping with the finding of Goldstein et al. (1996), Young et al. (1995) (Table 28–5) found that although the geriatric group with TBI performed better overall than did the group with AD, the only significant between-group differences were on measures of memory (HVLT, learning and delayed recall) and executive functioning (Trails B), with worse performance in the group with AD.

Does neuropsychiatric functioning differ with age following traumatic brain injury?   Among young adults, neuropsychiatric complaints are frequent in the month following a TBI and can include physical changes (e.g., headache, dizziness, sensitivity to light and noise), cognitive difficulties (e.g., concentration, memory), and alterations in mood (e.g., depression, posttraumatic anxiety) and behavior (e.g., impulsivity, irritability) (Binder 1986; Bohnen and Jolles 1992; Bohnen et al. 1992). For most patients, these symptoms resolve in 3–6 months. Among the elderly, preliminary evidence suggests that neurobehavioral recovery may be different and slightly more complicated.

Levin (1995) reported on a preliminary study using the Neurobehavioral Rating Scale to assess the functioning of elderly patients with TBI or AD and elderly control subjects. One month following their injury, patients with TBI

TABLE 28–5.   Comparison of neuropsychological test performance of geriatric patients with traumatic brain injury (*n* = 33) versus patients with mild dementia (*n* = 35)

Test	Geriatric patients with TBI	Patients with dementia	*P* value
Digit span forward	7.8	6.9	
Digit span backward	5.0	4.5	
Trails A	69.1	97.6	
Trails B	193.8	266.4	$P < .01$
Hopkins Verbal Learning Test			
Learning score	6.7	4.8	$P < .001$
Delayed score	5.2	1.8	$P < .001$

Note.   TBI = traumatic brain injury.
Source.   Reprinted from Young L, Fields RB, Lovell M: "Neuropsychological Differentiation of Geriatric Head Injury From Dementia" (abstract). *Journal of Neuropsychiatry* 7:414, 1995.

reported difficulties in the areas of cognition, meta-cognition, and language. When a subsample of this group was reassessed 6 months following their injury, no significant change in overall symptomatology was reported.

Similar results were found in another study of the natural history of post-TBI complaints in which the self-reports of older patients (ages 50–95, $n = 49$) were compared with the self-reports of younger patients (ages 18–45, $n = 139$) acutely and 4 months following their injury (Fields et al. 1993). For this study, a 29-item questionnaire (Post-Traumatic Neurobehavioral Screening Inventory [PTNSI]) (Fields and Coffey 1994), which assesses symptoms commonly reported following TBI, was used (C. A. Taylor et al. 1993). The two age groups were comparable in terms of severity of head injury and severity of other non-brain injuries. One month following the injury, neurobehavioral complaints were common among both younger and older patients, and the overall symptom profiles were quite similar, although symptoms of posttraumatic stress disorder were more common among the younger group and fatigue was reported more often in the older group. At the 4-month follow-up, however, age-related differences began to emerge (Table 28–6). The older patients endorsed fatigue, difficulty processing information, dysphoric mood, dizziness, and sensitivity to noise significantly more than did the younger patients. In addition, there was an age by time interaction found on three of the six subscales of the test (cognitive, behavior, posttraumatic stress) such that the older patients reported similar, or greater, distress in these areas at 4 months than they had 3 months earlier, whereas the younger patients reported improvement in all of these areas across the same time period. Thus, although preliminary, these findings suggest that the course of neurobehavioral recovery following TBI in elderly patients may be different, and somewhat worse, than that in younger patients.

Summary

To summarize, although limited, the available data on neuropsychiatric outcome suggest that TBI in the elderly produces neuropsychological effects that are qualitatively similar to the effects of TBI in young adults and that are distinguishable from the effects of normal aging and dementia. One important implication of these data is that if elderly are evaluated with age-appropriate tests and norms, a significant percentage (perhaps a majority) perform in a manner that is not significantly worse than that of younger adults, suggesting that not all elderly are at greater risk for negative outcome. With regard to the differentiation of geriatric TBI from dementia, the available data suggest that learning, delayed recall, semantic processing, and executive functioning are cognitive domains that may differentiate these two syndromes. With regard to neuropsychiatric outcome, in addition to the general finding that older adults are less likely to return to their preinjury level of functioning, there is now preliminary evidence that the course of recovery for older patients following a TBI may be different, and somewhat worse, than the course for younger patients.

Diagnosis and Management of Neuropsychiatric Sequelae

The neuropsychiatric assessment and treatment of patients who sustain TBIs will be more straightforward once diagnosis becomes more accurate, double-blind medication trials for specific syndromes have been completed, and the role of factors, such as age, in mediating response to treatment is understood. Until then, the literature suggests a number of potential principles that may provide guides for developing assessment and treatment strategies.

TABLE 28–6. Age differences in symptom report at 1 and 4 months following traumatic brain injury using the Posttraumatic Neurobehavioral Screening Inventory

Percentage of sample endorsing symptom	Age 18–45	Age 50–95	P
1 month	($n = 139$)	($n = 49$)	
Fatigue	48.6	66.0	$P < .05$
4 months	($n = 54$)	($n = 25$)	
Fatigue	30.9	72.0	$P < .001$
Difficulty processing information	12.0	44.0	$P < .005$
Dysphoric mood	20.1	45.8	$P < .05$
Dizziness	5.4	24.0	$P < .05$
Sensitivity to noise	5.4	20.0	$P < .05$

Diagnosis

The general assessment of symptoms following TBI can be a difficult process, given the ambiguity present in the symptom presentation, as well as the conflicting reports of the accident. As Parker and Rosenblum (1996) discuss, relevant information is often incomplete or inaccurate following traumatic injuries. This incomplete or incorrect information may be the result of a variety of factors. Many individuals with TBI may have presenting symptomatology (e.g., memory loss) that prevents them from accurately reporting the traumatic incident and resulting effects. In addition, the treatments that are used to prevent secondary problems (e.g., paralyzing drugs, intubation, pain management) may also hinder the information-gathering process. Lastly, patients may experience embarrassment or anxiety about re-experiencing the traumatic event, which may result in a reluctance to accurately report the incident and subsequent symptoms (Parker and Rosenblum 1996). As a result, many individuals with TBIs may not be adequately assessed, and thus not properly treated.

The diagnosis of a specific psychiatric disturbance in patients following TBI is often problematic as well (Coffey 1987; Ross and Rush 1981). For example, valid and reliable historical information may be difficult to obtain in patients with language deficits (e.g., aphasia) or neglect syndromes (e.g., unawareness or denial or illness). In addition, brain disorders may distort the signs and symptoms of psychiatric disturbances (e.g., complaints of hopelessness and helplessness secondary to depression may appear unconvincing in a patient with aprosody). Behavioral disturbances that result from TBI may be misdiagnosed as a psychiatric disorder, or, conversely, the behavioral disturbances that often accompany psychiatric illness may be mistakenly attributed to a brain disorder (e.g., psychomotor retardation of depression attributed to posttraumatic parkinsonism). These difficulties in recognizing psychiatric illness in patients with TBI impede efforts to determine the neuroanatomical correlates of behavior and may lead to inappropriate diagnosis and treatment.

Diagnostic process and tools.   Accurate diagnosis requires an understanding of the neuropsychiatric sequelae and the course of recovery of traumatic injuries of different types, locations, and severities. In addition, because there are multiple possible causes of neuropsychiatric symptoms, the evaluation of the patient with a TBI should include a review of prior head trauma, developmental and academic history, occupational history, and social history as well as a comprehensive psychiatric, medical, and substance abuse assessment. Because discrepancies between the reports of patients and families are common following TBI (Oddy et al. 1985), the importance of collateral history from relatives and hospital records is also critical.

With these general guidelines in mind, the assessment of specific disorders may require flexible strategies. Regarding the assessment of depression, for example, Ross and Rush (1981) suggest that, in addition to obtaining history from the patient and a reliable informant, clinical cues such as a complicated recovery from the brain injury, multiple "vegetative signs" of depression, atypical emotional outbursts, aprosody, and an abrupt deterioration in the patient's neurological status can be used to make a diagnosis. Among elderly patients, additional factors that must be considered include the presence of systemic medical conditions, preexisting neurodegenerative disorders, and possible developmental changes in the phenomenology of depressive symptoms related to aging (Caine et al. 1993).

Comprehensive assessment is further complicated by the lack of assessment tools and an inadequate classification system. Although current psychiatric diagnostic systems provide a useful starting point for studying patients with TBIs, it is possible that neuropsychiatric symptomatology following such injuries may be better classified by other approaches. For example, the "bottom up" approach of the Schedules for Clinical Assessment in Neuropsychiatry (SCAN) (World Health Organization 1992) is promising in that it assesses the presence and severity of a comprehensive list of symptoms rather than (or in addition to) the traditional method of establishing a specific diagnosis. This approach allows for the generation of clusters of symptoms that may have clinical significance but that do not meet diagnostic criteria.

A related issue pertains to the limits of the current diagnostic classification system for patients with neuropsychiatric disorders. Following TBIs, patients may have an identifiable pattern of symptoms but may not meet criteria for a DSM-IV disorder (American Psychiatric Association 1994). Furthermore, even when diagnostic criteria are met, it may be difficult to determine whether the brain disease is causal of the neuropsychiatric symptoms. Such etiological judgments may at times be unreliable and invalid, and it has been suggested that Axis I diagnoses such as major depression be kept purely phenomenological, with relevant causal or contributory organic factors identified on Axis III (Fogel 1991).

Imaging.   An improved diagnostic classification system for patients with TBIs will ultimately depend on the sensitivity of neuropsychiatric and neuropsychological assessment instruments and the correlation between these measures and indices of brain structure and function. Brain imaging is critical for the assessment of most patients who sustain a TBI, particularly for those with severe injuries (GCS 3–8). Although controversy remains about performing CT scans after mild and moderate TBIs, evidence suggests that approximately one-fifth of patients with mild TBIs have abnormal CT scans (Wald 1995). Therefore, routinely performing this procedure on individuals diagnosed with TBIs is still advisable. CT scanning is widely used and the modality of choice for its ability to detect intracranial hematomas, delineate bony structures of the craniofacial skeleton, and identify skull fractures in the acute (1–3 days) posttrauma period (Chakares and Bryan 1986; Pieper et al. 1996; Wald 1995; Yoshino and Seeger 1989).

Brain MRI is more sensitive than CT for assessing parenchymal damage, including the diffuse axonal "shear" lesions, and providing information about subcortical structures and the brainstem (Alavi 1989; Levin et al. 1985, 1987; Wald 1995). MRI also provides a better view of brain tissue adjacent to the skull (e.g., inferior frontal regions and temporal lobes) because, unlike CT, MRI is not subject to beam-hardening artifact. However, because MRI does not image bone, it is not helpful in assessing possible fractures, nor can MRI be used in patients attached to metal respirators or in those who have metal fragments (e.g., bullets or shrapnel) in their heads (Levin et al. 1992; Pieper et al. 1996; Wald 1995). In addition, the use of MRI may be impractical in the initial assessment because it tends to be time-consuming and often unavailable for immediate use (Pieper et al. 1996). However, increased sensitivity of MRI to the presence of brain lesions is particularly apparent among patients with mild-to-moderate TBIs (Levin et al. 1992), and follow-up MRI studies have been shown to be more predictive of eventual outcome (Wilson et al. 1988). Structural brain imaging studies of elderly patients must be interpreted within the context of changes that occur with normal aging (see Chapter 9 in this volume).

Functional brain imaging studies (e.g., regional cerebral blood flow [rCBF], single photon emission computerized tomography [SPECT], positron-emission tomography [PET], and functional MRI) have not yet found a role in the routine assessment of patients with TBI. Cerebral blood flow and metabolism are reduced acutely after brain injury, and the degree of metabolic suppression may be related to the severity of injury (Fieschi et al. 1974; Obrist et al. 1979). Metabolic imaging techniques appear to be more sensitive than either CT or MRI in detecting areas of brain abnormalities after TBI (Alavi 1989; Alavi et al. 1986; Langfitt et al. 1986; Ruff et al. 1989a), and such abnormalities correlate more closely with neuropsychological per-

formance postinjury than do the structural changes seen on CT or MRI (Ruff et al. 1989a). The clinical use of these metabolic imaging techniques and their particular characteristics in elderly patients must await further research (see Chapters 10 and 11 in this volume).

Management

Early considerations.

Based on age-related differences in the occurrence, pathophysiology, and sequelae of TBI in elderly individuals, Fogel and Duffy (1994) recommended guidelines for the acute and subacute assessment and treatment of older adults. In the acute postinjury phase, these recommendations include increased vigilance regarding possible early or delayed vascular complications (e.g., subdural hematoma and intracranial hemorrhage); identification and management of neuropsychiatric comorbidities (e.g., preexisting cognitive impairment, depression, and alcoholism); and ongoing monitoring of neuropsychiatric status if other medical problems predominate (e.g., serial assessment of mental status or functional capacity during treatment for orthopedic injuries). In the postacute phase, neuropsychiatric input is recommended for determining capacity to benefit from formal rehabilitation (e.g., based on degree of cognitive impairment, as well as physical deficits); assessing and managing functional deficits (e.g., capacity to take medication, live independently, or drive); and treating the behavioral and psychosocial consequences of the TBI (Fogel and Duffy 1994).

Acute pharmacological treatment of brain injury.

The diverse nature of TBIs and the need for acute management of multiple problems have made it difficult to conduct double-blind studies of potentially beneficial pharmacological strategies for TBI. In the absence of clinically proven algorithms of care, a number of studies have offered suggestions for treatment, as well as avenues for further research. These treatment strategies include the use of antioxidants or free-radical scavengers, as well as gangliosides and cyclooxygenase inhibitors, to prevent secondary brain damage (Faden 1996; Wald 1995). Gangliosides have been used with some success in patients with acute strokes, subarachnoid hemorrhages, and spinal cord injuries (Wald 1995).

The use of nimodipine, a calcium channel antagonist, is also being investigated in the treatment of TBI. It has been hypothesized that calcium channel blockers may moderate the influx of calcium that occurs following traumatic injuries, thereby reducing secondary excitotoxic damage. Although initial studies using nimodipine were favorable, subsequent studies demonstrated no significant differences when compared with an untreated control group (Wald 1995). The efficacy of other potential strategies (e.g., narcotics, barbiturates, corticosteroids, and *N*-methyl D-aspartate [NMDA] receptor antagonists) has yet to be established in humans.

Finally, as discussed above, approximately 5% of patients with TBI develop posttraumatic seizures. As a result, the use of anticonvulsants as a prophylactic measure has been examined. Although some research suggests that the use of prophylactic anticonvulsants reduces the occurrence of seizures during the first week following head injury, there is no demonstrated effect on reducing seizures after the initial week (Malec and Basford 1996; Schierhout and Roberts 1998; Temkin et al. 1990; Wald 1995).

Pharmacological treatment of neuropsychiatric disorders.

With regard to the neuropsychiatric sequelae of TBI, a number of studies offer suggestions for treatment, as well as avenues for further research. Reviews of the literature (Dubovsky 1992; Silver et al. 1992) (Chapter 34 in this volume) make several general points regarding the pharmacological treatment of younger and older adults with neuropsychiatric symptoms. First, until therapeutic interventions are able to limit the initial brain damage from the traumatic injury, a primary role for medication remains the control of certain target symptoms such as depression, anergia, mania, mood lability, agitation, anxiety, psychosis, and aggression (Silver et al. 1992). Control of such symptoms will have the additional beneficial effect of increasing the patient's capacity to participate in other ongoing therapies, including psychotherapy and cognitive rehabilitation (Silver et al. 1992) (also see Chapters 36 and 39 in this volume).

Second, patients who have experienced TBIs and patients who are elderly may be more sensitive to the effects of many psychotropic medications including heterocyclic antidepressants, monoamine oxidase inhibitors, lithium, antianxiety agents, and neuroleptics (Dubovsky 1992; Silver et al. 1992). As a result, starting with lower doses, titrating medications in smaller increments, and ultimately using lower maintenance doses have been recommended (Dubovsky 1992; Silver et al. 1992). Sedative and anticholinergic side effects are of particular concern (Dubovsky 1992; Silver et al. 1992). Other side effects include the risk of lowering seizure threshold among patients with TBI (Silver et al. 1992) and the risk of cardiovascular changes among elderly patients (Dubovsky 1992). To date, the extent to which the interaction between a TBI and an older brain alters sensitivity to medication is not known.

One example of the process of balancing efficacy with the possible complications associated with pharmacotherapy after brain injury concerns the treatment of depressive and anergic-abulic states. As noted above, one important limiting factor in this type of treatment is the risk of lowering seizure threshold in patients who are already at greater risk for seizures because of their brain injury (Silver et al. 1991, 1992). Tricyclic antidepressants, for example, have been reported to increase the likelihood of seizures after severe brain injuries (Wroblewski et al. 1990), whereas methylphenidate apparently does not (Wroblewski et al. 1992). Therefore, methylphenidate may be a consideration in retarded depressive and apathetic states following brain injury.

Rummans et al. (1999) reviewed the world's literature for controlled blinded treatment trials in neuropsychiatry and identified one study of TBI that met their criteria. In that study, Wroblewski et al. (1996) randomly selected 10 patients with major depression, diagnosed according to DSM-III-R, and recent TBI for a 3-month trial of desipramine (105–300 mg/day) (*n* = 4) or placebo (*n* = 6). Response was defined by a 50% reduction in number of DSM-III-R depression symptoms. All four patients on placebo were blindly crossed over to desipramine after 1 month because of nonresponse. Three of the six patients on desipramine and three of the four patients on placebo crossed over to desipramine responded to the active drug. Two patients receiving desipramine dropped out as a result of adverse effects.

Uncontrolled studies have reported variable findings. Modest improvement in depressive symptoms has been reported among patients with TBI following trials of carbamazepine (Varney et al. 1987) and fluoxetine (Cassidy 1989). In contrast, Dinan and Mobayed (1992) reported improvement in depressive symptoms in only 4 of 13 patients with mild TBI who met DSM-III criteria for depression and who were treated with amitriptyline, compared with 11 of the 13 patients with DSM-III major depression without TBI. Similarly, Saran (1985) found no significant improvement in mood in a sample of 10 patients with mild brain injury who were treated with phenelzine or amitriptyline.

Variability in responsiveness to treatment for depression across studies may be a result of several factors including differences in degree of structural brain changes (Coffey et al. 1989) and differences in diagnostic criteria (Silver et al. 1991). It is also possible that different subtypes of depression exist among this population. For example, Silver et al. (1991) hypothesized that depressive symptoms related to stroke-like focal disruption of neurotransmitter receptors may be more responsive to selective serotonin reuptake inhibitors than those symptoms that may be caused by the release of neurotoxins during more diffuse and severe injuries. Similarly, as discussed above, Jorge et al. (1993b) proposed subtypes of depression based, in part, on the point at which symptoms develop (e.g., early-onset depression was associated with lesion location; delayed-onset depression, with social factors). Until issues relating to diagnostic subtypes have been resolved and effective treatment strategies have been established, the focus of pharmacotherapy for posttraumatic neuropsychiatric disorders among elderly patients will remain the application of conventional treatment strategies for symptom management.

With regard to the cognitive sequelae of TBI, a recent case study (Taverni et al. 1998) of two patients (ages 21 and 46) suggested that donepezil (an acetylcholine-esterase inhibitor approved for use with patients with AD) may be helpful in reducing memory dysfunction following TBI. Figure 28–4 includes three clock drawings from a 79-year-old patient (with a doctoral-level education) who was started on donepezil and placed in a personal care facility after his fourth known TBI in 3 years. In this patient, who also had a history of lacunar infarctions, the addition of donepezil to his previous medication regimen (which included methylphenidate [Ritalin]) resulted in a generalized improvement in the areas of orientation, attention, short-term memory, and visuospatial capacities.

Psychotherapeutic strategies. For most of this century, a brain injury was considered to be an exclusionary criterion for psychotherapy. However, a number of authors have now argued convincingly for the role of psychotherapy following TBI (Burke 1995; Cicerone 1991; Cicerone et al. 1996; Lewis 1991; Lewis et al. 1992; Prigatano 1991a; Prigatano and Klonoff 1990). As with pharmacological strategies, this literature has focused on younger patients and lacks well-controlled studies.

In a review of the literature, Starratt and Fields (1991) suggested that two major themes are consistently emphasized by those conducting psychotherapy with patients with brain injury: 1) maintenance of self-identity and self-esteem in the face of loss and 2) the management of anxiety and affect. Attempts to adjust to the emotional dysregulation and to the cognitive, physical, vocational, and interpersonal losses that often accompany TBI are complicated by factors such as embarrassment, guilt, and premorbid attitudes and beliefs about persons with disabilities. The process of therapy, therefore, includes efforts to help patients understand their changed experience of the world, to facilitate the process of mourning over personal and other losses, and to promote adaptation to different types of existence (Lewis et al. 1992).

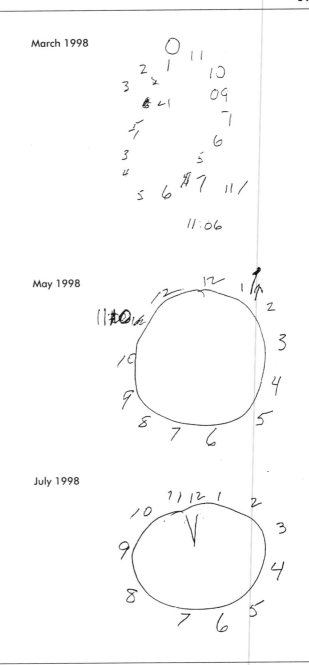

FIGURE 28–4. Serial clock drawings from a 79-year-old patient with four known traumatic brain injuries before (3/98) and after (5/98 and 7/98) starting donepezil and moving to a personal care facility.

Although psychotherapeutic strategies for patients with brain injury range from psychoanalytical to social learning and behavioral, a common denominator has been the need to depart from traditional approaches (Forrest 1992). The importance of this point cannot be overstated, as the demands and process of traditional psychotherapy can make some patients more distressed. Prigatano et al. (1988), for example, warned of increased paranoia among delusional patients with brain injury in "insight-oriented" groups and of behavior modification programs that may be perceived by patients as overly intrusive or controlling.

Based on the degree to which patients with brain injury are able to tolerate individual therapy sessions, the length, frequency, and location of these sessions may need to be modified. Barth and Boll (1981) suggested a number of such modifications. First, the behavior of patients with brain injury should not necessarily be equated with that of other therapy patients. For example, failure to keep an appointment may reflect a cognitive deficit rather than "avoidance."

Second, the type(s) of therapy will differ based on the nature and the severity of the injury. Some patients with significant cognitive and memory deficits may have limited awareness of their deficits (Prigatano 1991b) and may become increasingly distressed when confronted with their impairments (e.g., patients with frontal lobe lesions who demonstrate "catastrophic" reactions during challenging neuropsychological testing). Others may be able to identify their deficits but may not have the executive functioning capacities necessary to deal with them in an insight-oriented manner, and, as a result, they may become overwhelmed by this approach. Psychoeducational approaches are often helpful in providing the context for promoting postinjury adjustment, but all approaches should be tailored to the needs and resources of the individual patient. Insight-oriented, interpersonal, supportive, and cognitive approaches may be useful with patients whose relatively mild injuries have resulted in narcissistic injuries, survival guilt, and adjustment disorders. In contrast, behavioral approaches may be more applicable for patients with significant cognitive impairment who display more severe behavioral disruption.

Third, the timing of the intervention is important. Early in the postinjury period, patients may deny or may be unaware of the existence of neuropsychiatric problems and may resist treatment. Fourth, the pace of therapy may need to be slower with more frequent sessions. Finally, the goals for therapy may be different for patients with brain injury. Rather than seeking a complete resolution of conflicts, more appropriate goals may include increasing tolerance for frustration, improving acceptance of deficits, and establishing contingency plans for daily stressors (Starratt and Fields 1991).

Psychotherapy with older adults who have sustained TBIs is similar to psychotherapy with older adults who have experienced other types of physical or cognitive losses (see Chapter 36 in this volume). Like patients with TBIs, some patients who have had strokes or signs of early dementia are distressed by their losses, whereas others have limited awareness of these changes in functioning. Dealing with issues such as loss, mortality, financial concerns, envi-

ronment change, and unresolved personal and family matters is common among older adults in distress. Among those patients who are less distressed, the focus of intervention is typically on the caregiver who may experience both the burden of caregiving and the loss of emotional support from the injured patient. A number of "barriers" exist that limit the use of mental health services by elderly individuals (Gatz et al. 1985). These barriers include those related to the patients themselves (e.g., lack of psychological sophistication and importance of self-reliance), their therapists (e.g., ageist stereotypes, countertransference issues, and economic considerations), and their environments (e.g., travel and accessibility of location).

Rehabilitation and family considerations. Because of the difficulties inherent in researching the effectiveness of rehabilitation on TBI populations, much controversy and skepticism exist in regard to the benefits of such programs. A number of these criticisms pertain to the lack of a physiological focus, the ambiguity of defining "success," and the difficulty in monitoring the quality of the programs (Cope 1995). However, evidence of the beneficial effects of rehabilitation is increasing (see Chapter 39 in this volume). For example, studies have demonstrated that early (less than 7 days postinjury) rehabilitation in the acute setting resulted in shorter hospital stays and better functional outcomes. Other studies have demonstrated the effectiveness of outpatient and vocational rehabilitation in increasing employment and productivity, while decreasing emotional distress and the need for supervision (Cope 1995; Eames et al. 1995; Malec and Basford 1996).

With regard to elderly patients with TBI, even less is known about the effect of rehabilitation. Although the conventional wisdom is that the elderly will not benefit as much from traditional rehabilitation methods, little research has been conducted in this area. As Malec and Basford (1996) point out, although many studies report a negative association between age and the outcome of rehabilitation, a majority of these studies do not include elderly patients. Therefore, questions still exist as to the benefits of incorporating such treatment into their medical care.

The treatment of patients with TBIs must also take into account the resources of the patient's social support network. Involvement with the family may need to include psychoeducational approaches, stress management, and episodic or prolonged grief therapy. Such involvement also needs to take into account the specific neurobehavioral deficits of the patient. For example, patients whose frontotemporal injuries affect their capacity to tolerate frustration, learn new information, and deal with ambiguity may do better if families provide them with highly structured, predictable, and low-stress environments. In contrast, patients with frontal or right-hemisphere lesions who are anergic and may not perceive, or who misperceive, subtle nuances of verbal and nonverbal communication may do better when family members exaggerate facial expressions and voice quality to increase the likelihood that they are understood accurately. Among elderly patients, intervention strategies such as these become problematic when social support systems are limited in size or capacity (e.g., spouse with dementia).

Summary

The diagnosis and management of the neurobehavioral consequences of TBI is still a relatively new endeavor. In the absence of clear diagnostic criteria and proven treatment algorithms, clinicians will benefit from an approach that is more comprehensive, open, and flexible and less reductionistic. For some patients, like Phineas Gage, changes in behavior can be explained by a specific acquired lesion. For most patients (like the patient who drew the clocks in Figure 28–4), however, diagnosis, and certainly treatment, is more complicated and needs to take into account multiple factors.

▌ Traumatic Brain Injury and Alzheimer's Disease

Findings From Dementia Pugilistica

A potential link between TBI and AD is a logical hypothesis, given the relatively high prevalence of dementia among former boxers who experienced repeated head injuries earlier in life (Corsellis et al. 1973; Roberts 1969; Roberts et al. 1990). Dementia pugilistica (DP), or "punch-drunk" syndrome, can develop late in a boxer's career or several years after retirement. Typically, DP includes parkinsonian-like symptoms such as dysarthria, tremor, ataxia, and bradykinesia as well as general cognitive deterioration and personality change (Roberts 1969). Neuroanatomically, abnormalities of the septum pellucidum, cerebellar scarring, and degeneration of the substantia nigra have been reported (Corsellis et al. 1973). Histopathologically, DP was initially described as including neurofibrillary tangles in the absence of senile neuritic plaques (Corsellis et al. 1973). However, studies (Roberts et al. 1990) have documented that patients with DP have β-amyloid deposits (i.e., plaques) that are comparable to those seen in AD, suggesting that AD and DP may result from similar pathogenetic processes (Allsop et al. 1990; Roberts et al. 1990).

Epidemiological Studies

The question of whether a single significant head injury in adulthood increases the risk of developing dementia in later life has been posed for some time (e.g., Corsellis and Brierly 1959) but has received increased attention over the past two decades, with somewhat conflicting results. In the majority of studies comparing patients with AD with matched elderly control subjects, TBI was found to be significantly more common in the histories of the patients (Graves et al. 1990; Henderson et al. 1992; Heyman et al. 1984; Mayeux et al. 1993a; Mortimer et al. 1985; O'Meara et al. 1997; Rasmusson et al. 1995; Salib and Hillier 1997; Schofield et al. 1997). Despite methodological differences between studies in areas such as how the TBI or "head injury" was defined, the odds ratio (OR), or estimate of relative risk for AD in patients with a history of TBI, was fairly comparable in several studies (e.g., Graves et al. 1990, OR = 3.5; Mayeux et al. 1993a, OR = 3.7; Mortimer et al. 1985, OR = 4.4). Not surprisingly, other studies have reported greater variability in risk for AD (e.g., Van Duijin et al. 1992, OR = 1.6; Rasmusson et al. 1995, OR = 13.75), and a minority of studies did not find a significant association between a history of TBI and AD (Broe et al. 1990; Chandra et al. 1987; Williams et al. 1991). In their meta-analysis of the literature in this area, Mortimer et al. (1991) pooled data from several studies and concluded that a history of TBI with loss of consciousness was significantly more common in patients with AD than it was in control subjects and that it appeared to be more of a risk factor for men than for women and for sporadic cases of AD than for familial cases. More recent studies have supported the conclusions that the association between TBI and AD is stronger 1) in men (O'Meara et al. 1997; Salib and Hillier 1997), 2) when the length of consciousness is longer (Mayeux et al. 1993a; Schofield et al. 1997), 3) when the patient is older (Mayeux et al. 1993a), and 4) when the injury occurred within 5 years of the onset of symptoms of AD (Mayeux et al. 1993a).

The sporadic versus familial genetic question remains an unresolved one. In one study, Rasmusson et al. (1995) found that although a history of TBI was reported in 29% of their cases with AD and in only 3% of their control subjects, the OR was higher for the sporadic cases of AD (25.4) than it was for the familial cases (8.25). Similarly, O'Meara et al. (1997) found an association between TBI and AD among the men in their sample, but no increased risk for AD among their patients who had a specific genotype that increases risk for AD (i.e., apolipoprotien e-4; see below). Dramatically different conclusions were reached by Mayeux et al. (1995) and Tang et al. (1996), who found that a history of TBI was associated with increased risk for AD only in the presence of the specific apolipoprotein E e-4 genotype. Increased risk for AD was not associated with a history of TBI in these studies but was increased 10-fold when there was a history of TBI and at least one e-4 allele. Mayeux et al. (1995) concluded that "the biological effects of head injury may increase the risk of AD, but only through a synergistic relationship with apolipoprotein E-4" (p. 555).

Role of β-Amyloid Deposition in Alzheimer's Disease and Traumatic Brain Injury

Deposition of β-amyloid is one of the central pathological events in the neuronal degeneration that occurs in AD (Hardy 1994; Hardy and Allsop 1991) (see Chapter 24 in this volume). βAP deposits are found at the core of the senile plaques that are common in AD and selected other neurodegenerative disorders, and abnormalities in the processing and deposition of β-amyloid have been linked to increased risk for AD (Hardy 1994). βAP is part of a large transmembrane β-amyloid precursor protein (βAPP) that is encoded by a gene on chromosome 21 (Kang et al. 1987). β-Amyloid originates in the metabolism of βAPP, and soluble βAP accumulates in the brains of patients with AD until it polymerizes into amyloid fibers (Tabaton 1994). Deposition of βAP as the result of this "amyloid cascade" (Hardy and Higgins 1992; Selkoe 1993) produces neuronal degeneration.

The high prevalence of AD and diffuse deposition of βAP in the brains of patients with Down's syndrome (trisomy 21) (Giaccone et al. 1989) and in patients with mutations of the βAPP gene on chromosome 21 (Murrel et al. 1991) provide strong evidence of the critical role that βAPP plays in the development of early-onset AD (Hardy 1994). These findings also provide a genetic model of how the apparently lifelong overexpression and metabolism of the βAPP may cause AD.

An environmental model of how this process occurs has been proposed based on the findings from patients with DP and young adults who die following severe TBIs. As noted above, the findings of β-amyloid deposits in patients with DP (Roberts et al. 1990) suggest a causative role of repeated brain injuries in producing a dementia that resembles AD neuropathologically. Furthermore, in a study of patients of various ages who died following a severe head injury, β-amyloid deposits were found in 30% of the patients and βAPP immunoreactivity was increased in all of the patients examined (Roberts et al. 1991, 1994). Although more common in older adults, βAP deposition in

this study was found in young adults and children as young as 10 years of age. Of relevance to the elderly was the finding that, in addition to increased likelihood of βAP deposition with advancing age, there was an increased likelihood of βAP deposition following an injury sustained in a fall than in any other type of injury.

These findings extended the conclusions based on the patients with DP and suggested that even one significant brain injury can have a significant effect on the process of amyloid deposition and that this process occurs rapidly following brain injury. Although the mechanism by which this process occurs is not yet clear, Roberts et al. (1994) hypothesized that increased expression of βAPP may be part of an acute phase response to neuronal injury in the human brain designed to stabilize damaged synaptic membranes, promote synaptic plasticity, and facilitate repair and regeneration. They suggest further that induction of βAPP in the brain may be a normal, and possibly protective, response to neuronal injury, which, in susceptible individuals, might initiate a disease process.

Role of Apolipoprotein E-4 Allele in Dementia Pugilistica, Alzheimer's Disease, Traumatic Brain Injury, and Cholinergic Function

Another apparently critical component in understanding both amyloid deposition specifically and neuronal repair in general is the now well-documented finding that risk for AD has been linked to a specific allele for apolipoprotein E (ApoE) on chromosome 19 (Saunders et al. 1993; Strittmatter et al. 1993) (see Chapter 24 in this volume). ApoE was previously identified as having a role in cholesterol metabolism and, as a result, related to risk for coronary artery disease and stroke (Mahley 1988). Of relevance to AD, ApoE also has been found to bind with high affinity to β-amyloid in the cerebrospinal fluid and to be present in the senile plaques and tangles that are the hallmark of AD (Saunders et al. 1993). One hypothesis is that ApoE contributes to the risk of AD by mediating amyloid deposition (Rebeck et al. 1993; Schmechel et al. 1993) via genetic variability of the ApoE allele, which has three common variants: e-2, e-3, and e-4. The e-3 allele is most common and accounts for approximately 78% of the ApoE alleles in American and European whites (vs. 15% for the e-4 allele and 7% for the e-2 allele) (Utermann et al. 1980). It now appears that the presence of the e-4 allele increases the risk for AD (Brousseau et al. 1994; Corder et al. 1993; Mayeux et al. 1993b; Myers et al. 1996; Poirier et al. 1993; Saunders et al. 1993; Strittmatter et al. 1993), whereas the presence of the e-2 allele may be protective against AD (Corder et al. 1993;

Myers et al. 1996; Talbot 1994). In one study (Mayeux et al. 1993b), for example, the OR for AD for older adults who were homozygous for the e-4 allele (i.e., two e-4 alleles) was 17.9 and the OR for those who were heterozygous (i.e., one e-4 allele and one other allele) was 4.2 compared with that in older adults with other ApoE alleles.

The role that ApoE plays following nervous system injury is not well understood. Following peripheral nervous system injury, it has been reported that ApoE levels increase 250-fold (Boyles et al. 1990), possibly to increase cholesterol acquisition by the regenerating nerve (Rubinsztein 1995). A similar process has been postulated for central nervous system injury (Mahley 1988) and has received significant support from the animal literature. An animal model of ApoE deficiency was developed via ApoE-targeted genetic disruption and recombination of embryonic stem cells (Thomas and Capecchi 1987). Initial studies of ApoE-deficient mice revealed specific impairments in behavioral (e.g., working memory) and neurochemical (e.g., reduced cortical and hippocampal choline acetyltransferase activity) functioning. Recently, the role of ApoE mediation in neuronal repair following experimentally induced TBI (i.e., via weight drop) was investigated (Chen et al. 1997). In this study, ApoE-deficient and control mice were compared on measures of susceptibility to injury, rate and extent of recovery from injury, degree of cognitive and neurological dysfunction, and histopathological changes in the hippocampus. Overall, the results suggested a clear role for ApoE in mediating neuronal repair and behavioral recovery following TBI. Specifically, although the initial effects of the TBI were equivalent among the two groups, the ApoE-deficient mice displayed: 1) greater cognitive and motor impairment, 2) markedly impaired learning, and 3) greater neuronal death of CA3 hippocampal cells relative to the control mice. The authors concluded that the increased vulnerability for negative consequences following TBI among ApoE-deficient mice appeared to be the result of defects in ApoE-dependent neuronal repair mechanisms.

In humans, a role for ApoE in neuronal repair and remodeling after neuronal injury has been suggested, wherein the apolipoprotein E e-3 genotype is more effective in promoting neuronal repair than is the e-4 genotype (Weisgraber and Mahley 1996). This hypothesis has received support from two recent studies. Jordan et al. (1997) reported an association between ApoE genotype and degree of chronic neurological deficits in boxers. Specifically, while "low-exposure" boxers had less severe neurological deficits regardless of ApoE status, the severity of neurological deficits among "high-exposure" boxers was significantly worse among those with the ApoE e-4 allele. Simi-

larly, Teasdale et al. (1997) found that negative outcome (e.g., death, vegetative state, or severe disability) 6 months following TBI was significantly worse among patients with an ApoE e-4 allele (57%) than among patients without an ApoE e-4 allele (27%). A limitation of this study was that 64% of the ApoE e-4 sample had moderate-to-severe injuries (GCS = 3–12), whereas only 34% of the non-ApoE e-4 sample had moderate-to-severe injuries. The authors pointed out, however, that the association between ApoE status and outcome remained significant even when adjustments were made to control for age, GCS, and CT findings.

Summary

Recent studies have suggested a link between TBI in adulthood and the development of AD in later life. Although more prospective longitudinal studies of this proposed association are needed, the available data are intriguing and provide a conceptual model for considering TBI as one piece of the pathogenetic puzzle of AD. In this model, a TBI at any age (but apparently more so in older men with less capacity for neuronal repair) can set into motion a response that may be protective at the time of the injury but that, for some patients, may lay the foundation for the beginning of AD. More research is needed to determine whether this occurs in a manner in which the TBI per se is an environmental risk factor for AD and therefore is more common in sporadic cases (as suggested by Rasmusson et al. 1995); interacts synergistically with a genetic predisposition (e.g., ApoE e-4), and therefore is more common in genetically vulnerable individuals (as suggested by Mayeux et al. 1993 and Tang et al. 1996), or occurs via some other mechanism. The results of such studies may tell us a great deal about the pathophysiology of both TBI and AD.

▌ Final Summary

Epidemiological studies consistently document that geriatric TBI in the elderly is a relatively common phenomenon with several unique features. Compared to TBI among young adults, the occurrence of geriatric TBI is associated with differences in gender distribution, mechanism of injury, history of TBI, role of alcohol, and severity of injuries. Although older adults are, as a group, more likely to experience negative outcome, not all elderly are at greater risk for negative outcome. Determining the role that age plays in mediating outcome requires an awareness of factors such as preexisting impairment, type of injury, and the severity of other (i.e., nonbrain) injuries.

The neuropsychiatric assessment and treatment of geriatric TBI in the elderly is in its infancy. There is preliminary evidence that the syndrome of geriatric TBI can be distinguished from normal aging and from dementia based on neuropsychological test performance and that neuropsychiatric recovery following TBI may take longer among older adults. The limited data on the neuropsychological effects of TBI in the elderly suggest that these effects are similar to the effects on younger adults following TBI; however, studies on the long-term neuropsychological effects of TBI among older adults do not exist. With regard to neuropsychiatric treatment, until better diagnostic criteria and treatment algorithms are established, clinicians may benefit from following principles such as 1) monitoring for specific age-related problems (e.g., subdural bleeds), 2) monitoring for increased sensitivity to medication side effects, 3) looking for possible altered responsiveness to treatment, 4) reducing seizure threshold, and 5) considering nontraditional pharmacological and psychotherapeutic strategies.

Finally, the proposed link between TBI and AD may lead to a better understanding of the pathogenesis of both TBI and AD. The hypothesis that TBI increases the risk for AD via early deposition of the βAP among individuals with deficient neuronal repair mechanisms is becoming more credible; however, additional work is needed to determine if this or some other hypothesis will provide the most convincing explanation of the available data.

References

Adams JH: The autopsy in fatal non-missile head injuries. Curr Top Pathol 76:1–22, 1988

Adams JH, Mitchell DE, Graham DI, et al: Diffuse brain damage of immediate impact type. Brain 100:489–502, 1977

Adams JH, Graham DI, Murray LS, et al: Diffuse axonal injury due to nonmissile head injury in humans: an analysis of 45 cases. Ann Neurol 12:557–563, 1982

Adams JH, Doyle D, Ford I, et al: Diffuse axonal injury in head injury: definition, diagnosis and grading. Histopathology 15:49–59, 1989

Aharon-Peretz J, Kliot D, Amyel-Zvi E, et al: Neurobehavioural consequences of closed head injury in the elderly. Brain Inj 11:871–875, 1997

Alavi A: Functional and anatomic studies of head injury. J Neuropsychiatry Clin Neurosci 1 (suppl):S45–S50, 1989

Alavi A, Langfitt T, Fazekas F, et al: Correlation studies of head trauma with PET, MRI, and XCT. J Nucl Med 27:919–920, 1986

Alberico AM, Ward JD, Choi SC, et al: Outcome after severe head injury: relationship to mass lesions, diffuse injury, and ICP course in pediatric and adult patients. J Neurosurg 67:648–656, 1987

Alexander MP: Neuropsychiatric correlates of persistent postconcussive syndrome. J Head Trauma Rehabil 7:60–69, 1992

Alexander MP: Mild traumatic brain injury: pathophysiology, natural history, and clinical management. Neurology 45:1253–1260, 1995

Allsop D, Haga S, Bruton C, et al: Neurofibrillary tangles in some cases of dementia pugilistica share antigens with amyloid β-protein of Alzheimer's disease. Am J Pathol 136:255–260, 1990

Amacher AL, Bybee DE: Toleration of head injury by the elderly. Neurosurgery 20:954–958, 1987

American Association for Automotive Medicine: Abbreviated Injury Scale (AIS), 1985 Revision. Arlington Heights, IL, American Association for Automotive Medicine, 1985

American Psychiatric Association: Diagnostic and Statistical Manual of Mental Disorders, 3rd Edition. Washington, DC, American Psychiatric Association, 1980

American Psychiatric Association: Diagnostic and Statistical Manual of Mental Disorders, 4th Edition. Washington, DC, American Psychiatric Association, 1994

Anderson SI, Housley AM, Jones PA, et al: Glasgow Outcome Scale: an inter-rater reliability study. Brain Inj 7:309–317, 1993

Annegers JF, Grabow JD, Kurland LT, et al: The incidence, causes, and secular trend of head trauma in Olmsted County, Minnesota, 1935–1974. Neurology 30:912–919, 1980a

Annegers JF, Grabow JD, Groover RV, et al: Seizures after head trauma: a population study. Neurology 30:683–689, 1980b

Army Individual Test Battery: Manual of Directions and Scoring. Washington, DC, War Department, Adjutant General's Office, 1944

Bachman DL: The diagnosis and management of common neurologic sequelae of closed head injury. J Head Trauma Rehabil 7:50–59, 1992

Baker SP, O'Neil B, Haddon WJ, et al: The injury severity score: a method of describing patients with multiple injuries and evaluating emergency care. J Trauma 14:187–196, 1976

Barth JT, Boll TJ: Rehabilitation and treatment of central nervous system dysfunction: a behavioral medicine perspective, in Medical Psychology: Contributions to Behavioral Medicine. Edited by Prokop CP, Bradley LA. New York, Academic Press, 1981, pp 241–266

Barth JT, Macciocchi SN, Giordani B, et al: Neuropsychological sequelae of minor head injury. Neurosurgery 13:529–533, 1983

Bigler ED: Neuropathology of traumatic brain injury, in Traumatic Brain Injury. Edited by Bigler ED. Austin, TX, Pro-Ed, 1990a, pp 13–49

Bigler ED: Traumatic Brain Injury. Austin, TX, Pro-Ed, 1990b

Bigler ED: Diagnostic Clinical Neuropsychology. Austin, TX, University of Texas Press, 1991

Binder LM: Persisting symptoms after mild head injury: a review of the postconcussive syndrome. J Clin Exp Neuropsychol 8:323–346, 1986

Bohnen N, Jolles J: Neurobehavioral aspects of postconcussive symptoms after mild head injury. J Nerv Ment Dis 180: 683–692, 1992

Bohnen N, Jolles J, Twijnstra A: Neuropsychological deficits in patients with persistent symptoms six months after mild head injury. Neurosurgery 30:692–696, 1992

Bornstein RA, Miller HB, Van Schoor JT: Neuropsychological deficit and emotional disturbance in head-injured patients. J Neurosurg 70:509–513, 1989

Boyles JK, Notterpek LM, Anderson LJ: Accumulation of apolipoproteins in the regenerating and remyelinating mammalian peripheral nerve. J Biol Chem 265: 17805–17815, 1990

Brandt J: The Hopkins Verbal Learning Test: development of a new memory test with six equivalent forms. Clinical Neurologist 5:125–142, 1991

Broderick JP, Brott T, Tomsick T, et al: Intracerebral hemorrhage more than twice as common as subarachnoid hemorrhage. J Neurosurg 78:188–191, 1993

Broe GA, Henderson AS, Creasey H, et al: A case-control study of Alzheimer's disease in Australia. Neurology 40: 1698–1701, 1990

Brousseau T, Legrain S, Berr C, et al: Confirmation of the e4 allele of the apolipoprotein E gene as a risk factor for late-onset Alzheimer's disease. Neurology 44:342–344, 1994

Burke DC: Models of brain injury rehabilitation. Brain Inj 9:735–743, 1995

Busch CR, Alpern HP: Depression after mild traumatic brain injury: a review of current research. Neuropsychol Rev 8:95–108, 1998

Caine ED, Lyness JM, King DA: Reconsidering depression in the elderly. Am J Geriatr Psychiatry 1:4–20, 1993

Carlsson CA, vonEssen C, Lofgren J: Factors affecting the clinical course of patients with severe head injuries. J Neurosurg 29:242–251, 1968

Cartlidge NEF, Shaw DA: Head Injury. London, WB Saunders, 1981

Cassidy JW: Fluoxetine: a new serotonergically active antidepressant. J Head Trauma Rehabil 4:67–69, 1989

Chakares DW, Bryan RN: Acute subarachnoid hemorrhage: in vitro comparison of MRI and CT. AJNR 7:223–228, 1986

Chandra V, Philipose V, Bell PA, et al: Case-control study of late onset "probable Alzheimer's disease." Neurol 37: 1295–1300, 1987

Chen Y, Lomnitoski L, Michaelson DM, et al: Motor and cognitive deficits in apolipoprotein E–deficient mice after closed head injury. Neuroscience 80:1255–1262, 1997

Choi D: Ionic dependence of glutamate neurotoxicity. J Neurosci 7:369–379, 1987

Cicerone KD: Psychotherapy after mild traumatic brain injury: relation to the nature and severity of subjective complaints. J Head Trauma Rehabil 6(4):30–43, 1991

Cicerone KD, Smith LC, Ellmo W, et al: Neuropsychological rehabilitation of mild traumatic brain injury. Brain Inj 10:277–286, 1996

Cifu DX, Kreutzer JS, Marwitz JH, et al: Functional outcomes of older adults with traumatic brain injury: a prospective, multicenter analysis. Arch Phys Med Rehabil 77:883–888, 1996

Cifu DX, Kyser-Marcus L, Lopez E, et al: Acute predictors of successful return to work 1 year after traumatic brain injury: a multicenter analysis. Arch Phys Med Rehabil 78:125–131, 1997

Clifton GL, Kreutzer JS, Choi SC, et al: Relationship between Glasgow Outcome Scale and neuropsychological measures after brain injury. Neurosurgery 33:34–39, 1993

Coffey CE: Cerebral laterality and emotion: the neurology of depression. Compr Psychiatry 28:197–219, 1987

Coffey CE, Figiel GS, Djang WT, et al: Subcortical white matter hyperintensity on magnetic resonance imaging: clinical and neuroanatomic correlates. J Neuropsychiatry Clin Neurosci 1:135–144, 1989

Combes P, Fauvage B, Colonna M, et al: Severe head injuries: an outcome prediction and survival analysis. Intensive Care Med 22:1391–1395, 1996

Cope DN: The effectiveness of traumatic brain injury rehabilitation. Brain Inj 9:649–670, 1995

Cope DN, Date ES, Mar EY: Serial computerized tomographic evaluations in traumatic head injury. Arch Phys Med Rehabil 69:483–486, 1988

Corder EH, Saunders AM, Strittmatter WJ, et al: Gene dose of apolipoprotein E type 4 allele and the risk of Alzheimer's disease in late onset families. Science 261:921–923, 1993

Corsellis JAN, Brierly JB: Observations on the pathology of insidious dementia following head injury. Journal of Mental Science 105:714–724, 1959

Corsellis JAN, Bruton CJ, Freeman-Browne D: The aftermath of boxing. Psychol Med 3:270–273, 1973

Cowen TD, Meythaler JM, DeVivo MJ, et al: Influence of early variables in traumatic brain injury on functional independence measure scores and rehabilitation length of stay and charges. Arch Phys Med Rehabil 76:797–803, 1995

Cullum CM, Bigler ED: Ventricle size, cortical atrophy and the relationship with neuropsychological status in closed head injury: a quantitative analysis. J Clin Exp Neuropsychol 8:437–452, 1986

Cullum CM, Kuck J, Ruff RM: Neuropsychological assessment of traumatic brain injury in adults, in Traumatic Brain Injury. Edited by Bigler ED. Austin, TX, Pro-Ed, 1990, pp 129–163

Cummings JL: Clinical Neuropsychiatry. Orlando, FL, Grune & Stratton, 1985

Cummings JL, Benson DF: Dementia: A Clinical Approach, 2nd Edition. Boston, MA, Butterworths, 1992

Dalmady-Israel C, Zasler ND: Post-traumatic seizures: a critical review. Brain Inj 7:263–273, 1993

Davis CS, Acton P: Treatment of the elderly brain-injured patient: experience in a traumatic brain injury unit. J Am Geriatr Soc 36:225–229, 1988

Delis D, Kramer J, Fridlund A, et al: California Verbal Learning Test. San Antonio, TX, Psychological Corporation, 1986

Desai BT, Whitman S, Coonley-Hoganson R, et al: Urban head injury: a clinical series. J Natl Med Assoc 75:875–881, 1983

Dikmen SS, Temkin N, Armsden G: Neuropsychological recovery: relationship to psychosocial functioning and postconcussional complaints, in Mild Head Injury. Edited by Levin HS, Eisenberg HM, Benton AL. New York, Oxford University Press, 1989, pp 229–241

Dinan TG, Mobayed M: Treatment resistance of depression after head injury: a preliminary study of amitriptyline response. Acta Psychiatr Scand 85:292–294, 1992

Diringer MN, Edwards DF: Does modification of the Innsbruck and the Glasgow Coma Scales improve their ability to predict functional outcome? Arch Neurol 54:606–611, 1997

Dries DJ, Gamelli RL: Issues in geriatric trauma, in Trauma 2000: Strategies for the Millennium. Edited by Gamelli RL, Dries DJ. Austin, TX, RG Landes, 1992, pp 191–197

Dubovsky SL: Psychopharmacological treatment in neuropsychiatry, in American Psychiatric Press Textbook of Neuropsychiatry, 2nd Edition. Edited by Yudofsky SC, Hales RE. Washington, DC, American Psychiatric Press, 1992, pp 663–701

Eames P, Cotterill G, Kneale TA, et al: Outcome of intensive rehabilitation after severe brain injury: a long-term follow-up study. Brain Inj 10:631–650, 1995

Edna TH: Risk factors in traumatic head injury. Acta Neurochir (Wien) 69:15–21, 1983

Edna TH: Head injuries admitted to hospital: epidemiology, risk factors and long-term outcome. Journal of Oslo City Hospitals 37:101–116, 1987

Faden AI: Pharmacological treatment of acute traumatic brain injury. JAMA 276:569–570, 1996

Fann JR, Katon WJ, Uomoto JM, et al: Psychiatric disorders and functional disability in outpatients with traumatic brain injuries. Am J Psychiatry 152:1496–1499, 1995

Federoff JP, Starkstein SE, Forrester AW, et al: Depression in patients with acute traumatic brain injury. Am J Psychiatry 149:918–923, 1992

Feeney DM, Walker AE: The prediction of posttraumatic epilepsy: a mathematical approach. Arch Neurol 36:8–12, 1990

Fields RB: The effects of head injuries on older adults (abstract). Clinical Neuropsychologist 5:252, 1991

Fields RB: Traumatic brain injury in the elderly. Paper presented at the annual meeting of the National Academy of Neuropsychology, Orlando, FL, November 1994

Fields RB: Geriatric head injury, in Handbook of Neuropsychology and Aging. Edited by Nussbaum PD. New York, Plenum, 1997, pp 280–297

Fields RB, Ackerman M: Differential outcome following mild head injury due to age and type of injury. Paper presented at the National Academy of Neuropsychology, Dallas, TX, October 1991

Fields RB, Coffey CE: CT scan predictors of outcome following geriatric head injury (abstract). Archives of Clinical Neuropsychology 9:127, 1994

Fields RB, Taylor C, Starratt GK: Neuropsychiatric complaints following geriatric head injury (abstract). Archives of Clinical Neuropsychology 8:223–224, 1993

Fieschi C, Battistini N, Beduschi A, et al: Regional cerebral blood flow and intraventricular pressure in acute head injuries. J Neurol Neurosurg Psychiatry 37:1378–1388, 1974

Fife D, Faich G, Hollinshead WI, et al: Incidence and outcome of hospital-treated head injury in Rhode Island. Am J Public Health 76:773–778, 1986

Finger S: Recovery From Brain Damage. New York, Plenum, 1978

Fogel BS: Major depression versus organic mood disorder: a questionable distinction. J Clin Psychiatry 51:53–56, 1991

Fogel BS, Duffy J: Elderly patients, in Neuropsychiatry of Traumatic Brain Injury. Edited by Silver JM, Yudofsky SC, Hales RE. Washington, DC, American Psychiatric Press, 1994, pp 412–441

Forrest DV: Psychotherapy of patients with neuropsychiatric disorders, in American Psychiatric Press Textbook of Neuropsychiatry, 2nd Edition. Edited by Yudofsky SC, Hales RE. Washington, DC, American Psychiatric Press, 1992, pp 703–739

Frankowski RF: Descriptive epidemiological studies of head injury in the United States: 1974–1984. Adv Psychosom Med 16:153–172, 1986

Gasparrini WG, Satz P, Heilman KM, et al: Hemispheric asymmetries of affective processing as determined by the Minnesota Multiphasic Personality Inventory. J Neurol Neurosurg Psychiatry 41:470–473, 1978

Gatz M, Popkin SJ, Pino CD, et al: Psychological interventions with older adults, in Handbook of the Psychology of Aging. Edited by Birren JE, Schaie KW. New York, Van Nostrand Reinhold, 1985, pp 755–785

Gennarelli TA: Mechanisms of brain injury. J Emerg Med 11:5–11, 1993

Gentilini M, Nichelli P, Schoenhuber R: Assessment of attention in mild head injury, in Mild Head Injury. Edited by Levin HS, Eisenberg HM, Benton AL. New York, Oxford University Press, 1989, pp 163–175

Giaccone G, Tagliavani F, Linoli G, et al: Down's patients: extracellular preamyloid deposits precede neuritic degeneration and senile plaques. Neurosci Lett 97:232–238, 1989

Goldstein FC, Levin HS: Epidemiology of traumatic brain injury: incidence, clinical characteristics, and risk factors, in Traumatic Brain Injury. Edited by Bigler ED. Austin, TX, Pro-Ed, 1990, pp 51–67

Goldstein FC, Levin HS, Presley RM, et al: Neurobehavioral consequences of closed-head injury in older adults. J Neurol Neurosurg Psychiatry 57:961–966, 1994

Goldstein FC, Levin HS, Roberts VJ, et al: Neuropsychological effects of closed head injury in older adults: a comparison with Alzheimer's disease. Neuropsychology 7:147–154, 1996

Graves AB, White E, Koepsell TD, et al: The association between head trauma and Alzheimer's disease. Am J Epidemiol 131:491–501, 1990

Gronwall D: Cumulative and persisting effects of concussion on attention and cognition, in Mild Head Injury. Edited by Levin HS, Eisenberg HM, Benton AL. New York, Oxford University Press, 1989, pp 153–162

Gronwall D: Minor head injury. Neuropsychology 5:253–265, 1991

Gualtieri CT: Neuropsychiatry and Behavioral Pharmacology. New York, Springer-Verlag, 1991

Gualtieri CT: The problem of mild brain injury. Neuropsychiatry Neuropsychol Behav Neurol 8:127–136, 1995

Gudeman SK, Kishore PR, Becker DP, et al: Computerized tomography in the evaluation of incidence and significance of post-traumatic hydrocephalus. Radiology 141:397–402, 1981

Hamm RJ, Jenkins LW, Lyeth BG, et al: The effect of age on outcome following traumatic brain injury in rats. J Neurosurg 75:916–921, 1991

Hamm RJ, White-Gbadebo DM, Lyeth BG, et al: The effect of age on motor and cognitive deficits after traumatic brain injury in rats. Neurosurgery 31:1072–1078, 1992

Hannay HJ, Levin HS: The Continuous Recognition Memory Test. Houston, TX, Neuropsychological Resources, 1998

Hardy J: Alzheimer's disease: clinical molecular genetics. Alzheimer's Disease Update 10:239–247, 1994

Hardy J, Allsop D: Amyloid deposition as the central event in the aetiology of Alzheimer's disease. Trends Pharmacol Sci 12:383–388, 1991

Hardy JA, Higgins GA: Alzheimer's disease: the amyloid cascade hypothesis. Science 256:184–185, 1992

Harlow JM: Recovery from the passage of an iron bar through the head. Publications of the Massachusetts Medical Society 2:327–347, 1868

Hathaway SR, McKinley JC: Minnesota Multiphasic Personality Inventory, Revised. Minneapolis, MN, University of Minnesota, 1970

Henderson AS, Jorm AF, Kortem BS, et al: Environmental risk factors for Alzheimer's disease: their relationship to age of onset and to familial or sporadic types. Psychol Med 22:429–436, 1992

Hendrick EB, Harris L: Post-traumatic epilepsy in children. J Trauma 8:547–556, 1968

Heyman A, Wilkinson WE, Stafford JA, et al: Alzheimer's disease: a study of epidemiological aspects. Ann Neurol 15:335–341, 1984

Hofer T: Glasgow scale relationships in pediatric and adult patients. J Neurosci Nurs 25:218–227, 1993

Ip RY, Dorman J, Schentag C: Traumatic brain injury: factors predicting return to work or school. Brain Inj 9:517–532, 1995

Jenkins A, Teasdale G, Hadley MDM, et al: Brain lesions detected by magnetic resonance imaging in mild and severe head injuries. Lancet 2:445–446, 1986

Jennett B: Epidemiology of head injury. J Neurol Neurosurg Psychiatry 60:362–369, 1996

Jennett B, Bond MR: Assessment of outcome after severe brain injury: a practical scale. Lancet 1:480–484, 1975

Jennett B, Teasdale G: Management of Head Injuries. Philadelphia, PA, FA Davis, 1981

Jordan BD, Relkin NR, Ravdin LD, et al: Apolipoprotein E e4 associated with chronic traumatic brain injury in boxing. JAMA 278:136–140, 1997

Jorge RE, Robinson RG, Arndt S: Are there symptoms that are specific for depressed mood in patients with traumatic brain injury? J Nerv Ment Dis 181(2):91–99, 1993a

Jorge RE, Robinson RG, Arndt S, et al: Comparison between acute- and delayed-onset depression following traumatic brain injury. J Neuropsychiatry Clin Neurosci 5:43–49, 1993b

Juarez VJ, Lyons M: Interrater reliability of the Glasgow Outcome Scale. J Neurosci Nurs 27:283–286, 1995

Kang J, Lemaire H-G, Unterbeck A, et al: The precursor of Alzheimer's disease amyloid A4 protein resembles a cell-surface receptor. Nature 325:733–736, 1987

Katz DI: Neuropathology and neurobehavioral recovery from closed head injury. J Head Trauma Rehabil 7:1–15, 1992

Katz DI, Kehs GJ, Alexander MP: Prognosis and recovery from traumatic head injury: the influence of advancing age (abstract). Neurology 40 (suppl):276, 1990

Kilaru S, Garb J, Emhoff T, et al: Long-term functional status and mortality of elderly patients with severe closed head injuries. J Trauma 41:957–963, 1996

Kirkpatrick JB, DiMaio V: Civilian gunshot wounds of the brain. J Neurosurg 49:185–198, 1978

Kishore PR, Lipper MH, Miller JD, et al: Post-traumatic hydrocephalus in patients with severe head injuries. Neuroradiology 16:261–265, 1978

Klonoff PS, Lamb DG: Mild head injury, significant impairment on neuropsychological test scores, and psychiatric disability. The Clinical Neuropsychologist 12:31–42, 1998

Knaus WA, Draper EA, Wagner DP, et al: APACHE II: a severity of disease classification system. Crit Care Med 13:818–829, 1985

Kotwica Z, Jakubowski JK: Acute head injuries in the elderly: an analysis of 136 patients. Acta Neurochir (Wien) 118:98–102, 1992

Kraus JF, Nourjah P: The epidemiology of mild, uncomplicated brain injury. J Trauma 28:1637–1643, 1989

Kraus JF, Black MA, Hessol N, et al: The incidence of acute brain injury and serious impairment in a defined population. Am J Epidemiol 119:186–201, 1984

Kraus JF, McArthur DL, Silberman TA: Epidemiology of mild brain injury. Semin Neurol 14:1–7, 1994

Kutner KC, Barth JT: Sports related head injury. National Academy of Neuropsychology Bulletin 14:19–23, 1998

Langfitt TW, Obrist WD, Alavi A, et al: Computerized tomography, magnetic resonance imaging and positron emission tomography in the study of brain trauma. J Neurosurg 64:760–767, 1986

Levin H: Closed head injury in older adults: assessment by the neurobehavioral rating scale. Paper presented at the annual meeting of the International Neuropsychological Society, Seattle, WA, February 1995

Levin HS, Grossman RG, Rose JE, et al: Long-term neuropsychological outcome of closed head injury. J Neurosurg 50:412–422, 1979

Levin HS, Meyers CA, Grossman RG, et al: Ventricular enlargement after closed head injury. Arch Neurol 38:623–629, 1981

Levin HS, Benton AL, Grossman RG: Neurobehavioral Consequences of Closed Head Injury. New York, Oxford University Press, 1982

Levin HS, Handel SF, Goldman AM, et al: Magnetic resonance imaging after "diffuse" nonmissile head injury: a neurobehavioral study. Arch Neurol 42:963–968, 1985

Levin HS, Amparo E, Eisenberg HM, et al: Magnetic resonance imaging and computerized tomography in relation to the neurobehavioral sequelae of mild and moderate head injuries. J Neurosurg 66:706–713, 1987

Levin HS, Gary HE, Eisenberg HM, et al: Neurobehavioral outcome 1 year after severe head injury. J Neurosurg 73:699–709, 1990

Levin HS, Williams DH, Eisenberg HM, et al: Serial MRI and neurobehavioral findings after mild to moderate closed head injury. J Neurol Neurosurg Psychiatry 55:255–262, 1992

Levy DB, Hanlon DP, Townsend RN: Geriatric trauma. Clin Geriatr Med 9:601–620, 1993

Lewis L: A framework for developing a psychotherapy treatment plan with brain-injured patients. J Head Trauma Rehabil 6:22–29, 1991

Lewis L, Athey GI, Eyman J, et al: Psychological treatment of adult psychiatric patients with traumatic frontal lobe injury. J Neuropsychiatry Clin Neurosci 4:323–330, 1992

Lezak MD: Neuropsychological Assessment, 3rd Edition. New York, Oxford University Press, 1995

Luerssen TG, Klauber MR, Marshall LF: Outcome from head injury related to patient's age: a longitudinal prospective study of adult and pediatric head injury. J Neurosurg 68:409–416, 1988

Mahley RW: Apolipoprotein E: cholesterol transport protein with expanding role in cell biology. Science 240:622–630, 1988

Malec JF, Basford JS: Postacute brain injury rehabilitation. Arch Phys Med Rehabil 77:198–207, 1996

Marion DW, Carlier PM: Problems with initial Glasgow Coma Scale assessment caused by prehospital treatment of patients with head injuries: results of a national survey. J Trauma 36:89–95, 1994

Marshall LF, Becker DP, Bowers SA, et al: The national traumatic coma data bank, I: design, purpose, goals, and results. J Neurosurg 59:276–284, 1983

Marshall LF, Marshall SB, Klauber MR, et al: A new classification of head injury based on computerized tomography. J Neurosurg 75 (suppl):S14–S20, 1991

Masson F, Maurette P, Salmi LR, et al: Prevalence of impairments 5 years after a head injury, and their relationship with disabilities and outcome. Brain Inj 10:487–497, 1996

Mattson AJ, Levin HS: Frontal lobe dysfunction following closed head injury. J Nerv Ment Dis 178:282–291, 1990

Mayeux R, Ottman R, Tang M, et al: Genetic susceptibility and head injury as risk factors for Alzheimer's disease among community-dwelling elderly persons and their first-degree relative. Ann Neurol 33:494–501, 1993a

Mayeux R, Stern Y, Ottman R, et al: The apolipoprotein E4 allele in patients with Alzheimer's disease. Ann Neurol 34:752–754, 1993b

Mayeux R, Ottman R, Maestre G, et al: Synergistic effect of traumatic head injury and apolipoprotein-E4 in patients with Alzheimer's disease. Neurology 45:555–557, 1995

Mazaux J-M, Masson F, Levin H, et al: Long-term neuropsychological outcome and loss of social autonomy after traumatic brain injury. Arch Phys Med Rehabil 78:1316–1320, 1997

Mazzucchi A, Cattelani R, Missale G, et al: Head-injured subjects aged over 50 years: correlations between variables of trauma and neuropsychological follow-up. J Neurol 239:256–260, 1992

McIntosh TK, Smith DH, Meaney DF, et al: Neuropathological sequelae of traumatic brain injury: relationship to neurochemical and biomechanical mechanisms. Lab Invest 74:315–342, 1996

Menegazzi JJ, Davis EA, Sucov AN, et al: Reliability of the Glasgow Coma Scale when used by emergency physicians and paramedics. J Trauma 34:46–48, 1993

Merskey H, Woodforde JM: Psychiatric sequelae of minor head injury. Brain 95:521–528, 1972

Miller JD, Pentland B: The factors of age, alcohol, and multiple injury in patients with mild and moderate head injury, in Mild to Moderate Head Injury. Edited by Hoff JT, Anderson TE, Cole TM. Boston, MA, Blackwell Scientific, 1989, pp 125–133

Mortimer JA, French LR, Hutton JT, et al: Head injury as a risk for Alzheimer's disease. Neurology 35:264–267, 1985

Mortimer JA, Van Duijin CM, Chandra VV, et al: Head trauma as a risk factor for Alzheimer's disease: a collaborative reanalysis of case control studies. Int J Epidemiol 20: S28–S35, 1991

Murrel J, Farlow M, Ghetti B, et al: A mutation in the amyloid protein associated with hereditary Alzheimer's disease. Science 254:97–99, 1991

Myers RH, Schaefer EJ, Wilson PWF, et al: Apolipoprotein E e4 association with dementia in a population-based study: the Framingham study. Neurology 46:673–677, 1996

Naugle RI: Epidemiology of traumatic brain injury in adults, in Traumatic Brain Injury. Edited by Bigler Ed. Austin, TX, Pro-Ed, 1990, pp 69–103

Needles DL, Nieto-Sampedro M, Whittemore SR, et al: Neuronotrophic activity for ciliary ganglion neurons: induction following injury to the brain of neonatal, adult, and aged rats. Developmental Brain Research 18:275–284, 1985

Obrist WD, Gennarelli TA, Segawa H, et al: Relation of cerebral blood flow to neurological status and outcome in head-injury patients. J Neurosurg 51:292–300, 1979

Oddy M, Coughlan T, Tyerman A, et al: Social adjustment after closed head injury: a further follow-up seven years after injury. J Neurol Neurosurg Psychiatry 48:564–568, 1985

Olver JH, Ponsford JL, Curran CA: Outcome following traumatic brain injury: a comparison between 2 and 5 years after injury. Brain Inj 10:841–848, 1996

O'Meara ES, Kukull WA, Sheppard L, et al: Head injury and risk of Alzheimer's disease by apolipoprotein E genotype. Am J Epidemiol 146:376–384, 1997

Ommaya AK, Grubb RL Jr, Naumann RA: Coup and contrecoup injury: observations on the mechanics of visible brain injuries in the rhesus monkey. J Neurosurg 35:503–516, 1971

Oster C: Signs of sensory deprivation versus cerebral injury in post-hip fracture patients. J Am Geriatr Soc 25:368–370, 1977

Parker RS: Traumatic Brain Injury and Neuropsychological Impairment. New York, Springer-Verlag, 1990

Parker R, Rosenblum A: IQ loss and emotional dysfunctions after mild head injury in a motor vehicle accident. J Clin Psychol 52:32–43, 1996

Parkinson D, Stephenson S, Phillips S: Head injuries: a prospective, computerized study. Can J Surg 28:79–83, 1985

Pentland B, Jones PA, Roy CW, et al: Head injury in the elderly. Age Aging 15:193–202, 1986

Pieper DR, Valadka AB, Marsch C: Surgical management of patients with severe head injuries. Association of Perioperative Registered Nurses Journal 63:854–864, 1996

Poirier J, Davignon J, Bouthellier D, et al: Apolipoprotein E polymorphism in Alzheimer's disease. Lancet 342: 697–699, 1993

Ponsford JL, Olver JH, Curran C: A profile of outcome: 2 years after traumatic brain injury. Brain Inj 9:1–10, 1995

Povlishock JT, Coburn TH: Morphopathological change associated with mild head injury, in Mild Head Injury. Edited by Levin HS, Eisenberg HM, Benton AL. New York, Oxford University Press, 1989, pp 37–53

Prasad K: The Glasgow Coma Scale: a critical appraisal of its clinometric properties. J Clin Epidemiol 49:755–763, 1996

Prigatano G: Neuropsychological Rehabilitation After Brain Injury. Baltimore, MD, Johns Hopkins University Press, 1986

Prigatano GP: Disordered mind, wounded soul: the emerging role of psychotherapy in rehabilitation after brain injury. J Head Trauma Rehabil 6(4):1–10, 1991a

Prigatano GP: Disturbances of self-awareness of deficit after traumatic brain injury, in Awareness of Deficit After Brain Injury. Edited by Prigatano GP, Schacter DL. New York, Oxford University Press, 1991b, pp 111–126

Prigatano GP: Personality disturbances associated with traumatic brain injury. J Consult Clin Psychol 60:360–368, 1992

Prigatano GP, Klonoff PS: Psychotherapy and neuropsychological assessment after brain injury, in Traumatic Brain Injury. Edited by Bigler ED. Austin, TX, Pro-Ed, 1990, pp 313–330

Prigatano GP, O'Brien KP, Klonoff PS: The clinical management of paranoid delusions in postacute traumatic brain injured patients. J Head Trauma Rehabil 3(3):23–32, 1988

Rakier A, Guilburd JN, Soustiel JF, et al: Head injuries in the elderly. Brain Inj 9:187–193, 1995

Raskin SA, Mateer CA, Tweeten R: Neuropsychological assessment of individuals with mild traumatic brain injury. The Clinical Neuropsychologist 12:21–30, 1998

Rasmusson DX, Brandt J, Martin DB, et al: Head injury as a risk factor in Alzheimer's disease. Brain Inj 9:213–219, 1995

Rebeck GW, Reiter JS, Strickland DK, et al: Apolipoprotein E in sporadic Alzheimer's disease: allelic variation and receptor interactions. Neuron 11:575–580, 1993

Richardson JTE: Clinical and Neuropsychological Aspects of Closed Head Injury. London, Taylor & Francis, 1990

Roberts AJ: Brain Damage in Boxers. London, Pitman, 1969

Roberts GW, Allsop D, Bruton C: The occult aftermath of boxing. J Neurol Neurosurg Psychiatry 53:373–378, 1990

Roberts GW, Gentleman SM, Lynch A, et al: BA4 amyloid protein deposition in brain after head trauma. Lancet 338: 1422–1423, 1991

Roberts GW, Gentleman SM, Lynch A, et al: Beta amyloid protein deposition in the brain after severe head injury: implications for the pathogenesis of Alzheimer's disease. J Neurol Neurosurg Psychiatry 57:419–425, 1994

Rosenthal M, Bond MR, Griffith ER, et al: Rehabilitation of the Adult and Child With Traumatic Brain Injury. Philadelphia, PA, FA Davis, 1990

Ross AM, Pitts LH, Kobayashi S: Prognosticators of outcome after major head injury in the elderly. J Neurosci Nurs 24:88–93, 1992

Ross ED, Rush MD: Diagnosis and neuroanatomical correlates of depression in brain-damaged patients. Arch Gen Psychiatry 38:1344–1354, 1981

Roy CW, Pentland B, Miller JD: The causes and consequences of minor head injury in the elderly. Injury 17:220–223, 1986

Rubinsztein DC: Apolipoprotein E: a review of its roles in lipoprotein metabolism, neuronal growth and repair and as a risk factor for Alzheimer's disease. Psychol Med 25:223–229, 1995

Ruff RM, Buchsbaum MS, Troster AI, et al: Computerized tomography, neuropsychology, and positron emission tomography in the evaluation of head injury. Neuropsychiatry Neuropsychol Behav Neurol 2:103–123, 1989a

Ruff RM, Levin HS, Mattis S, et al: Recovery of memory after mild head injury: a three center study, in Mild Head Injury. Edited by Levin HS, Eisenberg HM, Benton AL. New York, Oxford University Press, 1989b, pp 176–188

Ruff RM, Marshall LF, Klauber MR, et al: Alcohol abuse and neurological outcome of the severely head injured. J Head Trauma Rehabil 5(3):21–31, 1990

Ruff RM, Marshall LF, Crouch J, et al: Predictors of outcome following severe head trauma: follow-up data from the traumatic coma data bank. Brain Inj 7:101–111, 1993

Rummans TA, Lauterbach E, Coffey CE, et al: Pharmacologic efficacy in neuropsychiatry: a review of placebo-controlled treatment trials. J Neuropsychiatry Clin Neurosci 11:176–189, 1998

Russell WR, Smith A: Post-traumatic amnesia in closed head injury. Arch Neurol 5:4–17, 1961

Rutherford WH: Post-concussion symptoms: relationship to acute neurological indices, individual differences, and circumstances of injury, in Mild Head Injury. Edited by Levin HS, Eisenberg HM, Benton AL. New York, Oxford University Press, 1989, pp 217–228

Salib E, Hillier V: Head injury and the risk of Alzheimer's disease: a case control study. Int J Geriatr Psychiatry 12:363–368, 1997

Saran AS: Depression after minor closed head injury: role of dexamethasone suppression test and antidepressants. J Clin Psychiatry 46:335–338, 1985

Saunders AM, Strittmatter WJ, Schmechel D, et al: Association of apolipoprotein E allele (e4) with late onset familial and sporadic Alzheimer's disease. Neurology 43:1467–1472, 1993

Schierhout G, Roberts I: Prophylactic antiepileptic agents after head injury: a systematic review. J Neurol Neurosurg Psychiatry 64:108–112, 1998

Schmechel DE, Saunders AM, Strittmatter WJ, et al: Increased amyloid β-peptide deposition in cerebral cortex as a consequence of apolipoprotein E genotype in late-onset Alzheimer disease. Proc Natl Acad Sci U S A 90:9649–9653, 1993

Schofield PW, Tang M, Marder K, et al: Alzheimer's disease after remote head injury: an incidence study. J Neurol Neurosurg Psychiatry 62:119–124, 1997

Sekino H, Nakamura N, Yuki K, et al: Brain lesions detected by CT scans in cases of minor head injury. Neurologica Medica Chirurgica 21:677–683, 1981

Selkoe DJ: Physiological production of the amyloid β-amyloid protein and the mechanism of Alzheimer's disease. Trends Neurosci 16:403–409, 1993

Silver JM, Yudofsky SC, Hales RE: Neuropsychiatric aspects of traumatic brain injury, in American Psychiatric Press Textbook of Neuropsychiatry. Edited by Hales RE, Yudofsky SC. Washington, DC, American Psychiatric Press, 1987, pp 179–190

Silver JM, Yudofsky SC, Hales RE: Depression in traumatic brain injury. Neuropsychiatry Neuropsychol Behav Neurol 4:12–23, 1991

Silver JM, Hales RE, Yudofsky SC: Neuropsychiatric aspects of traumatic brain injury, in American Psychiatric Press Textbook of Neuropsychiatry, 2nd Edition. Edited by Yudofsky SC, Hales RE. Washington, DC, American Psychiatric Press, 1992, pp 363–395

Sims ACP: Head injury, neurosis and accident proneness. Adv Psychosom Med 13:49–70, 1985

Sorenson SB, Kraus JF: Occurrence, severity, and outcomes of brain injury. J Head Trauma Rehabil 6(2):1–10, 1991

Sosin DM, Sacks JJ, Smith SM: Head injury associated deaths in the United States from 1979 to 1986. JAMA 262:2251–2255, 1989

Starmark JE, Stalhammar D, Holmgren E, et al: A comparison of the Glasgow Coma Scale and the Reaction Level Scale (RLS85). J Neurosurg 69:699–706, 1988

Starratt C, Fields R: Psychotherapy following brain injury. Allegheny General Hospital Neuroscience Journal 2(3):32–36, 1991

Steadman J, Graham J: Rehabilitation of the brain injured. Proceedings of the Royal Society of Medicine 63:23–27, 1970

Strittmatter WJ, Saunders AM, Smechel D, et al: Apolipoprotein E: high avidity binding to β-amyloid and increased frequency of type 4 allele in late-onset familial Alzheimer's disease. Proc Natl Acad Sci U S A 90:1977–1981, 1993

Tabaton M: Research advances in the biology of Alzheimer's disease. Alzheimer's Disease Update 10:249–255, 1994

Talbot C, Lendon C, Craddock N, et al: Protection against Alzheimer's disease with apoE-e2. Lancet 343:1432–1433, 1994

Tang M-X, Maestre G, Tsai W-Y, et al: Effect of age, ethnicity, and head injury on the association between ApoE genotypes and Alzheimer's disease. Ann N Y Acad Sci 802:6–15, 1996

Taverni JP, Seliger G, Lichtman SW: Donepezil mediated memory improvement in traumatic brain injury during post acute rehabilitation. Brain Inj 12:77–80, 1998

Taylor CA, Fields RB, Starratt G, et al: Neuropsychiatric complaints following traumatic injury: patients with head vs. non-head injuries (abstract). J Neuropsychiatry Clin Neurosci 5:450, 1993

Teasdale GM: Head injury. J Neurol Neurosurg Psychiatry 58:526–539, 1995

Teasdale G, Jennett B: Assessment of coma and impaired consciousness: a practical scale. Lancet 2:81–84, 1974

Teasdale GM, Nicoll JAR, Murray G, et al: Association of apolipoprotein E polymorphism with outcome after head injury. Lancet 350:1069–1071, 1997

Temkin NR, Dikmen SS, Wilensky AJ, et al: A randomized, double-blind study of phenytoin for the prevention of post-traumatic seizures. N Engl J Med 323:497–502, 1990

Tennant A, Macdermott N, Neary D: The long-term outcome of head injury: implications for service planning. Brain Inj 9:595–605, 1995

Thomas KR, Capecchi MR: Site-directed mutagenesis by gene targeting in mouse embryo-derived stem cells. Cell 51:503–512, 1987

Utermann G, Langenbeck U, Beisiegel U, et al: Genetics of the apolipoprotein E system in man. Am J Hum Genet 32:339–347, 1980

Van Duijin CM, Tanja TA, Haaxma R, et al: Head trauma and the risk of Alzheimer's disease. Am J Epidemiol 135:775–781, 1992

Varney NR, Martzke JS, Roberts RJ: Major depression in patients with closed head injury. Neuropsychology 1:7–9, 1987

Vollmer DG, Torner JC, Jane JA, et al: Age and outcome following traumatic coma: why do older patients fare worse? J Neurosurg 75 (suppl):S37–S49, 1991

Wagner D, Draper E, Knaus W, et al: APACHE III study design: development of APACHE III. Crit Care Med 17:S199–S203, 1989

Wald SL: Advances in the early management of patients with head injury. Horizons in Trauma Surgery 75:225–242, 1995

Weisgraber KH, Mahley RW: Human apolipoprotein E: the Alzheimer's disease connection. FASEB J 10:1485–1494, 1996

Wechsler D: Weschler Adult Intelligence Scale—Revised. San Antonio, TX, Psychological Corporation, 1981

Wechsler D: The Weschler Memory Scale, Revised Manual. San Antonio, TX, Psychological Corporation, 1987

Whittemore SR, Nieto-Sampedro M, Needles DL, et al: Neuronotrophic factors for mammalian brain neurons: injury induction in neonatal, adult, and aged rat brain. Developmental Brain Research 20:169–178, 1985

Williams DB, Annegers JF, Kokmen E, et al: Brain injury and neurologic sequelae: a cohort study of dementia, parkinsonism and amyotrophic lateral sclerosis. Neurology 41:1554–1557, 1991

Wilson JTL, Wiedman KD, Hadley DM, et al: Early and late magnetic resonance imaging and neuropsychological outcome after head injury. J Neurol Neurosurg Psychiatry 51:391–396, 1988

Wing JK, Cooper JE, Sartorius N: The Measurement and Classification of Psychiatric Symptoms. New York, Cambridge University Press, 1974

Wood RL: Neurobehavioral Sequelae of Traumatic Brain Injury. New York, Taylor & Francis, 1990

World Health Organization: Schedules for Clinical Assessment in Neuropsychiatry. Geneva, World Health Organization, 1992

Wroblewski BA, McColgan K, Smith K, et al: The incidence of seizures during tricyclic antidepressant drug treatment in a brain-injured population. J Clin Psychopharmacol 10:124–128, 1990

Wroblewski BA, Leary JM, Phelan AM, et al: Methylphenidate and seizure frequency in brain injured patients with seizure disorders. J Clin Psychiatry 53(3):86–89, 1992

Wroblewski BA, Joseph AB, Cornblatt RR: Antidepressant pharmacotherapy and the treatment of depression in patients with severe traumatic brain injury: a controlled, prospective study. J Clin Psychiatry 57:582–587, 1996

Yoshino MT, Seeger JF: CT still exam of choice in closed head trauma. Diagnostic Imaging 11:88–92, 1989

Young L, Fields RB, Lovell M: Neuropsychological differentiation of geriatric head injury from dementia (abstract). J Neuropsychiatry Clin Neurosci 7:414, 1995

Youngjohn JR, Burrows L, Erdal K: Brain damage or compensation neurosis? the controversial post-concussion syndrome. The Clinical Neuropsychologist 9:112–123, 1995

Zafonte RD, Hammond FM, Mann NR, et al: Relationship between Glasgow Coma Scale and functional outcome. Am J Phys Med Rehabil 13:364–369, 1996

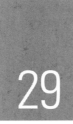

Epilepsy

Mario F. Mendez, M.D., Ph.D.

Epilepsy is associated with a variety of behavioral conditions that may be especially severe in elderly patients (Table 29–1). Seizure disorders can have psychosocial consequences, neuropsychological effects, seizure-related behavioral manifestations, and medication-induced behavioral changes. Moreover, throughout much of recorded history, patients with epilepsy have been considered to be prone to psychopathology during their seizure-free periods (Kraepelin 1923). In modern times, the belief in a universal epileptic predisposition to psychopathology has declined in favor of a specific predisposition of patients with temporal lobe epilepsy (TLE) to psychosis, depression, and other psychopathology (Gibbs et al. 1948). Although not systematically studied in the elderly population, this psychopathology can persist in later years. In this chapter, I explore the behavioral aspects of epilepsy that might affect elderly patients and conclude with a discussion of management issues.

▌ Demography and Definitions

Seizures result from abnormal neuronal discharges in the brain. They are sudden, involuntary behavioral events caused by excessive or hypersynchronous electrical discharges, often from hyperexcitable neurons. Seizures can be primary, secondary to a brain lesion, or symptomatic from acute, situational conditions such as sleep deprivation or drug withdrawal. The term *epilepsy* refers specifically to recurrent unprovoked seizures and includes primary and secondary epileptic seizures, but excludes symptomatic ones. The International Classification of Epileptic Seizures (Commission on Classification and Terminology of the International League Against Epilepsy 1981) further divides epileptic seizures into generalized (characterized by an initial widespread bihemispheric involvement) and partial (characterized by an initial focal onset in part of one hemisphere) (Table 29–2).

Epilepsy is a common neurological disorder. It affects up to 2 million people in the United States, has prevalence rates of 5–8 per 1,000, and has an overall annual incidence of about 30–50/100,000 person-years (Annegers 1997). The incidence of new-onset epilepsy is highest in the first year, drops to a minimum in individuals in their 30s through 50s, and increases again in those over age 60 to an annual incidence of 77–92/100,000 (Annegers 1997; Hauser 1992). Although two-thirds of epilepsy in young adults is idiopathic, more than half of elderly patients with epilepsy have a known cause (Hauser 1992). In those over age 65, about one-third have a cerebrovascular etiology for their seizures, approximately 10%–15% have brain tu-

TABLE 29–1. Behavioral disorders in epilepsy

Psychosocial

Low self-esteem, dependency, helplessness

Fear of loss of control

Stigmatization

Loss of independence

Associated marital, job, transportation, and related problems

Neuropsychological

From seizures

From underlying lesions/disease

From antiepileptic drugs (AEDs)

Ictally related

Prodromal symptoms: dysphoria, apprehension, etc.

Ictal automatisms and psychic symptoms

Nonconvulsive status: simple partial seizures, complex partial seizures, absence, and periodic lateralizing epileptiform discharges

Postictal confusion and other postictal behaviors

Ictal/postictal intermixed behaviors: twilight states, etc.

Psychotic episodes related to the ictus

Interictal

Chronic schizophrenic psychosis

Depression

Suicide

"Heightened significance" and other personality changes

Miscellaneous: hyposexuality, aggression, dissociative states, etc.

TABLE 29–2. The International Classification of Epileptic Seizures

I. Partial (focal, local) seizures

   A. Simple partial seizures (SPSs)

      Motor, somatosensory, autonomic, or psychic symptoms

   B. Complex partial seizures (CPSs)

      1. Begin with symptoms of simple partial seizure but progress to impairment of consciousness

      2. Begin with impairment of consciousness

   C. Partial seizures with secondary generalization

      1. Begin with simple partial seizure

      2. Begin with complex partial seizure (including those with symptoms of simple partial seizures at onset)

II. Generalized seizures (convulsive or nonconvulsive)

   A. Absence (typical and atypical)

   B. Myoclonus

   C. Clonic

   D. Tonic

   E. Tonic-clonic (GTCSs)

   F. Atonic/akinetic

III. Unclassified

Source. Adapted from Commission on Classification and Terminology of the International League Against Epilepsy 1981.

---

mors, and up to 23% have infections, trauma, or other secondary lesions (Luhdorf et al. 1986; Sanders and Murray 1991). Furthermore, in a study of elderly people with unexplained seizures, small vascular changes occurred more commonly in those with epilepsy than in nonepileptic control subjects (Shorvon et al. 1984).

■ Clinical Aspects of Epilepsy

In adults, the three most common types of seizures are 1) generalized tonic-clonic seizures (GTCSs), with convulsions (also known as *grand mal seizures*); 2) complex partial seizures (CPSs), with an alteration of consciousness; and 3) simple partial seizures (SPSs), with isolated motor, somatosensory, autonomic, or psychic symptoms (Table 29–2). SPSs that evolve to CPSs are considered *auras*, and CPSs that evolve to GTCSs are *secondarily generalized.* Al-

though about one-third of all patients with epilepsy have CPSs, about one-half of elderly patients with epilepsy have CPSs, reflecting the increased specific focal causes of their epilepsy (Hauser 1992). On electroencephalography (EEG), these seizure disorders may have interictal spikes and other markers of abnormal electrical activity, most commonly emanating from a temporal lobe. In addition, variants of childhood absence (*petit mal*) seizures, which result in brief lapses of consciousness, occur occasionally in elderly patients.

The evaluation of new-onset seizures in the elderly includes the identification of cerebrovascular, neoplastic, and other acquired neuropathology; the exclusion of acute, symptomatic seizures; and the characterization of any epileptiform discharges. These patients need neuroimaging of the brain, preferably magnetic resonance imaging with its superior resolution for most parenchymal lesions. Routine X-ray and laboratory studies help exclude the presence of symptomatic seizures. In addition, a lumbar puncture is indicated in the presence of a persistent alteration of consciousness, especially if accompanied by fever and meningeal signs. EEGs are more likely to define the type of epileptiform changes if the patient attains drowsiness or sleep during the tracing. However, computerized EEG techniques, which may help in mapping a structural lesion, are not very useful for evaluating these discharges.

Epileptic seizures must be differentiated from syncope and from nonepileptic seizures. Patients with brief lapses of consciousness but without typical ictal features or postictal confusion usually have syncope from a cardiovascular, toxic-metabolic, or cerebrovascular cause; however, these lapses could be atypical seizures, particularly if they are of frontal lobe origin. Some elderly patients may have syncope-like ictal events such as brief periods of amnesia or falling episodes (Godfrey 1989). Nonepileptic seizures, or pseudoseizures, are the most frequent conversion reaction among patients with seizures. Patients with nonepileptic seizures are most commonly young women with psychological stressors and poor coping skills, but nonepileptic seizures may occur in elderly patients. Nonepileptic seizures are characterized by a sudden collapse or by motor activity that does not fit a typical CPS or GTCS, ictal durations of two or more minutes, occurrence in the presence of a witness, possible induction with injections or suggestion, poor responsiveness to antiepileptic drugs (AEDs), and lack of a seizure-induced rise in serum prolactin levels (Kuyk et al. 1997; Lesser 1996).

The neuropsychiatric aspects of epilepsy include four categories: psychosocial, neuropsychological, ictally related behavioral alterations, and interictal psychopathology (Table 29–1). Psychosocial aspects are those directly the result of the stress of having a seizure disorder, and neuropsychological aspects refer to persistent disturbances in cognitive abilities. Temporary behavior changes also occur either before, during, or after a seizure as a direct result of ictal or seizure discharges. A final group of behaviors manifest as sustained psychopathology during the interictal or seizure-free period. Although these categories overlap and some behaviors are eventually reclassified as underlying mechanisms are identified, these categories are useful for discussing the neuropsychiatric aspects of epilepsy (D. B. Smith et al. 1991).

Psychosocial Impact of Seizures

The presence of a seizure disorder in later life has important psychosocial implications (Table 29–1). Epilepsy is associated with low self-esteem, a sense of decreased control and self-efficacy, and the perception of being stigmatized (Collings 1994; Tedman et al. 1995). Patients with epilepsy are subject to low self-esteem particularly arising from the greater dependency that the disorder engenders.

Self-esteem problems can be greater in elderly individuals, who already may be heavily reliant on family and others. The possibility of having a seizure at any time results in feelings of loss of control (Hermann and Wyler 1989). Elderly subjects tend to be cautious and conservative, and the potential for public loss of control can be particularly distressing. In addition to an overall increased sense of vulnerability is a very real fear of falling and sustaining incapacitating hip fractures or other trauma. There also is continued stigmatization from the disorder, and people often misunderstand and fear those with epilepsy. This can lead to housing problems; some nursing homes do not accept elderly patients with seizures.

The independence of elderly patients may already be impaired or tenuous, and epilepsy further narrows their ability to function independently (Luhdorf et al. 1986). Seizures may critically compromise the function of the elderly individuals who are still able to keep a job, provide their own transportation, maintain their economic status, and perform other independent activities. Although seizures by themselves rarely result in institutionalization, in an already impaired elder, seizures may be the final condition that terminates independent living. In addition, given the higher frequency of secondary epilepsy in the elderly, older patients are often already disabled from underlying neurological disorders such as stroke or dementia.

Neuropsychological Impact of Seizures

Neuropsychological functions are vulnerable to the effects of seizures. Prolonged seizures can result in metabolic and direct electrical injury to the brain. By age 70, significant loss of neuronal tissue has occurred, as well as a decline in cognitive efficiency, particularly on time-dependent tasks and in memory retrieval (Botwinick 1981). With this decreased neuronal reserve, elderly patients have a greater neuropsychological decline from neuronal damage as a result of ongoing seizure activity than do younger patients. For this reason alone, seizure duration and rate of recurrence of seizures are important clinical variables in the elderly.

In older patients with secondary epilepsy, seizures are often associated with disorders that impair cognition. Seizures can temporarily exacerbate stroke- or tumor-related deficits such as aphasias (Godfrey 1989). Furthermore, seizures occur in dementing disorders including Alzheimer's disease, vascular dementia, frontotemporal dementia, and other neurodegenerative disorders (McAreavey et al.

1992). Alzheimer's disease, the most prevalent dementia, may have seizures (usually GTCSs) in 10%–20% of patients, particularly late in the course (Mendez et al. 1994; Romanelli et al. 1990).

Although most seizures can be controlled with AEDs, these medications have potential neuropsychological side effects. Elderly patients have a slowed elimination of these drugs, require lower doses, are often on multiple interacting medications, and are, therefore, more likely to experience AED toxicity (Leppik 1992). With the already significant susceptibility to confusional states of the aged brain, the addition of AEDs greatly adds to the possibility of drug-induced delirium. Even at therapeutic levels, some drugs can cause specific problems. For example, barbiturates may need discontinuation because of drug-induced depression, suicidal ideation, sedation, psychomotor slowing, and paradoxical hyperactivity. The added susceptibility for AED-induced toxicity in elderly patients indicates the need for closer monitoring, especially of AED serum levels such as free phenytoin or carbamazepine epoxide levels, renal and liver function test values, and AED-induced hyponatremia.

▌ Ictally Related Behavioral Alterations

Ictally related behavioral alterations occur immediately before, during, and soon after seizures (Table 29–1). First, a prodrome of dysphoria, insomnia, anxiety, or buildup of tension may precede seizures or be relieved by them. Second, ictal discharges can produce both reactive automatisms involving semipurposeful activity and psychic manifestations producing affective, cognitive, language, memory, and perceptual changes. Examples of automatisms include ictal laughter from left-hemisphere discharges and ictal crying from right-hemisphere discharges (Dark et al. 1996). Examples of psychic manifestations include affective changes such as ictal fear and depression and cognitive changes such as derealization and depersonalization. Even a recurrent, uninvited thought can be a seizure manifestation (Mendez et al. 1996a). Moreover, prolonged alterations of responsiveness may result from nonconvulsive status epilepticus or from recurrent electrical discharges with EEG complexes known as *periodic lateralizing epileptiform discharges* (PLEDs) (Engel et al. 1978). Third, the postictal period includes a confusional state lasting minutes to hours or, occasionally, days. The postictal period can be particularly prolonged in elderly patients, who may take longer to recover from the disruption of seizures (Godfrey 1989). Although semidirected ictally related aggression is extremely rare, nondirected de-

structive behavior frequently occurs during the postictal confusional state as a response to attempts at restraint (Treiman 1991). Finally, occasional protracted periods with intermixed ictal and postictal changes can produce twilight states; compulsive wandering, or poriomania; an agitated state; and depressive delirium (Betts 1981).

One final class of ictally related behavioral manifestations is comprised of brief psychotic episodes, which usually follow a flurry of seizures, but may occasionally alternate with seizures (Devinsky et al. 1995; Kanemoto et al. 1996; Sachdev 1998). These episodes involve days to weeks of agitated, hallucinatory, paranoid, and impulsive behaviors often with sudden mood swings and suicide attempts. Most patients develop their psychotic episodes 12–48 hours after a flurry of seizures and may occasionally continue to display psychotic symptoms for an extended period of time. Another group develops psychotic episodes after seizures are controlled, and this "alternating psychosis" promptly resolves once the seizures recur (Pakalnis et al. 1987). *Forced* (or *paradoxical*) *normalization* refers to this subgroup with an antagonism between psychotic episodes and the seizures or EEG discharges (Landolt 1958).

▌ Interictal Psychopathology

Patients with epilepsy are susceptible to psychopathology during the seizure-free periods (Table 29–1). These behavioral disorders usually occur in patients with long-standing, incompletely controlled seizures, and, although not specifically studied in the elderly, these disorders can occur in older patients. Community epidemiological studies have shown a high prevalence of interictal psychiatric problems among patients with epilepsy (Gudmundsson 1966; Pond and Bidwell 1959/1960). The percentage of patients with epilepsy in psychiatric hospitals has ranged from 5% to 10%, significantly higher than the prevalence of epilepsy in the general population (Betts 1981; Mendez et al. 1986). Of patients attending epilepsy clinics, about 30% have had a prior psychiatric hospitalization (Stevens 1975), and about 18% were on at least one psychotropic drug (Wilensky et al. 1981). Studies report more psychopathology among patients with epilepsy than among control subjects with other neurological disorders (Mendez et al. 1993a, 1993d). Moreover, patients with epilepsy with CPSs of temporolimbic origin, particularly in the presence of psychic auras, may have a greater predisposition to psychopathology than other patients with epilepsy (Mendez et al. 1996b). In summary, although most patients with epilepsy do not have psychiatric disease, about one-quarter of patients with epilepsy, particularly those with long-standing CPSs and auras, have interictal psychosis, depression, suicidality, hyposexuality, and other psychopathology.

Interictal Psychosis

The best-known psychiatric disorder in epilepsy is the chronic "schizophreniform" psychosis (Sachdev 1998; Trimble 1991). The influential study by Slater and Beard (1963) reported 69 patients with both epilepsy and an interictal schizophrenic disorder and concluded that these two disorders occurred together more frequently than expected by chance. Although some investigators have interpreted this association as reflecting selective sampling (Stevens 1991), most subsequent studies indicate that 7%–12% of patients with epilepsy develop a psychotic disorder, usually a chronic, interictal schizophrenic illness (Trimble 1991). For example, in a controlled investigation of 1,611 outpatients with epilepsy, interictal schizophrenic disorders were 9–10 times more common among patients with epilepsy than among control subjects with other neurological disorders (Mendez et al. 1993d). Moreover, on the Minnesota Multiphasic Personality Inventory (MMPI), patients with epilepsy had more elevated schizophrenia and paranoia scale scores than did patients with other neurological disabilities (Dikmen et al. 1983).

The schizophrenic disorder may be especially associated with CPSs. One study found psychosis in 12% of 1,675 patients with CPSs of TLE origin, especially those with left-sided foci, compared with less than 1% of 6,671 patients with generalized epilepsy (Gibbs 1951), and a psychotic illness occurred in 9 (10%) of 87 children with TLE epilepsy followed for up to 30 years (Lindsay et al. 1979). In conclusion, patients with epilepsy have a severalfold greater risk for a chronic schizophrenic illness than does the general population, and the risk is particularly high for patients with CPSs, regardless of age.

Unlike ictally related psychotic episodes, the chronic interictal schizophrenic disorder has no direct relationship to individual seizures (Mendez et al. 1993d; Trimble 1991). Although the exact relationship of seizure activity and schizophrenia is debated (Sachdev 1998), these patients often have an 11- to 15-year history of poorly controlled seizures (Slater and Beard 1963). Furthermore, the schizophrenic symptoms commonly increase with increased CPS activity or with AED withdrawal (Mendez et al. 1993d) (Figure 29–1). Although removal of the seizure focus does not prevent the development of psychosis (Manchanda et al. 1996), left temporal mediobasal lesions are particularly associated with this psychotic disorder (Sherwin et al. 1982).

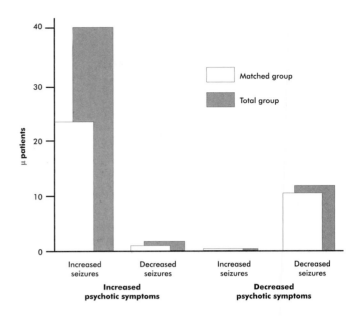

FIGURE 29–1. Correspondence of psychotic symptoms to seizure frequency. *Increased psychotic symptoms:* Total schizophrenic epilepsy group ($n = 149$): increased seizures in 42 and decreased seizures in 2 ($\chi^2 = 40.56$, df = 1, $P < .001$). Matched schizophrenic epilepsy group ($n = 62$): increased seizures in 24 and decreased seizures in 1 ($\chi^2 = 24.25$, df = 1, $P < .001$). *Decreased psychotic symptoms:* Total group: increased seizures in 9 and decreased seizures in 0 ($\chi^2 = 7.33$, df = 1, $P < .007$). Matched group: increased seizures in 8 and decreased seizures in 0 ($\chi^2 = 6.55$, df = 1, $P < .011$).
Source. Reprinted with permission from Mendez MF, Grau R, Doss RC, et al.: "Schizophrenia in Epilepsy: Seizure and Psychosis Variables." *Neurology* 43:1073–1077, 1993d.

The schizophrenic disorder resembles an episodic schizoaffective psychosis with prominent paranoia, positive symptoms, relatively preserved affect, and normal premorbid personality (Perez and Trimble 1980; Slater and Beard 1963; Trimble 1991). Compared with idiopathic schizophrenia, there may be more hallucinations and religiosity and less social withdrawal, systematized delusions, schneiderian first-rank symptoms, and family history of schizophrenia. However, these features are not clearly atypical or unique, and most schizophrenic syndromes in epilepsy can correspond to typical schizophrenic disorder categories (Mendez et al. 1993d).

Depression

Less well-known than the interictal psychosis is the problem of depression in epilepsy. Depression is undoubtedly a frequent neuropsychiatric disturbance in older patients with seizures. Depression occurs in up to 75% of patients in mixed epilepsy groups (Standage and Fenton 1975), and there are elevations in depressive traits in patients with epilepsy compared with those in control subjects (Robertson 1991). Depression is also the main reason for the psychiatric hospitalization of patients with epilepsy (Betts 1981; Mendez et al. 1986). Furthermore, most investigations report a twofold greater frequency of interictal depression among patients with seizures than among comparably disabled individuals (Kogeorgos et al. 1982; Mendez et al. 1986; Rodin and Schmaltz 1984; Standage and Fenton 1975). Depression is particularly prevalent among those with CPSs and ranges from 19% to 65% among patients with CPSs (Currie et al. 1971; Dongier 1959/1960; Roy 1979; Victoroff et al. 1994).

Patients with depression with epilepsy most commonly have a chronic interictal depression or dysthymia that is distinct from ictal depression (Devinsky and Bear 1991; Robertson et al. 1994). This interictal depression frequently has endogenous features, paranoia, and other symptoms suggesting a continuum with schizoaffective disorder (Mendez et al. 1986). According to most investigators, seizures relieve depression in patients with epilepsy (similar to the effects of electroconvulsive therapy [ECT]), whereas better seizure control or decreased secondarily generalized seizures make it worse (Mendez et al. 1993a; Robertson 1991). A few investigators have also reported depression with increased seizure activity or no relationship (Dodrill and Batzel 1986; Roy 1979). Depression is specifically associated with CPSs from left-sided temporal foci, suggesting neurobiologically based organic mood disorder rather than a nonspecific psychosocial reaction to a chronic disability (Altshuler et al. 1990; Mendez et al. 1986; Perini and Mendius 1984; Victoroff et al. 1994). Conversely, most studies have not confirmed the proposed association of right-hemisphere foci with the much rarer cases of mania found in epilepsy (Flor-Henry 1969).

Suicide

Elderly individuals with epilepsy are at greater risk for suicide than those without epilepsy. Among all patients with epilepsy, the estimated risk of death by suicide is 3%–22% or 4–5 times higher than that for the general population (Mathews and Barabas 1981). Among those with CPSs of TLE origin, the risk of suicide is as much as 25 times greater (Barraclough 1981). Furthermore, as many as one-third of all patients with epilepsy have attempted suicide at some point in time. A comparison of suicide attempts among patients with epilepsy and comparably impaired control subjects without epilepsy revealed suicide attempts in 30% of the subjects with epilepsy compared with only 7% of the control subjects (Mendez et al. 1986),

and this increased risk of suicide continued even long after temporal lobectomy and successful control of seizures (Jensen 1975).

Patients with epilepsy are likely to attempt suicide not only from psychosocial stress, but also because of the increased interictal psychopathology such as depression, psychosis, and borderline personality characteristics (Mendez et al. 1989). They are most likely to complete suicide when they have psychosis with paranoid hallucinations, agitated compunction to kill themselves, and occasional ictal command hallucinations to commit suicide (Mendez and Doss 1992). Ictal depression also has resulted in successful suicide attempts (Mendez and Doss 1992).

Personality Characteristics

Patients with epilepsy have a high prevalence of personality disorders (Mendez et al. 1993c; Perini et al. 1996; Swanson et al. 1995). Patients with epilepsy with personality disorders show dependent and avoidant personality traits. Those with epilepsy are stigmatized, feared, and subject to difficulties in obtaining a job, driving an automobile, and maintaining a marriage. These psychosocial difficulties along with underlying neurobiological factors may predispose patients with epilepsy to personality disorders.

Although no specific epileptic personality exists, a group of traits termed the Gastaut-Geschwind syndrome occur in a subset of patients with CPSs. Because most studies with the MMPI proved insensitive to the personality traits attributed to epilepsy, the Bear-Fedio Inventory was developed to assess these traits (Bear and Fedio 1977). Bear and Fedio found that patients with CPSs of TLE origin had a personality characterized by a sense of "heightened significance" indicated by sobriety and humorlessness, tenaciousness or "viscosity" in interpersonal encounters, a deepened affect, a pronounced sense of personal destiny, and an intense interest in religious, moral, and philosophical issues. Such patients are circumstantial, give overly detailed background information, and write copiously about their thoughts and feelings (Rao et al. 1992). In addition, patients with left-sided temporal foci tended to maximize their problems, whereas those with right-sided foci minimized them (Bear and Fedio 1977). Conclusive proof that patients with CPSs are prone to the Gastaut-Geschwind syndrome has remained illusive. Other applications of the Bear-Fedio Inventory found the same "personality" characteristics in patients without epilepsy who had psychiatric disorders or comparable physical disabilities (Rodin and Schmaltz 1984). Some patients with CPSs of TLE origin are explosive and dyscontrolled with emotional lability and poor impulse control (Blumer 1991).

Hyposexuality and Other Behavioral Disorders

Surveys suggest that incompletely treated patients with epilepsy experience hyposexuality (Toone 1987), a problem that can still affect elderly patients. Both men and women experience disturbances of sexual arousal and a lowered sexual drive (Morrell and Guldner 1996; Murialdo et al. 1995). Patients with epilepsy appear to lack libido and may experience impotence or frigidity. This hyposexuality improves after seizures are controlled (Toone 1987). Other patients with epilepsy experience physiological signs of decreased sexual arousal and possible subclinical hypogonadotropic hypogonadism (Murialdo et al. 1995).

The association of epilepsy with other conditions is less certain. Most directed aggression in epilepsy correlates less with seizures than with psychosis, "episodic dyscontrol" (intermittent explosive disorder with ictal-like features), subnormal intelligence, lower socioeconomic status, prior head injuries, and possible orbital frontal damage (Herzberg and Fenwick 1988; Mendez et al. 1993b). Case reports describe dissociative states in epilepsy (i.e., multiple personality disorder, possession and fugue states, and psychogenic amnesia) (Ahern et al. 1993); however, the relationship with epilepsy is not clear.

Etiology and Pathology

Although the mechanisms of psychopathology are not established, current theories of the psychopathology of epilepsy emphasize a physiological disturbance in the temporal limbic system rather than psychodynamic processes. As previously described, psychosis, depression, personality disorders, and hyposexuality are two to three times more common in patients with CPSs (most of whom have a temporal lobe focus) compared with patients with GTCSs. The most common pathological findings in patients with epilepsy are mediobasal temporal lobe lesions involving limbic structures. Stimulation and ablation studies in animals and humans link these temporal limbic structures to emotional behavior. Psychotic-like behavior in animal subjects has followed repeated application of epileptic agents to *kindle* limbic structures (Adamec 1990; P. F. Smith and Darlington 1996), patients with schizophrenia have had limbic discharges on depth electrode monitoring (Heath 1982), and disinhibition of the mesolimbic dopamine system has resulted from kindling in the limbic system (Stevens and Livermore 1978).

Several specific mechanisms are potentially responsible for psychiatric disturbances in epilepsy (Table 29–3). First, the underlying brain lesions could be the source of both seizures and behavioral changes. Psychosis may be more common with left temporal lobe pathology such as hamartomas or gangliogliomas (Taylor 1972), and depression is associated with strokes and other hypoactive lesions in the left hemisphere (Robinson and Szetela 1981). Second, ictal discharges could kindle behavioral changes by facilitating limbic-sensory associations and other neuronal connections. The schizophrenic psychosis is associated with increased frequencies of CPSs, and personality disorders may occur in those with auras (Mendez et al. 1993c). Third, decreased function, such as the focal interictal hypometabolism observed on positron-emission tomography (PET) (Bromfield et al. 1992), may lead to interictal behavioral changes. Depression often follows seizure control sufficient to inhibit secondary generalization to GTCSs (i.e., the surrounding hypometabolism may result in depression by preventing the spread of temporal limbic epileptic foci). Fourth, seizures may result in neuroendocrine or neurotransmitter changes including increased dopaminergic or inhibitory transmitters, decreased prolactin, increased testosterone, and increased endogenous opioids. These changes probably explain, at least in part, the hyposexuality found in some patients with

TABLE 29–3. Proposed relationships of psychiatric disturbances to epilepsy

Common neuropathology, genetics, or developmental disturbance

Ictal or subictal discharges potentiating abnormal behavior

Kindling or facilitation of a distributed neuronal matrix

Changes in spike frequency or inhibitory-excitatory balance

Altered receptor sensitivity (e.g., dopamine receptors)

Secondary epileptogenesis

Absence of function at the seizure focus

Inhibition and hypometabolism surrounding the focus

Release or abnormal activity of remaining neurons

Dysfunction or downregulation of associated areas

Neurochemical alterations

    Dopamine and other neurotransmitters

    Endorphins

Gonadotrophins and other neuroendocrinological changes

Psychodynamic influences

Dependence, learned helplessness, low self-esteem

Disruption of reality testing

Weakening of defense mechanisms

Organic and psychodynamic factors potentiating each other

Sleep disturbance

Drug-induced neurophysiological changes

epilepsy. Finally, physiological factors may be potentiated by psychodynamic factors. For example, a proposed role for auras in personality disorders or psychosis may relate to their impact on reality testing (Mendez et al. 1993c).

Treatment

Most epileptic seizures respond to AEDs. Phenytoin, carbamazepine, and valproate are primary drugs for partial seizures and GTCSs, the main seizures of adulthood (Table 29–4). Side effects and elimination half-lives are important considerations in choosing among AEDs. Monitoring of blood levels helps avoid dose-dependent side effects, but clinical monitoring of patients for idiosyncratic side effects is also necessary. The more sedating AEDs are considered secondary drugs in the management of seizures.

Another important property of AEDs is the time it takes for their serum concentrations to be reduced by half. For example, one may choose to use phenytoin over carbamazepine because it has a consistently longer half-life and can be potentially given once per day. The use of multiple AEDs affects efficacy, side effects, and half-lives; therefore, it is preferable to treat seizures with one AED rather than with several. For those patients who do not respond to

the primary AEDs, several newer drugs (e.g., gabapentin, lamotrigine, tiagabine, topiramate, vigabatrin) are available. Ultimately, when drug therapy fails to control seizures, patients may be considered for epilepsy surgery.

In the treatment of patients with epilepsy who are psychiatrically disturbed, a first consideration is the use of psychoactive AEDs (Pollack and Scott 1997) (Table 29–5). These medications may relieve some behavioral symptoms either through direct psychotropic properties or through their effects on seizure control (Post et al. 1985). The psychotropic properties of AEDs are particularly important in the management of depression (Robertson and Trimble 1985). If possible, discontinue phenobarbital and other barbiturates, which may promote depression in elderly patients, and use carbamazepine, valproate, or lamotrigine, which stabilize mood and provide prophylaxis against recurrent depressive episodes. Carbamazepine, valproate, gabapentin, and lamotrigine have significant antimanic properties, probably through mood stabilization effects. Carbamazepine, valproate, and gabapentin may also ameliorate some dyscontrolled, aggressive behavior in patients with brain injury. Clonazepam (Klonopin), in addition to its anxiolytic properties, can serve as a supplement to other antimanic therapies. Gabapentin also decreases anxiety and improves general well-being in some

TABLE 29–4. Antiepileptic drugs (AEDs)

AEDs (trade name)	Indications	Half-life (hours)	Therapeutic level (mg/L)	Usual adult dose (mg/day)	Dosing regimens
Primary drugs					
Phenytoin (Dilantin)	CPS, SPS, GTCS	10–34	10–20	300–500	bid–qd
Carbamazepine (Tegretol, Epitol)	CPS, SPS, GTCS	11–32	4–12	600–1200	tid
Valproic acid (Depakene), divalproex sodium (Depakote)	CPS, SPS, GTCS absence, atonic myoclonic	5–20	40–50	1000–3000	tid–qid bid (Depakote only)
Ethosuximide (Zarontin)	Absence	30–60	40–100	1000–2000	tid–qid
Secondary drugs					
Gabapentin (Neurontin)	CPS, SPS, 2°GTCS	4–7	2–20	900–3600	tid
Lamotrigine (Lamictal)	CPS, SPS 2°GTCS	15–24	2–20	75–600	bid
Topiramate (Topamax)	CPS, SPS, 2°GTCS	12–30	NE	200–400	bid
Tiagabine[a] (Gabitril)	CPS, SPS, 2°GTCS	6–8	NE	32–56	bid
Vigabatrin[a] (Sabril)	CPS, SPS, 2°GTCS	4–8	NE	1000–6000	bid–qd
Phenobarbital (various)	CPS, SPS, GTCS	46–140	15–40	90–120	bid–qd
Primidone (Mysoline)	CPS, SPS, GTCS	5–18	5–12	750–1000	tid–qid
Clonazepam (Klonopin)	Absence, atonic, myoclonic	20–40	.005–.07	2–6	tid–qid

Note. NE = not established.
[a]Pending approval.

TABLE 29–5. Psychiatric effects of antiepileptic drugs (AEDs)

Anticonvulsant	Psychiatric effects
Carbamazepine	Mood stabilizer, antimanic, mild antidepressant
Phenytoin	May cause depression
Valproic acid	Antimanic, possibly a mild antidepressant
Gabapentin	Mood stabilizer; treatment for bipolar, panic, and general anxiety disorders
Lamotrigine	Mood stabilizer, treatment for bipolar disorder and depression, may cause psychosis
Topiramate	May cause depression and psychosis
Tiagabine	May cause depression and psychosis
Vigabatrin	May cause depression and psychosis
Phenobarbital/primidone	May cause depression, hyperactivity, conduct disorder, and additional deficits
Ethosuximide	May cause psychosis
Clonazepam	May cause hyperactivity and additional deficits

patients with epilepsy. Both carbamazepine and ethosuximide may have value for borderline personality disorder.

Encephalopathic changes occur at toxic levels of all anticonvulsant drugs. Even at therapeutic levels, barbiturates may need discontinuation because of drug-induced depression, suicidal ideation, sedation, psychomotor slowing, and paradoxical hyperactivity in the very young and the very old. Gabapentin may induce aggressive behavior or hypomania, and vigabatrin may precipitate depression and psychosis. In addition, clinicians need to be aware of the potential emergence of psychopathology on withdrawal of anticonvulsant medications (Ketter et al. 1994). Anxiety and depression are the most common emergent symptoms, but psychosis and other behaviors may also occur.

Another therapeutic consideration is the seizure threshold–lowering effect of psychotropic medications (Itil and Soldatos 1980; Luchins et al. 1984; Oliver et al. 1982) (Table 29–6). This is usually not a problem, but can occasionally reach clinical significance. Psychotropic drugs are most convulsive when introduced rapidly or given in high doses. Clozapine and bupropion, particularly in combination, may be especially convulsant. When initiating psychotropic therapy, it is best to start low and go slow while monitoring anticonvulsant levels and EEGs. For example, clozapine has induced seizures in 1%–4.4% of patients when the dose was rapidly increased.

A potential exists for interaction of anticonvulsant and psychotropic medications. Attention to drug interactions is particularly important in elderly patients, who are often on multiple medications. In addition to increasing the metabolism of other AEDs, the addition of an AED most commonly increases the metabolism of psychotropic drugs with a consequent decrease in their therapeutic effective-

ness (Linnoila et al. 1980). The exception is the addition of valproic acid, which can increase psychotropic levels, rarely to a toxic range. Withdrawal of AEDs can precipitate rebound elevations in psychotropic levels. Alternatively, the initiation of a psychotropic can result in competitive inhibition of anticonvulsant metabolism with elevations of AED levels to toxicity (Vincent 1980).

Other therapeutic considerations that can affect the neuropsychiatric aspects of epilepsy include epilepsy surgery, ECT, and allowing patients to experience occasional partial or generalized seizures. Although epilepsy surgeries such as temporal lobectomy or corpus callosotomy are rarely performed in elderly patients, the removal of a secondary epileptogenic lesion such as a tumor may ameliorate seizures and associated behavioral disturbances (Krahn et al. 1996). Unfortunately, some patients with epilepsy continue to develop psychosis, personality changes, and suicidal behavior even long after primary epilepsy surgery (Falconer 1973; Jensen 1975; Koch-Weser et al. 1988). In addition to the occasional behavior alleviated by strict seizure control, allowing seizures under carefully controlled conditions, much like ECT, can relieve interictal depression, some cases of ictally related psychotic episodes, episodic dyscontrol, and, less frequently, other behaviors.

Summary

The neuropsychiatric aspects of epilepsy include a broad range of behavioral changes that can occur in elderly patients. The incidence of seizure disorders in those over age 65 is higher than at any time since infancy; consequently, understanding the particular psychosocial impact of seizures on older people is beneficial. In later life, neuro-

TABLE 29–6.   Seizure threshold effect of psychotropic medications

Potential	Antipsychotic	Antidepressant	Other psychotropic
Proconvulsant			
High	Clozapine	Bupropion	
	Chlorpromazine	Imipramine	
		Maprotiline	
		Amitriptyline	
		Amoxapine	
		Nortriptyline	
Moderate	Most piperazines	Protriptyline	Lithium
	Thiothixene	Clomipramine	
Low	Fluphenazine	Doxepin	Ethchlorvynol
	Haloperidol	Desipramine	Glutethimide
	Loxapine	Fluoxetine	Hydroxyzine
	Molindone	Sertraline	Meprobamate
	Pimozide	Trazodone	Methaqualone
	Thioridazine	Trimipramine	
	Risperidone	Other selective serotonin reuptake inhibitors	
	Olanzapine		
Anticonvulsant			
Low		Monoamine oxidase inhibitors	Oral benzodiazepine
	Methylphenidate		
	Dextroamphetamine		
High		Barbiturates	

psychological effects from seizures, from the causative brain lesions, and from anticonvulsant medications increase. There can be an increased severity of ictally related behavioral disturbances such as prolonged periods of postictal confusion. Moreover, patients with epilepsy have an increased frequency of interictal psychiatric disturbances, such as depression, psychosis, suicide, personality disorders, hyposexuality, and others. Management of these behavioral disorders requires attention to the behavioral effects of anticonvulsant medications, the convulsant effects of psychotropic medications, and the interactions between them.

References

Adamec RE: Does kindling model anything clinically relevant? Biol Psychiatry 27:249–279, 1990

Ahern GL, Herring AM, Tackenberg J, et al: The association of multiple personality and temporolimbic epilepsy. Intracarotid amobarbital test observations. Arch Neurol 50:1020–1025, 1993

Altshuler LL, Devinsky O, Post RM, et al: Depression, anxiety, and temporal lobe epilepsy: laterality of focus and symptoms. Arch Neurol 47:284–288, 1990

Annegers JF: Epidemiology of epilepsy, in The Treatment of Epilepsy: Principles and Practice, 2nd Edition. Edited by Wyllie E. Baltimore, MD, Williams & Wilkins, 1997, pp 157–164

Barraclough B: Suicide and epilepsy, in Epilepsy and Psychiatry. Edited by Reynolds E, Trimble MR. New York, Churchill Livingstone, 1981, pp 72–76

Bear D, Fedio P: Quantitative analysis of interictal behavior in temporal lobe epilepsy. Arch Neurol 34:454–467, 1977

Betts TA: Epilepsy and the mental hospital, in Epilepsy and Psychiatry. Edited by Reynolds E, Trimble MR. New York, Churchill Livingstone, 1981, pp 175–184

Blumer D: Personality in epilepsy. Semin Neurol 11:155–166, 1991

Botwinick J: Neuropsychology of aging, in The Handbook of Clinical Neuropsychology. Edited by Fiskov SB, Boll TJ. New York, Wiley, 1981, pp 135–171

Bromfield EB, Altshuler L, Leiderman BD, et al: Cerebral metabolism and depression in patients with complex partial seizures. Arch Neurol 49:617–623, 1992

Collings JA: International differences in psychosocial well-being: a comparative study of adults with epilepsy in three countries. Seizure 3:183–190, 1994

Commission on Classification and Terminology of the International League Against Epilepsy: Proposal for revised clinical and electroencephalographic classification of epileptic seizures. Epilepsia 22:489–501, 1981

Currie S, Heathfield KWG, Henson RA, et al: Clinical course and prognosis of temporal lobe epilepsy: a survey of 666 patients. Brain 92:173–190, 1971

Dark FL, McGrath JJ, Ron MA: Pathological laughing and crying. Aust N Z J Psychiatry 30:472–479, 1996

Devinsky O, Bear DM: Varieties of depression in epilepsy. Neuropsychiatry Neuropsychol Behav Neurol 4:49–61, 1991

Devinsky O, Abramson H, Alper K, et al: Postictal psychosis: a case control series of 20 patients and 150 controls. Epilepsy Res 20:247–253, 1995

Dikmen S, Hermann BP, Wilensky AJ, et al: Validity of the Minnesota Multiphasic Personality Inventory (MMPI) to psychopathology in patients with epilepsy. J Nerv Ment Dis 171:114–122, 1983

Dodrill CB, Batzel LW: Interictal behavioral features of patients with epilepsy. Epilepsia 27 (suppl 2):S64–S76, 1986

Dongier S: Statistical study of clinical and electro-encephalographic manifestations of 536 psychotic episodes occurring in 516 epileptics between clinical seizures. Epilepsia 1:117–142, 1959/1960

Engel J, Ludwig B, Fetell M: Prolonged partial complex status epilepticus: EEG and behavioral observations. Neurology 28:863–866, 1978

Falconer MA: Reversibility by temporal-lobe resection of the behavioral abnormalities of temporal-lobe epilepsy. N Engl J Med 289:451–455, 1973

Flor-Henry P: Depressive-like reactions and affective psychosis associated with temporal lobe epilepsy: etiologic factors. Am J Psychiatry 126:400–403, 1969

Gibbs FA: Ictal and non-ictal psychiatric disorders in temporal lobe epilepsy. J Nerv Ment Dis 113:522–528, 1951

Gibbs FA, Gibbs EL, Fuster B: Psychomotor epilepsy. Archives of Neurology and Psychiatry 60:331–339, 1948

Godfrey JBW: Misleading presentation of epilepsy in elderly people. Age Ageing 18:17–20, 1989

Gudmundsson G: Epilepsy in Iceland: a clinical and epidemiological investigation. Acta Neurol Scand Suppl 25:1–124, 1966

Hauser WA: Seizure disorders: the changes with age. Epilepsia 33 (suppl 4):S6–S14, 1992

Heath RG: Psychosis and epilepsy: similarities and differences in the anatomic-physiologic substrate. Advances in Biological Psychiatry 8:106–116, 1982

Hermann BP, Wyler AR: Depression, loss of control, and the effects of epilepsy surgery. Epilepsia 30:332–338, 1989

Herzberg JL, Fenwick PB: The aetiology of aggression in temporal lobe epilepsy. Br J Psychiatry 153:50–55, 1988

Itil TM, Soldatos C: Epileptogenic side effects of psychotropic drugs. JAMA 244:1460–1463, 1980

Jensen I: Temporal lobe epilepsy: late mortality in patients treated with unilateral temporal lobe resections. Acta Neurol Scand 52:374–380, 1975

Kanemoto K, Kawasaki J, Kawai I: Postictal psychosis: a comparison with acute interictal and chronic psychoses. Epilepsia 37:551–556, 1996

Ketter TA, Malow BA, Flamini R, et al: Anticonvulsant withdrawal-emergent psychopathology. Neurology 44:55–61, 1994

Koch-Weser M, Garron DC, Gilley DW, et al: Prevalence of psychological disorders after surgical treatment of seizures. Arch Neurol 45:1308–1313, 1988

Kogeorgos J, Fonagy P, Scott DF: Psychiatric symptom patterns of chronic epileptics attending a neurological clinic: a controlled investigation. Br J Psychiatry 140:236–243, 1982

Kraepelin E: Psychiatrie, 8th Edition. Leipzig, Germany, Johann Ambrosius Barltz, 1923

Krahn LE, Rummans TA, Peterson GC: Psychiatric implications of surgical treatment of epilepsy. Mayo Clin Proc 71:1201–1204, 1996

Kuyk J, Leiten F, Meinardi H, et al: The diagnosis of psychogenic non-epileptic seizures: a review. Seizure 6:243–253, 1997

Landolt H: Serial electroencephalographic investigations during psychotic episodes in epileptic patients and during schizophrenic attacks, in Lectures on Epilepsy. Edited by de Haas L. New York, Elsevier Science, 1958, pp 91–133

Leppik IE: Metabolism of antiepileptic medication: newborn to elderly. Epilepsia 33 (suppl 4):S32–S40, 1992

Lesser RP: Psychogenic seizures. Neurology 46:1499–1507, 1996

Lindsay J, Ounsted C, Richards P: Long-term outcome in children with temporal lobe seizures, III: psychiatric aspects in childhood and adult life. Dev Med Child Neurol 21:630–636, 1979

Linnoila M, Viukari M, Vaisanen K, et al: Effect of anticonvulsants on plasma haloperidol and thioridazine levels. Am J Psychiatry 137:819–821, 1980

Luchins DH, Oliver AP, Wyatt RJ: Seizures with antidepressants: an in vitro technique to assess relative risk. Epilepsia 25:25–32, 1984

Luhdorf K, Jensen LK, Plesner AM: Etiology of seizures in the elderly. Epilepsia 27:458–463, 1986

Manchanda R, Schaefer B, McLachlan RS, et al: Psychiatric disorders in candidates for surgery for epilepsy. J Neurol Neurosurg Psychiatry 61:82–89, 1996

Mathews WS, Barabas G: Suicide and epilepsy: a review of the literature. Psychosomatics 22:515–524, 1981

McAreavey MJ, Ballinger BR, Fenton GW: Epileptic seizures in elderly patients with dementia. Epilepsia 33:657–660, 1992

Mendez MF, Doss RC: Ictal and psychiatric aspects of suicide among epileptics. Int J Psychiatry Med 22:231–237, 1992

Mendez MF, Cummings JL, Benson DF: Depression in epilepsy, significance and phenomenology. Arch Neurol 43:766–770, 1986

Mendez MF, Lanska DJ, Manon-Espaillet R, et al: Causative factors for suicide attempts by overdose in epileptics. Arch Neurol 46:1065–1068, 1989

Mendez MF, Doss RC, Taylor JL, et al: Interictal depression in epilepsy: relationship to seizure variables. J Nerv Ment Dis 181:444–447, 1993a

Mendez MF, Doss RC, Taylor JL: Interictal violence in epilepsy. Relationship to behavior and seizure variables. J Nerv Ment Dis 181:566–569, 1993b

Mendez MF, Doss RC, Taylor JL, et al: Relationship of seizure variables to personality disorders in epilepsy. J Neuropsychiatry Clin Neurosci 5:283–286, 1993c

Mendez MF, Grau R, Doss RC, et al: Schizophrenia in epilepsy: seizure and psychosis variables. Neurology 43:1073–1077, 1993d

Mendez MF, Catanzaro P, Doss RC, et al: Seizures in Alzheimer's disease: a clinicopathological study. J Geriatr Psychiatry Neurol 7:53–58, 1994

Mendez MF, Cherrier M, Perryman KM: Epileptic forced thinking from left frontal lesions. Neurology 47:79–83, 1996a

Mendez MF, Engebrit B, Doss R, et al: The relationship of epileptic auras and psychological attributes. J Neuropsychiatry Clin Neurosci 8:287–292, 1996b

Morrell MJ, Guldner GT: Self-reported sexual function and sexual arousability in women with epilepsy. Epilepsia 37:1204–1210, 1996

Murialdo G, Galimberti CA, Fonzi S, et al: Sex hormones and pituitary function in male epileptic patients with altered or normal sexuality. Epilepsia 36:360–365, 1995

Oliver AP, Luchins DH, Wyatt RJ: Neuroleptic-induced seizures. Arch Gen Psychiatry 39:206–209, 1982

Pakalnis A, Drake ME, John K, et al: Normalizations: acute psychosis after seizure control in seven patients. Arch Neurol 44:289–292, 1987

Perez MM, Trimble MR: Epileptic psychosis-diagnostic comparison with process schizophrenia. Br J Psychiatry 37:245–249, 1980

Perini G, Mendius R: Depression and anxiety in complex partial seizures. J Nerv Ment Dis 172:287–290, 1984

Perini GL, Tosin C, Carraro C, et al: Interictal personality disorders in temporal lobe epilepsy and juvenile myoclonic epilepsy. J Neurol Neurosurg Psychiatry 61:601–605, 1996

Pollack MH, Scott EL: Gabapentin and lamotrigine: novel treatments for mood and anxiety disorders. CNS Spectrums 2:56–61, 1997

Pond DA, Bidwell BH: A survey of epilepsy in 14 general practices, II: social and psychological aspects. Epilepsia 1:285–299, 1959/1960

Post RM, Uhde TW, Joffe RT: Anticonvulsant drugs in psychiatric illness: new treatment alternatives and theoretical implications, in The Psychopharmacology of Epilepsy. Edited by Trimble MR. New York, Wiley, 1985, pp 141–171

Rao SM, Devinsky O, Grafman J, et al: Viscosity and social cohesion in temporal lobe epilepsy. J Neurol Neurosurg Psychiatry 55:149–152, 1992

Robertson MM: Depression in patients with epilepsy: an overview. Semin Neurol 11:182–189, 1991

Robertson MM, Trimble MR: The treatment of depression in patients with epilepsy: a double blind trial. J Affect Disord 9:127–136, 1985

Robertson MM, Channon S, Baker J: Depressive symptomatology in a general hospital sample of outpatients with temporal lobe epilepsy: a controlled study. Epilepsia 35:771–777, 1994

Robinson RG, Szetela B: Mood change following left hemisphere brain injury. Ann Neurol 9:447–453, 1981

Rodin E, Schmaltz S: The Bear-Fedio personality inventory and temporal lobe epilepsy. Neurology 34:591–596, 1984

Romanelli M, Morris JC, Ashkin K, et al: Advanced Alzheimer's disease is a risk factor for late-onset seizures. Arch Neurol 47:847–850, 1990

Roy A: Some determinants of affective symptoms in epileptics. Can J Psychiatry 24:554–556, 1979

Sachdev P: Schizophrenia-like psychosis and epilepsy: the status of the association. Am J Psychiatry 155:325–336, 1998

Sanders KM, Murray GB: Geriatric epilepsy: a review. J Geriatr Psychiatry Neurol 4:98–105, 1991

Sherwin I, Peron-Magnon P, Bancaud J, et al: Prevalence of psychosis in epilepsy as a function of laterality of the epileptogenic lesion. Arch Neurol 39:621–625, 1982

Shorvon SD, Gilliatt RW, Cox TCS, et al: Evidence of vascular disease from CT scanning in late onset epilepsy. J Neurol Neurosurg Psychiatry 47:225–230, 1984

Slater E, Beard A: The schizophrenia-like psychosis of epilepsy: psychiatric aspects. Br J Psychiatry 109:95–150, 1963

Smith DB, Treiman DM, Trimble MR: Neurobehavioral Problems in Epilepsy. New York, Raven, 1991

Smith PF, Darlington CL: The development of psychosis in epilepsy: a re-examination of the kindling hypothesis. Behav Brain Res 75:59–66, 1996

Standage KF, Fenton GW: Psychiatric symptom profiles of patients with epilepsy: a controlled investigation. Psychol Med 5:152–160, 1975

Stevens JR: Interictal clinical manifestations of complex partial seizures, in Advances in Neurology Series, Vol 2. New York, Raven, 1975, pp 85–112

Stevens JR: Psychosis and the temporal lobe, in Neurobehavioral Problems in Epilepsy. Edited by Smith DB, Treiman DM, Trimble MR. New York, Raven, 1991, pp 79–96

Stevens JR, Livermore A: Kindling of the mesolimbic dopamine system: animal model of psychosis. Neurology 28:36–46, 1978

Swanson SJ, Rao SM, Grafman J, et al: The relationship between seizure subtype and interictal personality. Results from the Vietnam Head Injury Study. Brain 118:91–103, 1995

Taylor D: Mental state and temporal lobe epilepsy: a correlative account of 100 patients treated surgically. Epilepsia 13:727–765, 1972

Tedman S, Thornton E, Baker G: Development of a scale to measure core beliefs and perceived self efficacy in adults with epilepsy. Seizure 4:221–231, 1995

Toone B: Sexual disorders in epilepsy, in Recent Advances in Epilepsy, 3rd Edition. Edited by Pedley TA, Meldrum BS. New York, Churchill Livingstone, 1987, pp 233–259

Treiman DM: Psychobiology of ictal aggression, in Neurobehavioral Problems in Epilepsy. Edited by Smith DB, Treiman DM, Trimble MR. New York, Raven, 1991, pp 341–356

Trimble MR: The Psychosis of Epilepsy. New York, Raven, 1991

Victoroff JI, Benson F, Grafton ST, et al: Depression in complex partial seizures: electroencephalographic and cerebral metabolic correlates. Arch Neurol 51:155–163, 1994

Vincent FM: Phenothiazine-induced phenytoin intoxication. Ann Intern Med 93:56–57, 1980

Wilensky AJ, Leal KW, Dudley DL, et al: Characteristics of psychotropic drug use in an epilepsy center population (abstract). Epilepsia 22:247, 1981

Neoplastic, Demyelinating, Infectious, and Inflammatory Brain Disorders

Douglas W. Scharre, M.D.

Acquired diseases of the brain are common in the elderly population. Neuropsychiatric disorders are frequent complications of these conditions and may be the sole manifestations of the brain dysfunction. In this chapter, I discuss the neuropsychiatric manifestations of the major neoplastic, demyelinating, infectious, and inflammatory disorders of the brain.

▌ Neoplastic Disorders

Demography

Primary and metastatic neoplasms of the central nervous system (CNS) are common in the geriatric population. The overall incidence of CNS tumors is 15/100,000 per year, and the age-specific incidence peaks between 60 and 80 years. Eighty-five percent of all primary CNS neoplasms occur intracranially; the rest are intraspinal. In clinical series, 45% of intracranial tumors are gliomas, 15% are meningiomas, 7% are pituitary adenomas, and 6% are metastatic (Tyler and Byrne 1992). However, many tumors go unrecognized during life, and in autopsy series meningiomas account for up to 40% and metastatic tumors for up to 18% of all intracranial neoplasms (Kurtzke and Kurland 1983). The most common cancers to metastasize to the brain are lung, breast, kidney, colon, testis, melanoma, and lymphoma (Alvord and Shaw 1991).

Physiology

There are multiple ways for CNS neoplasms to alter brain function. Direct invasion and compression will produce focal neurological deficits such as aphasia, hemiparesis, amnesia, or visual field deficits. Vasogenic brain edema is produced in many neoplasms secondary to capillary leakage across a defective blood-brain barrier (Adams et al. 1997). This edema in conjunction with the mass effect of the tumor often leads to increased intracranial pressure. The typical signs and symptoms of increased intracranial pressure are headache, nausea, vomiting, papilledema, sixth cranial nerve palsy, and mental status changes. Neuropsychiatric evaluation often shows diminished arousal, impaired attention, impaired cognition, irritability, emotional lability, and psychomotor retardation. Eventually, with continued increased intracranial pressure, bradycardia, hypertension, and herniation syndromes develop.

Tumors located near the ventricular system often cause obstructive hydrocephalus. Headache, cognitive decline, incontinence, and gait disturbances are frequent sequela. Tumors may also cause vascular obstruction, particularly of the venous system, resulting in ischemic infarctions, hemorrhages, and increased intracranial pressure. Thirty percent of all brain tumors will produce focal or generalized seizures.

Pathology

Intracranial neoplasms consist of rapidly growing tumor cells, tumor-related blood vessels, and necrotic tissue. Astrocytomas are classified as low grade, intermediate grade, or high grade (glioblastoma multiforme) according to the degree of nuclear atypism, mitosis, endothelial proliferation, and necrosis exhibited. Elderly individuals tend to have higher-grade astrocytomas. Oligodendrogliomas frequently contain calcifications and may bleed. Meningiomas are derived from cells of the arachnoid, pia mater, and dura mater and do not invade the brain parenchyma. Pituitary adenomas arise from one of several cell types in the anterior lobe of the pituitary. Most of the adenomas in the geriatric age range are nonfunctional chromophobe types (Alvord and Shaw 1991).

Laboratory Evaluations

Lumbar puncture is generally avoided because of the risk of precipitating a herniation syndrome when there is a mass lesion in the brain. When cerebrospinal fluid (CSF) is collected, it typically reveals a mild pleocytosis, elevated protein, and normal glucose (Cummings and Benson 1992). CSF cytology is helpful in cases of meningeal carcinomatosis.

Electroencephalography (EEG) in patients with brain tumors is usually abnormal, revealing either focal or generalized slowing, sharp waves and spikes, or frank epilepti-

form activity. Angiography demonstrates the amount of tumor vascularity, which, in gliomas, is often correlated to tumor growth rate. Angiography of meningiomas often shows a meningeal blood supply and a distinct vascular blush (Tyler and Byrne 1992).

Magnetic resonance imaging (MRI) and computed tomography (CT) reveal evidence of mass processes, edema, midline shifts, hydrocephalus, and hemorrhage. Contrast enhancement greatly improves tumor detection. MRI is more sensitive than is CT in the detection of small tumors, but CT can demonstrate calcifications and bony erosions better. Unfortunately, neither CT nor MRI can accurately define intraparenchymal tumor boundaries. For most intracranial tumors, MRI shows increased signal on T2-weighted and gadolinium-enhanced T1-weighted images. Meningiomas exhibit an extra-axial location, dural base, and marked enhancement with contrast agents. MRIs of a glioblastoma multiforme and a meningioma are shown in Figures 30–1 and 30–2, respectively. Cerebral metastases often appear as multiple ring-enhancing nodular masses (Tyler and Byrne 1992).

Magnetic resonance angiography (MRA), single photon emission computed tomography (SPECT), and positron-emission tomography (PET) can now provide infor-

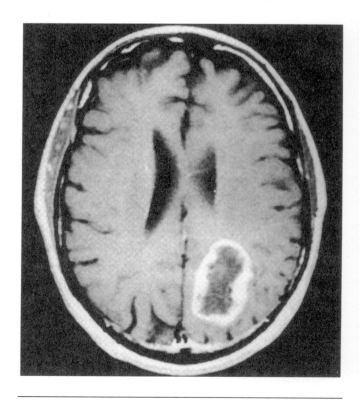

FIGURE 30–1. Gadolinium-enhanced, T1-weighted magnetic resonance image (MRI) of a 56-year-old man with a left parieto-occipital glioblastoma multiforme. The MRI reveals a ring-enhancing mass with a necrotic center.

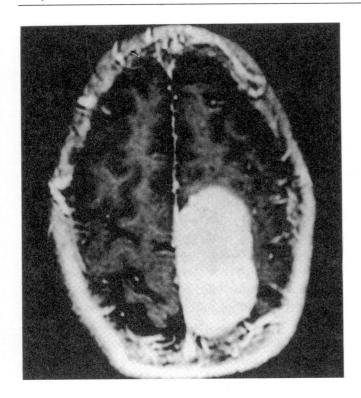

FIGURE 30–2. T1-weighted magnetic resonance image (MRI) of a 56-year-old woman with a left-sided posterior falx meningioma. A large, dural-based, extra-axial mass homogeneously enhances with gadolinium.

mation on tumor blood flow, grade, recurrence, and response to treatment (Tyler and Byrne 1992).

Treatment and Prognosis

The location and type of CNS neoplasms determines the approach to treatment. Surgical removal, debulking, chemotherapy, or radiation therapy are often used in some combination. Chemotherapy agents depend on the breakdown of the blood-brain barrier at the tumor site for selective drug delivery. The complications of radiation therapy include hypothalamic-pituitary dysfunction with resultant hypothyroidism, hypogonadism, or panhypopituitarism (Constine et al. 1993). Radiation-induced and chemotherapy-related leukoencephalopathy is discussed in the demyelinating disorders section below.

Corticosteroids are useful in reducing cerebral edema secondary to CNS neoplasms and thereby also aid in reduction of any associated increased intracranial pressure. Anticonvulsants are given to prevent seizures. Treatment of neuropsychiatric symptoms should avoid aggravating cognitive deficits. Psychosis is treated with very low dose haloperidol (0.5–1 mg/day) or with an atypical antipsychotic agent and increased slowly until an adequate re-

sponse is achieved. Depression is treated with antidepressants, usually a selective serotonin reuptake inhibitor. Mania is treated with divalproex sodium, carbamazepine, or a benzodiazepine; lithium is usually avoided because of its potential for exacerbating seizures (T. R. P. Price et al. 1992). Apathy and psychomotor retardation may be helped with methylphenidate or pemoline.

Astrocytomas and oligodendrogliomas are treated with surgery, radiation therapy, and chemotherapy, depending on their degree of malignancy. Meningiomas can be completely removed surgically in approximately 90% of cases but have a high rate of recurrence. Pituitary microadenomas are removed through a transphenoidal approach or treated with chemotherapy. Macroadenomas with extensive extraglandular extension often require craniotomies for removal, and postsurgical hormonal replacement is often required. Thirty percent of metastases are solitary and are candidates for surgical removal (Alvord and Shaw 1991). The 5-year survival rate for meningiomas is 60%, for gliomas 20%, and the median survival for glioblastoma multiforme is about 1 year (Kurtzke and Kurland 1983).

Neuropsychiatric Manifestations of Neoplastic Disorders

Frontal lobe tumors. Frontal lobe tumors produce mental status and personality changes in 90% of cases and frank dementia in 70% of cases, but few focal neurological findings (Cummings and Benson 1992). Apathy, disinhibition, or impulsivity are the hallmarks of frontal involvement. Euphoria or depression, irritability, lack of concern, poor judgment, disorientation, and poor attention are additional frequent early findings. Patients with right frontal tumors may display more euphoria, whereas those with left frontal tumors may display more depression and abulia (Belyi 1987). Psychosis with paranoia, delusions, and hallucinations can also be observed. The dementia is characterized by impaired word list generation and aphasia with dominant hemisphere tumors, decreased design fluency with nondominant hemisphere tumors, constructional deficits, motor programming deficits, perseveration, forgetfulness, poor abstraction, and psychomotor retardation. Large subfrontal meningiomas, gliomas spreading to both frontal lobes, and metastatic tumors frequently result in severe dementia. Fifty percent of patients with frontal lobe tumors develop seizures, usually focal motor (jacksonian) type, and a few develop hydrocephalus as a result of obstruction of the interventricular foramen. Tumors located in the posterofrontal region produce hemiparesis, olfactory groove meningiomas produce anosmia, sphenoid ridge meningiomas produce unilateral exophthalmos and cranial nerve palsies, prefrontal tumors often produce a grasp reflex, and involvement of the frontal eye fields produces a conjugate deviation of the eyes to the side of the tumor.

Temporal lobe tumors. Temporal lobe tumors may cause personality changes, irritability, euphoria, depression, anxiousness, psychosis, hallucinations (auditory, formed visual, and simple olfactory or gustatory), or cognitive impairment early in their course. Dominant hemisphere tumors can produce aphasia and verbal memory deficits (amnesia), whereas nondominant hemisphere tumors produce nonverbal memory deficits. Hydrocephalus may result from obstruction of the third ventricle or compression of the midbrain with obstruction of the cerebral aqueduct. Partial complex seizures are frequent and manifest with staring, blinking, complex motor activity, déjà vu phenomena, visual distortions, hallucinations, and other psychomotor disturbances (see Chapter 29 in this volume).

Parietal lobe tumors. Tumors that are located in the anterior parietal area may produce somatosensory disturbances including deficits in two-point discrimination; identification of finger writing (agraphesthesia); identification of objects by their shape, size, texture, or weight (astereognosis); simultaneous identification of bilateral stimulation (inattention); and localization of tactile stimuli (atopognosia). Parietal lobe tumors may cause a contralateral lower-quadrant field cut resulting from disruption of the superior optic radiations. Difficulties in drawing, apraxia, and focal sensory seizures may also occur with parietal lobe lesions.

Tumors involving the right parietal lobe are most likely to cause a neglect syndrome of the contralateral body and extrapersonal space (inattention). In the full-blown condition, patients will not see, dress, shave, or groom the neglected side of the body and do not respond to stimuli in the neglected hemispace. They may deny a contralateral hemiparesis (anosognosia). Left parietal lobe tumors in the angular gyrus region cause Gerstmann syndrome, including difficulties with writing (dysgraphia), finger identification, calculations (acalculia), and the ability to distinguish right from left. Often, aphasia and constructional disturbances are also present.

Occipital lobe tumors. Occipital lobe tumors commonly produce contralateral homonymous visual field deficits, simple visual seizures with generalization, and visual hallucinations consisting of unformed images such as flashes, streaks, or simple geometric patterns. Bilateral medial occipitotemporal tumors may cause a disturbance in visual recognition of objects (visual agnosia), identification of familiar faces (prosopagnosia), or recognition of familiar environments (environmental agnosia). Occasionally right-sided lesions alone may produce some of these syndromes.

Deep midline tumors. Deep midline tumors often lead to bihemispheric dysfunction as a result of invasion or brain compression by surrounding edema. Tumors within or near the third ventricle can obstruct the interventricular foramen or the cerebral aqueduct and cause hydrocephalus. Tumors within the ventricle can cause intermittent obstruction resulting in severe headaches and vomiting that are position dependent.

Pituitary and hypothalamic area tumors often cause bitemporal hemianopsia, optic atrophy, endocrine disturbances, diabetes insipidus, somnolence, personality changes, and cognitive decline. Excessive somnolence, rage attacks, and hyperphagia are occasionally seen with direct hypothalamic involvement.

Thalamic tumors produce memory loss, confusional states, emotional lability, hemiparesis, and hemihypesthesia with hemianesthesia. Basal ganglia tumors result in impaired attention, memory loss, personality changes, depression, and movement disorders including chorea, dystonia, or rigidity.

Pineal tumors compress the superior colliculus, producing aqueduct occlusion, hydrocephalus, and Parinaud's syndrome with paralysis of upward gaze and ptosis. Brainstem tumors produce cranial nerve deficits, long tract signs, cerebellar symptoms, and hydrocephalus. Personality changes, lethargy, disorientation, memory impairment, and mutism may also occur (Cummings and Benson 1992).

Posterior fossa tumors. Tumors in the posterior fossa can obstruct the fourth ventricle or the outflow into the basal cisterns, resulting in hydrocephalus. Prominent signs and symptoms include headache, vomiting, mental status changes, cranial nerve palsies, nystagmus, ataxia, dysmetria, hypotonia, and intention tremor.

Paraneoplastic Syndromes

The remote effects of carcinoma on the nervous system are poorly understood. The symptoms usually develop rapidly over a few weeks; they may occur before the discovery of the neoplasm. The production of onconeuronal autoantibodies directed against antigens shared by both the cancer and the nervous system is the most likely pathogenesis of these syndromes (Posner 1997). There are several syndromes affecting the brain that have been described.

Subacute cerebellar degeneration syndrome features ataxia, dysarthria, nystagmus, and diplopia as a result of antibodies against Purkinje cell cytoplasm (anti-Yo or anti-Tr) or neuronal nuclei (anti-Hu, also known as antineuronal nuclear antibody [ANNA-1]) of Purkinje cells. Opsoclonus paraneoplastic syndrome is characterized by uncontrolled eye movements as a result of antibodies against neuronal nuclei (Anti-Ri, also known as anti-neuronal nuclear antibody [ANNA-2]) probably directed to brainstem regions. Retinal degeneration paraneoplastic syndrome typically produces scotomas, blindness, and visual hallucinations as a result of anti-Recoverin antibodies of retina photoreceptors (Posner 1997).

Limbic encephalopathy, of all the paraneoplastic syndromes, is the one most associated with neuropsychiatric symptoms. Limbic encephalopathy has been seen most commonly with small-cell lung carcinoma and Hodgkin's disease. Other associations include carcinoma of the breast, uterus, ovary, prostate, and kidney; multiple myeloma; lymphosarcoma; reticulum cell sarcoma; neuroblastoma; and acute leukemia. The age at onset is typically 50–80 years, and men are more commonly affected. The condition may last several years. The syndrome is characterized by an amnestic memory disturbance, cognitive decline, depression, anxiety, personality changes, paranoia, hallucinations, and diminished alertness. Often a severe sensory neuropathy is present. Occasionally complex partial seizures, cerebellar deficits, brainstem signs, myelopathy, and autonomic failure are observed (Dalmau et al. 1992).

Neuronal loss and perivascular inflammatory infiltrates, particularly in the medial temporal areas, are found at autopsy (Newman et al. 1990). Sometimes the cerebellum, brainstem, spinal cord, dorsal root ganglia, and autonomic ganglia are involved. Neuroimaging is typically unrevealing. Rarely, MRI demonstrates increased signal on T2-weighted images in the frontal and temporal lobes (Kodama et al. 1991). CSF examination usually shows mild transient lymphocytic pleocytosis and persistent elevated protein, increased immunoglobulin G (IgG), and oligoclonal banding. Anti-Hu antibodies are seen in many cases and found in the nuclei of neurons (Dalmau et al. 1992). A new antibody to a subset of glial cells (anti-CV2) has been discovered in some patients with paraneoplastic encephalomyelitis (Honnorat et al. 1996). Treatments are being tested, but most have not shown great effect on the neurological symptoms. On the other hand, small-cell lung cancers with the Hu antigens appear more susceptible to therapy than those without (Posner 1997).

Demyelinating Disorders

Although demyelinating conditions are more common in young individuals, many examples of these disorders appear with late survival or presentation in the elderly population. A comprehensive list of common and rare white matter disorders is presented in Table 30–1. Primary demyelination involves the loss of the myelin sheath, leaving the axon intact but denuded. Dysmyelinating conditions reflect impairment in the formation or development of the myelin sheath. These two types of myelin disease give similar clinical and neuropsychiatric features.

Multiple Sclerosis

Multiple sclerosis (MS) is the most common demyelinating disorder of the CNS. Typically it presents in young adults, but 0.6% of the patients do not have their first symptom until age 60 or later (Hooge and Redekop 1992). The prevalence at age 70 is about 50/100,000 (Kurtzke and Kurland 1983). MS is rare in the tropics; its frequency increases in more northern latitudes. Women are affected more often than men by a 2 to 1 ratio.

Clinical features. The clinical course of MS has three forms: relapsing-remitting, acute progressive, and chronic progressive. Relapsing-remitting type is characterized by symptoms that may evolve over a few days and then partially or totally resolve over weeks. Rarely the course is an acute, rapidly progressive one over a few weeks or months to death. The most common pattern, particularly in those with onset over age 40, is a chronic, slowly progressive course.

Brainstem and spinal cord regions are frequently affected and may cause internuclear ophthalmoplegia, diplopia, trigeminal neuralgia, vertigo, myelopathy, acute transverse myelitis, bladder dysfunction, urinary frequency and urgency, urinary incontinence, constipation, autonomic dysfunction, sensory disturbances, paresthesias, loss of vibratory and position sense, gait imbalance, and pain syndromes, particularly of the back and lower extremities. Brain demyelination often results in optic neuritis, spastic weakness, gait imbalance, appendicular and truncal ataxia, intention tremor, dysmetria, sensory dysfunction, paroxysmal disorders, and neuropsychiatric syndromes. Treatment with steroids and other medications can complicate and contribute to the cognitive and psychiatric disturbances. Most patients with the onset of symptoms after age 50 or 60 have a slowly progressive myelopathy with spastic paraparesis, gait imbalance, and bladder impairment (Hooge and Redekop 1992; Noseworthy et al. 1983).

TABLE 30–1. Causes of demyelinating disorders in elderly patients

Autoimmune

Multiple sclerosis (MS)

Behçet's syndrome

Systemic lupus erythematosus (SLE)

Sjögren's syndrome

Acute disseminated encephalomyelitis

Vogt-Koyanagi-Harada syndrome

Postinfectious encephalomyelitis

Vascular

Binswanger's disease (subcortical arteriosclerotic encephalopathy)

Metabolic-toxic

Marchiafava-Bignami disease

Central pontine myelinolysis

Subacute combined degeneration (vitamin B_{12} deficiency)

Thiamine deficiency (vitamin B_1)

Vitamin B_6 deficiency

Vitamin E deficiency

Postanoxic/posthypoxic state

Radiation leukoencephalopathy

Chemotherapy-related leukoencephalopathy

Hereditary-metabolic

Metachromatic leukodystrophy (MLD)

Adrenoleukodystrophy (ALD)

Adrenomyeloneuropathy

Cerebrotendinous xanthomatosis

Membranous lipodystrophy

Hereditary adult-onset leukodystrophy

Globoid cell leukodystrophy, late onset

Infectious

Human immunodeficiency virus type 1 (HIV-1)–associated cognitive/motor complex

Progressive multifocal leukoencephalopathy (PML)

Lyme disease

Neoplastic

Lymphoma of the central nervous system

Paraneoplastic syndromes

Neuropsychiatric aspects. Neuropsychiatric symptoms may be the presenting complaint and, like other MS symptoms, may exacerbate and remit or may be continuously present after onset. Treatment with steroids or other medications can contribute to these symptoms. Table 30–2 lists the principal neuropsychiatric manifestations of MS and their approximate frequencies.

Fatigue—a sense of tiredness or lack of energy that is greater than expected for the effort required for a task or the degree of disability evidenced by the patient (The Canadian MS Research Group 1987)—occurs in approximately 75% of patients with MS, often preventing normal activities (Murray 1985). It must be differentiated from symptoms of depression, weakness, lack of rest, or excessive exercise. Fatigue in patients with MS is exacerbated by heat and improves with cooler temperatures (Krupp et al. 1988).

Approximately 75% of men and 50% of women with MS report sexual dysfunction (Stenager et al. 1992). In men, two-thirds have erectile dysfunction, and one-third report decreased libido. In women, painful genital dysesthesias, inability to achieve orgasm, and decreased libido are common. Nearly 90% of the men have neurogenic causes for their erectile dysfunction (Kirkeby et al. 1988). Hypersexuality is uncommon, but has been reported in 4% of patients with MS (Mahler 1992).

Sleep disturbances are seen in a quarter of patients with MS (Clark et al. 1992). Most have problems with sleep initiation or maintenance and do not awaken feeling rested. The sleep disturbance may be associated with depression, fatigue, spasticity, bladder difficulties, or periodic leg movements.

It is important to distinguish between how the patient subjectively feels (mood) and the outward expression of his emotion (affect). Approximately 11% of patients with MS have difficulties regulating their emotional expression, resulting in rapid mood swings or inappropriate emotional responses (Minden and Schiffer 1990). Many patients have depressed moods in spite of a euphoric affect.

TABLE 30–2. Frequency of neuropsychiatric manifestations in multiple sclerosis

Neuropsychiatric manifestation	Frequency
Fatigue	75%
Sexual dysfunction	50% (women)
	75% (men)
Hypersexuality	4%
Sleep disturbance	25%
Emotional lability	11%
Depression	50%
Euphoria	25%
Mania	13%
Personality changes	40%
Psychosis	1%–3%
Cognitive dysfunction	30%–50%

Compared with patients with other chronic neurological diseases, patients with MS have significantly more depression. Approximately half of all patients with MS experience at least one episode of major depression during their illness. No association has been found between their depression and a family history of depression, duration of illness, age, gender, or socioeconomic status (Minden et al. 1987). Depression is associated with recent exacerbations of MS symptoms requiring steroid therapy, but not with severity of disability or cognitive impairment in most studies (Good et al. 1992; Schiffer and Caine 1991).

Euphoria—a cheerful affect inappropriate to the situation—occurs in about 25% of patients with MS (Rabins 1990). It is not associated with steroid use and does not have other features of hypomania. In fact, many patients with euphoria have a depressed mood. Euphoria appears to be produced by bilateral subfrontal demyelination (Minden and Schiffer 1990), and patients with euphoria have more neurological and cognitive deficits than those without euphoria (Rabins 1990).

Mania occurs in up to 13% of patients with MS (Joffe et al. 1987), and patients with MS have twice the risk of developing bipolar disorder as the general population. Human leukocyte antigen (HLA) analysis and family history studies suggest a genetic predisposition for bipolar disorder in patients with MS who manifest manic behavior (Schiffer et al. 1988).

Apathy, lack of concern over their disabilities, lack of initiation, impaired insight, irritability, and poor judgment are personality changes observed in as many as 40% of patients with MS (Mahler 1992) and may be related to frontal lobe dysfunctioning (Mendez 1995).

Psychosis in MS—including auditory or visual hallucinations, delusions, or paranoia—is seen in approximately 1%–3% of patients, and it occurs at a later age than in idiopathic schizophrenia (Feinstein et al. 1992; Ron and Logsdail 1989). Psychosis can occur without steroid use and without a family history of schizophrenia. Psychosis in MS is associated with increased temporal and temporoparietal lobe abnormalities on MRI (Feinstein et al. 1992; Honer et al. 1987; Ron and Logsdail 1989).

Cognitive dysfunction occurs in 40%–65% of patients with MS (Fennell and Smith 1990; Rao 1996), with most investigators emphasizing memory impairment. Approximately 20%–30% of patients with MS meet criteria for a dementia syndrome with deficits primarily involving poor retrieval memory, slowed information processing, visuospatial abnormalities, and frontal-executive dysfunctioning: a pattern suggestive of a subcortical dementia syndrome (Huber et al. 1987; Rao 1986). Corpus callosal atrophy on MRI and increased plaque volume correlate with the severity of cognitive impairment (Huber et al. 1992b; Swirsky-Sacchetti et al. 1992). The cognitive changes do not correlate with duration of disease or depression, but may be more severe in the chronic progressive type of MS typical of that in elderly patients (Minden et al. 1990; Rao et al. 1991). The cognitive changes weakly correlate with physical disability in some studies (Rao et al. 1991), but not in others (Maurelli et al. 1992).

Both verbal and nonverbal memory are impaired, with spatial memory being more severely affected in most studies (Beatty et al. 1988; Grafman et al. 1990). The memory deficit is a retrieval abnormality and not a true amnesia (Rao 1986). Remote memory is usually spared (Rao et al. 1991). Verbal IQ is generally better preserved than is performance IQ (Rao 1986). However, word list generation, also called *verbal fluency* (the number of words beginning with a certain letter produced in 1 minute or the number of animals named per minute), is often decreased (Beatty et al. 1988; Rao et al. 1991). Rarely, aphasic syndromes have been described (Achiron et al. 1992). Executive functions including planning, abstraction, concept formation, set shifting, sustained attention, and organization skills are affected in MS (Fennell and Smith 1990) and suggest frontal lobe dysfunction (Mendozzi et al. 1993). Frontal white matter lesions on MRI correlate with these disturbances (Comi et al. 1995; Huber et al. 1992a). Signs of corpus callosal disconnection have been identified with dichotic listening tasks (Rubens et al. 1985), with tachistoscopic object-naming tasks (Rao et al. 1989), and from the clinical examination demonstrating left-hand apraxia, agraphia, and astereognosis (Schnider et al. 1993). Corpus callosal atrophy on MRI has been demonstrated in these patients.

Pathophysiology and diagnosis. MS is believed to be caused by an immune-mediated response triggered by exposure to an unknown environmental agent in the genetically predisposed individual. This response results in multifocal discrete inflammatory demyelinated areas scattered throughout the white matter, including the arcuate U-fiber regions. MRI shows these plaques in the white matter as areas of high signal on T2-weighted images (Figure 30–3), and gadolinium contrast can distinguish active from inactive plaques (Bastianello et al. 1990). Diagnosis is aided by finding increased immunoglobulin production and oligoclonal bands in the CSF (Table 30–3) and prolonged latencies on evoked potential testing (Poser et al. 1983).

Treatment. Oral prednisone, intravenous methylprednisolone, and intramuscular adrenocorticotropic hormone (ACTH) appear to speed the recovery of an acute

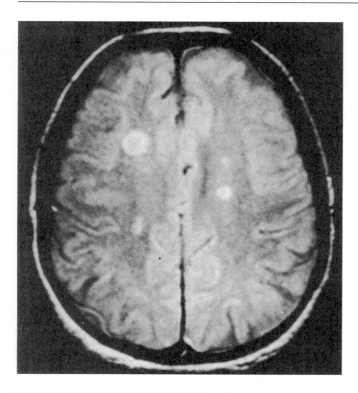

FIGURE 30–3.   Magnetic resonance image (MRI) of a 65-year-old woman with chronic progressive multiple sclerosis. MRI shows multiple areas of increased signal on the proton-density–weighted image in the right and left centrum semiovale regions.

exacerbation. Immunosuppressive drugs such as azathioprine, cyclophosphamide, and cyclosporin might have the potential to slow down the progression of MS, but their use is limited by potentially serious side effects. Intravenous immune globulin has also been recently tried (Achiron et al. 1996).

New therapies for relapsing-remitting MS, including interferon beta-1b given subcutaneously on alternate days (IFNB Multiple Sclerosis Study Group 1993; IFNB Multiple Sclerosis Study Group and University of British Columbia MS/MRI Analysis Group 1995; Lublin et al. 1996; Paty et al. 1993), interferon beta-1a given intramuscularly once weekly (Jacobs et al. 1996), and glatiramer acetate given subcutaneously daily (K. P. Johnson et al. 1995, 1998), are aimed at modifying the immune processes thought to be responsible for the pathogenesis of MS. These agents have had some effect on reducing the frequency and severity of relapses in patients with relapsing-remitting MS, reducing the progression of disability, and diminishing the number and size of MRI lesions. Combination therapies with corticosteroids, interferon beta, and glatiramer are being tried, but no formal results are available. Interferon beta products can produce antibodies

that may be associated with loss of efficacy under some circumstances in some patients, but this has not been consistent. Those with high titers may be more likely to become treatment nonresponders. Glatiramer, so far, has not been noted to produce antibodies associated with loss of efficacy.

Unfortunately, many of the immunotherapies can produce neuropsychiatric and other adverse effects. If used longer term, adrenocorticosteroids may cause serious infections, electrolyte disturbances, peptic ulcers, osteoporosis, myopathy, cataracts, and Cushing's habitus. Behavior disturbances include nervousness, insomnia, depression, mania, and psychosis. Immunosuppressive agents may also cause serious infections, increase risk of neoplasia, and cause multiple organ toxicities. The most common side effects of the immune modifying agents (interferon betas and glatiramer) are the injection site reactions. Postinjection flushing, palpitations, throat constriction, urticaria, and dyspnea can also occur. Dizziness, hypertonia, and tremor are seen with glatiramer, and seizures have been reported with the interferons. Neuropsychiatric side effects include fatigue, anxiety, depression, psychotic depression, and suicidality. Depression is a common reason for discontinuation of the interferon betas and glatiramer (Copaxone prescribing insert; Neilley et al. 1996). Although only 1% of patients spontaneously report depression after taking interferon beta-1b, as many as 40% in one study were actually experiencing new or increased symptoms of depression within 6 months of initiating therapy (Mohr et al. 1997). Treatment of the depression significantly reduced discontinuation of the interferon beta-1b (Mohr et al. 1997).

Management of specific symptoms may contribute to improved patient functioning. Spasticity is treated with a combination of physical therapy, tizanidine (Nance et al. 1997), baclofen, benzodiazepines, botulinum toxin, or dantrolene. Paroxysmal disorders respond to anticonvulsants. Bladder disorders and urinary tract infections are reduced by anticholinergics, self-catheterization, and prophylactic antibiotics.

Treatments for the neuropsychiatric manifestations are also available. Cognitive impairment may be helped with cholinesterase inhibitors (Leo and Rao 1988) or the use of memory aids, lists, routinization of daily activities, and other cognitive retraining strategies (LaRocca 1990). Pathological laughing or crying can be treated with low-dose amitriptyline (Schiffer et al. 1985) or fluoxetine (Seliger et al. 1992). Depression is treated with selective serotonin reuptake inhibitors with low side effects and very high response rates (Scott et al. 1996). Bipolar disorder is treated with lithium (Schiffer 1990) or sodium valproate. Anticholinergic agents may impair cognition but aid blad-

TABLE 30–3. Cerebrospinal fluid profiles of various conditions

Infection	White cells	Protein (mg/dL)	Glucose (mg/dL)	Miscellaneous
Multiple sclerosis	0–20 lymphocytosis	Normal, 100	Normal	Oligoclonal bands, IgG increase
Acute disseminated encephalomyelitis	10–4000 PMN, lymphocytes	Normal, 344	Normal	Increased pressure, occasional oligoclonal bands
Creutzfeldt-Jakob disease	0–15 lymphocytosis	Normal, 50–120	Normal	Occasional IgG increase, 14–3–3 brain protein
Herpes simplex encephalitis	50–1000 lymphocytosis	50–400	Normal	Culture, serology
Aseptic meningoencephalitis	5–1000 lymphocytosis	45–80	20–40, normal	Culture
HIV-1 dementia complex	0–8 lymphocytosis	< 80	Occasional decrease	IgG increase, culture
PML	0–8 lymphocytosis	< 80	Normal	PCR for JC virus DNA
Acute bacterial meningitis	100–60,000 PMN	100–1000	5–40	Culture, antigen detection
Brain abscess	0–500 PMN, lymphocytes	40–100	Occasional decrease	
Fungal meningitis	5–800 lymphocytosis	45–500	10–40, normal	Culture, cryptococcal antigen
Neurosyphilis	5–1000 lymphocytosis	50–100	< 40, normal	VDRL test, IgG increase
Neuroborreliosis (Lyme disease)	0–150 lymphocytosis	40–100	Normal	IgG increase, serology
Isolated angiitis of the CNS	0–800 lymphocytosis	40–600	Occasional decrease	Occasional IgG increase
Lymphomatoid granulomatosis	0–225 atypical lymphocytes	40–780	Normal	Occasional oligoclonal bands
Behçet's syndrome	0–500 lymphocytosis	Normal to 160	Normal	Occasional IgG increase, blood-brain barrier breakdown
SLE	0–50 lymphocytosis	Normal to 100	Normal	Oligoclonal bands, IgG increase, antineuronal antibodies, blood-brain barrier breakdown
Sjögren's syndrome	Mild lymphocytosis	Normal to 100	Normal	Oligoclonal bands, IgG increase

Note. CNS = central nervous system; IgG = immunoglobulin G; HIV-1 = human immunodeficiency virus type 1; PCR = polymerase chain reaction; PML = progressive multifocal leukoencephalopathy; PMN = polymorphonuclear cells; SLE = systemic lupus erythematosus; VDRL = Venereal Disease Research Laboratory.

Sources. From Alexander 1993; Ashwal 1995; Bale 1991; Brink and Miller 1996; Bushunow et al. 1996; Fishman 1992; Geerts et al. 1991; Halperin et al. 1991; Hsich et al. 1996; Kirschbaum 1968; Kleinschmidt-DeMasters et al. 1992; Levy et al. 1985; Marshall et al. 1988; McLean et al. 1995; Navia et al. 1986b; Pachner 1995; Schmidt 1989; West et al. 1995; Whitley and Lakeman 1995; and Younger et al. 1988.

der symptoms; the choice of treatment in any individual will depend on the relative anticholinergic effect desired. Fatigue may be ameliorated by amantadine (The Canadian MS Research Group 1987; Murray 1985) or pemoline (Weinshenker et al. 1992) or with steroids if associated with an acute exacerbation. Pharmacotherapy reassessment is essential to eliminate agents no longer needed. Support groups and psychotherapy are useful for information exchange, social interaction, stress reduction, and emotional support (Minden and Moes 1990).

Acute Disseminated Encephalomyelitis

Acute necrotizing hemorrhagic, postinfectious, and postvaccinal encephalomyelitis are forms of acute disseminated encephalomyelitis, an immune-mediated condition resulting in CNS demyelination. It can occur at any age. It is typically, but not exclusively, a monophasic illness presenting with fever, headache, and altered consciousness and typically preceded days or weeks earlier by either viral illness or vaccination (Geerts et al. 1991). The hemorrhagic form is usually, but not always, rapidly fatal (Huang et al. 1988). If the individual survives the acute condition, gradual recovery over days to weeks ensues. Hemiparesis, sensory deficits, seizures, dysarthria, or dysphasia may be present initially (Geerts et al. 1991). The neuropsychiatric residua vary depending on the degree of injury and extent of recovery. A subcortical dementia syndrome similar to that seen in multiple sclerosis is typical. Inflammation, demyelination, and variable hemorrhage occurs in the white matter. Neuroimaging studies show multifocal abnormalities and large lesions that often involve the cortex with very little periventricular or callosal involvement (Kesselring et al. 1990). CSF cultures are negative (Table 30–3). A brain biopsy may be required to rule out infection or tumor. Treatment is supportive and may require reduction of increased intracranial pressure. Surgical decompression has been recommended for the hemorrhagic form (Huang et al. 1988). Immunosuppression has been used with some success (Seales and Greer 1991).

Binswanger's Disease

Binswanger's disease, also called *subcortical arteriosclerotic encephalopathy*, is a vascular dementia resulting from hypoxic ischemia involving the small penetrating vessels supplying the deep white matter of the cerebral hemispheres. It occurs in elderly individuals, most with a history of chronic hypertension. A gradually progressive course of dementia with frontal features and personality change is typical. Neuropsychiatric findings include memory deficits, executive impairment, decreased attention, poor judgment, lack of spontaneity, reduced drive, apathy, perseveration, pseudobulbar palsy, emotional incontinence, and at times euphoria, elation, and aggressiveness (Babikian and Ropper 1987; McPherson and Cummings 1996). Weakness, ataxia, rigidity, small-stepped gait, frequent falls, frontal release signs, dysarthria, and urinary incontinence are typical neurological abnormalities. White matter demyelination is seen pathologically, and MRI reveals hyperintensities on T2-weighted images in the periventricular and deep white matter regions. Binswanger's disease and lacunar state commonly co-occur.

Marchiafava-Bignami Disease

Marchiafava-Bignami disease is characterized by demyelination of the corpus callosum and adjacent white matter. It is rare and occurs mostly in middle to late adult life in men who are chronically alcoholic. Many individuals exhibit a chronic dementia syndrome that progresses over months to years. Remissions are possible. Severe cases

present in stupor or coma, and the patient dies rapidly.

The neuropsychiatric features vary widely from case to case. The CNS manifestations include dementia, aphasia, slow information processing, frontal release signs, dysarthria, incontinence, hemiparesis, seizures, apraxic gait, and signs of corpus callosum interhemispheric disconnection such as left-sided limb apraxia, left-hand anomia, and agraphia (Lechevalier et al. 1977; Victor 1993). Personality changes, apathy, violence, and sexual deviations have also been reported.

Demyelination of the corpus callosum with relative sparing of the splenium and absence of inflammatory changes is the characteristic pathology. Less often, the anterior or posterior commissures, centrum semiovale, superior cerebellar peduncles, or the white matter of the pons are involved. MRI scans show demyelination essentially limited to the callosum (Chang et al. 1992). Alcoholic abstinence and proper nutrition is recommended.

Subacute Combined Degeneration

Subacute combined degeneration is caused by vitamin B_{12} (or rarely folate) deficiency, which produces demyelination in the spinal cord and brain. This condition can occur at any age and may be secondary to pernicious anemia, malabsorption syndromes, acquired immunodeficiency, stomach or small bowel resections, stomach acid–reducing agents, or rarely from a dietary B_{12} deficiency (Swain 1995). Clinical features of subacute combined degeneration are variable from case to case, but may include peripheral neuropathy, myelopathy, gait disturbance, incontinence, visual impairment, megaloblastic anemia, dementia, and neuropsychiatric syndromes.

Confusion, memory impairment, slow reaction time, and perseveration are common cognitive findings (Cummings and Benson 1992). The dementia may occasionally precede other systemic manifestations of the vitamin deficiency (Karnaze and Carmel 1990). Neuropsychiatric manifestations include apathy, depression, personality changes, agitation, aggression, paranoia, delusions, and hallucinations (Clementz and Schade 1990; Lindenbaum et al. 1988). Numbness, tingling, lower-extremity weakness, and gait disturbance may progress to flaccid paralysis and incontinence.

The dorsal and lateral columns of the spinal cord and the white matter in the brain show areas of spongiform degenerative demyelination. EEG reveals generalized slowing in those with dementia. A low serum B_{12} level is usually diagnostic. Serum methylmalonic acid and homocysteine are good confirmatory tests, and malabsorption is demonstrated by performing a Schilling test. Administration of vitamin B_{12} may reverse or stop the progression of the neurological symptoms and dementia.

Postanoxic/Posthypoxic States

Elderly individuals are particularly prone to anoxia/hypoxia from cardiopulmonary failure or sleep apnea. Chronic hypoxia results in a slowly progressive dementia syndrome, whereas acute anoxia can lead to profound neuronal injury and death. Rarely, patients may develop extensive white matter demyelination a few weeks after apparent recovery from an acute anoxic insult. The delayed symptoms include slowed responses, somnolence, irritability, depression, inattentiveness, disorientation, forgetfulness, pseudobulbar palsy, mutism, incontinence, gait disturbances, and spasticity (Plum et al. 1962). Death often occurs, but moderate recovery has been observed. Postanoxic demyelination is seen diffusely over both cerebral hemispheres on MRI.

Radiation and Chemotherapy-Related Leukoencephalopathy

Neoplastic conditions are very common in the geriatric population, and both radiation therapy and chemotherapy are often used either alone or in combination to treat the tumors. These therapies can be used either to reduce the tumor burden or as a prophylactic to reduce the likelihood of potential brain or spinal cord metastases. However, both may also lead to delayed demyelination of the CNS occurring from 3 months to 5 years after the treatment. The neurological complications of cranial irradiation include memory loss, cognitive decline, abulia, gait disturbance, ataxia, pyramidal tract signs, and tremors. Patients may become severely disabled with dementia and paresis (B. E. Johnson et al. 1985).

Chemotherapeutic agents cause a delayed demyelination thought to be secondary to oligodendrocyte neurotoxicity. The neurological findings are similar to the delayed effects of radiation treatment. Methotrexate is the most notable example of such an agent, especially when given intrathecally (Ojeda 1982). Cyclosporine (de Groen et al. 1987), cytosine arabinoside (Lee et al. 1986), and 5-fluorouracil combined with levamisole (C. C. Hook et al. 1992) have all been reported to cause demyelination. The combination of radiation therapy and chemotherapy, particularly when using methotrexate, cisplatin, lomustine, or amphotericin B, appears to enhance the neurotoxicity (So et al. 1987; Walker and Rosenblum 1992).

Demyelination with necrosis is the pathological finding seen with the delayed effects of radiation on the CNS.

Demyelination with or without necrosis has also been reported with the use of chemotherapeutic agents (C. C. Hook et al. 1992; Ojeda 1982). Diffuse symmetric white matter low attenuation, cerebral atrophy, ventricular dilation, and occasionally mass effect are seen with CT scanning of the head (So et al. 1987). MRI reveals increased signal on the T2-weighted images in the periventricular white matter in a diffuse, symmetric, and confluent pattern. Scattered focal lesions that enhance with gadolinium are also common (C. C. Hook et al. 1992; So et al. 1987).

Metachromatic Leukodystrophy

Metachromatic leukodystrophy (MLD) is a dysmyelinating disorder with infantile, juvenile, and adult forms. The adult form may present from ages 16 to 40 and will usually last from 5 to 20 years, but occasionally as long as 40 years. The enzyme deficient in this autosomal recessive inheritable disorder is arylsulfatase A. Personality changes and cognitive decline mark the insidious onset of the adult form (Baumann et al. 1991). Disinhibition, poor judgment, dishevelment, inappropriate affect, emotional lability, looseness of associations, diminished attention span, memory deficits, abstraction and calculation difficulties, spatial disorientation, and constructional problems are seen (Merriam et al. 1990). This progresses to psychosis (present in more than 50% of cases), occasionally mania, and dementia (Hyde et al. 1992). Spasticity, ataxia, and seizures are often present. Resting and postural tremors and choreoathetosis have occasionally been described (Merriam et al. 1990). Peripheral neuropathy, in the adult form, may not be clinically evident though present electrophysiologically. Sulfatide deposits are present around both central and peripheral nerves and in viscera. Demyelination sparing the arcuate fibers (U-fibers) is present in the cerebral hemispheres and evident on neuroimaging. Motor and sensory nerve conduction velocities are mildly slowed, and increased CSF protein is occasionally found. Diagnosis is made by measuring the enzyme deficiency in leukocytes or measuring the amount of sulfatide in urine (Baumann et al. 1991). Genetic counseling is indicated.

Adrenoleukodystrophy

Adrenoleukodystrophy (ALD) is an X-linked dysmyelinating disorder featuring a deficiency of a peroxisomal enzyme that results in the excessive storage of very long chain fatty acids (VLCFAs) (Naidu and Moser 1990). There are neonatal, juvenile, adolescent, and adult cerebral forms as well as an X-linked adrenomyeloneuropathy (AMN) form. The adult cerebral form, representing approximately 3% of all cases, may present from ages 18 to 57 (Weller et al. 1992). The AMN form, found in 21% of all cases, typically has its onset between ages 20 and 35 and rarely occurs in later adult life. Approximately 10%–15% of the women who are ALD carriers develop neurological deficits resembling AMN with onset between age 15 and 76 (Naidu and Moser 1990).

The initial finding in the adult cerebral form of ALD is usually dementia. Other neurological findings include upper motor neuron signs, paresis, ataxia, gait apraxia, dysarthria, homonymous hemianopsia, impaired visual acuity leading to cortical blindness, ocular movement disorders, and hearing loss. Seizures are a late finding. Psychiatric features are seen in nearly 40% of patients, often occur early in the course, and include hypomania, emotional lability, depression, hyperactivity, physical and sexual aggression, and psychosis (Kitchin et al. 1987). Adrenal insufficiency and a bronze discoloration of the skin typically become evident after the neurological symptoms begin. The AMN form begins with a progressive spastic paraparesis and a mild peripheral neuropathy, with 20% of patients eventually developing dementia. Emotional lability and depression have also been observed (Naidu and Moser 1990). In ALD, there is demyelination of cerebral white matter sparing the arcuate fibers. Increased signal on T2-weighted images is present in the periventricular white matter on MRI scanning, typically starting occipitally and progressing anteriorly. CSF protein is increased. Diagnosis is made by assaying VLCFAs in plasma or skin fibroblasts. A low cortisol level or a reduced adrenal response to stimulation indicates adrenal insufficiency. Treatment includes a low-VLCFA diet with erucic and oleic acid; adrenal steroids are used for the adrenal dysfunction.

Cerebrotendinous Xanthomatosis

Cerebrotendinous xanthomatosis is an autosomal recessive disorder resulting in impaired hepatic synthesis of bile salts, leading to markedly increased levels of cholestanol. Age at onset ranges from infancy to the seventh decade. Clinical features include cataracts, tuberous and tendon xanthomas, dementia, ataxia, pyramidal tract signs, spasticity, dysarthria, seizures, depression, and a demyelinating neuropathy. Early atherosclerosis with coronary artery disease is also common. The tendon xanthomas often begin between ages 20 and 40. Cognitive decline can appear in childhood or be delayed well past middle age. Spasticity and ataxia progress, and, in the terminal stage, incontinence and pseudobulbar palsy are present. Pathology shows extensor tendon xanthomas and brain deposi-

tion of high-density lipoprotein. CSF examination demonstrates a mildly elevated protein. CT and MRI scanning reveal atrophy, focal tuberous xanthomas, and demyelination in the cerebellum and cerebrum (Hokezu et al. 1992). Diagnosis is confirmed by finding elevated levels of cholestanol in plasma or bile. Early treatment with chenodeoxycholic acid to reduce the formation of cholestanol may reverse and prevent the clinical findings (Bjorkhem and Skrede 1990).

Infectious Disorders

Infectious conditions producing neuropsychiatric signs and symptoms are common at all ages. In the elderly population, diagnosis is more difficult because certain systemic signs such as fever may not be present, whereas other nonspecific symptoms such as confusion, headache, malaise, generalized weakness, and diminished appetite may be more prominent. Progression to an acute confusional state or delirium with hallucinations, delusions, paranoia, impaired attention, disorientation, cognitive deficits, sleep disturbance, and tremors may occur rapidly. Consideration of infectious etiologies at an early stage enables prompt diagnosis and treatment. Neuroimaging with MRI or CT followed by lumbar puncture and, potentially, brain biopsy are often necessary to determine the specific pathogen. Common CNS infections of the geriatric age group are listed in Table 30–4.

Prion Infections

Prions are *pro*teinaceous *in*fectious particles consisting of protein without nucleic acid. They can cause transmissible diseases, can be inherited on chromosome 20 in 10%–15% of cases, or may occur sporadically (DeArmond and Prusiner 1995; Prusiner 1995). The normal prion protein is hypothesized to be converted posttranslationally from an α-helix to an abnormal β-sheet conformation that is insoluble to detergents, tends to aggregate, and can induce normal prion proteins to change their conformation to the abnormal form, causing accumulation of prions to sufficient levels to cause a progressive neurodegenerative disease state (Prusiner and Hsiao 1994).

Creutzfeldt-Jakob disease. Creutzfeldt-Jakob disease (CJD) has a worldwide incidence of approximately 1 per 1 million. Approximately 90% of CJD cases arise sporadically without evidence of any infectious source, 5%–15% are familial, with an autosomal dominant inheritance, and rare iatrogenically transmitted cases have oc-

TABLE 30–4. Causes of central nervous system infections in elderly patients

Prions

   Creutzfeldt-Jakob disease (CJD)

   Gerstmann-Straüssler-Scheinker syndrome (GSS)

   Fatal familial insomnia

   Kuru

   New variant CJD

Virus

   Acute viral encephalitis

      Herpes simplex encephalitis

      Other meningoencephalitides

   Slow viral encephalitis

      Human immunodeficiency virus type 1 (HIV-1)

      Progressive multifocal leukoencephalopathy (PML)

Bacteria

   Acute bacterial meningitis

   Brain abscess

   Subdural empyema

   Epidural abscess

   Tuberculosis (meningitis)

   Whipple's disease

Fungus

   Chronic meningitis

   Spirochetes

   Syphilis

   Lyme disease

Parasites

   Toxoplasma

   Cysticercosis

   Amoeba

curred in humans from corneal transplants, depth electrodes, neurosurgical instrumentation, a cadaveric dura mater graft, and human growth hormone that was extracted from human cadaveric pituitaries (Rappaport 1987; Wasielewski et al. 1997).

The usual age at onset is between 50 and 70, with a range from 20 to 79 (Cummings and Benson 1992). The clinical course is typically very rapid: death usually comes within several months to 1 year. Occasionally, individuals have survived for several years. The familial forms have an earlier age at onset and a longer duration of illness (Brown et al. 1992).

Initially, the patient has complaints of generalized fatigue, anxiety, sleep disturbance, appetite change, depression, impaired concentration, and forgetfulness. After a few weeks, a progressive dementia ensues with aphasia, amnesia, apraxia, and agnosia. Myoclonus, chorea, tremor, ataxia, cerebellar signs, pyramidal signs, spasticity, rigidity, and seizures typically occur after the dementia has started. Hallucinations and delusions are also seen. Mutism, incontinence, decerebrate rigidity, and akinesis occur in the final phases (Brown et al. 1986; Cummings and Benson 1992).

Pathology shows a spongiform state in the cortical and subcortical gray matter with loss of neurons and gliosis (Masters et al. 1981). The spongiform changes reflect the occurrence of intracellular vacuoles. Occasionally, white matter gliosis and demyelination are also seen. Some patients with CJD have amyloid plaques in the cerebellum and cerebrum similar to those found in kuru. MRI results may be normal or reveal mild atrophy and areas of increased signal on T2-weighted images (Milton et al. 1991). PET and SPECT show multiple diffuse areas of hypometabolism/hypoperfusion in both cortical and subcortical regions (Goldman et al. 1993; Watanabe et al. 1996) (Figure 30–4). CSF showing a positive immunoassay for the 14-3-3 brain protein is strongly supportive of CJD (Hsich et al. 1996) (Table 30–3). The EEG shows background slowing and a characteristic periodic polyspike discharge (Chiofalo et al. 1980); this EEG pattern may be absent in the familial forms of CJD (Brown et al. 1992). Diagnosis can be made by the clinical features, EEG, and CSF and is confirmed by brain biopsy if the features are atypical. Treatment is not available except for supportive care.

Other prion diseases.   Gerstmann-Straüssler-Scheinker (GSS) syndrome is a rare autosomal dominant disorder with onset between ages 40 and 60. Seven known point mutations in the prion protein gene can result in the GSS syndrome (Prusiner 1996), which is characterized by a mild dementia with pyramidal, extrapyramidal, and cerebellar signs (Farlow et al. 1989). Ataxia is the usual presenting manifestation followed by dementia. Gaze palsies, deafness, and blindness may occur.

Fatal familial insomnia (FFI), sometimes referred to as familial thalamic dementia, is caused by a point mutation on the prion protein gene at codon 178 combined with a polymorphism at codon 129 (Medori et al. 1992; Petersen et al. 1992). FFI does not appear to be transmissible and has a course and presentation similar to CJD with the addition of progressive insomnia and dysautonomia. Onset is usually at about age 50 with a 12- to 13-month course to death. Patients often develop dysarthria, ataxia, myoclonus, pyramidal tract signs, insomnia, and autonomic disturbances including hyperhidrosis, hyperthermia, tachycardia, and hypertension. Although the neuropathology in FFI of neuronal loss and gliosis seems mostly restricted to the anterior and dorsal medial thalamic nuclei, these nuclei have tremendous connections with specific frontal lobe regions, and neuropsychological evaluation of these patients reveals significant executive dysfunctioning with difficulties with working memory, attention, sequencing, and planning abilities (Gallassi et al. 1992). Confusion, disorientation, and hallucinations can also be seen.

Kuru and new variant CJD are transmissible prion diseases affecting humans. Kuru is seen in certain New Guinea tribes who practice ritualistic cannibalism. New variant CJD appears to be a novel epidemic caused by the spread of bovine spongiform encephalopathy (BSE), a prion disease affecting cattle, to humans who consume BSE-contaminated cattle-derived products (Epstein and Brown 1997; Schonberger 1998).

Viral Infections

Viral infections can be classified as either acute, with a rapid onset of symptoms, or slow, with a chronic course over months to years (Table 30–4). The clinical features of the

infection relate to the selective vulnerability of certain cell types to the particular virus (R. T. Johnson 1982).

Herpes simplex encephalitis.   Herpes simplex encephalitis, an acute infection, is a common cause of encephalitis in elderly patients and is often treatable, but mortality is high. Incidence is about 1/400,000 per year, with half of all cases occurring in those over age 50 (Whitley 1991).

Initial clinical features include headache, fever, stiff neck, and photophobia. These symptoms progress over a few days to produce lethargy, mental status changes, memory impairment, aphasia, focal neurological deficits, seizures, and eventually coma (Whitley 1991). Recovery may be complete or partial. Frontal and temporal lobe involvement are common (Kapur et al. 1994). Frontal lobe injury often results in grasp reflexes, frontal release signs, motor impersistence, disinhibition, impulsivity, psychomotor hyperactivity, hyperoral behavior, apathy, echolalia, mutism, anomia, inattention, and utilization behaviors (Brazzelli et

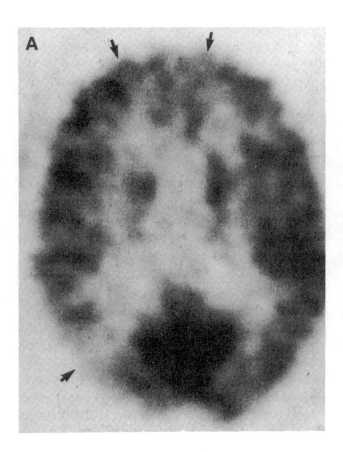 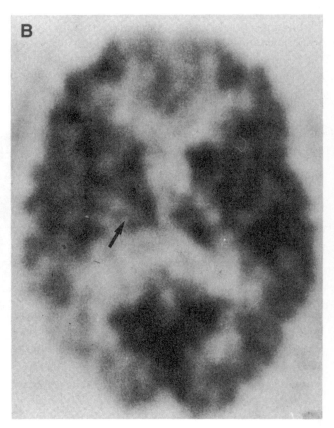

FIGURE 30–4.   Positron-emission tomography (PET) image of a 63-year-old man with autopsy-proven Creutzfeldt-Jakob disease. *Panel A:* PET shows multifocal areas of cortical hypometabolism involving the right parieto-occipital region and the bilateral frontal areas (*arrows*). *Panel B:* A slightly caudal PET slice revealing the relative hypometabolism seen in the right basal ganglia region (*arrow*).

al. 1994). Temporal lobe damage often causes amnesia, hallucinations, and, if bilateral, the Klüver-Bucy syndrome, which is characterized by hyperoral behavior, dietary changes, hypersexuality, placidity, visual agnosia, and hypermetamorphosis (excessive tactile exploration of the environment). Aphasia or dementia syndrome may be permanent (Cummings and Benson 1992).

Hemorrhagic necrosis and petechial hemorrhages are seen in the brain at autopsy. The medial temporal, insular, cingulate, and orbitotemporal regions are the areas most commonly involved (Okazaki 1983). Periodic lateralizing epileptiform discharges (PLEDs) are the usual focal EEG abnormality, seen in 80% of patients (Bale 1991). MRI often shows focal areas of increased T2 signal in the temporal/insular or frontal regions (Schroth et al. 1987). An imaging study is often necessary before the lumbar puncture to rule out a mass lesion. The lumbar puncture usually suggests a viral infection, and application of polymerase chain reaction (PCR) can confirm a specific diagnosis of herpes simplex virus infection in the brain (Whitley and Lakeman 1995) (Table 30–3). Brain biopsy is diagnostic, but is not always accurate, and it has an acute morbidity of at least 3% (Whitley 1991). Therapy with acyclovir (30 mg/kg body weight per day in three divided doses for 10 days) is started empirically and immediately because the toxic effects are minimal and mortality is reduced from 70% to 19% (Whitley 1991).

Other meningoencephalitides. The arboviruses are frequent causes of meningoencephalitis in the elderly population (Ho and Hirsch 1985). All are mosquito borne, and all have seasonal and geographic preferences. St. Louis encephalitis is the most common type in the United States. In a study of eastern equine encephalitis, 40% of all cases occurred in patients over age 50 (Przelomski et al. 1988). Western equine encephalitis is common particularly in young children and the elderly. Rubella, mumps, measles, Coxsackieviruses, polio, and adenoviruses typically occur in younger age groups (Bale 1991).

The acute prodromes of viral meningoencephalitides are all similar to that described for herpes simplex encephalitis above. The specific neurological deficits depend on the extent and distribution of the infection. Lethargy, mental status changes, focal neurological deficits, seizures, and coma may occur. The syndrome of inappropriate antidiuretic hormone (SIADH) secretion is common with St. Louis encephalitis (Ho and Hirsch 1985). Permanent postencephalitic intellectual deficits have been observed with several arbovirus infections including western equine, eastern equine, Japanese, and St. Louis encephalitis (Cummings and Benson 1992).

Human immunodeficiency virus type 1. Human immunodeficiency virus type 1 (HIV-1) is a retrovirus that preferentially infects helper T cells (Pantaleo et al. 1993). As the number of helper T cells declines, acquired immunodeficiency syndrome (AIDS) occurs, making the individual susceptible to numerous opportunistic infections (Centers for Disease Control 1992). The virus is constantly mutating, and certain virus types are able to enter the CNS easily and early in the course of the infection, making neurological symptoms common. High-risk groups include homosexual men, intravenous drug users, users of crack cocaine, individuals who receive contaminated blood products, heterosexual partners of HIV-1–infected individuals, and children of HIV-1–infected mothers (Rosenblum et al. 1988). Although this disease is most prevalent among men between ages 25 and 44, undoubtedly an increasing number of cases will be identified in the geriatric population.

It is estimated that 30 million people worldwide are infected with HIV-1 (Kahn and Walker 1998). Nearly everyone infected is expected to eventually develop AIDS. In 1996, more than 235,000 cases of AIDS in the United States alone were recorded (Centers for Disease Control 1997). The median period of time between the initial infection and the development of AIDS is 10 years. Elderly individuals, however, have a more rapid course.

Only 40%–90% of new HIV-1 infections are associated with symptomatic illness (Kahn and Walker 1998). The most common signs and symptoms of HIV-1 infection include fever, lethargy, rash, headache, lymphadenopathy, pharyngitis, myalgias, arthralgias, diarrhea, vomiting, and night sweats (Kahn and Walker 1998). Neurological and neuropsychiatric symptoms occur early, and opportunistic infections account for many additional clinical syndromes (Table 30–5).

Diagnosis of HIV-1 infection itself is made by detecting serum antibodies to HIV-1 proteins using HIV-1 enzyme-linked immunosorbent assay (ELISA) testing (Kahn and Walker 1998). At the time of seroconversion, some individuals develop a primary HIV-1 meningitis consisting of fever, headache, meningismus, and CSF pleocytosis (Cooper et al. 1985). Individuals may then become asymptomatic and have either mild (Bornstein et al. 1992) or no (McArthur et al. 1989) abnormalities on neuropsychological testing. However, once systemic findings appear (lymphadenopathy syndrome or AIDS-related complex [ARC]), 50% of these individuals have neurological signs or symptoms, and 50% have abnormalities on neuropsychological testing (Janssen et al. 1988). Mental and motoric slowness (Kieburtz and Schiffer 1989), referred to as the *HIV-1 associated minor cognitive/motor disorder*, is the most

TABLE 30–5.   Neurological disorders in human immunodeficiency virus–type 1 (HIV-1) infection

Primary HIV-1 infection
    Aseptic meningitis
    HIV-1–associated minor cognitive/motor disorder
    HIV-1–associated dementia complex
    HIV-1–associated myelopathy
    HIV-1–associated acute inflammatory demyelinating polyradiculoneuropathy (HIV-1–associated Guillain-Barré syndrome)
    Chronic inflammatory demyelinating polyneuropathy
    HIV-1–associated predominantly sensory polyneuropathy
    Mononeuritis multiplex
    HIV-1–associated myopathy
    Vasculitis (stroke)

Opportunistic infections
    Viral
        Cytomegalovirus (meningoencephalitis, retinitis, myelitis)
        Papovavirus (progressive multifocal leukoencephalopathy)
        Herpes simplex virus (myelitis, encephalitis)
        Varicella zoster virus (myelitis, encephalitis)
    Nonviral
        Toxoplasma gondii (meningoencephalitis)
        Mycobacteria (meningitis)
        Cryptococcus neoformans (meningitis, brain abscess)
        Aspergillus fumigatus (meningitis, brain abscess)
        Histoplasma capsulatum (meningitis, brain abscess)
        Candida albicans (meningitis, brain abscess)
        Coccidioides immitis (meningitis, brain abscess)
        Nocardia asteroides (brain abscess)
        Mucormycosis (brain abscess)
        Listeria monocytogenes (meningitis)
        Escherichia coli (meningitis)
        Syphilis (meningovascular)
        Amebic infections (brain abscess)

Opportunistic neoplasms
    Primary central nervous system lymphoma
    Metastatic systemic lymphoma
    Metastatic Kaposi's sarcoma

Other conditions
    Stroke (endocarditis, tumor hemorrhage)
    Drug intoxication or withdrawal

common abnormality (American Academy of Neurology AIDS Task Force 1991). Impaired memory, poor reasoning skills, and slow information processing speed are common (Rao 1996). By the time AIDS has been diagnosed, neurological complications are seen in 60% of individuals, and at autopsy neurological damage is found in 70%–90% (Kieburtz and Schiffer 1989).

HIV-1–associated dementia (subacute encephalopathy, HIV encephalopathy, or AIDS dementia complex) is the initial manifestation of AIDS in 7% of all patients with AIDS, but in those over age 74 it is the initial manifestation in 19% (Janssen et al. 1992). It affects 15%–20% of all patients with AIDS (Power and Johnson 1995). It is characterized by progression over weeks to months of a subcortical dementia syndrome with mental slowness, impaired concentration, forgetfulness, cognitive abnormalities, apathy, social withdrawal, slowed motor skills, ataxia, and weakness, potentially resulting in severe global cognitive dysfunction, paraplegia, mutism, and incontinence (American Academy of Neurology AIDS Task Force 1991; R. W. Price et al. 1988). Agitation, delusions, and hallucinations occur in a few patients (Cummings and Benson 1992). Neuropsychological testing reveals deficits particularly in nonverbal tasks and frontal lobe tasks including Trails B and verbal fluency (Hestad et al. 1993; Power and Johnson 1995). CT and MRI scans show generalized cerebral atrophy and periventricular white matter abnormalities (Ekholm and Simon 1988; Navia et al. 1986b). EEG results are either normal or show moderate diffuse slowing (Koppel et al. 1985). CSF is abnormal but nonspecific (Marshall et al. 1988; Navia et al. 1986b) (Table 30–3). The pathology of the HIV-1–associated dementia consists of reactive gliosis and microglial nodules, especially in the subcortical white and gray matter (Masliah et al. 1992; Navia et al. 1986a). Since the advent of zidovudine and other antiviral agents, HIV-1–associated dementia occurs less frequently and its progression is slowed (Atkinson and Grant 1994; Bartlett and Moore 1998; Schmitt et al. 1988).

Using combinations of newer antiviral agents, treatment of the neurological complications of AIDS has dramatically improved (Henry 1995). Currently the most effective treatments involve three of four drugs: two nucleoside analogues that inhibit reverse transcriptase and one or two protease inhibitors that prevents cleavage of HIV proteins (Bartlett and Moore 1998). Neuropsychiatric side effects of these treatments include fatigue, malaise, myopathy, and confusion with zidovudine; dose-related, occasionally painful, peripheral neuropathy with stavudine, didanosine, and zalcitabine; and paresthesias with ritonavir (The Medical Letter 1997).

Opportunistic infections and neoplasms involving the CNS are listed in Table 30–5 (Bale 1991; Kieburtz and Schiffer 1989; Levy and Bredesen 1988). Progressive multifocal leukoencephalopathy (PML) and cryptococcal meningitis are discussed below. CMV encephalitis in its severe forms causes diffuse, bilateral cerebral dysfunction with impaired alertness. Neuroimaging can occasionally show subependymal enhancement (Price 1996). Cerebral toxoplasmosis and primary CNS lymphoma can be diagnosed by clinical presentation, neuroimaging, and a treatment trial or occasionally a brain biopsy (Bale 1991). Cerebral toxoplasmosis evolves in only a few days, with focal neurological findings and enhancing lesions with mass effect and edema on MRI (Figure 30–5). Primary CNS lymphoma also causes focal neurological deficits but progresses more slowly, and MRI lesions are more diffuse in the deep white matter. Treatment with zidovudine and other antiviral agents lowers the frequency and mortality of opportunistic infections (Bartlett and Moore 1998; Schmitt et al. 1988). Specific treatments are also available for many of the opportunistic infections and neoplasms (Bale 1991).

Intracerebral hemorrhages, embolic infarctions from nonbacterial thrombotic endocarditis, strokes resulting from vasculitis, and medication effects also contribute to the neurological deficits seen with HIV-1 infection (Engstrom et al. 1989; Ochitill and Dilley 1988) (Table 30–5).

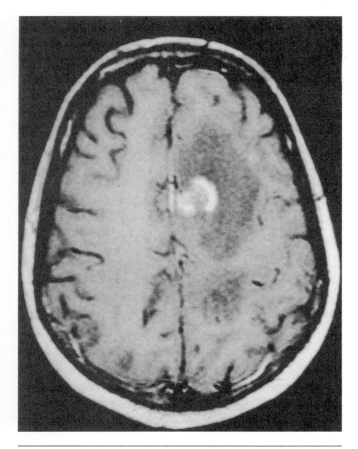

FIGURE 30–5. Gadolinium-enhanced T1-weighted magnetic resonance image (MRI) of an individual with acquired immunodeficiency syndrome (AIDS) and a cerebral abscess resulting from toxoplasmosis. MRI reveals a mass lesion in the left medial frontal region with surrounding edema.

Progressive multifocal leukoencephalopathy. PML caused by the papovavirus, JC virus, typically occurs in patients with deficits in cell-mediated immunity, particularly in association with AIDS or lymphoproliferative diseases or in those receiving immunosuppressive therapy (Holman et al. 1991). Onset is usually between ages 30 and 70, but can range from ages 6 to 84 (Stoner et al. 1988). The disease typically progresses over several weeks or months to death in less than 1 year (Bale 1991).

The neurological manifestations are multifocal. Impaired concentration, visuospatial deficits, memory impairment, speech disturbance, aphasia, calculation deficits, cognitive decline, hemianopsia, slowing of motor speed, paresis, sensory deficits, incoordination, and ataxia are common (Berger et al. 1987; Cummings and Benson 1992). Depression and agitation have been reported (Stagno et al. 1990). Fever or other systemic signs are not present.

Pathologically, multifocal demyelination is found in the subcortical white matter, particularly in the frontal and parieto-occipital regions (Whiteman et al. 1993). In these subcortical regions, axons are spared, but the oligodendrocytes and myelin are destroyed. Circling the demyelinative foci, enlarged oligodendrocytes with intranuclear inclusions consisting of papovavirus are present (R. T. Johnson 1982). MRI shows areas of demyelination without mass effect or contrast enhancement (Berger et al. 1987; Brink and Miller 1996), and PET studies show diminished metabolism in the same areas (Kiyosawa et al. 1988). CSF may confirm PML by detection of the CSF JC virus DNA (Brink and Miller 1996) (Table 30–3). Diagnosis is also made by brain biopsy, and treatment is supportive (Greenlee 1998).

Bacterial Infections

Acute bacterial meningitis. The incidence of bacterial meningitis is 5/100,000 per year. Mortality can be as high as 35% in those over age 65 (Behrman et al. 1989). Common organisms causing acute bacterial meningitis in the elderly population are *Streptococcus pneumoniae*, *Neisseria meningitidis*, *Listeria monocytogenes*, *Haemophilus influenzae* type B, and other Gram-negative bacilli (Ashwal 1995; Behrman et al. 1989; Durand et al. 1993; Stacy and Roeltgen 1991). Predisposing conditions such as diabetes, cancer, recent craniotomy, sinus surgery, skull fractures, or immunosuppressive therapy are present in about 35% of cases, and concurrent infections occur in approximately 40% of cases (Behrman et al. 1989).

Initial symptoms of a bacterial meningitis include

fever, headache, stiff neck, photophobia, nausea, and vomiting. Agitation, lethargy, and often, especially in the elderly, acute confusional states follow. Mental status changes are more common than are meningismus or headache (Behrman et al. 1989). Focal neurological deficits including hemiparesis, visual field defects, aphasia, cranial nerve palsies, and seizures are usually the results of cerebrovascular complications or acute obstructive hydrocephalus (Durand et al. 1993). Long-term sequela include dementia, aphasia, hydrocephalus, seizures, and persistent focal neurological deficits. Personality changes are common.

Purulent meningitis and brain edema are seen at autopsy. CT or MRI may show evidence of hydrocephalus, edema, or infarct. CSF is diagnostic, revealing increased intracranial pressure, polymorphonuclear pleocytosis, elevated protein, hypoglycorrhachia, positive cultures, and bacterial antigen detection (Ashwal 1995) (Table 30–3). Antibiotics are required for treatment. Adjunctive steroid use is now being considered more frequently for bacterial meningitis at any age (Ashwal 1995). Vaccination for some of the more common pathogens (*Streptococcus pneumoniae*) protects against disease and is cost-effective in the elderly (Monto and Terpenning 1996).

Brain abscess and epidural abscess. Abscesses consist of collections of purulent material that may be present in brain parenchyma, subdural space, or epidural space. The incidence of brain abscess is 4/1 million per year. Fifteen percent of all brain abscesses and 25% of all spinal epidural abscesses occur in patients over age 60. Typical organisms for brain abscesses include aerobic and anaerobic *Streptococcus*, *Bacteroides*, *Fusobacterium*, and *Clostridium* species. In immunocompromised individuals, various fungal species, cysticercosis, and toxoplasmosis are prevalent (Wispelwey and Scheld 1992). *Staphylococcus aureus*, anaerobic bacteria, and Gram-negative organism infections are frequent causes of brain abscesses after extension of a frontal sinusitis or middle ear infection (Luby 1992).

Headache, fever, mental status changes, and focal neurological signs are common initial symptoms (Wispelwey and Scheld 1992). Seizures and increased intracranial pressure may occur. Long-term sequela include late seizures and persistent focal neurological deficits. Enhanced MRI is very helpful in diagnosing brain abscesses (Sze and Zimmerman 1988), and EEG usually shows focal delta activity. Lumbar puncture may precipitate a herniation syndrome and is contraindicated in brain abscesses (Table 30–3). Treatments for brain abscesses include broad coverage antibiotics and occasionally surgical drainage (Wispelwey and Scheld 1992).

Fungal Infections

Half of all chronic fungal meningitis infections occur in individuals with depressed immune systems or chronic debilitation (Cummings and Benson 1992), making these infections frequent among the geriatric population. Cryptococcal meningitis is the most common of these infections (Jones and Nathwani 1995). Other causative organisms include *Coccidioides*, *Histoplasma*, *Candida*, *Blastomyces*, and *Aspergillus*.

Fungal infections begin insidiously and progress slowly over weeks to months. Headache, fever, and stiff neck are common, but may not always be present. Mental status changes occur more frequently and include lethargy, apathy, disorientation, poor concentration, memory deficits, and aphasia. Focal neurological deficits, cranial nerve dysfunction, gait imbalance, dementia, or hydrocephalus may also occur (Cummings and Benson 1992). CSF examination reveals lymphocytic pleocytosis, increased protein, and hypoglycorrhachia. Cryptococcal antigen in the CSF is specific for cryptococcal meningitis (Fishman 1992) (Table 30–3). Cultures or titers are necessary for diagnosis of other infections. Fluconazole and other new azole antifungal agents are safe and effective as first-line therapies without the severe toxicity seen with amphotericin B (Slavoski and Tunkel 1995).

Spirochete Infections

Syphilis. Syphilis, caused by the spirochete *Treponema pallidum*, is spread by sexual contact, and CNS invasion occurs in many patients, although most are asymptomatic (Scheck and Hook 1994). Syphilis recently is increasing in frequency, especially in patients with HIV-1 (Hook 1989). The annual incidence of syphilis of all types was 20/100,000 in the United States in 1990 (Hook and Marra 1992); for neurosyphilis it is estimated to be 2/100,000 (Simon 1985). Primary syphilis presents as a chancre that heals in several weeks and is followed by a diffuse skin rash indicative of the bacteremia of secondary syphilis. Meningeal neurosyphilis may be seen at this early stage. Tertiary syphilis occurs 2–50 years after the primary infection and occurs in various forms, including cardiovascular (aortitis), meningovascular, paretic, and tabetic. Because of the long incubation times, neurosyphilis frequently begins between ages 30 and 60 (Cummings and Benson 1992).

General paresis results from syphilitic invasion into the brain parenchyma. Before penicillin treatment, general paresis accounted for up to 20% of all admissions to mental hospitals (Hook and Marra 1992), but now it is extremely uncommon. The frontal lobes are classically involved in general paresis. Clinical features, many of which suggest frontal region impairment, include inattention, memory and cognitive deficits, dementia, tremulous speech, anomia, impaired judgment, irritability, pseudobulbar palsy, paralysis, tremor, ataxia, incontinence, optic atrophy, and Argyll Robertson pupils. Mania is seen in 20%–40% of patients, depression in 6%, and peculiar deportment, grandiose delusions, paranoia, and hallucinations in 3%–6% (Cummings and Benson 1992).

The pathology of syphilis is varied and includes meningitis, stroke, vasculitis, inflammatory infiltrates, neuronal loss, gliosis, and rarely gumma formation. MRI shows bilateral frontal and/or temporal lobe atrophy and subcortical abnormalities (Zifko et al. 1996). Screening for neurosyphilis should be done with the fluorescent treponemal antibody absorption (FTA-ABS) test because other screening tests may be nonreactive in tertiary syphilis (Simon 1985). False positives can occur with systemic lupus erythematosus and some infectious conditions (Hook and Marra 1992). If the FTA-ABS is positive, a lumbar puncture is indicated. CSF in neurosyphilis shows lymphocytic pleocytosis, elevated protein, positive Venereal Disease Research Laboratory (VDRL) test, occasional hypoglycorrhachia, and increased IgG (Table 30–3). Penicillin is the treatment of choice for all forms of syphilis, with the intravenous route and longer duration of treatments required for patients with neurosyphilis and syphilis associated with HIV-1 (Hook and Marra 1992). Desensitization is recommended for those with penicillin allergies (Centers for Disease Control 1989).

Lyme disease.   Lyme disease is caused by the tick-borne spirochete *Borrelia burgdorferi*. Age at onset ranges from 7 to 86 (Halperin et al. 1991). After the tick bite, an acute localized erythema chronicum migrans (ECM) rash and a viral-like syndrome occur. Dissemination occurs within a few weeks to months, with symptoms including a multifocal ECM rash, acute arthritis, cardiac conduction block, myocarditis, myositis, hepatitis, or meningoradiculoneuritis. Some individuals develop a chronic course leading to chronic arthritis, radiculoneuritis, encephalomyelitis, or encephalopathy.

Early neurological manifestations occur in 10% of patients and can include bilateral seventh nerve palsies, oculomotor disturbances, other cranial neuropathies, radiculopathies, mononeuritis multiplex, myopathy, and an acute lymphocytic meningitis with headache, photophobia, and meningismus (Finkel and Halperin 1992). Chronic neurological features typically include memory loss, anomia, cognitive deficits, and mild dementia. Deficits in executive function, attention, organization, initia-

tion, abstract concept formation, and verbal fluency are also typical and suggest frontal lobe dysfunction (Fallon and Nields 1994; Waniek et al. 1995). Behavioral disturbances include depression, emotional lability, sleep disturbances, anorexia nervosa, fatigue, irritability, psychosis with paranoia and hallucinations, and violent outbursts (Fallon and Nields 1994). Rarely, patients develop focal CNS deficits including paresis, ataxia, seizures, or a severe dementia with CSF evidence of an encephalitis (Halperin et al. 1991).

Neuropathological findings include peripheral neuritis, vasculitis, focal demyelination, and, in the late stages, neuronal loss, gliosis, and signs of brain parenchyma infection. MRI may reveal multifocal regions of increased signal in the white matter consistent with demyelination (Halperin et al. 1991). Diagnosis is made with a positive serology in the setting of appropriate clinical findings. Demonstration of intrathecal antibody production and CSF PCR for the spirochete may help with diagnosis (Pachner 1995) (Table 30–3). Intravenous antibiotics can prevent or halt the neurological complications and may lead to significant improvement.

Inflammatory Disorders

The inflammatory disorders include the vasculitides, the collagen vascular diseases, and certain other conditions. Most of these diseases can present at any age, but some are particularly prevalent in elderly individuals. Causes of inflammatory disorders involving the CNS in the geriatric age group are listed in Table 30–6. Some of these conditions have already been addressed.

Vasculitides

Giant cell (temporal) arteritis.   Giant cell (temporal) arteritis is a systemic vasculitis seen predominantly in the geriatric population. Nearly all patients are over age 50, and women are affected twice as often as are men. The incidence is as high as 7/100,000 per year (Boesen and Sorensen 1987), and it rises dramatically with increasing age to over 25/100,000 per year over age 80. Systemic symptoms are rarely absent and include fever, weight loss, anorexia, and malaise. The classic features of polymyalgia rheumatica syndrome, including pain and stiffness in the muscles of the neck, shoulders, and pelvis, are seen in 50% of those with giant cell arteritis. Headache, jaw claudication, scalp tenderness, and tenderness and nodularity of the superior temporal artery are common (Berlit

TABLE 30–6. Causes of inflammatory disorders involving the central nervous system in elderly patients

Vasculitides

　　Temporal arteritis

　　Polyarteritis nodosa

　　Allergic granulomatosis

　　Granulomatous angiitis

　　Wegener's granulomatosis

　　Takayasu's arteritis

　　Lymphomatoid granulomatosis

　　Eales' disease (idiopathic retinal vasculitis)

Collagen vascular diseases

　　Systemic lupus erythematosus (SLE)

　　Antiphospholipid antibody syndrome

　　Behçet's syndrome

　　Scleroderma

　　Rheumatoid arthritis

　　Sjögren's syndrome

　　Dermatomyositis

　　Cogan's syndrome

　　Mixed connective tissue disease

Other

　　Vogt-Koyanagi-Harada syndrome

　　Paraneoplastic disorders

1992; Chmelewski et al. 1992). The headache is characterized by a stabbing or throbbing pain, which is centered over the temple and radiates over the scalp and face. Scalp necrosis, muscular wasting, and angina occur infrequently.

Except for visual disturbance, CNS involvement is infrequent. Blurred vision, amaurosis fugax, and diplopia are reported, with blindness occurring, usually without warning, in 8%–23% of cases (Caselli and Hunder 1993). Multiple infarcts, more common in the posterior circulation territories, have been reported, but dementia syndromes unexplained by strokes are also seen (Caselli 1990). Less frequently, facial neuralgia, vertigo, and neuropathy occur (Nadeau and Watson 1990). Depression is the most common psychiatric manifestation.

Pathology shows a patchy giant cell arteritis frequently involving the branches of the external carotid, ophthalmic, and vertebral arteries. The large- and medium-sized arteries throughout the body are also involved, but are rarely symptomatic. Involvement of the intracranial arteries is uncommon. Multinucleated giant cells with destruction of the internal elastic lamina are seen. Anemia is common, and an elevated Westergren sedimentation rate (more than 50 mm/hour and often more than 100 mm/hour) is almost always found. A superior temporal artery biopsy is positive in approximately 70% of cases and should be done in all suspected cases (Nadeau and Watson 1990). Negative biopsies should not dissuade treatment in those with the typical clinical features. Prednisone, typically in doses of 40–60 mg/day, is an effective treatment and should be initiated without waiting for biopsy confirmation (Berlit 1992).

Polyarteritis nodosa.　Polyarteritis nodosa (PAN) characterizes a group of acute systemic necrotizing vasculitides, which includes Churg-Strauss angiitis. Immune complex deposition in PAN causes a relapsing and remitting vasculitis, which eventually leads to infarction or hemorrhage in multiple organs. The incidence of polyarteritis nodosa is approximately 0.2/100,000 per year, with males affected twice as often as females. Age at onset ranges from 6 to 80, with a mean of about 45. Common systemic findings include fever, weight loss, headache, anorexia, asthma, dyspnea, proteinuria, hypertension, arthralgias, skin rash, congestive heart failure, and gastrointestinal pain.

Neurological manifestations occur in up to 80% of cases, mostly resulting from peripheral nervous system involvement, giving rise to mononeuritis multiplex, polyneuropathy, cranial neuropathy, or myopathy. CNS involvement is seen in approximately 40% of cases and typically occurs later in the course with dementia, encephalopathy, psychosis, seizures, or strokes (Moore and Calabrese 1994). Specific neuropsychiatric symptoms occur in approximately 20% of cases and include disorientation, attentional deficits, memory impairment, cognitive deterioration, visual hallucinations, mania, paranoia, and hypoarousal progressing to coma. Hemiparesis, homonymous hemianopia, and ataxia occur secondary to the strokes.

Pathology shows a necrotizing vasculitis of the small and medium muscular arteries. Elevated sedimentation rate, anemia, leukocytosis, and thrombocytosis are common. Angiography reveals aneurysms and arteriopathy. MRI and CT may reveal evidence of infarction. CSF shows increased pressure, elevated protein, lymphocytic pleocytosis, and occasionally subarachnoid bleeding. Diagnosis is made clinically and confirmed by tissue biopsy (muscle, skin, sural nerve, or kidney) and angiography. Corticosteroids and immunosuppressive agents are the treatments of choice and often lead to remissions or recovery (Nadeau and Watson 1990).

Isolated angiitis of the central nervous system.　Isolated angiitis of the CNS, also known as *granulomatous angiitis*, is a rare vasculitis of unknown etiology and is confined to the CNS. It occurs at any age, with age at onset ranging from 3 to 96. Lymphoma, sarcoidosis, and herpes zoster conditions are occasionally associated with this vasculitis. Fever and weight loss are noted in 25% of cases. Usually, an initial subacute presentation with severe headache and encephalopathy is followed gradually by focal deficits, including strokes, and progressing to a vascular dementia syndrome affecting medium and small vessels (Vollmer et al. 1993).

Other common manifestations include seizures, aphasia, hemiparesis, supranuclear cranial nerve palsies, cerebellar signs, and myelopathy. Increased intracranial pressure may occur, leading to papilledema and potentially coma and brainstem herniation. Behavioral changes and psychosis are commonly seen.

A segmental vasculitis with fibrinoid necrosis and giant cells is found in the medium and small arteries, capillaries, and veins of the CNS. The sedimentation rate is increased in 60% of the patients but only to a mean of about 35 mm/hour. CT or MRI may be normal or reveal focal, occasionally enhancing, lesions, hemorrhage, or edema, which are found most commonly in the temporal and frontal cortical regions (Vollmer et al. 1993). Angiography may show vasculopathy, but usually does not. CSF findings are nonspecific (Table 30–3). Diagnosis is made clinically and confirmed by brain biopsy. Treatment with prednisone and cyclophosphamide is often ineffective, and there is an 87% mortality rate, with deaths occurring a mean of 6 months after onset of symptoms (Younger et al. 1988).

Wegener's granulomatosis.

Wegener's granulomatosis is a granulomatosis systemic necrotizing vasculitis that always affects the respiratory tract and often the kidneys. Typical systemic clinical manifestations include fever, weight loss, sinusitis, otitis media, saddle-nose deformity, cough, hemoptysis, pleuritis, glomerulonephritis, visual symptoms, ulcerative or papular skin lesions, arthralgias, myalgias, and pericarditis (Duna et al. 1995).

Neurological involvement consists mostly of cranial and peripheral neuropathies, including mononeuritis multiplex. The brain can be affected by infarction, hemorrhage, diffuse periventricular white matter lesions, meningeal inflammation, or granulomatous mass lesions causing seizures, focal deficits, and encephalopathy (Duna et al. 1995). Contiguous extension of granulomatous inflammation from the paranasal sinuses to the brain and often the frontal lobes is typical (Geiger et al. 1992).

Vasculitis, necrosis, and granulomas are seen pathologically on biopsy. Diagnosis is made by cytoplasmic antineutrophil cytoplasmic antibodies (c-ANCA) with a sensitivity and specificity of about 90% (Duna et al. 1995).

Angiography is not helpful, neuroimaging is useful but nonspecific, and CSF can rule out infection. Corticosteroids and cytotoxic agents are needed for successful treatment.

Lymphomatoid granulomatosis.

Lymphomatoid granulomatosis, a rare condition typically affecting the lungs, skin, and nervous system, is characterized by a perivascular mature T-cell lymphocytic infiltrate suggestive of a lymphomatous condition. In 60% of cases, a malignant lymphoma develops (Bushunow et al. 1996). Common manifestations include fever, weight loss, cough, chest pain, skin ulcers and papules, and peripheral neuropathies.

CNS dysfunction occurs in 20%–40% of cases and includes a broad spectrum of deficits such as monocular blindness, internuclear ophthalmoplegia, dysphagia, dysarthria, spasticity, paraparesis, hemiparesis, ataxia, aphasia, encephalopathy, and dementia. Behavioral symptoms reported include personality change, irritability, disinhibition, impulsivity, distractibility, and mood disturbance (Bushunow et al. 1996; Kleinschmidt-DeMasters et al. 1992).

CSF shows pleocytosis with atypical cells (Bushunow et al. 1996) (Table 30–3). Angiography can show a vasculitic pattern, and neuroimaging can show mass lesions, enhancement, or white matter changes. Treatment with prednisone and cyclophosphamide is usually necessary to maintain prolonged remissions. Adjunctive radiotherapy or chemotherapy can also be effective.

Behçet's syndrome.

Behçet's syndrome is an inflammatory disorder of uncertain etiology characterized by recurrent oral and genital ulcers, uveitis, thrombophlebitis, and arthritis (Moore and Calabrese 1994). Fever and gastrointestinal complaints are also common. Prevalence is uncertain, with reports ranging from 4 to 100 per 100,000. Cases have been reported from ages 6 to 72.

Up to 40% of cases have neurological symptoms. A relapsing focal meningoencephalitis affecting the brainstem, with headache, cranial neuropathies, dysarthria, long tract signs, and bulbar and pseudobulbar palsies, is the most common neurological manifestation. A dementia syndrome with memory deficits, aphasia, and cognitive impairment can occur. Seizures, increased intracranial pressure, and peripheral neuropathy have also been reported (Serdaroglu et al. 1989). Personality changes, disinhibition, emotional disturbances, apathy, and akinetic mutism are frequently described behaviors (Yamamori et al. 1994).

A chronic small vessel vasculitis is seen pathologically, often involving the brainstem, spinal cord, globus pallidus, hypothalamus, cerebral white matter, retina, and skin (Totsuka et al. 1985; Yamamori et al. 1994). Meningeal inflammation is also common. MRI sometimes reveals venous thrombosis and frequently shows deep subcortical and brainstem abnormalities (Al Kawi et al. 1991). Angiography is usually normal, and CSF examination shows a nonspecific lymphocytic pleocytosis with elevated protein (McLean et al. 1995) (Table 30–3). Diagnosis is based on clinical features. Treatment for CNS disease includes high-dose steroids and immunosuppressive agents.

Collagen Vascular Diseases

Systemic lupus erythematosus. Systemic lupus erythematosus (SLE) is a multisystem immunological disorder of uncertain etiology. The incidence of SLE is about 5/100,000 per year, and the prevalence is about 45/100,000 (Nadeau and Watson 1990). Women are much more often affected. Although SLE is a disease primarily of young to middle-aged adults, it can occur in the very old. Systemic manifestations may include fever, anorexia, rash, lymphadenopathy, arthralgias, pericarditis, valvular disease, pleuritis, Raynaud's phenomenon, alopecia, renal insufficiency, nephrotic syndrome, and hypertension (Nadeau and Watson 1990).

SLE has the highest incidence of neuropsychiatric and focal CNS manifestations of any of the collagen vascular disorders. CNS dysfunction may occur from primary involvement of the brain or secondarily from complications of the disease including infection, embolism from endocarditis, steroid treatment toxicity, and severe hypertension.

Neuropsychiatric manifestations are seen in 40%–75% of cases and often occur early in the disease course. More than 60% of cases develop memory and cognitive deficits (Carbotte et al. 1986), whereas 35%–60% have symptoms of impaired attention, an acute confusional state or delirium, psychosis with hallucinations and delusions, depression, hypomania, mania, phobias, or anxiety (West 1994). Neuropsychological testing shows deficits in information processing, cognitive flexibility, working memory, attention, and verbal fluency (Denburg et al. 1993). Focal CNS involvement, including seizures, strokes, supranuclear cranial nerve deficits, chorea, ataxia, parkinsonism, transverse myelitis, and focal paresis, is present in 10%–35% of cases (West 1994).

Occasionally associated with SLE is the antiphospholipid antibody syndrome consisting of the presence of antiphospholipid antibodies (particularly lupus anticoagulant and anticardiolipin antibodies), venous or arterial thrombotic strokes or ischemia, recurrent abortions, and thrombocytopenia (Brey et al. 1993; Lockshin 1992; Rosove and Brewer 1992). Myelopathy, deep vein thrombosis, Guillain-Barré syndrome, migraine, chorea, and seizures have also been associated with this syndrome (Levine and Welch 1987). Antiphospholipid antibodies are present in up to 50% of patients with SLE.

The main pathological feature of SLE is a small vessel vasculopathy with fibrinoid degeneration and endothelial proliferation of the small vessels, resulting in microinfarcts and microhemorrhages. Less commonly, a true vasculitis is seen. Angiography usually is unable to identify the microangiopathy of SLE. MRI is useful in localizing strokes, but is often normal even in those with neuropsychiatric symptoms and CNS involvement (neuropsychiatric lupus) (West et al. 1995). Nearly all individuals with neuropsychiatric lupus have abnormal CSF findings, including IgG index, oligoclonal bands, and/or CSF antineuronal antibodies, which may improve with response to therapy (West et al. 1995) (Table 30–3). An autoimmune process with these antineuronal antibodies may be an important cause of neuropsychiatric lupus and CNS involvement. Serum antiribosomal P protein antibodies are often seen in patients with neuropsychiatric lupus with psychosis and depression (Teh and Isenberg 1994). Diagnosis of SLE is based on clinical features, a positive antinuclear antibody test, and other specific antibody tests (Tan et al. 1982). Treatments include nonsteroidal anti-inflammatory agents, steroids, and immunosuppressive agents. Oral anticoagulants are advisable to prevent the recurrent thrombotic events seen with antiphospholipid antibodies (Khamashta et al. 1995). Neuroleptics are used for psychosis; anticonvulsants, for seizures.

Sjögren's syndrome. Sjögren's syndrome, seen mostly in women, is a systemic autoimmune disorder characterized by symptoms of dry eyes and dry mouth and may involve the lung, liver, kidney, heart, blood vessels, skin, muscles, joints, peripheral nerves, spinal cord, and brain. CNS manifestations, reported in up to 25% in some centers (Alexander 1993) and rarely observed in others (Moutsopoulos et al. 1993), include migraine, focal neurological deficits, intracerebral hemorrhage, subarachnoid hemorrhage, seizures, myelitis, aseptic meningitis, dementia, and psychiatric symptoms (Alexander 1993). The dementia syndrome has subcortical features, and the psychiatric symptoms include mood disturbances, depression, and obsessive-compulsive traits (Alexander 1993; Moutsopoulos et al. 1993).

Lymphocytic infiltration of the exocrine glands causes dry eyes and dry mouth. In the CNS, Sjögren's causes a vasculopathy of the small vessels, and so angiography shows a vasculitis in only 20% of cases (Alexander 1993). Laboratory evaluations are frequently positive for antinuclear antibodies and occasionally for anti-SS-A (Ro) (seen with more serious CNS disease) and anti-SS-B (La) antibodies. CSF often is abnormal but nonspecific (Table 30–3). Biopsy of a minor salivary gland is diagnostic. MRI shows subcortical and periventricular white matter lesions in 80%. SPECT, however, can show cortical hypoperfusion in patients with neuropsychiatric dysfunction without cortical MRI lesions (Alexander 1993). Corticosteroids and rarely other immunosuppressive agents are used for treatment.

Summary

Most acquired brain disorders occur in the geriatric population. Some conditions have their onset in late life, whereas other conditions have chronic courses and persist into advanced age. Diagnosis and treatment of these disorders in the elderly patient is influenced by the frequent co-occurrence of other chronic medical conditions, multiple medication regimens, and the normal physiological changes that accompany aging.

Neoplastic disorders involving the CNS occur frequently in elderly individuals, and they present as primary tumors, metastatic tumors, or paraneoplastic syndromes. MS often begins in early adulthood, but many patients survive well past 70. Neuropsychiatric features of MS include depression, psychosis, and mania. Toxic and metabolic causes of demyelination may begin in elderly patients. Both common and rare infectious disorders affecting the CNS have characteristic presentations in the elderly population, and most are treatable. Giant cell arteritis occurs almost exclusively in patients over age 50. Finally, SLE is a common disorder with frequent late survival and significant CNS manifestations.

References

Achiron A, Ziv I, Djaldetti R, et al: Aphasia in multiple sclerosis: clinical and radiologic correlations. Neurology 42:2195–2197, 1992

Achiron A, Barak Y, Goren M, et al: Intravenous immune globulin in multiple sclerosis: clinical and neuroradiological results and implications for possible mechanisms of action. Clin Exp Immunol 104 (suppl 1):67–70, 1996

Adams RD, Victor M, Ropper AH: Principles of Neurology, 6th Edition. New York, McGraw-Hill, 1997

Al Kawi MZ, Bohlega S, Banna M: MRI findings in neuro-Behçet's disease. Neurology 41:405–408, 1991

Alexander EL: Neurologic disease in Sjögren's syndrome: mononuclear inflammatory vasculopathy affecting central/peripheral nervous system and muscles, a clinical review and update of immunopathogenesis. Rheum Dis Clin North Am 19:869–908, 1993

Alvord EC Jr, Shaw C-M: Neoplasms affecting the nervous system of the elderly, in The Pathology of the Aging Human Nervous System. Edited by Duckett S. Philadelphia, PA, Lea & Febiger, 1991, pp 210–286

American Academy of Neurology AIDS Task Force: Nomenclature and research case definitions for neurologic manifestations of human immunodeficiency virus-type 1 (HIV-1) infection. Neurology 41:778–785, 1991

Ashwal S: Neurologic evaluation of the patient with acute bacterial meningitis. Neurol Clin 13:549–577, 1995

Atkinson JH, Grant I: Natural history of neuropsychiatric manifestations of HIV disease. Psychiatr Clin North Am 17:17–33, 1994

Babikian V, Ropper AH: Binswanger's disease: a review. Stroke 18:2–12, 1987

Bale JF Jr: Encephalitis and other virus-induced neurologic disorders, in Clinical Neurology. Edited by Baker AB, Joynt RJ. New York, Harper & Row, 1991, pp 1–86

Bartlett JG, Moore RD: Improving HIV therapy. Sci Am 279:84–87, 89, 91–93, 1998

Bastianello S, Pozzilli C, Bernardi S, et al: Serial study of gadolinium-DPTA MRI enhancement in multiple sclerosis. Neurology 40:591–595, 1990

Baumann N, Masson M, Carreau V, et al: Adult forms of metachromatic leukodystrophy: clinical and biochemical approach. Dev Neurosci 13:211–215, 1991

Beatty WW, Goodkin DE, Monson N, et al: Anterograde and retrograde amnesia in patients with chronic progressive multiple sclerosis. Arch Neurol 45:611–619, 1988

Behrman RE, Myers BR, Mendelson MH, et al: Central nervous system infections in the elderly. Arch Intern Med 149:1596–1599, 1989

Belyi BI: Mental impairment in unilateral frontal tumors: role of the laterality of the lesion. Int J Neurosci 32:799–810, 1987

Berger JR, Kaszovitz B, Post JD, et al: Progressive multifocal leukoencephalopathy associated with human immunodeficiency virus infection. Ann Intern Med 107:78–87, 1987

Berlit P: Clinical and laboratory findings with giant cell arteritis. J Neurol Sci 111:1–12, 1992

Bjorkhem I, Skrede S: Familial diseases with storage of sterols other than cholesterol: cerebrotendinous xanthomatosis and phytosterolemia, in The Metabolic Basis of Inherited Disease, 6th Edition. Edited by Scriver CR, Beaudet AL, Sly WS, et al. New York, McGraw-Hill, 1990, pp 1283–1293

Boesen P, Sorensen SF: Giant cell arteritis, temporal arteritis, and polymyalgia rheumatica in a Danish county: a prospective investigation, 1982–1985. Arthritis Rheum 30:294–299, 1987

Bornstein RA, Nasrallah HA, Para MF, et al: Neuropsychological performance in asymptomatic HIV infection. J Neuropsychiatry Clin Neurosci 4:386–394, 1992

Brazzelli M, Colombo N, Della Sala S, et al: Spared and impaired cognitive abilities after bilateral frontal damage. Cortex 30:27–51, 1994

Brey RL, Gharavi AE, Lockshin MD: Neurologic complications of antiphospholipid antibodies. Rheum Dis Clin North Am 19:833–850, 1993

Brink NS, Miller RF: Clinical presentation, diagnosis and therapy of progressive multifocal leukoencephalopathy. J Infect 32:97–102, 1996

Brown P, Cathala F, Castaigne P, et al: Creutzfeldt-Jakob disease: clinical analysis of a consecutive series of 230 neuropathologically verified cases. Ann Neurol 20:597–602, 1986

Brown P, Goldfarb LG, Kovanen J, et al: Phenotypic characteristics of familial Creutzfeldt-Jakob disease associated with the codon 178Asn PRNP mutation. Ann Neurol 31:282–285, 1992

Bushunow PW, Casas V, Duggan DB: Lymphomatoid granulomatosis causing central diabetes insipidus: case report and review of the literature. Cancer Invest 14:112–119, 1996

The Canadian MS Research Group: A randomized controlled trial of amantadine in fatigue associated with multiple sclerosis. Can J Neurol Sci 14:273–278, 1987

Carbotte RM, Denburg SD, Denburg JA: Prevalence of cognitive impairment in systemic lupus erythematosus. J Nerv Ment Dis 174:357–364, 1986

Caselli RJ: Giant cell (temporal) arteritis: a treatable cause of multi-infarct dementia. Neurology 40:753–755, 1990

Caselli RJ, Hunder GG: Neurologic aspects of giant cell (temporal) arteritis. Rheum Dis Clin North Am 19:941–953, 1993

Centers for Disease Control: Sexually transmitted diseases treatment guidelines. MMWR Morb Mortal Wkly Rep 38 (S-8):5–15, 1989

Centers for Disease Control: 1993 revised classification system for HIV infection and expanded surveillance case definition for AIDS among adolescents and adults. MMWR Morb Mortal Wkly Rep 41 (RR-17):1–19, 1992

Centers for Disease Control: Update: trends in AIDS incidence—United States, 1996. MMWR Morb Mortal Wkly Rep 46:861–867, 1997

Chang KH, Cha SH, Han MH, et al: Marchiafava-Bignami disease: serial changes in corpus callosum on MRI. Neuroradiology 34:480–482, 1992

Chiofalo N, Fuentes A, Galvez S: Serial EEG findings in 27 cases of Creutzfeldt-Jakob disease. Arch Neurol 37:143–145, 1980

Chmelewski WL, McKnight KM, Agudelo CA, et al: Presenting features and outcomes in patients undergoing temporal artery biopsy: a review of 98 patients. Arch Intern Med 152:1690–1695, 1992

Clark CM, Fleming JA, Li D, et al: Sleep disturbance, depression, and lesion site in patients with multiple sclerosis. Arch Neurol 49:641–643, 1992

Clementz GL, Schade SG: The spectrum of vitamin B_{12} deficiency. Am Fam Physician 41:150–162, 1990

Comi G, Filippi M, Martinelli V, et al: Brain MRI correlates of cognitive impairment in primary and secondary progressive multiple sclerosis. J Neurol Sci 132:222–227, 1995

Constine LS, Woolf PD, Cann D, et al: Hypothalamic-pituitary dysfunction after radiation for brain tumors. N Engl J Med 328:87–94, 1993

Cooper DA, Gold J, MacLean P, et al: Acute AIDS retrovirus infection. Lancet 1:537–540, 1985

Cummings JL, Benson DF: Dementia: A Clinical Approach, 2nd Edition. Stoneham, MA, Butterworth, 1992

Dalmau J, Graus F, Rosenblum MK, et al: Anti–Hu-associated paraneoplastic encephalomyelitis/sensory neuronopathy: a clinical study of 71 patients. Medicine (Baltimore) 71:59–72, 1992

de Groen PC, Aksamit AJ, Rakela J, et al: Central nervous system toxicity after liver transplantation: the role of cyclosporine and cholesterol. N Engl J Med 317:861–866, 1987

DeArmond SJ, Prusiner SB: Etiology and pathogenesis of prion diseases. Am J Pathol 146:785–811, 1995

Denburg SD, Denburg JA, Carbotte RM, et al: Cognitive deficits in systemic lupus erythematosus. Rheum Dis Clin North Am 19:815–831, 1993

Duna GF, Galperin C, Hoffman GS: Wegener's granulomatosis. Rheum Dis Clin North Am 21:949–986, 1995

Durand ML, Calderwood SB, Weber DJ, et al: Acute bacterial meningitis in adults: a review of 493 episodes. N Engl J Med 328:21–28, 1993

Ekholm S, Simon JH: Magnetic resonance imaging and the acquired immunodeficiency syndrome dementia complex. Acta Radiol 29:227–230, 1988

Engstrom JW, Lowenstein DH, Bredesen DE: Cerebral infarctions and transient neurologic deficits associated with acquired immunodeficiency syndrome. Am J Med 86:528–532, 1989

Epstein LG, Brown P: Bovine spongiform encephalopathy and a new variant of Creutzfeldt-Jakob disease. Neurology 48:569–571, 1997

Fallon BA, Nields JA: Lyme disease: a neuropsychiatric illness. Am J Psychiatry 151:1571–1583, 1994

Farlow MR, Yee RD, Dlouhy SR, et al: Gerstmann-Sträussler-Scheinker disease, I: extending the clinical spectrum. Neurology 39:1446–1452, 1989

Feinstein A, du Boulay G, Ron MA: Psychotic illness in multiple sclerosis. A clinical and magnetic resonance imaging study. Br J Psychiatry 161:680–685, 1992

Fennell EB, Smith MC: Neuropsychological assessment, in Neurobehavioral Aspects of Multiple Sclerosis. Edited by Rao SM. New York, Oxford University Press, 1990, pp 63–81

Finkel MJ, Halperin JJ: Nervous system Lyme borreliosis—revisited. Arch Neurol 49:102–107, 1992

Fishman RA: Cerebrospinal Fluid in Diseases of the Nervous System, 2nd Edition. Philadelphia, PA, WB Saunders, 1992

Gallassi R, Morreale A, Montagna P, et al: Fatal familial insomnia: neuropsychological study of a disease with thalamic degeneration. Cortex 28:175–187, 1992

Geerts Y, Dehaene I, Lammens M: Acute hemorrhagic leucoencephalitis. Acta Neurol Belg 91:201–211, 1991

Geiger WJ, Garrison KL, Losh DP: Wegener's granulomatosis. Am Fam Physician 45:191–196, 1992

Goldman S, Liard A, Flament-Durand J, et al: Positron emission tomography and histopathology in Creutzfeldt-Jakob disease. Neurology 43:1828–1830, 1993

Good K, Clark CM, Oger J, et al: Cognitive impairment and depression in mild multiple sclerosis. J Nerv Ment Dis 180:730–732, 1992

Grafman J, Rao SM, Litvan I: Disorders of memory, in Neurobehavioral Aspects of Multiple Sclerosis. Edited by Rao SM. New York, Oxford University Press, 1990, pp 102–117

Greenlee JE: Progressive multifocal leukoencephalopathy—progress made and lessons relearned. N Engl J Med 338:1378–1380, 1998

Halperin JJ, Volkman DJ, Wu P: Central nervous system abnormalities in Lyme neuroborreliosis. Neurology 41:1571–1582, 1991

Henry K: Management of HIV infection: a 1995–96 overview for the clinician. Minnesota Medicine 78:17–24, 1995

Hestad K, McArthur JH, Dal Pan GJ, et al: Regional brain atrophy in HIV-1 infection: association with specific neuropsychological test performance. Acta Neurol Scand 88:112–118, 1993

Ho DD, Hirsch MS: Acute viral encephalitis. Med Clin North Am 69:415–429, 1985

Hokezu Y, Kuriyama M, Kubota R, et al: Cerebrotendinous xanthomatosis: cranial CT and MRI studies in eight patients. Neuroradiology 34:308–312, 1992

Holman RC, Janssen RS, Buehler JW, et al: Epidemiology of progressive multifocal leukoencephalopathy in the United States: analysis of national mortality and AIDS surveillance data. Neurology 41:1733–1736, 1991

Honer WG, Hurwitz T, Li DKB, et al: Temporal lobe involvement in multiple sclerosis patients with psychiatric disorders. Arch Neurol 44:187–190, 1987

Honnorat J, Antoine JC, Derrington E, et al: Antibodies to a subpopulation of glial cells and a 66 kDa developmental protein in patients with paraneoplastic neurological syndromes. J Neurol Neurosurg Psychiatry 61:270–278, 1996

Hooge JP, Redekop WK: Multiple sclerosis with very late onset. Neurology 42:1907–1910, 1992

Hook CC, Kimmel DW, Kvols LK, et al: Multifocal inflammatory leukoencephalopathy with 5-fluorouracil and levamisole. Ann Neurol 31:262–267, 1992

Hook EW III: Syphilis and HIV infection. J Infect Dis 160:530–534, 1989

Hook EW III, Marra CM: Acquired syphilis in adults. N Engl J Med 326:1060–1069, 1992

Hsich G, Kenny K, Gibbs CJ Jr, et al: The 14-3-3 brain protein in cerebrospinal fluid as a marker for transmissible spongiform encephalopathies. N Engl J Med 335:924–930, 1996

Huang C-C, Chu N-S, Chen T-J, et al: Acute haemorrhagic leucoencephalitis with a prolonged clinical course. J Neurol Neurosurg Psychiatry 51:870–874, 1988

Huber SJ, Paulson GW, Shuttleworth EC, et al: Magnetic imaging correlates of dementia in multiple sclerosis. Arch Neurol 44:732–736, 1987

Huber SJ, Bornstein RA, Rammohan KW, et al: Magnetic resonance imaging correlates of executive function impairments in multiple sclerosis. Neuropsychiatry Neuropsychol Behav Neurol 5:33–36, 1992a

Huber SJ, Bornstein RA, Rammohan KW, et al: Magnetic resonance imaging correlates of neuropsychological impairment in multiple sclerosis. J Neuropsychiatry Clin Neurosci 4:152–158, 1992b

Hyde TM, Ziegler JC, Weinberger DR: Psychiatric disturbances in metachromatic leukodystrophy: insights into the neurobiology of psychosis. Arch Neurol 49:401–406, 1992

IFNB Multiple Sclerosis Study Group: Interferon beta-1b is effective in relapsing-remitting multiple sclerosis, I: clinical results of a multicenter, randomized, double-blind, placebo-controlled trial. Neurology 43:655–661, 1993

IFNB Multiple Sclerosis Study Group and University of British Columbia MS/MRI Analysis Group: Interferon beta-1b in the treatment of multiple sclerosis: final outcome of the randomized controlled trial. Neurology 45:1277–1285, 1995

Jacobs LD, Cookfair DL, Rudick RA, et al: Intramuscular interferon beta-1a for disease progression in relapsing multiple sclerosis. Ann Neurol 39:285–294, 1996

Janssen RS, Saykin AJ, Kaplan JE, et al: Neurological complication of human immunodeficiency virus infection in patients with lymphadenopathy syndrome. Ann Neurol 23:49–55, 1988

Janssen RS, Nwanyanwu OC, Selik RM, et al: Epidemiology of human immunodeficiency virus encephalopathy in the United States. Neurology 42:1472–1476, 1992

Joffe RT, Lippert GP, Gray TA, et al: Mood disorder and multiple sclerosis. Arch Neurol 44:376–378, 1987

Johnson BE, Becker B, Goff WB II, et al: Neurologic, neuropsychologic and computed cranial tomography scan abnormalities in 2- to 10-year survivors of small-cell lung cancer. J Clin Oncol 3:1659–1667, 1985

Johnson KP, Brooks BR, Cohen JA, et al: Copolymer 1 reduces relapse rate and improves disability in relapsing-remitting multiple sclerosis: results of a phase III multicenter, double-blind, placebo-controlled trial. Neurology 45: 1268–1276, 1995

Johnson KP, Brooks BR, Cohen JA, et al: Extended use of glatiramer acetate (Copaxone) is well tolerated and maintains its clinical effect on multiple sclerosis relapse rate and degree of disability. Neurology 50:701–708, 1998

Johnson RT: Viruses and chronic neurologic diseases. Johns Hopkins Medical Journal 150:132–140, 1982

Jones GA, Nathwani D: Cryptococcal meningitis. British Journal of Hospital Medicine 54:439–445, 1995

Kahn JO, Walker BD: Acute human immunodeficiency virus type 1 infection. N Engl J Med 339:33–39, 1998

Kapur N, Barker S, Burrows, et al: Herpes simplex encephalitis: long term magnetic resonance imaging and neuropsychological profile. J Neurol Neurosurg Psychiatry 57:1334–1342, 1994

Karnaze DS, Carmel R: Neurologic and evoked potential abnormalities in subtle cobalamin deficiency states, including deficiency without anemia and with normal absorption of free cobalamin. Arch Neurol 47:1008–1012, 1990

Kesselring J, Miller DH, Robb SA, et al: Acute disseminated encephalomyelitis. MRI findings and the distinction from multiple sclerosis. Brain 113:291–302, 1990

Khamashta MA, Cuadrado MJ, Mujic F, et al: The management of thrombosis in the antiphospholipid-antibody syndrome. N Engl J Med 332:993–997, 1995

Kieburtz K, Schiffer RB: Neurologic manifestations of human immunodeficiency virus infections. Neurol Clin 7: 447–468, 1989

Kirkeby HJ, Poulsen EU, Petersen T, et al: Erectile dysfunction in multiple sclerosis. Neurology 38:1366–1371, 1988

Kirschbaum WR: Jakob-Creutzfeldt Disease. New York, American Elsevier, 1968, p 132

Kitchin W, Cohen-Cole SA, Mickel SF: Adrenoleukodystrophy: frequency of presentation as a psychiatric disorder. Biol Psychiatry 22:1375–1387, 1987

Kiyosawa M, Bosley TM, Alavi A, et al: Positron emission tomography in a patient with progressive multifocal leukoencephalopathy. Neurology 38:1864–1867, 1988

Kleinschmidt-DeMasters BK, Filley CM, Bitter MA: Central nervous system angiocentric, angiodestructive T-cell lymphoma (lymphomatoid granulomatosis). Surg Neurol 37:130–137, 1992

Kodama T, Numaguchi Y, Gellad FE, et al: Magnetic resonance imaging of limbic encephalitis. Neuroradiology 33:520–523, 1991

Koppel BS, Wormser GP, Tuchman AJ, et al: Central nervous system involvement in patients with acquired immune deficiency syndrome (AIDS). Acta Neurol Scand 71:337–353, 1985

Krupp LB, Alvarez LA, LaRocca NG, et al: Fatigue in multiple sclerosis. Arch Neurol 45:435–437, 1988

Kurtzke JF, Kurland LT: The epidemiology of neurologic disease, in Clinical Neurology. Edited by Baker AB, Joynt RJ. New York, Harper & Row, 1983, pp 1–143

LaRocca NG: A rehabilitation perspective, in Neurobehavioral Aspects of Multiple Sclerosis. Edited by Rao SM. New York, Oxford University Press, 1990, pp 215–229

Lechevalier B, Andersson JC, Morin P: Hemispheric disconnection syndrome with a "crossed avoiding" reaction in a case of Marchiafava-Bignami disease. J Neurol Neurosurg Psychiatry 40:483–497, 1977

Lee Y-Y, Nauert C, Glass JP: Treatment-related white matter changes in cancer patients. Cancer 57:1473–1482, 1986

Leo GJ, Rao SM: Effects of intravenous physostigmine and lecithin on memory loss in multiple sclerosis: report of a pilot study. Journal of Neurological Rehabilitation 2:123–129, 1988

Levine SR, Welch KMA: The spectrum of neurologic disease associated with antiphospholipid antibodies: lupus anticoagulants and anticardiolipin antibodies. Arch Neurol 44:876–883, 1987

Levy RM, Bredesen DE: Central nervous system dysfunction in acquired immunodeficiency syndrome, in AIDS and the Nervous System. Edited by Rosenblum ML, Levy RM, Bredesen DE. New York, Raven, 1988, pp 29–63

Levy RM, Bredesen DE, Rosenblum ML: Neurological manifestations of the acquired immunodeficiency syndrome (AIDS): experience at UCSF and review of the literature. J Neurosurg 62:475–495, 1985

Lindenbaum J, Healton EB, Savage DG, et al: Neuropsychiatric disorders caused by cobalamin deficiency in the absence of anemia or macrocytosis. N Engl J Med 318:1720–1728, 1988

Lockshin MD: Antiphospholipid antibody syndrome. JAMA 268:1451–1453, 1992

Lublin FD, Whitaker JN, Eidelman BH, et al: Management of patients receiving interferon beta-1b for multiple sclerosis: report of a consensus conference. Neurology 46:12–18, 1996

Luby JP: Southwestern internal medicine conference: infections of the central nervous system. Am J Med Sci 304:379–391, 1992

Mahler ME: Behavioral manifestations associated with multiple sclerosis. Psychiatr Clin North Am 15:427–438, 1992

Marshall DW, Brey RL, Cahill WT, et al: Spectrum of cerebrospinal fluid findings in various stages of human immunodeficiency virus infection. Arch Neurol 45:954–958, 1988

Masliah E, Achim CL, Ge N, et al: Spectrum of human immunodeficiency virus–associated neocortical damage. Ann Neurol 32:321–329, 1992

Masters CL, Gajdusek DC, Gibbs CJ Jr: Creutzfeldt-Jakob disease virus isolation from the Gerstmann-Sträussler syndrome with an analysis of the various forms of amyloid plaque deposition in the virus-induced spongiform encephalopathies. Brain 104:559–588, 1981

Maurelli M, Marchioni E, Cerretano R, et al: Neuropsychological assessment in MS: clinical, neurophysiological and neuroradiological relationships. Acta Neurol Scand 86:124–128, 1992

McArthur JC, Cohen BA, Selnes OA, et al: Low prevalence of neurological and neuropsychological abnormalities in otherwise healthy HIV–1-infected individuals: results from the multicenter AIDS cohort study. Ann Neurol 26:601–611, 1989

McLean BN, Miller D, Thompson EJ: Oligoclonal banding of IgG in CSF, blood-brain barrier function, and MRI findings in patients with sarcoidosis, systemic lupus erythematosus, and Behçet's disease involving the nervous system. J Neurol Neurosurg Psychiatry 58:548–554, 1995

McPherson SE, Cummings JL: Neuropsychological aspects of vascular dementia. Brain Cogn 31:269–282, 1996

The Medical Letter: Drugs for HIV infection. Med Lett Drugs Ther 39:111–116, 1997

Medori R, Tritschler H-J, LeBlanc A, et al: Fatal familial insomnia: a prion disease with a mutation at codon 178 of the prion protein gene. N Engl J Med 326:444–449, 1992

Mendez MF: The neuropsychiatry of multiple sclerosis. Int J Psychiatry Med 25:123–130, 1995

Mendozzi L, Pugnetti L, Saccani M, et al: Frontal lobe dysfunction in multiple sclerosis as assessed by means of Lurian tasks: effect of age at onset. J Neurol Sci 115 (suppl): S42–S50, 1993

Merriam AE, Hegarty AM, Miller A: The mental disabilities of metachromatic leukodystrophy: implications concerning the differentiation of cortical, subcortical gray, and white matter dementias. Neuropsychiatry Neuropsychol Behav Neurol 3:217–225, 1990

Milton WJ, Atlas SW, Lavi E, et al: Magnetic resonance imaging of Creutzfeldt-Jakob disease. Ann Neurol 29:438–440, 1991

Minden SL, Moes E: A psychiatric perspective, in Neurobehavioral Aspects of Multiple Sclerosis. Edited by Rao SM. New York, Oxford University Press, 1990, pp 230–250

Minden SL, Schiffer RB: Affective disorders in multiple sclerosis: review and recommendations for clinical research. Arch Neurol 47:98–104, 1990

Minden SL, Orav J, Reich P: Depression in multiple sclerosis. Gen Hosp Psychiatry 9:426–434, 1987

Minden SL, Moes EJ, Orav J, et al: Memory impairment in multiple sclerosis. J Clin Exp Neuropsychol 12:566–586, 1990

Mohr DC, Goodkin DE, Likosky W, et al: Treatment of depression improves adherence to interferon beta-1b therapy for multiple sclerosis. Arch Neurol 54:531–533, 1997

Monto AS, Terpenning MS: The value of influenza and pneumococcal vaccines in the elderly. Drugs Aging 8:445–451, 1996

Moore PM, Calabrese LH: Neurologic manifestations of systemic vasculitides. Semin Neurol 14:300–306, 1994

Moutsopoulos HM, Sarmas JH, Talal N: Is central nervous system involvement a systemic manifestation of primary Sjögren's syndrome? Rheum Dis Clin North Am 19:909–912, 1993

Murray TJ: Amantadine therapy for fatigue in multiple sclerosis. Can J Neurol Sci 12:251–254, 1985

Nadeau SE, Watson RT: Neurologic manifestations of vasculitis and collagen vascular syndromes, in Clinical Neurology. Edited by Baker AB, Joynt RJ. New York, Harper & Row, 1990, pp 1–166

Naidu S, Moser HW: Peroxisomal disorders. Neurol Clin 8:507–519, 1990

Nance PW, Sheremata WA, Lynch SG, et al: Relationship of the antispasticity effect of tizanidine to plasma concentration in patients with multiple sclerosis. Arch Neurol 54:731–736, 1997

Navia BA, Cho E-S, Petito CK, et al: The AIDS dementia complex, II: neuropathology. Ann Neurol 19:525–535, 1986a

Navia BA, Jordan BD, Price RW: The AIDS dementia complex, I: clinical features. Ann Neurol 19:517–524, 1986b

Neilley LK, Goodin DS, Goodkin DE, et al: Side effect profile of interferon beta 1-b (Betaseron). Neurology 46:552–554, 1996

Newman NJ, Bell IR, McKee AC: Paraneoplastic limbic encephalitis: neuropsychiatric presentation. Biol Psychiatry 27:529–542, 1990

Noseworthy J, Paty D, Wonnacott T, et al: Multiple sclerosis after age 50. Neurology 33:1537–1544, 1983

Ochitill HN, Dilley JW: Neuropsychiatric aspects of acquired immunodeficiency syndrome, in AIDS and the Nervous System. Edited by Rosenblum ML, Levy RM, Bredesen DE. New York, Raven, 1988, pp 315–325

Ojeda VJ: Necrotizing leucoencephalopathy associated with intrathecal/intraventricular methotrexate therapy. Med J Aust 2:289–293, 1982

Okazaki H: Fundamentals of Neuropathology, 1st Edition. New York, Igaku-Shoin, 1983, pp 134–136

Pachner AR: Early disseminated Lyme disease: Lyme meningitis. Am J Med 98 (suppl 4A):30S–37S, 1995

Pantaleo G, Graziosi C, Fauci AS: The immunopathogenesis of human immunodeficiency virus infection. N Engl J Med 328:327–335, 1993

Paty DW, Li DKB, the UBC MS/MRI Study Group, et al: Interferon beta-1b is effective in relapsing-remitting multiple sclerosis, II: MRI analysis results of a multicenter, randomized, double-blind, placebo-controlled trial. Neurology 43:662–667, 1993

Petersen RB, Tabaton M, Berg L, et al: Analysis of the prion protein gene in thalamic dementia. Neurology 42:1859–1863, 1992

Plum F, Posner JB, Hain RF: Delayed neurologic deterioration after anoxia. Arch Intern Med 110:18–25, 1962

Poser CM, Paty DW, Scheinberg L, et al: New diagnostic criteria for multiple sclerosis: guidelines for research protocols. Ann Neurol 13:227–231, 1983

Posner JB: Paraneoplastic syndromes affecting the central nervous system. Annu Rev Med 48:157–166, 1997

Power C, Johnson RT: HIV-1 associated dementia: clinical features and pathogenesis. Can J Neurol Sci 22:92–100, 1995

Price RW: Neurological complications of HIV infection. Lancet 348:445–452, 1996

Price RW, Sidtis JJ, Navia BA, et al: The AIDS dementia complex, in AIDS and the Nervous System. Edited by Rosenblum ML, Levy RM, Bredesen DE. New York, Raven, 1988, pp 203–219

Price TRP, Goetz KL, Lovell MR: Neuropsychiatric aspects of brain tumors, in The American Psychiatric Press Textbook of Neuropsychiatry, 2nd Edition. Edited by Yudofsky SC, Hales RE. Washington, DC, American Psychiatric Press, 1992, pp 493–494

Prusiner SB: The prion diseases. Sci Am 272:48–51, 54–57, 1995

Prusiner SB: Human prion diseases and neurodegeneration. Curr Top Micrpbiol Immunol 207:1–17, 1996

Prusiner SB, Hsiao KK: Human prion diseases. Ann Neurol 35:385–395, 1994

Przelomski MM, O'Rourke E, Grady GF, et al: Eastern equine encephalitis in Massachusetts: a report of 16 cases, 1970–1984. Neurology 38:736–739, 1988

Rabins PV: Euphoria in multiple sclerosis, in Neurobehavioral Aspects of Multiple Sclerosis. Edited by Rao SM. New York, Oxford University Press, 1990, pp 180–185

Rao SM: Neuropsychology of multiple sclerosis: a critical review. J Clin Exp Neuropsychol 8:503–542, 1986

Rao SM: White matter disease and dementia. Brain Cogn 31:250–268, 1996

Rao SM, Bernardin L, Leo GJ, et al: Cerebral disconnection in multiple sclerosis: relationship to atrophy of the corpus callosum. Arch Neurol 46:918–920, 1989

Rao SM, Leo GJ, Bernardin L, et al: Cognitive dysfunction in multiple sclerosis, I: frequency, patterns, and prediction. Neurology 41:685–691, 1991

Rappaport EB: Iatrogenic Creutzfeldt-Jakob disease. Neurology 37:1520–1522, 1987

Ron MA, Logsdail SJ: Psychiatric morbidity in multiple sclerosis: a clinical and MRI study. Psychol Med 19:887–895, 1989

Rosenblum ML, Levy RM, Bredesen DE: Overview of AIDS and the nervous system, in AIDS and the Nervous System. Edited by Rosenblum ML, Levy RM, Bredesen DE. New York, Raven, 1988, pp 1–12

Rosove MH, Brewer PMC: Antiphospholipid thrombosis: clinical course after the first thrombotic event in 70 patients. Ann Intern Med 117:303–308, 1992

Rubens AB, Froehling B, Slater G, et al: Left ear suppression on verbal dichotic tests in patients with multiple sclerosis. Ann Neurol 18:459–463, 1985

Scheck DN, Hook EW III: Neurosyphilis. Infect Dis Clin North Am 8:769–795, 1994

Schiffer RB: Disturbances of affect, in Neurobehavioral Aspects of Multiple Sclerosis. Edited by Rao SM. New York, Oxford University Press, 1990, pp 186–195

Schiffer RB, Caine ED: The interaction between depressive affective disorder and neuropsychological test performance in multiple sclerosis patients. J Neuropsychiatry Clin Neurosci 3:28–32, 1991

Schiffer RB, Herndon RM, Rudick RA: Treatment of pathologic laughing and weeping with amitriptyline. N Engl J Med 312:1480–1482, 1985

Schiffer RB, Weitkamp LR, Wineman NM, et al: Multiple sclerosis and affective disorder: family history, sex, and HLA-DR antigens. Arch Neurol 45:1345–1348, 1988

Schmidt RP: Neurosyphilis, in Clinical Neurology. Edited by Baker AB, Joynt RJ. New York, Harper & Row, 1989, pp 1–23

Schmitt FA, Bigley JW, McKinnis R, et al (and the AZT Collaborative Working Group): Neuropsychological outcome of zidovudine (AZT) treatment of patients with AIDS and AIDS-related complex. N Engl J Med 319:1573–1578, 1988

Schnider A, Benson DF, Rosner LJ: Callosal disconnection in multiple sclerosis. Neurology 43:1243–1245, 1993

Schonberger LB: New variant Creutzfeldt-Jakob disease and bovine spongiform encephalopathy. Infect Dis Clin North Am 12:111–121, 1998

Schroth G, Gawehn J, Thron A, et al: Early diagnosis of herpes simplex encephalitis by MRI. Neurology 37:179–183, 1987

Scott TF, Allen D, Price TRP, et al: Characterization of major depression symptoms in multiple sclerosis patients. J Neuropsychiatry Clin Neurosci 8:318–323, 1996

Seales D, Greer M: Acute hemorrhagic leukoencephalitis. A successful recovery. Arch Neurol 48:1086–1088, 1991

Seliger GM, Hornstein A, Flax J, et al: Fluoxetine improves emotional incontinence. Brain Inj 6:267–270, 1992

Serdaroglu P, Yazici H, Ozdemir C, et al: Neurologic involvement in Behçet's syndrome: a prospective study. Arch Neurol 46:265–269, 1989

Simon RP: Neurosyphilis. Arch Neurol 42:606–613, 1985

Slavoski LA, Tunkel AR: Therapy of fungal meningitis. Clin Neuropharmacol 18:95–112, 1995

So NK, O'Neill BP, Frytak S, et al: Delayed leukoencephalopathy in survivors with small cell lung cancer. Neurology 37:1198–1201, 1987

Stacy M, Roeltgen D: Infection of the central nervous system in the elderly, in The Pathology of the Aging Human Nervous System. Edited by Duckett S. Philadelphia, PA, Lea & Febiger, 1991, pp 374–392

Stagno SJ, Naugle RI, Roca C, et al: Progressive multifocal leukoencephalopathy appearing as language disturbance. Neuropsychiatry Neuropsychol Behav Neurol 3:283–289, 1990

Stenager E, Stenager EN, Jensen K: Sexual aspects of multiple sclerosis. Semin Neurol 12:120–124, 1992

Stoner GL, Walker DL, Webster HDF: Age distribution of progressive multifocal leukoencephalopathy. Acta Neurol Scand 78:307–312, 1988

Swain R: An update of vitamin B_{12} metabolism and deficiency states. J Fam Prac 41:595–600, 1995

Swirsky-Sacchetti T, Mitchell DR, Seward J, et al: Neuropsychological and structural brain lesions in multiple sclerosis: a regional analysis. Neurology 42:1291–1295, 1992

Sze G, Zimmerman RD: The magnetic resonance imaging of infections and inflammatory diseases. Radiol Clin North Am 26:839–859, 1988

Tan EM, Cohen AS, Fries JF, et al: The 1982 revised criteria for the classification of systemic lupus erythematosus. Arthritis Rheum 25:1271–1277, 1982

Teh L-S, Isenberg DA: Antiribosomal P protein antibodies in systemic lupus erythematosus. A reappraisal. Arthritis Rheum 37:307–315, 1994

Totsuka S, Hattori T, Yazaki M, et al: Clinicopathologic studies on neuro-Behçet's disease. Folia Psychiatrica et Neurologica Japonica 39:155–166, 1985

Tyler JL, Byrne TN: Neoplastic disorders, in Clinical Brain Imaging: Principles and Applications. Edited by Mazziotta JC, Gilman S. Philadelphia, PA, FA Davis, 1992, pp 166–216

Victor M: Persistent altered mentation due to ethanol. Neurol Clin 11:639–661, 1993

Vollmer TL, Guarnaccia J, Harrington W, et al: Idiopathic granulomatous angiitis of the central nervous system. Arch Neurol 50:925–930, 1993

Walker RW, Rosenblum MK: Amphotericin B–associated leukoencephalopathy. Neurology 42:2005–2010, 1992

Waniek C, Prohovnik I, Kaufman MA, et al: Rapidly progressive frontal-type dementia associated with Lyme disease. J Neuropsychiatry Clin Neurosci 7:345–347, 1995

Wasielewski PG, Scharre DW, Mendell JR: Inherited neurological disorders: relevant considerations and new aspects, in Clinical Neurology. Edited by Baker AB, Joynt RJ. New York, Harper & Row, 1997, pp 1–48

Watanabe N, Seto H, Shimizu M, et al: Brain SPECT of Creutzfeldt-Jakob disease. Clin Nucl Med 21:236–241, 1996

Weinshenker BG, Penman M, Bass B, et al: A double-blind, randomized, crossover trial of pemoline in fatigue associated with multiple sclerosis. Neurology 42:1468–1471, 1992

Weller M, Liedtke W, Petersen D, et al: Very-late-onset adrenoleukodystrophy: possible precipitation of demyelination by cerebral contusion. Neurology 42:367–370, 1992

West SG: Neuropsychiatric lupus. Rheum Dis Clin North Am 20:129–158, 1994

West SG, Emlen W, Wener MH, et al: Neuropsychiatric lupus erythematosus: a 10-year prospective study on the value of diagnostic tests. Am J Med 99:153–163, 1995

Whiteman MLH, Post MJD, Berger JR, et al: Progressive multifocal leukoencephalopathy in 47 HIV-seropositive patients: neuroimaging with clinical and pathologic correlation. Radiology 187:233–240, 1993

Whitley RJ: Herpes simplex virus infections of the central nervous system: encephalitis and neonatal herpes. Drugs 42:406–427, 1991

Whitley RJ, Lakeman F: Herpes simplex virus infections of the central nervous system: therapeutic and diagnostic considerations. Clin Infect Dis 20:414–420, 1995

Wispelwey B, Scheld WM: Brain abscess. Semin Neurol 12:273–278, 1992

Yamamori C, Ishino H, Inagaki T, et al: Neuro-Behçet disease with demyelination and gliosis of the frontal white matter. Clin Neuropathol 13:208–215, 1994

Younger DS, Hays AP, Brust JCM, et al: Granulomatous angiitis of the brain: an inflammatory reaction of diverse etiology. Arch Neurol 45:514–518, 1988

Zifko U, Wimberger D, Lindner K, et al: MRI in patients with general paresis. Neuroradiology 38:120–123, 1996

Medical Therapies

Karen Blank, M.D.

James D. Duffy, M.D., Ch.B.

Physicians caring for older patients aim to follow the Hippocratic promise to "First do no harm." However, although medications are vital for the treatment of disease, the balance between benefits and risks of their use in elderly patients becomes precarious. In particular, the adverse behavioral effects of prescription medications can be devastating. Unfortunately, when physicians fail to recognize the drug-related etiology of these behavioral changes and prescribe psychotropic medications, they precipitate a pattern of escalating use of medications, increased side effects, and drug interactions.

Although the elderly (defined as those over age 65) represent 12% of the population in the United States, they are the largest group of users of pharmaceuticals, accounting for 34% of all pharmaceutical expenditures, almost three times that of the general population (Mueller et al. 1997). Multiple medication use is prevalent in elderly patients because they often have multiple chronic illnesses. Thirty-six percent of the elderly have three or more chronic conditions and account for 57% of drug expenditures for this group (Mueller et al. 1997). Among community-dwelling elderly, 83% consume at least one medica-

tion (Ostrom et al. 1985), with the average being 3.1 prescription drugs (Ouslander 1981; Rogowski et al. 1997). Medication usage rises drastically each time an elderly patient is hospitalized, with the typical elderly patient receiving 8–15 medications (Piraino 1995). Multiple medication use increases both the risk of adverse drug events and noncompliance (Graves et al. 1997). The elderly are two to three times more likely to experience adverse reactions compared with younger patients (Vestal and Cusack 1990). Rates of adverse drug reactions vary widely and have risen in recent surveys—perhaps as a reflection of adverse drug reaction monitoring mandated by the Joint Commission of the Accreditation of Healthcare Organizations. Hospitalizations attributable to adverse drug reactions have been estimated to account for 1.7%–16.8% of medical hospitalizations and 0.6%–7.5% of psychiatric admissions (Popli et al. 1997; Salzman 1995).

When considering drug use in the elderly population, it is important to remember that elderly patients frequently self-medicate with nonprescription drugs, buying 40% of all over-the-counter (OTC) drugs (Mueller et al. 1997; Piraino 1995). These drugs include nonsteroidal anti-inflammatory drugs (NSAIDs), antihistamines, analgesics,

H₂ blockers, and psychostimulants including caffeine or phenylpropanolamine. In addition, only sometimes with their physicians' recommendation, older patients consume alternative medications including melatonin, ginseng, Chinese herbal preparations, and vitamins in excess of recommended daily allowances. Many OTC and alternative agents have significant behavioral side effects, can cause drug interactions, or contain contaminants known to cause neuropsychiatric syndromes. A complete OTC and alternative therapies usage history must be obtained to anticipate and diagnose neurobehavioral changes (see discussion below) (Ernst 1998).

Although some drug reactions are idiosyncratic and unexpected, most can be appreciated as resulting from high-risk prescribing. A Canadian study (Tamblyn et al. 1994) found that 52.6% of the elderly patients in their sample received "high risk" prescriptions. McLeod and colleagues (1997) outline inappropriate or risk-laden practices as the prescription of medications that 1) are contraindicated for elderly people because of unacceptable risk/benefit ratios, 2) can cause drug-drug interactions, or 3) can cause drug-illness interactions. (Significant drug-drug interactions are shown in Appendix 31–1.) Considerable overlap exists between the drugs most frequently used by elderly patients and those known to cause neurobehavioral side effects. The most prevalent conditions among the elderly in the 1987 National Medical Expenditure Survey (Mueller et al. 1997) were arthritis and hypertension. Among elderly diabetics, 34% of drug expenditures were for cardiovascular and renal drugs, 21% for hormonal drugs, and 12% for pain relievers (Mueller et al. 1997). The Boston Collaborative Drug Surveillance Program (1971), which examined 90,000 drug exposures occurring during 10,600 hospital admissions, found the following drugs to be most frequently associated with behavioral side effects: prednisone, isoniazid, methyldopa, insulin, diazepam, furosemide, phenobarbital, chlordiazepoxide, and aminophylline. Hanlon and colleagues (1997) found that among ambulatory patients taking five scheduled medications per day, 35% had an adverse drug reaction over a 1-year period—many requiring emergency room and in-hospital care. Twenty-nine percent of these were central nervous system (CNS) reactions, with cardiovascular medications (33.3%) and CNS medications (17.8%) the most common offending agents. Table 31–1 lists some patient risk factors for interactions.

In this chapter, we review the pharmacodynamic and pharmacokinetic alterations in normal aging, their interactions with pathological processes, and the implications of polypharmacy. We also review the neuropsychiatric effects of prescribed and OTC medications in elderly patients and summarize how these medical therapeutic agents can interfere with a wide range of neurobehavioral functions including cognition, mood, arousal, sleep, ambulation, and sexual function.

Special Considerations in Geriatric Medical Therapy

Elderly patients are particularly susceptible to the neuropsychiatric complications of medical therapies because of age-related changes in CNS vulnerability, as well as changes in the body's ability to absorb, distribute, metabolize, and excrete drugs. Aging also increases the likelihood of multiple intercurrent illnesses and consequent drug interactions. In addition, aging may be associated with changes in drug-taking behaviors. The failure to recognize drug misuse and abuse in the elderly population can contribute to the development of neuropsychiatric complications of medical therapy. Rational medical treatment depends on an understanding of the interrelationships between these factors. Catterson et al. (1997) suggest conceptualizing these interactions as the "magnitude of effect" (the clinical response, both desired and untoward). Magnitude of effect is the product of the pharmacodynamics (the

TABLE 31–1. Patient risk factors for drug interactions

Multiple chronic conditions

Multiple medications

Female gender

Previous adverse drug reaction

Very young or old age

Obesity

Dehydration

Hypoproteinemia

Hypotension

Postresuscitation

Congestive heart failure

Liver dysfunction

Slow acetylators phenotype

Renal dysfunction

Hypothyroidism

Hypothermia

Source. Adapted with permission from Mills KC: "Essential Emergency Medicine Pharmacokinetics: Prevention of Iatrogenic Patient Poisoning." *Topics in Emergency Medicine* 15:18–29, 1993; Anastasio GD, Cornell KO, Menscer D: "Drug Interactions: Keeping It Straight (review)." *American Family Physician* 56:883–894, 1997.

action of the drug at the targets), the pharmacokinetics (the manner in which the drug is handled by the body and distributed to its target sites), and the biological variance (the individual biology of the patient and nature of the disease process). The following provides a brief review of some of the pertinent factors involved in the expected and undesired magnitude of effect of drug therapies in aging patients.

Pharmacodynamic Alterations in Normal Aging and in Common Diseases

The normal aging process is associated with predictable physiological alterations that influence the elderly person's response to medications. Although substantial interindividual and intraindividual variability in the extent and type of changes is associated with the aging process, certain characteristic neurochemical and neurophysiological changes have been well documented.

Age-related alterations in the major neurotransmitter systems contribute to the increased pharmacodynamic sensitivity of the elderly. Although some of the data remain contradictory, these predictable age-related changes include alterations in neuronal cell numbers and neurotransmitter production and breakdown, selective changes in the number of presynaptic and postsynaptic receptors with age, and alterations in the receptor binding site–second messenger system (Sunderland 1992). Functionally, these changes result in both reduced transmission of neuronal messages in the aging brain and reduced ability for the receptor to upregulate or downregulate in response to drugs. These CNS changes are believed to be responsible for many of the neuropsychiatric syndromes that occur in old age (Sunderland 1992) as well as the more prevalent toxic neuropsychiatric reactions secondary to medical treatments. The age-related pharmacodynamic changes in the major neurotransmitters are reviewed below and are summarized in Table 31–2 (Catterson et al. 1997).

Cholinergic system. Normal aging involves loss and shrinking of the cholinergic neurons in the basal forebrain (Mesulam et al. 1987) with resulting decreases of cholinergic innervation throughout the brain and reduced amount of the acetylcholine-synthesizing enzyme choline acetyltransferase (CAT) (Catterson et al. 1997). The cholinergic cell loss and decreases in CAT activity are thought to be responsible for some of the memory decline in normal aging. Because acetylcholine plays a vital role in memory storage and retrieval, drugs with anticholinergic properties cause further disruption of acetylcholine transmission, resulting in mild to severe cognitive impairment.

Dementia of the Alzheimer type is characterized by a dramatic degradation of cholinergic systems, with pronounced cholinergic cell loss and decreased CAT activity in the cerebral cortex, pyramidal cells of the hippocampus, and nucleus basalis of Meynert (Catterson et al. 1997; Sunderland 1992). Anticholinergic drugs commonly have a deleterious effect on the already compromised memory of these patients, frequently causing delirium with relatively low doses. In addition to changes in the cholinergic system, persons with dementia of the Alzheimer type exhibit alterations in adrenergic and serotonergic systems. The impact of these changes on drug response remains to be determined.

Patients with Parkinson's disease also demonstrate an increased sensitivity to anticholinergic agents. One study found the development of an acute confusional state in 93% of patients with Parkinson's disease who were taking anticholinergic medications (De Smet et al. 1982).

Dopaminergic system. In normal aging, reduced dopamine synthesis and transmission can result from declines in the activity of the enzymes tyrosine hydroxylase and dopa decarboxylase (Jeste and Wyatt 1987; Sunderland 1992). In addition, the number of dopamine neurons in the nigrostriatal tract decreases with age. The most frequent manifestation of this reduction in dopamine activity is the occurrence of movement and gait disorders and in the older patient's (often exquisite) sensitivity to neuro-

---

TABLE 31–2. Neurotransmitter pharmacodynamic changes with aging

Dopaminergic system
  ↓Dopamine D_2 receptors in the striatum
Cholinergic system
  ↓Choline acetyltransferase
  ↓Cholinergic cell numbers
Adrenergic system
  ↓cAMP production in response to β agonists
  ↓β-Adrenoceptor numbers
  ↓β-Receptor affinity
  ↓α_2-adrenoceptor responsiveness
Gabaminergic system
  ↓Psychomotor performance in response to benzodiazepines
?↑Postsynaptic receptor response to γ = aminobutyric acid

Source. Reprinted from Catterson ML, Preskorn SH, Martin RL: "Pharmacodynamic and Pharmacokinetic Considerations in Geriatric Psychopharmacology." *Geriatric Psychiatry* 20:215–218, 1997.

leptic-induced extrapyramidal symptoms. Significant changes also develop in the ratio of the subtypes of dopamine receptors with a progressive loss of D_2 receptors (Catterson et al. 1997; Sunderland 1992). These receptor changes may help explain the increased incidence of drug-induced extrapyramidal syndromes (Catterson et al. 1997) and the susceptibility of older persons to chronic effects of dopamine blockers and resultant high rates of tardive dyskinesia (Sunderland 1992). In this regard, is important to appreciate the dopamine blocking action of nonpsychotropic medications such as metoclopramide, which frequently produce extrapyramidal side effects in elderly patients.

The profound dopamine depletion (and subsequent neuroleptic supersensitivity) associated with Parkinson's disease often poses a therapeutic dilemma because these patients frequently develop delusional disorders and/or hallucinations as a consequence of dopamine agonist treatment (Cummings 1991). The selective dopamine subtype 4 (D_4), receptor blocking agents clozapine and olanzapine provide viable therapeutic options in such situations (Rabey et al. 1995; Rosenthal et al. 1992; Wolters et al. 1996; Young et al. 1997). Patients with Alzheimer's disease also experience reduction in dopaminergic function, which accounts for their increased susceptibility to the extrapyramidal effects of neuroleptics prescribed for control of their agitated behavior (Cross et al. 1984).

Serotonin system. Research has yielded contradictory results regarding age-related alterations in 5-hydroxytryptamine (5-HT, serotonin) CNS characteristics. However, most evidence indicates decreased function and sensitivity of the 5-HT_1 and frontal cortex 5-HT_2 receptors with aging (Sunderland 1992). A decrease in both serotonin production (Shih and Young 1978) and serotonin receptor number and sensitivity (Lawlor et al. 1989) has been linked to the alterations in appetite and sleep seen in elderly patients and may explain their apparently reduced response to serotonergic drugs (Sunderland 1992).

Adrenergic system. Studies of the noradrenergic system reveal, as yet unexplained, age-related reductions in responses mediated by β-adrenergic and α_2-adrenergic receptors. Drugs such as propranolol (β-adrenergic blocker) and clonidine (α_2-adrenergic agonist) may be therefore less effective in older patients (Catterson et al. 1997).

Gabaminergic system. Within the CNS, γ-aminobutyric acid (GABA) functions as an inhibitory neurotransmitter and therefore plays a major role in modulating neuronal transmission. Reduced GABA neurotrans-

mission is thought to be important in Huntington's disease, Parkinson's disease, and some forms of epilepsy, but the changes with normal aging are less understood (Sunderland 1992). Research suggests a role for the benzodiazepine-GABA receptor complex in the etiology of anxiety. Increased density and sensitivity of the benzodiazepine binding sites with age may explain the heightened sensitivity of the aging CNS to benzodiazepine sedating effects and to their deleterious effects on psychomotor performance (Catterson et al. 1997; Sunderland 1992).

Additional physiological changes of pharmacodynamic significance. In addition to alterations in the specific neurotransmitters described above, other age-related physiological changes can have significant implications for drug effects. These changes render the older person more susceptible to the adverse side effects of many medications and involve neurodegenerative changes in the autonomic nervous system that predispose to orthostatic hypotension and thermal dysregulation (Brocklehurst 1974; Caird et al. 1987; Nemeroff 1989).

Although these age-related physiological and pathological changes make the elderly more sensitive to the CNS effects of medical therapies, older patients may actually be less sensitive to the peripheral effects of some drugs (e.g., the chronotropic effects of isoproterenol, β-adrenergic blockage by propranolol, PR prolongation by verapamil and diltiazem, and the hypoglycemic effect of tolbutamide [Vestal and Cusack 1990]). The clinician must carefully balance these altered central and peripheral pharmacodynamics when prescribing for elderly patients.

Pharmacokinetics

Aging causes several changes that alter drug pharmacokinetics, the manner in which the drug is handled by the body and distributed to its target sites of action. The expected processes of normal aging, as well as an increased incidence of comorbid disease states, result in physiological and environmental changes that alter the absorption, distribution and transport, metabolism, and excretion of drugs.

Absorption. In theory, age-related changes of the gastrointestinal track would be expected to result in impairments of absorption of orally ingested drugs. These changes include reductions in stomach acid and mesenteric blood flow, decreases in the number of absorptive cells, decrease in the size of the absorbing surface, and impaired transport across the intestinal epithelial membrane. However, there appears to be little clinical impact of these changes in healthy older persons (Abernethy 1992; Greenblatt 1993). Thus, in normal aging, the rate of absorption (generally described as the time required for the drug to reach maximum plasma concentration [T_{max}]) is not significantly altered for most medications. Exception to this, however, are the absorption characteristics of levodopa and clorazepate. The increased gastric pH can contribute to decreased steady-state concentrations of clorazepate, and decreased dopa decarboxylase activity in the gastric mucosa can cause a threefold increase in the bioavailability of levodopa in elderly patients (Wood and Castleden 1991). When certain pathological processes and medications are present, however, the age-related changes become significant. Antacids can cause considerable decrements in the absorption of medications, and drugs and anticholinergics can impair intestinal motility and impair absorption. When these interactions lead to treatment failure, drug dosage escalation and toxicity can result.

Distribution. The physicochemical properties of a drug substantially influence how it is distributed. Lipophilicity greatly influences how rapidly a given drug will reach targets in the brain and how extensively it will distribute through the body (Greenblatt 1993). Increases in the volume of distribution of lipophilic drugs result in part from the general increase in total body fat (with decreased lean muscle mass) with aging. At age 25, the total body fat of the average 70-kg person is approximately 20%. By age 70, it is 30% or even higher in sedentary persons (Piraino 1995). Conversely, total body water content declines with age, from 60% to 54% in men and from 52% to 46% in women. The decline in body water tends to be exacerbated by a diminished sense of thirst and reduced fluid intake (Piraino 1995). As a result, hydrophilic medications, such as digoxin and lithium, will have smaller volumes of distribution and higher serum levels.

The most important clinical implication of these age-related changes stems from the relationship of volume of distribution (V_d) to clearance. Lipid-soluble drugs with high volumes of distribution accumulate more extensively in the elderly, and the time required for elimination of the drug is prolonged, often substantially. Another clinical effect of this change in V_d is that a single dose of medication may have diminished effect because of lowered presence in the plasma as a result of dilution into peripheral tissues. In chronic drug therapy, this effect is of little clinical importance (Abernethy 1992).

Another drug characteristic that strongly affects its volume of distribution is the extent to which it binds to plasma proteins. Albumin, the most important binding protein, typically decreases with age, particularly in the

face of poor nutrition or renal failure. Even small reductions in albumin significantly increase the free fraction of drugs that normally would be extensively protein bound (Piraino 1995). The result will be higher concentrations of free, unbound drug to diffuse to CNS receptors. Elderly patients receiving several highly protein-bound medications will have increased drug-free fractions resulting from competition for limited binding sites. Changes in albumin and α_1 acid glycoprotein with aging will, in addition, make the interpretation of total plasma drug concentration assays more complicated (Greenblatt 1993).

Metabolism and excretion. After absorption, the first-pass extraction by the liver (or presystemic extraction) often substantially reduces the amount of drug that reaches the systemic circulation. Aging results in decreased liver size, decreased blood flow, generally decreased activity of the hepatic microsomal enzymes, at least those involved in phase I metabolism (Catterson et al. 1997), and increased prevalence of slow acetylator status. For drugs typically highly metabolized by first-pass effects, less drug is removed from the splanchnic circulation, resulting in increased bioavailability in the systemic circulation. Low flow conditions and congestive heart failure can further diminish this first-pass effect.

Once a drug reaches the systemic circulation in an elderly patient, it tends to be cleared more slowly than that in a younger patient. Phase I enzymatic reactions (oxidation, reduction, and hydrolysis of drugs) are affected by aging far more than are the conjugation of drugs and metabolites (phase II enzymatic reactions). Drugs requiring oxidation for biotransformation will have a greatly prolonged half-life in elderly patients (Erwin 1993). Because the elimination half-life is dependent on clearance and volume of distribution, those drugs with an increased volume of distribution and a decreased hepatic clearance (e.g., diazepam) will have a significantly prolonged half-life in elderly patients. Because lorazepam and oxazepam are metabolized by phase II reactions, they are the most appropriate benzodiazepines for older patients.

Important drug interactions occur through induction or inhibition of hepatic enzymes. Advances have been made in understanding the family of hepatic microsomal drug-metabolizing enzymes known as cytochromes. Two cytochrome P450 systems, the P450 IID6 and P450 IIIA4, appear to be responsible for the biotransformation of more than 90% of the drugs used in clinical practice that undergo hepatic metabolism. These systems have come under particular scrutiny since the introduction of the selective serotonin reuptake inhibitor (SSRI) medications and the observation that coadministration of fluoxetine with a considerable number of other medications caused significant elevations of the plasma levels and the effects of the latter drugs (Anastasio et al. 1997; Greenblatt 1993) (Table 31–3).

Regarding excretion, although there is significant individual variation in renal function in elderly individuals, renal functioning begins a linear decline at age 40, and, by age 60, the decline becomes exponential (Catterson et al. 1997). Renal blood flow and glomerular filtration decrease as a function of age. On average, in those over age 65, renal clearance is reduced approximately 35% compared with that of the young. The function of the aging kidney is further diminished by congestive heart failure, diabetes, hypertension, and the concomitant use of sodium-depleting diuretics, nonsteroidal antiinflammatory medications and β-blockers. Thus, plasma clearance of water-soluble drugs and metabolites is often substantially compromised in elderly patients.

Compliance Concerns

In general, little evidence suggests that older patients, as a group, are less compliant than other patients. However, because the risks of noncompliance are more serious, greater emphasis on strict compliance is required to properly treat these patients (Lamy et al. 1992). Also, the causes of noncompliance may be different from those in younger age groups. Reasons for noncompliance in the elderly include 1) greater medication use and multiple simultaneous medication use; 2) unintentional noncompliance because of forgetting or not understanding the dosage schedule or reasons for medication; 3) intentional noncompliance because of cost or side effects; and 4) higher rates of adverse drug reactions (Salzman 1995).

The likelihood of noncompliance rises with the number of prescribed drugs and the disability of the patient (Ostrom et al. 1985). Noncompliance has been found to increase dramatically among the elderly when four or more medications are prescribed and/or when dosing more than twice a day is required (Salzman 1995). Bergman and Wilholm (1981) showed that in patients over age 65 the rate of noncompliance doubles when more than three drugs are prescribed (32% versus 69%). Cost appears to account for noncompliance in 10% of elderly patients, with higher noncompliance rates occurring when monthly medication costs exceed $90 (Salzman 1995). Patients with cognitive impairment require extra monitoring (Kennedy 1992). Those elderly patients who use several physicians and who may provide inconsistent medication histories (Jackson et al. 1989) are at risk for increased adverse events.

TABLE 31–3. Examples of drugs[a] that might interact with an antidepressant

CYP 1A2	CYP 2C19	2C9	CYP 2D6[b]	CYP 3A3/4
Acetaminophen	Barbiturates	Diclofenac	Chlorpheniramine	Benzodiazepines, alprazolam, clonazepam, diazepam, triazolam
Clozapine	Citalopram	Ibuprofen	Codeine	
Haloperidol	Diazepam	Naproxen	Desipramine, secondary TCAs	
Phenacetin	Mephenytoin	Omeprazole		Cisapride
Phenothiazines	Moclobemide	Phenytoin	Dextromethorphan	Corticosteroids
R-Warfarin (minor)	Propranolol	Piroxicam	Flecainide/encainide	Cyclosporine
Tacrine	Tertiary TCAs	S-Warfarin	Haloperidol	Dapsone
Tertiary TCAs		Tolbutamide	Hydrocodone	Estrogens
Theophylline			Phenothiazines	Ketoconazole, itraconazole
Thiothixene			Propranolol, timolol, metoprolol	Lovastatin
			Reduced haloperidol	Macrolide antibiotics
			Risperidone	Nonsedating antihistamines[c]
			Quinidine	Paclitaxel
				Quinidine
				Tamoxifen
				Zolpidem

Note. CYP = cytochrome P450; TCA = tricyclic antidepressant.
[a]Drug can be substrate and/or inhibitor of a given enzyme system.
[b]Inhibitor at 2D6, not a substrate.
[c]Terfenadine and astemizole contraindicated with CYP3A inhibitors; loratadine not contraindicated.
Source. Reprinted with permission from *The 1996 Black Book of Psychotropic Dosing and Monitoring.*

A benefit that may result from technological advances in health care delivery may be that physicians will have ready access to computerized databases and pharmacy records and with them be better able to orchestrate the patient's care.

Underrecognition of Drug Abuse and Misuse

Substance misuse and abuse in elderly patients can lead to a variety of neuropsychiatric complications of medical therapy (Gambert 1992; Lawson 1989). Alcohol, prescription sedatives and analgesics, OTC medications, and caffeine are the most frequent substances of abuse. Significant symptomatology can result from both their use and also from abrupt withdrawal (Graves et al. 1997). One study found that the presence of benzodiazepines in the admission urine of cognitively intact elderly patients accounted for 29% of the cases of delirium that occurred in hospital (Foy et al. 1995). Many patients will conceal their OTC drug use or may not consider them as drugs. Only one-sixth of patients will inform their physicians of their OTC use, and those with cognitive impairment are particularly vulnerable to OTC misuse (Atkinson et al. 1992).

The anticholinergic effects of diphenhydramine and other antihistamines found in most OTC sleep and cold remedies can cause significant cognitive effects, delirium, and psychosis in elderly patients, even in therapeutic doses. There is also an age-associated increased sensitivity to caffeine and other stimulants such as phenylpropanolamine, ephedrine, and pseudoephedrine found in OTC allergy and cold preparations. Elderly patients can also be at increased risk from the neuropsychiatric effects of NSAIDs in OTC preparations. These effects include aseptic meningitis, psychosis, and cognitive dysfunction (Hoppmann et al. 1991). (The neuropsychiatric aspects of drug abuse and misuse in the elderly population are discussed further in Chapter 16 in this volume.)

▍Drug-Induced Neuropsychiatric Syndromes

Appendix 31–2 summarizes the drugs associated with specific neuropsychiatric syndromes in elderly patients. These are further discussed below.

Delirium and Cognitive Impairment

Delirium occurs at rates ranging from 14% to 56% of elderly hospitalized patients, with associated hospital mortality rates of 10%–65%. Delirium results in longer, cost-lier hospitalizations and increased rates of nursing home placements (Inouye 1994). Drugs, particularly anticholinergic agents, represent the most common cause of confusional states across all age groups (Hodkinson 1973). (Delirium is discussed further in Chapter 19, and dementia, in Chapter 24 in this volume.) Identified factors predisposing to the development of delirium are 1) age greater than 60 years (Lipowski 1984; Liston 1982) and 2) brain dysfunction (Erkinjuntti et al. 1986; Lipowski 1990). Other independent risk factors for its development include severe illness or sudden change in neurological, cardiac, pulmonary, or metabolic state; dehydration; malnutrition; infection; withdrawal from sedative-hypnotics or alcohol; and vision impairment. Independent precipitating factors appear to be the use of physical restraints, use of bladder catheter, and the rapid addition of three or more medications in a short time period (Inouye and Charpentier 1996; Rummans et al. 1995).

Many of the same drugs that produce delirium can also cause chronic cognitive impairment in elderly patients. Katzman et al. (1988) reviewed nine published series and found drug-induced states to be the most common of the reversible causes of dementia, and Larson et al. (1987) implicated drugs as either a primary or contributing cause in 35 of their 300 patients evaluated for dementia. The sedative-hypnotic agents, especially long-acting benzodiazepines, were the drugs most commonly associated with cognitive impairment. Appendix 31–2 indicates the various medical therapies reported to be associated with the development of delirium and dementia. The most important agents causing cognitive impairment are discussed below.

Anticholinergic agents. A postulated mechanism of drug-induced delirium is the accumulation of anticholinergic effects (Tune et al. 1992). Narcotic analgesics, antiparkinsonian drugs, neuroleptics, tricyclic antidepressants, antispasmodics, and OTC cold and sleep preparations containing antihistamines all have significant anticholinergic effects. Anticholinergic agents are particularly likely to induce delirium and are postulated to induce an imbalance in the cholinergic and adrenergic pathways of the reticular activating system and thalamocortical projections, thereby disrupting the attentional matrix (Itil and Fink 1966).

As discussed above, the elderly brain is likely to be more sensitive to the anticholinergic effects of drugs, particularly if there is associated neurodegenerative disease. Indeed, the neurologically compromised elderly patient may develop delirium even after receiving 1% scopolamine eye drops or transdermal patches (Danielson et al. 1981; MacEwan et al. 1985). The extent of this hazard faced by elderly patients is highlighted by the finding that 60% of nursing home residents and 23% of elderly community dwellers are receiving at least one anticholinergic drug at any one time (Blazer et al. 1983). Of the 25 most commonly prescribed medications in elderly patients, 14 were found to have detectable anticholinergic effects (Tune et al. 1992). P. S. Miller et al. (1988) evaluated the effects of low-dose scopolamine (0.005 mg/kg body weight) versus placebo in presurgical elderly patients and found the degree of impairment on the Saskatoon Delirium Symptom Checklist and performance on the Rey Auditory-Verbal Learning test (Lezak 1983) to relate to both serum and cerebrospinal fluid anticholinergic levels. It is important to recognize that elderly patients may experience the central muscarinic toxicity that produces a confusional state or a dementia-like syndrome without necessarily manifesting the characteristic autonomic (nicotinic) changes of urinary retention, tachycardia, piloerection, or pupillary dilation (Crawshaw and Mullen 1984).

Although the mechanisms by which corticosteroids alter cognition and cause delirium are not clearly understood, these agents are known to have high anticholinergic potency. Corticosteroid-induced neuropsychiatric side effects occur in 5% of patients. The larger the corticosteroid dose or the more rapidly changes in dose are made, the higher the prevalence of delirium and other neuropsychiatric complications. Other mechanisms by which corticosteroids are postulated to exert neurobehavioral effect are through altered serotonergic, somatostatin, and GABA agonist activity. Changes in hippocampal activity have also been implicated (Vincent 1995). Factors that predispose to corticosteroid-induced delirium include advanced age, intercurrent illness, and female gender (Stoudemire et al. 1996).

The cognitive impairment and delirium that occur with tricyclic antidepressants are primarily a result of their anticholinergic effect. Although tricyclics continue to be used for depression and pain management, their use for depression has been diminished by the SSRIs and novel antidepressants. Most of the SSRIs, norepinephrine reuptake inhibitors, and reversible inhibitors of monoamine oxidase are essentially devoid of anticholinergic activity and have either no memory effect or may improve cognition (Oxman 1996). The minimal anticholinergic effects of these agents are likely to present a significant clinical advantage over the tricyclic agents. However, their use is still associated with delirium in isolated case reports (Bonne et al. 1995) through drug interactions (Rothschild 1995), development of hyperserotonergic states (Amir et al. 1997) (see serotonergic syndrome below), development of the syndrome of inappropriate antidiuretic hormone (SIADH)

with resultant hyponatremia, and possibly through withdrawal (although the latter is reported only in case reports) (Kasantikul 1995).

Recent reports of delirium with, and after, clozapine therapy hypothesized mechanisms mediated through the cholinergic system with withdrawal delirium caused by a central cholinergic rebound (Pitner et al. 1995; Stanilla et al. 1997; Wilkins-Ho and Hollander 1997).

Cardiovascular medications. Several antihypertensives have been reported to produce delirium. β-blockers in particular have been implicated in producing not only delirium (Kuhr 1979), but also hallucinosis, sleep disruption, and chronic fatigue (McGahan et al. 1984). The topical β-blocker timolol, used to treat glaucoma, can also produce delirium (Shore et al. 1987). Other antihypertensives implicated in the production of delirium include calcium channel blockers, clonidine, and methyldopa (Adler 1981; Hoffman and Ladogana 1981; Jacobsen et al. 1987). Methyldopa, propranolol, hydrochlorothiazide, and reserpine can also produce significant global cognitive impairment in the elderly (Larson et al. 1987).

Delirium can occur with therapeutic blood levels (Eisendrath and Sweeney 1987) of digoxin and herald the onset of potentially fatal cardiac arrhythmias (Sagel and Matisonn 1975). In addition to alterations in attention, digoxin can produce hallucinosis, sleep disruption, dysphoria, and irritability (Eisendrath and Sweeney 1987). Siberian ginseng has been reported to lead to increased digoxin levels (Ernst 1998). The muscarinic-blocking properties of the antiarrhythmics quinidine and disopyramide can also result in cognitive impairment in elderly patients.

Nonsteroidal anti-inflammatory drugs and other analgesic medications. Any of the NSAIDs can produce delirium and cognitive impairment in elderly patients (Allison and Shantz 1987; J. S. Goodwin and Regan 1982; Thornton 1980). NSAIDs are widely prescribed (in 1991 more than 70 million prescriptions were filled), and four NSAIDs, ibuprofen, ketoprofen, naproxen, and aspirin are available without prescription. The adverse effects of indomethacin are best recognized, but systematic information about the newer NSAIDs has been sparse. There are many case reports implicating most of the NSAIDs in causing delirium, mania, paranoid psychosis, and other depressive disorders with suicidal ideation (Browning 1996). Another case report describes a tacrine ibuprofen combination as causing delirium (Hooten and Pearlson 1996). As interest grows in using

NSAIDs for delaying onset and progression of Alzheimer's disease, delirium may become a treatment-limiting side effect. Elderly individuals are particularly susceptible to acute or chronic salicylate toxicity that can occur at "therapeutic levels" and frequently presents with delirium (Cupit 1982). Although the opiate analgesics are less likely to produce delirium, the anticholinergic effects of normeperidine (a metabolite of meperidine) can result in a syndrome characterized by agitation, hallucinosis, and confusion (Eisendrath et al. 1987), and meperidine, in combination with MAO inhibitors, can cause a fatal serotonin syndrome.

Histamine subtype 2 receptor antagonists. The histamine subtype 2 (H$_2$) receptor blockers cimetidine, ranitidine, and famotidine are available over the counter and generally have been considered to have a benign side-effect profile. Adverse CNS reactions including malaise, dizziness, somnolence, and headaches occur in less than 3% of adult patients. However, serious neuropsychiatric complications including mental confusion, agitation, depression, and hallucinations have been reported, predominantly in geriatric patients with impaired renal or hepatic function (Picotte-Prillmayer et al. 1995), causing delirium in as many as 17% of these patients (Schentag et al. 1979). Whereas cimetidine has traditionally been implicated in most cases of CNS side effects, no clear evidence supports a higher incidence of adverse reactions with cimetidine compared with the other H$_2$ blocking agents. A recent study (Kim et al. 1996) showed no significant difference between cimetidine and ranitidine in the occurrence of postoperative delirium. The observation that physostigmine can reverse cimetidine-induced delirium (Jenike and Levy 1983) suggests that there may be indirect cholinergic involvement.

Antiparkinsonian medications. Patients with Parkinson's disease receiving levodopa are at risk for developing delirium. Patients of advanced age with Parkinson's disease, those with dementia, and those with significant cortical atrophy appear to be at most risk for developing not only delirium, but other behavioral side effects such as hallucinosis and psychosis (Celesia and Barr 1970; Fennelly 1987; Young et al. 1997). Not surprisingly, the anticholinergics often prescribed to treat the tremor of Parkinson's disease also frequently produce confusion and cognitive impairment. The dopamine agonists bromocriptine and amantadine have also been reported to produce delirium in as many as 20% of patients (Cummings 1991; Lieberman et al. 1979; Postma and Vantilburg 1975).

Anesthesia. Postoperative delirium and less severe cognitive impairments are not uncommon in elderly patients. Several possible etiologies should be considered including anticholinergic preoperative preparations, hypoxia, metabolic disturbances, infection, fat embolism, hemodynamic disturbances, meperidine intoxication, pulmonary embolism, and sedative-hypnotic withdrawal (Irvin 1995; Lipowski 1990; Tzabar et al. 1996).

Serotonergic drugs. The serotonin syndrome is a potentially fatal complication of serotonergic drug therapy and is characterized by the triad of altered mental status, autonomic dysfunction, and neuromuscular abnormalities (Martin 1996). Clinical manifestations include agitation, delirium, mutism, ataxia, mydriasis, diaphoresis, hyperthermia, shivering, fluctuating blood pressure, tremor and myoclonus, cardiovascular collapse, coma, seizures, and death. The serotonin syndrome is sometimes mistaken for the neuroleptic malignant syndrome but, in all but the most severe cases, lacks the serious muscle breakdown of the latter (Gelenberg 1995; Martin 1996; Stahl 1997; Sternbach 1991). The syndrome occurs because of toxic amounts of serotonin, rarely caused by a single serotonergic medication (Kolecki 1997), but more often by drug combinations of serotonergic acting medications or when MAO inhibitors are combined with an SSRI or with meperidine. Clinical features of serotonin syndromes are shown in Table 31–4.

Other drugs causing delirium and cognitive impairment. Low doses of benzodiazepines, relating to the plasma concentration, can also cause significant cog-

TABLE 31–4. Most common clinical features of the serotonin syndrome in 38 patients in 12 reports

Clinical Feature	N	%
Mental status changes		
Confusion	16	42
Hypomania	8	21
Restlessness	17	45
Myoclonus	13	34
Hyperreflexia	11	29
Diaphoresis	10	26
Shivering	10	26
Tremor	10	26
Diarrhea	6	16
Incoordination	5	13

Source. Reprinted with permission from Sternbach H: "The Serotonin Syndrome." *American Journal of Psychiatry* 48:705–713, 1991.

nitive impairment in elderly patients (Pomara et al. 1984). The ability of benzodiazepines to impair the acquisition of new information (anterograde amnesia) and impair attention has been clearly documented. Deleterious effects on vigilance and encoding have been observed (Coenen and van Luijtelaar 1997). Several studies have confirmed improved memory, cognitive functioning, energy, and sense of well-being in elderly nursing home residents after discontinuation of benzodiazepines (Griffiths and Weerts 1997). The long-acting benzodiazepines are worrisome because of their increased accumulation and the persistence of side effects. But the ultra-short acting benzodiazepines used as hypnotics have also been shown to have substantial cognitive impact including anterograde amnesia and delirium in susceptible individuals (Patterson 1987; Reynolds et al. 1985). After news that triazolam causes amnestic episodes was disseminated through the popular press, its sales dropped dramatically. Recently, Lobo and Greene (1997) have concluded from their literature review that the new and popular hypnotic zolpidem is strikingly similar to triazolam. Although not a benzodiazepine, zolpidem binds with the GABA receptor (although selective for subtype 1) and shares triazolam's pharmacokinetic properties. Zolpidem has been found to cause confusion, visual hallucinations, and amnestic periods occurring during the night and sometimes persisting into the next day.

The Veterans Affairs cooperative study of the cognitive effects of anticonvulsants in 622 patients with epilepsy reported that patients on phenobarbital, primidone, and phenytoin exhibit significant cognitive impairment compared with matched control subjects receiving carbamazepine (Smith et al. 1987). Carbamazepine and sodium valproate have shown less tendency to induce cognitive impairment in most studies, although the latter has been implicated as causing a dementia-like syndrome associated with reversible cerebral atrophy (McLachlan 1987). In a study of 36 patients with epilepsy who were on long-term valproate therapy, 32 were found to have reversible parkinsonism with cognitive impairment that had developed insidiously (Armon et al. 1996). Willmore (1995) cautions that elderly patients with declining intellectual function, motor impairments, or altered sensory function may be especially susceptible to dose-related CNS side effects of antiepileptic drugs and delineates the special cautions of polypharmacy and drug interactions in the elderly.

Other drugs reported to cause cognitive impairment include lithium, various antibiotics, radio-contrast agents, interferon, heavy metals, organic solvents, cyclosporine, various antineoplastic agents, phenylpropanolamine, and caffeine. (For an excellent review, see Morrison and Katz 1989.)

Anxiety

Anxiety can be caused by a variety of pharmacological agents (Appendix 31–2). There is an increased sensitivity to stimulants with aging, and the elderly may be particularly susceptible to caffeinism—even without a history of excessive intake (Williams and Caranasos 1992). Caffeine may also be taken unknowingly in various OTC cold and allergy preparations. Sympathomimetic amines, which may be present in such OTC preparations, are common causes of secondary anxiety in elderly patients (Lader 1982). Elderly individuals, particularly those with cognitive impairment, are susceptible to paradoxical excitement manifested by anxiety and agitation as a result of alcohol, benzodiazepines, barbiturates, and other sedative-hypnotics. Short-acting benzodiazepines can cause rebound anxiety, precipitating escalating use of the drug. Erratic use of sedative-hypnotics can cause withdrawal insomnia and daytime anxiety. Tricyclic antidepressants, bupropion, and fluoxetine have all been reported to produce restlessness, anxiety, and insomnia (Williams and Caranasos 1992).

The withdrawal effects of narcotics, alcohol, benzodiazepines, and other sedative-hypnotics are also frequent causes of anxiety. Other drugs implicated as causing anxiety include corticosteroids, theophylline, thyroxine, antiparkinsonian drugs (particularly levodopa and bromocriptine), various cardiac drugs (disopyramide and nifedipine), cycloserine, anticonvulsants, antihistamines, anticholinergics, and various respiratory drugs. Ten percent to 15% of patients treated with dopaminergic agents will develop anxiety symptoms (Cummings 1991).

Depression, Mania, and Psychosis

Drugs implicated in causing affective and psychotic disorders are listed in Appendix 31–2. In this section, we discuss the most important of these as they pertain to elderly patients.

Cardiac medications. Cardiac glycosides, antiarrhythmics, and antihypertensives have all been associated with the development of psychotic and affective symptoms. The long-known catecholamine-depleting effects of reserpine account for the frequent association of depression with the use of this antihypertensive (F. K. Goodwin and Bunney 1971). α-Methyldopa has also long been associated with depressive symptoms, acting primarily via its metabolite α-methylnorepinephrine, a potent α_2-adrenergic agonist. In their extensive review of the literature, Paykel et al. (1982) also found an incidence of depression of 1.5% for clonidine, another α_2-adrenergic agonist; 1.1% for the β-adrenoreceptor blocker propranolol; and 1.9% for guanethidine.

The association between β-blockers and the development of a major depressive disorder is inconclusive (Patten et al. 1997), but propranolol has been reported to cause other neuropsychiatric side effects including visual hallucinations and psychosis (Fleminger 1978; Fraser and Carr 1976). Fleminger (1978) found that 17.5% of 115 patients had visual hallucinations and/or illusions with propranolol. Although the incidence of depression with propranolol is probably much less than originally thought, atenolol, being less lipophilic than propranolol and thus crossing the blood-brain barrier less easily, is probably the preferable β-blocker to use in those susceptible to the development of depression.

Digitalis has a very narrow therapeutic index, and toxic levels can produce delirium, aphasia, and hallucinations (Levenson 1979). Depression can occur as a side effect at therapeutic levels, particularly in elderly patients (Pascualy and Veith 1989). The psychiatric side effects of digoxin are associated with elevated serum levels, and the susceptibility of elderly patients is probably related to decreased clearance of the drug. Patten et al. (1996) found an association of the use of angiotensin-converting enzyme (ACE) inhibitors and the presence of depression, particularly in women and subjects over age 65. Although case reports have suggested an association of calcium channel blockers with depression, this association was not observed in two more systematic studies (Patten et al. 1995, 1996).

The antiarrhythmics quinidine, procainamide, and disopyramide have all been associated with the development of hallucinations and psychosis. This may relate to their anticholinergic effects, although their psychiatric side effects are frequently associated with polypharmacy (K. A. Wood et al. 1988).

Corticosteroids. The Boston Collaborative Drug Surveillance Program study (1971) found prednisone to be the most frequent drug-related cause of moderate or severe psychiatric side effects, occurring in 2.6% of patients. Lewis and Smith (1983), in an extensive review of the literature, reported a 5% incidence of serious psychiatric symptoms in patients receiving corticosteroids, with higher rates in oncology patients (Vincent 1995). This association was found to be dose-related, with doses of prednisone greater than 80 mg causing psychiatric disturbances at a rate of 18.4%. In patients who develop psychosis, 77% are receiving more than the dose equivalent of 40 mg daily (Vincent 1995). Most patients develop neuropsychiatric complications early in their course of treatment, 43% during the first week and 93% during the first 6 weeks. In a review of cases of steroid-induced psychiatric disorders, depression was seen in 40% of patients, 28% experienced hypomania (with 8% having a combination of depression

and mania), 14% were acutely psychotic, and 10% were delirious. Suicidal ideation has been reported in 17%–33% of patients with steroid psychosis, and the suicide rate in these cases is approximately 2%. Minor psychiatric syndromes occur commonly and include anxiety, irritability, and panic reactions. Most cases of steroid-induced psychiatric disorders last 2–6 weeks (Vincent 1995). Female sex, systemic lupus erythematosus, and high doses of prednisone are risk factors. Decreasing the steroid dose (slowly to avoid precipitating a steroid withdrawal syndrome) and administering neuroleptics, benzodiazepines, valproate, or electroconvulsive therapy are generally effective treatments. Lithium has been found to be effective prophylaxis for those patients known to be at risk (Vincent 1995). Tricyclic antidepressants do not appear to be as effective and, in fact, can exacerbate steroid-induced mania.

Nonsteroidal anti-inflammatory drugs. Hoppmann et al. (1991) reviewed the neuropsychiatric reports of side effects of NSAIDs. Elderly patients have been suspected as being particularly susceptible, especially with NSAIDs that are mostly protein bound, although one review found no data to support age alone as being an independent risk factor, but rather comorbidities and co-medications confer the heightened risk (Solomon and Gurwitz 1997). Psychosis has been reported as a side effect of both indomethacin and sulindac, agents that are structurally related. The mechanism of inducing psychosis could relate to the indolic moiety of indomethacin, similar to serotonin. Ibuprofen, naproxen, salicylates, and other NSAIDs have also been associated with depression and cognitive impairment, particularly in elderly patients. Browning's report (1996) of four patients who developed severe exacerbations of underlying psychiatric disorders emphasizes the need for caution when NSAIDs are used in patients with psychiatric histories.

Antiparkinsonian drugs. In a review of antiparkinsonian drug treatment, Young and colleagues (1997) found that the most prominent neuropsychiatric adverse effects were psychosis and delirium. Cummings (1991) reviewed the neuropsychiatric complications of the treatment of Parkinson's disease. He found that 30% of patients treated with dopaminergic agents develop visual hallucinations; 10% have delusional syndromes; 10%, euphoria; 1%, mania; and 10%–15%, anxiety symptoms. Elderly patients and patients with dementia appear more susceptible to these complications. Younger patients can be more susceptible to depression and insomnia (Wagner et al. 1996). Clozapine and olanzapine can be effective in treating psychotic symptoms if they do not resolve with dosage reduction (Friedman and Lannon 1989; Rabey et al. 1995; Rosenthal et al. 1992; Wolters et al. 1996). However, patients with Parkinson's disease are exquisitely sensitive to the anticholinergic side effects of clozapine and can become encephalopathic at even small doses (i.e., >25 mg daily) (Duffy and Kant 1996). Anticholinergics used in Parkinson's disease are more frequently associated with delirium, but can also present with delusions and/or hallucinations.

H₂ blockers. The H_2 blockers cimetidine and ranitidine have been reported to cause depression, mania, and psychosis (Billings and Stein 1986; Billings et al. 1981; Hubain et al. 1982; Russell and Lopez 1980). Both have also been found to induce neurobehavioral symptoms when discontinued. In this situation, the symptoms have been found to be associated with a drop in prolactin levels and ameliorated by treatment with domperidone, an agent that causes hyperprolactinemia (Rampello et al. 1997). Cimetidine has traditionally been viewed as more neuroactive, but a recent study by Kim et al. (1996) found postoperative patients on cimetidine or ranitidine to be equally likely to experience decrements in their Mini-Mental State Exam scores (Folstein et al. 1975). As the role of histamine as a central neurotransmitter is still unclear, the mechanism of action of these neurobehavioral effects is not certain. Jenike and Levy (1983) reported that physostigmine can reverse cimetidine-induced delirium, suggesting that there may be indirect cholinergic involvement. Cimetidine interacts significantly with a number of other medications (Appendix 31–1), and care must be taken in patients taking numerous drugs. Because cimetidine and ranitidine are both excreted primarily by the kidney, the clinician should be particularly cautious in prescribing H_2 blockers in elderly patients with diminished renal function.

Psychotropics. Reports of benzodiazepine-induced depression and psychosis are difficult to evaluate because the patients often had preexisting psychiatric illness and/or concomitant therapies. In a retrospective review, Greenblatt et al. (1976) reported that 3% of more than 2,000 patients on flurazepam manifested depression, although almost half of these were on other drug therapy as well. (The extremely long half-life of flurazepam makes it unsuitable for use in the elderly.) Confusion, hallucinations, and seizures also occur with benzodiazepine withdrawal. Also, a number of cases of mania with antidepressant therapy and withdrawal, as well as with stimulants and sympathomimetics, have been reported (Sultzer and Cummings 1989). (The neuropsychiatric aspects of psychotropic medication are discussed further in Chapter 34 in this volume.)

Gait and Mobility Disorders and Falls

Disorders of gait, particularly those that result in a fall, represent a significant source of hazard and subsequent disability in elderly people. As many as 15% of people over age 65 have a gait disorder (Newman et al. 1960); the incidence rises to 25% after age 79 (Lundgren-Lindquist et al. 1983). The annual incidence of falls in the elderly is approximately 220 per 1000, resulting in approximately 7 million falls annually (Monane and Avorn 1996). The magnitude of the problem is highlighted by the finding that, in people over age 75 in the community, more than one-third of them fall each year (Tinetti 1977), and as many as 10% of these falls result in serious (sometimes fatal) injury (Smallegan 1983). The psychological and physical repercussions of these falls frequently necessitate placement in a nursing home (Kellogg International 1987). The problem in nursing homes reaches catastrophic proportions where the annual incidence of falls is 1,600 per 1,000 residents (Sudarsky 1990). Medications are important contributors to these statistics and profoundly influence the ability of elderly patients to ambulate safely and efficiently.

Normal changes in ambulation associated with aging include 1) shorter, broader strides; 2) decreased speed; 3) diminished pelvic rotation; and 4) a decreased capacity for adjusting posture in response to environmental demands (MacDonald and MacDonald 1977). In addition to these expected changes, the elderly person can also develop gait abnormalities as a consequence of some other identifiable pathology such as musculoskeletal changes, Parkinson's disease, myelopathies (e.g., cervical spondylosis), cerebellar degeneration, normal pressure hydrocephalus, and subcortical atherosclerotic disease (Sudarsky 1990). Medications can aggravate these pathological processes or can produce gait abnormalities independently.

A large-scale study of "frequent fallers" in St. Louis found the following drugs to be associated with falls: diazepam, laxatives (may have reflected the more frail and inactive contingent), diuretics, and diltiazem (Cumming et al. 1991). Other medications that have been conclusively demonstrated to increase the risk of falling include psychotropic medications, especially long-acting benzodiazepines (Monane et al. 1996), barbiturates, tricyclic antidepressants, neuroleptics (particularly phenothiazines), antihypertensives, including diuretics and calcium channel blockers (J. B. Schwartz 1996), digitalis (Koski et al. 1996), levodopa, and NSAIDs (Davie et al. 1981; MacDonald 1983; MacDonald and MacDonald 1977; Prudnam and Evans 1981; Ray et al. 1989). The risk of falls in an elderly person rises proportionally to the number of medications he or she is taking. Particularly hazardous are combinations of medications that have additive side effects (e.g., antihypertensives in combination with sedative-hypnotics) (MacDonald 1983).

The age-related changes in CNS vulnerability in elderly patients discussed above may predispose them to drug-induced movement disorders. (The problems of hyperkinetic movement disorders and tardive dyskinesia are discussed further in Chapter 25 in this volume.) Neuroleptics are the most common cause of drug-induced movement disorders, but dopamine agonists also frequently produce dyskinesias, and a variety of other medical therapies have been associated with movement abnormalities (Table 31–5). Elderly patients are at an increased risk particularly for drug-induced parkinsonism from antiemetic and antipsychotic medications, related, perhaps, to the diminished number of nigral dopaminergic neurons associated with aging (Friedman 1992). This can be a significant cause of immobility, gait disturbance, falls, and mortality in elderly patients (Wilson and MacLennen 1989). Parkinsonism has also been reported with chronic valproate treatment (Armon et al. 1996) and has infrequently been reported with the SSRIs (Leo et al. 1995). (For excellent reviews, see Lang and Weiner 1992 and L. G. Miller and Jankovic 1992.)

Sleep Disorders Produced by Medical Therapies

The predictable alterations in sleep architecture associated with aging are reviewed in Chapter 17 in this volume. The incidence of insomnia increases as a function of age and physical status (Gillin and Byerly 1990). Many elderly persons complain of poor sleep and/or unacceptable daytime drowsiness and frequently seek treatment—either from their physician or via OTC medications. In the context of neurodegenerative disorders, sleep problems frequently exhaust relatives and precipitate the family's decision to seek institutionalization of a loved one (Berry and Webb 1985). Medications can play a significant role in producing sleep disturbances in the elderly. In addition, the particular vulnerabilities of the aging brain demand the judicious selection of appropriate treatment strategies for sleep disorders. A failure to do so may result in escalating sleep and behavioral problems.

The use of benzodiazepines, which are frequently prescribed for elderly patients, presents particular hazards (Closser 1991). The elderly are more sensitive to benzodiazepines secondary to their altered pharmacokinetics and enhanced postsynaptic receptor sensitivity (Swift 1986). Benzodiazepines are frequently administered to elderly patients who complain of insomnia. The extent of benzodiazepine use is highlighted by studies that reported that half of all elderly medical admissions were receiving benzodiazepines (Foy et al. 1986), and among institutionalized elderly, more than 90% were prescribed sedative-hypnotic drugs (Reynolds et al. 1985).

Ironically, although benzodiazepines are usually initially prescribed to treat insomnia, they are a frequent cause of deteriorating sleep quality (Schneider-Heimert 1988). Sustained use results in diminished slow-wave and rapid-eye-movement (REM) sleep, with no alteration in total sleep time (Schneider-Heimert 1988). The problem

TABLE 31–5. Drug-induced movement disorders

Movement disorders	Drugs
Accentuated physiological tremor	Epinephrine, isoproterenol, caffeine, theophylline, lithium, tricyclic antidepressants, thyroid hormone, hypoglycemic agents, sodium valproate, nicotinic acid, cyclosporine
Cerebellar ataxia and tremor	Phenytoin, barbiturate, lithium, 5-fluorouracil, cimetidine-triazolam interaction
Chorea-dyskinesia	Neuroleptics, levodopa, bromocriptine, phenytoin, ethosuximide, carbamazepine, oral contraceptives, chloroquine, antidepressants, metoclopramide, lithium, antidepressants, benzodiazepines, antihistamines, calcium channel blockers, cocaine, methyldopa, cimetidine
Dystonia	Neuroleptics, levodopa, bromocriptine, lithium, metoclopramide, carbamazepine, cimetidine, chlorzoxazone, calcium channel blockers
Myoclonus and tics	Neuroleptics, amphetamines, methylphenidate, fenfluramine, levodopa, bromocriptine, antidepressants, pemoline, cocaine
Parkinsonism	Neuroleptics, reserpine, tetrabenazine, methyldopa, α-methyltyrosine, lithium, diazoxide, physostigmine, metoclopramide, trazodone, meperidine, etretinate, cimetidine, cinnarizine, flunarizine
Akathisia	Neuroleptics, reserpine, tetrabenazine, metoclopramide, antidepressants, calcium channel blockers, buspirone, methysergide, cimetidine

may be further compounded when the elderly person develops rebound insomnia after missing even a single dose of a short-acting preparation, often resulting in escalating hypnotic use (Gillin et al. 1989). Patients receiving ultra-short–acting benzodiazepines such as triazolam can experience this rebound phenomenon within a few hours of their last dose and can require more than one dose per evening to maintain sleep and avoid becoming agitated or confused. In addition, the ultra-short–acting benzodiazepines have been reported to produce in susceptible individuals myriad behavioral changes, including anterograde amnesia, delirium, anxiety, and dysphoria (Patterson 1987; Reynolds et al. 1985). The deleterious effects of triazolam and zolpidem have been shown to occur during the night and sometimes persist into the next day (Lobo et al. 1997).

The long half-life benzodiazepines (e.g., flurazepam) should be avoided in elderly patients because these drugs are likely to produce prolonged daytime drowsiness, cognitive disturbances, and potentially hazardous ataxia (Carskadon et al. 1982). Sleep apnea increases with age and may be significantly aggravated by the use of sedative-hypnotics, thereby creating a potentially serious risk (Ancoli-Israel et al. 1985; Reynolds et al. 1985). Overall, the use of benzodiazepines for insomnia in elderly patients remains controversial. Their administration should probably be limited to the brief use of the intermediate benzodiazepines in stressful situations.

Several cardiovascular drugs have been reported to exert a powerful influence on sleep architecture. β-blockers (particularly lipophilic agents such as propranolol, metoprolol, and pindolol) and reserpine have been associated with nightmares, hallucinations, fatigue, and diminished sleep quality (Henningsen and Mattiason 1979). Clonidine causes REM suppression with decreased time in deep sleep and more awakenings (i.e., decreased quality of sleep) (Spiegel and Devos 1980). Several antiarrhythmics including amiodarone, lorcainide, and quinidine have been reported to produce insomnia (Greene et al. 1983; Guillemenault and Silvestri 1982; Karacan et al. 1976).

Methylxanthines, found in theophylline, theobromine, and caffeine, are common causes of insomnia. Caffeine, available in beverages such as tea or coffee and frequently found in OTC preparations, produces difficulty initiating sleep and delays the onset of REM sleep to the latter part of the night (Karacan et al. 1976). Psychostimulants such as methylphenidate that are sometimes used to treat depression in the elderly produce a significant reduction in slow-wave and REM sleep (Kay et al. 1976).

Corticosteroids also cause sleep disturbances, with insomnia commonly reported. Nightmares, excessively morbid or vivid dreams, and even psychosis can also occur (Force et al. 1997; Vincent 1995). Melatonin, popularly used for sleeplessness and aging and sold over the counter in the United States (though not in Europe), has been reported to cause nightmares, fatigue, hypotension, and sleep disorders with highly irregular sleep-wake cycles (Middleton et al. 1996). There is particular concern when melatonin is taken on an inappropriate time schedule, at high doses, or over long periods (Guardiola-Lemaitre 1997).

Finally, nonspecific causes of diminished sleep quality should be considered. These include prolonged confinement to bed, physical discomfort caused by medical illness (e.g., arthritis, Parkinson's disease, and orthopnea), and the alteration in sleep cycle characteristic of confusional states.

Sexual Disorders

Sexuality in older people is a subject of considerable misunderstanding. Older people do experience some age-associated alterations in sexual function, but these do not preclude an active and satisfying sex life. Sexual activity continues well into later life. A national survey reported that more than half of married persons between ages 66 and 70 report having sex at least four times per month. More than one-quarter of married people over age 76 report an active sex life, with an average frequency of sex of more than twice per month (Marsiglio and Donnelly 1991). It is important to note that, unless physical disability intervenes, the sexual behavior of older people tends to remain consistent over time (George and Weiler 1981). These statistics highlight the importance of obtaining a sexual history in all older patients. Any change from their premorbid baseline may herald recent physical or psychosocial stressors.

Although growing older does not mandate an abandonment of sexuality, predictable age-related physiological changes do affect the elderly person's sexual functioning (Grenshaw 1985). The older male is likely to experience some decrease in libido and a slowing of sexual arousal that may delay ejaculation. The postmenopausal woman is likely to experience a number of physiological changes that may reduce the pleasure of sexual intercourse. These changes include decreased vaginal lubrication, atrophic changes in the mucosal lining of the vaginal wall, and decreased turgidity of the vaginal outlet. In addition, physical disability is likely to exert a powerful negative influence on the older person's sexual activity (Marsiglio and Donnelly 1991). As a consequence, elderly people are likely to be more vulnerable to the drug-induced disorders in sexual functioning outlined in Table 31–6.

The SSRIs are well known to induce sexual dysfunction. Data are not yet available from studies of this complication specifically in the elderly population, but extrapolation from data on younger patients gives reason for concern. In a prospective Spanish study of outpatients (Montejo-Gonzalez et al. 1997) with a mean age of 39.6, researchers found SSRI-induced sexual dysfunction in a majority (58%) of the patients, with a significant increase in the incidence when physicians asked the patients direct questions about decreased libido, delayed orgasm or anorgasmia, delayed ejaculation, inability to ejaculate, and

TABLE 31–6. Effects of commonly prescribed drugs on sexual function

Drugs	Libido	Effects on sexual function, arousal, or erection	Orgasm or ejaculation
Psychotropic agents			
Amphetamines and cocaine	Enhanced with low doses; decreased with high doses	Decreased with chronic use	Increased with low doses; diminished with high doses
Monoamine oxidase–inhibiting antidepressants	–	–	Impaired
Tricyclic antidepressants	May be impaired	May be impaired	May be impaired; may cause spontaneous seminal emission
Bupropion	Increased	–	–
Trazodone	Increased	May cause priapism	–
Fluoxetine	Increased	–	–
Lithium carbonate	Impaired	Impaired	–
Neuroleptic agents	May be decreased	Impaired (rare priapism)	Retrograde ejaculation rarely
Sedative-hypnotics	Reduced	Reduced	–
Benzodiazepines	–	Impaired with chronic usage	–
Buspirone	Increased	–	–
Narcotics	Impaired in high doses	Impaired in high doses	Impaired in high doses
Antihypertensive agents			
Reserpine, 97-methyldopa	Decreased	Decreased (common)	May be impaired
Diuretics	–	May be impaired	–
Clonidine	–	–	May block emission in males
Propranolol	May be decreased	May be decreased	–
Anticholinergic agents	–	May be impaired	–
Sympathomimetics			
Phendimetrazine	Increased	–	–
Fenfluramine	Increased	–	–
Hormonal agents			
Androgens	Increased	Increased (men)	Increased (men)
Estrogens	Decreased (men) Variable (women)	May cause impotence in men	Delayed
Thyroxine	Increased	–	–
Adrenal steroids	Decreased in high doses	–	–
Miscellaneous			
Levodopa	May be increased	–	–
Cholestyramine	Increased	–	–
Disulfiram	–	Occasional impotence	Delayed

impotence versus when sexual dysfunction was spontaneously reported (14%). This finding is of special note for geriatric care because older patients are less frequently asked about their sexual functioning and are less likely to volunteer the information. Sexual dysfunction was found to correlate with dose and have a higher incidence in men. Retrospective chart studies show lower incidence (16.3%), but still involving significant numbers of patients treated with SSRIs (Keller Ashton et al. 1997).

A recent study revealed that, although erectile dysfunction is a frequent disorder in hyperlipidemia, hypolipidemic drugs additionally increase the incidence of impotence (Bruckert et al. 1996). Other medications reported to induce a variety of sexual dysfunctions include apomorphine, carbamazepine, metoclopramide, chlorthalidone, hydrochlorothiazide, and other antidepressants. A more complete listing is outlined in Table 31–6.

Disturbances in Taste and Smell

The loss or distortion of sense of smell or taste significantly compromises a person's nutritional status and enjoyment of his or her environment. Drug-induced disturbances are common and include anosmia and ageusia (absence of smell and taste, respectively), dysosmia (distortion and misinterpretation of smells), parageusia (misinterpretation of tastes as foul), parosmia (perception of an odorant that is not present), and dysgeusia (the distortion or misinterpretation of a taste while eating). The medical disorders associated with impairments of olfaction and the sense of taste are lengthy. (The reader is referred to the excellent review by Ackerman and Kasbekar 1997.) Symptoms require a careful differential diagnosis. Anosmia occurs in 90% of patients with Alzheimer's disease and Huntington's chorea and 70% of those with idiopathic Parkinson's disease (Ackerman and Kasbekar 1997). For such patients, and other frail elderly, further interference with their sense of smell or taste may cause them to avoid eating. Drugs associated with anosmia are levodopa, alpha interferon, chemotherapeutic agents, nifedipine, and diltiazem. Distortions in taste (dysgeusia) or loss of the sense of taste (ageusia) have been reported to occur with the ACE inhibitors (oral and topical), nifedipine, and medications with sulfhydryl groups (propylthiouracil, penicillamine, and captopril). Captopril is considered to be the agent most commonly associated with dysgeusia. The ACE inhibitors are reported to cause dysgeusia in 8.4% of patients. Dysgeusia has, in rare instances, been reported to become persistent and permanent (Ackerman and Kasbekar 1997). Xerostomia, or dry mouth, a common side effect of anticholinergics, commonly interferes with taste, dentition, and oral intake.

Herbal Remedies

Recent years have witnessed an explosive rise in the popularity of alternative therapies—most particularly herbal and so-called natural remedies. The market for botanical therapies continues to grow rapidly and has become a multibillion dollar industry. Unfortunately, despite the enormity of this burgeoning financial trade in herbs, their clinical efficacy and safety remain unproved and untested. Adding to this confusion, most clinicians fail to question their patients about alternative therapy use, and most patients remain embarrassed to broach the subject with their physician. As evidenced in a recent survey of 400 users of herbal remedies who reported an 8% incidence of adverse effects, although the incidence of adverse effects from herbal remedies is probably comparatively low, they do occur (Abbot et al. 1996).

Adverse effects from herbs may result as a consequence of 1) allergic reactions, 2) toxic effects, 3) drug interactions, 4) mutagenic effects, and 5) the toxicity associated with contaminants (Ernst 1998). Drug interactions are particularly important in the context of elderly patients who are already consuming many prescription medications. Recognized drug interactions include coagulation abnormalities in patients using warfarin concurrently with Chinese herbal teas (Tam et al. 1995). The Ayurvedic remedy shankhapushpi has been reported to lower phenytoin levels, thereby placing the patient at increased risk for seizures. Undoubtedly, many other drug interactions will be recognized as the popularity of herbal remedies increases. Currently recognized direct toxic effects of herbal remedies are outlined in Table 31–7.

Poor quality control over the preparation of herbal remedies results in unacceptable contamination of these products. Identified contaminants in Ayurvedic preparations have included lead, mercury, arsenic, aluminium, tin, aspirin, and acetaminophen (Bayly et al. 1995). Heavy metal and prescription medication contamination of Chinese herbal remedies has also been frequently reported. Kelp, a popular and presumably benign remedy, may contain toxic levels of arsenic that may produce clinical toxicity (Gertner et al. 1995).

Summary

Medical therapies not uncommonly cause neuropsychiatric morbidity in elderly patients. These complications can become serious enough to warrant hospitalization, with 8% or more of geriatric admissions attributable to adverse drug reactions. The increased susceptibility of the elderly

TABLE 31–7. Adverse effects with likely cause-effect relationship

Name of plant/constituent	Adverse effect	Reason for assuming causality
Aconite	Palpitations, arrhythmias, nausea, abdominal pain	Adverse effect reported frequently
Aristolochic acid	Nephrotoxic	Adverse effect reported often
Ayurvedic remedies	Heavy metal poisoning	Heavy metals used in processing and found in preparations
Broom	Oxytocic properties	Documented adverse effect of sparteine (a constituent of broom)
Chaparral	Liver damage	Case reports
Chinese herbal mixtures	Heavy metal poisoning	Case reports; heavy metals found in preparations
Comfrey	Liver damage	Case reports
Flavonoids	Hemolytic anemia, renal damage	Case reports
Germander	Liver damage	Case reports
Guar gum	Gastrointestinal obstruction	Case reports
Licorice root	Hypokalemia, hypertension, arrhythmias, edema	Case reports
Pennyroyal	Liver damage	Case reports
Pyrrolizine	Liver damage	Case reports

Source. Adapted from Ernst 1998.

to the CNS side effects of medical therapies should always be considered when neurobehavioral changes occur in older medical patients. Medical therapies may cause depression, mania, psychosis, sexual disorders, delirium, dementia, anxiety, sleep disturbances, movement disorders, falls, and changes in olfaction and the sense of taste. To minimize the risk of these adverse effects, one must consider the following factors in prescribing medications to elderly patients:

1. Understand alterations in pharmacokinetics and neurochemistry associated with aging.
2. Identify the presence of any neurodegenerative process and understand the possible ramifications of these diseases for drug effects and sensitivity.
3. Identify social and physical determinants that make medication compliance problematic (e.g., living alone, financial constraints, vision and hearing loss).
4. Always consider the possible involvement of OTC medications and herbal therapies or misuse of prescription medication.
5. Obtain a baseline mental status examination. If patients are treated with high-risk medications or combinations, follow the mental status carefully.
6. Always consider drug toxicity when the patient exhibits an alteration in attention or cognition or any behavioral change.

7. Be aware of inappropriate medication practices for the treatment of elderly patients.
8. Have a table of drug-drug interactions readily available for use when polypharmacy is required.

References

Abbot NC, White AR, Ernst E: Complementary medicine (letter). Nature 381:386, 1996

Abernethy DR: Psychotropic drugs and the aging process: pharmacokinetics and pharmacodynamics, in Clinical Geriatric Psychopharmacology, 2nd Edition. Edited by Salzman C. Baltimore, MD, Williams & Wilkins, 1992, pp 61–76

Ackerman BH, Kasbekar N: Disturbances of taste and smell induced by drugs (review). Pharmacotherapy 17:482–496, 1997

Adler S: Methyldopa-induced decrease in mental activity. JAMA 230:1428–1429, 1981

Allison N, Shantz I: Delirium due to tiaprofenic acid. Canadian Medical Association Journal 137:1022–1023, 1987

Amir I, Dano M, Joffe A: Recurrent toxic delirium in a patient treated with SSRIs: is old age a risk factor? Isr J Psychiatry Relat Sci 34:119–121, 1997

Anastasio GD, Cornell KO, Menscer D: Drug interactions: keeping it straight (review). Am Fam Physician 56: 883–888, 891–894, 1997

Ancoli-Israel S, Kripke DF, Mason W, et al: Sleep apnea and periodic movements in an aging sample. J Gerontol 40: 419–425, 1985

Armon C, Shin C, Miller P: Reversible parkinsonism and cognitive impairment with chronic valproate use. Neurology 47:626–635, 1996

Atkinson RM, Ganzini L, Bernstein MJ: Alcohol and substance-use disorders in the elderly, in Handbook of Mental Health and Aging. Edited by Birren JE, Sloane R, Cohen GD. San Diego, CA, Academic Press, 1992, pp 515–555

Bayly GR, Braithwaite RA, Sheehan TMT: Lead poisoning from Asian traditional remedies in the West Midlands: report of a series of five cases. Hum Exp Toxicol 14:4–28, 1995

Bergman U, Wilholm BE: Patient medication on admission to a medical clinic. Eur J Clin Pharmacol 20:185–191, 1981

Berry DTR, Webb WB: Sleep and cognitive functions in normal older adults. J Gerontol 40:331–335, 1985

Billings R, Stein M: Depression associated with ranitidine. Am J Psychiatry 143:915–916, 1986

Billings R, Tang SW, Rafkoff VM: Depression associated with cimetidine. Can J Psychiatry 26:260–261, 1981

Blazer DG, Fedrespiel CF, Ray WA, et al: The risk of anticholinergic toxicity in the elderly: a study of prescribing practices in two populations. J Gerontol 38:31–35, 1983

Bonne O, Shalev AY, Bloch M: Delirium associated with mianserin. Eur Neuropsychopharmacol 5:147–149, 1995

Boston Collaborative Drug Surveillance Program: Psychiatric side effects of nonpsychiatric drugs. Seminars in Psychiatry 3(4):406–420, 1971

Brocklehurst JC: Aging in the autonomic nervous system. Aging 4 (suppl):7, 1974

Browning CH: Nonsteroidal anti-inflammatory drugs and severe psychiatric side effects. Int J Psychiatry Med 26:25–34, 1996

Bruckert E, Giral P, Heshmati HM, et al: Men treated with hypolipidemic drugs complain more frequently of erectile dysfunction. J Clin Pharm Ther 21:89–94, 1996

Caird FI, Andrews GR, Kennedy RD: Effect of posture on blood pressure in the elderly. British Heart Journal 35:448, 1987

Carskadon MA, Seidel WF, Greenblatt DJ, et al: Daytime carryover of triazolam and flurazepam, elderly insomniacs. Sleep 5:361–371, 1982

Catterson ML, Preskorn SH, Martin RL: Pharmacodynamic and pharmacokinetic considerations in geriatric psychopharmacology. Geriatric Psychiatry 20:215–218, 1997

Celesia GG, Barr AN: Psychosis and other psychiatric manifestations of levodopa therapy. Arch Neurol 23:193–200, 1970

Closser MH: Benzodiazepines and the elderly. J Subst Abuse Treat 8:35–41, 1991

Coenen AM, van Luijtelaar EL: Effects of benzodiazepines, sleep and sleep deprivation on vigilance and memory. Acta Neurol Belg 97:123–129, 1997

Crawshaw JA, Mullen PEW: A study of benzhexol abuse. Br J Psychiatry 145:300–303, 1984

Cross AJ, Crow TJ, Johnson JA, et al: Studies on neurotransmitter receptor systems in neocortex and hippocampus in senile dementia of the Alzheimer type. J Neurol Sci 64: 109–117, 1984

Cumming RG, Miller JR, Kelsey JL, et al: Medications and multiple falls in elderly people: the St. Louis OASIS study. Age Ageing 20:455–461, 1991

Cummings JL: Behavioral complications of drug treatment of Parkinson's disease. J Am Geriatr Soc 39:708–716, 1991

Cupit GC: The use of non-prescription analgesics in an older population. J Am Geriatr Soc 30 (suppl):76–80, 1982

Danielson DA, Porter JB, Lawson DH, et al: Drug induced psychiatric disturbances in medical inpatients. Psychopharmacology 74:105–108, 1981

Davie JW, Blumenthal MD, Robinson-Hawkins S: A model of risk of falling for psychogeriatric patients. Arch Gen Psychiatry 38:463–467, 1981

De Smet Y, Ruberg M, Serdaru M, et al: Confusion, dementia and anticholinergics in Parkinson's disease. J Neurol Neurosurg Psychiatry 45:1161–1164, 1982

Duffy JD, Kant R: Clinical utility of clozapine in 16 patients with neurological disease. J Neuropsychiatry Clin Neurosci 8:92–96, 1996

Eisendrath SJ, Sweeny MA: Toxic neuropsychiatric effects of digoxin at therapeutic serum concentrations. Am J Psychiatry 144:506–507, 1987

Eisendrath SJ, Goldman B, Douglas J, et al: Meperidine-induced delirium. Am J Psychiatry 144:1062–1065, 1987

Erkinjuntti T, Wikstrom J, Palo J: Dementia among medical inpatients. Arch Intern Med 146:1923–1926, 1986

Ernst E: Harmless herbs? a review of the recent literature. Am J Med 104:170–178, 1998

Erwin WG: Geriatrics, in Pharmacotherapy: A Pathophysiologic Approach. Edited by Kepiro JT, Talbert RL, Hayes PE, et al. Norwalk, CT, Appleton & Lange, 1993, pp 2064–2070

Fennelly ME: Ranitidine-induced mental confusion. Crit Care Med 15:1165–1166, 1987

Fleminger R: Visual hallucinations and illusions with propranolol. BMJ 1:1182, 1978

Folstein MF, Folstein SE, McHugh PR: Mini-Mental State: a practical method for grading the cognitive state of patients for the clinician. J Psychiatr Res 12:189–198, 1975

Force RW, Hansen L, Bedell M: Psychotic episode after melatonin (letter). Ann Pharmacother 31:1408, 1997

Foy A, Drinkwater V, March S: Confusion after admission to hospital in elderly patients using benzodiazepines. BMJ 293:1072, 1986

Foy A, O'Connell D, Henry D, et al: Benzodiazepine use as a cause of cognitive impairment in elderly hospital inpatients. J Gerontol A Biol Sci Med Sci 50:M99–M106, 1995

Fraser HS, Carr AC: Propranolol psychosis. Br J Psychiatry 129:508–509, 1976

Friedman JH: Drug-induced parkinsonism, in Drug-Induced Movement Disorders. Edited by Lang AE, Weiner WJ. Mount Kisco, NY, Futura, 1992, pp 41–84

Friedman JH, Lannon MC: Clozapine in the treatment of psychosis in Parkinson's disease. Neurology 39:1219–1221, 1989

Gambert SR: Substance abuse in the elderly, in Substance Abuse: A Comprehensive Textbook, 2nd Edition. Edited by Lawison JH, Ruit P, Millman RB, et al. Baltimore, MD, Williams & Wilkins, 1992, pp 213–234

Gelenberg AJ: "Serotonin Syndrome" and an antiserotonin drug. Biologic Therapies in Psychiatry Newsletter 18:18–19, 1995

George LK, Weiler SJ: Sexuality in middle and late life. Arch Gen Psychiatry 38:912–992, 1981

Gertner E, Marshall PS, Filandrinos D: Complications resulting from the use of Chinese herbal medications containing undeclared prescription drugs. Arthritis Rheum 38:614–617, 1995

Gillin JC, Byerly WF: The diagnosis and management of insomnia. N Engl J Med 322:239–248, 1990

Gillin JC, Spinweber CL, Johnson LC: Rebound insomnia: a critical review. J Clin Psychopharmacol 9:161–172, 1989

Goodwin FK, Bunney WE: Depressions following reserpine: a reevaluation. Seminars in Psychiatry 3(4):435–448, 1971

Goodwin JS, Regan M: Cognitive dysfunction associated with naproxen and ibuprofen in the elderly. Arthritis Rheum 25:1013–1015, 1982

Graves T, Hanlon JT, Schmader EK, et al: Adverse events after discontinuing medications in elderly outpatients. Arch Intern Med 157:2205–2210, 1997

Greenblatt DJ: Basic pharmacokinetic principles and their application to psychotropic drugs. J Clin Psychiatry 54:S8–S13, 1993

Greenblatt D, Allen M, Shader R: Toxicity of high dose flurazepam in the elderly. Clin Pharmacol Ther 21:355, 1976

Greene HL, Graham EL, Werner JA, et al: Toxic and therapeutic effects of amiodarone in the treatment of cardiac arrhythmias. J Am Coll Cardiol 2:1114–1128, 1983

Grenshaw TL: Age-related changes in sexual function. Geriatric Consultant 3(5):26–29, 1985

Griffiths RR, Weerts EM: Benzodiazepine self-administration in humans and laboratory animals—implications for problems of long-term use and abuse. Psychopharmacology 134:1–37, 1997

Guardiola-Lemaitre B: Toxicology of melatonin (review). J Biol Rhythms 12:697–706, 1997

Guillemenault C, Silvestri R: Aging, drugs and sleep. Neurobiol Aging 3:379–386, 1982

Hanlon JT, Schmader KE, Koronkowski MJ, et al: Adverse drug events in high risk older outpatients. J Am Geriatr Soc 45:945–948, 1997

Henningsen NC, Mattiason I: Long-term clinical experience with atenolol—a new selective beta-1-blocker with few side-effects from the central nervous system. Acta Medica Scandinavica 205:61–66, 1979

Hodkinson HM: Mental impairment in the elderly. J R Coll Physicians Lond 7:305–317, 1973

Hoffman WF, Ladogana L: Delirium secondary to clonidine therapy. New York State Journal of Medicine 81:382–383, 1981

Hooten WM, Pearlson G: Delirium caused by tacrine and ibuprofen interaction (letter). Am J Psychiatry 153:842, 1996

Hoppmann RA, Peden JG, Ober K: Central nervous system side effects of nonsteroidal anti-inflammatory drugs: aseptic meningitis, psychosis, and cognitive dysfunction. Arch Intern Med 151:1309–1313, 1991

Hubain P, Sobolski J, Mendlewicz J: Cimetidine-induced mania. Neuropsychobiology 8:223–224, 1982

Inouye SK: The dilemma of delirium: clinical research controversies regarding diagnosis and evaluation of delirium in hospitalized elderly medical patients. Am J Med 97:278–288, 1994

Inouye SK, Charpentier PA: Precipitating factors for delirium in hospitalized elderly persons: predictive model and interrelationship with baseline vulnerability. JAMA 275:852–857, 1996

Irvin SM: Identification of potential problems for elderly outpatients after preoperative medication: a case study. Journal of Post Anesthesia Nursing 10:159–162, 1995

Itil T, Fink M: Anticholinergic drug-induced delirium: experimental modification, quantitative EEG and behavioral correlations. J Nerv Ment Dis 143:492–507, 1966

Jackson JE, Ramsdell JW, Renvall M, et al: Reliability of drug histories in a specialized geriatric outpatient clinic. J Gen Intern Med 4:39–43, 1989

Jacobsen FM, Sack DA, James SP: Delirium induced by verapamil (letter). Am J Psychiatry 144:248, 1987

Jenike MA, Levy JC: Physostigmine reversal of cimetidine-induced delirium and agitation. J Clin Psychopharmacol 3:43–44, 1983

Jeste DV, Wyatt RJ: Aging and tardive dyskinesia, in Schizophrenia and Aging. Edited by Miller NE, Cohen GD. New York, Guilford, 1987, pp 275–286

Karacan I, Thornby JI, Anch AM, et al: Dose related sleep disturbance produced by coffee and caffeine. Clin Pharmacol Ther 20:682–689, 1976

Kasantikul D: Reversible delirium after discontinuation of fluoxetine. J Med Assoc Thai 78:53–54, 1995

Katzman R, Lasker B, Bernstein N: Advances in the diagnosis of dementia accuracy of diagnosis and consequences of misdiagnosis of disorders causing dementia. Aging and the Brain 32:17–62, 1988

Kay DC, Blackburn AB, Buckingham JA: Human pharmacology of sleep, in Pharmacology of Sleep. Edited by Williams RL, Karacan I. New York, Wiley, 1976, pp 83–210

Keller Ashton A, Hamer R, Rosen RC: Serotonin reuptake inhibitor–induced sexual dysfunction and its treatment: a large-scale retrospective study of 596 psychiatric outpatients. J Sex Marital Ther 23:165–175, 1997

Kellogg International Work Group on the Prevention of Falls by the Elderly: The prevention of falls in later life. Dan Med Bull 34 (suppl 4):1–24, 1987

Kennedy JS: Adverse drug effects in the older adult, in Drug-Induced Dysfunction in Psychiatry. Edited by Kesharen MS, Kennedy JS. New York, Hemisphere, 1992, pp 93–101

Kim KY, McCartney JR, Kaye W, et al: The effect of cimetidine and ranitidine on cognitive function in postoperative cardiac surgical patients. Int J Psychiatry Med 26:295–307, 1996

Kolecki P: Isolated venlafaxine-induced serotonin syndrome. J Emerg Med 15:491–493, 1997

Koski K, Luukinen H, Laippala P, et al: Physiological factors and medications as predictors of injurious falls by elderly people: a prospective population-based study. Age Ageing 25:29–38, 1996

Kuhr BM: Prolonged delirium with propranolol. J Clin Psychiatry 40:194–195, 1979

Lader M: Differential diagnosis of anxiety in the elderly. J Clin Psychiatry 43 (9 [sec 2]):4–7, 1982

Lamy PP, Salzman C, Nevis-Olesen J: Drug prescribing patterns, risks, and compliance guidelines, in Clinical Geriatric Psychopharmacology, 2nd Edition. Edited by Salzman S. Baltimore, MD, Williams & Wilkins, 1992, pp 15–37

Lang AE, Weiner WJ: Drug-Induced Movement Disorder. Mount Kisco, NY, Futura, 1992

Larson EB, Kukull WA, Buchner D, et al: Adverse drug reactions associated with global cognitive impairment in elderly persons. Ann Intern Med 107:169–173, 1987

Lawlor BA, Sunderland T, Mellow AM, et al: A preliminary study of the effects of intravenous m-chlorphenylpiperazine, a serotonin, in elderly subjects. Biol Psychiatry 25:679–686, 1989

Lawson AW: Substance abuse problems of the elderly: considerations for treatment and prevention, in Alcoholism and Substance Abuse in Special Populations. Edited by Lawson GW, Lawson AW. Rockville, MD, Aspen, 1989, pp 95–133

Leo RJ, Lichter DG, Hershey LA: Parkinsonism associated with fluoxetine and cimetidine: a case report. J Geriatr Psychiatry Neurol 8:231–233, 1995

Levenson JJ: Neuropsychiatric Side Effects of Drugs in the Elderly. New York, Raven, 1979

Lewis DA, Smith RE: Steroid-induced psychiatric syndromes. J Affect Disord 5:319–332, 1983

Lezak MD: Neuropsychological Assessment. New York, Oxford University Press, 1983, pp 422–429

Lieberman AN, Kupersmith M, Gopinathan G, et al: Bromocriptine in Parkinson's disease: further studies. Neurology 29:363–369, 1979

Lipowski ZJ: Acute confusional states in the elderly, in Clinical Neurology of Aging. Edited by Albert ML. New York, Oxford University Press, 1984, pp 277–297

Lipowski ZJ: Delirium: Acute Confusional States. New York, Oxford University Press, 1990

Liston EH: Delirium in the aged. Psychiatr Clin North Am 5:49–66, 1982

Lobo BL, Greene WL: Zolpidem: distinct from triazolam? Ann Pharmacother 31:625–632, 1997

Lundgren-Lindquist B, Aniansson A, Rundgren A: Functional studies in 79 year olds, III: walking performance and climbing capacity. Scand J Rehabil Med 15:125–131, 1983

MacDonald JB: The role of drugs in falls in the elderly. Clin Geriatr Med 1:3:621–636, 1983

MacDonald JB, MacDonald ET: Nocturnal femoral fracture and continuing widespread use of barbiturate hypnotics. BMJ 2:483–485, 1977

MacEwan GW, Remick RA, Noone JA: Psychosis due to transdermally administered scopolamine. Canadian Medical Association Journal 133:431–432, 1985

Marsiglio W, Donnelly D: Sexual relations in later life: a national study of married persons. J Gerontol 46 (suppl 6):338–344, 1991

Martin TG: Serotonin syndrome (review). Ann Emerg Med 28:520–526, 1996

McGahan DJ, Wojslaw A, Prasad V, et al: Propranolol-induced psychosis. Drug Intelligence and Clinical Pharmacy 18:601–603, 1984

McLachlan RS: Pseudoatrophy of the brain with valproic acid monotherapy. Can J Neurol Sci 14:294–296, 1987

McLeod PJ, Huang AR, Tamblyn RM, et al: Defining inappropriate practices in prescribing for elderly people: a national consensus panel. Canadian Medical Association Journal 156:385–391, 1997

Mesulam M-M, Mufson EJ, Rogers J: Age-related shrinkage of cortically projecting cholinergic neurons: a selective effect. Ann Neurol 22:31–36, 1987

Middleton BA, Stone BM, Arendt J: Melatonin and fragmented sleep patterns. Lancet 348:551–552, 1996

Miller LG, Jankovic J: Drug-induced movement disorders: an overview, in Movement Disorders in Neurology and Neuropsychiatry. Edited by Joseph AB, Young RR. Oxford, England, Blackwell Scientific, 1992, pp 5–32

Miller PS, Richardson S, Jyu CA, et al: Association of low serum anticholinergic levels and cognitive impairment in elderly presurgical patients. Am J Psychiatry 145:342–345, 1988

Mills KC: Essential emergency medicine pharmacokinetics: prevention of iatrogenic patient poisoning. Topics in Emergency Medicine 15:18–29, 1993

Monane M, Avorn J: Medications and falls. Causation, correlation and prevention. Clin Geriatr Med 12:847–858, 1996

Montejo-Gonzalez AL, Llorca G, Izquierdo JA, et al: SSRI-induced sexual dysfunction: fluoxetine, paroxetine, sertraline and fluvoxamine in a prospective multicenter, and descriptive clinical study of 344 patients. J Sex Marital Ther 23:176–194, 1997

Morrison RL, Katz IR: Drug-related cognitive impairment: current progress and recurrent problems, in Annual Review Gerontology and Geriatrics, Vol 9. Edited by Lawton MP. New York, Springer, 1989, pp 232–279

Mueller C, Schur C, O'Connell J: Prescription drug spending: the impact of age and chronic disease status. Am J Public Health 87:1626–1629, 1997

Nemeroff CB: Chemical messengers of the brain, in Geriatric Psychiatry. Edited by Busse E, Blazer DG. Washington DC, American Psychiatric Press, 1989, pp 97–134

Newman G, Dovenmuehle RH, Busse EW: Alterations in neurological status with age. J Am Geriatr Soc 8:915–917, 1960

Ostrom JR, Hammarlund ER, Christensen DB, et al: Medication use in the elderly population. Med Care 23:157–164, 1985

Ouslander J: Drug therapy in the elderly. Ann Intern Med 95:711–722, 1981

Oxman TE: Antidepressants and cognitive impairment in the elderly. J Clin Psychiatry 57:S38–S44, 1996

Pascualy M, Veith RC: Depression as an adverse drug reaction, in Aging and Clinical Practice: Depression and Coexisting Disease. Edited by Robinson RG, Rabins PV. New York, Igaku-Shoin, 1989, pp 132–151

Patten SB, Love EJ: Drug-induced depression. Psychother Psychosom 66:63–73, 1997

Patten SB, Williams JV, Love EJ: Self-reported depressive symptoms in association with medication exposures among medical inpatients: a cross-sectional study. Can J Psychiatry 40:264–269, 1995

Patten SB, Williams JV, Love EJ: Case-control studies of cardiovascular medications as risk factors for clinically diagnosed depressive disorders in a hospitalized population. Can J Psychiatry 41:469–476, 1996

Patterson JF: Triazolam syndrome in the elderly. South Med J 80:1425–1426, 1987

Paykel ES, Flemingero RF, Watson JP: Psychiatric side effects of antihypertensives other than reserpine. J Clin Psychopharmacol 2:14–39, 1982

Picotte-Prillmayer D, DiMaggio JR, Baile WF: H$_2$ blocker delirium. Psychosomatics 36:74–77, 1995

Piraino AJ: Managing medication in the elderly. Hosp Pract (Off Ed) 30:59–64, 1995

Pitner JK, Mintzer JE, Pennypacker LC, et al: Efficacy and adverse effects of clozapine in four elderly psychotic patients. J Clin Psychiatry 56:180–185, 1995

Pomara N, Stanley B, Block R, et al: Adverse effects of single therapeutic doses of diazepam on performance in normal geriatric subjects: relationship to plasma concentration. Psychopharmacology 84:342–346, 1984

Popli AP, Hegarty JD, Siegel AJ, et al: Transfer of psychiatric inpatients to a general hospital due to adverse drug reactions. Psychosomatics 38:35–37, 1997

Postma JU, Vantilburg W: Visual hallucinations and delirium during treatment with amantadine. J Am Geriatr Soc 23:212–215, 1975

Prudnam D, Evans JG: Factors associated with falls in the elderly: a community study. Age Aging 10:141–146, 1981

Rabey JM, Treves TA, Neutfeld MY, et al: Low-dose clozapine in the treatment of levodopa-induced mental disturbances in Parkinson's disease. Neurology 43:432–434, 1995

Rampello L, Raffaele R, Nicoletti G, et al: Neurobehavioral syndrome induced by H$_2$-receptor blocker withdrawal: possible role of prolactin. Clin Neuropharmacology 20:49–54, 1997

Ray WA, Griffin MR, Downey W: Benzodiazepines of long and short half-life and the risk of hip fracture. JAMA 262:3303–3307, 1989

Reynolds CF, Kupfer DJ, Hoch CC, et al: Sleeping pills in the elderly: are they ever justified? J Clin Psychiatry 46:9–12, 1985

Rogowski J, Lillard LA, Kington R: The financial burden of prescription drug use among elderly persons. Gerontologist 37:475–482, 1997

Rosenthal SH, Fenton ML, Harnett DS: Clozapine for the treatment of levodopa-induced psychosis in Parkinson's disease. Gen Hosp Psychiatry 14:285–286, 1992

Rothschild A: Delirium: an SSRI-benztropine adverse effect? (letter). J Clin Psychiatry 56:537, 1995

Rummans TA, Evans JM, Krahn LE, et al: Delirium in elderly patients: evaluation and management. Mayo Clin Proc 70:989–998, 1995

Russell WL, Lopez LM: Cimetidine-induced mental status changes: case report and literature review. American Journal of Hospital Pharmacy 37:1667–1671, 1980

Sagel J, Matisonn R: Neuropsychiatric disturbance as the initial manifestation of digitalis toxicity. S Afr Med J 46:512–521, 1975

Salzman C: Medication compliance in the elderly. J Clin Psychiatry 56 (suppl 1):18–23, 1995

Schentag J, Cerra F, Calleri G, et al: Pharmacokinetics and clinical studies in patients with cimetidine-associated confusion. Lancet 1:117–181, 1979

Schneider-Heimert D: Why low-dose-benzodiazepine dependent insomniacs can't escape their sleeping pills. Acta Psychiatr Scand 78:706–711, 1988

Schwartz JB: Calcium antagonists in the elderly. A risk-benefit analysis (review). Drugs Aging 9:24–36, 1996

Shih JC, Young H: The alteration of serotonin binding sites in aging human brain. Life Sci 23:1441–1448, 1978

Shore JH, Fraunfelder FT, Meyer SM: Psychiatric side effects from topical ocular timolol, a beta-adrenergic blocker. J Clin Psychopharmacol 7:264–267, 1987

Smallegan M: How families decide on nursing home admission. Geriatric Consultant 1:21–24, 1983

Smith DF, Mattson RH, Cramer JA, et al: Results of a nationwide VA cooperative study comparing the efficacy and toxicity of carbamazepine, phenobarbital phenytoin and primidone. Epilepsia 28 (suppl 3):S50–S58, 1987

Solomon DH, Gurwitz JH: Toxicity of nonsteroidal anti-inflammatory drugs in the elderly: is advanced age a risk factor? (review). Am J Med 102:208–215, 1997

Spiegel R, Devos JE: Central effects of guanfacine and clonidine during wakefulness and sleep in healthy subjects. British Journal of Clinical Psychopharmacology 10 (suppl): 165–158, 1980

Stahl SM: Serotonin: it's possible to have too much of a good thing. J Clin Psychiatry 58:520–521, 1997

Stanilla JK, de Leon J, Simpson GM: Clozapine withdrawal resulting in delirium with psychosis: a report of three cases. J Clin Psychiatry 58:252–255, 1997

Sternbach H: The serotonin syndrome. Am J Psychiatry 148:705–713, 1991

Stoudemire A, Anfinson T, Edwards J: Corticosteroid-induced delirium and dependency (clinical conference). Gen Hosp Psychiatry 18:196–202, 1996

Sudarsky L: Geriatrics: gait disorders in the elderly. N Engl J Med 20:1441–1445, 1990

Sultzer DL Cummings JL: Drug-induced mania: causative agents, clinical characteristics and management: a retrospective analysis of the literature. Medical Toxicology and Adverse Drug Experience 4:127–143, 1989

Sunderland T: Neurotransmission in the aging central nervous system, in Clinical Geriatric Psychopharmacology, 2nd Edition. Edited by Salzman S. Baltimore, MD, Williams & Wilkins, 1992, pp 41–60

Swift CG: Special problems relating to the use of hypnotics in the elderly. Acta Psychiatr Scand Suppl 73:92–98, 1986

Tam LS, Chan TYK, Leung WK: Warfarin interaction with traditional Chinese medicines: danshen and methyl salicylate medicated oil. Aust N Z J Med 25:258, 1995

Tamblyn RM McLeod PJ, Abrahamowicz M, et al: Questionable prescribing for elderly patients in Quebec. Canadian Medical Association Journal 150:1801–1809, 1994

Thornton TL: Delirium associated with sulindac. JAMA 243: 1630–1631, 1980

Tune L, Carr S, Hoag E, et al: Anticholinergic effects of drugs commonly prescribed for the elderly: potential means of assessing risk of delirium. Am J Psychiatry 149:1393–1394, 1992

Tzabar Y, Asbury AJ, Millar K: Cognitive failures after general anesthesia for day-case surgery. Br J Anaesth 76:194–197, 1996

Vestal RE, Cusack BJ: Pharmacology and aging, in Handbook of the Biology of Aging. Edited by Schneider EL, Roew JW. San Diego, CA, Academic Press, 1990, pp 349–383

Vincent FM: The neuropsychiatric complications of corticosteroid therapy (review). Compr Ther 21:524–528, 1995

Wagner ML, Fedak MN, Sage JI, et al: Complications of disease and therapy: a comparison of younger and older patients with Parkinson's disease. Ann Clin Lab Sci 26:389–395, 1996

Wilkins-Ho M, Hollander Y: Toxic delirium with low-dose clozapine (letter). Can J Psychiatry 42:429–430, 1997

Williams L, Caranasos GJ: Neuropsychiatric effects of drugs in the elderly. J Fla Med Assoc 79(6):371–375, 1992

Willmore LJ: The effect of age on pharmacokinetics of antiepileptic drugs. Epilepsia 36(S5):S14–S21, 1995

Wilson JA, MacLennen WJ: Review: drug-induced parkinsonism in elderly patients. Age Ageing 18:208–210, 1989

Wolters EC, Jansen EN, Tuynman-Qua HG, et al: Olanzapine in the treatment of dopaminomimetic psychosis in patients with Parkinson's disease. Neurology 47:1085–1087, 1996

Wood KA, Harris MJ, Morreale A, et al: Drug-induced psychosis and depression in the elderly. Psychiatr Clin North Am 11:167–189, 1988

Wood P, Castleden CM: Psychopharmacology in the elderly, in Psychiatry in the Elderly. Edited by Jacob R, Oppenheimer C. Oxford, England, Oxford University Press, 1991, pp 339–372, 1991

Young BK, Camicioli R, Ganzini L: Neuropsychiatric adverse effects of antiparkinsonian drugs. Characteristics, evaluation and treatment (review). Drugs Aging 10:367–383, 1997

APPENDIX 31–1.   Significant potential drug-drug interactions in psychogeriatrics

Drugs	Interacting drugs	Consequences
Salicylates	β-Adrenergic blockers	Decreased antihypertensive action
	Hypoglycemics (chlorpropamide)	Large acetylsalicylic acid doses may cause hypoglycemia
	Lithium	Possible lithium toxicity
	Valproate	Possible valproate toxicity
Nonsteroidal anti-inflammatory drugs	β-Blockers	Decreased antihypertensive action
	Captopril	Indomethacin-decreased antihypertensive action
	Furosemide	Decreased diuretic action and antihypertensive effect
	Haloperidol	Possible severe sedation with indomethacin
	Potassium	Indomethacin-induced hyperkalemia
	Thiazide diuretics	Hyponatremia
Antidepressants, tricyclic	Clonidine	Decreased antihypertensive effect
	Disulfiram	Organic mental disorder
	Guanethidine	Decreased antihypertensive
	Hypoglycemics (chlorpropamide)	Doxepin-induced hypoglycemia
	Nitroglycerin (sublingual; tolazamide)	Nortriptyline-induced hypoglycemia
	Trimethoprim-sulfamethoxazole	Nitroglycerine may not dissolve; loss of antidepressant effect
Antidepressants, nontricyclic	Tricyclic antidepressants	Fluoxetine, fluvoxamine, and other stressors may inhibit metabolism of some tricyclic antidepressants
	Digoxin	Trazodone may increase risk of digoxin toxicity
	Phenothiazines	Trazodone combined may produce severe hypotension
	Triazolam, alprazolam, haloperidol	Nefazodone may inhibit metabolism of triazolo benzodiazepines and haloperidol
Carbamazepine	Anticoagulants	Prothrombin time decreased
	Cimetidine	Carbamazepine levels increased
	Desipramine	Carbamazepine and desipramine levels increased
	Diltiazem	Neurotoxicity
	Metoclopramide	Neurotoxicity
	Theophylline	Theophylline concentration decreased
	Thiazide diuretics	Hyponatremia
	Verapamil	Carbamazepine levels increased
β-Adrenergic blockers	Alcohol	May block signs of delirium tremens
	Cimetidine	Decreased β-adrenergic blocker metabolism
	Clonidine	Paradoxical hypertension
	Diltiazem	Heart failure
	Haloperidol	Profound hypotension
	Sulfonylureas	Prolonged hypoglycemia with hypoglycemic overdose
	Insulin	Prolonged hypoglycemia with hypoglycemic overdose
	Maprotiline	Decreased maprotiline metabolism
	Methyldopa	Hypertensive reaction
	Nifedipine	Heart failure
	Chlorpromazine	Levels increased of both medications
	Thioridazine	Thioridazine levels increased

(continued)

APPENDIX 31–1.   **Significant potential drug-drug interactions in psychogeriatrics** *(continued)*

Drugs	Interacting drugs	Consequences
	Sympathomimetic bronchodilators	Decreased bronchodilation
	Theophyllines	Theophylline toxicity
	Thiazide diuretics	Cardiac arrhythmias
	Verapamil	Heart failure
Lithium	Methyldopa	Lithium toxicity
	Phenytoin	Lithium toxicity
	Verapamil	Neurotoxicity, bradycardia

Source.   Reprinted with permission from Kennedy JS: "Adverse Drug Effects in the Older Adult," in *Drug-Induced Dysfunction in Psychiatry.* Edited by Ketharen MS, Kennedy JS. New York, Hemisphere, 1992, pp. 93–101.

APPENDIX 31–2. Drug- and toxin-induced neuropsychiatric disorders

	Depression	Mania	Anxiety or agitation	Delirium	Psychosis	Visual hallucinations	Dementia-like syndrome
Antihypertensive drugs							
Clonidine	✔	✔	✔	✔			✔
Oxprenolol	✔						
Propranolol	✔	✔		✔	✔	✔	
Reserpine	✔						
Methyldopa	✔			✔	✔		
Guanethidine	✔						
Hydralazine	✔			✔			
Bethanidine	✔						
Captopril		✔	✔				
Nifedipine	✔						
Prazosin	✔						
Cardiac glycosides	✔	✔		✔	✔	✔	✔
Antiarrhythmics							
Procainamide	✔	✔		✔	✔		
Lidocaine	✔			✔	✔		
Quinidine				✔			
Disopyramide				✔	✔		
Antiparkinsonian drugs							
Amantadine	✔		✔	✔	✔	✔	
Bromocriptine	✔	✔	✔	✔	✔	✔	
Levodopa	✔	✔	✔	✔	✔	✔	✔
Pergolide					✔		
Lisuride		✔			✔		
Piribedil		✔					
Trihexyphenidyl				✔		✔	
Procyclidine				✔		✔	
Biperiden				✔		✔	
Analgesics							
NSAIDs	✔			✔	✔		
Salicylates			✔	✔	✔		
Narcotics	✔		✔	✔		✔	
Ibuprofen					✔		
Phenacetin	✔				✔		
Naproxen					✔		
Indomethacin	✔	✔			✔	✔	
Anticonvulsants							
Carbamazepine	✔	✔		✔	✔		
Valproate				✔			✔
Phenytoin	✔			✔	✔	✔	✔
Barbiturates	✔		✔	✔			✔
Ethosuximide	✔		✔		✔	✔	
Clonazepam					✔		✔
Phenacemide					✔		

APPENDIX 31–2. Drug- and toxin-induced neuropsychiatric disorders *(continued)*

	Depression	Mania	Anxiety or agitation	Delirium	Psychosis	Visual hallucinations	Dementia-like syndrome
Sedative-hypnotics							
Benzodiazepines	✔	✔	✔	✔	✔		✔
Chloral hydrate	✔			✔			✔
Ethanol	✔			✔			✔
Clomethiazole	✔			✔			✔
Clorazepate	✔			✔			✔
Meprobamate				✔	✔		✔
Anticholinergics/antispasmodics							
Atropine				✔	✔	✔	✔
Benztropine				✔	✔	✔	✔
Propantheline				✔	✔	✔	✔
Scopolamine				✔	✔	✔	✔
Dicyclomine				✔	✔	✔	✔
Hyoscyamine				✔	✔	✔	✔
Lithium		✔		✔			✔
Antidepressants							
TCAs		✔	✔	✔	✔	✔	✔
MAOIs		✔			✔		
Bupropion			✔				
Trazodone		✔			✔		
Fluoxetine		✔	✔	✔			
Sertraline		✔					
Maprotiline						✔	
Neuroleptics							
Butyrophenones	✔			✔			✔
Phenothiazines	✔			✔	✔		✔
Clozapine				✔			
Thiothixene				✔			
Molindone				✔			
Antidiarrheals							
Diphenoxylate/atropine				✔			
Loperamide				✔			
Antimicrobial agents							
Podophyllin					✔		
Penicillins	✔		✔			✔	
Sulfamethoxazole	✔			✔			
Clotrimazole	✔						
Cycloserine	✔		✔	✔	✔		
Dapsone	✔	✔	✔				
Ethionamide	✔						
Tetracycline	✔					✔	
Griseofulvin	✔						
Metronidazole	✔						
Streptomycin	✔						

APPENDIX 31–2. Drug- and toxin-induced neuropsychiatric disorders *(continued)*

	Depression	Mania	Anxiety or agitation	Delirium	Psychosis	Visual hallucinations	Dementia-like syndrome
Antimicrobial agents *(continued)*							
Nitrofurantoin	✔						
Nalidixic acid	✔						
Antimalarials					✔	✔	
Sulfonamides	✔		✔			✔	
Procaine penicillin	✔		✔	✔	✔		
Thiocarbanilide	✔						
Acyclovir	✔			✔			
Isoniazid	✔	✔	✔		✔	✔	
Mefloquine				✔			
Iproniazid		✔			✔	✔	
Cephalosporins				✔	✔		
Ciprofloxacin				✔			
Amphotericin B				✔			
Antihistamines (H$_1$ blocking agents)							
Diphenhydramine				✔			
Chlorpheniramine				✔			
H$_2$ blockers							
Cimetidine	✔	✔		✔	✔	✔	
Ranitidine	✔			✔			
Drugs for urinary incontinence							
Oxybutynin				✔			
Flavoxate				✔			
Hyoscyamine				✔			
Withdrawal syndromes							
Barbiturates			✔	✔		✔	
Alcohol	✔		✔	✔	✔	✔	
Benzodiazepines			✔	✔	✔	✔	
Amphetamines	✔	✔	✔	✔	✔		
Chloral hydrate			✔	✔		✔	
Corticosteroids	✔		✔	✔			
Propranolol		✔	✔				
Reserpine		✔	✔				
MAOIs		✔	✔				
TCAs		✔	✔				
Caffeine			✔				
Meprobamate			✔			✔	
Opiates			✔		✔	✔	
Hallucinogens							
Phencyclidine		✔			✔	✔	
Indole hallucinogens	✔	✔			✔	✔	

APPENDIX 31–2. Drug- and toxin-induced neuropsychiatric disorders *(continued)*

	Depression	Mania	Anxiety or agitation	Delirium	Psychosis	Visual hallucinations	Dementia-like syndrome
Hallucinogens *(continued)*							
Cannabinols			✔		✔	✔	
Ketamine						✔	
Nitrous oxide						✔	
Antineoplastic drugs							
Azathioprine	✔						✔
C-Asparaginase	✔			✔	✔		
Plicamycin (mithramycin)	✔						
Vincristine	✔						
6-Azauridine	✔						
Bleomycin	✔						
Trimethoprim	✔						
Interferon	✔		✔	✔			
Endocrine agents							
Corticosteroids	✔	✔		✔	✔	✔	
ACTH		✔					
Oral contraceptives	✔						
Thyroid hormones		✔	✔		✔	✔	
Triamcinolone	✔						
Norethisterone	✔						
Danazol	✔						
Clomiphene citrate					✔		
Central nervous system stimulants							
Cocaine		✔	✔				
Sympathomimetics		✔	✔		✔	✔	
Amphetamine	✔	✔	✔		✔		
Fenfluramine	✔		✔				
Diethylpropion	✔		✔		✔		
Phenmetrazine	✔		✔				
Caffeine			✔	✔			
Methylphenidate		✔	✔		✔		
Pseudoephedrine		✔	✔		✔		
Pemoline		✔	✔				
Isoetharine		✔	✔				
Phenylpropanolamine		✔	✔		✔		
Ephedrine		✔	✔		✔		
Phenylephrine		✔	✔		✔		
Epinephrine			✔				
Isoproterenol			✔				
Miscellaneous drugs							
Acetazolamide	✔						
Albuterol					✔		
Anticholinesterase	✔		✔	✔			
Aprindine					✔		

APPENDIX 31–2. Drug- and toxin-induced neuropsychiatric disorders *(continued)*

	Depression	Mania	Anxiety or agitation	Delirium	Psychosis	Visual hallucinations	Dementia-like syndrome
Miscellaneous drugs *(continued)*					✔		
Arsenic			✔		✔	✔	✔
Aspartame		✔					
Baclofen	✔	✔			✔		
Benzene			✔				
Bromide		✔			✔	✔	✔
Calcium		✔					
Carbon disulfide			✔		✔		✔
Carbon monoxide					✔		✔
Choline	✔						
Cocaine		✔	✔		✔		
Cyclobenzaprine		✔		✔			
Cyclosporin A		✔					
Cyproheptadine	✔	✔					
Diethyl-*m*-toluamide		✔					
Diltiazem	✔	✔					
Diphenoxylate	✔						
Disulfiram	✔	✔		✔	✔	✔	✔
Flutamide		✔					
Halothane	✔						
Heavy metals			✔		✔	✔	✔
Isosafrole					✔		
L-Glutamine		✔					
Manganese					✔		✔
Mebeverine	✔						
Meclizine	✔						
Mepacrine		✔					
Mercury			✔		✔		✔
Methoserpidine	✔						
Methysergide	✔						
Metoclopramide	✔	✔		✔			
Metrizamide		✔			✔	✔	
Organophosphates			✔				✔
Oxandrolone		✔					
Oxymetholone		✔					
Pentazocine					✔		
Phenindione	✔						
Phosphorous			✔				
Pizotifen	✔						
Procaine	✔			✔			
Procarbazine		✔					
Procyclidine		✔					
Propafenone		✔					
Salbutamol	✔						

APPENDIX 31–2. Drug- and toxin-induced neuropsychiatric disorders *(continued)*

	Depression	Mania	Anxiety or agitation	Delirium	Psychosis	Visual hallucinations	Dementia-like syndrome
Miscellaneous drugs *(continued)*							
Tetrabenazine	✔						
Thallium					✔		✔
Theophylline		✔	✔				
Tryptophan		✔					
Veratrum	✔						
Yohimbine		✔	✔				
Zidovucine (AZT)		✔					

Note. NSAIDs = nonsteroidal anti-inflammatory drugs; TCAs = tricyclic antidepressants; MAOIs = monoamine oxidase inhibitors; H_1 = histamine subtype 1 receptor; H_2 = histamine subtype 2 receptor; ACTH = adrenocorticotropic hormone.
Source. Adapted from Callahan (1992); Cummings (1985b, 1986); Estroff and Gold (1986); Hall et al. (1980); Levinson (1979); Morrison and Katz (1989); Pascualy and Veith (1989); Sultzer and Cummings (1989); Williams and Caranasos (1992); K. A. Wood et al. (1988).

Neurobehavioral Syndromes

Mark D'Esposito, M.D.

A wide variety of neurobehavioral syndromes can arise from focal or diffuse damage to the cerebral cortex. The mental status examination, as reviewed in Chapter 6 in this volume, is an examination of the cerebral cortex and subcortical structures with cognitive functions. It is helpful heuristically to organize disorders of cognition in a fashion similar to how the mental status examination is organized, that is, by the principal cognitive domains—attention, language, memory, visuospatial perception, and executive function. One goal of this chapter is to review clinicoanatomical relationships by describing the neuroanatomical correlates of each of the cognitive domains. Knowledge of these syndromes and their anatomical basis will allow the clinician to accurately characterize the cognitive impairments found in age-related disorders, leading to more accurate diagnosis. For example, although Alzheimer's disease and Pick's disease are both dementia syndromes, they differ dramatically in their clinical presentation. Alzheimer's disease, which predominantly affects temporoparietal cortex, presents as a disorder of memory, language, and visuospatial skills, whereas Pick's disease, which affects frontotemporal cortex, presents as a disorder of executive function and behavior.

■ Disorders of Attention

Attention is not a unitary concept, but rather it likely is comprised of many related processes. For example, normal attention requires 1) awareness of stimuli presented in one's environment, 2) the ability to voluntarily focus one's attention on a specific stimulus, 3) the ability to resist other stimuli by suppressing an involuntary shift of attention, 4) the ability to shift attention quickly and smoothly and the ability to decide which of many competing stimuli should be the focus of one's attention, and 5) the ability to redirect that focus by voluntary control (Geschwind 1982). It is not currently possible to attribute each of these processes to specific regions of the brain. Attention can be impaired after focal or diffuse insults to the brain. If focal, damage will be within a network of brain regions that includes the ascending pathways of the mesencephalic reticular activating system or thalamocortical projections

Supported by National Institute of Neurological Disorders and Stroke Grant NS 01762, National Institute of Aging Grant AG13483, and the American Federation for Aging Research.

to association areas within parietal and prefrontal cortex (Mesulam 1985). If diffuse, the spectrum of etiologies causing impaired attention is broad, such as ingestion of prescription or nonprescription drugs, metabolic derangements, or infections (Lipowski 1990).

Acute Confusional State

Acute confusional state, also referred to as delirium, is defined as a disorder of attention. This syndrome is described in detail in Chapter 19 in this volume. In brief, the onset of this syndrome is sudden, and the level to which a patient can maintain attention often fluctuates, either from minute to minute or hour to hour. The patient may concurrently have altered alertness, but attentional difficulties can be present in the setting of completely intact alertness. Because attention is critical for all other types of information processing, patients will often exhibit deficits in other cognitive domains such as memory, perception, and executive function, even though there is not focal damage to the anatomical structures that support these abilities.

As mentioned, acute confusional states typically arise from diffuse damage to the brain. Rarely, focal damage will cause acute confusion. A middle cerebral artery causing right parietal lobe damage (Mesulam et al. 1976) or unilateral posterior cerebral artery strokes involving the parahippocampal-fusiform-lingual gyri (Medina et al. 1974) can present as confusion. On the surface, patients with Wernicke's aphasia secondary to a middle cerebral artery stroke will appear confused, although the deficit is of language and not attention. These patients will not be making any sense when they speak and will not understand what other people are saying to them. Attributing the deficit to a confusional disorder is a common misinterpretation of the patient's clinical problem, especially among family members or friends who are the first to encounter the patient at the time of the stroke.

Syndrome of Neglect

The most important function subserved by the right hemisphere is the ability of individuals to direct their attention into their environment. It is postulated that the right hemisphere can direct attention into both the left and right half of space, whereas the left hemisphere mostly directs attention into the right half of space (Mesulam 1985). Thus, damage to the right hemisphere will cause a deficit directing attention into the left visual space. This deficit is known as neglect and is defined as the inability to respond to or acknowledge stimuli present in the left hemispace (Heilman and Valenstein 1991). Although neglect can also occur after

left hemisphere lesions, it is much more common and more severe after right hemisphere damage. Neglect is one of several impairments that are more commonly found after damage to the right hemisphere (Table 32–1).

Studies of patients with right hemisphere damage have demonstrated that there are at least three forms of neglect: attentional, representational, and intentional (Heilman and Valenstein 1991). Evidence indicates that four major cerebral regions (Figure 32–1) provide an integrated network for directing attention within extrapersonal space and inner representations (Mesulam 1981). *Attentional* neglect is the failure to attend to stimuli in the left hemispace. This type of neglect is easily demonstrated on the clinical examination. The patient seems to ignore people on their left side or will not eat items on the left side of their plate. On formal mental status testing, the patient will showed marked rightward deviation when attempting to bisect a line in half. Another easy test for neglect is to place a number of lines on a blank page and ask the patient to cross off all of the lines. The patient will cross off lines on only the right side of the page and fail to acknowledge that there are lines on the left side of the page. A writing sample, line cancellation test, and clock drawing from a patient with neglect are provided in Figure 32–2.

It is vital that the clinician be able to recognize the difference between left visual neglect and left visual hemianopia, that is, the inability to see in the left visual field. The latter is a result of damage to the visual system, usually at the level of the optic radiations in the temporal and parietal lobes or primary visual cortex in the occipital lobes. When the line bisection or line cancellation test is given to patients with neglect or a visual field deficit, performance may be identical. One way to distinguish between these two possibilities is to move the piece of paper with target stimuli into the right visual field of the patient. The patient with the left visual field deficit should now be able to see the targets and bisect or cross them off correctly.

TABLE 32–1. Clinical characteristics of the right hemisphere syndrome

Cognitive impairment
Neglect
Visuospatial impairment
Aprosody
Motor impersistence
Behavioral impairment
Denial of illness (anosognosia)
Variety of behavioral deficits including agitation and delusions

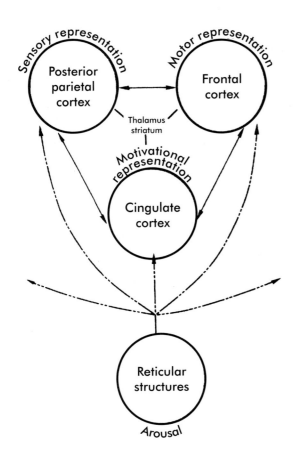

FIGURE 32–1. Neural network subserving neglect.

The patient with neglect will continue to avoid the left side of the page regardless of where the target stimulus is in their field of view. Unfortunately, some patients with extensive right hemisphere damage will demonstrate both neglect and a visual field deficit. In these patients, it may be impossible to disentangle these two phenomena.

Another important point for clinicians is that neglect may not be limited to the visual modality. When visual stimuli are presented simultaneously in opposite visual fields, patients with neglect will extinguish stimuli presented in the left visual field. That is, patients will fail to acknowledge stimuli in the left field only under simultaneous conditions, not during single presentation in the left field. This same phenomenon can occur with simultaneous presentation of auditory or tactile stimuli. The most common site of damage causing attentional neglect is in the posterior parietal lobe (Heilman et al. 1983). However, attentional neglect can also occur after subcortical lesions such as in the posterior thalamus (Watson and Heilman 1979).

A second type of neglect is called *representational* neglect. This type of neglect is manifested as a loss of the internal mental representation of the space opposite the side of the lesion. For example, when a group of patients with right hemisphere lesions were asked to imagine that they were facing a well-known cathedral in a square in Milan, they were unable to recall details regarding the left side of the square. However, when they were asked to imagine themselves facing away from the cathedral (i.e., their backs toward the cathedral), they were able to recall those left-sided details that were now on their right (Bisiach and Luzzatti 1978). Like patients with attentional neglect, patients with representation neglect also tend to have posterior lesions.

A third type of neglect, *action-intentional* neglect, is a unilateral deficit of motor program activation that causes reduced and delayed movements to the contralesional side (Coslett et al. 1990). Thus, despite being aware of stimuli in the left side of space, patients will fail to respond to stimuli on the left side. For example, if patients were blindfolded and asked to find all the items that were spread across a table, they would be reluctant to move their right hand into the left side of the table for exploration. Intentional neglect is most common after frontal (or anterior) lesions.

Disorders of Language

Distinction Between Speech and Language

Damage to the frontal, temporal, and/or parietal cortex will usually cause aphasia (Alexander and Benson 1991). *Aphasia* is defined as a disturbance of language, that is, the set of symbols that humans use as a means for communication. In contrast, speech is defined as the mechanical processes of language production, such as articulation and phonation. The major difference in the neural substrate for these disorders is that a lesion in the left hemisphere generally causes impairments in language, whereas damage to any component of the motor system for vocalization can cause impairment in speech. For example, a motor neuron disease such as amyotrophic lateral sclerosis or a muscle disease such as myasthenia gravis can cause a speech disturbance leaving language completely intact. A language disturbance, or aphasia, is specifically a result of cortical or subcortical brain damage.

Left Hemisphere Is Dominant for Language—With a Few Exceptions

It is believed that in as many as 99% of right-handers and 70% of left-handers, language is subserved by the left

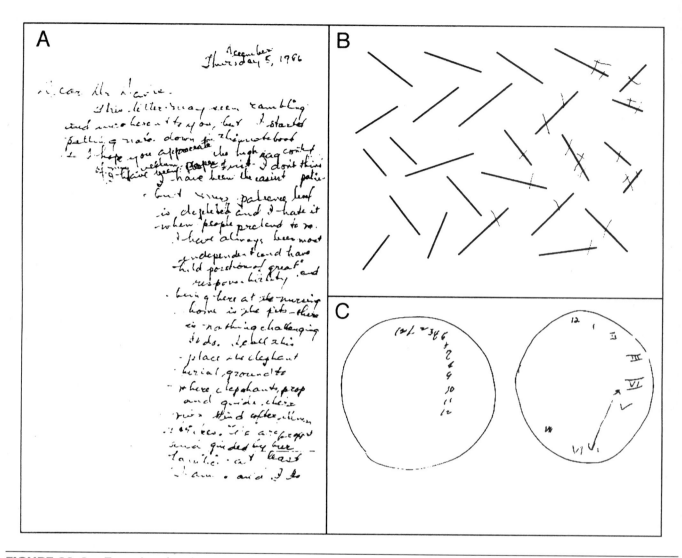

FIGURE 32–2. Examples of performance of a patient with neglect from right hemisphere lesions on handwriting sample (*panel A*), line cancellation test (*panel B*), and clock drawing (*panel C*). In each of the samples, the left side of the page is ignored.

hemisphere and brain injury on that side will cause aphasia (Benson and Geschwind 1985). Because more than 90% of the population reports themselves as right-handed, the vast majority of patients encountered with aphasia will have left hemisphere damage. In contrast, a very small percentage of right-handers, less than 1%, and up to 30% of left-handers have language subserved by the right hemisphere and can develop an aphasic syndrome from damage to the right hemisphere. Because aphasias resulting from right hemisphere lesions are fairly uncommon, they have not been studied extensively, but a few clinical observations have been made (Alexander et al. 1989). First, right-hemisphere lesions can cause two types of aphasia. In the first situation, the aphasia appears to manifest the identical clinical manifestations as if it were a result of damage in the left hemisphere. For example, right anterior lesions will cause a

nonfluent aphasia. Alternatively, aphasia resulting from a right hemisphere lesion can appear quite anomalous. For example, anterior lesions may cause a fluent aphasia. Second, although the right hemisphere, especially in left-handers, sometimes subserves language, right hemisphere functions such as directed attention and visuospatial skills often can be retained on that side. As one can envision, a large lesion in the right hemisphere in some left-handers can cause a profound cognitive disorder.

Anatomy of Language

The left hemisphere contains an organized distributed network for language function. Lesions in anterior portions of the brain, or in the frontal cortex, will cause impairments in the ability to produce fluent output, yet auditory comprehension of language is relatively preserved. The classic anterior aphasia is Broca's aphasia. Alternatively, damage to posterior portions of the brain, in the temporal and parietal lobes, will not cause a problem with producing fluent output but will cause a significant deficit in auditory comprehension of language. The classic posterior aphasia is Wernicke's aphasia. Large lesions that extend both anteriorly and posteriorly result in global aphasia, that is, that demonstrated in patients who are nonfluent and have a significant comprehension impairment. Damage to the arcuate fasciculus, the white matter bundle connecting Wernicke's and Broca's areas, will cause deficits in repetition of spoken language, called a conduction aphasia. Each of these aphasias is usually a result of occlusion of branches of the middle cerebral artery that supplies the lateral surface of the cerebral hemispheres. Damage in watershed territories of the brain (borderzones between the middle cerebral artery and the anterior or posterior cerebral artery), which leaves Broca's area, Wernicke's area, and the arcuate fasciculus intact, will cause transcortical aphasias, which are characterized by a perseveration of the ability to repeat spoken language. Damage almost anywhere in the left hemisphere will cause anomia, or a word-finding deficit. Also, many aphasic syndromes will recover into an anomic aphasia. These clinicoanatomical relationships are illustrated in Figure 32–3. It is also important to note that isolated subcortical lesions involving the striatum or the thalamus can cause each of the principal aphasic syndromes (D'Esposito and Alexander 1995; Mega and Alexander 1994). The characteristic features of each of the classic aphasic syndromes are presented in Table 32–2.

Aphasic Syndromes: Nonfluent Versus Fluent

Nonfluent aphasic syndromes. *Broca's aphasia* is a result of a lesion in the posterior portion of the inferior frontal gyrus, or frontal operculum. The most common cause of Broca's aphasia is a stroke in the territory of the superior division of the middle cerebral artery. Poor fluency, good comprehension, and poor repetition define it. These patients use short phrases (less than four to five words), have reduced grammatical form, poor articulation, and prosody. It is important to know that even though these patients have good functional comprehension, they may have problems understanding syntactically complex utterances such as interpreting the following sentence: The boy was chased by the girl who was fast. Who is being chased?

Broca's aphasia is usually accompanied by a right-sided sensorimotor deficit as well as buccofacial and left limb

ideomotor apraxia. Ideomotor apraxia is defined as the inability to produce a learned motor activity in the absence of sensorimotor impairments or a failure to understand the task (Geschwind 1975). Most patients will perform better when they are asked to carry out whole-body or eye movements. Buccofacial apraxia usually suggests damage to frontal opercular cortex in the left hemisphere, whereas limb apraxia usually suggests left parietal damage (Alexander and Benson 1991).

Global aphasia is a result of a large lesion that includes both Broca's and Wernicke's areas and is usually caused by a compete middle cerebral artery territory stroke. Poor fluency, poor comprehension, and poor repetition define it. Patients' deficits may range from a complete lack of output and understanding to the ability to produce a few stereotyped phrases that carry no meaning and understanding of some gestures. Interestingly, even patients with aphasia with severe comprehension deficits may understand an examiner's gestures. These preserved abilities can sometimes lead to an underestimation of the severity of their comprehension deficit. Also, the patient may retain many pragmatic skills that are involved in everyday conversation, such as knowing when to speak and when to pause and listen. Global aphasia is usually accompanied by a right-sided sensorimotor deficit, as well as a visual field deficit.

Transcortical motor aphasia is a result of a lesion in the watershed territory between the anterior and middle cere-

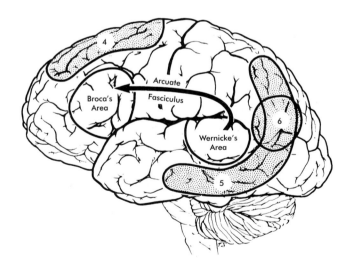

FIGURE 32–3. Schematic diagram of the anatomical location of lesions that cause each of the classic aphasic syndromes. Combined damage to Broca's and Wernicke's area = global aphasia; damage to arcuate fasciculus = conduction aphasia; 4 = transcortical motor aphasia; 5 = transcortical sensory aphasia; 6 = anomic aphasia.

TABLE 32–2. Characteristic features of classic aphasic syndromes

Aphasia syndrome	Fluency	Comprehension	Repetition
Anomic	Good	Good	Good
Conduction	Good	Good	Poor
Transcortical sensory	Good	Poor	Good
Wernicke's	Good	Poor	Poor
Transcortical motor	Poor	Good	Good
Broca's	Poor	Good	Poor
Global	Poor	Poor	Poor

bral artery or to a medial left frontal lesion. Poor fluency yet good comprehension and repetition define it. The striking finding in these patients, in contrast to patients with Broca's aphasia, is their ability to repeat phrases that they cannot produce spontaneously, called echolalia. Patients often repeat the examiner's utterance. Transcortical motor aphasia is usually accompanied by right hemiakinesia, that is, a lack of initiation of movement of the right side despite adequate strength.

Fluent aphasic syndromes.   *Wernicke's aphasia* is a result of a lesion that causes extensive damage to the posterior region of the left superior temporal gyrus (Wernicke's area). The most common cause is a stroke in the territory of the inferior division of the middle cerebral artery. Good fluency, poor comprehension, and impaired repetition define it. These patients have normal articulation and prosody and can produce sentence-length phrases effortlessly. Their spontaneous speech can be filled with phonemic paraphasias, semantic paraphasias, or neologisms. Paraphasias are substitutions for or within words. Semantic paraphasias are substitutions of words of similar meaning (e.g., "knife" for "spoon"). Phonemic paraphasias are sound substitutions (e.g., "scoon" for "spoon"). A neologism is a nonsense word such as "platin." Comprehension deficit can be mild, as when the patient has difficulty only at the sentence level, or severe, as when the patient is impaired even at attempting to understand single words. These patients may have similar impairments in reading and writing. Unlike many patients with nonfluent aphasia, patients with fluent aphasia may have several profound behavioral impairments such as anosognosia (unawareness of one's illness), perseveration, and agitation. Because the lesion is in posterior portions of the brain, a sensorimotor deficit is rarely found. Visual pathways are usually interrupted as they course through the temporal lobe on their way to the visual cortex, manifesting as a visual field deficit in the right upper quadrant of space.

Conduction aphasia is a result of a lesion that causes

damage to the arcuate fasciculus as it courses through the left inferior parietal lobe (supramarginal gyrus). Good fluency, good comprehension but poor repetition define it. The output of patients with conduction aphasia consists of abundant phonemic paraphasic errors especially during repetition. These patients often do not have any other neurological deficits.

Transcortical sensory aphasia is a result of a lesion in the watershed territory between the posterior and middle cerebral artery. It is defined as good fluency, good repetition, but poor comprehension. This syndrome is similar to Wernicke's aphasia with spared repetition. These patients usually do not have a sensorimotor deficit but may have a visual field cut.

Anomic aphasia is usually a result of a small lesion in the temporoparieto-occipital junction. It is defined as good fluency, repetition, and comprehension, but with a word-finding deficit. Essentially all patients with aphasia are anomic, but anomic aphasia refers to a syndrome in which word finding is the only deficit. It is also important to realize that many aphasic syndromes can recover into an anomic aphasia.

Related Syndromes

Aphemia refers to an isolated speech (not language) disturbance resulting from a cortical lesion restricted to the lower motor cortex (Schiff et al. 1983). Another term that is used is cortical dysarthria. *Gerstmann syndrome* is a clinical concept of limited usefulness but is commonly referred to in the clinical world. It refers to the tetrad of agraphia, acalculia, right-left disorientation, and finger agnosia (Strub and Geschwind 1974). Finger agnosia generally refers to the inability to name fingers. Damage to the inferior parietal lobule can cause this syndrome. However, because many of these signs are seen in many types of aphasia, its utility in clinicoanatomical correlation is limited. *Alexia* refers to acquired inability to read; *agraphia* refers to the inability to write. Most aphasic syndromes with a deficit in spoken language also have a similar deficit in reading and writing. Alexia without agraphia refers to the syndrome in which patients cannot read despite the preserved ability to write. Alexia results from a lesion in the left posterior cerebral artery territory, which includes the left occipito-temporal lobe and splenium of the corpus callosum (Damasio and Damasio 1983). Alexia is accompanied by a right hemianopia and, because of the splenial lesion, visual information projected to the right occipital cortex is cut off from the left hemisphere language center.

Disorders of Memory

Theoretical Model of Memory

A better understanding of memory disorders can be derived from a proper understanding of the theoretical distinctions of memory that have been developed by psychologists studying healthy humans. Such work has led to the proposal of several subdivisions of *long-term memory* (Squire 1987). One of the most widely accepted is a dichotomous classification of *declarative* versus *procedural* memory as illustrated in Figure 32–4.

Declarative memory represents memories of episodes and facts that can be consciously accessed, and *procedural memory* represents memory for skills. Unlike declarative memory, procedural memory is not available to our consciousness. Procedural memories can be either motor skills or mental procedures such as performing complex arithmetic. Declarative memory can be further subdivided into *episodic* and *semantic* memory (Tulving 1985). *Episodic memory* represents memories for specific personally experienced episodes. In contrast, *semantic memory* represents memories of facts, principles, and rules that make up our general knowledge of the world. It is proposed that semantic memories have evolved from specific episodes when such information was first encountered, but with the passage of time these episodes lose their temporal context (Cermak 1984). An illustration of these distinctions is that you may recall when you last rode your bicycle (episodic memory), know what a bicycle is (semantic memory), or know how to ride a bicycle (procedural memory) (Parkin 1993).

Another proposed classification of memory is a division between *explicit* and *implicit* memory (Schacter 1987). *Explicit memory* includes conscious recollection of any type of memory encompassing both episodic and semantic memories. *Implicit memory* does not require conscious recollection and would include procedural memory, but the implicit memory domain would also account for the phenomena of priming and classical conditioning. Priming is the phenomenon that previously encountered information has an increased probability of being recalled later even if there is no explicit recall of the earlier ("priming") experience (Tulving and Schacter 1990). For example, in a prototypical priming experiment, the subject is first presented with a list of words to read (e.g., motel, abstain, house). Subsequently, the subject is given three-letter stems (e.g, mot-) and is asked to produce the first word that comes to mind. The probability of generating a previously encountered word (e.g., motel) is increased compared with the probability of generating words not on the original list.

In clinical practice, the usage of the terms to describe memory processes has become imprecise and has not always followed these theoretical constructs. Many clinicians use the terms short-term memory to refer to learning new episodic information and long-term memory to refer to remote memories. This clinically sensible distinction does not, however, conform to experimental models of memory structure and only creates confusion when used in clinical reports. *Short-term memory* is properly defined as a system that temporarily (for seconds) stores information before becoming consolidated into long-term memory. Short-term memory (or working memory) can be tested with a span task such as digit span or pointing span, and long-term memory is tested by asking the subject to learn items that must be retrieved after an interval with distraction. The term *amnesic syndrome* properly refers to the loss of long-term memory only. *Remote memory* is information that has been consolidated in the past and may now be considered episodic, semantic, or procedural, depending upon its structure. Each of these systems (short-term memory, long-term memory, and remote memory) has a distinct anatomical basis.

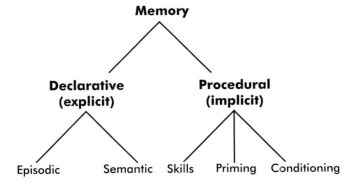

FIGURE 32–4. Proposed divisions of long-term memory.

Anatomy of Memory

The report of the patient H.M. in 1957 demonstrated conclusively that the hippocampus was critical for long-term memory (Scoville and Milner 1957). H.M. had intractable epilepsy and underwent bilateral surgical excision of the hippocampus and amygdala. After surgery, H.M. was left with a dense and isolated amnesia that has not changed in severity to this day. Anatomical studies in nonhuman primates with experimental lesions of the medial temporal lobe support the importance of this region in declarative memory (Squire and Zola-Morgan 1991). These studies and correlative lesion studies in humans have shown that the hippocampus and amygdala are part of a critical neural network that exists to subserve memory functioning (Zola-Morgan and Squire 1993). The anatomical structures supporting memory are illustrated in Figure 32–5.

This memory network has two anatomical loops or circuits (Mishkin 1978, 1982). The first circuit, called the Papez circuit, includes the hippocampus that projects via the fornices to the mammillary bodies. Via the mammillothalamic tract, the mammillary bodies project to the anterior nuclei of the thalamus, which in turn send projections to the posterior cingulate cortex. The circuit is completed by projections from the cingulate back to the hippocampus. Within this circuit are also important reciprocal connections between the hippocampus and basal forebrain, via the fornix. The basal forebrain is a term that includes the septal nucleus, diagonal band of Broca, and nucleus basalis of Meynert. The second circuit includes the amygdala that projects to the dorsomedial nucleus of the thalamus via amygdala fugal pathways. The dorsomedial nucleus sends projections to the prefrontal cortex that has direct reciprocal connections with the amygdala, completing the loop. In nonhuman primates, damage to either pathway alone does not result in amnesia, but damage to both of these two memory circuits will produce profound amnesia (Mishkin 1978). Memory deficits may be caused by a lesion anywhere within this neural network, including pathways that connect critical structures (e.g., the fornix) (D'Esposito et al. 1995; Gaffan and Gaffan 1991).

Thus, three main regions with critical pathways that interconnect them form a network for memory functioning. These are the medial temporal lobes, the diencephalon, and the basal forebrain. Human studies have consistently supported this anatomical model. For example, H.M. demonstrates the classic example of damage to medial temporal lobes. The best-studied example of amnesia resulting from damage of the diencephalon is Korsakoff's syndrome (KS), which causes damage to both the mammillary bodies and the dorsomedial nucleus of the thalamus (Victor et al. 1971). Isolated lesions of the basal forebrain occur most commonly after anterior communicating artery aneurysm rupture and can result in dense amnesia (Alexander and Freedman 1984; D'Esposito et al. 1996). This region has strong reciprocal connections with the medial temporal lobe. Also, the nucleus basalis projects widely to the cortex and is the primary source of cortical cholinergic input. Patients with Alzheimer's disease have early and profound memory loss and a marked reduction of neurons in this region (Whitehouse et al. 1981). Thus, damage to the medial temporal lobes, diencephalon, basal forebrain, or the pathways that interconnect these regions can cause severe impairments in long-term memory, also called anterograde amnesia. An important target of the medial temporal lobes and the diencephalon is the prefrontal cortex, which has emerged as an important region that also contributes to long-term memory function, but its main function is to subserve short-term memory.

Other types of memory processes are not dependent on these circuits. For example, isolated impairments in remote memory, also called retrograde amnesia, are caused by extensive damage to the anterior temporal lobes and not the medial temporal lobes (Kapur 1993). Procedural memory impairments are found in patients with damage to the basal ganglia and cerebellum (Gabrieli 1998).

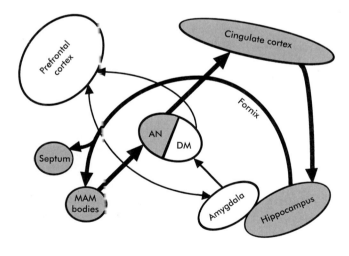

FIGURE 32–5. Neuroanatomical structures involved in memory function. *Gray-shaded* structures are part of the hippocampal circuit; *white* structures are part of the amygdala circuit. AN = anterior nucleus of the thalamus; DM = dorsomedial nucleus of the thalamus; Mam bodies = mammillary bodies.

Patterns of Amnesia

Specification of lesion sites associated with amnesia has led to investigation of possible differences in the pattern of memory loss with different lesion sites. Although each of the regions that, when damaged, cause amnesia is part of the same functional network subserving memory, it is possible that damage to different regions in the network affects different stages of memory processes, leading to different patterns of deficits (Parkin 1984).

Amnesia produced by *bilateral medial temporal amnesia* has the following characteristics. Short-term memory is normal. Long-term memory is severely impaired (anterograde amnesia). Once learned, information in long-term memory is very rapidly forgotten. Semantic memory is generally preserved, although acquisition of new semantic knowledge is deficient (Gabrieli et al. 1988) and retrieval of general semantic knowledge can be subtly defective after medial temporal damage (Barr et al. 1990). Remote memory of personal events (retrograde amnesia) is variably affected, but in cases with damage limited to the hippocampus the retrograde deficit is usually restricted to a brief period (weeks to a few years) before the injury (Corkin 1984). All implicit memory tasks are performed normally (Corkin 1968).

The classic contrasting example of *diencephalic amnesia* has been KS. Patients with KS have many similarities to patients with medial temporal damage (Butters and Stuss 1989). They also have normal short-term memory, severe anterograde amnesia, rapid rates of forgetting, normal semantic memory, and normal implicit memory. The major differences between KS and medial temporal lesions are in retrograde amnesia. Patients with KS have a more severe retrograde amnesia, often showing a temporal gradient with better recall of more remote information (Albert et al. 1979).

Patients with *frontal lobe damage* have long-term memory impairments. They differ from those with medial temporal damage in obvious ways; they are not amnesic as defined above. The impairments in memory seem to be a result of inefficiencies caused by poor attention or poor executive function (Hecaen and Albert 1978). The most consistent finding in patients with frontal lesions is impairment in multiple-trial list learning tasks (Janowsky et al. 1989). On this task, they fail on recall measures but have generally normal performance on recognition measures. This has been interpreted as defective retrieval, a function that requires strategy and effort, as opposed to normal storage, a function that is more passive. Patients with frontal lesions also have a number of specific impairments in memory (Shimamura 1995). They are defective in recall of temporal order, that is, recalling the context of learned items, even when they can remember these items. Finally, they have defective metamemory, that is, they are poor judges of knowing what they remember and how well their

memory functions. Damage to the prefrontal cortex will also cause a severe deficit in working memory (or short-term memory), which refers to the ability to temporarily store and manipulate information (Baddeley 1986). Elegant investigations in monkeys have shown that the prefrontal cortex is critical for the formation and storage of representations for short periods of time (Fuster 1997; Goldman-Rakic 1987).

Disorders of Visuoperception

The visual system extends from early striate and extrastriate cortex within the occipital lobe to the temporal and parietal association cortex. The visual system is organized into two streams, dorsal and ventral. The dorsal stream includes posterior parieto-occipital regions, whereas the ventral stream includes inferior medial temporo-occipital regions (Figure 32–6). Connections among these visual streams allow for progressively more complex processing of visual stimuli. Nonhuman primate lesion studies (Ungerleider and Mishkin 1982) as well as studies of patients with focal brain injury (Newcombe et al. 1987) have supported the notion that the dorsal stream supports spatial processing of stimuli ("Where is it?"), whereas the ventral stream supports the recognition of stimuli ("What is it?"). Bilateral damage to the earliest stages of visual processing within striate cortex will cause cortical blindness. Sometimes accompanying cortical blindness is Anton's syndrome, which is characterized by a patient's unawareness and denial of visual loss. This phenomenon is similar to the unawareness of left hemiplegia that is seen in patients with neglect resulting from right hemisphere lesions.

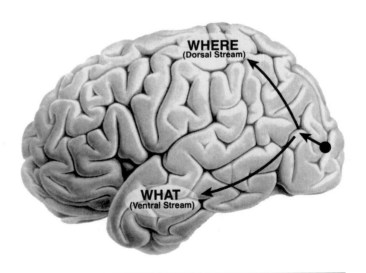

FIGURE 32–6.   Dorsal and ventral visual streams.

Dorsal Visual Systems

Damage within the posterior parietal cortex will cause deficits in spatial processing. Patients with right hemisphere damage perform more poorly than those with left hemisphere damage on tests of spatial processing such as judgment of line orientation (Benton et al. 1975) or mental rotation (Dizunno and Mann 1990). However, there is evidence that the left hemisphere also plays a role in spatial processing (Mehta and Newcombe 1991). A common way at the bedside to demonstrate the spatial deficit in patients with brain damage is to ask them to copy a drawing. Damage to either the left or right parietal lobe can cause a patient to produce an accurate copy of a figure, but the nature of the impairment differs. For example, a patient with left hemisphere damage will likely produce a figure that lacks details and is oversimplified but that retains its overall spatial configuration. In contrast, a patient with right hemisphere damage will likely produce a figure that is disorganized, possibly with parts in isolation but without an appropriate overall spatial configuration (Patterson and Zangwill 1944). An example of a copy of a drawing by a patient with focal injury is shown in Figure 32–7.

Balint's syndrome is a striking example of a disorder of spatial processing and refers to the triad of optic ataxia, ocular apraxia, and simultagnosia (Pierrot-Deseilligny et al. 1986). This syndrome typically occurs after bilateral damage to the parieto-occipital junction as a result of a watershed infarction between the middle and posterior cerebral arteries. Inferior visual field deficits can accompany these deficits. Optic ataxia is the inability to reach for a target under visual guidance. Ocular apraxia is the inability to visually scan one's environment by shifting gaze toward new visual stimuli. Simultagnosia refers to the inability to perceive the environment as a whole (Coslett and Saffran 1991). For example, if a patient was shown a complex scene in a magazine, he or she would be able to point out the details or parts of the scene (e.g., a bicycle) but would be unable to describe the entire scene (e.g., a bicycle race up a large hill in the mountains). In severe forms of this syndrome, patients are functionally disabled and essentially act as if they are blind.

Ventral Visual Systems

Damage within inferomedial temporo-occipital cortex will cause deficits in recognition of stimuli. *Visual object agnosia* refers to the inability to recognize objects through the visual modality despite intact elementary visual perception and other cognitive abilities (Farah 1990). This rare and unusual disorder has been further subdivided into apperceptive and associative types. Patients with apperceptive agnosia cannot "see" objects (Benson and Greenberg 1969). They cannot describe, match, or draw a picture of an object. Patients with associative agnosia can "see" the object but cannot recognize it (Rubens and Benson 1971). These patients can make perfect copies of the objects that they are unable to recognize (Figure 32–8). Presumably, in apperceptive agnosia, the visual image has been processed within striate cortex to extract the most elementary features, but a useful visual image cannot be formed because of a failure at the perceptual level. In associative visual agnosia, damage to the visual system presumably occurs after a stable visual image has been formed, but this percept cannot be used to access the knowledge of the object. Associative agnosia is caused by bilateral temporo-occipital damage typically a result of basilar

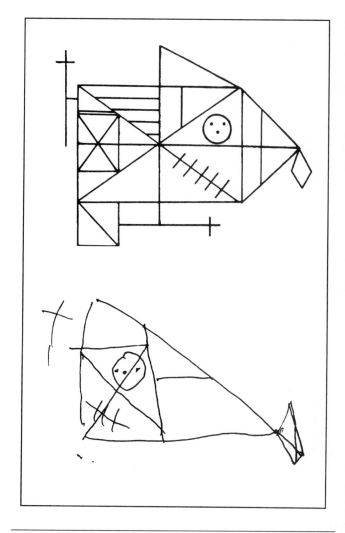

FIGURE 32–7. Illustration of impaired Rey figure copy (*bottom panel*) as compared with the target figure (*top panel*) from a patient with a right parietal lesion.

artery occlusion or embolic events to both posterior cerebral arteries, although visual agnosia can occur after unilateral damage to either hemisphere (Levine 1978; McCarthy and Warrington 1986). In addition to object agnosia, these patients usually have bilateral upper visual field deficits and can also have prosopagnosia, alexia, achromatopsia (i.e., inability to perceive color), or topographical disorientation. Apperceptive agnosia more typically occurs after diffuse injuries, such as cerebral hypoxia.

Patients with visual agnosia can recognize an object by other modalities such as touching it or from its spoken definition, demonstrating that they have not lost the meaning of the object. The deficit in visual agnosia is also not merely a deficit in naming the object since patients cannot identify the object by nonverbal means such as pantomiming its use. Alternatively, optic aphasia refers to a syndrome that occurs when a patient cannot name an object when presented only visually but can clearly identify it through another means (Coslett and Saffran 1989).

Prosopagnosia refers to the selective inability to recognize faces and can be considered a distinct form of visual agnosia. Patients are able to recognize familiar faces such as relatives via other means such as their voice, clothes, or body shape. In some patients the impairment has not been limited to human faces in that patients can have difficulty recognizing other classes of visually similar objects such as specific types of cars or cows in a dairy herd (Damasio et al. 1982). Prosopagnosia arises after lesions of the inferomedial temporo-occipital lobe develop, usually as a result of a posterior cerebral artery infarction. Most early, large clinical surveys of prosopagnosia have concluded that bilateral lesions are necessary (Damasio et al. 1982), but more recent reviews have demonstrated that prosopagnosia can occur with damage confined to the right hemisphere (De Renzi et al. 1994).

Disorders of Executive Function

Anatomy of Executive Function

The frontal lobes can be divided into three major subdivisions: the motor/premotor cortex, the limbic cortex, and the prefrontal cortex. The prefrontal cortex, which is multimodal association cortex, has afferent and/or efferent connections to practically all areas of association cortex in the parietal, temporal, and occipital lobes (Fuster 1997). In addition, there are connections to the premotor cortex (and therefore indirect connections to primary motor cortex); the limbic cortex (including the cingulate gyrus, amygdala, and hippocampus); the basal ganglia (the caudate and putamen); the thalamus (predominantly the dorsomedial nucleus); the hypothalamus; and the brainstem. Also, a number of connections exist within the frontal cortex, but these pathways are still poorly understood. Therefore, it is clear that the prefrontal cortex is in direct communication with almost every area of the brain (sensory, motor, and limbic systems) and plays a vital role in almost every function of the brain. Damage to prefrontal cortex causes impairment in behavior as well as high-level cognitive abilities, which have collectively been called executive function (Stuss and Benson 1986).

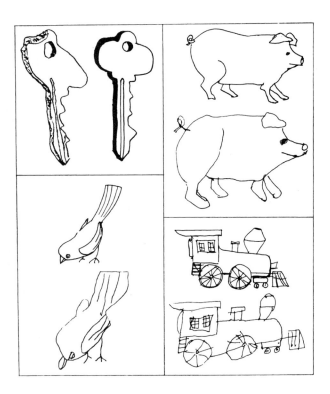

FIGURE 32–8. Copies of various figures from a patient with apperceptive agnosia. Each of these figures, which were copied accurately, could not be recognized visually.

Behavioral Deficits After Prefrontal Damage

A number of behavioral alterations can occur as a result of damage to prefrontal cortex. Such damage usually results in socially inappropriate behavior and difficulty in performing actions that require appropriate decisions and planning. Of course, the normal variation and range of human behavior must be taken into account when making any determination of impairment. The patient's age, educational level, social and cultural group, and previous achievements are important factors to consider. Many of the alterations in behavior overlap with the range of normal behavior, and big lesions may appear silent unless a comparison is made to the patient's previous state. It is also important to keep in mind that any combination of these behaviors can be observed in any single patient.

Patients with prefrontal damage can show a lack of appreciation for and disregard of social rules and restrictions. Patients can appear impulsive, disinhibited, or, in the extreme, out of control, exhibiting short periods of anger or rage. An example of this behavior was the change noted in the famous patient Phineas Gage. Before his accident, he was a religious, family-loving, honest, and hardworking man who was described after his frontal injury as "fitful, irreverent, indulging at times in the grossest profanity . . . impatient of restraint or advice when it conflicts with his desires . . . obstinate, devising many plans of operation, which are no sooner arranged than they are abandoned in turn for others appearing more feasible" (Harlow 1868). In contrast, patients with prefrontal damage may show a flat affect, blunted emotional response, and decrease in drive. An example of this behavior is evident in the following description of a different patient with a frontal injury: "He was quiet, did not initiate conversation, and appeared remote and withdrawn. Although frequently incontinent, he was unconcerned and almost never initiated an attempt to remedy the status" (Benson 1994). Self-awareness may be considered one of the highest cognitive attributes of the frontal lobes.

Although patients with frontal damage have little impairment of basic cognitive functions such as language and visuoperception, they can have difficulty using these skills. This problem is illustrated in the following case history: "While being evaluated for the presence of diabetes insipidus, the patient was instructed, 'Don't drink any water; don't go near the water fountain.' Within a few minutes he was observed having a drink at the water fountain. When asked by the examiner what he had just been told, he immediately replied: 'Don't drink any water; don't go near the water fountain.' " He had understood and remembered the instructions, but this knowledge could not be used to control his actions (Benson 1994). His actions were clearly separated from his knowledge.

Cognitive Deficits After Prefrontal Damage

Interestingly, extensive frontal lobe damage may have little impact on the abilities measured by standardized intelligence tests or other neuropsychological tests (see Chapter 7 in this volume), but these findings are in marked contrast to the way that these patients perform in unintelligent ways in real life (Shallice and Burgess 1991). Based on this observation, it is obvious that neuropsychological tests designed for the laboratory do not always capture the abilities that are necessary for success in real life. For example, "real-life behavior requires heavy time processing demands (working memory) and a core system of values based on both inherited (drives, instincts) and acquired (education, socialization) information that is probably not necessary for most artificial problems posed by neuropsychological tasks" (Damasio and Anderson 1993).

Executive function, which is used to describe the type of abilities that are impaired after prefrontal damage, is difficult to conceptualize and difficult to develop tasks to examine directly, especially at the bedside. The following impairments are characteristic of executive dysfunction:

1. *Inability to initiate, stop, and modify behavior in response to changing stimuli.* An impairment of this type is illustrated when patients with frontal injury perform the Wisconsin Card Sorting Test (Heaton 1985). In this test, a deck of cards is presented one at time to a patient who must sort each one according to various stimulus dimensions (color, form, or number). Each card from the deck contains from one to four identical figures (stars, triangles, crosses, or circles) in one of four colors. The patient is told after each response whether the response is correct or not and must infer from this information only (the sorting principle is not given by the examiner) what the next response should be. After 10 correct sorts, the sorting principle is changed without warning. During this test, patients with frontal injury usually understand and can repeat the rules of the test but are unable to follow them or use knowledge of incorrect performance to alter their behavior (Milner 1963).
2. *Inability to handle sequential behavior necessary for organization, planning, and problem solving.* Patients with frontal injury often have no difficulty with the basic operations of a given task. For example, when performing complex mathematical problems requiring multiple steps, the patient may initially respond impulsively to an early step and will be unable to string together and execute the component steps required for solving the problem (Stuss and Benson 1984). However, the ability to perform each of the mathematical operations in isolation (e.g., adding and subtracting) required to complete the complex task might be intact. The problem "The price of canned peas is two cans for 31 cents; what is the price of one dozen cans?" is almost impossible for patients with

frontal damage even though these patients perform the direct arithmetical task of multiplying 6 times 31 with ease (Stuss and Benson 1984).

3. *Inability to inhibit responses.* This impairment can be demonstrated with a measure called the Stroop paradigm (Stroop 1935). It is based on the observation that it takes longer to name the color of a series of conflicting color words (e.g., "red" printed in blue ink) than to name the color of a series of color blocks.

This phenomenon is exaggerated in patients with frontal lesions (Perret 1974). A related phenomenon is that these patients may display a remarkable tendency to imitate the examiner's gestures and behaviors even when no instruction has been given to do so, and even when this imitation entails considerable personal embarrassment. The mere sight of an object may also elicit the compulsion to use it, although the patient has not been asked to do so and the context is inappropriate—as in a patient who sees a pair of glasses and puts them on, even though he is already wearing his own pair (Figure 32–9). These symptoms have been called the "environmental dependency syndrome." It has been postulated that the frontal lobes may promote distance from the environment and the parietal lobes foster approach toward one's environment. Therefore, loss of frontal inhibition may result in overactivity of the parietal lobes. Without prefrontal cortex, our autonomy from our environment would not be possible. A given stimulus would automatically call up a predetermined response regardless of context (Lhermitte 1986; Lhermitte et al. 1986).

4. *Perseveration.* This is defined as an abnormal repetition of a specific behavior. It can be present after frontal damage in a wide range of tasks including motor acts, verbalizations, sorting tests, drawing, or writing (Figure 32–10).

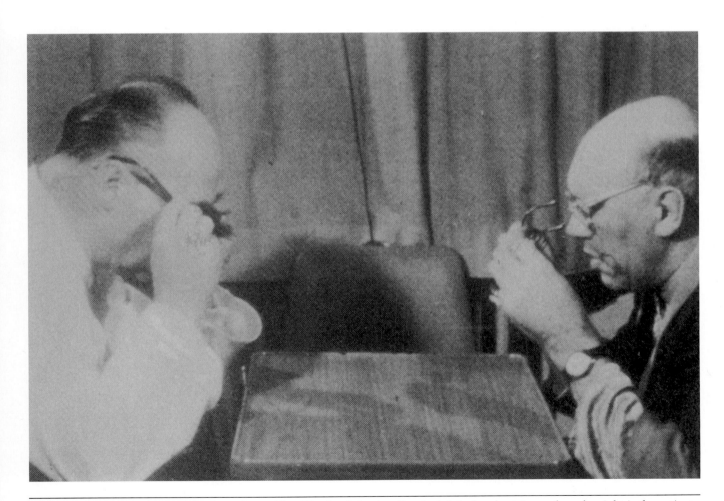

FIGURE 32–9. A photograph of a patient with utilization behavior. On the left is the physician and on the right is the patient. A pair of glasses were placed on the table in front of the patient without any instructions from the physician to do anything with them. Nevertheless, the patient put the glasses on his face even though he had another pair of glasses already on.

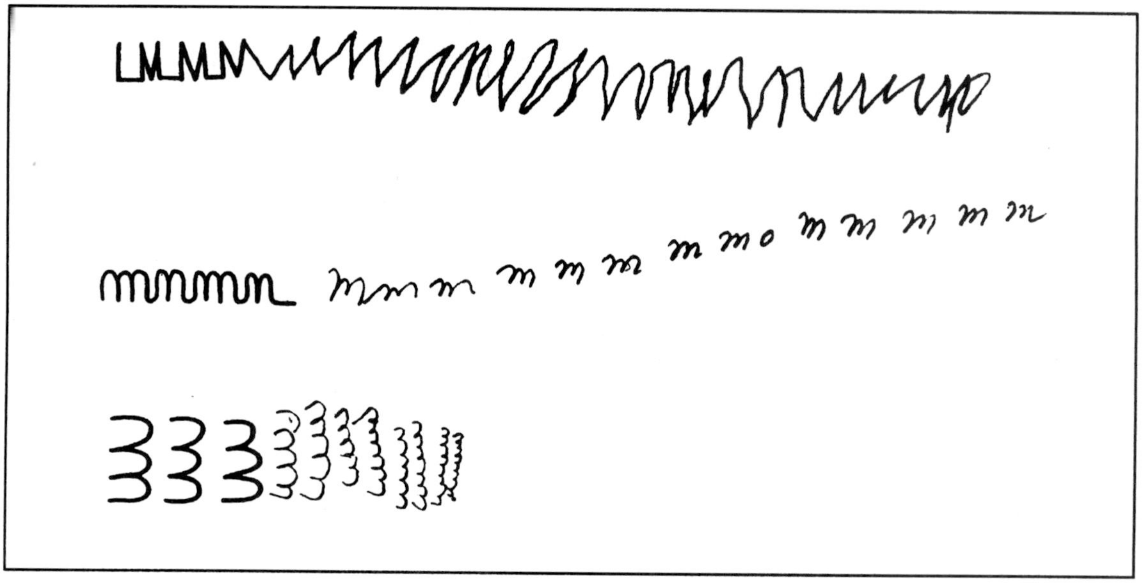

FIGURE 32–10.   Several examples of perseverative behavior from patients with frontal pathology.

Frontal Lobe Syndromes

At least three signature behavioral/cognitive syndromes (Cummings 1993) occur after damage to different regions of the prefrontal cortex (Figure 32–11). These syndromes reflect separable circuits of connection of the prefrontal cortex with subcortical structures (see Chapter 4 in this volume). First, damage to the dorsolateral prefrontal circuit causes executive dysfunction. These patients have difficulty generating hypotheses and flexibly maintaining and shifting sets as required by changing task demands. Second, damage to the orbitofrontal circuit causes disinhibited, irritable, and labile behavior. This type of lesion also results in imitation and utilization behavior. Unlike patients with dorsolateral damage, these patients may not have significant executive impairments. Third, damage to the medial frontal/anterior cingulate circuit causes akinesia, apathy, and unconcern. Of course, patients may have damage to more than one of these frontal circuits that can lead to a mixture of clinical deficits.

▌ Summary

Injury to the cerebral cortex can cause a wide range of neurobehavioral syndromes with a characteristic profile of deficits in attention, language, memory, visuoperception, or executive function. These syndromes can occur in isolation as a result of a stroke causing very focal damage (e.g., posterior cerebral artery infarction causing alexia) or combinations of each of these syndromes can be seen in more

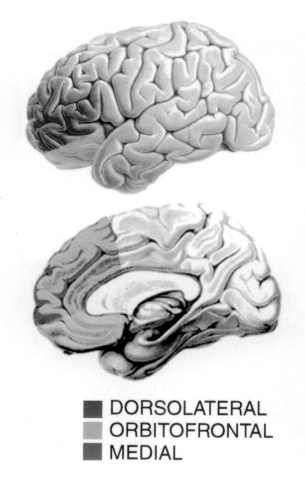

■ DORSOLATERAL
■ ORBITOFRONTAL
■ MEDIAL

FIGURE 32–11.   Functional subdivisions of the frontal lobes corresponding to dissociable behavioral syndromes.

widespread damage to the brain (e.g., Alzheimer's disease causing amnesia, aphasia, and visuospatial deficits). Knowledge of the clinicoanatomical relationships described in this chapter is critical for diagnosis, treatment, management, and rehabilitation of patients with injury to the cerebral cortex.

▌ References

Albert M, Butters N, Levin J: Temporal gradients in the retrograde amnesia of patients with alcoholic Korsakoff's disease. Arch Neurol 36:211–216, 1979

Alexander MP, Benson DF: The aphasias and related disturbances, in Clinical Neurology, Vol 1. Edited by Joynt R. Philadelphia, PA, JB Lippincott, 1991, pp 1–58

Alexander MP, Freedman M: Amnesia after anterior communicating artery aneurysm. Neurology 34:752–757, 1984

Alexander MP, Fischette MR, Fischer RF: Crossed aphasias can be mirror image or anomalous. Case reports, review and hypothesis. Brain 112:953–973, 1989

Baddeley A: Working Memory. New York, Oxford University Press, 1986

Barr WB, Goldberg E, Wasserstein J, et al: Retrograde amnesia following unilateral temporal lobectomy. Neuropsychologia 28:243–255, 1990

Benson D: The Neurology of Thinking. New York, Oxford University Press, 1994

Benson DF, Geschwind N: Aphasia and related disorders: a clinical approach, in Principles of Behavioral Neurology. Edited by Mesulam MM. Philadelphia, PA, FA Davis, 1985, pp 193–238

Benson DF, Greenberg JP: Visual form agnosia. A specific defect in visual discrimination. Arch Neurol 20:82–89, 1969

Benton AL, Hannay HJ, Varney NR: Visual perception of line direction in patients with unilateral brain disease. Neurology 25:907–910, 1975

Bisiach E, Luzzatti C: Unilateral neglect of representational space. Cortex 14:129–133, 1978

Butters N, Stuss DT: Diencephalic amnesia, in Handbook of Neuropsychology. Edited by Boller F, Grafman J. New York, Elsevier Science, 1989, pp 107–148

Cermak LS: The episodic-semantic distinction in amnesia, in Neuropsychology of Memory. Edited by Squire L, Butters N. New York, Guilford, 1984, pp 55–62

Corkin S: Acquisition of motor skill after bilateral medial temporal lobe excision. Neuropsychologia 6:255–265, 1968

Corkin S: Lasting consequences of bilateral medial temporal lobectomy: clinical course and experimental findings in H.M. Semin Neurol 4:249–259 1984

Coslett HB, Saffran EM: Preserved object recognition and reading comprehension in optic aphasia. Brain 112:1091–1110, 1989

Coslett HB, Saffran E: Simultanagnosia. To see but not two see. Brain 114:1523–1545, 1991

Coslett HB, Bowers D, Fitzpatrick E, et al: Directional hypokinesia and hemispatial inattention in neglect. Brain 113:475–486, 1990

Cummings JL: Frontal-subcortical circuits and human behavior. Arch Neurol 50:873–880, 1993

Damasio A, Damasio H, Van Hoesen G: Prosopagnosia: anatomic basis and anatomical mechanisms. Neurology 32:331–341, 1982

Damasio AR, Anderson SW: The frontal lobes, in Clinical Neuropsychology. Edited by Heilman K, Valenstein E. New York, Oxford University Press, 1993, pp 409–460

Damasio AR, Damasio H: The anatomic basis of pure alexia. Neurology 33:1573–1583, 1983

De Renzi E, Perani D, Carlesimo GA, et al: Prosopagnosia can be associated with damage confined to the right hemisphere—an MRI and PET study and a review of the literature. Neuropsychologia 32:893–902, 1994

D'Esposito M, Alexander MP: Subcortical aphasia: distinct profiles following left putaminal hemorrhage. Neurology 45:38–41, 1995

D'Esposito M, Verfaellie M, Alexander MP, et al: Amnesia following traumatic bilateral fornix transection. Neurology 45:1546–1550, 1995

D'Esposito M, Alexander MP, Fischer R, et al: Recovery of memory and executive function following anterior communicating artery aneurysm rupture. J Int Neuropsychol Soc 2:565–570, 1996

Ditunno PL, Mann VA: Right hemisphere specialization for mental rotation in normals and brain damaged subjects. Cortex 26:177–188, 1990

Farah MJ: Visual Agnosia: Disorders of Object Recognition and What They Tell Us About Normal Vision. Cambridge, MA, MIT Press, 1990

Fuster J: The Prefrontal Cortex: Anatomy, Physiology, and Neuropsychology of the Frontal Lobes, 3rd Edition. New York, Raven, 1997

Gabrieli JD: Cognitive neuroscience of human memory. Annu Rev Psychol 49:87–115, 1998

Gabrieli JDE, Cohen NJ, Corkin S: The impaired learning of semantic knowledge following bilateral medial temporal-lobe resection. Brain 7:157–177, 1988

Gaffan D, Gaffan EA: Amnesia in man following transection of the fornix: a review. Brain 114:2611–2618, 1991

Geschwind N: The apraxias: neural mechanisms of disorders of learned movement. Am Sci 63:188–195, 1975

Geschwind N: Disorders of attention: a frontier in neuropsychology. Philos Trans R Soc Lond B Biol Sci 298:173–185, 1982

Goldman-Rakic PS: Circuitry of the prefrontal cortex and the regulation of behavior by representational memory, in Handbook of Physiology. Sec 1. The Nervous System, Vol 5. Edited by Plum F, Mountcastle V. Bethesda, MD, American Physiological Society, 1987, pp 373–417

Harlow J: Recovery from the passage of an iron bar through the head. Proceedings of the Massachusetts Medical Society 2: 725–728, 1868

Heaton RK: Wisconsin Card Sorting Test. Odessa, FL, Psychological Assessment Resources, 1985

Hecaen H, Albert ML: Human Neuropsychology. New York, Wiley, 1978

Heilman K, Valenstein E: Neglect and related disorders, in Clinical Neuropsychology. Edited by Heilman K, Valenstein E. New York, Oxford University Press, 1991, pp 279–336

Heilman KM, Watson RT, Valenstein E, et al: Localization of lesions in neglect, in Localization in Neuropsychology. Edited by Kertesz A. New York, Academic Press, 1983, pp 455–470

Janowsky JS, Shimamura AP, Kritchevsky M, et al: Cognitive impairment following frontal lobe damage and its relevance to human amnesia. Behav Neurosci 103:548–560, 1989

Kapur N: Focal retrograde amnesia in neurological disease: a critical review. Cortex 29:217–234, 1993

Levine DN: Prosopagnosia and visual object agnosia: a behavioral study. Brain Lang 5:341–365, 1978

Lhermitte F: Human autonomy and the frontal lobes, Part II: patient behavior in complex and social situations: the "environmental dependency syndrome." Ann Neurol 19: 335–343, 1986

Lhermitte F, Pillon B, Serdaru M: Human autonomy and the frontal lobes, Part I: imitation and utilization behavior: a neuropsychological study of 75 patients. Ann Neurol 19: 326–334, 1986

Lipowski ZJ: Delirium: Acute Confusional States. New York, Oxford University Press, 1990

McCarthy RA, Warrington EK: Visual associative agnosia: a clinico-anatomical study of a single case. J Neurol Neurosurg Psychiatry 49:1233–1240, 1986

Medina JL, Rubino FA, Ross E: Agitated delirium caused by infarctions of the hippocampal formation and fusiform and lingual gyri: a case report. Neurology 24:1181–1183, 1974

Mega MS, Alexander MP: Subcortical aphasia: the core profile of capsulostriatal infarction. Neurology 44:1824–1829, 1994

Mehta Z, Newcombe F: A role for the left hemisphere in spatial processing. Cortex 27:153–167, 1991

Mesulam MM: A cortical network for directed attention and unilateral neglect. Ann Neurol 10:309–325, 1981

Mesulam MM: Attention, confusional states and neglect, in Principles of Behavioral Neurology. Edited by Mesulam M. Philadelphia, PA, FA Davis, 1985, pp 125–168

Mesulam MM, Waxman SG, Geschwind N, et al: Acute confusional states with right middle cerebral artery infarctions. J Neurol Neurosurg Psychiatry 39:84–89, 1976

Milner B: Effects of different brain regions on card sorting. Arch Neurol 9:90–100, 1963

Mishkin M: Memory in monkeys severely impaired by combined but not separate removal of the amygdala and hippocampus. Nature 273:297–298, 1978

Mishkin M: A memory system in the monkey. Philos Trans R Soc Lond B Biol Sci 298:85–92, 1982

Newcombe F, Ratcliff G, Damasio H: Dissociable visual and spatial impairments following right posterior cerebral lesions: clinical, neuropsychological and anatomical evidence. Neuropsychologia 25:149–161, 1987

Parkin A: Memory: Phenomenon, Experiment and Theory. Oxford, England, Blackwell Scientific, 1993

Parkin AJ: Amnesic syndrome: a lesion-specific disorder? Cortex 20:479–508, 1984

Patterson LR, Zangwill OL: Disorders of visual space perception associated with lesions of the right cerebral hemisphere. Brain 67:331–358, 1944

Perret E: The left frontal lobe of man and the suppression of habitual responses in verbal categorical behaviour. Neuropsychologia 12:323–330, 1974

Pierrot-Deseilligny C, Gray F, Brunet P: Infarcts of both inferior parietal lobules with impairment of visually guided eye movements, peripheral visual inattention and optic ataxia. Brain 109:81–97, 1986

Rubens AB, Benson DF: Associative visual agnosia. Arch Neurol 24:305–316, 1971

Schacter DL: Implicit memory: history and current status. J Exp Psychol Learn Mem Cogn 13:501–518, 1987

Schiff HB, Alexander MP, Naeser MA, et al: Aphemia. Clinical-anatomic correlations. Arch Neurol 40:720–727, 1983

Scoville WB, Milner B: Loss of recent memory after bilateral hippocampal lesions. Neuropsychologia 20:11–21, 1957

Shallice T, Burgess PW: Deficits in strategy application following frontal lobe damage in man. Brain 114:727–741, 1991

Shimamura AP: Memory and frontal lobe function, in The Cognitive Neurosciences. Edited by Gazzaniga MS. Cambridge, MA, MIT Press, 1995, pp 803–813

Squire LR: Memory and Brain. New York, Oxford University Press, 1987

Squire LR, Zola-Morgan S: The medial temporal lobe memory system. Science 253:1380–1386, 1991

Stroop JR: Studies of interference in serial verbal reactions. Journal of Experimental Psychology 18:643–662, 1935

Strub R, Geschwind N: Gerstmann syndrome without aphasia. Cortex 10:378–387, 1974

Stuss DT, Benson DF: Neuropsychological studies of the frontal lobes. Psychol Bull 95:3–28, 1984

Stuss DT, Benson DF: The Frontal Lobes. New York, Raven, 1986

Tulving E: How many memory systems are there? Am Psychol 40:385–398, 1985

Tulving E, Schacter DL: Priming and human memory systems. Science 247:301–306, 1990

Ungerleider LG, Mishkin M: Two cortical systems, in Analysis of Visual Behavior. Edited by Ingle D, Goodale M, Mansfield R. Cambridge, MA, MIT Press, 1982, pp 549–586

Victor M, Adams RD, Collins GH: The Wernicke-Korsakoff syndrome. Philadelphia, PA, FA Davis, 1971

Watson RT, Heilman KM: Thalamic neglect. Neurology 29:690–694, 1979

Whitehouse PJ, Price DL, Clark AW, et al: Alzheimer's disease: evidence for selective loss of cholinergic neurons in the nucleus basalis. Ann Neurol 10:122–126, 1981

Zola-Morgan S, Squire LR: Neuroanatomy of memory. Annu Rev Neurosci 16:547–563, 1993

SECTION V

Principles of Neuropsychiatric Treatment of the Elderly

C. Edward Coffey, M.D., Section Editor

33

Geriatric Neuropsychopharmacology

Why Does Age Matter?

George S. Zubenko, M.D., Ph.D.

Trey Sunderland, M.D.

Older adults respond less predictably to most medications than younger adults, typically requiring lower daily doses to achieve desired therapeutic effects while minimizing adverse effects and toxicity. This unpredictability is particularly evident among the frail elderly who carry a significant burden of comorbid medical problems and central neurodegenerative disorders or are at the upper extreme of the life cycle. Yet this population has a burgeoning need for clinical services and in recent years has become an increasingly important focus of attention for practitioners. Our goal with this chapter is to provide clinicians with a conceptual framework for understanding and responding to aging and age-related events that influence pharmacotherapeutics in older patients with neuropsychiatric disorders. Limitations and gaps in our knowledge base are also highlighted. This chapter includes a phenomenological overview of the aging process, a consideration of age-related factors that influence the pharmacokinetic and pharmacodynamic properties of psychotropic drugs, methods of enhancing medication compliance, and a brief conclusion.

Phenomenological Overview

Although aging is most easily defined by the passage of time, the number and extent of physiological changes asso-

Helpful comments provided by Dr. James M. Perel are gratefully acknowledged. This work was supported by Research Grants MH43261 and MH/AG47346, and Independent Scientist Award MH00540 for the National Institute of Mental Health and the National Institute on Aging.

ciated with aging are complex and highly variable among individuals. Moreover, within individuals, decrements in physiological functions often do not develop at the same rate or extent across all tissues and organ systems. When they do emerge, functionally significant changes occur predictably in the directions of decreased efficiency and decreased maximal capacity. Useful general relationships have emerged between chronological age and physiological variables that are relevant to assessments of health and the practice of pharmacotherapeutics. However, intra-individual and interindividual heterogeneity limits the informativeness of chronological age alone as an indicator of physiology. A complete history, physical and mental status examinations, functional assessment, and appropriate laboratory testing can provide a more accurate and comprehensive picture in this regard.

Age-related medical disorders, whether a reflection of a pathological acceleration of the normal aging process or novel derangements, often have an important impact on the pharmacotherapy of neuropsychiatric disorders in the elderly. In fact, the consequences of age-related illnesses often overshadow those of normative aging by rendering patients less responsive to treatment, less tolerant of adverse medication effects, or both. For example, even when adequate treatment is provided, comorbid medical burden is a predictor of poorer response of major depression to acute treatment (Katz et al. 1990; Popkin et al. 1985; Zubenko et al. 1994). This phenomenon also contributes to suboptimal responsiveness of patients with neuropsychiatric disorders by limiting the spectrum of medications and other treatment modalities that can be employed. Moreover, the medical disorders of late life are often chronic, contributing to an accumulating burden of medical problems with advancing age. Finally, complex relationships of chronic illness, pain, disability, and depression lead to the co-occurrence of these conditions at rates that are greater than expected from chance alone.

As a consequence of this age-related increase in medical comorbidity, older Americans fill an average of 13 prescriptions each year, greater than twice the national average and nearly three times that of individuals under 65 (Baum et al. 1988; Chrischilles et al. 1992). The use of prescription medications continues to further increase with age within this segment of the population. In a rural community survey, 13% of those between 65 and 70 took no medications compared with 7% of those 85 and older (Helling et al. 1987). Nonprescription drug use also increases with age with about two-thirds of seniors using over-the-counter medications (Lamy 1980). These values underestimate the use of medications by hospitalized patients and those in residential settings such as personal care

or nursing homes. In a study of 868 older psychiatric inpatients with a mean age of 62, this population had an average of six active ICD-9-CM (International Classification of Diseases, 9th Revision, Clinical Modification, 4th Revision 1993) medical problems and were taking an average of three to four nonpsychotropic prescription medications (Zubenko et al. 1997).

The common use of multiple prescription and nonprescription drugs by older Americans may contribute significantly to reduced effectiveness and increased toxicity of medications in this population by multiple interacting mechanisms. Reduced rates of metabolism and excretion of drugs among the elderly place them at risk for adverse effects if daily dosages are not adjusted accordingly. The use of multiple medications increases the likelihood of adverse drug interactions. Furthermore, the greater number of medications increases the likelihood of an adverse reaction with age-associated physiological changes or age-related medical conditions. Finally, polypharmacy invites noncompliance with prescribed medications. Increasing the number of medications and overall complexity of the medication regimen decreases the likelihood that any of the medications will be taken as prescribed. The result is reduced overall therapeutic effectiveness, greater burden of adverse effects, and greater likelihood of discontinuation of prescribed medications altogether.

Aging and the Pharmacokinetic Properties of Psychotropic Drugs

A rich literature describes numerous physiological changes that accompany normative aging and their impact on the pharmacokinetic properties of psychotropic drugs. A general summary of these physiological alterations and their effects on drug absorption, distribution, plasma protein binding, hepatic metabolism and clearance, and renal clearance is presented in Table 33–1. Common clinical implications of these relationships for pharmacotherapeutics are also described.

Absorption

Aging and age-related alterations occur throughout the gastrointestinal tract. Difficulties with swallowing are relatively common among elderly patients with neuropsychiatric disorders, especially those that are associated with neurodegenerative or cerebrovascular diseases (Jost 1997; Ribeiro et al. 1998; Sonies 1992; Zubenko et al. 1997). Dysphagia complicates the administration of medications, often rendering the dosing schedule erratic and necessitat-

TABLE 33–1. Age-related physiologic changes that influence the pharmacokinetics of psychotropic drugs

	Pharmacokinetic effects	Clinical implications
Absorption ↓ Swallowing ↑ Gastric pH ↓ Gastric emptying ↓ Intestinal motility ↑ Transit time ↓ Absorptive surface area ↓ Mesenteric blood flow	Decreased rate of absorption, especially when compounded by anticholinergic effects, antacids, or coadministration with food. May reduce bioavailability in some cases.	Delayed onset of action and reduced clinical effect if incomplete absorption occurs. Minimize factors that reduce absorption.
Distribution ↓ Muscle mass ↓ Total body water ↑ Total body fat	Increased total body fat leads to the increased volume of distribution of most (lipophilic) psychotropic drugs, resulting in increased half-life without change in steady-state plasma concentration. Effect of decreased total body water on decreased half-life for lithium is outweighed by age-associated reduction in renal clearance.	Increased treatment interval is required to reach steady-state plasma concentrations of psychotropic drugs. Decreased duration of action of single doses of these agents as a result of redistribution into fat stores.
Plasma protein binding ↓ Albumin (↓ ↓ malnutrition) ↑ α₁-acid glycoprotein (↑ ↑ illness)	Effects on the plasma concentration of free drug vary, depending on whether the drug is protein bound (all but lithium), whether it binds preferentially to albumin (benzodiazepines and neuroleptics) or α₁-acid glycoprotein (heterocyclic antidepressants), and whether hepatic clearance is restricted to unbound drug (sedative hypnotics) or not (most heterocyclic antidepressants, selective serotonin reuptake inhibitors, and neuroleptics). Competition for protein binding site by coadministered drugs can produce transient increases in the plasma concentrations of free drug.	On average, modest increase in the potency and toxicity of neuroleptics can result along with modest decrease in the potency and toxicity of heterocyclic antidepressants. Greater effects can occur in malnourished patients or those with comorbid medical illnesses. Increase surveillance for adverse effects when adding new medications to regimen.
Hepatic metabolism and clearance ↓ Liver volume ↓ Hepatic blood flow ↓ Oxidative metabolism ↓ N-Demethylation → Conjugation	Decreased metabolism of many psychotropic drugs results in increased peak and steady-state plasma levels. Increased ratios of parent drug to demethylated (often active) derivatives can occur. Modest effect of age on biotransformation by glucuronide, sulfate, or acetyl conjugation.	Reductions in the specific activities of cytochrome P450 isoenzymes can result from genetic polymorphism, age-related diseases, and inhibition by coadministered medications. Modest if any effects of age alone. Anticipate the need for reduced dosages of psychotropic drugs, especially on initial administration, to avoid excessive peak and steady-state plasma concentrations that produce toxicity. Advance dosages and introduce additional medications with caution. Monitor carefully for the emergence of adverse effects and toxicity. When indicated, employ benzodiazepines cleared by glucuronide conjugation (oxazepam, lorazepam, temazepam).

(continued)

TABLE 33–1. Age-related physiologic changes that influence the pharmacokinetics of psychotropic drugs *(continued)*

	Pharmacokinetic effects	Clinical implications
Renal clearance ↓ Renal blood flow ↓ Glomerular filtration rate	Decreased renal clearance leads to increased half-life and increased steady-state plasma concentration for lithium and active water-soluble metabolites of other psychotropic drugs. Diuretics and nonsteroidal anti-inflammatory drugs may further increase half-life and steady-state plasma concentration for lithium.	Evaluate renal function before initiating therapy with lithium or other drugs cleared primarily by the kidneys. Age-related decrements in renal clearance can be worsened by common chronic diseases, including hypertension, congestive heart failure, and diabetes. Initiate lithium therapy at a reduced daily dosage and titrate dosage cautiously using plasma levels while monitoring for adverse effects. Toxicity can occur in elderly patients at plasma lithium levels at or below the usual therapeutic range (0.8–1.2 mEq/L). Diuretics and nonsteroidal anti-inflammatory drugs may lead to lithium retention. Monitor potential toxicity in patients with renal failure who may retain water-soluble active metabolites such as cardiotoxic metabolites of heterocyclic antidepressants.

ing the coadministration of medications with food substances that may alter absorption. Most studies have documented age-associated decreases in gastric emptying and intestinal motility, although some reports suggest that these functions are preserved in healthy elders in the absence of intercurrent illness or medication effects (Altman 1990; Annesley 1989; Pilotto et al. 1995; Russell 1992; Schmucker 1985). Increases in gastric pH can also delay absorption by altering the ionization of drugs and further retarding gastric emptying (Altman 1990; Annesley 1989; Russell 1992; Schmucker 1985; Trey et al. 1997). These factors along with reductions in absorptive surface area and mesenteric blood flow may contribute to a reduced rate of drug absorption (Altman 1990; Annesley 1989; Holt and Balint 1993; Pilotto et al. 1995; Russell 1992; Schmucker 1985; Trey et al. 1997). This outcome can be compounded by anticholinergic drug effects, the administration of antacids, and the ingestion of food. Diseases of the liver, pancreas, and intestine are more common in the elderly and may also lead to impaired absorption (Altman 1990; Annesley 1989; Holt and Balint 1993; Pilotto et al. 1995; Russell 1992; Schmucker 1985; Trey et al. 1997). The clinical result of incomplete absorption is a delay in the onset of action and reduced clinical effect.

Distribution

Age-related alterations in drug distribution result from reductions in lean muscle mass and total body water, along with an increase in total body fat (Borkan et al. 1983; Forbes and Reina 1970; Novak 1972). Because most psychotropic drugs are lipophilic, their volumes of distribution increase commensurate with their degree of lipophilicity and the increase in body fat that occurs with aging. This pharmacokinetic effect leads to increased drug half-lives without changing steady-state plasma concentrations. The clinical consequence is that a longer treatment interval is required to reach steady-state plasma concentrations of most psychotropic drugs, which are typically administered regularly over months to years. In contrast, a reduced duration of action of single doses of these agents can result from redistribution into fat stores. Intermediate effects of these age-related changes in body composition can occur for drugs that have water-soluble metabolites that are pharmacologically active.

In contrast to most psychotropic drugs, lithium is not lipophilic and distributes into total body water. However, the potential reduction in half-life for lithium as a result of an age-related reduction in total body water is outweighed by decreases in renal clearance.

The blood-brain barrier partitions the brain parenchyma from substances in the systemic circulation, including medications. Although lipophilic psychotropic drugs distribute into the brain by passive diffusion, the blood-brain barrier is likely to regulate the passage of drugs that contain charged moieties, drugs that are protein-bound, and active hydrophilic drug metabolites into the brain. The contribution of this phenomenon to the distribution of centrally acting drugs to their sites of action remains a potentially important but understudied area of investigation. Available evidence suggests that the integrity of the blood-brain barrier decreases with age, especially in the context of central neurodegenerative disorders such as Alzheimer's disease (AD) (Kalaria 1996; Kleine and Hackler 1994; Shah and Mooradian 1997; Skoog et al. 1998). Such age-related changes may contribute to increased sensitivity to psychotropic medications.

Plasma Protein Binding

After absorption in the blood, virtually all psychotropic medications with the exception of lithium bind at least partially to plasma proteins, chiefly albumin and α_1-acid glycoprotein. This phenomenon is important because only unbound drug is able to cross the blood-brain barrier and interact with its intended target in the brain. Unbound drug may also interact with peripheral sites of action that result in unwanted side effects.

Protein binding characteristics of psychotropic drugs are largely determined by their chemical and structural properties (Loi and Vestal 1988). Although heterocyclic antidepressants bind to both albumin and α_1-acid glycoprotein, the free fractions (concentration of free drug/total drug concentration) of these agents in plasma depend primarily on the concentration of α_1-acid glycoprotein. In contrast, the free fractions of benzodiazepines and most neuroleptics depend primarily on albumin levels.

Aging is typically associated with modest reductions in plasma albumin levels (Adir et al. 1982; Greenblatt 1979; Loi and Vestal 1988). However, chronic debilitation from medical problems including dementia often results in malnutrition, with more significant reductions in plasma albumin levels. In contrast, most studies suggest that aging is accompanied by moderate elevations in plasma α_1-acid glycoprotein levels (Abernathy and Kerzner 1984; Amitai et al. 1993; Loi and Vestal 1988). Because α_1-acid glycoprotein is an acute-phase reactant, illnesses that are accompanied by inflammation and activation of the immune system produce greater elevations in the levels of this protein. On average, moderate age-associated changes occur in plasma albumin (decreased) and α_1-acid glycoprotein levels (increased), along with increased age-related variance that is attributable in part to an accumulating burden of medical illness.

Protein binding has a variable effect on hepatic metabolism and clearance that is also drug specific (von Moltke et al. 1998). For several commonly prescribed sedative-hypnotics (chlordiazepoxide, diazepam, lorazepam, alprazolam), hepatic clearance is restricted by protein binding. As a result, increases in the free fractions of these compounds that are attributable to age-associated reductions in albumin result in proportionate increases in their hepatic clearance and only a minimal increase in the concentration of free drug under steady-state conditions. However, for many psychotropic medications (most tricyclic antidepressants, selective serotonin reuptake inhibitors [SSRIs], neuroleptics), hepatic clearance is unaffected by protein binding.

The extent and characteristics of protein binding, and their clinical significance, are highly variable. They depend in important ways on the age, gender, health, and specific medications taken by each patient. On average, modest increases in the potency and toxicity of neuroleptics and modest decreases in the potency and toxicity of antidepressant medications would be expected from age-associated changes in the levels of albumin and α_1-acid glycoprotein because the hepatic clearance of these compounds is unrestricted by protein binding. Increased sensitivity of the elderly to the sedating effects of benzodiazepines depends to a greater extent on age-related reductions in hepatic and renal clearance as well as on increased tissue sensitivity.

Although significant clinical manifestations of altered protein binding appear to be uncommon, they are more likely to occur among the frail elderly who manifest the greatest perturbations in the levels of albumin and α_1-acid glycoprotein as the result of extreme age or comorbid medical burden. Competition for protein binding sites by coadministered drugs can also produce transient increases in the free concentrations of the competing compounds. These considerations warrant greater surveillance for adverse effects, especially when adding new medications to a regimen.

Hepatic Metabolism and Clearance

Most psychotherapeutic drugs other than lithium are cleared by hepatic biotransformation. After oral administration and intestinal absorption, these medications are transported to the liver through the portal and hepatic veins before entering the systemic circulation. Drug metabolism that occurs in the intestinal mucosa and during the first pass through the liver substantially reduces the bioavailability of many orally administered psychotropic drugs.

Biotransformation in the liver is most commonly accomplished through a series of oxidative reactions. The first step in this process is often demethylation, which typically produces an active metabolite. As an example, the tricyclic antidepressants amitriptyline and imipramine are demethylated to nortriptyline and desipramine, respectively. Subsequent oxidative conversions yield progressively more water-soluble compounds with varying degrees of pharmacological activity that are more readily excreted by the kidneys and gut. A second mechanism of biotransformation relies on the conjugation of drugs or their metabolites with glucuronide, sulfate, or acetyl moieties. Such conjugation reactions produce more polar, hydrophilic compounds that are usually devoid of pharmacological activity.

These oxidative reactions are catalyzed by the cytochrome P450 (CYP 450) family of isoenzymes that are localized to hepatic microsomes. They are divided into several subfamilies: CYP 1A2, CYP 2C9/10, CYP 2C19, CYP 2D6, and CYP 3A3/4. Subfamilies CYP 1A2, CYP 2D6, and CYP 3A3/4 account for the metabolism of most psychotropic drugs. A list of commonly prescribed psychotropic drugs and the CYP 450 isoenzymes that contribute to their metabolism is presented in Table 33–2. Not surprisingly, the substrate specificity of these isoenzymes often overlaps. When more than one isoenzyme family is involved, the predominant route of metabolism is indicated by the boldface drug name.

Aging is accompanied by reductions in the rate of metabolism of many psychotropic drugs by the liver. This decreased metabolism results in higher peak and steady-state plasma drug levels compared with those of younger patients receiving the same dosing regimen. Reduced hepatic metabolism associated with normative aging in humans appears to result, at least partially, from reductions in total liver volume and hepatic blood flow (Le Couteur and McLean 1998; Woodhouse and James 1990; Yuen 1990). Reduced uptake into hepatocytes as well as functional shunting as a result of the saturation of particular isoenzymes remain potential, but largely unexplored, contributors as well. Age-related diseases such as congestive heart can further reduce hepatic metabolism by compromising hepatic blood flow.

Most studies of humans have revealed little or no reductions in the specific activities or substrate affinities of the CYP 450 isoenzymes with advancing age in the absence of histopathological changes in the liver (Hunt et al. 1992; Le Couteur and McLean 1998; Pollock et al. 1992; Schmucker et al. 1990; Woodhouse and James 1990; Yuen 1990). However, reductions in the activities of these isoenzymes can result from genetic polymorphisms (e.g.,

CYP 2D6), age-related diseases, and inhibition by coadministered medications. Aging has only a modest effect on biotransformation by glucuronide, sulfate, or acetyl conjugation. Rather than age-related factors, an inherited polymorphism that affects the rate of acetylation accounts for more of the population variance in this phenotype.

Because the elderly often take multiple medications, they are at risk for the development of drug interactions that arise from the inhibition of one or more of the CYP 450 isoenzymes. Such interactions do not necessarily result in significant clinical consequences, especially when modest initial doses are employed and cautiously adjusted to achieve the desired therapeutic effect. A list of common or clinically significant inhibitors of CYP 450 isoenzymes is presented in Table 33–3. As an example, the comparison of Tables 33–2 and 33–3 reveals that both paroxetine and fluoxetine inhibit CYP 2D6. As a result, they would be expected to increase the steady-state plasma levels of tricyclic antidepressants in patients receiving stable doses of the latter. Paroxetine and fluoxetine also inhibit their own metabolism. Therefore, increases in the oral dosages of paroxetine and fluoxetine produce disproportionately larger increases in the corresponding steady-state plasma levels of these agents.

So far, these pharmacokinetic considerations have focused on the effects of coadministered drugs on the metabolism of psychotropic agents. In turn, psychotropic drugs can slow the metabolism of nonpsychotropic medications through their inhibitory effects on CYP 450 isoenzymes. As shown in Table 33–4, inhibitors of CYP 1A2 such as fluvoxamine can interfere with the metabolism of acetaminophen, propafenone, propranolol, warfarin, and theophylline. Inhibitors of CYP 2D6 such as paroxetine can slow the metabolism of several narcotic analgesics, antiarrhythmics, and β-blockers. Inhibitors of CYP 3A3/4 such as nefazodone may result in increased plasma levels of many drugs including narcotic and nonnarcotic analgesics, antibiotics, antihistamines, antitumor agents, antiarrhythmics, calcium channel blockers, immunosuppressants, steroids, and agents used to treat gastroesophageal reflux. All of these classes of drugs are commonly prescribed for age-related medical conditions.

Less commonly, some agents induce increases in hepatic enzyme activity, potentially resulting in subtherapeutic plasma levels of medications (see references for Tables 33–2 through 33–4). For example, cigarette smoking is an inducer of CYP 1A2 activity, whereas phenobarbital and phenytoin induce CYP 3A3/4. Carbamazepine induces its own metabolism (CYP 3A3/4; Table 33–2) and that of haloperidol, requiring upward adjustment of dosages to maintain therapeutic plasma levels. Some evidence

TABLE 33–2. Some common psychotropic drugs metabolized by cytochrome P450 (CYP 450) isoenzymes

	CYP 1A2	CYP 2D6	CYP 3A3/4
Antidepressants			
	Amitriptyline	Amitriptyline	Amitriptyline
			Citalopram
	Clomipramine	Clomipramine	Clomipramine
		Deprenyl	
		Desipramine	
		Fluoxetine	Fluoxetine
			Fluvoxamine
	Imipramine	Imipramine	Imipramine
			Nefazodone
		Nortriptyline	
		Paroxetine	
		Sertraline	Sertraline
		Trimipramine	
		Venlafaxine	
Antipsychotics			
		Chlorpromazine	
	Clozapine	Clozapine?	Clozapine
		Haloperidol	
	Olanzapine		
		Perphenazine	
		Risperidone	
		Sertindole	Sertindole
		Thioridazine	
Anxiolytics			
			Alprazolam
			Buspirone
			Clonazepam
			Diazepam[a]
			Midazolam
			Triazolam
Anticonvulsants/mood stabilizers[b]			
		Carbamazepine	
	Phenytoin		Phenytoin
Cognitive enhancers[c]			
		Donepezil	Donepezil
	Tacrine		

[a]Predominantly metabolized by CYP 2C19 with a smaller contribution from CYP 2C9/10.
[b]Valproic acid is primarily conjugated and excreted as a glucuronide derivative (minor contribution from CYP 2C19). Neurontin is excreted largely unchanged.
[c]Metrifonate is conjugated and excreted as a glucuronide derivative.
Source. Adapted from Gelenberg 1995; Intek Labs 1999; Michalets 1998; Micromedex 1999; Nemeroff et al. 1995–1996, 1996; Patel and Salzman 1998; Pollock 1994.

TABLE 33-3. Some common or significant inhibitors of cytochrome P450 (CYP 450) isoenzymes

CYP 1A2	CYP 2D6	CYP 3A3/4
		Astemizole
Cimetidine	Cimetidine	Cimetidine
	Desipramine	
	Diltiazem	Diltiazem
		Erythromycin
	Flecainide	
		Fluconazole
	Fluoxetine	
Fluvoxamine		Fluvoxamine
		Itraconazole
		Ketoconazole
		Nefazodone
	Norfluoxetine	Norfluoxetine
	Paroxetine	
	Propafenone	
	Quinidine	
	Sertraline (high doses)	
Theophylline		
		Troleandomycin
		Verapamil

Source. Adapted from Gelenberg 1995; Intek Labs 1999; Michalets 1998; Micromedex 1999; Nemeroff et al. 1995–1996, 1996; Patel and Salzman 1998; Pollock 1994.

suggests that the capacity for CYP 450 isoenzyme induction may be blunted in late life (Pearson and Roberts 1984; Schmucker 1979; Vestal 1989).

Tables 33–2 through 33–4 do not include comprehensive lists of medications. Instead, they are intended to illustrate common or clinically important drug properties and interactions that occur at the level of hepatic metabolism. This topic is currently receiving considerable attention, leading to a rapidly growing number of drugs whose metabolic profiles have been examined. Furthermore, published studies of drug metabolism performed using animal models of aging may not always provide data that are relevant to humans. When discrepancies were identified, we relied on results from human studies for inclusion in this section. Finally, the results of human in vitro studies of drug metabolism have not always been readily reconcilable with the results of human studies performed in vivo, reflecting the limitations of experimental designs and our current understanding of this complex topic.

Renal Clearance

Renal blood flow and glomerular filtration rate decline with age (Annesley 1989; Pollock et al. 1992; von Moltke et al. 1998; and see references to Tables 33–2 through 33–4). As a result, the renal clearance of lithium as well as active water-soluble metabolites of lipophilic parent compounds is reduced. Elevated and potentially toxic steady-state levels of lithium and cardiotoxic metabolites of tricyclic antidepressants may develop in elderly patients if doses that are used in younger adults are not adjusted downward.

Clinically, it is important to recognize that plasma creatinine concentrations overestimate the actual glomerular filtration rate in elderly subjects as a result of the reduction in muscle mass that occurs with aging. Congestive heart failure can further impair renal clearance by reducing renal blood flow, and hypertension and diabetes reduce glomerular filtration rate by producing microvascular damage. Moreover, the treatments for hypertension and congestive heart failure often include sodium-depleting diuretics. These agents along with nonsteroidal anti-inflammatory drugs are commonly prescribed for the elderly, further inhibit lithium excretion, and thereby enhance the potential for toxicity.

Aging and the Pharmacodynamic Properties of Psychotropic Drugs

Reports of increased susceptibility of the elderly to the adverse effects of psychotropic medications are commonplace in the literature. A list of some of these common adverse effects is presented in Table 33–5. However, the relative contributions of age-dependent changes in tissue sensitivity to the action of a drug (pharmacodynamics) and those that arise from alterations in pharmacokinetic characteristics are often difficult to determine unambiguously, especially in humans. Paradigms for simultaneously measuring pharmacokinetic variables while monitoring clinical effects have been developed for this purpose. However, these approaches do not readily lend themselves to the repeated dosing strategies that are typically used for psychotherapeutic drugs over weeks, months, and years. Moreover, such studies relate clinical effects to plasma levels of active drugs and metabolites that may not always reflect the concentrations of these compounds at their sites of action in the central nervous system.

The capacity for the brain to remodel itself at intercellular, cellular, and subcellular levels in response to endogenous and external stimuli appears to diminish in late life, especially among individuals who have central neurodegenerative disorders (Zubenko 1997) (Tables 33–6

TABLE 33–4. Common nonpsychotropic drugs metabolized by cytochrome P450 (CYP 450) isoenzymes

	CYP 1A2	CYP 2D6	CYP 3A3/4
Analgesics			
	Acetaminophen		Acetaminophen
			Alfentanil
		Codeine	Codeine
			Lidocaine
		Meperidine	
		Oxycodone	
		Tramadol	
Antibiotics			
			Clarithromycin
			Dapsone
			Erythromycin
			Ketoconazole
			Triacetyloleandomycin
Antihistamines			
			Astemizole
			Loratadine
			Terfenadine
Antitumor drugs			
			Adriamycin
			Paclitaxel
			Tamoxifen
			Vinblastine
Cardiovascular drugs			
Antiarrhythmics			
			Amiodarone
			Disopyramide
		Encainide	
		Flecainide	
		Lidocaine	Lidocaine
		Mexiletine	
	Propafenone	Propafenone	Propafenone
			Quinidine
β-Blockers			
		Metoprolol	
	Propranolol	Propranolol	
		Timolol	
Calcium channel blockers			
			Diltiazem

(continued)

TABLE 33–4. Common nonpsychotropic drugs metabolized by cytochrome P450 (CYP 450) isoenzymes (*continued*)

	CYP 1A2	CYP 2D6	CYP 3A3/4
			Felodipine
			Nicardipine
			Nifedipine
			Nimodipine
			Verapamil
Other			
		Warfarin	
			Lovastatin
Steroids			
			Androstenedione
			Cortisol
			Dexamethasone
			Estradiol
			Ethinyl estradiol
			Progesterone
			Testosterone
Other			
			Caffeine
			Cisapride
			Cyclosporin
			Ethosuximide
			Omeprazole
	Theophylline		

Source. Adapted from Gelenberg 1995; Intek Labs 1999; Michalets 1998; Micromedex 1999; Nemeroff et al. 1995–1996, 1996; Patel and Salzman 1998; Pollock 1994.

through 33–9. This age-associated reduction in plasticity can account for the decreased average rate of response of depressed elders to antidepressant therapy compared with that of younger adults. It can also account for the association of cognitive impairment with a somewhat poorer acute response to antidepressant treatment among elderly patients with major depression. Recovery from drug-induced toxicity also appears to be slower in this segment of the population. As an example, residual symptoms of lithium-induced encephalopathy can persist for a substantive period after drug discontinuation when lithium levels are no longer detectable in plasma.

Benzodiazepines

The elderly fill more prescriptions for benzodiazepines (Balter et al. 1974; Baum et al. 1986) and experience more

adverse effects from these drugs than their younger counterparts (Boston Collaborative Drug Surveillance Program 1973; Castleden et al. 1977; Cook et al. 1984; Giles et al. 1978; Greenblatt et al. 1991; Pomara et al. 1984; Ray et al. 1989; Reidenberg et al. 1978; Thompson et al. 1983). The increased magnitude of pharmacological effects in the elderly, including sedation as well as memory and psychomotor impairment, is partially attributable to age-related reductions in the rates of clearance and elimination that predispose the elderly to the development of elevated plasma levels of these compounds (Greenblatt et al. 1991; Herings et al. 1995; Kroboth et al. 1990; Pomara et al. 1984). However, the increased sensitivity of the elderly to these effects remains evident even when similar plasma concentrations are maintained in younger and older individuals (Bertz et al. 1997; Castleden et al. 1977; Cook et al. 1984; Greenblatt et al. 1991; Herings et al. 1995; Kroboth

TABLE 33–5. **Common adverse effects of psychotropic drugs in the elderly**

- Central nervous system (sedation, confusion, disorientation, memory impairment, delirium)
- Anticholinergic, peripheral (constipation, dry mouth, blurred vision, urinary retention)
- Motor (extrapyramidal symptoms, tremor, impaired gait, increased body sway, falling)
- Cardiovascular (hypotension, cardiac conduction delay)
- Other (agitation, mood and perceptual disturbances, headache, sweating, sexual dysfunction, gastrointestinal disturbances [nausea, anorexia, changes in weight or bowel habits], hyponatremia)

et al. 1990; Nikaido et al. 1990; Pomara et al. 1985; Reidenberg et al. 1978; Swift et al. 1985). The elderly can also experience paradoxical excitement from benzodiazepines, a qualitatively different effect. Although the mechanisms that underlie these age-dependent pharmacodynamic alterations have not been elucidated, age-associated reductions in the numbers of GABAergic neurons (Allen et al. 1983) and the specific activity of the biosynthetic enzyme glutamic acid decarboxylase in selected brain regions (McGeer 1981) have been reported from autopsy studies, along with lower γ-aminobutyric acid (GABA) levels in cerebrospinal fluid (Bareggi et al. 1985; Hare et al. 1982). Together, these pharmacokinetic and pharmacodynamic changes render elderly patients who take benzodiazepines more vulnerable on average to excessive sedation, to memory and psychomotor impairment, and to falls and resulting skeletal fractures.

Lithium

Unlike dosages of most other psychotropic drugs, oral dosages of lithium salts are typically adjusted to achieve target plasma levels of lithium ion in the range of 0.8–1.2 mEq/L. This approach should minimize the contributions of age-related pharmacokinetic changes (chiefly reduced renal clearance) to the development of therapeutic or adverse effects. Yet, at this relatively narrow range of plasma lithium levels, elderly patients develop adverse effects more commonly, and those adverse effects that develop tend to be more debilitating than those experienced by younger patients (Satlin and Liptzin 1998). These effects include cognitive impairment, tremor, muscle rigidity, abnormalities of gait, gastrointestinal distress (nausea, diarrhea), polydipsia, polyuria, and electrocardiogram changes. In fact, it is not uncommon to encounter elderly patients who develop intolerable adverse effects, including delirium, at steady-state plasma levels below 0.8 mEq/L. It is unclear

whether aging is associated with increased risk of lithium-induced hypothyroidism or renal disease that occur with longer-term treatment.

These common clinical observations strongly suggest that aging is accompanied by sensitization of target tissues to the adverse effects of lithium. However, the neurobiological substrates and mechanisms that are responsible for this phenomenon are unknown. Whether the age-associated increase in the sensitivity of the elderly to the adverse effects of lithium is likewise accompanied by increased therapeutic potency is uncertain.

Cholinergic Antagonists

Many psychotropic drugs have significant anticholinergic (antimuscarinic) potency, especially antidepressant and antipsychotic medications. Less appreciated is that numerous medications prescribed for indications other than behavioral disorders among the elderly also possess clinically meaningful anticholinergic potencies (Tune et al. 1992). Some common examples include cimetidine and ranitidine; dipyridamole, warfarin, isosorbide, nifedipine, and digoxin; codeine, theophylline, and prednisolone. Over-the-counter medications taken by the elderly for various indications also frequently include ingredients that have significant anticholinergic properties (e.g., diphenhydramine hydrochloride [Benadryl]). These agents alone and in combination contribute to the development of clinically important anticholinergic effects both centrally and in the periphery (Table 33–5).

The relative contributions of pharmacokinetic and pharmacodynamic phenomena to the increased vulnerability of the elderly to the anticholinergic effects of medications have not been clearly defined and probably differ in relative importance depending on the particular drug(s) involved. Challenge studies employing single intravenous doses of the antimuscarinic agent scopolamine have demonstrated greater cognitive impairment with aging (Table 33–6). These results suggest that aging is associated with greater intrinsic sensitivity of the central nervous system to cognitive impairment induced by anticholinergic agents.

Numerous age-related neurobiological changes in the central cholinergic nervous system can contribute to the increased sensitivity of the elderly to the anticholinergic effects of psychotropic and other medications. As shown in Table 33–6, all of these effects of aging are in the direction of decreased cholinergic function. Advancing age is accompanied by a reduction in the number of cholinergic neurons in the basal forebrain that innervate the cortex. The basis for this selective loss of cholinergic neurons in aging individuals is unclear. One factor may be related to

TABLE 33–6. Age-related changes in the cholinergic system

Cholinergic markers[a]	Location	Techniques	Findings
Cholinergic neurons			
Mesulam et al. (1987)	Basal forebrain	Cell counts, autopsy	Decreased
Choline uptake			
Cohen et al. (1995)	Brain	MR in vivo spectroscopy	Decreased
Choline acetyltransferase			
Court et al. (1993)	Cortex and hippocampus	Specific activity, autopsy	Decreased
Allen et al. (1983)	Cerebellum	Specific activity, autopsy	Normal
Acetylcholinesterase			
Nakano et al. (1986)	Cerebrospinal fluid	Specific activity, autopsy	Increased
M_1, M_2 receptors			
Lee et al. (1996)	Cortex	^{11}C-Labeled TRB PET	Normal
Suhara et al. (1993)	Cortex	^{11}C-Labeled NMPB PET	Decreased
Nordberg et al. (1992)	Cortex and thalamus	^{3}H-Labeled QNB/carbachol	M_1 decreased
		^{3}H-Labeled QNB/pirenzepine	M_2 increased
G-protein coupling			
Cutler et al. (1994)	Basal ganglia	Carbachol stimulation, autopsy	Decreased
Nicotinic receptor			
Nordberg et al. (1992)	Cortex	^{3}H-Labeled nicotine binding, autopsy	Decreased
Flynn and Mash (1986)	Cortex	^{3}H-Labeled nicotine binding, autopsy	Decreased
Scopolamine infusion			
Molchan (1992)	Cognitive-behavioral	Drug challenge	Increased sensitivity

Note. MR = magnetic resonance; NMPB = *N*-methyl-4-piperidylbenzilate; PET = positron-emission tomography; QNB = quinuclidinyl benzilate; TRB = tropanyl benzilate.
[a]Complete reference citations are at the end of the chapter.
Source. Adapted from Allen et al. 1983; Court et al. 1993; Cutler et al. 1994; Flynn and Mash 1986; Lee et al. 1996; Mesulam et al. 1987; Molchan et al. 1992; Muller et al. 1991; Nakano et al. 1986; Nordberg et al. 1992; Suhara et al. 1993; Sunderland et al. 1995.

their need to draw on a limited supply of choline for multiple purposes, including the synthesis of structural components of cell membranes, second-messenger molecules, and the neurotransmitter acetylcholine. Despite its key role of choline in neuronal metabolism, brain cells lack the capacity to synthesize choline de novo. The significant decline in the uptake of circulating choline into brain that develops with age can disproportionately compromise cholinergic neurons whose need for choline is the greatest (Cohen et al. 1995).

Aging is also associated with a decrease in the specific activity of the biosynthetic enzyme choline acetyltransferase in the cortex and an increase in the activity of the catabolic enzyme acetylcholinesterase in cerebrospinal fluid. These biochemical changes can reduce the synthesis of acetylcholine while enhancing its rate of degradation once released into the synaptic cleft. Studies of age-related changes in the densities of muscarinic receptors have yielded inconsistent results, possibly because reduced numbers of presynaptic muscarinic receptors are accompanied by a compensatory increase in the density of postsynaptic muscarinic receptors. Reductions in the density of nicotinic receptors in the brain have been reported with aging, although the functional significance of these receptors is unclear.

AD is the most common cause of mental impairment among the elderly (Bachman et al. 1992; Evans et al. 1989; Jorm et al. 1987) (see Chapter 24 in this volume). The pathophysiology of this disorder is complex, and numerous neuronal types and neurotransmitter systems are affected (Zubenko 1997). One of the most consistently reported and profound pathological changes in AD is the loss of cholinergic neurons from the basal forebrain that innervate the neocortex and hippocampus (Arendt et al. 1983; Saper et al. 1985; Whitehouse et al. 1982). This process substantially exceeds that expected for age and is reflected in a loss of choline acetyltransferase as well as decreases in acetylcholinesterase, choline uptake, and the synthesis and release of acetylcholine from cortical tissue slices (Bird et al. 1983; Bowen et al. 1983; Davies and Maloney 1976; Pope at al. 1964; Rossor et al. 1982; Sims et al. 1983). Because the cholinergic system plays an important role in memory and learning (Drachman and Leavitt 1974), its degeneration in AD seems likely to contribute to the development of dementia.

Inconsistent changes or only modest reductions in total, M_1, and M_2 muscarinic receptor binding have been reported in neocortical, hippocampal, and subcortical brain regions from patients with AD (Greenamyre and Maragos 1993). As with normative aging, these inconsistencies in autopsy findings can result from a complex sequence of events including the progressive loss of presynaptic cholinergic afferents accompanied by the transient upregulation of cholinergic receptors or postsynaptic neurons. Some studies also suggest reduced coupling of the M_1 receptor to its corresponding G protein (Flynn et al. 1991; Smith et al. 1987). Altered regulation of muscarinic binding and cerebral perfusion after low-dose chronic scopolamine administration has been demonstrated in vivo by single photon emission computed tomography (SPECT) scans of patients with AD and elderly control subjects (Sunderland et al. 1995). Nicotine receptor binding has consistently been reported to be substantially reduced in the cortices of patients with AD (Araujo et al. 1988; Flynn and Mash 1986; Perry et al. 1987; Rinne and Myllykylä 1991; Shimohama et al. 1986; Whitehouse et al. 1986), although the functional significance of this finding is unclear.

These findings are consistent with the common observation that patients with AD are even more sensitive to the central effects of anticholinergic and other drugs than older adults who have normal cognition (Molchan et al. 1992). The subgroup of patients with AD with Lewy body pathology (AD Lewy body variant, ADLBV) have been reported to have even greater cholinergic and dopaminergic deficits and can be the most prone to central toxicity from anticholinergic and antidopaminergic drugs (Förstl et al. 1993; Hansen et al. 1990; Langlais et al. 1993; Lippa et al. 1994; Perry et al. 1990, 1991, 1993) (see Chapter 24 in this volume).

Dopaminergic Antagonists

The elderly are at increased risk of developing extrapyramidal symptoms from the antidopaminergic actions of psychotropic drugs, chiefly the conventional antipsychotic medications. These adverse effects typically consist of parkinsonian symptoms (rigidity, tremor, bradykinesia), akathisia, and tardive dyskinesia (Kalish et al. 1995; Sweet et al. 1995). For reasons that are unclear, neuroleptic-induced dystonic reactions appear to be less common in the elderly than in younger patients. The coadministration of heterocyclic antidepressants or lithium may exacerbate neuroleptic-induced extrapyramidal symptoms by an unknown mechanism.

The relative contributions of pharmacokinetic and pharmacodynamic phenomena to the increased susceptibility of the elderly to extrapyramidal symptoms have not been clearly delineated. However, numerous age-related neurobiological changes can render the central dopaminergic system more sensitive to pharmacological antagonists in later life. As shown in Table 33–7, the number of

TABLE 33–7. Age-related changes in the dopaminergic system

Dopaminergic markers[a]	Location	Techniques	Findings
Dopaminergic neurons			
Morgan et al. (1987)	Substantia nigra	Cell counts, autopsy	Decreased
Tyrosine hydroxylase			
McGeer (1981)	Basal ganglia	Specific activity, autopsy	Decreased
Robinson et al. (1977)	Caudate	Specific activity, autopsy	Unchanged
Monoamine oxidase[b]			
Oreland and Gottfries (1986)	Cortical, subcortical areas	Specific activity, autopsy	MAO-A, unchanged; MAO-B, increase
Dopamine D$_1$ receptor			
DeKeyser et al. (1990)	Striation	^{3}H-Labeled SCH-23390, autopsy	Unchanged
Dopamine D$_2$ receptor			
Volkow et al. (1998); Rinne et al. (1993)	Basal ganglia	^{11}C-Labeled raclopride PET	Decreased
Wang et al. (1995)	Basal ganglia	^{18}F-Labeled NMS PET	Decreased
Roth and Joseph (1994)	Striatum (rat)	mRNA, in situ hybridization	Decreased
DeKeyser et al. (1990)	Striatum	^{3}H-Labeled spiperone, autopsy	Unchanged
Dopamine transporter			
Volkow et al. (1998)	Basal ganglia	^{11}C-Labeled methylphenidate PET	Decreased
Van Dyck et al. (1995)	Striatum	^{123}β-CIT SPECT	Decreased
Volkow et al. (1994)	Basal ganglia	^{11}C-Labeled cocaine PET	Decreased
Bannon et al. (1992)	Striatum	mRNA, nuclease protection, autopsy	Decreased
DeKeyser et al. (1990)	Striatum	^{3}H-Labeled GBR 12935, autopsy	Decreased
Homovanillic acid			
Hartikainen et al. (1991)	Cerebrospinal fluid	HPLC	Unchanged
Bareggi et al. (1985)	Cerebrospinal fluid	HPLC	Increased

Note. β-CIT = β-carbomethoxy-3β-(4-iodophenyl) tropane; HPLC = high performance liquid chromatography; NMS = *N*-methylspiperone; PET = positron–emission tomography; SPECT = single photon emission computed tomography.
[a]Complete reference citations are at the end of the chapter.
[b]Dopamine is metabolized by both MAO-A and MAO-B.
Source. Adapted from Bannon et al. 1992; Bareggi et al. 1985; DeKeyser et al. 1990; McGeer 1981; Morgan et al. 1987; Oreland and Gottfries 1986; Rinne et al. 1993; Robinson et al. 1977; Roth and Joseph 1994; Van Dyck et al. 1995; Volkow et al. 1994, 1998; Wang et al. 1995.

neurons in the substantia nigra, the largest collection of dopaminergic nerve cell bodies in the brain, declines with age. Reduction in the specific activity of the biosynthetic enzyme tyrosine hydroxylase, along with increased activity of the catabolic enzyme monoamine oxidase B, can result in reduced synthesis and steady-state levels of dopamine in the dopaminergic neurons that remain. Reductions in the density of dopamine D_2 receptors, at least some of which are located on presynaptic neurons, may reflect the same age-related cell loss. In contrast, the density of D_1 receptors may increase with age as a compensatory mechanism. Age-related reductions in the activity of the dopamine transporter, which serves to recover and inactivate dopamine that is released into the synaptic cleft, may also facilitate dopaminergic neurotransmission across the synapses that remain or may simply reflect the loss of presynaptic dopaminergic neurons. The concentration of homovanillic acid, a major metabolite of dopamine, has been reported to increase in cerebrospinal fluid with age. The last finding may reflect a compensatory increase in the firing rates of surviving dopaminergic neurons.

Postsynaptic denervation supersensitivity has been suggested as a mechanism that contributes to the sensitivity of some patients with Parkinson's disease to dopaminergic agents, including L-dopa preparations ((+)-carbidopa) used to treat this condition. In such cases, psychotic symptoms (delusions, hallucinations) can emerge alone or in the context of delirium. If the use of other antiparkinsonism drugs is not a viable alternative, this clinical scenario can often be managed by reducing the dosage of L-dopa to the extent possible while adding an atypical antipsychotic medication with reduced tendencies to worsen extrapyramidal symptoms and hypotension.

The mechanism of action of L-dopa in the treatment of Parkinson's disease appears to depend on the conversion of this precursor to dopamine in surviving dopaminergic neurons. The progressive degeneration of these neurons that occurs in Parkinson's disease may contribute to the loss of efficacy of L-dopa in the late stages of this disorder.

Noradrenergic Effects

Age-related changes in the central noradrenergic system are summarized in Table 33–8. Consistent with observations from the cholinergic and other aminergic systems, the transition into late life is accompanied by neurobiological changes that tend to reduce central noradrenergic tone. These changes include a reduced number of cells in the locus ceruleus, the largest collection of noradrenergic nerve cell bodies in the brain, along with a decrease in the specific activity of the biosynthetic enzyme

tyrosine hydroxylase. Unlike dopamine, norepinephrine is preferentially metabolized by monoamine oxidase A, whose activity does not appear to increase with age. These changes are accompanied by decreases in the densities of α_2, β_1, and β_2 receptors in the projection areas of the locus ceruleus. Moreover, signal transduction across these receptors may be reduced as a result of less efficient G-protein coupling. In spite of these changes, the concentration of methoxyhydroxyphenylglycol, a major metabolite of norepinephrine, appears to increase with age in cerebrospinal fluid. This may result from a compensatory increase in the firing rate of the reduced number of noradrenergic neurons whose postsynaptic sites include fewer, less efficient receptors.

These age-related changes in the central aminergic nervous system may contribute to the vulnerability of older adults to the development of neuropsychiatric syndromes, especially when the degree of neurodegeneration is marked, as occurs in AD and Parkinson's disease (Zubenko 1996; Zubenko and Moossy 1988; Zubenko et al. 1990, 1991). Moreover, these changes can result in a blunted acute response of such patients to antidepressant medications, prolong the time required for a therapeutic response, and contribute to relapse as degenerative changes progress (Zubenko et al. 1994).

Selective Serotonin Reuptake Inhibitors

As a drug class, the SSRIs have a more benign side-effect profile than the heterocyclic antidepressants and monoamine oxidase inhibitors (MAOIs). Their common adverse effects include headache, gastrointestinal disturbances (chiefly nausea, anorexia, and diarrhea), increased sweating, and sexual dysfunction. Their lack of significant anticholinergic (except paroxetine) and adverse cardiovascular effects has increasingly led to their preferred use in depressed patients who have a significant burden of comorbid medical problems, including the neurodegenerative disorders (see Chapter 13 in this volume). The SSRIs have become especially popular as first-line antidepressants in primary care settings.

Evidence of increased sensitivity of the elderly to the effects of SSRIs is largely limited to interactions with other drugs through inhibition of the CYP 450 isoenzymes (see section on hepatic metabolism and clearance). Little direct evidence implicates age-dependent pharmacodynamic changes in this regard. Instead, age-associated decreases in function of the central serotonergic nervous system may predispose elderly patients to behavioral syndromes, especially in the context of the neurodegenerative diseases. These pathological changes may also contribute to a

TABLE 33–8. Age-related changes in the noradrenergic system

Noradrenergic markers[a]	Location	Techniques	Findings
Noradrenergic neurons			
Mann (1991)	Locus ceruleus	Cell counts, autopsy	Decreased
Tyrosine hydroxylase			
McGeer (1981)	Basal ganglia	Specific activity, autopsy	Decreased
Robinson et al. (1977)	Caudate	Specific activity, autopsy	Unchanged
Monoamine oxidase[b]			
Oreland and Gottfries (1986)	Cortical, subcortical areas	Specific activity, autopsy	MAO-A, Unchanged; MAO-B, Increased
α_2 receptor			
Sastre and Garcia-Sevilla (1994); Supiano and Hogikyan (1993)	Cortex	^{3}H-Labeled clonidine, autopsy	Decreased
Pascual et al. (1992)	Cortex	^{3}H-Labeled bromoxidine, autopsy	Decreased
Kalaria and Andorn (1991)	Cortex	^{3}H-Labeled p-aminoclonidine, autopsy	Decreased
β receptors			
Arango et al. (1990);	Cortex	^{125}I-Labeled pindolol, autopsy	Unchanged
Kalaria et al. (1989)	Cortex	^{125}I-Labeled pindolol, autopsy	Decreased
G-protein coupling			
Insel (1993)	Animal cortex	Forskolin stimulation	Decreased
MHPG			
Hartikainen et al. (1991)	Cerebrospinal fluid	HPLC	Unchanged
Gottfries (1990)	Cerebrospinal fluid	HPLC	Increased

Note. HPLC = high performance liquid chromatography; MAO = monoamine oxidase; MHPG = methoxyhydroxyphenylglycol.
[a]Complete reference citations are at the end of the chapter. [b]Norepinephrine is preferentially metabolized by MAO-A.
Source. Adapted from Arango et al. 1990; Gottfries 1990; Hartikainen et al. 1991; Insel 1993; Kalaria et al. 1989; Mann 1991; McGeer 1981; Mendelsohn and Paxinos 1991; Oreland and Gottfries 1986; Pascual et al. 1992; Robinson et al. 1977; Sastre and Garcia-Sevilla 1994; Supiano and Hogikyan 1993.

blunted response to short-term treatments for these behavioral syndromes, delay the rate of recovery, and contribute to relapse as progression occurs.

Age-related changes in the central serotonergic system are presented in Table 33–9. These changes include reductions in the numbers of serotonergic nerve terminals in the neocortex, as reflected by the decreased density of the serotonin transporter. The specific activity of the biosynthetic enzyme tryptophan hydroxylase has also been reported to decline with advancing age. Age-related changes in central serotonergic receptors are complex as a result of differential effects reported for various characteristics of multiple receptor subtypes. Decreased densities of the serotonin transporter may reflect the age-related reduction in the number of serotonergic neurons. The level of 5-hydroxyindoleacetic acid, the major metabolite of serotonin, increases with age. The last finding may reflect a compensatory increase in the firing rates of surviving serotonergic neurons.

Cardiovascular Effects and Orthostatic Hypotension

The prevalence of orthostatic hypotension increases with age to become a common condition in late life, where it affects as many as 30% of community-dwelling elders (Patel et al. 1993). Its clinical importance is reflected by its link to syncope, recurrent falling, skeletal fractures, and related sources of morbidity and mortality.

The etiology of orthostatic hypotension among the elderly is typically multifactorial (Mets 1995; Verhaeverbeke and Mets 1997). Although age-related autonomic dysfunction plays an important role in the pathogenesis of orthostatic hypotension, this condition is often induced by the use of psychotropic or other medications in the elderly. Perhaps even more commonly, subclinical cases of orthostatic hypotension are rendered symptomatic by the administration of drugs that aggravate the underlying pathophysiology of this condition. This latter observation highlights the predictive value and clinical importance of pretreatment measurements of postural changes in blood pressure and heart rate before administering medications whose side-effect profiles include postural hypotension.

The pathophysiology of orthostatic hypotension is complex and incompletely understood (Abernathy 1990; Feely and Coakley 1990; Hämmerlein et al. 1998; Mets 1995; Verhaeverbeke and Mets 1997). Common factors that contribute to the development of orthostatic hypotension are listed in Table 33–10. As described in previous sections, aging is associated with functional decrements in several central aminergic systems that participate

in the regulation of blood pressure and other fundamental processes. In the periphery, aging is also associated with a decrease in the baroreceptor reflex response to reductions in blood pressure. Reductions that occur in arterial compliance (elasticity) with aging may contribute to the decreased sensitivity of the baroreceptor region to changes is blood pressure. Decreased compliance of the arterial wall may also render the systemic circulation more vulnerable to changes in blood pressure that result from small reductions in circulating blood volume. In addition to these effects, aging is associated with decreased responsiveness of the heart and vasculature to the chronotropic and inotropic effects of adrenergic stimulation, especially those medicated through β-adrenergic receptors. Finally, reduced activity of the renin-angiotensin-aldosterone system becomes manifest in the elderly. These physiological changes that occur during the course of normative aging contribute to the increased prevalence of orthostatic hypotension in the elderly and to their sensitivity to this common adverse effect of psychotropic and other medications.

Age-related diseases also predispose the elderly to orthostatic hypotension. Heart disease can lead to reduced cardiac output both at rest and in response to exercise or other stimuli. Diabetes mellitus often causes disturbances of fluid and electrolyte balance as well as impairments of the peripheral autonomic nervous system that produce or worsen orthostatic hypotension. Parkinson's disease can lead to peripheral manifestations of autonomic dysregulation, including orthostatic hypotension, that result from the degeneration of central aminergic systems (see Chapter 26 in this volume). Orthostatic hypotension is also commonly associated with dehydration, immobility, or prolonged bedrest, which accompany chronic, debilitating medical disorders in late life. Eating, urination, and defecation all transiently worsen orthostasis.

Not surprisingly, drugs used to lower blood pressure in the treatment of hypertension or congestive heart failure aggravate orthostatic hypotension. These agents include calcium channel blockers, α- and β-adrenergic blockers, angiotensin-converting enzyme inhibitors, and nitrates. In addition, many psychotropic drugs induce or worsen postural hypotension. Their hypotensive actions reflect their potency as α_1 antagonists and to a lesser extent their antimuscarinic potency. These effects can be magnified by age-related decreases in metabolism, clearance, and elimination if dosing is not adjusted accordingly.

Heterocyclic antidepressants typically produce some degree of orthostatic hypotension at the usual doses used to treat elderly patients with depression. The tertiary amines (amitriptyline and imipramine) are the worst, whereas nortriptyline produces less of this adverse effect. Tricyclic

TABLE 33–9. Age-related changes in the serotonergic system

Serotonergic markers[a]	Location	Techniques	Findings
5-HT transporter			
Marcussen et al. (1987)	Cortex	^{123}β-CIT SPECT	Decreased
Tryptophan hydroxylase			
Meek et al. (1977)	Selected brain areas	Specific activity, autopsy	Decreased
Monoamine oxidase[b]			
Oreland and Gottfries (1986)	Cortical, subcortical areas	Specific activity, autopsy	MAO-A, Unchanged; MAO-B, Increased
5-HT$_{1A}$ receptor			
Burnet et al. (1994)	Hippocampus	mRNA, RT-PCR, autopsy	Increased
Marcussen et al. (1984, 1987)	Striatum	^{3}H-Labeled IMI binding, autopsy	Unchanged
Middlemiss et al. (1986)	Frontal cortex	^{3}H-Labeled 8-OH-DPAT, autopsy	Decreased
5-HT$_{2A}$ receptor			
Baeken et al. (1998)	Cortex	^{123}I-5-I-R91150, SPECT	Decreased
Meltzer et al. (1998)	Cortex	^{18}F-Labeled altanserin, PET	Decreased
Wang et al. (1995); Sparks (1989)	Frontal, occipital	^{18}F-Labeled NMS PET	Decreased
Burnet et al. (1994)	Hippocampus	mRNA, RT-PCR, autopsy	Unchanged
5-HIAA			
Hartikainen et al. (1991)	Cerebrospinal fluid	HPLC	Unchanged
Bareggi et al. (1985)	Cerebrospinal fluid	HPLC	Increased

Note. β-CIT = β-carbomethoxy-3β-(4-iodophenyl) tropane; 5-HIAA = 5-hydroxyindoleacetic acid; 5-HT = hydroxytryptamine (serotonin); IMI = imipramine; 8-OH-DPAT = 8-hydroxy-2(di-*N*-propylamino) tetralin; MAO = monoamine oxidase; NMS = *N*-methylspiperone; PET = positron-emission tomography; RT-PCR = reverse transcriptase–polymerase chain reaction assay of mRNA levels; SPECT = single photon emission computed tomography.
[a]Complete reference citations are at the end of the chapter.
[b]Serotonin is preferentially metabolized by MAO-A.

Source. Adapted from Baeken et al. 1998; Bareggi et al. 1985; Burnet et al. 1994; Marcussen et al. 1984, 1987; Meek et al. 1977; Meltzer et al. 1998; Middlemiss et al. 1986; Oreland and Gottfries 1986; Sparks 1989; Wang et al. 1995.

TABLE 33–10. Common contributors to orthostatic hypotension in the elderly

Central homeostatic mechanisms (decreased)

Autonomic regulation (decreased baroreceptor response, decreased vascular compliance, decreased response to adrenergic stimuli)

Renin-angiotensin-aldosterone system (decreased response of juxtaglomerular cells)

Age-related diseases (e.g., heart disease, diabetes, Parkinson's disease)

Medications

  Antihypertensives/congestive heart failure (calcium channel blockers, α- and β-adrenergic blockers, angiotensin-converting enzyme inhibitors, nitrates)

  Psychotropic drugs

   Antidepressants (heterocyclic antidepressants, monoamine oxidase inhibitors)

   Antipsychotics (conventional antipsychotics, especially low potency phenothiazines)

   Lithium

   Anti-parkinsonism drugs (L-dopa, bromocriptine, selegiline, anticholinergics)

---

antidepressants also prolong cardiac conduction, another adverse effect that worsens with age, to a varying degree among individual patients and may preclude their use in predisposed patients. Although MAOIs may be better known for hypertensive crises that result from interactions with tyramine-containing foods, sympathomimetic drugs, and meperidine, treatment with MAOIs typically produces some degree of hypotension, especially among the elderly. This adverse effect is shared by selegiline, which is relatively selective for the B form of monoamine oxidase that is preferentially localized to the brain. By contrast, the SSRIs do not induce significant hypotension or prolongation of cardiac conduction, a feature that has contributed to their popularity in the treatment of depression in the elderly.

Orthostatic hypotension is also a common adverse effect of antipsychotic medications. The phenothiazines with the lowest antipsychotic potency possess the greatest α_1-antiadrenergic and antimuscarinic potency (e.g., chlorpromazine, thioridazine). These properties make them unsuitable for the treatment of most elderly patients. Higher potency neuroleptic agents such as haloperidol produce less hypotension and are better tolerated by elderly patients at modest doses (usually less than 4 mg/day). However, at higher doses, significant parkinsonian symptoms usually emerge. Newer atypical antipsychotic drugs that possess fewer hypotensive and extrapyramidal effects

are likely to play an increasingly important role in the pharmacotherapy of neuropsychiatric disorders in the elderly (see Chapters 14 and 34 in this volume).

Lithium can contribute to postural hypotension by inducing diuresis through direct effects on the kidney (diabetes insipidus). As already discussed, the degeneration of central aminergic systems that occurs in Parkinson's disease may be accompanied by manifestations of autonomic dysregulation in the periphery, including orthostatic hypotension (among others). Moreover, the common treatments for Parkinson's disease, that is, L-dopa ((+)-carbidopa), bromocriptine, selegiline, and anticholinergic agents, all share hypotension among their side-effect profiles.

Drug-Related Falls

Aging is an important risk factor for accidental falls (Cumming 1998). About one-third of community-dwelling individuals over 65 fall at least once each year and nearly 10% have recurrent falls (Tinetti et al. 1988). The incidence of falling increases progressively in this population after the age of 65, nearly doubling by age 90 (Campbell et al. 1989, 1990). Not surprisingly, the risk of accidental falls is greater among nursing home residents and hospitalized patients than community-dwelling individuals of similar age (Tinetti and Speechley 1989).

Hip fractures are among the most common consequences of falling, and the incidence of hip fractures also increases with age. Among women over age 80, the annual incidence of hip fractures is about 3% per year, nearly twice that for men (Cummings et al. 1985). This gender difference may reflect greater osteoporosis and lower bone density among women compared with that of men. Hip fractures are often important harbingers of functional decline. The majority of people who have hip fractures never return to their previous level of physical functioning. About a fifth of such individuals die within a year of the hip fracture and another fifth transition to a residential care setting (Cumming et al. 1996; Katelaris and Cumming 1996). Sequelae of hip fractures can also include myocardial infarctions, strokes, excessive bleeding in patients taking anticoagulants, and pneumonia during the recovery phase. Other fall-related fractures can involve the wrist, humerus, ankle, and other bony structures that contribute to disability but typically have less serious consequences than hip fractures (Ray et al. 1987).

Patients who take psychotropic medications, including antidepressants, benzodiazepines, and antipsychotic drugs, are at increased risk of falling and having hip fractures. The evidence implicating antidepressants is the most compelling. Antidepressant medications have been associated with falls and hip fractures among elderly individuals who reside in a variety of settings (community, nursing homes, and acute care and rehabilitation hospitals), and this association remains robust in studies that controlled for numerous potentially confounding variables (Lipsitz et al. 1991; Ray et al. 1987, 1991; Ruthazer and Lipsitz 1993). Interestingly, SSRIs have been reported in one study to be more strongly related to falls than were tricyclic antidepressants (Ruthazer and Lipsitz 1993). Although this result is somewhat surprising, it may result from impairments in balance produced by some SSRIs or may reflect the use of SSRIs in patients with greater medical comorbidity. Heterocyclic antidepressants have several pharmacological effects that probably contribute to accidentals falls. These effects include sedation, psychomotor retardation, postural hypotension, and anticholinergic properties that may cause blurred vision and cognitive impairment. The risk of falling appears to be the greatest during the first 90 days of antidepressant treatment (Ray et al. 1991), when initial dosages are being adjusted and before physiological adaptation to these adverse effects has fully occurred.

Although sedative/hypnotic/anxiolytic agents have been reported to increase the risk of falling, the most convincing evidence involves the use of benzodiazepines (Aisen et al. 1992; Cumming and Klineberg 1993; Cumming et al. 1991; Gales and Menard 1995; Lord et al. 1995; Luukinen et al. 1995; Ray et al 1987, 1989; Ryynanen et al. 1993; Sorock and Thimkin 1988; Yip and Cumming 1994). The level of increased risk of falling is related to the use of elevated dosages, long-acting agents, and the coadministration of more than one benzodiazapine. Patients taking excessive doses of benzodiazepines are at substantially greater risk of hip fracture regardless of the benzodiazepine prescribed (Herings et al. 1995). The increased risk of falling associated with benzodiazepine usage appears to result from sedation and related psychomotor retardation.

Antipsychotic drugs, chiefly phenothiazines, also increase the risk of falls (Mion et al. 1989; Prudham and Evans 1981; Ray et al. 1987; Sorock 1983; Yip and Cumming 1994). Most of this evidence has resulted from studies of patients in nursing homes and rehabilitation settings. Little evidence exists on the relative risk of falling associated with specific antipsychotic drugs. These agents may increase the risk of falling by producing sedation, orthostatic hypotension, extrapyramidal gait disturbances, and anticholinergic effects that impair cognition or vision. If so, the risk of falling would be expected to be lower among patients receiving modest doses of high-potency neuroleptics or atypical antipsychotic drugs that produce fewer of these adverse effects.

Evidence for the role of cardiovascular medications in contributing to falls is less conclusive than for psychotropic medications. This may be a result of the common practice of grouping various cardiovascular medications together into a single classification rather than analyzing their individual contributions. Some studies have reported an association of the use of antihypertensives with falls (Campbell et al. 1989; Lord et al. 1994; Wells et al. 1985), an effect that may be a result of symptomatic postural hypotension (Ensrud et al. 1992). However, thiazide diuretics have the potential to confer a protective effect against fractures through a positive effect on bone density (Jones et al. 1995; Middler et al. 1973). The use of digoxin, nitrates, and calcium channel blockers have also been reported to be associated with falls (Cumming et al. 1991; Gales and Menard 1995; Koski et al. 1996; Luukinen et al. 1995).

Several studies have reported that analgesics and nonsteroidal anti-inflammatory drugs (NSAIDs) are associated with an increased risk of falling (Cummings et al. 1991; Lipsitz et al. 1991; Myers et al. 1991). The extent to which potential confounding effects of arthritis contributed to these findings is uncertain. NSAIDs have also been reported to cause cognitive dysfunction (Hoppmann et al. 1991), but they also increase bone density and may confer some degree of protection against hip fractures (Bauer et al. 1996). Narcotic analgesics can increase the risk of fall-related hip fractures by producing sedation, cognitive impairment, and postural hypotension (Shorr et al. 1992).

Table 33–11 includes a variety of additional risk factors for falls that result from aging, age-related diseases, medications, or environmental conditions (Robbins et al. 1989; Thapa et al. 1995). Many of these risk factors are influenced by contributions from multiple sources. The elderly often take multiple medications, which increases the risk of adverse effects, including falls. Lower extremity weakness and pain may result from a variety of common medical conditions of the elderly including arthritis, heart failure, vascular insufficiency, and stroke, as well as decreased activity itself. Decrements in gait and balance occur with aging, medication exposure, and many of the same medical conditions that produce weakness of the lower extremities. Neurodegenerative conditions such as AD and Parkinson's disease may likewise contribute to disturbances of gait and balance. Symptomatic postural hypotension is also an important risk factor for falls, and its evolution is addressed in the previous section. Cognitive impairment and depression contribute to the risk of falling through multiple mechanisms. Cognitive impairment often involves impairments of memory, planning, visuospatial function, judgment, and praxis and the development of extrapyramidal symptoms, all of which predispose to falling. Depression slows cognitive and motor skills; antidepressant medications further increase the risk of falling. Impairments in vision and hearing occur with normal aging and can be exacerbated by conditions such as cataract formation, glaucoma, macular degeneration, and diabetes, as well as medications with anticholinergic properties. Also, proprioceptive and other sensory deficits can arise from B_{12} deficiency and diabetes (peripheral neuropathy). The development of functional impairment is usually related to the multiple risk factors and conditions listed in Table 33–11. Finally, environmental hazards such as stairs and poor lighting increase the risk of falling among the elderly. Assessments of such environmental hazards often identify risks that are readily eliminated.

Therapeutic Compliance

Ensuring patient adherence to a prescribed treatment plan (medication compliance) is a complex longitudinal task that is influenced by many factors (Table 33–12). Estimates of the extent of medication noncompliance among the elderly have ranged from 40% to 75% (Cooper et al. 1982; Jackson et al. 1989; Lamy et al. 1992; Ostrum et al. 1988). Inappropriate discontinuation of prescribed medications may occur in as many as 40% of older adults, usually within the first year of treatment (Cooper et al. 1982; Jackson et al. 1989; Lamy et al. 1992; Ostrum et al. 1988).

Effective ongoing communication is essential for the

TABLE 33–11. Reported risk factors for accidental falls among the elderly

Psychotropic medication (heterocyclic antidepressants, selective serotonin reuptake inhibitors, benzodiazepines, antipsychotic drugs)

Cardiovascular drugs (antihypertensives, calcium channel blockers, nitrates, digoxin)

Analgesics and nonsteroidal anti-inflammatory drugs

Polypharmacy

Lower extremity weakness or pain

Gait and balance impairment

Postural hypotension

Cognitive impairment or depression

Perceptual deficits

Functional impairment

Specific medical conditions and overall burden of medical problems (arthritis, heart disease, incontinence, neurological disorders)

Environmental hazards

TABLE 33–12. Factors that influence medication compliance in the elderly

Doctor-patient relationship and patient education

Ethnic and cultural background

Complexity of regimen (numbers of medications and daily doses)

Isolation and cognitive impairment

Disturbances of mood, thought, and behavior

Perceived benefit

Medical comorbidity

Adverse effects

Cost

Follow-up

development of a successful doctor-patient relationship. For older individuals who live independently, this dyadic relationship does not differ significantly from that developed between younger adults and their physicians. However, much of the practice of geriatric neuropsychiatry requires broadening the conceptualization of the doctor-patient relationship to include a spouse or other family member who serves as the primary caregiver, as well as the patient's primary care physician. For patients in residential care settings, this collaboration best includes a clinician from the facility. Although the geriatric psychiatrist must remain mindful of confidentiality issues, the short-term and sustained effectiveness of neuropsychiatric interventions is dependent on the successfulness of these collaborators in implementing a consensual treatment plan.

Guided by the diagnostic assessment, a clearly articulated treatment plan, including what medications are being prescribed for specific indications, the dosing regimen, and a review of potential side effects, must be discussed with the patient and relevant caregivers. In general, in-person or verbal communications are superior to written materials alone in encouraging compliance. Sensitivity to ethnic and cultural diversity also enhances compliance. Formulation of the medication regimen should include attention to the age-related pharmacokinetic and pharmacodynamic principles described in this chapter including complications that might arise from the use of over-the-counter medications. Because increasing numbers of medications and daily doses of medications discourage compliance (Col et al. 1990; Lamy 1986; Lamy et al. 1992), efforts should be directed at arriving at the simplest regimen possible without sacrificing effectiveness. Issues of cost are also important for elderly patients who are often supported by fixed incomes.

These efforts should also include a follow-up plan for

assessing treatment response and monitoring for the potential development of adverse effects. Office calls by the patient or his or her caregivers to clarify questions or to address newly emergent adverse effects should be encouraged, especially at times of medication changes or dosage adjustments. This approach reduces anxiety in the patient and other caregivers, reduces adverse outcomes, provides an opportunity to respond to emergent adverse reactions at the earliest time, builds trust in the doctor-patient-family relationship, and enhances both compliance and positive outcomes.

Elders who live independently and lack a network of family or social supports are at increased risk of missed dosages and irregular dosing schedules. Unfortunately, this results in decreased therapeutic efficacy and can lead to increased side effects. Incorrect guesses about the source of particular side effects that are made without consultation with the physician can result in alterations in the dose or schedule of the wrong drug. When memory or other cognitive impairment is among the side effects that develop, compliance is further compromised. As a result, this pattern of partial compliance often progresses to complete discontinuation of medications. Discontinuation can include medications used to treat general medical conditions along with psychotherapeutic agents, a circumstance that can further compromise the health of the patient. Abrupt discontinuation can also precipitate toxic withdrawal states, including delirium.

For patients with cognitive impairment or who have disturbances of mood, thought, or behavior, the importance of family or other caregivers in encouraging treatment compliance is essential. Memory and other impairments of cognition can lead to underdosing and subtherapeutic responses, as well as overdosing and toxicity. Major depression is often associated with excessive guilt or therapeutic nihilism that undermines compliance, as well as increased somatic complaints that are often difficult to distinguish from drug-induced adverse effects. In contrast, mania and elated mood may preclude accurate self-perception and the need for treatment altogether. Paranoid delusions that frequently accompany mood and neurodegenerative disorders often lead to medication refusal, at least intermittently. The participation and encouragement from family members or other trusted caregivers who support the treatment plan is indispensable in these circumstances.

The burden of comorbid medical problems also threatens compliance. Greater numbers of medical problems complicate and can limit the effectiveness of psychotherapeutic drugs, lead to the need for more prescribed medications, and increase the risk of adverse ef-

fects. All of these factors highlight the importance of optimizing the patient's complete medication regimen in consultation with his or her primary care physician. This should include an ongoing dialogue between the psychiatrist and primary care physician as the health care needs of the patient evolve with time.

Conclusion

Neuropsychiatric syndromes are common disorders among the elderly that produce suffering, functional disability, and loss of independence and hasten death. This burden is born not only by older individuals who have these syndromes, but also by the families who care for them and the substantial health care resources that are consumed in the process. Pharmacotherapy can play an important role in ameliorating these maladies along with the increases in morbidity and mortality that they cause.

In this chapter, we illustrate various mechanisms that contribute to the increased variance and decreased predictability in the responses of older adults to medications, with a focus on psychotherapeutic drugs. These mechanisms are numerous, complex, interactive, and drug-specific. Moreover, the picture is incomplete. Much remains to be learned about the age-related metabolism, clearance, and excretion of these agents and metabolites, as well as their accessibility to their presumed sites of action in the brain. Even less systematic information is available about the organismal, systemic, cellular, subcellular, and molecular mechanisms that contribute to age-related alterations in tissue sensitivity to the pharmacological actions of psychotropic drugs. Although the increased sensitivity of the elderly to the adverse effect of psychotherapeutic drugs is well-established, little evidence exists to demonstrate that aging is accompanied by a similar increase in the therapeutic potency of these agents. This last observation can result in a reduced margin of safety.

The difficulty in carrying out experiments designed to elucidate these areas of human biology has been limiting. Animal paradigms have not always accurately modeled their human counterparts, and the results of human in vitro and in vivo studies have not always been easily reconcilable. Furthermore, adults over 65 have been underrepresented in clinical studies. Clinical and preclinical data on elderly individuals over 75, the most rapidly growing segment of the United States population, are especially lacking.

The recommendation to "start low and go slow" remains sound practical advice, while monitoring therapeutic response and potential adverse effects in collaboration with the patient and other caregivers. Newly emergent signs and symptoms that correspond temporally to the initiation of medications or changes in dosage are often medication related, even if they seem to be outside of the usual spectrum of side effects for the particular drugs being manipulated. They may indeed represent unusual side effects or they may represent more common adverse effects of coadministered medications whose previously stable plasma levels were altered as the result of a drug interaction.

To this appropriate recommendation of caution, one might add the virtues of patience and persistence. Once initiated, the physician should be patient and resist the urge to rapidly increase low starting doses of medications in the elderly. Unlike most medications used in general medical practice whose peak actions occur in hours or a few days, the peak therapeutic effects of most psychotropic drugs typically occur over weeks to months. This interval is longer for the elderly than for younger adults. Overly rapid advancement of dosages, in response to unrealistic expectations that this will hasten therapeutic response, often results in excessive drug levels in plasma and tissue, with associated toxicity.

The consequences of aging and age-related factors, including medical comorbidity, can blunt therapeutic responses and restrict the spectrum of psychotherapeutic agents that are appropriate for use in particular elderly patients. Persistence in the pursuit of therapeutic response and willingness to try alternative pharmacological strategies is often rewarded by remarkable clinical responses that surprise even family members. The continual development of novel efficacious psychotherapeutic medications with increasingly benign side-effect profiles will also contribute to the successful treatment of neuropsychiatric disorders in the elderly.

Finally, the achievement of an optimal acute therapeutic response of neuropsychiatric disorders as well as the maintenance of this response over time may require different pharmacological agents or combinations of agents, different treatment modalities (e.g., medications, electroconvulsive therapy, psychotherapy), and combinations of these modalities over the remaining life-span of older adults. These issues are the appropriate subject of future controlled studies of efficacy as well as intervention studies that evaluate their effectiveness in nonpsychiatric specialty and primary care settings.

■ References

Abernathy DR: Altered pharmacodynamics of cardiovascular drugs and their relation to altered pharmacokinetics in elderly patients. Clinical Pharmacology, Clinics in Geriatric Medicine 6:285–292, 1990

Abernathy DR, Kerzner L: Age effects on alpha-1-acid glycoprotein concentration and imipramine plasma protein binding. J Am Geriatr Soc 32:705–708, 1984

Adir J, Miller AK, Vestal RE: Effects of total plasma concentration and age on tolbutamide plasma protein binding. Clin Pharmacol Ther 31:488–493, 1982

Aisen PS, Deluca T, Lawlor BA: Falls among geropsychiatry inpatients are associated with PRN medications for agitation. Int J Geriatr Psychiatry 7:709–712, 1992

Allen SJ, Benton JS, Goodhardt MJ, et al: Biochemical evidence of selective nerve cell changes in the normal aging human and rat brain. J Neurochem 41:256–265, 1983

Altman DF: Changes in gastrointestinal, pancreatic, biliary, and hepatic function with aging. Gastrointestinal Disorders in the Elderly, Gastroenterology Clinics of North America 19(2):227–234, 1990

Amitai Y, Kennedy EJ, DeSandre P, et al: Distribution of amitriptyline and nortriptyline in blood: role of α-1-glycoprotein. Ther Drug Monit 15:267–273, 1993

Annesley TM: Special considerations for geriatric therapeutic drug monitoring. Clinical Chemistry 35(7):1337–1341, 1989

Araujo DM, Lapchak PA, Robitaille Y, et al: Differential alteration of various cholinergic markers in cortical and subcortical regions of human brain in Alzheimer's disease. J Neurochem 50:1914–1923, 1988

Arendt T, Bigl V, Arendt A, et al: Loss of neurons in the nucleus basalis of Meynert in Alzheimer's disease, paralysis agitans, and Korsakoff's disease. Acta Neuropathol (Berl) 61:101–108, 1983

Bachman DL, Wolf PA, Linn R, et al: Prevalence of dementia and probable senile dementia of the Alzheimer type in the Framingham Study. Neurology 42:115–119, 1992

Balter MB, Levine J, Manheimer D: Cross-national study of the extent of anti-anxiety sedative drug use. N Engl J Med 290:766–774, 1974

Bareggi SR, Franceschi M, Smirne S: Neurochemical findings in cerebrospinal fluid in Alzheimer's disease, in Normal Aging, Alzheimer's Disease, and Senile Dementia: Aspects on Etiology, Pathogenesis, Diagnosis, and Treatment. Edited by Gottfries CG. Brussels, Editions de l'Université de Bruxelles, 1985, pp 203–212

Bauer DC, Orwoll ES, Fox KM, et al: Aspirin and NSAID use in older women: effect on bone mineral density and fracture risk. J Bone Miner Res 111:29–35, 1996

Baum C, Kennedy DL, Knapp DE, et al: Drug utilization in the U.S.: 1985, Seventh Annual Review. Rockville, MD, Food and Drug Administration, Center for Drugs and Biologics, 1986, pp 1–411

Baum C, Kennedy DL, Knapp DE, et al: Prescription drug use in 1984 and changes over time. Med Care 26:105–114, 1988

Bertz RJ, Kroboth PD, Kroboth FJ, et al: Alprazolam in young and elderly men: sensitivity and tolerance to psychomotor, sedative and memory effects. J Pharmacol Exp Ther 281(3):1317–1329, 1997

Bird TD, Stranahan S, Sumi SM, et al: Alzheimer's disease: choline acetyltransferase activity in brain tissue from clinical and pathological subgroups. Ann Neurol 14:284–293, 1983

Borkan GA, Hults DE, Gerzof SG, et al: Age changes in body composition revealed by computed tomography. J Gerontol 38:673–677, 1983

Boston Collaborative Drug Surveillance Program: Clinical depression of the central nervous system due to diazepam and chlordiazepoxide in relation to cigarette smoking and age. N Engl J Med 288:277–280, 1973

Bowen DM, Allen SJ, Benton JS, et al: Biochemical assessment of serotonergic and cholinergic dysfunction and cerebral atrophy in Alzheimer's disease. J Neurochem 41:266–272, 1983

Campbell AJ, Borrie MJ, Spears GF: Risk factors for falls in a community-based prospective study of people 70 years and older. J Gerontol 44:M112–M117, 1989

Campbell AJ, Borrie MJ, Spears GF, et al: Circumstances and consequences of falls experienced by a community population 70 years and over during a prospective study. Age Ageing 19:136–141, 1990

Castleden CM, George CF, Marcer D, et al: Increased sensitivity to nitrazepam in old age. BMJ 1:10–12, 1977

Chrischilles EA, Foley DJ, Wallace RB, et al: Use of medications by persons 65 and over: data from the established populations for epidemiologic studies of the elderly. J Gerontol A Biol Sci Med Sci 47(5):137–144, 1992

Cohen BM, Renshaw PF, Stoll AL, et al: Decreased brain choline uptake in older adults. JAMA 274:903–907, 1995

Col N, Fanale JE, Kronholm P: The role of medication non-compliance and adverse drug reactions in hospitalizations of the elderly. Arch Intern Med 150:841–845, 1990

Cook PJ, Flanagan R, James IM: Diazepam tolerance: effect of age, regular sedation, and alcohol. BMJ 289:351–353, 1984

Cooper JK, Love DW, Raffoul PR: Intentional prescription nonadherence (noncompliance) by the elderly. J Am Geriatr Soc 30:329–333, 1982

Cumming RG: Epidemiology of medication-related falls and fractures in the elderly. Epidemiology, Drugs and Aging 12(1):43–53, 1998

Cumming RG, Klineberg RJ: Psychotropics, thiazide diuretics and hip fractures in the elderly. Med J Aust 158:414–417, 1993

Cumming RG, Miller JP, Kelsey JL, et al: Medications and multiple falls in elderly people: the St. Louis OASIS study. Age Ageing 20:455–461, 1991

Cumming RG, Klineberg R, Katelaris A: Cohort study of institutionalization after hip fracture. Aust N Z J Public Health 20:579–582, 1996

Cummings SR, Kelsey JL, Nevitt MC, et al: Epidemiology of osteoporosis and osteoporotic fractures. Epidemiol Rev 7:178–208, 1985

Davies P, Maloney AJF: Selective loss of central cholinergic neurons in Alzheimer's disease (letter). Lancet 2:1403, 1976

Drachman DA, Leavitt J: Human memory and the cholinergic system. Arch Neurol 30:113–121, 1974

Ensrud KE, Nevitt MC, Yunis C, et al: Postural hypotension and postural dizziness in elderly women. Arch Intern Med 152:1058–1064, 1992

Evans DA, Funkenstein HH, Albert MS, et al: Prevalence of Alzheimer's disease in a community population of older persons: higher than previously reported. JAMA 262:2551–2556, 1989

Feely J, Coakley D: Altered pharmacodynamics in the elderly. Clinical Pharmacology, Clinics in Geriatric Medicine 6(2):269–283, 1990

Flynn DD, Mash DC: Characterization of L-[³H]nicotine binding in human cerebral cortex: comparison between Alzheimer's disease and normal. J Neurochem 47:1948–1954, 1986

Flynn DD, Weinstein DA, Mash DC: Loss of high-affinity agonist binding to M_1 muscarinic receptors in Alzheimer's disease: implications for the failure of cholinergic replacement therapies. Ann Neurol 29:256–262, 1991

Forbes GB, Reina JC: Adult lean body mass declines with age: some longitudinal observations. Metabolism 19:653–663, 1970

Förstl H, Burns A, Luthert P, et al: The Lewy-body variant of Alzheimer's disease: clinical and pathological findings. Br J Psychiatry 162:385–392, 1993

Gales BJ, Menard SM: Relationship between the administration of selected medications and falls in hospitalized elderly patients. Ann Pharmacother 29:354–358, 1995

Giles HG, MacLeod SM, Wright JR, et al: Influence of age and previous use on diazepam dosage required for endoscopy. Canadian Medical Association Journal 118:513–514, 1978

Greenamyre JT, Maragos WF: Neurotransmitter receptors in Alzheimer disease. Cerebrovascular and Brain Metabolism Reviews 5:61–94, 1993

Greenblatt DJ: Reduced albumin concentration in the elderly: a report from the Boston Collaborative Surveillance Program. J Am Geriatr Soc 27:20–22, 1979

Greenblatt DJ, Harmatz JS, Shader RI: Clinical pharmacokinetics of anxiolytics and hypnotics in the elderly: therapeutic considerations. Clin Pharmacokinet 21(4):165–177, 262–273, 1991

Hämmerlein A, Derendorf H, Lowenthal DT: Pharmacokinetic and pharmacodynamic changes in the elderly: clinical implications. Clin Pharmacokinet 35(1):49–64, 1998

Hansen L, Salmon D, Galasko D, et al: The Lewy body variant of Alzheimer's disease: a clinical and pathologic entity. Neurology 40:1–8, 1990

Hare TA, Wood JH, Manyam BV, et al: Central nervous system gamma-aminobutyric acid activity in man: relationship to age and sex as reflected in CSF. Arch Neurol 39:247–249, 1982

Helling DR, Lemke JH, Semla TP, et al: Medication use characteristics in the elderly: the Iowa 65+ Rural Health Study. J Am Geriatr Soc 35:4–12, 1987

Herings RMC, Stricker BH, deBoer A, et al: Benzodiazepines and the risk of falling leading to femur fractures: dosages more important than elimination half-life. Arch Intern Med 155:1801–1807, 1995

Holt PR, Balint JA: Effects of aging on intestinal lipid absorption. Am J Physiol 264 (Gastrointestinal and Liver Physiology 27):G1–G6, 1993

Hoppmann RA, Peden JG, Ober SK: Central nervous system side effects of nonsteroidal anti-inflammatory drugs. Arch Intern Med 151:1309–1313, 1991

Hunt CM, Westerkam WP, Stave GM, et al: Hepatic cytochrome P-4503A (CYP3A) activity in the elderly. Mech Ageing Dev 64:189–199, 1992

International Classification of Diseases, 9th Revision, Clinical Modification, 4th Revision. Los Angeles, CA, Practice Management Information Corporation, 1993

Jackson JE, Ramsdell JW, Renvall M, et al: Reliability of drug histories in a specialized geriatric outpatients clinic. J Gen Intern Med 4(1):39–43, 1989

Jones G, Nguyen T, Sambrook PN, et al: Thiazide diuretics and fractures: can meta-analysis help? J Bone Miner Res 10:106–111, 1995

Jorm AF, Korten AE, Henderson AS: The prevalence of dementia: a quantitative integration of the literature. Acta Psychiatr Scand 76:465–479, 1987

Jost WH: Gastrointestinal motility problems in patients with Parkinson's disease: effects of antiparkinsonian treatment and guidelines for management. Disease Management, Drugs and Aging 10(4):249–258, 1997

Kalaria RN: Cerebral vessels in ageing and Alzheimer's disease. Pharmacol Ther 72(3):193–214, 1996

Kalish SC, Bohn RL, Mogun H, et al: Antipsychotic prescribing patterns and the treatment of extrapyramidal symptoms in older people. J Am Geriatr Soc 43:969–973, 1995

Katelaris AG, Cumming RG: Health status before and mortality after hip fracture. Am J Public Health 86:557–560, 1996

Katz IR, Simpson GM, Curlik SM, et al: Pharmacologic treatment of major depression for elderly patients in residential care settings. J Clin Psychiatry 51:41–47, 1990

Kleine TO, Hackler R: Age-related changes in the blood-brain barrier of humans. Neurobiol Aging 15(6):763–764, 1994

Koski K, Luukinen H, Laippala P, et al: Physiological factors and medications as predictors of injurious falls by elderly people: a prospective population-based study. Age Ageing 25:29–38, 1996

Kroboth PD, McAuley JW, Smith RB: Alprazolam in the elderly: pharmacokinetics and pharmacodynamics during multiple dosing. Psychopharmacology (Berl) 100:477–484, 1990

Lamy PP: Prescribing for the Elderly. Litteton, MA, PSG 1980

Lamy PP: Compliance in long-term care. Geriatric Medicine Today 5(9):61–75, 1986

Lamy PP, Salzman C, Nevis-Olesen J: Drug prescribing patterns, risks, and compliance guidelines, in Clinical Geriatric Psychopharmacology, 2nd Edition. Edited by Salzman C. Baltimore, MD, Williams & Wilkins, 1992, pp 15–37

Langlais PJ, Thal L, Hansen L, et al: Neurotransmitters in basal ganglia and cortex of Alzheimer's disease with and without Lewy bodies. Neurology 43:1927–1934, 1993

Le Couteur DG, McLean AJ: The aging liver: drug clearance and an oxygen diffusion barrier hypothesis. Clin Pharmacokinet 34(5):359–373, 1998

Lippa CF, Smith TW, Swearer JM: Alzheimer's disease and Lewy body disease: a comparative clinicopathological study. Ann Neurol 35:81–88, 1994

Lipsitz LA, Jonsson PV, Kelley MM, et al: Causes and correlates of recurrent falls in ambulatory frail elderly. J Gerontol 46:M114–M122, 1991

Loi CM, Vestal RE: Drug metabolism in the elderly. Pharmacol Ther 36:131–149, 1988

Lord SR, Sambrook PN, Gilbert C, et al: Postural stability, falls and fractures in the elderly: results from the Dubbo Osteoporosis Epidemiology Study. Med J Aust 160:684–691, 1994

Lord SR, Anstey KJ, Williams P, et al: Psychoactive medication use, sensory-motor function and falls in older women. Br J Clin Pharmacol 39:227–234, 1995

Luukinen H, Koski K, Laippala P, et al: Predictors of recurrent falls among the home-dwelling elderly. Scand J Prim Health Care 13:294–299, 1995

McGeer EG: Neurotransmitter system in aging and senile dementia. Progress in Neuro-psychopharmacology 5:435–445, 1981

Mets TF: Drug-induced orthostatic hypotension in older patients. Drugs Aging 6(3):219–228, 1995

Middler S, Pak CY, Murad F, et al: Thiazide diuretics and calcium metabolism. Metabolism 22:139–146, 1973

Mion LC, Gregor S, Buettner M, et al: Falls in the rehabilitation setting: incidence and characteristics. Rehabilitation Nursing 14:17–22, 1989

Molchan SE, Martinez RA, Hill JL, et al: Increased cognitive sensitivity to scopolamine with age and a perspective on the scopolamine model. Brain Res Rev 17:215–226, 1992

Myers AH, Baker SP, Van Natta ML, et al: Risk factors associated with falls and injuries among elderly institutionalized persons. Am J Epidemiol 133:1179–1190, 1991

Nikaido AM, Ellinwood EH, Heatherly DG, et al: Age-related increase in CNS sensitivity to benzodiazepines as assessed by task difficulty. Psychopharmacology (Berl) 100:90–97, 1990

Novak LP: Aging, total body potassium, fat-free mass, and cell mass in males and females between ages 18 and 95 years. J Gerontol 27:438–443, 1972

Ostrum FE, Hammarlund ER, Christensen DB, et al: Medication usage in an elderly population (1985). Med Care 23:157–170, 1988

Patel A, Maloney A, Damato AN: On the frequency and reproducibility of orthostatic blood pressure changes in healthy community-dwelling elderly during 60-degree head-up tilt. Am Heart J 126:184–188, 1993

Pearson MW, Roberts CJC: Drug induction of hepatic enzymes in the elderly. Age Ageing 13:313, 1984

Perry EK, Perry RH, Smith CJ, et al: Nicotinic receptor abnormalities in Alzheimer's and Parkinson's diseases. J Neurol Neurosurg Psychiatry 50:806–809, 1987

Perry EK, Marshall E, Perry RH, et al: Cholinergic and dopaminergic activities in senile dementia of Lewy body type. Alzheimer Dis Assoc Disord 4:87–95, 1990

Perry EK, McKeith I, Thompson P, et al: Topography, extent, and clinical relevance of neurochemical deficits in dementia of Lewy body type, Parkinson's disease, and Alzheimer's disease. Ann N Y Acad Sci 640:197–202, 1991

Perry EK, Irving D, Kerwin JM, et al: Cholinergic transmitter and neurotrophic activities in Lewy body dementia: similarity to Parkinson's and distinction from Alzheimer disease. Alzheimer Dis Assoc Disord 7:69–79, 1993

Pilotto A, Franceschi M, Del Favero G, et al: The effect of aging on oro-cecal transit time in normal subjects and patients with gallstone disease. Aging Clinical Experimental Research 7(4):234–237, 1995

Pollock BG, Perel JM, Altieri LP, et al: Debrisoquine hydroxylation phenotyping in geriatric psychopharmacology. Psychopharmacol Bull 28(2):163–168, 1992

Pomara N, Stanley B, Block R, et al: Adverse effects of single therapeutic doses of diazepam on performance in normal geriatric subjects: relationship to plasma concentrations. Psychopharmacology (Berl) 84:342–346, 1984

Pomara N, Stanley B, Block R, et al: Increased sensitivity of the elderly to the central depressant effects of diazepam. J Clin Psychiatry 46:185–187, 1985

Pope A, Hess HH, Lewin E: Microchemical pathology of the cerebral cortex in pre-senile dementias. Transactions of the American Neurological Association 89:15–16, 1964

Popkin MK, Callies AL, Mackenzie TB: The outcome of antidepressant use in the medically ill. Arch Gen Psychiatry 42:1160–1163, 1985

Prudham D, Evans JG: Factors associated with falls in the elderly: a community study. Age Ageing 10:141–146, 1981

Ray WA, Griffin MR, Schaffner W, et al: Psychotropic drug use and the risk of hip fracture. N Engl J Med 316:363–369, 1987

Ray WA, Griffin MR, Downey W: Benzodiazepines of long and short elimination half-life and the risk of hip fracture. JAMA 262:3303–3307, 1989

Ray WA, Griffin MR, Malcolm E: Cyclic antidepressants and the risk of hip fracture. Arch Intern Med 151:754–756, 1991

Reidenberg MM, Levy M, Warner H, et al: Relationship between diazepam dose, plasma level, age and central nervous system depression. Clin Pharmacol Ther 23:371–374, 1978

Ribeiro AC, Klingler PJ, Hinder RA, et al: Esophageal manometry: a comparison of findings in younger and older patients. Am J Gastroenterology 93(5):706–710, 1998

Rinne JO, Myllykylä P: A postmortem study of brain nicotinic receptors in Parkinson's and Alzheimer's disease. Brain Res 547:167–170, 1991

Robbins AS, Rubenstein LZ, Josephson KR, et al: Predictors of falls among elderly people: results of two population-based studies. Arch Intern Med 149:1628–1633, 1989

Rossor MN, Garrett NJ, Johnson AL, et al: A post-mortem study of the cholinergic and GABA systems in senile dementia. Brain 105:313–330, 1982

Russell RM: Changes in gastrointestinal function attributed to aging. Am J Clin Nutr 55:1203S–1207S, 1992

Ruthazer R, Lipsitz LA: Antidepressants and falls among elderly people in long-term care. Am J Public Health 83:746–749, 1993

Ryynanen OP, Kivela SL, Honkanen R, et al: Medications and chronic diseases as risk factors for falling injuries in the elderly. Scand J Soc Med 21:264–271, 1993

Saper CB, German DC, White CL: Neuronal pathology in the nucleus basalis and associated cell groups in senile dementia of the Alzheimer's type: possible role in cell loss. Neurology 35:1089–1095, 1985

Satlin A, Liptzin B: Diagnosis and treatment of mania, in Clinical Geriatric Psychopharmacology, Third Edition. Edited by Salzman C. Baltimore, MD, Williams & Wilkins, 1998, pp 310–330

Schmucker DL: Age related changes in drug disposition. Pharmacol Rev 30:445–456, 1979

Schmucker DL: Aging and drug disposition: an update. Pharmacol Rev 37(2):133–148, 1985

Schmucker DL, Woodhouse KW, Wang RK, et al: Effects of age and gender on in vitro properties of human liver microsomal monooxygenases. Clin Pharmacol Ther 48:365–374, 1990

Shah GN, Mooradian AD: Age-related changes in the blood-brain barrier. Exp Gerontol 32(4/5):501–519, 1997

Shimohama S, Taniguchi T, Fujiwara M, et al: Changes in nicotinic and muscarinic cholinergic receptors in Alzheimer-type dementia. J Neurochem 46:288–293, 1986

Shorr RI, Griffin MR, Daugherty JR, et al: Opioid analgesics and the risk of hip fracture in the elderly: codeine and propoxyphenic. J Gerontol 47:M111–M115, 1992

Sims NR, Bowen DM, Allen SJ, et al: Presynaptic cholinergic dysfunction in patients with dementia. J Neurochem 40:503–509, 1983

Skoog I, Wallin A, Fredman P, et al: A population study on blood-brain barrier function in 85-year-olds: relation to Alzheimer's disease and vascular dementia. Neurology 50: 966–971, 1998

Smith CJ, Perry EK, Perry RH, et al: Guanine nucleotide modulation of muscarinic receptor binding in postmortem human brain—a preliminary study in Alzheimer's disease. Neurosci Lett 82:227–232, 1987

Sonies BC: Oropharyngeal dysphagia in the elderly. Clin Geriatr Med 8(3):569–577, 1992

Sorock GS: A case-control study of falling incidents among the hospitalized elderly. Journal of Safety Research 14:47–52, 1983

Sorock GS, Thimkin EE: Benzodiazepine sedatives and the risk of falling in a community dwelling elderly cohort. Arch Intern Med 148:2441–2444, 1988

Sunderland T, Esposito G, Molchan SE, et al: Differential cholinergic regulation in Alzheimer's patients compared to controls following chronic blockade with scopolamine: a SPECT study. Psychopharmacology (Berl) 121:231–241, 1995

Sweet RA, Mulsant BH, Gupta B, et al: Duration of neuroleptic treatment and prevalence of tardive dyskinesia in late life. Arch Gen Psychiatry 52:478–486, 1995

Swift CG, Ewen JM, Clarke P, et al: Responsiveness to oral diazepam in the elderly: relationship to total and free plasma concentrations. Br J Clin Pharmacol 20:111–118, 1985

Thapa PB, Gideon P, Fought RL, et al: Psychotropic drugs and risk of recurrent falls in ambulatory nursing home residents. Am J Epidemiol 142(2):202–211, 1995

Thompson TL, Moran MG, Nies AS: Psychotropic drug use in the elderly. N Engl J Med 308:134–138, 193–199, 1983

Tinetti ME, Speechley M: Prevention of falls among the elderly. N Engl J Med 320:1055–1059, 1989

Tinetti ME, Speechley M, Ginter SF: Risk factors for falls among elderly persons living in the community. N Engl J Med 319:1701–1707, 1988

Trey G, Marks IN, Louw JA, et al: Changes in acid secretion over the years: a 30-year longitudinal study. J Clin Gastroenterol 25(3):499–502, 1997

Tune L, Carr S, Hoag E, et al: Anticholinergic effects of drugs commonly prescribed for the elderly: potential means for assessing risk of delirium. Am J Psychiatry 149(10): 1393–1394, 1992

Verhaeverbeke I, Mets T: Drug-induced orthostatic hypotension in the elderly: avoiding its onset. Pharmacoepidemiology, Drug Safety (2):105–118, 1997

Vestal RE: Aging and determinants of hepatic drug clearance. Hepatology 9:331–334, 1989

von Moltke LL, Abernathy DR, Greenblatt DJ: Kinetics and dynamics of psychotropic drugs in the elderly, in Clinical Geriatric Psychopharmacology, Third Edition. Edited by Salzman C. Baltimore, MD, Williams & Wilkins, 1998, pp 70–93

Wells BG, Middleton B, Lawrence G, et al: Factors associated with the elderly falling in intermediate care facilities. Drug Intelligence and Clinical Pharmacy 19:142–145, 1985

Whitehouse PJ, Price DL, Struble RG, et al: Alzheimer's disease and senile dementia: loss of neurons in the basal forebrain. Science 215:1237–1239, 1982

Whitehouse PJ, Martino AM, Antuono PG, et al: Nicotinic acetylcholine binding sites in Alzheimer's disease. Brain Res 371:146–151, 1986

Woodhouse KW, James OFW: Hepatic drug metabolism and ageing. Br Med Bull 46(1):22–35, 1990

Yip YB, Cumming RG: The association between medications and falls in Australian nursing-home residents. Med J Aust 160:15–18, 1994

Yuen GJ: Altered pharmacokinetics in the elderly. Clinical Pharmacology, Clinics in Geriatric Medicine 6(2): 257–267, 1990

Zubenko GS: Clinicopathological and neurochemical correlates of major depression and psychosis in primary dementia. Int Psychogeriatr 98:219–223, 1996

Zubenko GS: Molecular neurobiology of Alzheimer's disease (syndrome?). Harv Rev Psychiatry 5:177–213, 1997

Zubenko GS, Moossy J: Major depression in primary dementia: clinical and neuropathologic correlates. Arch Neurol 45: 1182–1186, 1988

Zubenko GS, Moossy J, Kopp U: Neurochemical correlates of major depression in primary dementia. Arch Neurol 47:209–214, 1990

Zubenko GS, Moossy J, Martinez AJ, et al: Neuropathological and neurochemical correlates of psychosis in primary dementia. Arch Neurol 48:619–624, 1991

Zubenko GS, Mulsant BH, Rifai AH, et al: Impact of acute psychiatric hospitalization on major depression in late life and prediction of response. Am J Psychiatry 51:987–994, 1994

Zubenko GS, Marino LJ, Sweet RA: Medical comorbidity in elderly psychiatric inpatients. Biol Psychiatry 41:724–736, 1997

■ References for Tables 33–2 through 33–4

Gelenberg AJ: The P450 family. Biological Therapies in Psychiatry Newsletter 18(8):29–31, 1995

Intek Labs: Reference Guide to Substrates, Inhibitor and Inducers of the Major Human Liver Cytochrome P450 Enzymes Involved in Xenobiotic Transformation. Research Triangle Park, NC, Intek Labs, 1999

Michalets EL: Update: clinically significant cytochrome P-450 drug interactions. Pharmacotherapy 18:84–112, 1998

Micromedex: Micromedex Computer and Clinical Information System, Vol 99. Englewood, CO, Micromedex, 1999

Nemeroff CB, Devane CL, Pollack BG: Summary and review of antidepressants and the cytochrome P450 system. American Society for Clinical Psychopharmacology Progress Notes 6(4):38–40, 1995–1996

Nemeroff CB, DeVane CL, Pollock BG: Newer antidepressants and the cytochrome P450 system. Am J Psychiatry 153: 311–320, 1996

Patel J, Salzman C: Enzyme metabolism and drug interaction, in Clinical Geriatric Psychopharmacology, Third Edition. Edited by Salzman C. Baltimore, MD, Williams & Wilkins, 1998, pp 547–552

Pollock BG: Recent developments in drug metabolism of relevance to psychiatrists. Harv Rev Psychiatry 2:204–213, 1994

References for Table 33–6

Allen SJ, Benton JS, Goodhardt MJ, et al: Biochemical evidence of selective nerve cell changes in the normal aging human and rat brain. J Neurochem 41:256–265, 1983

Cohen BM, Renshaw PF, Stoll AL, et al: Decreased brain choline uptake in older adults. JAMA 274:903–907, 1995

Court JA, Perry EK, Johnson M, et al: Regional patterns of cholinergic and glutamate activity in the developing and aging human brain. Dev Brain Res 74:73–82, 1993

Cutler R, Joseph JA, Yamagami K, et al: Area specific alterations in muscarinic stimulated low K_m GTPase activity in aging and Alzheimer's disease: implications for altered signal transduction. Brain Res 664:54–60, 1994

Flynn DD, Mash DC: Characterization of L-[³H]nicotine binding in human cerebral cortex: comparison between Alzheimer's disease and the normal. J Neurochem 47:1948–1954, 1986

Lee KS, Frey KA, Koeppe RA, et al: In vivo quantification of cerebral muscarinic receptors in normal human aging using positron emission tomography and [¹¹C]-tropanyl benzilate. J Cereb Blood Flow Metab 16:303–310, 1996

Mesulam M-M, Mufson EJ, Rogers J: Age-related shrinkage of cortically projecting cholinergic neurons: a selective effect. Ann Neurol 22:31–36, 1987

Molchan SE, Martinez RA, Hill JL, et al: Increased cognitive sensitivity to scopolamine with age and a perspective on the scopolamine model. Brain Res Rev 17:215–226, 1992

Muller WE, Stoll L, Schubert T, et al: Central cholinergic functioning and aging. Acta Psychiatr Scand 366 (suppl):34–43, 1991

Nakano S, Kato T, Nakamura S, et al: Acetylcholinesterase activity in cerebrospinal fluid of patients with Alzheimer's disease and senile dementia. J Neurol Sci 75:213–223, 1986

Nordberg A, Alafuzoff I, Winblad B: Nicotinic and muscarinic subtypes in the human brain: changes with aging and dementia. J Neurosci Res 31:103–111, 1992

Suhara T, Inoue O, Kobayashi K, et al: No age-related changes in human benzodiazepine receptor binding measured by PET with [¹¹C]R513. Neurosci Lett 159:207–210, 1993

Sunderland T, Esposito G, Molchan SE: Differential cholinergic regulation in Alzheimer's patients compared to controls following chronic blockade with scopolamine: a SPECT study. Psychopharmacology (Berl) 121:231–241, 1995

References for Table 33–7

Bannon MJ, Poosch MS, Xia Y, et al: Dopamine transporter mRNA content in human substantia nigra decreases precipitously with age. Proc Natl Acad Sci U S A 89: 7095–7099, 1992

Bareggi SR, Franceschi M, Smirne S: Neurochemical findings in cerebrospinal fluid in Alzheimer's disease, in Normal Aging, Alzheimer's Disease, and Senile Dementia: Aspects on Etiology, Pathogenesis, Diagnosis, and Treatment. Edited by Gottfries CG. Brussels, Editions de l'Université de Bruxelles, 1985, pp 203–212

DeKeyser J, Ebinger G, Vauquelin G: Age-related changes in the human nigrostriatal dopaminergic system. Ann Neurol 27:157–161, 1990

Hartikainen R, Soininen H, Reinihainen KJ, et al: Neurotransmitter markers in the cerebrospinal fluid of normal subjects: effects of aging and other confounding factors. Journal of Neural Transmission General Section 84:103–117, 1991

McGeer EG: Neurotransmitter systems in aging and senile dementia. Progress in Neuro-psychopharmacology 5: 435–445, 1981

Morgan DG, May PC, Finch CE: Dopamine and serotonin systems in human and rodent brain: effects of age and neurodegenerative disease. J Am Geriatr Soc 35:334–345, 1987

Oreland L, Gottfries CH: Brain and brain monoamine oxidase in aging and in dementia of Alzheimer's type. Prog Neuropsychopharmacol Biol Psychiatry 10:533–540, 1986

Rinne JO, Heitala J, Ruotsalainen U, et al: Decrease in human striatal dopamine D_2 receptor density with age: a PET study with [¹¹C]raclopride. J Cereb Blood Flow Metab 13: 310–314, 1993

Robinson DS, Sourkes TL, Nies A, et al: Monoamine metabolism in human brain. Arch Gen Psychiatry 34:89–92, 1977

Roth GS, Joseph JA: Age-related changes in the translational and posttranscriptional regulation of the dopaminergic system. Life Sci 55:2031–2035, 1994

Van Dyck CH, Seibyl JP, Malison RT, et al: Age-related decline in striatal dopamine transporter binding with Iodine-123-β-SPECT. J Nucl Med 36:1175–1181, 1995

Volkow ND, Fowler JS, Wand GJ, et al: Decreased dopamine transporters with age in healthy human subjects. Ann Neurol 36:237–239, 1994

Volkow ND, Wang GJ, Fowler JS, et al: Parallel loss of presynaptic and postsynaptic dopamine markers in normal aging. Ann Neurol 44:143–147, 1998

Wang GJ, Volkow ND, Logan J, et al: Evaluation of age-related changes in serotonin 5-HT$_2$ and dopamine D$_2$ receptor availability in healthy human subjects. Life Sci 56:249–253, 1995

Sastre M, Garcia-Sevilla JA: Density of alpha-2A adrenoceptors and G$_i$ proteins in the human brain: ratio of high-affinity agonist sites to antagonist sites and effect of age. J Pharmacol Exp Ther 269:1062–1072, 1994

Supiano MA, Hogikyan RV: High affinity platelet α$_2$-adrenergic receptor density is decreased in older humans. J Gerontol A Biol Sci Med Sci 48:173–179, 1993

▋ References for Table 33–8

Arango V, Ernsberger P, Marzuk PM, et al: Autoradiographic demonstration of increased 5-HT$_2$ and β-adrenergic receptor binding sites in the brains of suicide victims. Arch Gen Psychiatry 47:1038–1047, 1990

Gottfries CG: Neurochemical aspects of aging and diseases with cognitive impairment. J Neurosci Res 27:541–547, 1990

Hartikainen R, Soininen H, Reinihainen KJ, et al: Neurotransmitter markers in the cerebrospinal fluid of normal subjects: effects of aging and other confounding factors. Journal of Neural Transmission General Section 84:103–117, 1991

Insel PA: Adrenergic receptor, G proteins, and cell regulation: implications for aging research. Exp Gerontol 28:341–348, 1993

Kalaria RN, Andorn AC: Adrenergic receptors in aging and Alzheimer's disease: decreased alpha 2–receptors demonstrated by [^{3}H]ρ-aminoclonidine binding in prefrontal cortex. Neurobiol Aging 12:131–136, 1991

Kalaria RN, Andorn AC, Tabaton M, et al: Adrenergic receptors in aging and Alzheimer's disease: increased beta 2–receptors in prefrontal cortex and hippocampus. J Neurochem 53:1772–1781, 1989

Mann DMA: Is the pattern of nerve cell loss in aging and Alzheimer's disease a real, or only an apparent, selectivity? Neurobiol Aging 12:340–343, 1991

McGeer EG: Neurotransmitter systems in aging and senile dementia. Progress in Neuro-psychopharmacology 5:435–445, 1981

Mendelsohn FAO, Paxinos G (eds): Receptors in the human nervous system. San Diego, CA, Academic Press, 1991

Oreland L, Gottfries CH: Brain and brain monoamine oxidase in aging and in dementia of Alzheimer's type. Prog Neuropsychopharmacol Biol Psychiatry 10:533–540, 1986

Pascual J, del Arco C, Gonzalez AM, et al: Quantitative light microscopic autoradiographic localization of α$_2$-adrenoreceptors in the human brain. Brain Res 585: 116–127, 1992

Robinson DS, Sourkes TL, Nies A, et al: Monoamine metabolism in human brain. Arch Gen Psychiatry 34:89–92, 1977

▋ References for Table 33–9

Baeken C, D'haenen H, Flanen P, et al: ^{123}I-5-I-R91150, a new single-photon emission tomography legend for 5-HT$_{2A}$ receptors: influence of age and gender in healthy subjects. Eur J Nucl Med 25(12):1617–1622, 1998

Bareggi SR, Franceschi M, Smirne S: Neurochemical findings in cerebrospinal fluid in Alzheimer's disease, in Normal Aging, Alzheimer's Disease, and Senile Dementia: Aspects on Etiology, Pathogenesis, Diagnosis, and Treatment. Edited by Gottfries CG. Brussels, Editions de l'Université de Bruxelles, 1985, pp 203–212

Burnet PWJ, Eastwood SL, Harrison PJ: Detection and quantification of 5-HT$_{1A}$ and 5-HT$_{2A}$ receptor mRNAs in human hippocampus using a reverse transcriptase-polymerase chain reaction (RT-PCR) technique and their correlation with binding site densities and age. Neurosci Lett 178:85–89, 1994

Hartikainen R, Soininen H, Reinihainen KJ, et al: Neurotransmitter markers in the cerebrospinal fluid of normal subjects: effects of aging and other confounding factors. Journal of Neural Transmission General Section 84:103–117, 1991

Marcussen J, Oreland L, Winblad B: Effect of age on human brain serotonin (S-1) binding sites. J Neurochem 43: 1699–1705, 1984

Marcussen JO, Alafuzoff I, Backstrom IT, et al: 5-Hydroxytryptamine-sensitive [^{3}H]imipramine binding of protein nature in the human brain, II: effect of normal aging and dementia disorders. Brain Res 425:137–145, 1987

Meek JL, Bertilsson L, Cheny DL, et al: Aging-induced changes in acetylcholine and serotonin content of discrete brain nuclei. J Gerontol 32:129–131, 1977

Meltzer CC, Smith G, Price JC, et al: Reduced binding of [^{18}F]altanscrin to serotonin type 2A receptors in aging: persistence of efficient after partial volume correction. Brain Res 813(1):167–171, 1998

Middlemiss DN, Palmer AM, Edel N, et al: Binding of the novel serotonin agonist 8-hydroxy-2-(di-n-propylamino)tetralin in normal and Alzheimer brain. J Neurochem 46:993–996, 1986

Oreland L, Gottfries CH: Brain and brain monoamine oxidase in aging and in dementia of Alzheimer's type. Prog Neuropsychopharmacol Biol Psychiatry 10:533–540, 1986

Severson JA, marcusson JO, Osterburg HH, et al: Elevated density of [^{3H}] binding in aged human brain. J Neurochem 45:1382–389, 1995

Sparks DL: Aging and Alzheimer's disease: altered cortical serotonergic binding. Arch Neurol 46:138–140, 1989

Wang GJ, Volkow ND, Fowler JS, et al: Evaluation of age-related changes in serotonin 5-HT$_2$ and dopamine D$_2$ receptor availability in healthy human subjects. Life Sci 56:249–253, 1995

34

Psychopharmacology

Steven L. Dubovsky, M.D.

Randall Buzan, M.D.

Accounting for 11% of the population, elderly individuals take 20%–25% of all prescribed medications (Sargenti et al. 1988). The average nursing home patient takes 9.3 medications (Pollock et al. 1992), at least 1 of which is likely to be a psychotropic medication (Avorn et al. 1992). Patients may continue for many years to take medications that contribute to neuropsychiatric morbidity (Salzman 1992).

A number of factors complicate the prescription of psychotropic medications for geriatric patients with neuropsychiatric illnesses (Ahronheim 1992; Salzman 1992; Sargenti et al. 1988). Adding these drugs to medications the patient already is taking—including over-the-counter substances that may not be reported to the physician—not only increases the risk of interactions but makes it difficult for a patient with memory impairment to keep track of which pills must be taken when. Further, patients with tremors, arthritis, visual problems, or confusion find it difficult to open the childproof containers that pharmacists are required to dispense medications in unless directed otherwise.

In this chapter, we review the pharmacological treatment of neuropsychiatric conditions in elderly patients. To facilitate an understanding of parameters that affect pharmacotherapy in older patients with neuropsychiatric disorders, we briefly review general principles of pharmacology and physiology applicable to geriatric neuropsychiatry. We then review the use of the major classes of psychotropic medications and the treatment of special problems such as agitation and dementia. Electroconvulsive therapy (ECT), which is clearly effective and well tolerated in geriatric patients (Philibert et al. 1995), is considered in detail in Chapter 35.

Changes in the Aging Nervous System Relevant to Psychopharmacology

Even in the absence of frank neurological disease, changes in brain structure and function as the nervous system ages make older patients more vulnerable to side effects of psychotropic medications (Ahronheim 1992; Rovner 1990; Salzman 1990; Sargenti et al. 1988) (see also Chapter 3). Loss of neurons in the cortex, locus coeruleus, and hippocampus makes sedative and psychomotor side effects more pronounced. A gradual decline in central cholinergic transmission increases sensitivity to anticholinergic side effects such as confusion and amnesia, which are even more marked in the presence of dementia. Reduced sensitivity of baroreceptors in the carotid artery and of hypothalamic blood pressure regulatory centers, along with decreased numbers of α_1-noradrenergic receptors, make it difficult to maintain blood pressure in the face of the hypotensive effects of antidepressants and neuroleptics. A decline in the number of neurons in the substantia nigra and dopamine receptors in the corpus striatum increases sensitivity to extrapyramidal side effects, which is usually a limiting side effect in the presence of Parkinson's disease.

Although it is clearly established that elderly patients are more sensitive to side effects of psychotropic medications, especially sedation, psychomotor impairment, orthostatic hypotension, and anticholinergic side effects (Abernathy 1992), there is no empirical support in most cases for the common assertion that geriatric patients are also more sensitive to therapeutic actions (Abernathy 1992; Young and Meyers 1991). Indeed, reduced sensitivity of β-adrenergic (Ahronheim 1992; Rovner 1990), benzodiazepine (Young and Meyers 1991), and other receptors may make some drugs less efficient in elderly patients. This issue is considered in more detail in discussions of specific medications.

The response to psychotropic medications in older patients with neurological illness changes as the disease evolves. For example, loss of dopaminergic neurons reduces the capacity of the parkinsonian brain to synthesize dopamine from L-dopa, resulting in reduced benefit from treatment as the disease progresses. Similarly, progressive loss of cholinergic neurons in Alzheimer's disease makes drugs that prolong the action of acetylcholine (e.g., cholinesterase inhibitors) less effective in the later stages of Alzheimer's disease. Loss of postsynaptic dopamine receptors with age makes agitated patients with neuropsychiatric illness more vulnerable to extrapyramidal side effects of neuroleptics. These issues are discussed when specific medications and illnesses are considered.

Psychopharmacological Principles

A few basic concepts are helpful in predicting medication actions in elderly patients with neuropsychiatric illness (Abernathy 1992; Ahronheim 1992). *Pharmacokinetics*, or what the body does to a drug, refers to factors influencing drug disposition, including absorption, distribution, metabolism, and excretion. *Pharmacodynamics*, the processes influencing the action of drugs at tissue sites, describes what the medication does to the body. The *volume of distribution* is the hypothetical volume in which a medication is in equilibrium, reflecting how widely a drug is distributed throughout the body.

The *elimination half-life* is the time required to eliminate half the amount of medication in the body. It takes four to five half-lives, which for many drugs administered to elderly patients is more than 2 weeks (Abernathy 1992), to eliminate about 90% of a drug. When the interval between doses is less than the elimination half-life, the medication accumulates until the amount entering the plasma equals the amount being cleared (Abernathy 1992). This resulting concentration is the *steady state concentration*, which is directly proportional to the dose and inversely proportional to the clearance (Young and Meyers 1991). It takes four to five half-lives to achieve about 90% of a steady state (Abernathy 1992).

Although gastrointestinal absorption is essentially unchanged in elderly patients (Abernathy 1992; Young and Meyers 1992), anticholinergic drugs and antacids frequently taken by older neurological patients delay absorption of other medications (Abernathy 1992). Once a medication is absorbed, its metabolism is altered in elderly individuals in several ways (Abernathy 1992; Sargenti et al. 1988; Young and Meyers 1991). First-pass metabolism, which occurs when a drug is carried from the gut to the liver after absorption, is slowed because hepatic blood flow decreases with age. As a result, the blood level and therefore the effect of drugs with extensive first-pass metabolism (e.g., triazolam, midazolam, calcium channel blocking agents, neuroleptics, and all antidepressants except trazodone) can be increased.

After entering the circulation following first-pass metabolism, medications undergo another series of metabolic transformations (Ahronheim 1992; Salzman 1990). Phase I (oxidative) metabolism is mediated by the cytochrome P450 oxidase system and produces demethylated biologically active metabolites. For example, diazepam is metabolized to desmethyldiazepam, desmethyldiazepam is metabolized to oxazepam, amitriptyline is metabolized to nortriptyline, and nortriptyline is metabolized to 11-hydroxynortriptyline. Because phase I metabolism slows with aging, blood levels and half-lives of parent compounds of many tricyclic antidepressants (TCAs), benzodiazepines, neuroleptics, and anticonvulsants tend to increase, causing more toxic, as well as therapeutic, effects at the same dose. On the other hand, individuals who are slow oxidative metabolizers when they are younger remain slow metabolizers as they age (Pollock et al. 1992). Phase II metabolism, which through glucuronidation, acetylation, or sulfation produces inactive water-soluble metabolites that are excreted by the kidney, is not altered by the aging process.

Slowed oxidative metabolism should result in a lower dose of most psychotropic medications being necessary to achieve the same blood level. However, metabolic rates vary substantially from person to person, and the number of individuals with slow metabolism by the P450 system does not increase with age (Pollock et al. 1992). Further, the age-associated decline in P450 activity that has been observed in animals may not be true of humans (Pollock et al. 1992). Some older patients therefore will continue to have rapid phase I metabolism and will need the same medication doses as those required by younger patients to achieve a therapeutic level (Pollock et al. 1992). In addition, many studies of pharmacokinetics and drug dosing in geriatric patients are complicated by the use of mixed-age samples, different age ranges, and older methodology, making application of findings to clinical practice difficult (Salzman 1992).

The distribution of psychotropic drugs changes substantially with age. Because all of these drugs—with the exception of lithium—are lipid soluble, they distribute into fatty tissue, which increases as a percentage of total body weight from 19% at age 25 to 35% at age 70 (Young and Meyers 1991). As a result, psychotropic medications distribute more widely in peripheral tissues and remain in the body longer, and the proportion diffusing into the brain diffuses more slowly because of increased distribution elsewhere (Abernathy 1992). Because equilibration in the body takes longer, it takes more time to reach a steady state and thus the onset of therapeutic effect may be delayed. Side effects and drug accumulation may also begin later than anticipated (Abernathy 1992). The reverse effects occur with lithium, which, being hydrophilic, has a decreased volume of distribution in elderly patients (Abernathy 1992).

All psychotropic medications except lithium are extensively bound to plasma protein, and only the unbound fraction is available both for pharmacological action and for metabolism (Abernathy 1992; Young and Meyers 1991). Changes in protein binding do not produce noticeable changes in drug action in healthy geriatric patients, but those with marked decreases in serum albumin concentration (e.g., because of inanition) may develop elevated levels of free benzodiazepines and anticonvulsants (Young and Meyers 1991). Acutely ill geriatric patients may have elevated levels of α_1-glycoprotein, which binds heterocyclic antidepressants (HCAs) and neuroleptics, leading to reduced therapeutic effects of these drugs at the same total blood level (Sargenti et al. 1988).

All psychotropic drugs are excreted by the kidneys, lithium directly and other medications after metabolic transformation in the liver to hydrophilic metabolites (Abernathy 1992; Young and Meyers 1991). As a result of reduced renal blood flow, creatinine clearance falls by as much as 60% in elderly patients (Abernathy 1992; Young and Meyers 1991). Reduced renal lithium clearance, combined with lithium's smaller volume of distribution, leads to higher lithium levels and a half-life that is increased by up to 50% (Abernathy 1992; Young and Meyers 1991). Diminished clearance of toxic water-soluble metabolites of TCAs (e.g., 11-hydroxynortriptyline) can enhance cardiac and other toxic effects of these drugs.

Longer half-lives, longer times to reach a steady state, larger volumes of distribution of lipid-soluble drugs, and slower elimination, along with hypersensitivity of the central nervous system (CNS) to many toxic effects, necessitate changes in prescribing practices for elderly neuropsychiatric patients. Initial doses should be lower than for younger patients, and more time should elapse between dose increases. Some patients may achieve therapeutic levels at lower final doses, but others may ultimately require the same or even higher doses as those required by younger patients. The appearance of toxicity, especially in the CNS, as well as therapeutic effects, may be delayed longer than in younger adults. Approaches to these problems are outlined in the following discussions of specific medication categories.

Omnibus Budget Reconciliation Act and Prescribing Practices

Concerns that 33%–74% of nursing home residents were receiving psychotropic medications led to regulations—outlined in the Omnibus Budget Reconciliation Act of 1987 (OBRA-87)—limiting the use of these medications in long-term care facilities (Hawes et al. 1997; Lantz et al. 1996). These regulations have been in effect since 1990 for Medicare- and Medicaid-certified nursing homes (Hawes et al. 1997). Among the changes instituted by OBRA-87 was regular functional assessment of nursing home patients using the Resident Assessment Instrument (RAI), which measures physical functioning, mood, behavior, activities of daily living, and other basic functions. Mandating use of the RAI tripled the amount of accurate patient data in nursing home charts, although data in the charts of 51% of residents are still incomplete (Hawes et al. 1997). Prescriptions of antipsychotic and antianxiety drugs declined after institution of OBRA regulations, although this decrease may have been related as much to changes in standards or practice as to OBRA (Hawes et al. 1997; Lantz et al. 1996). At the same time, antidepressant prescriptions increased, which suggests that depression is being treated more appropriately (Lantz et al. 1996). Formal educational programs reduce the inappropriate use of psychotropics in nursing homes, without producing more disruptive behavior or distress (Avorn et al. 1992).

Despite these advances, many older residents of nursing homes and elderly patients in general hospitals continue to receive one or more psychotropic medications, and for questionable indications (Avorn et al. 1992; O'Reilly and Rusnak 1990). For example, amitriptyline—which has anticholinergic, sedative, and hypotensive side effects that can be dangerous to older patients—and long-acting benzodiazepines—which increase the risk of falls—are still prescribed frequently (Avorn et al. 1992). A community survey in Australia indicated that 40% of elderly people who complained of insomnia were receiving hypnotic medications, but so were 10% of elderly people living at home and more than one-third of older people living in institutions who did not have trouble sleeping (S. Henderson et al. 1995).

Heterocyclic Antidepressants

Depression, the most common psychiatric disorder in elderly patients, is often a neuropsychiatric condition in this population in that it is more likely than other psychiatric problems in the same age group to be associated with cognitive complaints (McMahon and DePaulo 1992), cortical and subcortical atrophy and basal ganglia lesions (Coffey et al. 1993; Rabins et al. 1991), and treatment resistance (Coffey et al. 1991; Rabins et al. 1991) (see also Chapter 13). Disruption of systems for affective expression caused by brain lesions can result in atypical presentations of depression that may include unusual course of the neurological illness, lack of initiative, pseudodementia, and toothache and other odd forms of pain (Ruegg et al. 1988; Salzman 1985).

The three best-studied forms of geriatric depression illustrate principles that apply to the general use of antidepressants in geriatric neuropsychiatry. Poststroke depression (see Chapters 13 and 27) is more likely to occur in patients with left-sided lesions; enlarged ventricles and poorer functioning on mental status examination are additional risk factors (Dagon 1990; Robinson et al. 1984). Further, depression following stroke may represent an interaction between premorbid risk factors such as previous depressive episodes, side of lesion, and location of lesion (frontal vs. nonfrontal and dorsal vs. ventral) (C. A. Ross 1992). No matter what the pathophysiology, poststroke depression may respond to antidepressants (Lipsey et al. 1984; Robinson et al. 1984).

The second common neuropsychiatric presentation of major depression occurs as a complication of Parkinson's disease. This syndrome also may respond to antidepressant therapy (Cummings 1992). In the third variety of neuropsychiatric depression, patients with dementias or other illnesses affecting the right side of the brain do not appear depressed because the full depressive syndrome is masked by aprosodia; such patients may nevertheless benefit from antidepressants (E. D. Ross and Rush 1981). Antidepressants appear to be less useful in elderly patients with dysphoria not meeting criteria for major depression (Salzman 1990).

Antidepressants produce about a 60% remission rate in elderly patients with depression, compared with a 13% rate of remission with placebo (Georgotas et al. 1986). However, relapse is common (Georgotas et al. 1988; Zis and Goodwin 1979), especially in patients with an incomplete remission, chronic depression, and three or more previous depressive episodes (Georgotas et al. 1988). Continuation therapy for 8 months to 2 years has been found to decrease relapse rates substantially, compared with placebo, in geriatric patients with unipolar depression (Flint 1994; Young and Meyers 1991).

Neurological Uses

Heterocyclic antidepressants (HCAs) include the tricyclic antidepressants (TCAs) and the tetracyclic antidepressant maprotiline. Second-generation antidepressants with diverse structures, such as trazodone, bupropion, venlafaxine, nefazodone, and mirtazepine, are the oldest and best studied of the antidepressants. Although the HCAs are still prescribed frequently, geriatric patients with CNS disease often cannot tolerate the anticholinergic, antihistaminic, and antiadrenergic side effects of these medications, which cause memory loss, sedation, weight gain, and postural hypotension. As a result, the HCAs have largely been replaced as treatments for primary depression in neurological patients by newer and better-tolerated antidepressants, discussed in subsequent sections of this chapter. However, HCAs and related antidepressants continue to have applications in some neurological and neuropsychiatric conditions and still play a major role in the treatment of psychotic depression.

HCAs have been used as primary treatments for some neurological disorders, but these applications have not been studied formally in elderly neuropsychiatric patients. Amitriptyline, imipramine, desipramine, doxepin, and trazodone have been found to reduce chronic pain in both the usual antidepressant doses and in lower doses (Hoogiverf 1985; Rosenblatt et al. 1984). Rectal doxepin at dosages of 25–150 mg/day has been found to ameliorate chronic pain in terminally ill cancer patients too weak to take the medication orally (Storey and Trumble 1992). Even though many patients with chronic pain are depressed, the antinociceptive effect does not seem to be dependent on an antidepressant action, in that one state may improve with an antidepressant but not the other. The finding that desipramine but not fluoxetine was as effective as amitriptyline for neuropathic pain suggests that a serotonergic mechanism may not be essential for pain relief by antidepressants, as is commonly assumed (Max et al. 1992).

In younger patients, amitriptyline is frequently used as a prophylactic agent for migraine headaches (Mathew 1981), and other TCAs are probably effective as well, although propranolol may be a more reliable antimigraine drug (Goodman and Charney 1985). Many patients find that migraine headaches become less frequent and less severe with age, permitting a reduction in migraine prophylaxis. Highly serotonergic antidepressants such as fluoxetine and sertraline often make migraine headaches worse or increase their frequency. On the other hand, the capacity of trazodone and nefazodone to antagonize 5-HT$_2$ receptors on blood platelets in a manner similar to that of antimigraine drugs such as the ergotamines may make these medications more useful for migraine headaches (Dubovsky 1994). Fluoxetine (Lauterbach and Schiveri 1991) and amitriptyline (Schiffer et al. 1985) have been noted to ameliorate pseudobulbar affect in some patients with cerebral disease. In addition to 5-HT$_2$ antagonist properties that can be helpful for patients with migraine headaches, mirtazepine has 5-HT$_3$ antagonist properties that can be useful for patients with intractable nausea. Dopamine reuptake inhibition may make venlafaxine, which is effective for refractory depression, a potential treatment for depression in patients with dementia.

Available Preparations

HCAs (Table 34–1) have different structures containing rings composed of carbon, nitrogen, and/or oxygen with varying side chains. Tertiary amine TCAs such as amitriptyline and imipramine are used as reference antidepressants in many studies, but they are poorly tolerated by older patients with organic brain disease. Secondary amine congeners of these drugs such as nortriptyline and desipramine, which have the additional advantage of demonstrated correlations between blood level and clinical response, are better choices for older patients (Young and Meyers 1991). Newer antidepressants are no more effective than the TCAs for nonpsychotic depression and may be less effective for psychotic depression (Rockwell et al.

TABLE 34–1. Heterocyclic and related antidepressants in use in the United States

Medication	Trade name(s)	Starting dose (mg)[a]	Daily dose (mg)[a]
Amitriptyline[b]	Elavil	10	25–100
Nortriptyline[b,c]	Pamelor, Aventyl	10	10–50[d]
Protriptyline[b]	Vivactil	5	5–20
Imipramine[b]	Tofranil	10	25–100[d]
Desipramine[b,c]	Norpramin, Pertofrane	10	25–100[d]
Trimipramine[b]	Surmontil	10	25–100
Clomipramine[b]	Anafranil	10	50–150
Doxepin[b]	Sinequan, Adapin	10	10–75
Amoxapine[b]	Asendin	10	25–300
Maprotiline	Ludiomil	10	25–75
Trazodone	Desyrel	25	25–200
Bupropion	Wellbutrin	75	75–450
Nefazodone	Serzone	50	200–600
Venlafaxine	Effexor	25	125–300
Mirtazepine	Remeron	7.5	15–30

[a]Geriatric dose.
[b]Tricyclic antidepressant.
[c]Secondary amine.
[d]Dose adjusted according to blood level.

1988), but they have fewer sedative, anticholinergic, cardiotoxic, and psychomotor side effects (Gottfries and Hesse 1990; Roose et al. 1991).

Metabolism and Dosing

Certain aspects of antidepressant metabolism that change with aging must be taken into consideration in prescribing these drugs to older neuropsychiatric patients (Abernathy 1992; Alexopoulos 1992; Cohn et al. 1990; Rockwell et al. 1988). Tertiary amine antidepressants are demethylated to secondary amines, and these and other antidepressants are hydrolyzed by the P450 system to water-soluble hydroxy metabolites that are cleared by the kidneys. Some of these metabolites (e.g., 10-hydroxynortriptyline, 2-hydroxydesipramine) have been linked to cardiac conduction defects and some (e.g., 2-hydroxydesipramine) may have antidepressant properties.

Because the efficiency of demethylation diminishes with age, conversion of tertiary amines to secondary amine metabolites is slower and the parent compounds, which have more adverse effects, tend to accumulate. In addition, reduced renal clearance of cardiotoxic hydroxy metabolites enhances cardiac side effects at therapeutic doses. These changes make tertiary amine TCAs poor choices for most elderly patients. Phase I clearance of newer antidepressants such as fluoxetine, sertraline and bupropion is also impaired by age, but less so than that of the TCAs. However, even in younger patients the half-life of fluoxetine is 1–3 days and the half-life of its active metabolite, norfluoxetine, can increase from 9 days to 3 weeks with chronic use (Pato et al. 1991). Slower metabolism of antidepressants results in longer half-lives, more time to reach a steady state, and higher blood levels of the parent drug. These factors are not affected by brain disease.

Although therapeutic and toxic blood levels may be achieved with lower antidepressant doses in elderly patients, the same blood levels and even the same doses as those in younger patients may be necessary for an antidepressant effect. Young et al. (1985) found a mean dose of 75 mg of nortriptyline per day to be effective for the treatment of geriatric depression. Roose et al. (1987) administered nortriptyline at dosages of 87–92 mg/day with mean serum nortriptyline levels of 92 ng/mL, and imipramine at dosages of 240–280 mg/day with mean serum imipramine plus desipramine levels greater than 300 ng/mL. Nortriptyline levels of 50–150 ng/mL and desipramine levels above 125 ng/mL have been found necessary for antidepressant efficacy in elderly patients in other reports (Dagon 1990; Young and Meyers 1991), and Georgotas et al. (1986) confirmed that the range of nortriptyline levels was roughly

the same in elderly patients (50–180 ng/mL) as that usually reported in younger adults (50–150 ng/mL [Rubin et al. 1985]).

In a study of desipramine in unipolar nonpsychotic depression in patients over age 60 (Nelson et al. 1985), the minimum effective desipramine level was 115 ng/mL, the same value found in a comparison group of patients under age 60. Dosages of 125–350 mg/day were necessary in this study, and geriatric patients who did not initially respond improved when the dose was increased until the blood level was in the therapeutic range. These findings suggest that although lower doses and blood levels might be used initially, the dose should be increased in nonresponding patients until the serum level is in the therapeutic range for imipramine, desipramine, nortriptyline, and possibly amitriptyline or until the patient responds. However, side effects are more likely to occur at higher doses, and adverse effects are not correlated with blood levels, especially of parent compounds.

Neuropsychiatric Side Effects

Some side effects of HCAs are particularly problematic in the neuropsychiatric setting. Examples are summarized in Table 34–2 (Ahronheim 1992; Alexopoulos 1992; Baldessarini and Marsh 1990; Bryner and Winograd 1992; Davidson 1989; Demuth et al. 1985; Flint 1994; Herman et al. 1990; Jick et al. 1992; Paradis et al. 1992; Rizos et al. 1988; Rockwell et al. 1988; Roose et al. 1987, 1991; Yassa et al. 1987; Young and Meyers 1991; Young et al. 1985).

Special Considerations

Before depression is treated in elderly patients with brain disease, an attempt should be made to discontinue medications and treat underlying illnesses. When antidepressants are indicated, tertiary amine TCAs should be avoided. Secondary amine TCAs and newer antidepressants such as bupropion, venlafaxine, and the selective serotonin reuptake inhibitors (SSRIs) are better tolerated. Whereas all TCAs can impair cognitive performance in elderly patients (Flint 1994), the dopaminergic effect of bupropion and venlafaxine may enhance cognition in some patients.

Dementia.   Patients with diffuse brain disease or with dysfunction of the right hemisphere may lose the capacity to express affect directly and may express coexisting depression as negativism, emotional lability, hostility, catatonia, or cognitive disturbance out of proportion to the actual lesion (E. D. Ross and Rush 1981) (see also Chapter 24). Although there is some controversy (discussed later in this

TABLE 34–2. Some neuropsychiatric side effects of heterocyclic and related antidepressants

Side effect(s)	Manifestations and comments	Medication(s)
Cardiovascular side effects	Orthostatic hypotension; may cause falls when patient goes to bathroom in middle of night.	TCAs, trazodone, maprotiline; less marked with secondary amines and newer antidepressants
	Type I antiarrhythmic effect causes suppression of ventricular arrhythmias and slowing of conduction. Conduction-repolarization abnormalities with nortriptyline correlated with concentration of E-10-hydroxynortriptyline.	TCAs
	Tachycardia not as marked in older patients as in younger patients.	Imipramine, amitriptyline, clomipramine, trimipramine, doxepin, maprotiline, mirtazepine
	Aggravation of ventricular tachyarrhythmias.	Trazodone, ?other serotonergic antidepressants
Sedation	Histamine, subtype 1 (H_1), receptor blockade causes oversedation, impaired memory and cognition, worsening of organic mental syndromes, and reduced new learning.	Amitriptyline, trimipramine, doxepin, maprotiline, trazodone, clomipramine, nefazodone, mirtazepine
Psychomotor impairment	Impaired driving. Tolerance may not develop.	Amitriptyline, imipramine, trimipramine, doxepin, clomipramine, trazodone
Central anticholinergic syndrome	Anxiety, agitation, confusion, restlessness, disorientation, assaultiveness, and psychosis.	Amitriptyline, imipramine, clomipramine, trimipramine, doxepin, maprotiline, paroxetine
Lowered seizure threshold	Usually involves aggravation of preexisting seizure disorders. Incidence of seizures probably <4 per 1,000 in nonepileptic patients taking therapeutic doses. Dose-related phenomenon for all antidepressants.	Bupropion, maprotiline, amoxapine, tertiary amine TCAs, but not sertraline
Extrapyramidal side effects	Parkinsonism caused by dopamine receptor blockade by amoxapine and inhibition of dopamine release resulting from serotonergic action of SSRIs.	Amoxapine, fluoxetine, ?other SSRIs, high doses of imipramine and amitriptyline
	Akathisia has mechanism similar to parkinsonism.	Amoxapine, fluoxetine, ?other SSRIs
	Tardive dyskinesia: orofacial dyskinesia reported in 18 patients, only 6 of whom were taking antidepressant > 4 months, suggesting chance association except for amoxapine.	Amoxapine, imipramine, amitriptyline, nortriptyline, clomipramine, trazodone, doxepin, nomifensine, tranylcypromine
Falls	Caused by sedation, orthostatic hypotension, and impaired balance.	Imipramine, amitriptyline, doxepin, trazodone, clomipramine, SSRIs
Neuromuscular side effects	Tremor and myoclonus.	TCAs, maprotiline
	Peripheral neuropathy.	Amitriptyline
	Proximal myopathy.	Imipramine
Sleep disorders	Vivid dreams, nightmares, and insomnia.	Desipramine, nortriptyline, protriptyline, fluoxetine
Auditory disturbance	Tinnitus.	Most TCAs
Urological side effects	Urinary retention.	Amitriptyline, imipramine, trimipramine, doxepin, maprotiline
	Priapism not yet reported in elderly patients.	Trazodone
	Sexual dysfunction may respond to yohimbine, cyproheptadine, trazodone.	SSRIs

Note. SSRI = selective serotonin reuptake inhibitors; TCA = tricyclic antidepressant.

chapter) about whether antidepressants can improve cognition and behavior in patients with dementia, a trial of an antidepressant or ECT may be the only means of determining how much disability may be attributable to unrecognized depression in these patients (see also Chapter 35). Antidepressants that should be considered first under these circumstances are those that might enhance cognition, such as bupropion and venlafaxine. Other antidepressant classes should be considered before the TCAs. Acute confusion after ECT may be greater in some patients with dementia, but the underlying dementia is not exacerbated (Dubovsky 1993).

Parkinson's disease.   The anticholinergic properties of tertiary amine antidepressants such as imipramine and amitriptyline could be useful in the treatment of Parkinson's disease; however, the same properties aggravate the cognitive deficits that are often present and have additive side effects with other anticholinergic drugs that patients with Parkinson's disease may be taking (see also Chapter 26). Because of its dopaminergic properties, bupropion improves parkinsonian symptoms in about one-third of patients (Cummings 1992). Venlafaxine could be useful in the treatment of the same group of patients, although its efficacy in parkinsonism has not been studied. The monoamine oxidase inhibitor (MAOI) L-deprenyl (selegiline), which is used as a primary treatment for Parkinson's disease, is also an appropriate choice. Stimulants have dopaminergic properties that could benefit some parkinsonian patients. The neuroleptic attributes of amoxapine contraindicate its use in the presence of Parkinson's disease. The use of SSRIs is discussed in a later section. Independent of its impact on depression, ECT has been shown to improve signs and symptoms of Parkinson's disease, especially in patients with the on-off phenomenon (Cummings 1992; Dubovsky 1993) (see also Chapter 35). Bromocriptine, an antiparkinsonian dopamine agonist, may have antidepressant effects in some patients, but this and other antiparkinsonian drugs also may cause depression.

Seizure disorders.   In sufficient doses, all antidepressants have the potential to lower the seizure threshold (Davidson 1989), an effect that only rarely causes spontaneous seizures in patients without neurological predisposing factors (Jick et al. 1992). For most antidepressants, the dose at which seizures may occur is considerably higher than the usually therapeutic range, but in the cases of bupropion and maprotiline, doses that can produce seizures (greater than 450 and 225 mg/day, respectively, in younger adults) overlap therapeutic doses (Davidson 1989). Doses of these drugs at which epilepsy may be ag-

gravated in older patients are not known, but because they may be close to the geriatric therapeutic range, it is wise to avoid prescribing bupropion and maprotiline to older patients with epilepsy. Amoxapine, which can cause intractable seizures in elderly patients and which has extrapyramidal side effects, should not be taken at all by these patients (Litovitz and Troutman 1983). Doxepin, secondary amine TCAs, and MAOIs are safer in epileptic patients, but trazodone, nefazodone, and the SSRIs are the best initial choices. In one study of younger adults (Cohn et al. 1990), sertraline at a mean dose of 117 mg/day did not lower the seizure threshold.

Interactions

HCAs interact with many other medications that are prescribed in geriatric neuropsychiatry. Some important examples are listed in Table 34–3 (Bailey et al. 1992; Dagon 1990; Rizos et al. 1988; Sargenti et al. 1988; Young and Meyers 1991).

Selective Serotonin Reuptake Inhibitors

Ease of use and lack of anticholinergic, cardiotoxic, and hypotensive side effects have made the selective serotonin reuptake inhibitors (SSRIs) the preferred initial treatment for primary geriatric depression. The SSRIs have been found to be as effective as the HCAs in the treatment of geriatric major depression (Flint 1994; Mendels 1993; F. T. Miller and Freilicher 1995).

Neurological Uses

SSRIs have been used to reduce the frequency of migraine headaches, although their tendency to increase serotonergic transmission may increase migraine frequency in some patients (Dubovsky 1994). A capacity to reduce dopaminergic transmission could be useful for some patients with tics.

Available Preparations and Dosing

Five SSRIs are available in the United States: fluoxetine, sertraline, fluvoxamine, paroxetine, and citalopram. Fluoxetine has a long elimination half-life and has an active metabolite with an even longer half-life (Dubovsky and Thomas 1995), making it a better choice for treatment in older patients. Paroxetine has slightly more anticholinergic properties than do other SSRIs and would not be

TABLE 34–3. Some potential tricyclic and heterocyclic antidepressant interactions

Medications	Interacting medication(s)	Interaction(s)
Tricyclic antidepressants (TCAs)	Anticholinergic drugs	Additive anticholinergic effects
	Tranquilizers, sedatives, low-potency neuroleptics	Increased sedation
	Low-potency neuroleptics, antihypertensive drugs	Increased orthostatic hypotension
	Antihypertensives (clonidine, guanethidine, bethanidine, and debrisoquin)	Decreased effect of both classes
	Antihypertensives	Hypertensive crisis
	Type I antiarrhythmics	Additive antiarrhythmic effect, prolonged QT, widened QRS, increased risk of bundle branch block
	Directly acting sympathomimetics	Potentiation of sympathomimetic
	Disulfiram	Increased activity of both classes
	Cimetidine	Increased TCA levels
All heterocyclic antidepressants	Neuroleptics other than flupenthixol	Increased levels of both classes; clinically relevant for antidepressant; increased intracardiac conduction delay
	Stimulants	Increased antidepressant levels
	Anticonvulsants	Decreased antidepressant levels
	Cholestyramine	Decreased antidepressant levels

used first in patients with dementia. Initial and final doses for elderly patients are summarized in Table 34–4 (Flint 1994).

Neuropsychiatric Side Effects

Stimulation of serotonin 5-HT$_2$ heteroreceptors by increased synaptic serotonin with SSRIs reduces release of dopamine, producing extrapyramidal side effects (Dubovsky 1994). Stiffness, tremor, bradykinesia, and akathisia caused by SSRIs can be particularly troublesome for patients with Parkinson's disease (Dubovsky and Thomas 1995). A few cases of tardive dyskinesia have been reported in younger patients taking SSRIs (Dubovsky and Thomas 1996). The syndrome of inappropriate secretion of antidiuretic hormone (SIADH), which can present as confusion or seizures, has also occasionally been reported (Flint 1994). SSRI-induced nausea, which can be a limiting side effect, can be treated with fresh gingerroot or a serotonin receptor 5-HT$_3$ antagonist such as ondansetron.

▌ Monoamine Oxidase Inhibitors

Currently undergoing a renaissance, monoamine oxidase inhibitors (MAOIs) are as effective as TCAs in the treat-

TABLE 34–4. Selective serotonin reuptake inhibitors in use in the United States

Medication	Trade name	Starting dose (mg)[a]	Daily dose (mg)[a]
Fluoxetine	Prozac	10	10–40
Sertraline	Zoloft	25	50–200
Paroxetine	Paxil	10	10–40
Fluvoxamine	Luvox	25	50–200
Citalopram	Celexa	10	10–40

[a]Geriatric dose.

ment of geriatric depression (Georgotas et al. 1986). Indeed, because activity of the B form of monoamine oxidase (MAO) increases with aging and is even higher in Alzheimer's patients and patients with Parkinson's disease (Alexopoulos 1992; Danielczyk et al. 1988; Flint 1994), MAOIs may be particularly appropriate choices in geriatric neuropsychiatry (Rockwell et al. 1988), especially in the presence of apathy and low motivation (Salzman 1990). Patients with depression and physical symptoms of anxiety that mimic symptoms of neurological disease, such as light-headedness, dizziness, numbness, and paresthesias, may be candidates for treatment with MAOIs, especially in the presence of rejection sensitivity, mood reactivity, and intolerance of or lack of response to HCAs (Pare 1985).

Neurological Uses

L-Deprenyl (selegiline) given at dosages of 5–10 mg/day is a treatment for Parkinson's disease. At these dosages, selegiline does not usually interact with other antiparkinsonian drugs or tyramine-containing foods, because it is selective for the A form of MAO. Increased MAO levels in Alzheimer's disease and other dementias may be an indication that MAOIs could be useful in these conditions, and selegiline was found in several open studies and one single-blind investigation to improve anxiety, depression, and cognitive dysfunction in patients with Alzheimer's disease (Schneider and Sobin 1992) (discussed later in this chapter). Because they suppress rapid eye movement (REM) sleep and have alerting properties, MAOIs can be used to treat narcolepsy.

Available Preparations

Three classes of MAOIs (Alexopoulos 1992) are now in use in the United States (Table 34–5). Tranylcypromine has amphetamine-like properties and is the most stimulating of the MAOIs. Inhibition of MAO does not persist as long after tranylcypromine is discontinued as it does after withdrawal of other MAOIs. The antidepressant dose of L-deprenyl (20–40 mg/day) is higher than the antiparkinsonian dose. However, side effects may be less troublesome than with other MAOIs. Moclobemide, a reversible inhibitor of MAO-A that at moderate doses does not interact with tyramine or serotonin reuptake inhibitors, has been found to be effective in the treatment of geriatric depression (Flint 1994). Because it does not cause postural hypotension or have anticholinergic side effects, moclobemide is an appropriate choice for older patients; however, because it was not deemed to be profitable in the United States, it will not be released here.

Metabolism and Dosing

MAOIs are metabolized by acetylation, which is not affected by aging; however, plasma levels in elderly patients are usually higher with a given dose, probably because of slowing of additional metabolic steps (Alexopoulos et al. 1992). Initial doses, rate of dose increment, and final doses therefore are lower for geriatric patients than for younger patients. However, the dose of MAOI necessary to inhibit MAO is not always lower than in younger patients (Alexopoulos 1992), and some elderly depressed patients require the same MAOI doses as do younger patients (Young and Meyers 1991). In addition, rapid acetylation of MAOIs is not attenuated by age. Patients who are "rapid acetylators" may require higher doses than those recommended by the manufacturer, which by and large are not based on prospective dose-response studies.

Neuropsychiatric Side Effects

MAOIs produce more side effects in elderly patients than do HCAs (Georgotas et al. 1988). Some examples are listed in Table 34–6 (Alexopoulos 1992; Georgotas et al. 1986, 1988; Lawrence 1985; Lieberman et al. 1985; Meyler and Herxheimer 1968; Pare 1985; Sargenti et al. 1988).

Special Considerations

Although seizures have occurred in nonepileptic patients after overdose of MAOIs, at therapeutic doses these drugs are safe for patients with epilepsy. Patients with carcinoid or pheochromocytoma should not be given MAOIs because of the risk of fatal serotonergic or hypertensive reactions. Selegiline is an appropriate first choice for the treatment of depressed patients with parkinsonism, although at higher doses (see the following section) it may interact with levodopa, bromocriptine, and dietary substances. Elderly patients often do not consider over-the-counter preparations to be medications, and therefore they do not necessarily avoid such drugs when warned about potential MAOI interactions. The major risk of MAOIs in dementia is that patients will not remember the dietary restrictions (Young and Meyers 1991). On the other hand, in a study of older patients with depression, Pancheri et al. (1994) found

TABLE 34–5. Monoamine oxidase inhibitors in use in the United States

Medication (by class)	Trade name	Starting dose (mg)[a]	Daily dose (mg)[a,b]
Hydrazines			
Phenelzine	Nardil	7.5	15–60
Isocarboxazid	Marplan	5	10–30[c]
Nonhydrazines			
Tranylcypromine	Parnate	5	10–40
Phenylethylamines			
Selegiline (L-deprenyl)	Eldepryl	5	10–40[e]

[a]Geriatric dose.
[b]Higher doses may be necessary.
[c]Experience in elderly patients limited.
[d]Withdrawn due to poor sales.
[e]Antiparkinsonian dose = 5–10 mg.

TABLE 34–6. Some neuropsychiatric side effects of monoamine oxidase inhibitors

Side effect	Manifestations	Comments
Altered brain function	Sedation, activation, headache, paradoxical reactions, memory loss, confusion, ataxia, irritability, insomnia, mania, psychosis	Abrupt withdrawal can cause insomnia, nightmares, mania, psychosis, and delirium.
Autonomic dysfunction	Postural hypotension, anticholinergic side effects, sexual dysfunction	Phenelzine and isocarboxazid most anticholinergic.
Peripheral nervous system dysfunction	Peripheral neuropathy, paresthesias, gait disturbance, falls	Caused by direct neurotoxicity or interference with B_6 metabolism. Pyridoxine replacement may be helpful.
Neuromuscular irritability	Twitching, myoclonus, muscle tension, tremor, muscle and joint pain	May reflect mild serotonin syndrome. Nocturnal myoclonus occurs in 10%–15% of patients taking phenelzine. No tolerance.
Sexual dysfunction	Anorgasmia, impotence	Cyproheptadine occasionally helpful. Avoid yohimbine.

that even though more patients stopped taking moclobemide than stopped taking imipramine, moclobemide but not imipramine produced improved cognition as well as improvement of anxiety and depression. MAOIs do not aggravate cardiac conduction delays (Young and Meyers 1991).

Interactions

MAOIs have two potentially dangerous interactions. The first is the hypertensive reaction that occurs with foods that are high in tyramine content and with certain adrenergic medications. Hypertensive reactions occur because MAOIs irreversibly inhibit both MAO-A, which is found in the gut and the brain, and MAO-B, which is found in the brain but not the gut. Because gastrointestinal MAO-A metabolizes ingested tyramine (a pressor amine found in many foods) before it can be absorbed into the bloodstream, inhibition of the enzyme results in increased intestinal absorption of tyramine and an amplified pressor response that is augmented by decreased tyramine metabolism in sympathetic nerve ganglia. Hypertensive crises are no more common in elderly patients than in other patients (Georgotas et al. 1986), but they are more dangerous in patients with fragile cerebral vasculature. Because selegiline is selective for MAO-B at antiparkinsonian doses and therefore does not inhibit intestinal MAO, tyramine in the gastrointestinal tract is degraded normally. However, at doses greater than 10 mg/day selegiline loses its selectivity and inhibits MAO-A, producing tyramine reactions.

In a study of traditionally proscribed foods, K. I. Shulman et al. (1989) found that the tyramine content of most of them is so low that massive amounts (e.g., 50 glasses of wine) would have to be ingested to produce a hypertensive reaction. The investigators suggested that a more real-

istic list would include all cheese except cottage cheese and cream cheese, concentrated yeast extract, sauerkraut, broad bean pods, aged meats, salami, air-dried sausage, old chicken liver, protein extracts, spoiled protein-containing foods, and pure soy products. Patients should refrain from taking sympathomimetic drugs, including most cold preparations, decongestants, and anorectics. Antihistamines, acetaminophen, Cepacol, Sucrets, and plain Alka Seltzer are safe, but Alka Seltzer Plus is not. Dextromethorphan, which has serotonergic properties, should be avoided because of the risk of serotonin syndrome (described shortly).

Experience with younger patients suggests that a 10-mg tablet of nifedipine chewed and placed under the tongue for rapid absorption can blunt the severity of hypertensive reactions (Clary and Schweitzer 1987) until the more definitive treatment of 2–5 mg of intravenous phentolamine can be administered. However, nifedipine is poorly absorbed from the buccal mucosa, and dangerous hypotension may occur. Chlorpromazine should not be used to treat hypertensive reactions in geriatric neuropsychiatric practice because of the risk of dangerous hypotensive and anticholinergic side effects.

Because serotonin is metabolized by MAO-A, the second type of dangerous MAOI interaction is with serotonergic substances such as L-tryptophan, meperidine, dextromethorphan, imipramine, clomipramine, SSRIs, and possibly buspirone (Salzman 1992; Sargenti et al. 1988). TCAs other than imipramine and clomipramine can be safely combined with MAOIs if the TCA is started first and low initial doses of each medication are used. Serotonin syndrome is a neurotoxic condition characterized by ataxia, hyperreflexia, myoclonus, excitation, diaphoresis, dysarthria, paresthesias, fever, confusion, delirium, seizures, coma, hypotension, and fatal cardiac arrhythmias (Lieberman et al. 1985).

MAOIs interact with a number of other kinds of compounds, some of which are listed in Table 34–7 (Lieberman et al. 1985; Meyler and Herxheimer 1968; Pare 1985; Salzman 1992; Sargenti et al. 1988).

▎ Stimulants

Stimulants increase central release of norepinephrine, dopamine, and serotonin and may have direct dopamine agonist properties (Hoffman and Lefkowitz 1990). Stimulants, available preparations of which are listed in Table 34–8 (Alexopoulos 1992; Salzman 1992), have been found superior to placebo in some double-blind studies of geriatric depression and depression in patients with dementia, especially those who are apathetic and unmotivated (Chiarello and Cole 1987; Rockwell et al. 1988; Warneke 1990). In addition, stimulants can improve negative symptoms such as apathy and withdrawal in geriatric patients with dementia (Galynker et al. 1997). Chiarello and Cole (1987) suggested that a preference for coffee may be an indication of a good response to a stimulant.

Depression in neurologically ill patients may respond within a few weeks to stimulants, although dose-finding studies have not been conducted. In one study (Holmes et al. 1989), cognitive deterioration was found to improve along with depression when human immunodeficiency virus (HIV) encephalopathy was treated with stimulants. Tolerance to the antidepressant effect generally has not been noted in older neuropsychiatric patients (Kaufman et al. 1984), and appetite and sleep improve when the depression remits. The medication can sometimes be withdrawn after a few months without return of symptoms (Kaufman et al. 1984), especially if the underlying neurological illness improves, but chronic treatment has been successful in some instances (Chiarello and Cole 1987).

Stimulants can also be used to augment HCA therapy in treatment-resistant geriatric depression (Warneke 1990). One strategy for patients who cannot tolerate therapeutic doses of HCAs is to administer a lower dose of HCA and increase the blood level of the HCA with a stimulant (discussion follows), avoiding side effects associated with products of first-pass metabolism. Intermittent treatment of bipolar depression with a stimulant can reduce the risk of antidepressant-induced hypomania or mood cycling. The major neurological uses of stimulants are in the treatment of narcolepsy and of apathy and cognitive deterioration in dementia.

Metabolism and Dosing

Until formal data have been collected concerning stimulant metabolism in elderly patients, low initial doses and gradual increments (e.g., in the case of methylphenidate, by 2.5 mg/day every week) are recommended (Table 34–8). Dosages of 5–15 mg/day are often successful in antidepressant augmentation, and administration of 10–40 mg/day is successful as primary treatment for depression in elderly neurologically ill patients. Adderall, a proprietary combination of *l*- and *d*-amphetamine used to treat attention-deficit disorder in children, has not been studied in elderly patients with neuropsychiatric illness.

Neuropsychiatric Side Effects

Stimulant side effects are usually dose related, toxicity being rare at doses less than 15 mg/day (Hoffman and Lefkowitz 1990). Many of the adverse effects noted in Ta-

TABLE 34–7. Some potential monoamine oxidase inhibitor interactions

Medication(s)	Interaction(s)
Hydrazine[a] plus nonhydrazine[b] MAOI	Fever, hypertension, convulsions, stroke, coma
Levodopa	Hypertension; less with carbidopa
Amantadine	Hypertension
General anesthetics, sedatives, narcotics, antihistamines, neuroleptics, antiparkinsonian drugs	Potentiation of central nervous system depression due to inhibition of hepatic metabolism
Antihypertensive drugs	Increased hypotension
Insulin	Increased hypoglycemic effect
Reserpine, tetrabenazine	Excitation
Aspartane	Headache, diaphoresis
Bupropion	Increased bupropion toxicity, serotonin syndrome

Note. MAOI = monoamine oxidase inhibitor.
[a]Phenelzine and isocarboxazid.
[b]Tranylcypromine and pargyline.

TABLE 34–8. Commonly used central nervous system stimulants

Medication	Trade name	Starting dose (mg)[a]	Usual daily dose (mg)[a]
d-Amphetamine	Dexedrine	2.5	2.5–60
Methylphenidate	Ritalin	2.5	2.5–60
Pemoline	Cylert	37.5	37.5–112.5

[a]Geriatric dose.

ble 34–9 represent excessive CNS and cardiovascular stimulation (Ahronheim 1992; Hoffman and Lefkowitz 1990; Rockwell et al. 1988; Young and Meyers 1991).

Special Considerations

The dopaminergic properties of stimulants could be useful for patients with depression and parkinsonism, but the same effect aggravates chorea and psychosis and may lower the seizure threshold. As discussed later in this chapter, a trial of stimulants in patients with dementia may help to identify the component that is attributable to depression.

Interactions

Stimulants increase blood levels of TCAs, neuroleptics, and other medications metabolized by the P450 system. Therefore, stimulants can be used to raise serum levels of another medication, with no dose increase of that drug required.

▮ Nonpharmacological Antidepressant Treatments

When interactions, side effects, or lack of efficacy limits the usefulness of antidepressants, or when the patient is se-

TABLE 34–9. Some neuropsychiatric side effects of stimulants

Side effect	Manifestations
Central nervous system stimulation	Agitation, restlessness, tremor, diaphoresis, hyperreflexia, confusion, cognitive deterioration, paranoia, hallucinations, suicidal and homicidal behavior, convulsions
Cardiovascular stimulation	Tachycardia, hypertension, hypotension, headache, palpitations, arrhythmias, angina, circulatory collapse, cerebral hemorrhage

verely ill, ECT is an obvious consideration, even in the presence of epilepsy, dementia, or delirium (see Chapter 35). Stimulants (discussed in the previous section) are useful in treating apathetic depression associated with neurological illness. At dosages of 40–90 mg/day, buspirone has antidepressant effects in younger patients (Rickels et al. 1991), and augmentation of HCAs with buspirone at dosages of 10–60 mg/day can be as effective as lithium augmentation, with fewer side effects in older patients with brain disease.

Exposure to 2,500–10,000 lux of light for ½–2 hours has been found to be an effective treatment for seasonal affective disorder and some cases of nonseasonal depression. Like any antidepressant, artificial bright light can induce hypomania. The incidence of seasonal affective disorder and the effectiveness of bright light in the geriatric population have not been studied formally, but consideration of this treatment is warranted in patients with a seasonal variation of mood who cannot tolerate antidepressant side effects. The use of artificial bright light to treat abnormalities of the sleep-wake cycle is discussed later in this chapter. Medications that sensitize the lens and retina of the eye to phototoxicity—including imipramine, fluoxetine, lithium, chlorpromazine, thioridazine, and propranolol—should be used with great caution, if at all, in elderly patients who are exposed to bright light or who spend much time in the sun (Roberts et al. 1992).

Repetitive transcranial magnetic stimulation (rTMS) is a method of regional magnetic stimulation of the brain that produces localized subconvulsant electrical discharges and that has been found to have antidepressant effects in a few animal studies, as well as in some pilot studies and small controlled comparisons to sham treatment (George et al. 1997; Markwort et al. 1997; Zyss et al. 1997). In a study in which subjects were informed of their treatment (Tom and Cummings 1998), rTMS produced temporary relief of depression in patients with Parkinson's disease. Like ECT, rTMS may improve the movement disorder of parkinsonism itself, separate from its antidepressant effect (Brandt et al. 1997). An advantage of rTMS is that it does not require the presence of seizures or high doses of electrical energy to be effective, and therefore it should be better tolerated by patients with dementia. A few patients with refractory depression have responded to rTMS to the left frontal cortex (Post et al. 1997). However, improvement of depression with rTMS is only transient, and relapse occurs as soon as the treatment is discontinued (Markwort et al. 1997; Post et al. 1997). Seizures and myoclonus have sometimes occurred in patients receiving rTMS (Jaggy and Koch 1997).

▌ Antimanic Drugs

The risk of mania does not increase with age (Young and Klerman 1992), but bipolar disorder does not "burn out" with age either (K. I. Shulman et al. 1992; Snowdon 1991; Young and Meyers 1991) (see also Chapter 13). Between 5% and 10% of elderly patients undergoing treatment for mood disorders have episodes of mania or hypomania (Young and Klerman 1992), and 5%–10% of bipolar patients become ill for the first time after age 50 (Yassa et al. 1988). Even in the geriatric population, having had previous episodes of depression without mania is no guarantee of a unipolar illness, because up to 25 years may elapse between the onset of depression and the first manic episode (Snowdon 1991).

As is true of depression, late-onset mania in elderly patients is frequently an expression of underlying neurological disease (Snowdon 1991). In addition, manifestations of early-onset primary bipolar disorder can be modified later in life by coexisting brain disease (Young and Klerman 1992). In various reports, 24%–36% of cases of late-onset bipolar disorder have been associated with overt neurological disease (K. I. Shulman et al. 1992; Young and Meyers 1991), which is often present before the onset of mania (Snowdon 1991). The severity of the neurological component is indicated by a retrospective study (K. I. Shulman et al. 1992) in which half of 50 elderly manic patients were dead from medical causes after 6 years of follow-up.

One common neurological precipitant of mania is stroke, especially in association with right-sided lesions of the frontal cortex, basal ganglia, thalamus, or basotemporal cortex or in association with preexisting subcortical atrophy. Other neurological causes of late-onset mania include adrenal steroids, calcium replacement, levodopa, antidepressants, bronchodilators, decongestants, vitamin B_{12} deficiency, hyperthyroidism, epilepsy, trauma, and degenerative, vascular, or neoplastic disease of the right hemisphere (Dagon 1990; Snowdon 1991; Yassa et al. 1988; Young and Klerman 1992).

The frequent association of geriatric mania with neurological disease leads to a high frequency of cognitive dysfunction (Young and Klerman 1992) and resistance to lithium (Hardy et al. 1987; Young and Klerman 1992). Treatment of neurological causes and withdrawal of medications that cause mania may lead to improvement, but additional antimanic treatments are often necessary.

Lithium

Lithium is the best-studied medication for the treatment and prophylaxis of mania in elderly patients. Lithium aug-

mentation can be useful in bipolar and, to a lesser extent, unipolar depression (Jefferson 1990; Roy and Pickar 1985); obsessive-compulsive disorder (Jefferson 1990; Jenike 1990); and schizophrenia (Jefferson 1990).

Neurological uses. Lithium has been noted in uncontrolled reports to ameliorate cluster headaches, Huntington's disease, and spasmodic torticollis. Lithium-induced leukocytosis is a treatment for leukopenia caused by chemotherapy for cancer and autoimmune disease. Reduced renal water conservation caused by lithium therapy may counteract the syndrome of inappropriate secretion of antidiuretic hormone (SIADH), which can complicate some tumors and infections of the CNS.

Metabolism and dosing. Because of age-related reduction of renal clearance and volume of distribution, only one-half to two-thirds of the usual adult doses are necessary to achieve the same plasma level as that in younger patients (Liptzin 1992; Young and Meyers 1991). In elderly patients, lithium half-life is usually (Ahronheim 1992; Liptzin 1992), but not always (Hardy et al. 1987), increased to about 40 hours, resulting in a longer time to reach a steady state (Liptzin 1992), with a corresponding delay in onset of therapeutic action as well as slower elimination after discontinuation. Because of the prolonged half-life, lithium doses should not be increased more frequently than once per week (Ahronheim 1992; Liptzin 1992). The risk of neurotoxic side effects probably warrants even slower dosage adjustments in elderly patients with neuropsychiatric illness.

Clinical lore holds that the therapeutic effect of lithium occurs at lower blood levels as well as lower doses in elderly patients (Salzman 1990). However, there is no empirical evidence for this assertion (Hardy et al. 1987; Young and Meyers 1991). Low starting doses (e.g., 75–150 mg/day) and maintenance doses (e.g., 600–1,200 mg/day) are appropriate (Ahronheim 1992; Liptzin 1992), but the dose should be increased if the patient does not respond and the blood level is not in the usual adult therapeutic range. Single daily doses of lithium enhance compliance, reduce adverse effects, and are safe in elderly patients (Hardy et al. 1987; Mellerup and Plenge 1990).

Neuropsychiatric side effects. Lithium toxicity is common at serum levels greater than 1.5–2.0 mEq/L, but toxicity may occur at therapeutic levels, especially in elderly patients with CNS disease (Hardy et al. 1987; Liptzin 1992). Toxicity produces a coarse tremor, ataxia, vertigo, dysarthria, disorientation, nausea, and vomiting. Severe intoxication is associated with muscle fasciculations, hyperreflexia, confusion, delirium, seizures, and coma. Irreversible memory loss, brain damage, cerebellar symptoms, and motor deficits may occur following lithium intoxication (Saxena and Maltikarjuna 1988).

Lithium side effects, which occur at therapeutic levels, are more frequent at blood levels above 0.8 mEq/L, although lithium is more reliably prophylactic at higher levels, at least in younger adults (Gelenberg et al. 1989; Vestergaard et al. 1988). As many as 50% of lithium-treated patients develop reversible impairment of memory and concentration, which is problematic for patients with dementia. Hypokalemia increases the risk of neurological side effects (Jefferson and Greist 1977). Common CNS side effects are summarized in Table 34–10 (Griffin 1992;

TABLE 34–10. Some neuropsychiatric side effects of lithium

Type of side effects	Manifestations and comments
Neuromuscular	Tremor, ataxia, dysarthria, incoordination, and myoclonus. Falls may result from ataxia and incoordination. Elderly patients more prone to tremor and myoclonus.
Mental	Impaired memory, concentration, and consciousness; anterograde amnesia; aphasia; confusion; dazed feeling; and flat affect.
Extrapyramidal	Parkinsonism.
Degenerative	Parkinsonism and Creutzfeldt-Jakob–like syndrome.
Intracranial	Pseudotumor cerebri.
Electroencephalo-graphically demonstrated	Generalized slowing, disorganization of background rhythm, discharges, rapid eye movement (REM) sleep suppression, and seizures.
Endocrinological	Hyperparathyroidism may produce mental and neuromuscular symptoms, especially depression or mania. Hypothyroidism may initiate rapid cycling or confusion.
Renal	Polyuria and polydipsia not more common in elderly patients. Lithium does not cause or accelerate renal failure in elderly patients. Nephrogenic diabetes insipidus may be reduced by amiloride, which reduces lithium transport into collecting duct.

Liptzin 1992; Rizos et al. 1988; Salzman 1990; Saul 1985; Schneider and Sobin 1992; Young and Meyers 1991).

Special considerations. Lithium can lower the seizure threshold and induce seizures in nonepileptic patients (Massey and Folger 1984). However, in one study (Shukla et al. 1988), lithium at therapeutic levels did not increase seizure frequency or anticonvulsant requirement in a small group of patients with epilepsy and bipolar disorder. The use of lithium in elderly patients with seizure disorders has not been investigated formally, but anticonvulsants with antimanic properties (discussed later in this chapter) should be considered for such patients.

Because lithium occasionally causes extrapyramidal side effects, it can be problematic in parkinsonian patients. Cognitive side effects of lithium are poorly tolerated by patients with dementia. Because lithium slows the rate of depolarization of the sinus node and conduction through the atrioventricular node, electrocardiograms should be obtained with dosage increases and cardiac function should be followed closely in elderly patients with heart disease who take lithium.

Interactions. Neurotoxic interactions between lithium and neuroleptics, which consist mainly of extrapyramidal and neuromuscular syndromes or delirium (F. Miller and Menninger 1987), may represent aggravation of lithium neurotoxicity by the neuroleptic, additive neurotoxic effects or a true interaction between the two classes of medication. Neurotoxicity is more common with higher neuroleptic doses and higher lithium levels and may be irreversible in a few cases (W. J. Cohen and Cohen 1974; Izzo and Brody 1985). A neurotoxic interaction of lithium with clozapine that included confusion, delirium, incoordination, dystonias, and myoclonus has also been reported (Blake et al. 1992). Because neuroleptics are mainly used to control agitation and psychosis until the antimanic action of lithium occurs, it has been recommended that the risk of neurotoxicity could be lessened by deferring lithium therapy until the patient's behavior is under control, at which point the neuroleptic can be gradually withdrawn (Chou 1991). Other interactions of lithium with drugs used in geriatric neuropsychiatry are summarized in Table 34–11 (Abernathy 1992; Ahronheim 1992; Chou 1991; Jefferson 1990; Liptzin 1992; P. J. Perry et al. 1984; Rizos et al. 1988; Salzman 1990; Young and Meyers 1991).

Alternatives to lithium. ECT is clearly effective for mania in elderly patients (Black et al. 1987; Dubovsky and Buzan 1997) (see also Chapter 35). None of the medications that have been used in younger patients with mania

TABLE 34–11. Some potential lithium interactions

Medication(s)	Interaction(s)
Neuroleptics, carbamazepine, clonazepam, calcium channel blockers	Neurotoxicity, increased extrapyramidal side effects
Thiazide diuretics, angiotensin-converting enzyme (ACE) inhibitors	Increase in serum lithium concentration by 35%
Furosemide, amiloride	No effect on lithium clearance
Theophylline, aminophylline, ?caffeine	Increased lithium clearance, decreased lithium half-life
Nonsteroidal anti-inflammatory drugs	Increase in serum lithium concentration by 50%
Tetracyclines, spectinomycin, metronidazole	Increased serum lithium concentration
Iodine	Increased risk of hypothyroidism
β-Blockers	Increased serum lithium concentration
Fluoxetine	Increased serum lithium concentration

as alternatives or adjuncts to lithium have been studied systematically in elderly patients for this indication (Young and Meyers 1991), but some anecdotal evidence exists.

Carbamazepine, the best studied of the alternatives to lithium, may be particularly useful in mixed, rapid-cycling, and lithium-resistant bipolar disorders, although tolerance to prophylaxis of mood disorders may develop (Post 1990). Carbamazepine is an obvious choice for bipolar patients with epilepsy or electroencephalograms (EEGs) showing nonspecific abnormalities, and the drug is better tolerated than lithium in elderly patients with brain damage. However, carbamazepine can cause confusion and neurotoxicity in some of these patients, especially when combined with other antimanic drugs or neuroleptics, and older patients may be unable to tolerate the sedation it causes. Carbamazepine can also be useful in trigeminal neuralgia but is less reliably effective for other kinds of neuropathic pain (Ahronheim 1992).

Because carbamazepine induces its own metabolism, the half-life tends to decrease over a month or so from 36 to 10–20 hours (Ahronheim 1992). Some therapeutic, as well as some toxic, effects of carbamazepine can be attributed to an active epoxy metabolite (Ahronheim 1992). The initial dose of carbamazepine in elderly patients should be 50–100 mg (Ahronheim 1992; Salzman 1990). The therapeutic

dosage for epilepsy, and presumably for mood disorders, in older patients is thought to be 300–1,200 mg/day (Liptzin 1992; Salzman 1990); higher doses may be necessary for pain control (Ahronheim 1992). Side effects and interactions are noted in Tables 34–12 and 34–13 (Ahronheim 1992; Liptzin 1992; Salzman 1990; Thomas 1997).

Valproic acid appears to be a most useful agent for some bipolar patients with EEGs showing abnormalities, rapid cycling, mixed affective states, and resistance to other medications (Chou 1991). In a few studies, valproate was found to be effective in elderly patients with bipolar disorder (Liptzin 1992). Starting dosages of 125 mg/day and total daily doses of 125–1,800 mg, with blood levels around 100 ng/mL, have been recommended (Bowden et al. 1994; Liptzin 1992; Salzman 1990), but these can only be considered estimates in neurologically ill geriatric patients. Some valproate side effects and interactions are noted in Tables 34–12 and 34–13.

Verapamil at dosages of 240–480 mg/day has been used in several elderly patients with dementia and bipolar disorder, with good results and minimal side effects (Dubovsky and Buzan 1997; Dubovsky et al. 1986). Nimodipine, which is used to treat some forms of stroke and which may have applications in dementia, has antimanic properties (Dubovsky and Buzan 1997) and could also be useful in geriatric bipolar illness complicated by dementia or cerebrovascular disease. It has also been observed (but not demonstrated in controlled studies) that nimodipine may be a useful antidepressant in patients with dementia (Riekkinen et al. 1997; Vry et al. 1997). Side effects and interactions of calcium channel blockers are included in Tables 34–12 and 34–13.

The anticonvulsants lamotrigine and gabapentin have recently been used as antimanic and mood-stabilizing drugs. However, there are as yet no published controlled studies of such indications (Dubovsky and Buzan 1997). Both medications are well tolerated by elderly patients, the primary interactions being reduction of the drugs' serum levels by carbamazepine and increase of serum levels by valproate (Thomas 1997). Lamotrigine may have neuroprotective properties related to reduction of excitatory amino acid transmission, making it potentially useful for bipolar patients with cerebrovascular disease (Thomas 1997).

In addition to being used as antimanic and mood-stabilizing medications, anticonvulsants are used to treat seizure disorders, the incidence of which increases between age 60 and 75 (see also Chapter 29). Most new episodes of epilepsy in elderly patients are secondary to cerebrovascular disease, brain tumors, neurodegenerative disease, and toxic-metabolic conditions (Thomas 1997). Certain

TABLE 34–12. Some neuropsychiatric side effects of alternatives to lithium

Alternative	Side effect/type of side effects	Manifestations
Carbamazepine	Neurotoxicity	Ataxia, dizziness, sedation, lethargy, diplopia, cognitive impairment, irritability, confusion, restlessness, seizures
	Neuroendocrinological	Syndrome of inappropriate secretion of antidiuretic hormone (SIADH), hypocalcemia
	Hematological	Transient leukopenia
	Hypersensitivity	Agranulocytosis, aplastic anemia, thrombocytopenia, rash, hepatitis, pneumonitis
Valproic acid	Neurotoxicity	Sedation, ataxia, tremor, impaired memory
	Dermatological	Rash, alopecia
	Gastrointestinal	Weight gain, anorexia, nausea, vomiting; hepatitis in 1 in 50,000 adults
Verapamil	Neurological	Sedation, dizziness, headache, occasional extrapyramidal symptoms

TABLE 34–13. Some potential interactions of alternatives to lithium

Alternative	Medication(s)	Interaction(s)
Carbamazepine	Lithium	Neurotoxicity
	Anticonvulsants, neuroleptics, benzodiazepines, warfarin sodium	Decreased blood level of other medication, caused by enzyme induction
	Fluoxetine	Increased carbamazepine levels
	Neuroleptics	Neurotoxicity
	Cimetidine, erythromycin, isoniazid	Increased carbamazepine levels
Valproic acid	Aspirin	Increased valproate levels
	Other anticonvulsants	Increased levels of other anticonvulsant
	Clonazepam	Absence status epilepticus
Verapamil	Carbamazepine, lithium	Increased carbamazepine and lithium levels, neurotoxicity
	Lithium, β-blockers	Additive cardiac slowing

adverse effects of antiepileptic drugs are more common in elderly patients (Table 34–14) (Thomas 1997).

Antianxiety Drugs

Benzodiazepines and azapirones are the primary treatments for generalized anxiety in elderly patients (see also Chapter 15). Benzodiazepines are most appropriately used to treat acute anxiety or insomnia in response to a discrete stress (Salzman 1990). Because generalized anxiety disorder is chronic and recurrent, ongoing treatment is often necessary. Azapirones are better tolerated by chronically anxious patients with brain disease, because these drugs do not impair higher cortical function, but their delayed onset of action makes them ineffective when used on an as-needed basis.

Alprazolam has been the most thoroughly studied as a treatment for panic disorder, but other benzodiazepines appear to be effective if administered in equivalent doses. Clonazepam has been used to treat mania (Chouinard and Penry 1985), although some of its apparent antimanic effect could be secondary to sedation, which is difficult for many older neuropsychiatric patients to tolerate. Alprazolam and perhaps other benzodiazepines may have antidepressant effects in mixed anxiety-depression, but antidepressants and azapirones have a wider margin of safety for this indication in neurologically ill elderly patients. Azapirones can be used to augment antidepressants in the treatment of depression and obsessive-compulsive disorder.

TABLE 34–14. Some side effects of anticonvulsants

Adverse effect	Comments
Megaloblastic anemia	Greater incidence of folate deficiency increases risk of anemia
Osteomalacia	Decreased calcium and vitamin D intake increases risk
Cognitive impairment	Reduced memory and aggravation of dementia
Depression	Anticonvulsants may precipitate or aggravate symptoms of depression
Falls	Especially with sedating anti-convulsants
Cardiac conduction defects	Carbamazepine and oxycarba-mazepine can worsen conduction defects and bradycardia

Benzodiazepines

Neurological uses.   Clonazepam is used to treat generalized, myoclonic, and absence seizures (Chouinard and Penry 1985) (see also Chapter 29). Clonazepam may also be useful in pain syndromes such as trigeminal neuralgia that are associated with paroxysmal dysesthesias, burning sensations and hyperesthesias (Bouckonis and Litman 1985) (see also Chapter 18) and with choroeoathetosis and neuroleptic-induced akathisia (Chouinard and Penry 1985). Intravenous diazepam is a well-known treatment for status epilepticus. Intravenous midazolam is used for severe agitation in delirium patients.

Available preparations.   Benzodiazepines can be divided into short– and long–half-life preparations. As a general rule, the long–half-life drugs are poorly tolerated by elderly patients with neuropsychiatric illness because accumulation leads to sedation, amnesia, psychomotor impairment, ataxia, and falls (Mustard and Mayer 1997; Ray 1992). Properties of benzodiazepines used to treat anxiety are summarized in Table 34–15 (Abernathy 1992; Ahronheim 1992; Regestein 1992; Salzman 1992; Salzman et al. 1983). (Benzodiazepine hypnotics are discussed in a later section.)

Metabolism and dosing.   Unlike antidepressants, anticonvulsants, and low-potency neuroleptics, benzodiazepines do not induce their own metabolism (Salzman 1992). Diazepam, chlordiazepoxide, clorazepate, praze-

pam, halazepam, and flurazepam have long elimination half-lives that are prolonged two to three times in elderly patients (Regestein 1992), resulting in a longer time to reach a steady state and drug accumulation over time (Salzman et al. 1983). Long–half-life benzodiazepines also have a complex hepatic oxidative metabolism that produces desmethyldiazepam, an active metabolite with a half-life in elderly patients of 80–130 hours (Salzman 1990, 1992; Salzman et al. 1983).

Hydroxylated benzodiazepines such as oxazepam, lorazepam, alprazolam, triazolam, and temazepam have intermediate and shorter half-lives and simpler metabolic pathways that are not affected as much by aging (Salzman 1990, 1992; Salzman et al. 1983). Such medications do not accumulate in elderly patients and are quicker to reach a steady state. Despite long half-lives in elderly patients, benzodiazepines are often given in divided doses to minimize periods of intoxication caused by blood level peaks. Recommended dose ranges for geriatric neuropsychiatry are noted in Table 34–15.

Neuropsychiatric side effects.   The older CNS may be more prone to benzodiazepine toxicity, perhaps because of increased sensitivity of the benzodiazepine receptor (Salzman 1992). Patients with disease of the brain may be even more vulnerable to adverse effects of CNS depression caused by benzodiazepines, such as excessive sedation, memory impairment, confusion, falls, or paradoxical reactions. As they grow older, geriatric patients may develop benzodiazepine toxicity at doses that were previously well tolerated (Regestein 1992). Common benzodiazepine side effects are presented in Table 34–16 (Ahronheim 1992; Hart et al. 1991; Ray 1992; Regestein 1992; Salzman 1991, 1992; Salzman et al. 1983; Young and Meyers 1991).

Dependence and withdrawal.   Physical dependence on benzodiazepines can occur after treatment for months with therapeutic doses, especially with shorter-half-life compounds (Salzman 1991). On abrupt discontinuation, three kinds of syndromes may occur, all of which are more severe and prolonged in elderly patients with impaired central nervous systems (Busto et al. 1986; Noyes et al. 1988; Salzman 1991). Relapse (return of the original anxiety symptoms) occurs gradually over weeks to months in 60%–80% of chronically anxious patients. Rebound (an intensification of the original symptoms, lasting several days) occurs within hours to days in 25%–75% of patients. Withdrawal, which occurs within hours to a day or two of stopping short–half-life benzodiazepines and within days to weeks of discontinuing longer–half-life preparations,

TABLE 34–15. Some benzodiazepine anxiolytics in use in the United States

Medication	Starting dose (mg)[a]	Therapeutic dose (mg)[a]	Half-life (hours)	Comments
Midazolam	2.5	5–15	1–3	Used intravenously for agitation and orally for sleep. Use for anxiety in elderly patients not studied.
Lorazepam	0.5	0.5–4	12–18	Does not accumulate in elderly patients.
Alprazolam	0.25	0.25–2.0	17–24	Increased half-life in elderly patients. Has 2 active metabolites.
Oxazepam	10	10–90	10–14	Active metabolite of diazepam with no active metabolites of its own. Slow onset of action due to slow absorption.
Clonazepam	0.125	0.25–2	>100	Very sedating. Accumulates with long-term use.
Diazepam	2	2–10	75–90	Metabolized to desmethyldiazepam, active metabolite with half-life of 194 hours.
Chlordiazepoxide	5	20–40	30	Metabolized to desmethyldiazepam and desmethylchlordiazepoxide, both active.
Prazepam	5	10–15	} See diazepam	These 3 prodrugs (precursors) are demethylated to desmethyldiazepam, the major active metabolite.
Clorazepate	3.75	7.5–30		
Halazepam	5	10–40		

[a]Geriatric dose.

TABLE 34–16. Some neuropsychiatric side effects of benzodiazepines

Side effect	Manifestation(s)	Comments
Central nervous system depression	Sedation, paradoxical excitement, disinhibition, suspiciousness, agitation, aggression, wandering, ataxia, falls, delirium	Sedation persists up to 2 weeks after discontinuation of long–half-life benzodiazepines. Tolerance may develop with careful dosage increases. Long-acting benzodiazepines are most likely to produce falls, the most common cause of injury in elderly patients.
Cognitive dysfunction	Confusion, anterograde amnesia, dementia-like syndrome, aggravation of dementia	Rebound insomnia more common with triazolam and other very short half-life benzodiazepines; less common with alprazolam.
Psychomotor impairment	Impaired driving	Elderly neuropsychiatric patients more vulnerable to psychomotor impairment. Benzodiazepines implicated more frequently than alcohol or other medications in accidents involving elderly patients. Automobile accidents second most common cause of injury in elderly patients.
Electroencephalographic changes	Decreased alpha, increased low-voltage fast activity, especially in frontal regions	Depressed patients with increased REM density may develop nightmares or vivid dreams due to further increased REM by benzodiazepines.

Note.   REM = rapid eye movement.

adds to anxiety autonomic symptoms and new CNS symptoms such as confusion, tremor, and myoclonus. Withdrawal symptoms may be even more delayed and prolonged in older patients who continue to take benzodiazepines or other CNS depressants intermittently. Withdrawal after a single dose of a benzodiazepine with a very short half-life such as triazolam and midazolam may produce rebound anxiety, confusion, and amnesia, especially in patients with brain disease (Regestein 1992; Salzman 1992).

Special considerations. Benzodiazepines are obvious choices for treatment of anxious patients with epilepsy, but many geriatric patients with dementia, cerebellar disease, or psychomotor impairment tolerate these drugs poorly. Benzodiazepines are often more effective for and better tolerated in neuroleptic-induced akathisia than are antiparkinsonian drugs.

Chronic use of benzodiazepines can aggravate existing cognitive deficits in patients with dementia and cause dementia in neurologically intact patients. The use of these and all CNS depressants should, therefore, be reviewed before diagnosis or treatment of primary dementia.

Withdrawal from benzodiazepines and other CNS depressants can produce a variety of neuropsychiatric syndromes (Table 34–17) that are easily mistaken for neurological illness in elderly patients. These syndromes often appear when a new physician becomes concerned about a patient's use of tranquilizers and discontinues them, when the patient runs out of medication, or when the medication is abruptly discontinued after admission to a hospital or other facility. The latter problem often develops because a patient does not consider use of the benzodiazepine important enough to report it to the physician or conceals use of the drug out of shame or fear of the physician's disapproval. The doctor then underestimates the patient's drug intake.

Family members can be important sources of information about the patient's use of medications prescribed by other doctors or obtained over the counter. Toxicology screening is usually negative when an abstinence syndrome is present, but it may reveal unsuspected use of other substances.

Withdrawal from any combination of CNS depressants can be diagnosed with the barbiturate tolerance test (D. E. Smith and Wesson 1970); however, experience with this test in elderly patients has not been reported in the literature. Specific dosage guidelines have not been formally addressed in studies involving geriatric patients, but one recommendation would be that if phenobarbital is used, 45- to 60-mg doses should be taken on an empty stomach once signs of withdrawal appear. These doses should be repeated every 2–6 hours until intoxication begins to develop. Signs of withdrawal and/or intoxication (e.g., decreased level of consciousness, dysarthria, postural hypotension, hyperreflexia, hyporeflexia, and nystagmus) should be recorded before and 1 hour after each dose to determine the next dose. Once definite intoxication occurs, or when 300–500 mg of phenobarbital has been administered in a 24-hour period, the total amount is divided into four doses, given every 6 hours, and the phenobarbital is withdrawn by about 10% per day. Each specific dose is determined by the patient's overall course and the patient's response to the last dose. Phenobarbital often begins to accumulate after 4–8 days, and it may be necessary to withdraw the drug more rapidly at this point. A pentobarbital withdrawal protocol can also be used in elderly patients (Dubin et al. 1986), although seizures are more likely if an individual dose is missed.

Interactions. As indicated in Table 34–18, benzodiazepines have pharmacokinetic as well as pharmacodynamic interactions with medications in common use in neuropsychiatry (Salzman 1992).

Alternatives to benzodiazepines. The only currently available azapirone is buspirone, which is effective

TABLE 34–17. Manifestations of central nervous system depressant withdrawal

Anxiety, panic, insomnia, agitation, restlessness, irritability

Hypersensitivity to light and noise

Headache, dizziness, diaphoresis

Myalgia, tremor, muscle twitching

Fever

Tinnitus, seasickness

Amnesia

Psychosis

Delirium

Seizures

TABLE 34–18. Some benzodiazepine interactions

Medication(s)	Interaction(s)
Central nervous system depressants	Increased sedation, confusion, amnesia, and psychomotor impairment
Opioids	Increased respiratory depression
Cimetidine	Increased benzodiazepine levels
Anticonvulsants, adrenal steroids	Decreased benzodiazepine levels

for generalized anxiety in older as well as younger patients (Salzman 1992). Because buspirone does not impair cognition or psychomotor function (Hart et al. 1991), it is preferable to benzodiazepines for treating anxiety in patients with dementia. However, buspirone is not effective when given intermittently. The use of buspirone to reduce agitation in patients with dementia is discussed in a later section.

Buspirone, gepirone, and ipsapirone have been shown to have primary antidepressant properties in younger patients, but the high doses that are necessary (40–90 mg/day) are difficult for many geriatric patients to tolerate. More moderate doses (e.g., 10–40 mg/day) may augment the antidepressant or antiobsessional effect of antidepressants, the only adverse reactions of concern being headache, nausea, dizziness, and mild serotonin syndrome when azapirones are combined with highly serotonergic antidepressants such as fluoxetine. Because buspirone inhibits presynaptic dopamine autoreceptors, it may enhance dopaminergic transmission and therefore could be useful for some parkinsonian patients. The same effect could produce abnormal movements, but there is no reason this drug should cause tardive dyskinesia, given that it does not block postsynaptic dopamine receptors.

TCAs, even if they are not sedating, have been found to be as effective as benzodiazepines in the treatment of generalized anxiety disorder; in many studies it was not clear whether patients might also have been depressed, but depression was excluded in at least one study (Hoehn-Saric et al. 1988). Because relatively high doses of benzodiazepines may be necessary to treat panic disorder, antidepressants other than bupropion are more appropriate choices for patients with panic disorder complicated by neurological syndromes who would be expected to be sensitive to benzodiazepine adverse effects and discontinuation syndromes. Venlafaxine and the SSRIs can be effective for generalized anxiety and are better tolerated by older patients than are benzodiazepines and TCAs. All other antidepressants except bupropion have also been noted to have anxiolytic properties.

Antihistamines (e.g., hydroxyzine or diphenhydramine, at a dose of 10–25 mg one to four times per day) are frequently used as anxiolytics or sleeping pills in elderly patients with dementia (Ahronheim 1992; Salzman 1992). However, the antianxiety effect is unpredictable, and tolerance to the sedative effect usually occurs rapidly. In addition, anticholinergic side effects aggravate memory loss. The most appropriate use of antihistamines in geriatric neuropsychiatry may be for sedating a patient for electroencephalography, because they have minimal effects on this measure.

Antipsychotic Drugs

Antipsychotic drugs are effective for all forms of psychosis. Well-established indications include schizophrenia, bipolar disorder, and psychotic unipolar depression. In low doses, antipsychotic drugs can be helpful in psychiatric syndromes commonly encountered in geriatric neuropsychiatry such as hallucinations and delusions caused by neurological factors, paraphrenia, and late-onset paranoia (Young and Meyers 1991). Pimozide with or without antidepressants has been found effective for monosymptomatic hypochondriacal delusions and delusions of parasitosis (Dagon 1990). The use of antipsychotic drugs to control agitation in patients with neurological illness is discussed later in this chapter.

Neurological Uses

Antipsychotic drugs can be used to treat interictal psychoses (Dagon 1990), as can ECT (Dubovsky 1993). Low doses of most neuroleptics other than thioridazine can ameliorate nausea and vomiting caused by cancer chemotherapy, autonomic dysfunction, vestibular syndromes, and related conditions (Richelson 1985), although serotonin 5-HT$_3$ receptor antagonists such as ondansetron and granisetron are more effective and have fewer adverse effects (Dubovsky 1994). Low doses of chlorpromazine can stop intractable hiccups, and the phenothiazine trimeprazine, which does not have antipsychotic properties, is an antipruritic agent. Haloperidol and pimozide are often used to control chorea and other involuntary movements in Huntington's disease and Tourette syndrome. (The uses of neuroleptics in delirium and dementia are discussed later in this chapter.)

Available Preparations

The older antipsychotic drugs are neuroleptics (from the Greek for "to clasp the neuron") in that they control psychosis and produce neurological side effects. In neuropsychiatric practice, antipsychotic drugs do not differ in efficacy. Older patients with schizophrenia, like their younger counterparts, seem to respond better to lower than to higher neuroleptic doses (Weisbard et al. 1997). However, older patients with schizophrenia may have a different pattern of response to neuroleptics than younger patients, with more improvement of negative symptoms (Weisbard et al. 1997). Regardless of diagnosis, older patients with neurological illnesses have a greater risk of neurological side effects from neuroleptics. These adverse effects are less problematic with the newer atypical antipsychotic medications such as clozapine, risperidone, olanzapine, quetiapine, and ziprasidone because 5-HT$_2$ receptor antagonism ameliorates the motor effects of dopamine, subtype 2 (D$_2$, receptor blockade. Like younger patients, older patients tolerate the atypical antipsychotic drugs better and those patients with schizophrenia have greater improvement of negative symptoms with these drugs (Tamminga and Lahti 1996). Some characteristics of antipsychotic drugs as used in geriatric neuropsychiatry are summarized in Tables 34–19 and 34–20 (Ahronheim 1992; Lohr et al. 1992; Salzman 1990).

Metabolism and Dosing

As with other lipid-soluble medications in elderly patients, the volume of distribution of neuroleptics is increased and metabolism is slowed, resulting in a longer time to reach steady state and prolonged therapeutic as well as toxic effects (Lohr et al. 1992; Wragg and Jeste 1988). Reduced dopaminergic transmission in elderly patients may contribute to the development of neurological and antipsychotic effects at lower blood levels (Lohr et al. 1992). Some low-potency neuroleptics (e.g., chlorpromazine and

TABLE 34–19. Neuroleptic medications in use in the United States

Medication (by class)	Starting dose[a]	Usual dosage[a]	Comments
Phenothiazines			
Chlorpromazine	10 mg	10–300 mg/day	Many active metabolites from complex hepatic and gastrointestinal metabolism. Hypotension prohibits parenteral use in elderly patients.
Thioridazine	10 mg	10–300 mg/day	Use in elderly patients limited by anticholinergic and cardiac side effects.
Triflupromazine	10 mg	10–75 mg/day	Moderate sedation, hypotension, and extrapyramidal side effects.
Acetophenazine	10 mg	10–100 mg/day	Moderate sedation, hypotension, and extrapyramidal side effects.
Mesoridazine	10 mg	10–200 mg/day	Thioridazine metabolite. May be useful in some treatment-resistant psychoses.
Perphenazine	2 mg	4–20 mg/day	Midrange in potency and side effects.
Trifluoperazine	1 mg	2–15 mg/day	More extrapyramidal side effects than with perphenazine
Fluphenazine	0.25 mg	0.5–6 mg/day	Most potent phenothiazine.
Fluphenazine decanoate and enanthate	0.25 ml	0.25–0.5 ml every 2–3 weeks	Erratic absorption due to decreased muscle mass in elderly individuals.
Thioxanthenes			
Thiothixene	1 mg	1–15 mg/day	Similar to trifluoperazine in potency and side effects.
Chlorprothixene	10 mg	10–100 mg/day	Similar to chlorpromazine in potency and side effects.
Butyrophenones			
Haloperidol	0.25 mg	0.25–8 mg/day	Intramuscular dose poorly tolerated by elderly patients.
Diphenylbutyl-piperidines			
Pimozide	0.25 mg	0.25–4 mg/day	Calcium channel and dopamine, subtype 2 (D$_2$), receptor blocking properties. Useful for atypical psychoses, but high incidence of cardiotoxicity.
Dihydroindolones			
Molindone	5 mg	10–100 mg/day	Not associated with weight gain or seizures.
Dibenzoxazepines			
Loxapine	10 mg	10–100 mg/day	Metabolized to amoxapine. May have special applications in psychotic depression and schizophrenia with secondary depression.

[a]Geriatric dose/dosage.

TABLE 34–20. Atypical antipsychotic medications in use in the United States

Medication	Starting dose (mg)[a]	Usual daily dose (mg)[a]	Comments
Clozapine	12.5	50–450	Sedation, salivation, and weight gain difficult to tolerate. Neuroleptic malignant syndrome occasionally reported.
Risperidone	1	2–6	Extrapyramidal side effects more common than with clozapine.
Quetiapine	25	50–100	Unclear risk of eye damage.
Olanzapine	0.5	5–15	Weight gain in 50% of patients

[a]Geriatric dose.

thioridazine) induce their own metabolism and have complex metabolic pathways with many active metabolites, making them problematic in older patients. Butyrophenones and thioxanthenes appear to have only inactive metabolites (Ko et al. 1985). In a few studies of patients with Alzheimer's disease, the effective plasma concentration of haloperidol to control agitation and psychosis was less than the 4–18 ng/mL range thought to represent the therapeutic range for schizophrenia, although most patients with Alzheimer's disease cannot tolerate higher levels (Devanand et al. 1992).

In acutely ill younger patients, intramuscular injection of neuroleptics avoids first-pass metabolism and increases bioavailability. However, this form of administration is usually too painful and absorption of drugs administered by this route is too unpredictable in older patients, who have decreased muscle mass (Lohr et al. 1992; Wragg and Jeste 1988). (Intravenous use of neuroleptics is discussed later in this chapter.)

Neuropsychiatric Side Effects

Antipsychotic drugs are frequently prescribed for older patients with agitation or psychosis, but these patients are particularly vulnerable to neurological side effects, summarized in Table 34–21 (Ahronheim 1992; Almeida 1991; Lohr et al. 1992; Satlin et al. 1992; Wragg and Jeste 1988; Yassa et al. 1991; Young and Meyers 1991). Elderly patients with dementia are at increased risk for extrapyramidal side effects, possibly as a result of degenerative changes in nigrostriatal pathways, higher blood levels with a given dose, and longer duration of treatment with greater cumulative neuroleptic exposure (Young and Meyers 1991). Tremor, rigidity, and bradykinesia are more common side effects in older patients, whereas dystonia occurs less frequently than in younger patients (Young and Meyers 1991). Acute and chronic extrapyramidal side effects are less frequent with risperidone, olanzapine, quetiapine, and

zaprasidone and are almost unheard of with clozapine.

Tardive dyskinesia occurs in 20%–40% of elderly patients taking neuroleptics (Ereshefsky et al. 1989; Saltz et al. 1991; Yassa et al. 1991). The risk of tardive dyskinesia in older patients is higher in women and in patients with a history of acute extrapyramidal side effects, brain damage, longer neuroleptic exposure, mood disorder, medical illness, concurrent use of antiparkinsonian drugs, and drug holidays (Almeida 1991; Lohr et al. 1992). Tardive dyskinesia in elderly patients must be distinguished from oral movements due to loose dentures and from spontaneous dyskinesias, which occur in 0.22%–5% of elderly individuals who have not been exposed to neuroleptics (Green et al. 1993; Yassa et al. 1991), the higher prevalence occurring in patients with brain disease.

Whereas tardive dyskinesia eventually resolves after drug discontinuation in 80% of younger adults, remission after the neuroleptic is withdrawn occurs in only one-third to one-half of geriatric patients (Almeida 1991; Yassa et al. 1991; Young and Meyers 1991). The best strategy for dealing with tardive dyskinesia in older neurologically ill patients, therefore, is to reduce the risk of its occurrence. Useful approaches to achieving this goal include using the lowest possible dose and avoiding drug holidays, antiparkinsonian drugs, and rapid dose escalations (Wragg and Jeste 1988). Compared with traditional neuroleptics, the atypical antipsychotic drugs clozapine, risperidone, olanzapine, and quetiapine all have a lower incidence of extrapyramidal side effects and tardive dyskinesia in older as well as younger individuals (Casey 1997).

Several experimental treatments for tardive dyskinesia have been introduced, with variable success. Calcium channel blockers ameliorate dyskinetic movements in animals and humans but have not been studied extensively (Dubovsky 1986). Vitamin E has been thought to improve tardive dyskinesia in 21%–45% of patients in whom symptoms have been present for less than 5 years (Egan et al. 1992). However, in a 6-week double-blind, pla-

TABLE 34–21.   **Some neuropsychiatric side effects of antipsychotic drugs**

Side effect	Manifestations	Comments
Central nervous system depression	Sedation, confusion, and memory impairment.	Tolerance may develop within 1–3 weeks if dose is increased slowly.
α-Adrenergic blockade	Orthostatic hypotension.	May produce falls, especially in patients with extrapyramidal side effects.
	Priapism.	Especially with chlorpromazine and thioridazine. Not yet reported in elderly patients.
Akathisia	May be acute or tardive. Subjective report of restlessness may be impaired in elderly patients.	Most common neuroleptic-induced movement disorder. Treat with decreased neuroleptic dose or addition of β-blocker or benzodiazepine.
Parkinsonism	Tremor, rigidity, bradykinesia, stiffness, shuffling gait, salivation, and loss of postural reflexes.	Occurs in 75% of elderly patients. May cause falls. Try to decrease dose before adding antiparkinsonian drug. Amantadine may produce less anticholinergic toxicity than other antiparkinsonian drugs.
Dystonia	Spasm of face, neck, and extraocular muscles. Less frequent in elderly than in younger patients. Not dose related in elderly patients.	Treat with lower neuroleptic dose, anticholinergic drug (e.g., benztropine 0.5–1 mg), or diphenhydramine 25 mg.
Pisa syndrome	Dystonic reaction in which body is flexed to one side.	Responds to same treatment as for dystonia.
Rabbit syndrome	Tardive orofacial dyskinesia with 5-Hz lip movements resembling rabbit chewing.	Responds to anticholinergic medications.
Tardive dyskinesia	Orofacial movements most common in elderly patients. Next in order of frequency are movements of feet, neck, shoulders, trunk, diaphragm, pharynx, and intercostal muscles. May be associated with cognitive impairment in elderly schizophrenic patients.	Acute extrapyramidal side effects may predict later tardive dyskinesia in geriatric patients. Tardive dyskinesia is more frequent and more persistent in elderly patients.
Catatonia	Waxy flexibility, catalepsy, negativism, mutism, staring, echolalia, and echopraxia.	Responds to withdrawal of neuroleptic and to amantadine or antiparkinsonian drugs.
Neuroleptic malignant syndrome	Extrapyramidal signs and dysfunction. Rigidity, dystonia, tremor, fever, tachycardia, unstable blood pressure, diaphoresis, increased serum creatine phosphokinase and white blood cell count, and myoglobinuria.	Has been reported in elderly as well as in younger patients.
Seizures	Spontaneous seizures or lowered seizure threshold.	Most frequent with clozapine, loxapine, and low-potency neuroleptics. Older patients more susceptible to seizures, especially patients with history of seizures, central nervous system disease, or recent electroconvulsive therapy.
Photosensitivity	Increased sensitivity of skin and eyes to sun. May persist for months after drug is discontinued.	May sensitize eyes to toxic effects of sun or bright light.
Pigmentary retinopathy	Irreversible pigment deposition in retina.	With daily doses of thioridazine of > 800 mg.
Syndrome of inappropriate secretion of antidiuretic hormone (SIADH)	Hyponatremia may produce confusion or seizures.	Water retention may be aggravated by additional direct effect of neuroleptic on kidney.
Hypothermia	Temperature dysregulation that does not progress to neuroleptic malignant syndrome.	Especially with clozapine and phenothiazines in hypothyroid patients.
Electrocardiographically demonstrated side effects	Electrocardiographic changes, sudden death rare.	Thioridazine and pimozide.

cebo-controlled study of the effects of 1,600 IU of vitamin E daily in 18 patients, one-third of whom were older than 53 years, meaningful improvement was found in only a few (Egan et al. 1992). Clozapine, which is technically not a neuroleptic, reduced tardive dyskinesia by 50% or more in 43% of cases, with the greatest efficacy occurring in tardive dystonia and severe tardive dyskinesia (Lieberman et al. 1991). This effect does not appear to represent temporary masking of tardive dyskinesia with eventual exacerbation of the syndrome, as occurs with neuroleptics.

Neuroleptic malignant syndrome, which has been reported in 0.5%–1.0% of patients taking neuroleptics (Guze and Baxter 1985), has been associated most frequently with high-potency neuroleptics but has also been reported with low-potency neuroleptics, clozapine, metoclopramide, carbidopa-levodopa, and withdrawal of amantadine and carbidopa-levodopa (Mueller 1985; Pelonero et al. 1985). Older patients seem to be somewhat less vulnerable to neuroleptic malignant syndrome, but the risk is increased in the elderly population by brain damage, other forms of neurological disease, and debilitation (Mueller 1985). Waiting more than 2 weeks before readministering neuroleptics after an episode of neuroleptic malignant syndrome, using low doses of low-potency neuroleptics of a different class, and carefully monitoring vital signs, mental status, and extrapyramidal side effects may decrease the risk of another episode of neuroleptic malignant syndrome (Rosebush and Stewart 1989).

Although neuroleptic malignant syndrome can occur with clozapine, it is much less frequent than it is with neuroleptics (Kane et al. 1988). However, clozapine is difficult to administer to elderly patients with neuropsychiatric illness for several reasons. The risk of agranulocytosis may increase with age, especially in Ashkenazi Jews (Gelenberg 1992). In addition, sedation, orthostatic hypotension, hypersalivation, hyperthermia, and akathisia are common side effects (Wilson 1992). The manufacturer-reported incidence of seizures with clozapine is 1%–2% at doses less than 300 mg/day and 4%–6% at doses of 300–600 mg/day. The manufacturer has reported 9 (incidence of 1 in 3,000 patients) nonfatal cases of respiratory or cardiac arrest with clozapine, in some instances in patients who were also taking benzodiazepines. Slower dose titration of clozapine is associated with better long-term results (Chengappa et al. 1995).

Special Considerations

Treatment with neuroleptics of behavioral problems associated with delirium and dementia are considered in later sections of this chapter (see also Chapters 19, 23, and 24).

Clozapine, loxapine, and low-potency neuroleptics should not be administered to patients with seizure disorders; haloperidol and molindone may be safer for such patients (Fenwick 1989). Because dopamine blockade by neuroleptics increases prolactin levels, great caution is necessary when these medications are administered to patients with prolactin-secreting pituitary tumors or, possibly, a history of breast cancer. Prolactinemia occurs more frequently with risperidone than with olanzapine.

Agitation and psychosis in patients with Parkinson's disease may be related to dementia or to toxicity of dopaminergic drugs (see also Chapter 26). If changing the medication does not relieve psychosis, administering clozapine at dosages of 6.25–275 mg/day can be effective (Bajulaize and Addonizio 1992; Lohr et al. 1992), even if dopamine agonists are continued (Wolk and Douglas 1992). Patients with Parkinson's disease tolerate neuroleptics poorly, but atypical antipsychotic drugs are sometimes useful. ECT may improve the neurological illness as well as the psychosis (Dubovsky 1993) (see also Chapter 35).

Interactions

Antipsychotic agents interact with many neurological and cardiovascular drugs. Some examples are listed in Table 34–22 (Ayd 1986; Bailey et al. 1992; Dagon 1990; Kahn et al. 1990; D. D. Miller 1991; Rizos et al. 1988; Sargenti et al. 1988; Sassim and Grohmann 1988).

Alternatives to Antipsychotic Drugs

In neurologically ill patients with catatonia; mania; depression; schizoaffective, schizophreniform, or some schizophrenic psychoses (Van Valkenberg and Clayton 1983); or delirium (Dubovsky 1993), ECT can be more rapidly effective and better tolerated than neuroleptics (see also Chapter 35). When neuroleptics are necessary, benzodiazepines, reserpine, baclofen, or droperidol may augment the antiagitation (but not the antipsychotic) effect, reducing the amount of neuroleptic needed for behavioral control (Bodkin 1990; Richelson 1985). Benzodiazepines alone may ameliorate catatonia (Fricchione 1989).

▌ Treatment of Insomnia

Complaints of disturbed sleep are more common in elderly patients than in younger patients (Spiegel 1990). Some complaints reflect diminished efficiency and more frequent interruptions of sleep (see also Chapter 17). A Dutch

TABLE 34–22.   Some antipsychotic drug interactions

Medication(s)	Interaction(s)
Central nervous system depressants	Increased sedation, confusion, falls
Guanethidine	Decreased antihypertensive effect
Lithium	Increased extrapyramidal side effects
Anticholinergic antiparkinsonian drugs, cimetidine, antacids	Decreased neuroleptic levels caused by inhibition of gastrointestinal absorption
Anticonvulsants	Decreased neuroleptic levels caused by increased metabolism
Tricyclic antidepressants	Increased levels of both; clinically significant only for tricyclic antidepressant
Levodopa	Decreased antiparkinsonian effect due to dopamine receptor blockade
Propranolol	Increased levels of both classes
Benzodiazepines	Physical collapse with clozapine
Carbamazepine	Increased risk of fatal bone marrow suppression with clozapine

study of 1,485 elderly individuals (Middelkoop et al. 1996) found that women had more trouble getting to sleep, had more interrupted sleep, and used sedative-hypnotics more frequently, whereas men complained of more daytime sleepiness. Worrying and nocturia were the most common causes of insomnia in this study. In other cases, neurological or medical disorders disrupt sleep (Regestein 1992; Salzman 1992; Spiegel 1990). Dementia and delirium are associated with reversal or fragmentation of the sleep-wake cycle, more awakenings, and decreased total, stage 4, and REM sleep. These changes are aggravated by sleeping pills and other CNS depressants but may be corrected by entrainment to normal light-dark cycles. Alzheimer's disease is associated with reversal of the sleep-wake cycle, and residence in long-term care facilities increases the risk of disordered sleep in older patients (Gottlieb 1990). Grief, depression, and anxiety are common causes of disturbed sleep in elderly patients that respond to specific therapies. Medical and neurological causes of insomnia in elderly patients include dementia with sundowning, chronic pain, nocturnal myoclonus, restless legs syndrome, sleep apnea, and gastroesophageal reflux. Many psychoactive substances

used by geriatric patients can produce insomnia (Table 34–23).

Although geriatric patients often request a drug for insomnia, frequently the best approach is to stop medications the patient is already taking, especially sleeping pills. Up to one-third of elderly people and 20%–40% of patients in intermediate care facilities take benzodiazepine sleeping pills regularly. However, these drugs lose their effectiveness after 20–30 days, after which time they are taken to prevent withdrawal insomnia. Sleep architecture may remain abnormal for some time after the hypnotic is withdrawn.

The initial approach to geriatric insomnia should include discontinuing substances such as caffeine and alcohol that disrupt sleep and treating illnesses that cause insomnia. Patients should improve sleep hygiene through such measures as increasing daytime activity, arising at the same time each morning, keeping the room at a comfortable temperature, setting aside a time to review the day's activities before getting into bed, and not spending time in bed when not asleep.

When these measures are not effective, a hypnotic medication may be appropriate. Benzodiazepine sleeping pills are best used for time-limited insomnia in reaction to identifiable stress; when these medications are to be given chronically, intermittent dosing may prolong their effectiveness. Short–half-life benzodiazepines (Table 34–24) (Greenblatt et al. 1991; Johnson et al. 1990; Regestein 1992; Salzman 1990; Spiegel 1990) do not accumulate in elderly patients, but they may produce early-morning awakening and rebound insomnia when used for more than 1–2 weeks. Longer–half-life preparations are more likely to produce daytime sedation and psychomotor impairment (Dubovsky 1993). In the standard geriatric dose (0.125 mg) triazolam does not appear to aggravate memory loss in patients with Alzheimer's disease, but it also seems not to be effective for disrupted sleep in these patients (McCarten et al. 1995).

Quazepam, a new hypnotic that is selective for the

TABLE 34–23.   Substances that cause sleep disturbances in elderly individuals

Caffeine (stimulant effect lasts 12–20 hours)
Nicotine
Alcohol
Activating antidepressants
Diuretics
Antiarrhythmics
β-Blockers
Chronic use of sleeping pills

TABLE 34–24. Benzodiazepine hypnotics

Medication	Dose (mg)	Half-life (hours)	Comments
Triazolam	0.125[a]	2–5	Clearance reduced in elderly. Even lowest dose may produce next-day anxiety, agitation, anterograde amnesia, irritability, and insomnia.
Midazolam	5–15	1–3	Minimal psychomotor impairment.
Temazepam	10–30	10–20	Higher doses occasionally helpful for some treatment-resistant patients. Peak plasma levels occur 1 hour after ingestion.
Flurazepam	15	100–200	Not recommended for elderly patients because of accumulation and central nervous system depression.
Quazepam	7.5–15	Not studied in elderly patients	Parent drug is selective for benzodiazepine type 1 receptor but desalkylflurazepam metabolite is nonselective and has long half-life.
Estazolam	0.5–1	Not studied in elderly patients	Similar to other high-potency benzodiazepines (e.g., triazolam).
Zolpidem	5–10	3–6	Nonbenzodiazepine structure but acts on benzodiazepine type 1 receptor. Less cognitive impairment than with benzodiazepines.

[a]This dose effective in older but not younger adults.

benzodiazepine type 1 receptor, should not produce as much daytime sedation, as much impairment of memory and psychomotor function (attributed in part to benzodiazepine type 2 receptors), or as many withdrawal syndromes (attributed in part to peripheral-type benzodiazepine receptors) as nonselective benzodiazepines. However, quazepam is metabolized to desalkylflurazepam, a nonselective flurazepam metabolite that accumulates with chronic treatment. Zolpidem, a benzodiazepine type 1 receptor selective agonist sleeping pill, has not yet been found to have a nonselective metabolite that might complicate continued treatment. In a study of zolpidem in geriatric insomnia, 5- and 10-mg doses were found to be equally effective, and both doses were as effective as 0.25 mg of triazolam (Roger et al. 1993). Given that confusion occurred only in patients taking triazolam and additional experience supports the finding of a lack of cognitive impairment with zolpidem (Scharf et al. 1991), zolpidem may be the first choice among medications acting on benzodiazepine receptors for geriatric insomnia.

Of the available alternatives to benzodiazepines for the treatment of insomnia in geriatric neuropsychiatry (Regestein 1992; Spiegel 1990; Salzman 1990), sedating antidepressants (e.g., trazodone or nefazodone, in doses of 25–75 mg) are most reliable, even in patients who are not depressed. However, these drugs may cause daytime hangover and sedation in older patients with neuropsychiatric illness. Antihistamines (e.g., diphenhydramine, in doses of 25–50 mg) can be useful sedatives in patients with pruritis, but in patients with brain disease, they may produce bothersome anticholinergic side effects and daytime sedation that increase impairment of memory and psychomotor performance. Aspirin at dosages of 325–650 mg/day can have mild hypnotic effects in some patients and may counteract sleep disruption caused by adrenal steroids and bronchodilators. In contrast, over-the-counter sleeping pills, which are frequently used by elderly patients, are not particularly effective and cause daytime sedation and have anticholinergic effects (Balter and Uhlenhuth 1991).

Treatment of Delirium

Agitation due to delirium in elderly patients requires urgent intervention when the patient is at risk of injury, dehydration, cardiovascular collapse, or gross noncompliance with essential medical therapy (see also Chapter 19). Emergency pharmacotherapy in such situations has never been the subject of controlled studies, but clinical experience has accumulated with a number of intravenous medications, particularly haloperidol, benzodiazepines, and droperidol. As discussed in Chapter 35, one to four ECT treatments can rapidly ameliorate delirium of virtually any etiology (Dubovsky 1995). The barbiturate tolerance test discussed earlier should be considered before any other treatment when delirium could be the result of withdrawal from CNS depressants.

Intravenous haloperidol can be useful for treating severe agitation in delirium patients. Therapy is started with a 1- to 5-mg dose. For patients of mixed ages on a coronary care unit, Tesar et al. (1985) recommended increasing haloperidol doses rapidly to 30–75 mg and administering them as frequently as necessary to control agitation. In patients who are unresponsive to repeated intravenous doses of haloperidol, an intravenous haloperidol drip at 5–25 mg/hour may be effective (Fernandez et al. 1988). Although extrapyramidal side effects are common with intramuscular administration of haloperidol, they are relatively rare with the intravenous route (Fernandez et al. 1988).

In their work with delirium patients with metastatic cancer of the brain, many of whom were elderly, Adams et al. (1986) first administered 3 mg of intravenous haloperidol and then followed with 0.5–1.0 mg of lorazepam. If the patient did not improve within 20 minutes, 5–10 mg of haloperidol was combined with or followed by 2–10 mg of lorazepam; individual doses of haloperidol did not exceed 10 mg. When pain was believed to contribute to delirium, Fernandez et al. (1988) added 0.5–4.0 mg of hydromorphone to each dose of the other intravenous medications. Patients unresponsive to other treatments have had amobarbital added to intravenous haloperidol and lorazepam, surprisingly without disinhibition or respiratory suppression (Adams et al. 1986). Hypercortisolemia, hypoxemia, and hypothyroidism may contribute to resistance to intravenous haloperidol or lorazepam (Adams et al. 1986).

According to these investigators, one of these regimens usually ameliorates severe agitation within 90 minutes. Many patients need no further treatment, whereas some require additional intravenous or oral doses of 5–10 mg of haloperidol, possibly augmented with 0.5 mg of lorazepam (Adams 1988; Fernandez et al. 1988). The longest reported duration of intravenous therapy was 3 months, in a terminally ill patient with an intractable behavioral disorder.

Through a survey of British practitioners, Pilowsky et al. (1992) found that initial intravenous doses of 10–60 mg of haloperidol per day or 10–80 mg of diazepam per day, followed by 20–40 mg of haloperidol and/or 10–40 mg of diazepam, respectively, were used most frequently for uncontrollable agitation in neurological and primary psychiatric illness. Intravenous droperidol, a butyrophenone used as an anesthetic, has also been found to be an effective antiagitation agent in delirium (Pilowsky et al. 1992; Szuba et al. 1992). Droperidol, which is associated with an 8% incidence of extrapyramidal side effects in emergency dosing, has higher potency, more rapid onset of action, and a shorter half-life than does haloperidol (Szuba et al. 1992). In an average dose of 7 mg, droperidol is equally effective intramuscularly with an equally low incidence of extrapyramidal syndromes, making it an appealing choice for patients who are so agitated or have such fragile veins

that intravenous dosing is not practical.

The tranquilizing effect of midazolam, a lipophilic high-potency benzodiazepine, occurs quickly with intravenous doses of 5–15 mg, and rapid elimination prevents accumulation and excessive sedation (Bond et al. 1989). Intravenous midazolam controls violent and self-destructive behavior in mentally retarded younger patients (Bond et al. 1989) (see also Chapter 21) but has not been studied in the geriatric population. Amnesia after a single intravenous dose is common, but this is not an issue for delirious patients.

Treatment of Lethal Catatonia

ECT is the treatment of choice for lethal catatonia, an unusual syndrome of catatonia, neurological signs, and fever (Mann et al. 1986) (see also Chapter 35). Intravenous dantrolene was helpful for two elderly patients taking imipramine or diazepam who developed catatonia, leukocytosis, and fever (Pennati et al. 1991). Because of the possible relationship of lethal catatonia to extrapyramidal syndromes, neuroleptics should not be administered.

Treatment of Problem Behaviors in Dementia Patients

Agitation is a nonspecific term for a group of disruptive behaviors that range from verbal perseveration, yelling, cursing, biting, and screaming to wandering, pacing, disinhibition, sexually inappropriate behavior, property destruction, and unpredictable attacks on self and others (Lantz and Marin 1996) (see also Chapter 22). The incidence of agitation in elderly residents of nursing homes and among patients with Alzheimer's disease ranges from 32% to 85% (Chandler and Chandler 1998; Yudofsky et al. 1997). More than half of a community sample of patients with dementia were verbally disruptive, and 45% were physically aggressive (Cohen-Mansfield 1989). The onset of agitation frequently leads to nursing home admission (Cohen-Mansfield 1995).

OBRA mandated that specific target behaviors be documented when neuroleptics are used for agitation in elderly patients (Yeager 1995). These behaviors must be dangerous or functionally impairing if they are to be treated pharmacologically, and attempts should be made at least every 6 months to taper medications unless there are compelling clinical reasons not to attempt drug withdrawal. Documenting agitation and its response to treatment can be difficult because agitation is often intermittent and subject to numerous environmental variables (Cohen-Mansfield 1995; Cohen-Mansfield et al. 1992). Obtaining 1-month baseline scores on an agitation scale (Overt Agitation Scale; Yudofsky et al. 1997) and then quantitatively tracking response over time permits clinicians to determine whether there is any measurable correlation of symptoms with intervention (Mulsant et al. 1997). The Overt Agitation Severity Scale is a reliable and valid instrument that can be easily and effectively used over a 15-minute observation period (Yudofsky et al. 1997). Some clinicians prefer individualized instruments using target symptoms developed in concert with staff members or family members who will be applying the ratings. However, global scores are less accurate than specific behavioral ratings in estimating the benefits of an intervention (Mulsant et al. 1997).

Before instituting drug therapy for agitation, it is important to address physiological, environmental, and psychiatric factors (Malone et al. 1993) that may cause or contribute to agitation (Table 34–25). It is particularly important to withdraw medications that may be disinhibiting, especially benzodiazepines. In addition to aggravating confusion, these medications cause hypotension, falls, and withdrawal syndromes and are poor choices as treatments for agitation in elderly patients (Mustard and Mayer 1997; "Practice Guideline" 1997). Useful behavioral interventions include keeping a clock and calendar in the room; providing a predictable routine; regular reorientation of the patient; encouraging concrete, repetitive conversations; reducing complex tasks like bathing to a series of steps; not confronting memory lapses and delusions; and installing locks that are difficult to operate, so that wandering is reduced. An ingenious approach was used with one patient who kept pulling fire alarms in her nursing home, apparently responding to the word *PULL* printed on the switches in bold type. Putting signs that said "Not You, Gladys!" on all alarms stopped this behavior (L. Robbins, personal communication, February 1998).

Neuroleptics

Molchan and Little (1995) reviewed 24 studies involving 2,200 patients with dementia and found that delusions were present in 11%–73% of patients, hallucinations occurred in 3%–67%, misidentifications of persons or places occurred in 5%–30%, and unspecified psychotic features were present in 5%–50%. However, psychosis is an uncommon cause of aggressive behavior in this population (Deutsch and Bylsma 1991). Most of the time, nonspecific sedative effects of antipsychotic drugs result in, at best, a modest and transient reduction in agitation and aggression

in patients with dementia who do not have a comorbid primary psychosis (Risse and Barnes 1986; Schneider and Sobin 1992).

In a review of 20 controlled studies of neuroleptics that included a total of 1,207 patients with dementia, Sunderland and Silver (1998) found that 60% of patients had positive short-term clinical outcomes; no neuroleptic appeared more efficacious than any other. However, after conducting a meta-analysis of all double-blind, placebo-controlled, parallel-group studies of neuroleptics in dementia from 1960 to 1982, Schneider and Pollock (1990) concluded that the benefit from neuroleptics was only 18% greater than that from placebo. In more recent double-blind comparisons in agitated patients with dementia, improvement with haloperidol, the most frequently ad-

TABLE 34–25. **Common causes of agitation in patients with dementia**

Medications
Sedative-hypnotics
Anxiolytics
Antihistamines
Antibiotics
Antihypertensives
Any medication, including aspirin

Intercurrent medical disorders
Sleep deprivation
Delirium
Urinary tract infection
Pneumonia
Hypoxemia
Sleep apnea
Subdural hematoma
Chronic pain

Intercurrent psychiatric disorders
Major depression
Bipolar disorder
Panic disorder
Psychotic disorders
Accentuation of maladaptive character traits

Environmental factors
Change of surroundings or roommate
Power struggles with family or staff
Frustration (catastrophic reaction)
Change of staff or personnel
Overstimulating or understimulating environment
Abuse by caretakers

ministered neuroleptic, was no greater than with oxazepam, diphenhydramine, or trazodone (Coccaro et al. 1990; Sultzer et al. 1997). Such results suggest that any benefit from neuroleptics may be attributable to nonspecific sedating and tranquilizing actions. In addition, the best results with neuroleptics have been obtained in shorter studies (R. Levy 1996), which conclude before there has been a chance for tolerance to the sedative effect to develop. In the long term, neuroleptics do not even influence the course of psychotic symptoms in patients with dementia, probably because such symptoms fluctuate spontaneously over time (Ballard and O'Brien 1997). Further, more than 20% of neuroleptic-treated dementia patients exhibit increased confusion and motor symptoms (Goldstein and Birnbom 1976; G. R. Smith et al. 1974).

The risk of tardive dyskinesia is five to six times greater in older individuals with dementia than in younger dementia patients (Jeste et al. 1996). In addition, neuroleptics may have adverse effects on cognitive function. In a prospective 2-year study of 71 patients with dementia, the mean decrease in cognitive scores was twice as great among the 16 patients who took neuroleptics as it was among patients not treated with these drugs ($P = .002$), and the rate of cognitive decline increased after neuroleptic therapy was begun (McShane et al. 1997). Cortical Lewy bodies on autopsy did not explain the differences between neuroleptic-treated and non–neuroleptic-treated patients. Although another autopsy study showed no correlation between neuroleptic use in 7 schizophrenic patients and the development of Alzheimer's pathology (Niizato and Ikeda 1996), additional clinical experience has reinforced the impression that neuroleptics can impair cognition as well as motor function (Ahronheim 1992; Risse and Barnes 1986; Wragg and Jeste 1988). Even if neuroleptics do not hasten cognitive deterioration, the risks of chronic neuroleptic therapy outweigh the benefits for most patients with dementia without comorbid primary psychotic illnesses.

Is it possible to withdraw neuroleptics in some patients as OBRA mandates and scientific data warrant? In a double-blind study of 22 patients with dementia, neuroleptic withdrawal was possible without any significant increase in aggression (Bridges-Parlet et al. 1997). Werner et al. (1994) performed a retrospective review of psychotropic medication use in 88 nursing home residents ages 66–102 years whose physical restraints were removed. These investigators found that neuroleptic use decreased, probably as a result of closer observation and interaction with the patients. Agitation has been shown to decrease and cognitive function to increase in nursing home patients in whom neuroleptic therapy was discontinued after educational interventions with the staff (Rovner et al. 1996).

Atypical Antipsychotic Drugs

Unlike the typical neuroleptics, atypical antipsychotic drugs with serotonin 5-HT$_2$ receptor antagonist properties have a specific antiaggressive effect that can be useful in patients with dementia, even if they are not psychotic (Dubovsky 1994). A lower incidence of extrapyramidal side effects makes these medications better tolerated by psychotic or agitated patients with Parkinson's disease because they are not as likely to cause extrapyramidal side effects. Because patients with parkinsonism and hallucinations have lower Mini-Mental State Exam (MMSE) scores and are more likely to require nursing home placement (Klein et al. 1997), finding a medication to manage agitation in these patients is a common and important challenge.

Risperidone is the best studied of the atypical antipsychotic drugs in elderly patients. Of 26 elderly patients without dementia (mean age, 70.4 years), 24 of whom had psychotic disorders and two of whom had bipolar disorder, 77% had moderate or marked improvement with a mean risperidone dose of 3.8 mg/day (Sajatovic et al. 1996). Extrapyramidal side effects occurred in only 4 patients. In a review of the use of risperidone in 122 hospitalized elderly patients, 53% of whom were treated for agitation or psychosis associated with dementia, Zarate et al. (1997) found the mean dose to be 1.6 mg/day. The drug appeared to be effective in 85% of cases. Patients undergoing rapid dose increases were more likely to discontinue risperidone because of adverse effects. Although 11% of patients developed extrapyramidal side effects with risperidone, 40% of patients experiencing preexisting extrapyramidal side effects with other neuroleptics were able to discontinue their use of antiparkinsonian agents after risperidone therapy was started.

In other case series, dosages of risperidone have ranged from 0.5 to 6 mg/day, for treatment of various forms of agitation, aggression, and screaming in patients with dementia due to Alzheimer's disease, cerebrovascular disease, and Lewy body dementia (Goldberg and Goldberg 1997; Herrmann et al. 1997; Jeanblanc and Davis 1995; Kopala and Honer 1997; Madhusoodanan et al. 1995; Raheja et al. 1995). In a double-blind, placebo-controlled trial of risperidone (Marder 1998), 625 dementia patients with Alzheimer's disease, vascular dementia, or mixed dementia were randomized to treatment with risperidone (0.5, 1, or 2 mg/day) or placebo (at the same dosages) for 12 weeks. Patients receiving 1 or 2 mg of risperidone per day showed significant improvement in psychosis as well as in severity and frequency of aggressive behaviors. Side effects were no more frequent than with the 1-mg dose of placebo but were significantly more frequent than with placebo at the 2-mg dose. Although risperidone is more expensive than conventional neuroleptics per dose, decreased hospital costs may make it a cost-effective treatment, at least in the treatment of schizophrenia (Aronson 1997).

It has been suggested that olanzapine, whose side effect profile is similar to that of risperidone, will be equally well tolerated and effective in patients with dementia or parkinsonism (Fava 1997; Glazer 1997). Although there are no published controlled studies of olanzapine in psychotic or agitated patients with dementia or Parkinson's disease, clinical experience suggests that this medication may be a reasonable alternative to risperidone in such patients. An advantage of olanzapine is that it has few interactions with other medications often prescribed for elderly patients (Ereshefsky 1996).

Despite the increased risk of confusion and orthostatic hypotension in elderly patients (Lake et al. 1997; Thorpe 1997), clozapine has been found to be useful for older patients with psychosis (Frankenburg and Kalunian 1994) or mania (R. W. Shulman et al. 1997). Patients ages 55–64 years may have a greater likelihood of benefit than patients 65 and over (Sajatovic et al. 1997). Clozapine at dosages of 6.25–75 mg/day has also been found to be effective in a number of patients with dementia or Parkinson's disease without increasing movement disorders (Pitner et al. 1995; Valldeoriola et al. 1997). In a prospective open-label study of 12 patients with psychosis associated with Parkinson's disease, Chacko et al. (1995) found significant improvement in psychosis and behavior in all patients and sustained improvement in 10 patients. Probably as a result of slow dose titration, clozapine was well tolerated in this study. In another prospective open trial of clozapine (Factor et al. 1994), involving administration to 17 patients with Parkinson's disease and psychosis at dosages ranging from 6.25 mg every other day to 150 mg/day, marked improvement of psychosis was observed during the first year, without any increase in the severity of the movement disorder. Improvement was not statistically significant during the second year of treatment, possibly because the benefits of clozapine were obscured by the effects of increasing doses of levodopa and by progression of dementia, part of the natural course of the illness. Agitated patients with dementia or parkinsonism and prominent psychosis or aggression that has proven nonresponsive to other interventions are appropriate candidates for treatment with clozapine (Salzman 1996).

Anticonvulsants

Anticonvulsants may be particularly useful in patients with dementia and comorbid mood disorders or with EEGs showing abnormalities (Fava 1997). Tariot et al. (1994) studied 17 patients with Alzheimer's disease and 8 patients with vascular dementia in a double-blind crossover study consisting of two 5-week periods of treatment with carbamazepine or placebo, each period separated by a 2-week washout interval. The mean carbamazepine dose was 300 mg/day, with a mean serum level of 5.7 μg/mL. The condition of 16 patients taking carbamazepine was considered to have improved, compared with the condition of 4 patients in the placebo group. Carbamazepine was generally well tolerated. Encouraged by their initial trial, Tariot and colleagues (1998) performed a 6-week multisite, randomized, placebo-controlled, double-blind, parallel-group trial involving 51 nursing home patients with agitation and dementia and using similar carbamazepine doses. The study was terminated after a planned interim analysis showed that carbamazepine was more beneficial than placebo (agitation and aggression were reduced in 77% of patients taking carbamazepine and 21% of those taking placebo). Although it is often well tolerated and effective, carbamazepine has the potential for interactions with many of the medications often taken by older patients.

Narayan and Nelson (1997) performed a retrospective chart review and reported that 56% of 25 agitated patients with dementia had improvement of behavioral disturbances with divalproex alone or in addition to neuroleptics (mean divalproex level, 1,650 mg/day). Only 1 patient had an increase in confusion. In a prospective open trial (Mellow et al. 1993), 50 of 88 patients had at least a partial response and 40 patients had moderate to marked benefit. Dosages ranged from 375 to 2,500 mg/day, and side effects were minimal. Although it may help patients sleep, valproate therapy in elderly patients has been associated with oversedation, parkinsonism, and reversible dementia (Walstra et al. 1997). No case series have been reported in which agitated patients with dementia were treated with gabapentin or lamotrigine. Although these new anticonvulsants may prove useful for some patients, experience with younger patients with brain damage suggests that these medications may be overstimulating in older patients with dementia, resulting in aggression (Anderson et al. 1996; Beran and Gibson 1998).

Antidepressants

In reviewing eight case reports and open trials, Tariot et al. (1997) found that 75–400 mg of trazodone per day improved agitation and aggression in 42 of 56 patients with dementia (44 with Alzheimer's disease and 12 with other causes of dementia). Sultzer et al. (1997) found trazodone to be as effective overall as haloperidol in 28 agitated patients with dementia. Trazodone caused sedation and balance problems in two patients but was better tolerated than haloperidol. In a placebo-controlled, double-blind trial comparing buspirone at dosages of 30 mg/day with trazodone dosages of 150 mg/day for 4 weeks in 10 patients with Alzheimer's disease, Lawlor et al. (1994) found that trazodone produced greater reductions in agitation, psychosis, and hostility. Experience with trazodone as a hypnotic suggests that it would be an appropriate treatment for agitated patients with dementia and disrupted sleep (Devanand 1997). Nefazodone, whose combined serotonin reuptake and 5-HT$_2$ antagonist properties might suggest the potential to reduce agitation and psychosis, has not been studied for these indications. Nefazodone shares with trazodone a metabolite that may reduce agitation in some patients with dementia (Lawlor et al. 1991).

Substances that enhance serotonergic transmission dampen unpredictable, impulsive aggressive behaviors of the kind that occur in patients with dementia (Dubovsky 1994). In relatively low doses, SSRIs in open trials have reduced stereotypical and aggressive behavior in elderly patients with dementia (Trappler and Vinuela 1997). Fluoxetine, sertraline, and paroxetine were found to reduce disinhibition, compulsive behavior, and depressive symptoms in patients with frontotemporal dementia (Swartz et al. 1997). Additional case series and open trials have demonstrated improvement in agitation with all available SSRIs, although well-controlled studies are lacking (Flint 1994; Herrmann and Lanctot 1997; Karlsson 1996; Lebert et al. 1994; Omar et al. 1995; Schneider and Sobin 1992). Drug interactions are important considerations. Metabolism of tacrine, which is primarily by cytochrome P450 1A2, may be increased substantially by fluvoxamine, which inhibits 1A2 (Becquemont et al. 1997). On the other hand, levels of donepezil, which is metabolized by cytochrome P450 2D6 and 3A4, may be increased by fluoxetine, paroxetine, and nefazodone.

Selegiline (L-deprenyl), an MAOI with antioxidant properties that may slow cognitive deterioration, has been noted to reduce agitation in some patients with dementia. However, other antidepressants are better tolerated and easier to administer to agitated patients.

Buspirone

In two open trials, 15–60 mg of buspirone per day significantly improved agitation in 10 of 26 patients with mixed dementias (Herrmann and Eryavec 1993). In a blinded trial comparing 15 mg of buspirone per day with 1.5 mg of haloperidol per day in 26 nursing home patients with Alzheimer's disease, both groups improved, but a greater reduction

of tension and anxiety occurred in the buspirone-treated patients (Cantillon et al. 1996). After a 1-week placebo washout interval, 2 weeks of treatment with 30 mg of buspirone per day improved delusions and anxiety as well as agitation in 12 patients with Alzheimer's disease (M. A. Levy et al. 1994). In an open study of 10 Alzheimer's disease patients (Sakauye et al. 1993), reduction of agitation began at a dose of 35 mg of buspirone per day and was maximal at a dose of 60 mg. Buspirone is well tolerated by patients with dementia (Markovitz 1993; Zayas and Grossberg 1996), although patients and their caretakers may find it difficult to keep track of the large number of pills necessary at higher doses.

β-Adrenergic Blocking Agents

In double-blind and open studies, propranolol at dosages of 10–600 mg/day has been shown to be effective in reducing pacing, assaultiveness, and agitation in elderly patients with dementia (Lohr et al. 1992; Salzman 1990; Schneider and Sobin 1992; Shankle et al. 1995; Weiler et al. 1988). Pindolol and nadolol also reduced impulsivity and assaultiveness in double-blind studies of patients with dementia (Schneider and Sobin 1992). Improvement with β-blockers may occur with 1–2 weeks but can be delayed 4–6 weeks (Risse and Barnes 1986; Silver and Yudofsky 1985). Elderly patients who do not have high levels of vagal tone may tolerate these medications without excessive cardiac slowing, but congestive heart failure, heart block, sinus bradycardia, insulin-dependent diabetes mellitus, asthma, and chronic obstructive pulmonary disease are contraindications (Lohr et al. 1992; Risse and Barnes 1986; Salzman 1990). High doses of β-blockers may cause hallucinations and depression and may aggravate aggression (Parker 1985; Schneider and Sobin 1992). A dementia syndrome may also occur (Fisher 1992). β-Blockers increase blood levels of neuroleptics and anticonvulsants.

Other Treatments

Some of the behavioral disturbances seen in patients with dementia are associated with fragmentation of sleep-wake and activity cycles (see also Chapter 17). In an innovative study of 22 patients with severe dementia (Van Someren 1997), exposure to bright ambient light (1,136 lux) but not dim light over the course of the day decreased daytime hyperactivity and nighttime wandering in patients without visual impairment. Briefer exposure to morning light of the intensity used to treat seasonal affective disorder (2,500–10,000 lux) might be even more effective in normalizing circadian rhythms and behavioral disorganization in dementia patients.

It appears, based on anecdotal reports, that stimulants sometimes reduce agitation in dementia patients, possibly as a result of paradoxical sedation (Chambers et al. 1982; Schneider and Sobin 1992). The serotonergic effect of dextromethorphan may explain a few reports of a calming effect of this substance in patients with dementia (Coccaro et al. 1990; Risse and Barnes 1986).

Drug Treatment of Cognitive Deterioration

The most common cause of dementia in elderly patients is Alzheimer's disease (E. Perry and Court 1992) (see also Chapter 24). However, at least 20% of cases of dementia have a reversible cause (Ahronheim 1992), one of the most important of which is depression. The intimate relationship between depressive "pseudodementia" (more accurately the dementia syndrome of depression) and neurological dementia makes it difficult to differentiate them (Christensen et al. 1997; Lundquist et al. 1997; Reifler 1997). Up to 89% of patients with the dementia syndrome of depression eventually develop Alzheimer's or other dementias (Gottfries and Hesse 1990), a far greater percentage than would be expected with the passage of time alone. This observation raises the possibility that in some cases depression may lower the threshold for the expression of cognitive deficits of dementia that later evolve on their own even if they improve temporarily when the depression remits.

Even when dementia is present, depression can make a substantial contribution to cognitive or behavioral decline (E. D. Ross 1981). A trial of an antidepressant may therefore be warranted in patients with dementia in whom other reversible causes are not found, even if a patient does not meet formal criteria for major depressive disorder (Nahas et al. 1997). Because sedating and anticholinergic effects further impair cognitive function (Bressler and Katz 1993), TCAs are less desirable for this indication than is bupropion, venlafaxine, SSRIs, or stimulants. Nefazodone has been reported to improve cognition, but sedation can limit this benefit. As noted earlier, L-deprenyl (selegiline) may improve cognitive function, but dietary restrictions that the patient may not be able to remember are necessary at antidepressant doses.

Medication Reduction

One of the most important interventions in the treatment of any dementia is to withdraw medications that can impair cognition. In a study of 1,810 residents of a district of Stockholm who were age 75 years or older, Wills et al. (1997) found that 85% of both dementia patients and individuals without dementia were taking at least one medication and that 34% of patients with dementia were taking four or more agents. Dementia patients took significantly more antipsychotic drugs but notably fewer sedative-hypnotics than did individuals without dementia (Wills et al. 1997). The amount of medication use may have been underestimated in the dementia population, because more of these patients did not know what medications, if any, they were taking.

Treatment of Associated Factors

Even minor medical problems can aggravate dementia. Treating anemia, hypothyroidism, urinary tract infections, and other conditions often improves cognition. Vascular risk factors such as hypertension often coexist with Alzheimer's disease, and treating these risk factors reduces the risk that Alzheimer's disease will be complicated by a component of vascular dementia (Rockwood et al. 1997). Sleep-related breathing disorders and movement disorders, which can further impair cognition, are more common in elderly dementia patients than in persons without dementia (Bader et al. 1996).

Cognitive-Enhancing Therapies

Most of the new medications that have been approved for treating the actual cognitive decline of primary degenerative dementia have been studied in Alzheimer's disease, but they may be useful in other dementias. These treatments have been found to produce either modest cognitive improvement (an increase of usually three to four points on the Alzheimer's Disease Assessment Scale [ADAS]) or less decline in cognition compared with placebo. Although this amount of improvement is noticeable to patients and caretakers, in other patients statistically significant improvement or slowing of deterioration may not be clinically meaningful (Bracco and Amaducci 1990), and important symptoms not reflected in rating scales may be unaffected (Gauthier et al. 1991; Lebowitz 1992).

Even though there is no definitive treatment for Alzheimer's disease, anything with even a slight chance of benefit is worth trying, if only for the purpose of providing a concrete representation of hope. In addition, it has been estimated that prevention of a two-point decrease in ADAS scores in patients with severe dementia who are living at home would save $3,700 per year and that increasing ADAS scores by two points in the same patients would save $7,100 per year (Ernst et al. 1997). Such savings must be balanced against the risk of disruption of a family that continues to live with a patient whose dementia is already too severe to permit reasonable functioning but who does not deteriorate enough to justify placement out of the home (Filley et al. 1996). In such situations, families may undergo more disruption than if deterioration progressed further.

A family member or other authorized agent usually provides informed consent for a patient with severe dementia who has impaired ability to understand the nature of the illness, the risks and benefits of a treatment, reasonable alternatives, and the consequences of consenting to or refusing the treatment (see also Chapter 41). The task of determining whether patients with mild or moderate dementia can provide informed consent can be more difficult. In a study of 17 older patients without dementia and 29 patients with mild Alzheimer's disease (mean MMSE score, 24), five specialists in geriatric medicine, neurology, or psychiatry demonstrated 98% agreement on the competence of the subjects without dementia to consent but only 56% agreement on the competence of the patients with Alzheimer's disease (Marson et al. 1997). The truism that informed consent is a dynamic process is particularly apt in dementia patients, whose capacity to understand their circumstances fluctuates along with their cognition. The validity of consent therefore should be reevaluated periodically in all patients with Alzheimer's disease.

Cholinergic Therapies

Because of acetylcholine's role as a neurotransmitter of memory, and the cognitive impairment produced by drugs that interfere with central cholinergic transmission, the selective loss of presynaptic cholinergic neurons and muscarinic receptors in Alzheimer's disease has been thought to have etiological importance (Branconnier et al. 1992; Bromidge et al. 1997; Farlow et al. 1992; Gauthier et al. 1991; Schneider 1996). Postsynaptic muscarinic M1 receptors remain intact in Alzheimer's disease, making receptor stimulation a potentially feasible approach (Bromidge et al. 1997). Activation of nicotinic receptors may produce a neuroprotective effect and muscarinic receptor stimulation may promote neural regeneration (Schneider 1996). Medications that increase brain acetylcholine levels may hold promise in the treatment of Lewy body dementia (E. Perry and Court 1992) but have produced inconsistent results in many cases of Alzheimer's disease (Bracco and Amaducci 1990; Tariot 1992). The lack of more consistently positive findings may reflect the heterogeneity of Alzheimer's disease, the involvement of other neurotransmitter systems, or perhaps such massive cholinergic neuronal destruction in some patients that the

system is no longer capable of responding to exogenous manipulation (Branconnier et al. 1992).

With the exception of lecithin (phosphatidylcholine), which produced positive results in one study, acetylcholine precursors have been found ineffective in Alzheimer's disease (Gottfries and Hesse 1990; Tariot 1992). This is not surprising in view of the loss of neurons capable of utilizing precursors. Even though cholinergic muscarinic receptors are preserved in Alzheimer's disease, trials of bethanechol and arecoline, nonselective muscarinic cholinergic agonists, have not yielded positive results (Gauthier et al. 1991). Xanomeline, a muscarinic agonist, did not improve cognition in one trial but did reduce agitation, delusions, and hallucinations (Knopman and Morris 1997). In a 6-month multicenter study of 343 Alzheimer's disease patients randomized to treatment with placebo or one of three doses of xanomeline, the higher dose was associated with substantially better scores on the ADAS and the Clinician's Interview-Based Impression of Change as well as marked reduction of agitation and psychosis (Bodick et al. 1997). Because efficacy was limited by notable gastrointestinal side effects, a transdermal preparation is being developed (Bodick et al. 1997). A muscarinic M1 agonist, SB202026, which has few peripheral effects, did improve cognition in preliminary trials (Bromidge et al. 1997; Knopman and Morris 1997) and is now in phase 3 trials (Bromidge et al. 1997).

Cholinesterase inhibitors have been more consistently successful in increasing cholinergic tone. Oral physostigmine at a dosage of 8 mg/day for 3 weeks improved performance on a test of auditory learning, but this effect was not clinically meaningful (Sevash et al. 1991). Because physostigmine has a half-life of only 30 minutes, it is not a practical chronic treatment (Bracco and Amaducci 1990). However, extended-release physostigmine has proven effective in double-blind clinical trials (Knopman and Morris 1997; Thal et al. 1996), with higher doses being more effective (Thal et al. 1996). Frequent gastrointestinal side effects may limit the use of extended-release physostigmine in clinical practice.

Tacrine (1,2,3,4-tetrahydro-9-acridinamine monochloride monohydrate [or THA]) is a reversible cholinesterase inhibitor with a duration of action longer than that of physostigmine. Findings of early studies with positive results suggested that 40%–50% of patients with Alzheimer's disease who tolerate tacrine, or 30% of all patients who take it, had some meaningful improvement, although it was not clear whether this improvement would last longer than 3 months (Small 1992). A multicenter phase 3 study supported by the manufacturer of tacrine (trade name Cognex) included 468 patients age 50 or older with probable Alzheimer's disease. After a 6-week placebo washout period, patients received one of the following treatments: placebo for 6 weeks followed by tacrine 20 mg/day for 6 weeks; tacrine 20 mg/day for 12 weeks; tacrine 20 mg/day for 6 weeks followed by tacrine 40 mg/day for 6 weeks; tacrine 40 mg/day for 12 weeks; or tacrine 40 mg/day for 6 weeks followed by tacrine 80 mg/day for 6 weeks. The longest trial therefore was 12 weeks. Patients taking 80 mg of tacrine per day demonstrated an average increase of 3.7 points on the ADAS, compared with an increase of 0.1 point with placebo. Assessments by physicians and caretakers of patients' cognitive and global functioning also increased with the higher tacrine dose.

Eagger et al. (1992) noted a two-point improvement in MMSE scores that was maximal at 4 weeks and sustained over 12 weeks in patients taking 150 mg of tacrine daily. Improvement was more marked when serum tacrine concentrations exceeded 8 ng/mL (Eagger and Levy 1992).

Although the clinical importance of findings of the first two studies was not addressed, Davis et al. (1992) did consider clinical correlations of test scores. To maximize the likelihood of finding patients who would respond to tacrine, these investigators enrolled only Alzheimer's disease patients older than 50 who demonstrated improvement in ADAS scores of at least four points after taking 40 or 80 mg of tacrine daily for 6 weeks. During a subsequent 6-week double-blind phase, these patients then received either placebo or the dose of tacrine that had seemed helpful during the preliminary phase. Patients taking tacrine had a smaller decrement of cognitive function than did patients taking placebo, one that was statistically significant mainly for word recognition. The difference could have been explained by a greater decline of cognitive functioning in the placebo group caused by withdrawal from tacrine given during the initial phase. The placebo group returned to previous levels of functioning when tacrine was reinstituted. However, none of the differences between tacrine and placebo was detectable clinically.

In an editorial on these studies, Growdon (1992) commented that tacrine probably does have a measurable effect on cognition but it is "clinically trivial." To the degree that tacrine is helpful for some patients, long-term benefits would be expected to be limited by continued degeneration of cholinergic neurons (Ahronheim 1992). Problems with tacrine in clinical practice include the need for dosing four times daily and the fact that 10%–25% of patients taking tacrine develop reversible increases in serum transaminase levels, especially alanine aminotransferase (Farlow et al. 1992; Small 1992), that require discontinuation of the drug. An economic analysis of tacrine, the results of which

are probably applicable to all cholinesterase inhibitors, showed that beginning treatment at an earlier stage of Alzheimer's disease results in more cost savings (because of later institutionalization, for example) than does starting treatment later (Wimo et al. 1997).

A number of second-generation cholinesterase inhibitors have been released that have a simpler dosing regimen, do not affect hepatic function, and are better tolerated because of more selective inhibition of brain cholinesterase. Donepezil (Aricept) has an elimination half-life of 60 hours, permitting once-daily dosing (Schneider 1996). Within the dosage range of 5–10 mg/day, higher doses produce more improvement (Schneider 1996). Because donepezil is metabolized by cytochrome P450 2D6 and 3A4, its levels may be increased by inhibitors of these enzymes such as fluoxetine or nefazodone (Barner and Gray 1998). E2020 (Exelon), which is administered twice a day, is also more effective at higher doses (Schneider 1996); the dosage range is 6–12 mg/day. E2020 enhances release of norepinephrine and dopamine at the same time that it increases cholinergic transmission (Giacobini et al. 1996).

Even though metrifonate has an elimination half-life of only a few hours, its inhibition of cholinesterase lasts up to 6 weeks, making dosing intervals of once a day to once a week possible (Schneider 1996). Metrifonate has been found to be safe as a treatment for schistosomiasis in 30 years of experience in various countries. In two recent placebo-controlled studies involving 888 patients with Alzheimer's disease, doses of 10–60 mg of metrifonate per day improved cognitive as well as behavioral symptoms, with higher doses being more effective (Cummings 1998; Morris 1998). Metrifonate performed significantly better than placebo in a 3-month double-blind study of 50 patients with Alzheimer's disease (Becker et al. 1996). Huperzine A, which is more selective for cerebral cholinesterase than are other cholinesterase inhibitors, has shown promise in animal studies (Cheng et al. 1996).

Given that all cholinesterase inhibitor study findings have suggested better results at higher doses, it seems appropriate to increase the dose to the highest tolerated level within the range that has been studied. A 3- to 6-month trial is indicated to determine whether the medication will slow deterioration and ameliorate behavioral disturbances even if meaningful cognitive improvement does not occur. Because controlled studies of cholinesterase inhibitors have not lasted more than 6 months, the duration of therapy with these medications remains uncertain. However, results of open studies suggest that the medication should be continued until deterioration becomes obvious despite high doses of the medication (Knopman and Morris 1997).

Adverse effects of cholinesterase inhibitors are primarily a result of peripheral cholinergic excess. Nausea, vomiting, and abdominal cramps, the most common of these adverse effects, can often be reduced by fresh gingerroot or over-the-counter antiemetics (e.g., Emetrol). As is discussed later, ondansetron may improve cognition and anxiety in addition to reducing nausea, but phenothiazines such as prochlorperazine have anticholinergic properties that may aggravate dementia. Cardiac slowing can be a limiting side effect. Hepatotoxicity has not been reported with any of the new cholinesterase inhibitors.

Calcium Antagonists and Antiexcitotoxins

Another promising line of investigation involves the role of the intracellular calcium ion (Ca^{2+}) in neuronal degeneration (Branconnier et al. 1992; Choi 1988). All known cytotoxic processes, including ischemia, toxins, immune mechanisms, and genetically programmed cell death (apoptosis), increase free intracellular Ca^{2+} concentration ($[Ca^{2+}]i$). Although Ca^{2+} stimulates many crucial cellular actions, including learning and gene activation, excessive elevations of $[Ca^{2+}]i$ activate enzymes such as phospholipases, which break down the cell membrane and liberate arachidonic acid and xanthine oxidase, and proteases that degrade structural proteins. Arachidonic acid can be oxidized to cytotoxic free radicals, and xanthine oxidase can facilitate the formation of superoxide radicals.

Elderly patients may be more vulnerable to Ca^{2+}-induced neurotoxicity because resting $[Ca^{2+}]i$ increases with age as a result of prolonged calcium influx through potential-dependent channels. As some people age, $[Ca^{2+}]i$ may gradually increase to the point at which apoptotic genes are activated, stimulating pathological processes that further promote the increase in $[Ca^{2+}]i$ until it reaches cytotoxic levels. If progression of the increase in resting $[Ca^{2+}]i$ with age could be delayed, $[Ca^{2+}]i$ might be slower to reach levels that promote neurotoxicity.

Sustained increases of $[Ca^{2+}]i$ can be produced by excitatory amino acids (excitotoxins) such as glutamate (Choi 1988; Garthwaite 1991; Manev et al. 1990). In moderate concentrations, excitatory amino acids facilitate learning and neuronal development; however, excessive release and decreased uptake inhibition of excitotoxins have been implicated in various forms of brain damage, including Alzheimer's disease. In one study, for instance (Pomara et al. 1992), cerebrospinal fluid levels of free glutamate were increased in 10 patients with early Alzheimer's disease compared with control subjects.

Through their interaction with specific receptors, the best studied of which is the N-methyl-D-aspartate (NMDA) receptor, glutamate and other excitotoxins produce sustained influx of Ca^{2+} through a receptor-operated calcium channel that persists after the excitotoxin is withdrawn. The NMDA receptor also facilitates translocation of the ubiquitous intracellular enzyme protein kinase C to the cell membrane, where Ca^{2+} activates it. Protein kinase C phosphorylates cytotoxic calcium-dependent proteins and enhances further Ca^{2+} influx by phosphorylating calcium channels.

One approach to reducing excitotoxicity involves the noncompetitive NMDA antagonists such as MK-801, ketamine, and dextromethorphan. These drugs bind to a phencyclidine (PCP) receptor linked to the NMDA complex to attenuate Ca^{2+} influx. In animals with ligated cerebral arteries, MK-801 improves learning and reduces neuronal death in regions such as the hippocampus and neocortex, where high concentrations of NMDA receptors are found and vulnerability to glutamate neurotoxicity seems greatest (Albers et al. 1989). Like all drugs that bind to the PCP receptor, noncompetitive NMDA antagonists could have psychotomimetic effects (Albers et al. 1989).

Another approach to reducing excitotoxicity and Ca^{2+}-stimulated neurotoxicity is to attenuate elevations of $[Ca^{2+}]i$ by reducing calcium influx through potential-dependent channels. In a 12-week preliminary analysis of a double-blind phase 3 study of Alzheimer's disease (supported by the manufacturer), nimodipine—a lipid-soluble dihydropyridine calcium channel blocking agent—was found to slow progression of memory impairment compared with placebo (Tollefson 1990). However, final results of the study failed to support statistically significant superiority of nimodipine to placebo.

Vasodilators

Vasodilators do not really increase cerebral perfusion and may even reduce circulation through the brain through a steal effect. Drugs that used to be thought of as vasodilators therefore may be more appropriately classified with the nootropics (metabolic enhancers) (Jenike et al. 1990). The best studied of the vasodilator-nootropics is Hydergine, a mixture of three hydrogenated ergot alkaloids, which was reported to be helpful in 18 studies of mild dementia (Bracco and Amaducci 1990; Gottfries and Hesse 1990; Tariot 1992). In these studies, the measure most consistently improved by Hydergine was mood (Jenike et al. 1990). In a double-blind study (Jenike et al. 1990), no difference was found between treatment with 3 mg and treatment with 12 mg of Hydergine per day over the course of a year, in terms of ratings of dementia and functioning; however, because there was no placebo control, it was impossible to state whether either dose was actually helpful. On the other hand, in a double-blind, placebo-controlled study, Thompson et al. (1990) found Hydergine to be of no benefit at all to patients with moderate dementia. None of the other available nootropics has been found helpful in Alzheimer's disease (Shrotriya et al. 1996). However, in a 4-month placebo-controlled trial of cyclandelate, a papaverine-like substance, in 127 patients with mixed dementias, slower deterioration was observed with active drug than with placebo (Schellenberg et al. 1997). As yet, there is no convincing evidence of the capacity of any vasodilator-nootropic to slow deterioration of Alzheimer's disease for more than a few months.

Ginkgo biloba is an extract of the ginkgo tree that is thought to have antioxidant properties that might reduce adverse effects of free radicals on the brain. In a 3-month double-blind study involving 20 patients (Maurer et al. 1997), 240 mg of one ginkgo extract (EGb 761) was administered daily. The ginkgo preparation was associated with significantly better improvement on a test of attention and memory compared with placebo, which was associated with decreased scores on the same test. However, the difference in ADAS scores between the ginkgo- and placebo-treated groups was not statistically significant. In a 1-year study of EGb 761 (Le Bars et al. 1997), 327 patients with Alzheimer's disease or multi-infarct dementia were randomly assigned to treatment with gingko or placebo. Mean ADAS scores of placebo-treated patients were 1.4 points lower than those of ginkgo-treated patients ($P = .04$). Clinically significant improvement (an increase of 4 points or more) occurred in 27% of patients taking the ginkgo preparation, compared with 14% of patients treated with placebo ($P = .027$). When clinician global assessments of improvement were performed, no differences were found between groups. The large number of dropouts (172 patients) and the mixtures of diagnoses make the results difficult to interpret.

Estrogen

Estrogen receptors have been identified on hippocampal, hypothalamic, and cholinergic neurons. In addition, estrogen may promote growth and survival of cholinergic neurons and synthesis and release of acetylcholine, promote synaptic plasticity, increase regional cerebral blood flow, decrease apolipoprotein E concentrations, and have antioxidant properties (Birge 1997; Gidal et al. 1996; Knopman and Morris 1997; McBee et al. 1997; Yaffe et al. 1998). Epidemiological study findings suggest that Alzheimer's disease is more frequent in menopausal women than in men of the same age (McBee et al. 1997) and that estrogen replacement therapy reduces the risk of Alzheimer's disease in postmenopausal women, with increasing estrogen dose and duration of treatment being associated with decreasing risk (Gidal et al. 1996; McBee et al. 1997) (see also Chapter 24). Postmenopausal women taking estrogen had better scores on tests of immediate recall than did women in a placebo-control group (McBee et al. 1997). Yaffe et al. (1998) performed a meta-analysis of 10 studies of risk factors for Alzheimer's disease and other dementias. In two prospective cohort studies and one case-control study, the risk of dementia was significantly lower in postmenopausal women taking estrogen; in the other studies, the risk in the estrogen groups was nonsignificantly decreased or increased. Overall, the results of the meta-analysis suggested a 29% reduction in the risk of dementia with hormone replacement therapy (HRT) (Yaffe et al. 1998). None of the studies controlled for the possible confounding influence of comorbid depression.

Results of initial trials of estrogen treatment in women with Alzheimer's disease have been contradictory (McBee et al. 1997). The only placebo-controlled trial was a small one in which estrogen therapy was associated with improvement on one of three dementia scales compared with placebo (Yaffe et al. 1998). As of March 1998, only 58 women had been studied in trials of HRT for Alzheimer's disease, and most of these trials were small, brief, or unblinded (Yaffe et al. 1998). However, several prospective double-blind studies of estrogen therapy in women with Alzheimer's disease are currently under way (Knopman and Morris 1997). The largest of these is the Women's Health Initiative–Memory Study, a 6- to 9-year prospective controlled study of HRT involving more than 8,000 women at 39 centers (McBee et al. 1997).

The modest but definite increased risk of breast cancer in women who have taken estrogen within the past 5 years must be taken into account when prescribing estrogen for prevention or treatment of Alzheimer's disease, especially in women with a personal or family history of breast cancer. In a meta-analysis of 51 studies in 21 countries involving a total of 52,705 women with invasive breast cancer and 108,411 women without breast cancer (overall median age at the start of HRT, 48 years) (Collaborative Group on Hormonal Factors in Breast Cancer 1997), the relative risk for breast cancer in women who had ever undergone HRT was 1.14 ($P = .001$). The risk of breast cancer in women who had received HRT for 5 years or more was increased 1.35 times compared with placebo, but the risk of breast cancer was not increased in women who had not undergone HRT for at least 5 years.

Nonsteroidal Anti-Inflammatory Drugs

Inflammatory processes in Alzheimer's disease have been implicated by findings of activated microglia and reactive astrocytes in neurofibrillary tangles (Lukiw and Bazan 1997). Such findings have promoted the hypothesis that amyloid deposition results in an acute-phase response that leads to the release of inflammatory substances such as prostaglandins, which further injure neurons (Lukiw and Bazan 1997). Prostaglandin synthesis is catalyzed by cyclooxygenase isoenzymes (Jouzeau et al. 1997), the activity of some of which is increased in some patients with Alzheimer's disease (Lukiw and Bazan 1997). Because nonsteroidal anti-inflammatory drugs (NSAIDs) inhibit cyclooxygenase, they could reduce some of the secondary damage in Alzheimer's disease. β-Amyloid peptide stimulates peripheral blood monocytes to release soluble neurotoxic factors that are inhibited by dexamethasone and NSAIDS (Dzenko et al. 1997). Findings of an epidemiological study (Knopman and Morris 1997) suggested that individuals who take NSAIDs have a lower risk of developing Alzheimer's disease than do persons who do not take them, theoretically because inflammatory processes may play a role in the progression of the disease. In a trial of indomethacin, the deterioration of Alzheimer's disease in patients receiving active treatment appeared to be slower than in subjects taking placebo (Schneider 1996). An approach for avoiding the gastrointestinal toxicity of NSAIDs is to develop selective cyclooxygenase-2 inhibitors, which inhibit the inducible enzyme associated with inflammation in the brain and elsewhere while sparing cyclooxygenase-1, which is thought to be responsible for gastrointestinal effects (Knopman and Morris 1997). These substances have not yet been subjected to clinical trials in dementia.

Antioxidants

Trials of medications with antioxidant properties (Knopman and Morris 1997; Schneider 1996) have been based on evidence of increased oxidative stress in Alzheimer's disease, which can disrupt neuronal DNA and neuronal membranes (Bozner et al. 1997; Schneider 1996), and of the mediation of amyloid neurotoxicity by free radicals (Bozner et al. 1997). In a 2-year placebo-controlled trial of vitamin E and selegiline (both of which are antioxidants) in Alzheimer's disease patients with moderate dementia, both of the active drugs delayed progression of Alzheimer's disease by about 8 months (Sano et al. 1997). For unclear reasons, outcome was worse with a combination of the two medications than with either one alone.

Vitamin E in particular seems to be a benign and possibly useful adjunctive treatment for Alzheimer's disease, although it can exacerbate some coagulopathies (Knopman and Morris 1997).

Selegiline reduces oxidative stress associated with dopamine breakdown and may slow degeneration of neuronal systems in patients with comorbid Parkinson's and Alzheimer's disease (Schneider 1996). In 8 of 11 controlled trials in patients with Alzheimer's disease, improvement of cognition was observed with selegiline, and in 2 of 5 controlled trials, selegiline had a positive effect on agitation, anxiety, and depression (Tolbert and Fuller 1996). In a 14-week randomized comparison of 10 mg of selegiline daily and placebo in Alzheimer's disease, selegiline was found to improve behavior and cognition without significantly affecting mood (Lawlor et al. 1997). In a 14-week randomized trial in 25 outpatients with Alzheimer's disease, significant improvement of agitation, mood, and cognition occurred with selegiline compared with placebo (Lawlor et al. 1997). However, in a 6-month trial, no differences were noted between placebo and selegiline in ratings of behavior or cognitive function (Freedman et al. 1998).

5-HT$_3$ Antagonists

Because serotonergic influences can inhibit some aspects of cognitive function, antagonists of the serotonin 5-HT$_3$ receptor may prove useful in Alzheimer's disease (Knopman and Morris 1997). A trial of ondansetron is currently under way. Ondansetron and zacopride, a 5-HT$_3$ antagonist used as an antipsychotic drug, are of particular interest to psychiatrists because they also have antianxiety properties and may be useful in the treatment of substance abuse (Dubovsky 1994). The antiemetic effect of 5-HT$_3$ antagonists makes these medications appropriate choices for the treatment of intractable nausea caused by cholinesterase inhibitors that does not respond to less expensive treatments.

Of the novel treatments for Alzheimer's disease being studied (Bracco and Amaducci 1990; Crapper McLachlan et al. 1991; Crook et al. 1991, 1992a, 1992b; Gottfries and Hesse 1990; V. W. Henderson et al. 1989; Knopman and Morris 1997; Lindvall et al. 1990; Parnetti et al. 1997; Rainer et al. 1997; Spagnoli et al. 1991; Tariot 1992; Weyer et al. 1997), the most innovative are therapies involving nerve growth factors, substances that inhibit β-amyloid accumulation, or apolipoprotein E analogues and genetic therapies (see also Chapter 38). Such approaches will substantially increase the number of options available for treating dementia.

Psychiatric Side Effects of Neurological Drugs

Psychiatric syndromes commonly are caused by the many medications taken by elderly neurologically ill patients. Some important reactions are noted in Table 34–26 ("Drugs That Cause Psychiatric Symptoms" 1984; Kulkarni et al. 1992; Lohr et al. 1992). Whenever possible, the offending medicine should be withdrawn before psychiatric treatments are initiated. (Further discussion of these medications can be found in Chapter 31.)

Summary

Many Axis I disorders in elderly patients are true neuropsychiatric syndromes in that psychiatric symptoms in this population are often produced or aggravated by neurological dysfunction. Treating such syndromes is complicated by the sensitivity of the older nervous system to the toxic but probably not the therapeutic effects of psychotropic medications, as well as by interactions of psychotropic medications with the many neurological drugs taken by elderly patients. Many of the more frequently used medicines for geriatric neuropsychiatric conditions are poorly tolerated, especially the sedating and anticholinergic TCAs and neuroleptics and the long–half-life benzodiazepines. SSRIs and other new-generation antidepressants and atypical antipsychotic drugs are better-tolerated alternatives. Short–half-life benzodiazepines are appropriate choices for some patients with acute anxiety, but anxiety and insomnia in patients with overt brain disease often is better managed with azapirones or antidepressants.

Severe agitation in delirium patients can be treated emergently with ECT or with intravenous haloperidol, droperidol, or benzodiazepines. Intermittent explosive outbursts and other behavioral disturbances can be managed with β-adrenergic blocking agents, buspirone, lithium, anticonvulsants, some antidepressants, cholinesterase inhibitors, and anticonvulsants. Atypical antipsychotic drugs such as risperidone have primary antiaggressive properties. Neuroleptics should be avoided for this indication unless nothing else is effective. There is no proven treatment for dementia itself, but the second-generation cholinesterase inhibitors produce at least some improvement. Selegiline, antioxidants, estrogen, and possibly NMDA antagonists may have some potential.

TABLE 34–26. Psychiatric side effects of neurological medications

Syndrome	Medication(s)
Depression	Adrenal steroids
	Amantadine
	Asparaginase
	Cimetidine
	Digoxin
	Indomethacin
	Levodopa
	Methyldopa
	Metoclopramide
	Narcotics
	Procainamide
	Propranolol
	Reserpine
	Thiazide diuretics
Mania	Adrenal steroids
	Baclofen
	Bromocriptine
	Captopril
	Cimetidine
	Dextromethorphan
	Indomethacin
	Isoniazid
	Levodopa
Confusion	Asparaginase
	Aspirin
	Cisplatin
	Cyclophosphamide
	Opiates
	Pentazocine
	Ranitidine
	Sulindac
	Any medication in patients with brain damage
Psychosis	Adrenal steroids
	Anticonvulsants
	Asparaginase
	Bromocriptine
	Cimetidine
	Cisplatin
	Cyclophosphamide
	Digoxin
	Isoniazid
	Levodopa

(continued)

TABLE 34–26. Psychiatric side effects of neurological medications *(continued)*

Syndrome	Medication(s)
Psychosis *(continued)*	Lisuride
	Pergolide
	Procainamide
	Propranolol
	Quinidine
	Ranitidine
	Sulindac
	Tocainide
Sleep disorder and bad dreams	Antidepressants
	Baclofen
	Bromocriptine
	Cimetidine
	Levodopa
	Lisuride
	Pergolide
	Propranolol

▌ References

Abernathy DE: Psychotropic drugs and the aging process: pharmacokinetics and pharmacodynamics, in Clinical Geriatric Psychiatry, 2nd Edition. Edited by Salzman C. Baltimore, MD, Williams & Wilkins, 1992, pp 61–76

Adams F: Emergency intravenous sedation of the delirious medically ill patient. J Clin Psychiatry 49 (suppl):22–26, 1988

Adams F, Fernandez F, Anderson BS: Emergency pharmacotherapy of delirium in the critically ill cancer patient. Psychosomatics 27 (suppl):33–37, 1986

Ahronheim JC: Handbook of Prescribing Medications for Geriatric Patients. Boston, MA, Little, Brown, 1992

Albers GW, Goldberg MP, Choi DW: N-methyl-D-aspartate antagonists ready for clinical trial in brain ischemia? Ann Neurol 25:398–403, 1989

Alexopoulos GS: Treatment of depression, in Clinical Geriatric Psychiatry, 2nd Edition. Edited by Salzman C. Baltimore, MD, Williams & Wilkins, 1992, pp 137–174

Almeida JH: Neuroleptic side-effects—the "rabbit syndrome." Int J Geriatr Psychiatry 6:537–539, 1991

Anderson GD, Yau MK, Gidal BE, et al: Bidirectional interaction of valproate and lamotrigine in healthy subjects. Clin Pharmacol Ther 60:145–156, 1996

Aronson SM: Cost-effectiveness and quality of life in psychosis: the pharmacoeconomics of risperidone. Clin Ther 19:139–147, 1997

Avorn J, Soumerai SB, Everitt DE, et al: A randomized trial of a program to reduce the use of psychoactive drugs in nursing homes. N Engl J Med 327:168–173, 1992

Ayd F: Prophylactic antiparkinsonian drug therapy: pros and cons. International Drug Therapy Newsletter 21:5–6, 1986

Bader GG, Turesson K, Wallin A: Sleep-related breathing and movement disorders in healthy elderly and demented subjects. Dementia 7:279–287, 1996

Bailey DN, Coffee JJ, Anderson B, et al: Interaction of tricyclic antidepressants with cholestyramine in vitro. Ther Drug Monit 14:339–342, 1992

Bajulaize R, Addonizio G: Clozapine in the treatment of psychosis in an 82-year-old woman with tardive dyskinesia (letter). J Clin Psychopharmacol 12:364–365, 1992

Baldessarini RJ, Marsh E: Fluoxetine and side effects (letter). Arch Gen Psychiatry 47:191–192, 1990

Ballard C, O'Brien J: A prospective study of psychotic symptoms in dementia sufferers: psychosis in dementia. Int Psychogeriatr 9:57–64, 1997

Balter MB, Uhlenhuth EH: The beneficial and adverse effects of hypnotics. J Clin Psychiatry 52 (suppl):16–23, 1991

Barner EL, Gray SL: Donepezil use in Alzheimer disease. Ann Pharmacother 32:70–77, 1998

Becker RE, Colliver JA, Markwell SJ, et al: Double-blind, placebo-controlled study of metrifonate, an acetylcholinesterase inhibitor, for Alzheimer disease. Alzheimer Dis Assoc Disord 10:124–131, 1996

Becquemont L, Ragueneau I, Le Bot MA, et al: Influence of the CYP1A2 inhibitor fluvoxamine on tacrine pharmacokinetics in humans. Clin Pharmacol Ther 61:619–627, 1997

Beran RG, Gibson R: Aggressive behaviour in intellectually challenged patients with epilepsy treated with lamotrigine. Epilepsia 39:280–282, 1998

Birge SJ: The role of estrogen in the treatment of Alzheimer's disease. Neurology 48 (suppl 7):S36–S41, 1997

Black DW, Winokur G, Nasrallah A: Treatment of mania: a naturalistic study of electroconvulsive therapy vs. lithium in 438 patients. J Clin Psychiatry 48:132–139, 1987

Blake LM, Marks RC, Luchins DJ: Reversible neurologic symptoms with clozapine and lithium. J Clin Psychopharmacol 12:297–299, 1992

Bodick NC, Offen WW, Shannon HE, et al: The selective muscarinic agonist xanomeline improves both the cognitive deficits and behavioral symptoms of Alzheimer disease. Alzheimer Dis Assoc Disord 11 (suppl 4):S16–S22, 1997

Bodkin JA: Emerging uses for high-potency benzodiazepines in psychotic disorders. J Clin Psychiatry 51 (suppl):41–46, 1990

Bond WS, Mandos LA, Kurtz MB: Midazolam for aggressivity and violence in 3 mentally retarded patients. Am J Psychiatry 146:925–926, 1989

Bouckonis AJ, Litman RE: Clonazepam in the treatment of neuralgic pain syndromes. Psychosomatics 26:933–936, 1985

Bowden CL, Brugger AM, Swann AC: Efficacy of divalproex vs lithium in the treatment of mania. The Depakote Mania Study Group. JAMA 271: 918–924, 1994

Bozner P, Grishko V, LeDoux SP, et al: The amyloid beta protein induces oxidative damage of mitochondrial DNA. J Neuropathol Exp Neurol 56:1356–1362, 1997

Bracco L, Amaducci L: Drug development for the treatment of dementia, in Clinical and Scientific Psychogeriatrics, Vol 2: The Interface of Psychiatry and Neurology. Edited by Bergener M, Finkel SI. New York, Springer, 1990, pp 260–287

Branconnier RJ, Branconnier ME, Wadshe TM, et al: Blocking the Ca2+ activated cytotoxic mechanisms of cholinergic neuronal death: a novel treatment strategy for Alzheimer's disease. Psychopharmacol Bull 28:175–181, 1992

Brandt SA, Ploner CJ, Meyer BU: Repetitive transcranial magnetic stimulation: possibilities, limits and safety aspects [in German]. Nervenarzt 68:778–784, 1997

Bressler R, Katz MD: Drug therapy for geriatric depression. Drugs Aging 3:195–219, 1993

Bridges-Parlet S, Knopman D, Steffes S: Withdrawal of neuroleptic medications from institutionalized dementia patients: results of a double-blind, baseline-treatment-controlled pilot study. J Geriatr Psychiatry Neurol 10: 119–126, 1997

Bromidge SM, Brown F, Cassidy F, et al: Design of [R-(Z)]-(+)-alpha-(methoxyimino)-1-azabicyclo[2.2.2]octane-3-acetonitrile (SB 202026), a functionally selective azabicyclic muscarinic M1 agonist incorporating the N-methoxy imidoyl nitrile group as a novel ester bioisostere. J Med Chem 40:4265–4280, 1997

Bryner C, Winograd CH: Fluoxetine in elderly patients: is there cause for concern? J Am Geriatr Soc 40:902–905, 1992

Busto V, Sellers EM, Naranjo C, et al: Withdrawal reaction after long-term therapeutic use of benzodiazepines. N Engl J Med 315:854–859, 1986

Cantillon M, Brunswick R, Molina D, et al: Buspirone vs haloperidol: a double-blind trial for agitation in a nursing home population with Alzheimer's disease. Am J Geriatr Psychiatry 4:263–267, 1996

Casey DE: Will the new antipsychotics bring hope of reducing the risk of developing extrapyramidal syndromes and tardive dyskinesia? Int Clin Psychopharmacol 12 (suppl 1): S19–S27, 1997

Chacko RC, Hurley RA, Harper RG, et al: Clozapine for acute and maintenance treatment of psychosis in Parkinson's disease. J Neuropsychiatry Clin Neurosci 7:471–475, 1995

Chambers CA, Bain J, Rosebottom R, et al: Carbamazepine in senile dementia and overactivity—a placebo controlled double blind trial. IRCS Medical Science 10:505–506, 1982

Chandler JD, Chandler JE: The prevalence of neuropsychiatric disorders in a nursing home population. J Geriatr Psychiatry Neurol 1:71–76, 1998

Cheng DH, Ren H, Tang XC: Huperzine A, a novel promising acetylcholinesterase inhibitor. Neuroreport 8:97–101, 1996

Chengappa KN, Baker RW, Kreinbrook SB, et al: Clozapine use in female geriatric patients with psychoses. J Geriatr Psychiatry Neurol 8:12–15, 1995

Chiarello RJ, Cole JO: The use of psychostimulants in general psychiatry: a reconsideration. Arch Gen Psychiatry 44: 286–295, 1987

Choi DW: Glutamate neurotoxicity and diseases of the nervous system. Neuron 1:623–634, 1988

Chou JCY: Recent advances in the treatment of acute mania. J Clin Psychopharmacol 11:3–21, 1991

Chouinard G, Penry JK: Neurologic and psychiatric aspects of clonazepam: an update. Psychosomatics 26 (suppl):1–37, 1985

Christensen H, Griffiths K, Mackinnon A, et al: A quantitative review of cognitive deficits in depression and Alzheimer-type dementia. J Int Neuropsychol Soc 3:631–651, 1997

Clary C, Schweitzer E: Treatment of MAOI hypertensive crisis with sublingual nifedipine. J Clin Psychiatry 48:249–250, 1987

Coccaro EF, Kramer E, Zemishlany A, et al: Pharmacologic treatment of noncognitive behavioral disturbances in elderly demented patients. Am J Psychiatry 147:1640–1645, 1990

Coffey CE, Weiner RD, Djang WT, et al: Brain anatomic effects of electroconvulsive therapy. Arch Gen Psychiatry 48: 1013–1021, 1991

Coffey CE, Wilkinson WE, Weiner RD, et al: Quantitative cerebral anatomy in depression: a controlled magnetic resonance imaging study. Arch Gen Psychiatry 50:7–16, 1993

Cohen WJ, Cohen NH: Lithium carbonate, haloperidol and irreversible brain damage. JAMA 230:1283–1287, 1974

Cohen-Mansfield J: Agitation in the elderly. Adv Psychosom Med 19:101–113, 1989

Cohen-Mansfield J: Assessment of disruptive behavior/agitation in the elderly: function, methods, and difficulties. J Geriatr Psychiatry Neurol 8:52–60, 1995

Cohen-Mansfield J, Marz MS, Werner P: Agitation in elderly persons: an integrative report of findings in a nursing home. Int Psychogeriatr 4:221–240, 1992

Cohn CK, Shrivastava R, Mendels J, et al: Double-blind, multicenter comparison of sertraline and amitriptyline in elderly depressed patients. J Clin Psychiatry 51 (suppl B): 28–33, 1990

Collaborative Group on Hormonal Factors in Breast Cancer: Breast cancer and hormone replacement therapy: collaborative reanalysis of data from 51 epidemiological studies of 52,705 women with breast cancer and 108,411 women without breast cancer. Lancet 350:1047–1059, 1997

Crapper McLachlan DR, Dalton AJ, Krick TPA, et al: Intramuscular desferrioxamine in patients with Alzheimer's disease. Lancet 337:1304–1308, 1991

Crook TH, Tinklenberg J, Yesavage J, et al: Effects of phosphatidylserine in age-associated memory impairment. Neurology 41:644–649, 1991

Crook T[H], Petrie W, Wells C, et al: Effects of phosphatidylserine in Alzheimer's disease. Psychopharmacol Bull 28:61–66, 1992a

Crook T[H], Wilner E, Rothwell A, et al: Noradrenergic intervention in Alzheimer's disease. Psychopharmacol Bull 28:67–70, 1992b

Cummings JL: Depression and Parkinson's disease: a review. Am J Psychiatry 149:443–454, 1992

Cummings JL: Metrifonate treatment of the cognitive deficits of Alzheimer's disease. Neurology 50:1214–1221, 1998

Dagon EM: Other organic mental syndromes, in Verwoerdt's Clinical Geropsychiatry, 3rd Edition. Edited by Bienenfeld D. Baltimore, MD, Williams & Wilkins, 1990, pp 85–105

Danielczyk W, Streifler M, Konradi C, et al: Platelet MAO-B activity and the psychopathology of Parkinson's disease, senile dementia and multi-infarct dementia. Acta Psychiatr Scand 78:730–736, 1988

Davidson J: Seizures and bupropion: a review. J Clin Psychiatry 50:256–261, 1989

Davis KL, Thal LJ, Gamzu ER, et al: A double-blind placebo-controlled multicenter study of tacrine for Alzheimer's disease. N Engl J Med 327:1953–1959, 1992

Demuth GW, Breslov RE, Drescher J: The elicitation of a movement disorder by trazodone: case report. J Clin Psychiatry 46:535–536, 1985

Deutsch LH, Eylsma FW: Psychosis and physical aggression in probable Alzheimer's disease. Am J Psychiatry 148:1159–1163, 1991

Devanand DP: Behavioral complications and their treatment in Alzheimer's disease. Geriatrics 52 (suppl 2):S37–S39, 1997

Devanand DP, Cooper MA, Sackeim HA, et al: Low dose oral haloperidol and blood levels in Alzheimer's disease: a preliminary study. Psychopharmacol Bull 28:169–173, 1992

Drugs that cause psychiatric symptoms. Med Lett Drugs Ther 26:75–78, 1984

Dubin WR, Weiss KJ, Dorn JM: Pharmacotherapy of psychiatric emergencies. J Clin Psychopharmacol 6:210–222, 1986

Dubovsky SL: Calcium antagonists: a new class of psychiatric drugs? Psychiatric Annals 16:724–728, 1986

Dubovsky SL: Approaches to developing new anxiolytics and antidepressants. J Clin Psychiatry 54 (suppl):75–83, 1993

Dubovsky SL: Beyond the serotonin reuptake inhibitors: rationales for the development of new serotonergic agents. J Clin Psychiatry 55 (suppl):34–44, 1994

Dubovsky SL: Electroconvulsive therapy, in Comprehensive Textbook of Psychiatry/VI, 6th Edition. Edited by Kaplan HI, Sadock BJ. Baltimore, MD, Williams & Wilkins, 1995, pp 2129–2140

Dubovsky SL, Buzan RD: Novel alternatives and supplements to lithium and anticonvulsants for bipolar affective disorder. J Clin Psychiatry 58:224–242, 1997

Dubovsky SL, Thomas M: Beyond specificity: effects of serotonin and serotonergic treatments on psychobiological dysfunction. J Psychosom Res 39:429–444, 1995

Dubovsky SL, Thomas M: Tardive dyskinesia associated with fluoxetine. Psychiatr Serv 47:991–993, 1996

Dubovsky SL, Franks RD, Allen S, et al: Calcium antagonists in mania: a double blind placebo control study of verapamil. Psychiatry Res 18:309–320, 1986

Dzenko KA, Weltzien RB, Pachter JS: Suppression of A beta-induced monocyte neurotoxicity by antiinflammatory compounds. J Neuroimmunol 80:6–12, 1997

Eagger S, Levy R: Serum levels of tacrine in relationship to clinical response in Alzheimer's disease. Int J Geriatr Psychiatry 7:115–119, 1992

Eagger S, Morant N, Levy R, et al: Tacrine in Alzheimer's disease: time course of changes in cognitive function and practice effects. Br J Psychiatry 160:36–40, 1992

Egan MF, Hyde TM, Albers GW, et al: Treatment of tardive dyskinesia with vitamin E. Am J Psychiatry 149:773–777, 1992

Ereshefsky L: Pharmacokinetics and drug interactions: update for new antipsychotics. J Clin Psychiatry 57 (suppl 11):12–25, 1996

Ereshefsky L, Watanabe MD, Tran-Johnson TK: Clozapine: an atypical antipsychotic agent. Clin Pharm 8:691–709, 1989

Ernst RL, Hay JW, Fenn C, et al: Cognitive function and the costs of Alzheimer disease: an exploratory study. Arch Neurol 54:687–693, 1997

Factor SA, Brown D, Molho ES, et al: Clozapine: a 2-year open trial in Parkinson's disease patients with psychosis. Neurology 44:544–546, 1994

Farlow M, Gracon SI, Hershey LA, et al: A controlled trial of tacrine in Alzheimer's disease. JAMA 268:2523–2529, 1992

Fava M: Psychopharmacologic treatment of pathologic aggression. Psychiatr Clin North Am 20:427–451, 1997

Fenwick P: The nature and management of aggression in epilepsy. J Neuropsychiatry Clin Neurosci 1:418–425, 1989

Fernandez F, Holmes VF, Adams F, et al: Treatment of severe refractory agitation with a haloperidol drip. J Clin Psychiatry 49:239–241, 1988

Filley CM, Chapman MM, Dubovsky SL: Ethical concerns in the use of palliative drug treatment for Alzheimer's disease. J Neuropsychiatry Clin Neurosci 8:202–205, 1996

Fisher CM: Amnestic syndrome associated with propranolol toxicity: a case report. Clin Neuropharmacol 15:397–403, 1992

Flint AJ: Recent developments in geriatric psychopharmacotherapy. Can J Psychiatry 39 (suppl 1):S9–S18, 1994

Frankenburg FR, Kalunian D: Clozapine in the elderly. J Geriatr Psychiatry Neurol 7:129–132, 1994

Freedman M, Rewilak D, Xerri T, et al: L-Deprenyl in Alzheimer's disease: cognitive and behavioral effects. Neurology 50:660–668, 1998

Fricchione G: Catatonia: a new indication for benzodiazepines? Biol Psychiatry 26:761–765, 1989

Galynker I, Ieronimo C, Miner C, et al: Methylphenidate treatment of negative symptoms in patients with dementia. J Neuropsychiatry Clin Neurosci 9:231–239, 1997

Garthwaite J: Glutamate, nitric oxide and cell-cell signalling in the nervous system. Trends Neurosci 14:60–67, 1991

Gauthier S, Gauthier L, Bouchard R, et al: Treatment of Alzheimer's disease: hopes and reality. Can J Neurol Sci 18:394–397, 1991

Gelenberg AJ: Clozapine agranulocytosis update. Biological Therapies in Psychiatry 15:37–40, 1992

Gelenberg AJ, Kane JM, Keller MB, et al: Comparison of standard and low serum levels of lithium for maintenance treatment of bipolar disorder. N Engl J Med 231:1489–1493, 1989

George MS, Wassermann EM, Kimbrell TA, et al: Mood improvement following daily left prefrontal repetitive transcranial magnetic stimulation in patients with depression: a placebo-controlled crossover trial. Am J Psychiatry 154:1752–1756, 1997

Georgotas A, McCue RE, Hapworth W, et al: Comparative efficacy and safety of MAOIs versus TCAs in treating depression in the elderly. Biol Psychiatry 21:1155–1166, 1986

Georgotas A, McCue RE, Cooper TB, et al: How effective and safe is continuation therapy in elderly depressed patients? Arch Gen Psychiatry 45:929–932, 1988

Giacobini E, Zhu XD, Williams E, et al: The effect of the selective reversible acetylcholinesterase inhibitor E2020 on extracellular acetylcholine and biogenic amine levels in rat cortex. Neuropharmacology 35:205–211, 1996

Gidal BE, Crismon ML, Wagner ML, et al: Current developments in neurology, part II: advances in the pharmacotherapy of Alzheimer disease, Parkinson's disease, and stroke. Ann Pharmacother 30:1446–1451, 1996

Glazer WM: Olanzapine and the new generation of antipsychotic agents: patterns of use. J Clin Psychiatry 58:18–21, 1997

Goldberg RJ, Goldberg J: Risperidone for dementia-related disturbed behavior in nursing home residents: a clinical experience. Int Psychogeriatr 9:65–68, 1997

Goldstein SE, Birnbom F: Piperacetazine versus thioridazine in the treatment of organic brain disease: a controlled double-blind study. J Am Geriatr Soc 24:355–359, 1976

Goodman WK, Charney DS: Therapeutic applications and mechanisms of monoamine oxidase and heterocyclic antidepressant drugs. J Clin Psychiatry 46:6–22, 1985

Gottfries CG, Hesse C: Pharmacotherapy in psychogeriatrics: an update, in Clinical and Scientific Psychogeriatrics, Vol 2: The Interface of Psychiatry and Neurology. Edited by Bergener M, Finkel SI. New York, Springer, 1990, pp 288–313

Gottlieb GL: Sleep disorders and their management: special considerations in the elderly. Am J Med 88:29S–33S, 1990

Green BH, Dewey ME, Copeland JR, et al: Prospective data on the prevalence of abnormal involuntary movements among elderly people living in the community. Acta Psychiatr Scand 87:418–421, 1993

Greenblatt DJ, Harmatz JS, Shapiro L, et al: Sensitivity to triazolam in the elderly. N Engl J Med 324:1691–1698, 1991

Griffin JP: A review of the literature on benign intracranial hypertension associated with medication. Adverse Drug React Toxicol Rev 11:41–57, 1992

Growdon JH: Treatment for Alzheimer's disease? (editorial) N Engl J Med 327:1306–1308, 1992

Guze BH, Baxter LR: Neuroleptic malignant syndrome. N Engl J Med 313:163–166, 1985

Hardy BG, Shulman KI, Mackenzie SE, et al: Pharmacokinetics of lithium in the elderly. J Clin Psychopharmacol 7:153–158, 1987

Hart RP, Colenda CC, Hamer RM: Effects of buspirone and alprazolam on the cognitive performance of normal elderly subjects. Am J Psychiatry 148:73–77, 1991

Hawes C, Mor V, Phillips CD, et al: The OBRA-87 nursing home regulations and implementation of the Resident Assessment Instrument: effects on process quality. J Am Geriatr Soc 45:977–985, 1997

Henderson S, Jorm AF, Scott LR, et al: Insomnia in the elderly: its prevalence and correlates in the general population. Med J Aust 162:22–24, 1995

Henderson VW, Roberts E, Wimer C, et al: Multicenter trial of naloxone in Alzheimer's disease. Ann Neurol 25:404–406, 1989

Herman JV, Brotman AW, Pollack MH, et al: Fluoxetine-induced sexual dysfunction. J Clin Psychiatry 51:27–29, 1990

Herrmann N, Eryavec G: Buspirone in the management of agitation and aggression associated with dementia. Am J Geriatr Psychiatry 1:249–253, 1993

Herrmann N, Lanctot KL: From transmitters to treatment: the pharmacotherapy of behavioural disturbances in dementia. Can J Psychiatry 42 (suppl 1):51S–64S, 1997

Herrmann N, Bremner KE, Naranjo CA: Pharmacotherapy of late life mood disorders. Clin Neurosci 4:41–47, 1997

Hoehn-Saric R, McLeod DR, Zimmerl WD: Differential effects of alprazolam and imipramine in generalized anxiety disorder. J Clin Psychiatry 49:293–301, 1988

Hoffman BB Lefkowitz RJ: Adrenergic receptor antagonists, in Goodman and Gilman's The Pharmacological Basis of Therapeutics, 8th Edition. Edited by Gilman AG, Rall TW, Nies AS, et al. New York, Pergamon, 1990, pp 187–243

Holmes VF, Fernandez F, Levy JK: Psychostimulant response in AIDS-related complex patients. J Clin Psychiatry 50:5–8, 1989

Hoogiverf B: Amitriptyline treatment of painful diabetic neuropathy: an inadvertent single-patient clinical trial. Diabetes Care 3:526–527, 1985

Izzo KL, Brody R: Rehabilitation in lithium toxicity. Arch Phys Med Rehabil 66:779–782, 1985

Jaggy H, Koch E: Chemistry and biology of alkylphenols from *Ginkgo biloba L.* Pharmazie 52:735–738, 1997

Jeanblanc W, Davis YB: Risperidone for treating dementia-associated aggression. Am J Psychiatry 152:1239–1240, 1995

Jefferson JW: Lithium: the present and the future. J Clin Psychiatry 51 (suppl):4–8, 1990

Jefferson JW, Greist JH: Primer of Lithium Therapy. Baltimore, MD, Williams & Wilkins, 1977

Jenike MA: Approaches to patients with treatment-refractory obsessive-compulsive disorder. J Clin Psychiatry 51 (suppl):15–21, 1990

Jenike MA, Albert M, Baer L, et al: Ergot mesylates for Alzheimer's disease: a year-long double blind trial of 3 mg vs. 12 mg daily. Int J Geriatr Psychiatry 5:375–380, 1990

Jeste DV, Eastham JH, Lacro JP, et al: Management of late-life psychosis. J Clin Psychiatry 57 (suppl 3):39–45, 1996

Jick SS, Jick H, Knauss TA, et al: Antidepressants and convulsions. J Clin Psychopharmacol 12:241–245, 1992

Johnson LC, Chernick DA, Sateia MJ: Sleep, performance, and plasma levels in chronic insomniacs during 14-day use of flurazepam and midazolam: an introduction. J Clin Psychopharmacol 10 (suppl):5S–9S, 1990

Jouzeau JY, Terlain B, Abid A, et al: Cyclo-oxygenase isoenzymes: how recent findings affect thinking about nonsteroidal anti-inflammatory drugs. Drugs 53:563–582, 1997

Kahn EM, Schulz C, Perel JM, et al: Change in haloperidol level due to carbamazepine: a complicatory factor in combined medication for schizophrenia. J Clin Psychopharmacol 10:54–57, 1990

Kane JM, Honigfeld G, Singer J, et al: Clozapine for treatment-resistant schizophrenia. Arch Gen Psychiatry 45:789–796, 1988

Karlsson I: Pharmacologic treatment of noncognitive symptoms of dementia. Acta Neurol Scand Suppl 165:101–104, 1996

Kaufman MW, Cassem N, Murray G, et al: The use of methylphenidate in depressed patients after cardiac surgery. J Clin Psychiatry 45:82–84, 1984

Klein C, Kompf D, Pulkowski U, et al: A study of visual hallucinations in patients with Parkinson's disease. J Neurol 244:371–377, 1997

Knopman DS, Morris JC: An update on primary drug therapies for Alzheimer disease. Arch Neurol 54:1406–1409, 1997

Ko GN, Korpi ER, Linnoila M: On the clinical relevance and methods of quantification of plasma concentrations of neuroleptics. J Clin Psychopharmacol 5:253–262, 1985

Kopala LC, Honer WG: The use of risperidone in severely demented patients with persistent vocalizations. Int J Geriatr Psychiatry 12:73–77, 1997

Kulkarni J, Horne M, Butler E, et al: Psychotic symptoms resulting from intraventricular infusion of dopamine in Parkinson's disease. Biol Psychiatry 31:1225–1227, 1992

Lake JT, Rahman AH, Grossberg GT: Diagnosis and treatment of psychotic symptoms in elderly patients. Drugs Aging 11: 170–177, 1997

Lantz MS, Marin D: Pharmacologic treatment of agitation in dementia: a comprehensive review. J Geriatr Psychiatry Neurol 9:107–119, 1996

Lantz MS, Giambanco V, Buchalter EN: A ten-year review of the effect of OBRA-87 on psychotropic prescribing practices in an academic nursing home. Psychiatr Serv 47: 951–955, 1996

Lauterbach EC, Schiveri MM: Amelioration of pseudobulbar affect by fluoxetine: possible alteration of dopamine-related pathophysiology by a selective serotonin reuptake inhibitor. J Clin Psychopharmacol 11:392–393, 1991

Lawlor BA, Sunderland T, Mellow AM, et al: A pilot placebo controlled study of chronic m-CPP administration in Alzheimer's disease. Biol Psychiatry 30:140–144, 1991

Lawlor BA, Radcliffe J, Molchan SE, et al: A pilot placebo-controlled study of trazodone and buspirone in Alzheimer's disease. Int J Geriatr Psychiatry 9:55–59, 1994

Lawlor BA, Aisen PS, Green C, et al: Selegiline in the treatment of behavioural disturbance in Alzheimer's disease. Int J Geriatr Psychiatry 12:319–322, 1997

Lawrence JM: Reactions to withdrawal of antidepressants, antiparkinsonian drugs, and lithium. Psychosomatics 11:869–877, 1985

Le Bars PL, Katz MM, Berman N, et al: A placebo-controlled, double-blind, randomized trial of an extract of *Ginkgo biloba* for dementia. North American EGb Study Group. JAMA 278:1327–1332, 1997

Lebert F, Pasquier F, Petit H: Behavioural effects of fluoxetine in dementia of Alzheimer type. Int J Geriatr Psychiatry 9:590–591, 1994

Lebowitz BD: Developments in treatment of Alzheimer's disease. Psychopharmacol Bull 28:59–60, 1992

Levy MA, Burgio LD, Sweet R, et al: A trial of buspirone for the control of disruptive behaviors in community-dwelling patients with dementia. Int J Geriatr Psychiatry 9:841–848, 1994

Levy R: Sedation in acute and chronic agitation. Pharmacotherapy 16:152S–159S, 1996

Lieberman JA, Kane JM, Reife R: Neuromuscular effects of monoamine oxidase inhibitors. J Clin Psychopharmacol 5:221–228, 1985

Lieberman JA, Saltz BL, Johns CA, et al: The effects of clozapine on tardive dyskinesia. Br J Psychiatry 158:503–510, 1991

Lindvall O, Brundin P, Widner H, et al: Grafts of fetal dopamine neurons survive and improve motor function in Parkinson's disease. Science 247:574–577, 1990

Lipsey JR, Robinson RG, Pearlson GD, et al: Nortriptyline treatment of post-stroke depression: a double-blind study. Lancet 1:297–300, 1984

Liptzin B: Treatment of mania, in Clinical Geriatric Psychiatry, 2nd Edition. Edited by Salzman C. Baltimore, MD, Williams & Wilkins, 1992, pp 175–188

Litovitz TL, Troutman WG: Amoxapine overdose: seizures and fatalities. JAMA 250:1069–1071, 1983

Lohr JB, Jeste DV, Harris MJ, et al: Treatment of disordered behavior, in Clinical Geriatric Psychiatry, 2nd Edition. Edited by Salzman C. Baltimore, MD, Williams & Wilkins, 1992, pp 80–113

Lukiw WJ, Bazan NG: Cyclooxygenase 2 RNA message abundance, stability, and hypervariability in sporadic Alzheimer neocortex. J Neurosci Res 50:937–945, 1997

Lundquist RS, Bernens A, Olsen CG: Comorbid disease in geriatric patients: dementia and depression. Am Fam Physician 55:2687–2694, 1997

Madhusoodanan S, Brenner R, Araujo L, et al: Efficacy of risperidone treatment for psychoses associated with schizophrenia, schizoaffective disorder, bipolar disorder, or senile dementia in 11 geriatric patients: a case series. J Clin Psychiatry 56:514–518, 1995

Malone ML, Thompson L, Goodwin JS: Aggressive behaviors among the institutionalized elderly. J Am Geriatr Soc 41:653–656, 1993

Manev H, Costa E, Wrobewski JT, et al: Abusive stimulation of excitatory amino acid receptors: a strategy to limit neurotoxicity. FASEB J 4:2789–2797, 1990

Mann SC, Caroff SN, Bleier HR: Lethal catatonia. Am J Psychiatry 143:1374–1378, 1986

Marder SR: Atypical antipsychotic agents in the treatment of schizophrenia and other psychiatric disorders, part I: unique patient populations. J Clin Psychiatry 59:259–265, 1998

Markovitz PJ: Treatment of anxiety in the elderly. J Clin Psychiatry 54:64–68, 1993

Markwort S, Cordes P, Aldenhoff J: Transcranial magnetic stimulation as an alternative to electroshock therapy in treatment resistant depressions: a literature review. Fortschr Neurol Psychiatr 65:540–549, 1997

Marson DC, McInturff B, Hawkins L, et al: Consistency of physician judgments of capacity to consent in mild Alzheimer's disease. J Am Geriatr Soc 45:453–457, 1997

Massey EW, Folger WN: Seizures activated by therapeutic levels of lithium carbonate. South Med J 77:1173–1175, 1984

Mathew NT: Prophylaxis of migraine and mixed headache: a randomized controlled study. Headache 21:105–109, 1981

Maurer K, Ihl R, Dierks T, et al: Clinical efficacy of *Ginkgo biloba* special extract EGb 761 in dementia of the Alzheimer type. J Psychiatr Res 31:645–655, 1997

Max MB, Lynch SA, Muir J, et al: Effects of desipramine, amitriptyline and fluoxetine on pain in diabetic neuropathy. N Engl J Med 326:1250–1256, 1992

McBee WL, Dailey ME, Dugan E, et al: Hormone replacement therapy and other potential treatments for dementias. Endocrinol Metab Clin North Am 26:329–345, 1997

McCarten JR, Kovera C, Maddox MK, et al: Triazolam in Alzheimer's disease: pilot study on sleep and memory effects. Pharmacol Biochem Behav 52:447–452, 1995

McMahon FJ, DePaulo JR: Clinical features of affective disorders and bereavement. Current Opinion in Psychiatry 5:580–584, 1992

McShane R, Keene J, Gedling K, et al: Do neuroleptic drugs hasten cognitive decline in dementia? Prospective study with necropsy follow up. BMJ 314:266–270, 1997

Mellerup ET, Plenge P: Side effects of lithium. Biol Psychiatry 28:464–465, 1990

Mellow AM, Solano-Lopez C, Davis S: Sodium valproate in the treatment of behavioral disturbance in dementia. J Geriatr Psychiatry Neurol 6:205–209, 1993

Mendels J: Clinical management of the depressed geriatric patient: current therapeutic options. Am J Med 94:13S–18S, 1993

Meyler L, Herxheimer A: Side Effects of Drugs. Baltimore, MD, Williams & Wilkins, 1968

Middelkoop HA, Smilde-van den Doel DA, Neven AK, et al: Subjective sleep characteristics of 1,485 males and females aged 50–93: effects of sex and age, and factors related to self-evaluated quality of sleep. J Gerontol A Biol Sci Med Sci 51: M108–M115, 1996

Miller DD: Effect of phenytoin on plasma clozapine concentration in two patients. J Clin Psychiatry 52:23–25, 1991

Miller F, Menninger J: Correlation of neuroleptic dose and neurotoxicity in patients given lithium and a neuroleptic. Hosp Community Psychiatry 38:1219–1221, 1987

Miller FT, Freilicher J: Comparison of TCAs and SSRIs in the treatment of major depression in hospitalized geriatric patients. J Geriatr Psychiatry Neurol 8:173–176, 1995

Molchan SE, Little JT: Psychosis, in Behavioral Complications of Alzheimer's Disease. Edited by Lawlor BHA. Washington, DC, American Psychiatric Press, 1995, pp 55–76

Morris JC: Metrifonate benefits cognitive, behavioral, and global function in patients with Alzheimer's disease. Neurology 50:1222–1230, 1998

Mueller PS: Neuroleptic malignant syndrome. Psychosomatics 26:654–662, 1985

Mulsant BH, Mazumdar S, Pollock BG, et al: Methodological issues in characterizing treatment response in demented patients with behavioral disturbances. Int J Geriatr Psychiatry 12:537–547, 1997

Mustard CA, Mayer T: Case-control study of exposure to medication and the risk of injurious falls requiring hospitalization among nursing home residents. Am J Epidemiol 145:738–745, 1997

Nahas Z, Kunik ME, Orengo CA, et al: Depression in male geropsychiatric inpatients with and without dementia: a naturalistic study. J Affect Disord 46:243–246, 1997

Narayan M, Nelson JC: Treatment of dementia with behavioral disturbance using divalproex or a combination of divalproex and a neuroleptic. J Clin Psychiatry 58:351–354, 1997

Nelson JC, Jatlow PI, Mazure C: Desipramine plasma levels and response in elderly melancholic patients. J Clin Psychopharmacol 5:217–220, 1985

Niizato K, Ikeda K: Long-term antipsychotic medication of schizophrenics does not promote the development of Alzheimer's disease brain pathology. J Neurol Sci 138:165–167, 1996

Noyes R, Garvey MJ, Cook BL: Benzodiazepine withdrawal: a review of the evidence. J Clin Psychiatry 49:382–389, 1988

Omar SJ, Robinson D, Davies HD, et al: Fluoxetine and visual hallucinations in dementia. Biol Psychiatry 38:556–558, 1995

O'Reilly R, Rusnak C: The use of sedative-hypnotic drugs in a university teaching hospital. CMAJ 142:585–589, 1990

Pancheri P, Delle CR, Donnini M, et al: Effects of moclobemide on depressive symptoms and cognitive performance in a geriatric population: a controlled comparative study versus imipramine. Clin Neuropharmacol 17 (suppl 1):S58–S73, 1994

Paradis CF, Stack JA, George CJ, et al: Nortriptyline and weight change in depressed patients over 60. J Clin Psychopharmacol 12:246–250, 1992

Pare CMB: The present status of monoamine oxidase inhibitors. Br J Psychiatry 146:576–584, 1985

Parker WA: Propranolol-induced depression and psychosis. Clin Pharm 4:214–218, 1985

Parnetti L, Senin U, Mecocci P: Cognitive enhancement therapy for Alzheimer's disease: the way forward. Drugs 53:752–768, 1997

Pato MT, Murphy DL, DeVane CL: Sustained plasma concentrations of fluoxetine and/or norfluoxetine four and eight weeks after fluoxetine discontinuation (letter). J Clin Psychopharmacol 11:224–225, 1991

Pelonero AL, Levenson JL, Silverman JL: Neuroleptic therapy following neuroleptic malignant syndrome. Psychosomatics 26:946–947, 1985

Pennati A, Sacchetti E, Calzeroni A: Dantrolene in lethal catatonia (letter). Am J Psychiatry 148:268, 1991

Perry E, Court J: Biological correlates of dementia. Current Opinion in Psychiatry 5:554–560, 1992

Perry PJ, Calloway RA, Cook BL, et al: Theophylline-precipitated alterations of lithium clearance. Acta Psychiatr Scand 69:528–539, 1984

Philibert RA, Richards L, Lynch CF, et al: Effect of ECT on mortality and clinical outcome in geriatric unipolar depression. J Clin Psychiatry 56:390–394, 1995

Pilowsky LS, Ring H, Shine PJ, et al: Rapid tranquilisation: a survey of emergency prescribing in a general psychiatric hospital. Br J Psychiatry 160:831–835, 1992

Pitner JK, Mintzer JE, Pennypacker LC, et al: Efficacy and adverse effects of clozapine in four elderly psychotic patients. J Clin Psychiatry 56:180–185, 1995

Pollock BG, Perel JM, Altieri LP, et al: Debrisoquine hydroxylation phenotyping in geriatric psychopharmacology. Psychopharmacol Bull 28:163–168, 1992

Pomara N, Singh R, Deptula D, et al: Glutamate and other CSF amino acids in Alzheimer's disease. Am J Psychiatry 149:251–254, 1992

Post RM: Non-lithium treatment for bipolar disorder. J Clin Psychiatry 51 (suppl):9–19, 1990

Post RM, Kimbrell TA, McCann U, et al: Are convulsions necessary for the antidepressive effect of electroconvulsive therapy: outcome of repeated transcranial magnetic stimulation [in French]. Encephale 23 (spec no 3):27–35, 1997

Practice guideline for the treatment of patients with Alzheimer's disease and other dementias of late life. American Psychiatric Association. Am J Psychiatry 154 (suppl):1–39, 1997

Rabins PV, Pearlson E, Aylward E, et al: Cortical magnetic resonance imaging changes in elderly inpatients with a major depression. Am J Psychiatry 148:617–620, 1991

Raheja RK, Bharwani I, Penetrante AE: Efficacy of risperidone for behavioral disorders in the elderly: a clinical observation. J Geriatr Psychiatry Neurol 8:159–161, 1995

Rainer M, Brunnbauer M, Dunky A, et al: Therapeutic results with Cerebrolysin in the treatment of dementia. Wien Med Wochenschr 147:426–431, 1997

Ray WA: Psychotropic drugs and injuries among the elderly: a review. J Clin Psychopharmacol 12:386–396, 1992

Regestein QR: Treatment of insomnia in the elderly, in Clinical Geriatric Psychiatry, 2nd Edition. Edited by Salzman C. Baltimore, MD, Williams & Wilkins, 1992, pp 235–253

Reifler BV: Diagnosing Alzheimer's disease in the presence of mixed cognitive and affective symptoms. Int Psychogeriatr 9 (suppl 1):59–64, 1997

Richelson E: Pharmacology of neuroleptics in use in the United States. J Clin Psychiatry 46:8–14, 1985

Rickels K, Amsterdam JD, Clary C, et al: Buspirone in major depression: a controlled study. J Clin Psychiatry 52:34–38, 1991

Riekkinen M, Schmidt B, Kuitunen J, et al: Effects of combined chronic nimodipine and acute metrifonate treatment on spatial and avoidance behavior. Eur J Pharmacol 322:1–9, 1997

Risse SC, Barnes R: Pharmacologic treatment of agitation associated with dementia. J Am Geriatr Soc 34:368–376, 1986

Rizos AL, Sargenti CJ, Jeste DV: Psychotropic drug interactions in the patient with late-onset depression or psychosis. Psychiatr Clin North Am 11:253–275, 1988

Roberts JE, Renne CE, Dillon J, et al: Exposure to bright light and the concurrent use of photosensitizing drugs. N Engl J Med 326:1500–1501, 1992

Robinson RG, Kubos KL, Starr LP, et al: Mood disorders in stroke patients: importance of location of lesion. Brain 107: 81–93, 1984

Rockwell E, Lam RW, Zisook S: Antidepressant drug studies in the elderly. Psychiatr Clin North Am 11:215–231, 1988

Rockwood K, Ebly E, Hachinski V, et al: Presence and treatment of vascular risk factors in patients with vascular cognitive impairment. Arch Neurol 54:33–39, 1997

Roger M, Attali P, Coquelin JP: Multicenter, double-blind, controlled comparison of zolpidem and triazolam in elderly patients with insomnia. Clin Ther 15:127–136, 1993

Roose SP, Glassman AH, Giardina EGV, et al: Tricyclic antidepressants in depressed patients with cardiac conduction disease. Arch Gen Psychiatry 44:273–275, 1987

Roose SP, Dalak GW, Glassman AH, et al: Cardiovascular effects of bupropion in depressed patients with heart disease. Am J Psychiatry 148:512–516, 1991

Rosebush P, Stewart T: Neuroleptic malignant syndrome. Am J Psychiatry 146:717–725, 1989

Rosenblatt RM, Reich J, Dehrung D: Tricyclic antidepressants in the treatment of depression and chronic pain: analysis of the supporting evidence. Anesth Analg 63:1025–1032, 1984

Ross CA: Alzheimer's disease and other neuropsychiatric disorders. Current Opinion in Psychiatry 5:561–566, 1992

Ross ED: The aprosodias: functional anatomic organization of the affective components of language in the right hemisphere. Arch Neurol 38:561–569, 1981

Ross ED, Rush AJ: Diagnosis and neuroanatomical correlates of depression in brain damaged patients. Arch Gen Psychiatry 38:1344–1354, 1981

Rovner BW: Aging and the central nervous system, in Verwoerdt's Clinical Geropsychiatry, 3rd Edition. Edited by Bienenfeld D. Baltimore, MD, Williams & Wilkins, 1990, pp 17–25

Rovner BW, Steele CD, Shmuely Y, et al: A randomized trial of dementia care in nursing homes. J Am Geriatr Soc 44:7–13, 1996

Roy A, Pickar D: Lithium potentiation of imipramine in treatment-resistant depression. Br J Psychiatry 148:528–533, 1985

Rubin EH, Biggs JT, Preshorn SH: Nortriptyline pharmacokinetics and plasma levels: implications for clinical practice. J Clin Psychiatry 46:418–424, 1985

Ruegg RG, Zosook S, Swerdlow NR: Depression in the aged: an overview. Psychiatr Clin North Am 11:83–94, 1988

Sajatovic M, Ramirez LF, Vernon L, et al: Outcome of risperidone therapy in elderly patients with chronic psychosis. Int J Psychiatry Med 26:309–317, 1996

Sajatovic M, Jaskiw G, Konicki PE, et al: Outcome of clozapine therapy for elderly patients with refractory primary psychosis. Int J Geriatr Psychiatry 12:553–558, 1997

Sakauye KM, Camp CJ, Ford PA: Effects of buspirone on agitation associated with dementia. Am J Geriatr Psychiatry 1:82–84, 1993

Saltz BL, Woerner MG, Kane JM, et al: Prospective study of tardive dyskinesia incidence in the elderly. JAMA 266: 2402–2406, 1991

Salzman C: Clinical guidelines for the use of antidepressant drugs in geriatric patients. J Clin Psychiatry 46 (10, part 2) :38–44, 1985

Salzman C: Principles of psychopharmacology, in Verwoerdt's Clinical Geropsychiatry, 3rd Edition. Edited by Bienenfeld D. Baltimore, MD, Williams & Wilkins, 1990, pp 234–249

Salzman C: The APA task force report on benzodiazepine dependence, toxicity and abuse. Am J Psychiatry 148: 151–152, 1991

Salzman C (ed): Clinical Geriatric Psychiatry, 2nd Edition. Baltimore, MD, Williams & Wilkins, 1992

Salzman C: Clozapine in elderly psychotic patients. J Clin Psychiatry 57:7–12, 1996

Salzman C, Shader RI, Greenblatt DJ, et al: Long vs short half-life benzodiazepines in the elderly: kinetics and clinical effects of diazepam and oxazepam. Arch Gen Psychiatry 40:293–297, 1983

Sano M, Ernesto C, Thomas RG, et al: A controlled trial of selegiline, alpha-tocopherol, or both as treatment for Alzheimer's disease. The Alzheimer's Disease Cooperative Study. N Engl J Med 336:1216–1222, 1997

Sargenti CJ, Rizos AL, Jeste DV: Psychotropic drug interactions in the patient with late-onset psychosis and mood disorder, part 1. Psychiatr Clin North Am 11:235–252, 1988

Sassim N, Grohmann R: Adverse drug reactions with clozapine and simultaneous application of benzodiazepines. Pharmacopsychiatry 21:306–307, 1988

Satlin A, Volicer L, Ross V, et al: Bright light treatment of behavioral and sleep disturbances in patients with Alzheimer's disease. Am J Psychiatry 149:1028–1032, 1992

Saul RF: Pseudotumor cerebri secondary to lithium carbonate. JAMA 253:2869–2871, 1985

Saxena S, Maltikarjuna P: Severe memory impairment with acute overdose lithium toxicity. Br J Psychiatry 152: 853–854, 1988

Scharf MB, Mayleben DW, Kaffeman M, et al: Dose response effects of zolpidem in normal geriatric subjects. J Clin Psychiatry 52:77–83, 1991

Schellenberg R, Todorova A, Wedekind W, et al: Pathophysiology and psychopharmacology of dementia—a new study design, 2: cyclandelate treatment—a placebo- controlled double-blind clinical trial. Neuropsychobiology 35:132–142, 1997

Schiffer RB, Herndon RM, Rudide RA: Treatment of pathological laughing and weeping with amitriptyline. N Engl J Med 312:1480–1482, 1985

Schneider LS: New therapeutic approaches to Alzheimer's disease. J Clin Psychiatry 57 (suppl 14):30–36, 1996

Schneider LS, Pollock VE: A metaanalysis of controlled trials of neuroleptic treatment in dementia. J Am Geriatr Soc 38:553–563, 1990

Schneider LS, Sobin PB: Non-neuroleptic treatment of behavioral symptoms and agitation in Alzheimer's disease and other dementia. Psychopharmacol Bull 28:71–79, 1992

Sevash S, Guterman A, Villalon AV, et al: Improved verbal learning after outpatient oral physostigmine therapy in patients with dementia of the Alzheimer type. J Clin Psychiatry 52:300–303, 1991

Shankle WR, Nielson KA, Cotman CW: Low-dose propranolol reduces aggression and agitation resembling that associated with orbitofrontal dysfunction in elderly demented patients. Alzheimer Dis Assoc Disord 9:233–237, 1995

Shrotriya RC Cutler NR, Sramek JJ, et al: Efficacy and safety of BMY 21,502 in Alzheimer disease. Ann Pharmacother 30:1376–1380, 1996

Shukla S, Mukherjee S, Decina P: Lithium in the treatment of bipolar disorders associated with epilepsy: an open study. J Clin Psychopharmacol 8:201–204, 1988

Shulman KI, Walker SE, Mackenzie S, et al: Dietary restriction, tyramine, and the use of monoamine oxidase inhibitors. J Clin Psychopharmacol 9:397–402, 1989

Shulman KI, Tohen M, Satlin A, et al: Mania compared with unipolar depression in old age. Am J Psychiatry 149:341–345, 1992

Shulman RW, Singh A, Shulman KI: Treatment of elderly institutionalized bipolar patients with clozapine. Psychopharmacol Bull 33:113–118, 1997

Silver JM, Yudofsky S: Propranolol for aggression: literature review and clinical guidelines. International Drug Therapy Newsletter 20:9–12, 1985

Small GW: Tacrine for treating Alzheimer's disease. JAMA 268:2564–2565, 1992

Smith DE, Wesson DR: A new method for treatment of barbiturate dependence. JAMA 213:294–295, 1970

Smith GR, Taylor CW, Linkous P: Haloperidol vs thioridazine for the treatment of psychogeriatric patients: a double-blind clinical trial. Psychosomatics 15:134–137, 1974

Snowdon J: A retrospective case-note study of bipolar disorder in old age. Br J Psychiatry 158:485–490, 1991

Spagnoli A, Cucca U, Menasce G, et al: Long-term acetyl-L-carnitine treatment in Alzheimer's disease. Neurology 41:1726–1732, 1991

Spiegel R: Sleep sleep disorders and the regulation of vigilance in physiological and pathological aging, in Clinical and Scientific Psychogeriatrics, Vol 1: The Holistic Approaches. Edited by Bergener M, Finkel SI. New York, Springer, 1990, pp 216–249

Storey P, Trumble M: Rectal doxepin and carbamazepine therapy in patients with cancer. N Engl J Med 327:1318–1319, 1992

Sultzer DL, Gray KF, Gunay I, et al: A double-blind comparison of trazodone and haloperidol for treatment of agitation in patients with dementia. Am J Geriatr Psychiatry 5:60–69, 1997

Sunderland T, Silver MA: Neuroleptics in the treatment of dementia. Int J Geriatr Psychiatry 3:79–88, 1998

Swartz JR, Miller BL, Lesser IM, et al: Frontotemporal dementia: treatment response to serotonin selective reuptake inhibitors. J Clin Psychiatry 58:212–216, 1997

Szuba MP, Bergman KS, Baxter LR Jr, et al: Safety and efficacy of high dose droperidol in agitated patients (letter). J Clin Psychopharmacol 12:144–146, 1992

Tamminga CA, Lahti AC: The new generation of antipsychotic drugs. Int Clin Psychopharmacol 11 (suppl 2):73–76, 1996

Tariot PN: Neurobiology and treatment of dementia, in Clinical Geriatric Psychiatry, 2nd Edition. Edited by Salzman C. Baltimore, MD, Williams & Wilkins, 1992, pp 277–299

Tariot PN, Erb R, Leibovici A, et al: Carbamazepine treatment of agitation in nursing home patients with dementia: a preliminary study. J Am Geriatr Soc 42:1160–1166, 1994

Tariot PN, Schneider L, Porsteinsson AP: Treating Alzheimer's disease: pharmacologic options now and in the near future. Postgrad Med 101:73–76, 1997

Tariot PN, Erb R, Podgorski CA, et al: Efficacy and tolerability of carbamazepine for agitation and aggression in dementia. Am J Psychiatry 155:54–61, 1998

Tesar GE, Murray GB, Cassem VH: Use of high-dose intravenous haloperidol in the treatment of agitated cardiac patients. J Clin Psychopharmacol 5:344–347, 1985

Thal LJ, Schwartz G, Sano M, et al: A multicenter double-blind study of controlled-release physostigmine for the treatment of symptoms secondary to Alzheimer's disease. Physostigmine Study Group. Neurology 47:1389–1395, 1996

Thomas RJ: Seizures and epilepsy in the elderly. Arch Intern Med 157:605–617, 1997

Thompson TL, Filley C, Mitchell D, et al: Lack of efficacy of Hydergine in patients with Alzheimer's disease. N Engl J Med 323:445–448, 1990

Thorpe L: The treatment of psychotic disorders in late life. Can J Psychiatry 42 (suppl 1):19S–27S, 1997

Tolbert SR, Fuller MA: Selegiline in treatment of behavioral and cognitive symptoms of Alzheimer disease. Ann Pharmacother 30:1122–1129, 1996

Tollefson G: Short-term effects of the calcium channel blocker nimodipine (bay-e-9736) in the management of primary degenerative dementia. Biol Psychiatry 27:1133–1142, 1990

Tom T, Cummings JL: Depression in Parkinson's disease: pharmacological characteristics and treatment. Drugs Aging 12:55–74, 1998

Trappler B, Vinuela LM: Fluvoxamine for stereotypic behavior in patients with dementia. Ann Pharmacother 31:578–581, 1997

Valldeoriola F, Nobbe FA, Tolosa E: Treatment of behavioural disturbances in Parkinson's disease. J Neural Transm Suppl 51:175–204, 1997

Van Someren EJW: Indirect bright light improves circadian rest-activity rhythm disturbances in demented patients. Biol Psychiatry 41:955–963, 1997

Van Valkenberg C, Clayton PJ: Electroconvulsive therapy and schizophrenia. Biol Psychiatry 20:699–700, 1983

Vestergaard P, Poulstrup I, Schou M, et al: Prospective studies in a lithium cohort. Acta Psychiatr Scand 78:434–441, 1988

Vry JD, Fritze J, Post RM: The management of coexisting depression in patients with dementia: potential of calcium channel antagonists. Clin Neuropharmacol 20:22–35, 1997

Walstra GJ, Teunisse S, van Gool WA, et al: Reversible dementia in elderly patients referred to a memory clinic. J Neurol 244:17–22, 1997

Warneke L: Psychostimulants in psychiatry. Can J Psychiatry 35:3–10, 1990

Weiler PG, Mungas D, Bernick C: Propranolol for the control of disruptive behavior in senile dementia. J Geriatr Psychiatry Neurol 1:226–230, 1988

Weisbard JJ, Pardo M, Pollack S: Symptom change and extrapyramidal side effects during acute haloperidol treatment in chronic geriatric schizophrenics. Psychopharmacol Bull 33:119–122, 1997

Werner P, Cohen-Mansfield J, Farley J, et al: Effects of removal of physical restraints on psychotropic medication in the nursing home. Journal of Geriatric Drug Therapy 8:59–71, 1994

Weyer G, Babej-Dolle RM, Hadler D, et al: A controlled study of 2 doses of idebenone in the treatment of Alzheimer's disease. Neuropsychobiology 36:73–82, 1997

Wills P, Claesson CB, Fratiglioni L, et al: Drug use by demented and non-demented elderly people. Age Ageing 26:383–391, 1997

Wilson WH: Clinical review of clozapine treatment in a state hospital. Hosp Community Psychiatry 43:700–703, 1992

Wimo A, Karlsson G, Nordberg A, et al: Treatment of Alzheimer disease with tacrine: a cost-analysis model. Alzheimer Dis Assoc Disord 11:191–200, 1997

Wolk SI, Douglas CJ: Clozapine treatment of psychosis in Parkinson's disease: a report of five consecutive cases. J Clin Psychiatry 53:373–376, 1992

Wragg RE, Jeste DV: Neuroleptics and alternative treatments: management of behavioral symptoms and psychosis in Alzheimer's disease and related conditions. Psychiatr Clin North Am 11:195–212, 1988

Yaffe K, Sawaya G, Lieberburg I, et al: Estrogen therapy in postmenopausal women: effects on cognitive function and dementia. JAMA 279:688–695, 1998

Yassa R, Camille Y, Belzile L: Tardive dyskinesia in the course of antidepressant therapy: a prevalence study and review of the literature. J Clin Psychopharmacol 7:243–246, 1987

Yassa R, Nair NPV, Iskandar H: Late-onset bipolar disorder. Psychiatr Clin North Am 11:117–129, 1988

Yassa R, Nastase C, Cvejic J, et al: The Pisa syndrome (or pleurothotonus): prevalence in a psychogeriatric population. Biol Psychiatry 29:942–945, 1991

Yeager B: Management of the behavioral manifestations of dementia. Arch Intern Med 155:250–260, 1995

Young RC, Klerman GL: Mania in late life: focus on age at onset. Am J Psychiatry 149:867–876, 1992

Young RC, Meyers BS: Psychopharmacology, in Comprehensive Review of Geriatric Psychiatry. Edited by Sadavoy J, Lazarus LW, Jarvik LF. Washington, DC, American Psychiatric Press, 1991, pp 435–467

Young RC, Alexopoulos GS, Shamoian CA, et al: Plasma 10-hydroxynortriptyline and ECG changes in elderly depressed patients. Am J Psychiatry 142:866–868, 1985

Yudofsky SC, Kopecky HJ, Kunik M, et al: The Overt Agitation Severity Scale for the objective rating of agitation. J Neuropsychiatry Clin Neurosci 9:541–548, 1997

Zarate CA Jr, Baldessarini RJ, Siegel AJ, et al: Risperidone in the elderly: a pharmacoepidemiologic study. J Clin Psychiatry 58:311–317, 1997

Zayas EM, Grossberg GT: Treating the agitated Alzheimer patient. J Clin Psychiatry 57:46–51, 1996

Zis AP, Goodwin FK: Major affective disorder as a recurrent illness. Arch Gen Psychiatry 36:835–839, 1979

Zyss T, Gorka Z, Kowalska M, et al: Preliminary comparison of behavioral and biochemical effects of chronic transcranial magnetic stimulation and electroconvulsive shock in the rat. Biol Psychiatry 42:920–924, 1997

35

Electroconvulsive Therapy

C. Edward Coffey, M.D.

Charles H. Kellner, M.D.

If major depression were not a serious public health problem in the elderly population, there would be no need to discuss electroconvulsive therapy (ECT) in this book. Yet, major depression is one of the most common and serious illnesses in the elderly (see Chapter 13). In addition to death from suicide, depressive illness is associated with substantial mortality from medical illness (Avery and Winokur 1976). ECT remains the "gold standard" treatment for serious depression and, as such, requires careful consideration as a therapeutic modality. Such consideration is particularly relevant because there is evidence that ECT is especially safe and effective in elderly patients (Consensus Conference 1985) and because of the sensitivity to the side effects of antidepressant medication experienced by the geriatric population. With the burgeoning of psychopharmacological treatments for depression over the past 35 years, many may have believed that ECT was well on its way to extinction; however, we are now no longer sanguine about the efficacy of antidepressant medications for all patients. Even with the

most sophisticated psychopharmacological treatment combinations, a substantial proportion of patients remains severely ill. For these patients, it is fortunate that ECT is still available.

The case for ECT is strengthened by its remarkable record of safety. ECT compares favorably with any procedure in all of medicine for its low morbidity and mortality. With recent advances in ECT technique, the safety profile of the treatment continues to be refined, and ECT has enjoyed a resurgence as a more mainstream treatment in the psychiatric armamentarium. Furthermore, it has a predictably rapid onset of effect and can be performed in both inpatient and outpatient settings.

It is widely known that ECT is most commonly used for the treatment of severe depression. We will discuss its use for this indication in depth here, but because this is a textbook of neuropsychiatry, we will also evaluate ECT as a treatment for mood disorders due to a general medical condition such as poststroke depression, as well as for neurological disorders such as Parkinson's disease. As the mind-body dualism separating the fields of psychiatry and neurology dissolves, investigators and clinicians will have further opportunities to explore the potent effects of ECT on functions of the brain as well as of the mind.

ECT in Geriatric Practice

Considerable evidence exists to demonstrate that a large proportion of patients receiving ECT is elderly. Kramer (1985) reviewed patterns of ECT use in California between 1977 and 1983 and found that the probability of receiving ECT increased with age of the patient. Patients 65 years and older were given ECT at a rate of 3.86/10,000 population, compared with 0.85/10,000 in those 25–44 years old. In an analysis of the data on ECT use in California between 1984 and 1994, Kramer (1999) found similar patterns. Lambourn and Barrington (1986) surveyed the use of ECT from 1972 to 1983 in a British population of 3 million and found that ECT was more common in patients (especially female patients) 60 years or older. In a study of 5,729 psychiatric admissions over 3 years, Malla (1988) found that patients who received ECT in general hospitals were significantly older than patients who did not receive ECT. Babigian and Guttmacher (1984) reviewed a massive data set from the Monroe County (New York) Psychiatric Case Register over three 5-year periods. They found that among patients who were being hospitalized for the first time, those who received ECT were older than those who did not. Thompson et al. (1994) analyzed data from the National Institute of Mental Health Sample Survey Program for 1980 and 1986, which included representative samples of psychiatric inpatients in the United States. These researchers found that approximately one-third of ECT recipients were 65 years or older, a figure far out of proportion to the representation of that age group in the sample (8.2%). In contrast, Hermann et al. (1995) reported that age was not related to ECT use as estimated from the American Psychiatric Association's 1988–1989 Professional Activities Survey.

Several features of the natural history of major depressive illness help to explain the frequent use of ECT in elderly patients. Post (1992) reviewed data suggesting that major affective disorders increase in both severity and cycle frequency with increasing age. In a review of the course of illness of late-onset depression, Alexopoulos (1990) cited evidence for an association between high relapse rates and later onset of illness (Zis and Goodwin 1979). Thus in the geriatric population, the frequency and severity of depressive illness, its impact on quality of life, and the increased sensitivity of the elderly to adverse effects of antidepressant medications, combine to make ECT an attractive and often-used treatment option (Benbow 1987, 1989; McCall et al. 1999; Weiner 1982).

Medical Physiology of ECT in Elderly Patients

The data on the physiology of ECT have been compiled largely from mixed-age samples, and to our knowledge, few data focus specifically on the physiology of ECT in elderly patients. Clearly, the myriad physiological changes that accompany an ECT seizure take on particular importance in elderly individuals, in whom medical illnesses involving multiple organ systems are so common. In a study of 33 elderly patients (mean age, 74 years) receiving ECT, Gaspar and Samarasinghe (1982) found the incidence of major or minor medical risk factors for ECT to be 75%. Of greatest importance are the physiological effects of ECT on the brain and the cardiovascular system. As described later in this chapter, modifications in ECT technique may be required in patients with brain or cardiovascular disease.

Cerebral Physiology

With ECT, an electrical stimulus is used to depolarize cerebral neurons and thereby produce a generalized cerebral seizure. The mechanism by which ECT seizures are propagated is not well understood. Bilateral ECT appears to lead to seizure generalization through direct stimulation of the diencephalon, whereas seizures induced with unilateral stimulation may begin focally in the stimulated cortex and then generalize via corticothalamic pathways (Staton 1981).

During the initial phase of the induced seizure, electroencephalographic activity is variable, consisting of patterns of low-voltage fast activity and polyspike rhythms. These patterns correlate with tonic or irregular clonic motor movements. With seizure progression, electroencephalographic activity evolves into a pattern of hypersynchronous polyspikes and waves that characterize the clonic motor phase. These regular patterns begin to slow and eventually disintegrate as the seizure ends, sometimes terminating abruptly in a flat electroencephalogram (EEG) (Weiner and Krystal 1993). The ictal EEG has been the focus of much research, by our group and others, aimed at identifying markers of therapeutic response (discussed in a later section). These studies indicate that age has a major impact on a number of ictal EEG measures and is associated with shorter seizure duration, shorter slow-wave–phase duration, weaker overall strength and patterning, and lower early ictal, midictal, and postictal amplitudes (Krystal et al. 1995, 1998; Nobler et al. 1993).

Transient cumulative changes are also evident on the interictal EEG during a course of ECT. Increased predominance of delta activity on the interictal EEG is seen as a function of the number of ECT treatments given in a course of ECT and their rate of administration (Fink 1979). Asymmetric (left greater than right) decreases in average EEG frequency after a course of ECT have been correlated with increasing age of the patient (Turek 1972; Volavka et al. 1972). (No such relation was reported by Bergman et al. [1953].) Strömgren and Juul-Jensen (1975) found an association between age and postictal slowing with bilateral ECT but not with unilateral nondominant ECT. By 30 days after the ECT course, EEGs resemble baseline EEGs in most patients (Abrams 1997a). The effects of aging on the severity and persistence of interictal electroencephalographic changes have not been extensively studied.

The ECT-induced seizure is also associated with a variety of transient and benign changes in cerebral physiology, including increases in cerebral blood flow, cerebral blood volume (resulting in a transient increase in intracranial pressure), and cerebral metabolism of oxygen and glucose (Bolwig et al. 1977; Brodersen et al. 1973; Prohovnik et al. 1986). The brief increase in intracranial pressure is rarely of clinical consequence, but it is the reason for the well-known proscription against ECT in patients with space-occupying mass lesions. Postictally, cerebral blood flow and metabolism are decreased globally and regionally for at least several hours, and then they return to normal values (Nobler et al. 1994; Rosenberg et al. 1988; Scott et al. 1994; Volkow et al. 1988). Conflicting data exist regarding the interictal effects of ECT, with both reduced (Nobler et al. 1994) and increased (Bonne et al. 1996) cerebral blood flow reported approximately 1 week after a course of ECT. The effects of age on these changes have not been described.

Transient disruptions in blood-brain barrier permeability also occur during the seizure (Bolwig et al. 1977) and may account for the short-lived increase in T_1 relaxation times demonstrated by brain magnetic resonance (MR) imaging after ECT (Mander et al. 1987; Scott et al. 1990). The effects of age and associated brain changes on these blood-brain barrier alterations have not been described in humans, but in animals age is associated with more pronounced blood-brain barrier changes after 10 electroconvulsive seizures (Oztas et al. 1990).

Cardiovascular Physiology

ECT results in a marked activation of the autonomic nervous system, and the relative balance of parasympathetic and sympathetic nervous system activity determines the observed cardiovascular effects (Applegate 1997). Vagal (parasympathetic) tone is increased during and immediately after administration of the electrical stimulus, and this may be manifested by bradycardia or even a brief period of asystole. With development of the seizure, activation of the sympathetic nervous system occurs, resulting in a marked increase in heart rate, blood pressure, and cardiac workload. Peripheral stigmata of sympathetic activation may also be observed and include piloerection and gooseflesh. The tachycardia and hypertension continue through the ictus and generally end along with the seizure. Shortly after the seizure, there may be a second period of increased vagal tone that may be manifested by bradycardia and various dysrhythmias, including ectopic beats. As the patient awakens from anesthesia, there may be an additional period of increased heart rate and blood pressure as a result of arousal and further sympathetic outflow (Welch and Drop 1989).

The cardiovascular responses during ECT combine to produce an increase in myocardial oxygen demand and a decrease in coronary artery diastolic filling time. Transient electrocardiographic changes in the ST segment and T waves are seen in some patients during the procedure, but it is unclear whether these findings are related to myocardial ischemia (Gould et al. 1983; McCall 1997; Wesner 1986; Zvara et al. 1997). A direct effect of central nervous system stimulation on cardiac repolarization has been proposed as an alternative mechanism (Welch and Drop 1989). No corresponding increase in levels of cardiac enzymes has been found to accompany these electrocardiographic changes (Braasch and Demaso 1980). In a study of patients receiving ECT, Messina et al. (1992) obtained echocardiograms during and after ECT treatments and found transient regional wall motion abnormalities more often in patients with ST-T changes on electrocardiograms (ECGs), suggesting a period of demand myocardial ischemia. The clinical importance of these findings remains to be evaluated.

The effects of age on the cardiovascular response to ECT have been examined in only a few modern studies. Shettar et al. (1989) randomly assigned 19 patients (mean age [± SD], 51 ± 21 years; range, 19–84 years) to ECT with pretreatment with glycopyrrolate or with placebo, the alternate pretreatment drug being used for the subsequent ECT treatment (i.e., each patient served as his or her own control). For both types of pretreatment, there was no correlation between age and length of poststimulus asystole. In two controlled studies of mixed-age samples that included elderly patients (Prudic et al. 1987; Webb et al. 1990), no relationship was found between age and ECT-induced changes in heart rate, blood pressure, or rate-pressure product. In a study of relatively younger patients (mean age, 43 years; range, 20–64 years), Huang et al. (1989) noted a significant inverse correlation between age and increases in blood pressure and rate-pressure product.

Although these results suggest that age, per se, is not associated with the extent of the cardiovascular response to ECT, these findings must be interpreted cautiously. Some of the subjects in these studies (especially those who were older) were also receiving antihypertensive drug therapy that may have attenuated their cardiovascular response to the treatments, and (as discussed later in this chapter) other clinical observations suggest that at least some elderly patients with cardiovascular disease may be at risk for marked increases in pulse and blood pressure during ECT (Applegate 1997; Bodley and Fenwick 1966; Gerring and Shields 1982; Zielinski et al. 1993).

Diagnostic Indications and Efficacy

Major Depression

The most common indication for ECT in the elderly population remains depression, both unipolar and bipolar. In elderly patients with depression, ECT is typically used as a second-line treatment, after patients have failed to respond to a trial of medication or have exhibited intolerance of the side effects of medication. ECT should be considered a first-line intervention, however, in certain situations: severe suicidality, inanition and malnutrition, history of previous response to ECT, or patient preference (American Psychiatric Association 2000).

Several clinical studies involving mixed-age samples and various diagnoses have found increasing age to be associated with a favorable outcome from ECT (Black et al. 1993; Carney et al. 1965; Coryell and Zimmerman 1984; Folstein et al. 1973; Gold and Chiarella 1944; Kahn et al. 1959; Mendels 1965; Roberts 1959; Strömgren 1973). Investigators in other studies involving older patients have reported a diminished response to unilateral but not bilateral ECT (Heshe et al. 1978; Pettinati et al. 1986; Strömgren 1973) or a requirement for longer courses of treatment (Ottosson 1960; Rich et al. 1984b).

The effects of ECT in elderly patients with depression have been directly examined in a small number of studies, but results are somewhat difficult to compare because of differences in patient samples (e.g., size and diagnosis), ECT technique (e.g., stimulus waveform and dosage and electrode placement), and assessment methodology (Table 35–1). Nevertheless, reported response rates range from

63% to 98%, clearly demonstrating that increasing age, per se, does not have a negative impact on the effectiveness of ECT for depressive illness. Indeed, other data (although uncontrolled) indicate that ECT is associated with reduced chronicity, decreased morbidity, and decreased mortality (Avery and Winokur 1976; Babigian and Guttmacher 1984; Wesner and Winokur 1989).

There are no controlled, prospective, randomized studies comparing the efficacy and side effects of ECT versus drug therapy for treatment of depression in elderly patients. In a retrospective chart review of 112 consecutive geriatric hospital admissions, Meyers and Mei-Tal (1985–1986) compared outcome in depressed patients who had received ECT with outcome in those who had received tricyclic antidepressants (nonrandom assignment) and found that ECT was associated with a better response rate (81% versus 62%) and a lower morbidity rate (0% versus 27%).

Because major depression in elderly patients appears to respond well to ECT, there may be little need to correlate specific clinical features with ECT response. However, in the case of data derived largely from mixed-age samples, a particularly good response to ECT has been associated with the presence of psychosis, catatonia, pseudodementia, pathological guilt, anhedonia, agitation, and neurovegetative signs (Greenberg and Fink 1992; Hickie et al. 1996; Salzman 1982; Zorumski et al. 1988). In a prospective study involving 29 elderly patients (Fraser and Glass 1980), guilt, anhedonia, and agitation were identified as positive prognostic signs. In multiple studies, response to ECT has been particularly good in patients with delusional depression, compared with a nonpsychotic group (Hickie et al. 1996; Mulsant et al. 1991; Pande et al. 1990; Wilkinson et al. 1993), although other studies have found no difference (O'Leary et al. 1995; Rich et al. 1984a, 1986; Sobin et al. 1995; Solan et al. 1988). The use of ECT in agitated or psychotic elderly patients may spare them exposure to neuroleptic agents. This consideration is important, given the high risk of tardive dyskinesia and drug-induced parkinsonism in elderly patients (Jenike 1985; see also Chapter 25).

Several authors have also attempted to identify predictors of nonresponse to ECT. In a retrospective study, Magni et al. (1988) compared elderly patients who responded to ECT and those who did not respond and found that physical illness during the index episode, fewer negative life events preceding the onset of the index episode, and prior depressive episodes of long duration were predictive of nonresponse to ECT. Other investigators have found that longer duration of the index episode predicts poorer outcome (Fraser and Glass 1980; Karlinsky and

TABLE 35–1. Studies of electroconvulsive therapy (ECT) as a treatment for geriatric depression

Study	Subjects	Methods	Findings
Fraser and Glass 1980	29 patients (8 men, 21 women) Age 64–86 years Depressive illness by Feighner criteria[a]	Prospective ECT two times/week; chopped sine wave; randomized assignment to bilateral (n = 16) or right unilateral (n = 13) electrode placement Blinded outcome rating	Both groups had significant reductions in HRSD scores 3 weeks after last treatment, at which point 28 patients (97%) showed "satisfactory" clinical outcome. No group differences in therapeutic response. Average time to reorientation after fifth ECT treatment was 32.8 minutes for bilateral ECT and 9.5 minutes for right unilateral ECT. WMS scores improved during ECT, and 3 weeks after ECT all scores were normal. No group differences.
Gaspar and Samarasinghe 1982	33 patients (9 men, 24 women) Age 66–88 years (mean ± SD, 73.9 ± 5.7 years) Depression in 28 (85%) of 33 patients; diagnostic criteria unspecified	Prospective ECT two times/week for 3–4 weeks, then one time/week; mean number of ECT treatments, 8.7 (range, 2–29); bilateral Outcome rated as good, intermediate, poor	Good outcome in 26 patients (79%), intermediate outcome in 3 (9%), poor outcome in 4 (12%).
Karlinsky and Shulman 1984	33 inpatients (11 men, 22 women) Age 62–85 years (mean ± SD, 73.2 ± 5.0 years) DSM-III major depression, single episode, in 12 patients (36.4%); major depression, recurrent, in 18 (54.5%); bipolar disorder in 3 (9.1%)	Retrospective ECT two or three times/week; sine wave; unilateral (n = 23, 69.7%), bilateral (n = 3, 9.1%), or both (n = 7, 21.2%) Nonblinded outcome rating by author consensus from clinical progress notes Follow-up at 3 and 6 months	Immediate "good" response in 14 patients (42.4%), "moderate" response in 12 (36.4%), "poor" response in 7 (21.2%). During 6-month follow-up, 23 patients (69.7%) remained out of hospital and 6 (18.2%) received more ECT. Only one complication (pneumonia), and even this patient was able to complete ECT course.
Burke et al. 1985	30 patients (7 men, 23 women) Age 60–82 years (mean, 72 years) DSM-III major depression in 24 patients, bipolar disorder in 5	Retrospective Average number of ECT treatments, 9 (range, 1–25); brief pulse; bilateral in 70% Outcome rating (four-point scale) determined by review of medical records	92% of patients with major depression improved, and 69% showed complete symptom resolution.
Burke et al. 1987	136 patients (39 men, 97 women) Mean age of total sample, 48 years; 96 subjects < 60 years (mean ± SD, 39 ± 12.19 years), 40 subjects > 60 years (mean ± SD, 69 ± 6.43 years) 81% of total sample had a major affective disorder; diagnoses of elderly subgroup unspecified	Sine wave; bilateral in 87%, unilateral in 73%; mean number (± SD) of ECT treatments, 9 ± 3.6	70% of total sample had complete resolution of affective symptoms (61% < 60 years, 75% > 60 years). Complication rates increased with age (35% in older group, 18% in younger group).
Kramer 1987	50 inpatients (9 men, 41 women) Age 61–88 years (mean, 74.1 years) DSM-III major depression in 49 patients, schizophrenia in 1	Retrospective ECT three times/week; brief pulse; bilateral all patients Nonblinded assessment by author's chart review	46 patients (92%) "much improved" after ECT. No serious medical complications.
Godber et al. 1987	163 patients (43 men, 120 women) Mean age, 86 years; all > 65 years Primary depression by Feighner criteria[a] in 153 patients (94%), psychotic symptoms in 80 (49%)	ECT two times/week for most patients, three times/week for those slow to respond; sine wave; right unilateral in 155 patients (95%); mean number of ECT treatments, 11.2	83 patients (51%) "fully recovered," 37 (23%) "much improved," 34 (21%) poor response.
Magni et al. 1988	30 patients (14 men, 16 women) Mean age, 73.9 years DSM-III major depression	Retrospective ECT two or three times/week initially, then once weekly; bilateral in all patients; minimum of 7 ECT treatments (range, 7–12) Independent clinical rating by two psychiatrists	19 patients (63%) responded to ECT.

(continued)

TABLE 35–1. Studies of electroconvulsive therapy (ECT) as a treatment for geriatric depression *(continued)*

Study	Subjects	Methods	Findings
Coffey et al. 1988	44 inpatients (18 men, 26 women) with leukoencephalopathy Age 60–86 years (mean, 73 years) DSM-III major depression in all patients	Retrospective ECT three times/week; brief-pulse, "moderately suprathreshold" stimulus; average number of ECT treatments, 9 (range, 6–14) Nonblinded global ratings of clinical response	"Excellent" response in 54%, "good" response in 44%.
Coffey et al. 1989	51 inpatients (15 men, 36 women) Age 60–90 years (mean, 71.3 years) DSM-III major or bipolar depression in 49 patients, organic affective disorder in 2	Prospective ECT three times/week; brief pulse; unilateral (*n* = 38), bilateral (*n* = 3), or both (*n* = 10); mean number of ECT treatments, 9 (range, 5–18) Nonblinded observer and patient self-rating	42 patients (82%) met criteria for full therapeutic response. No association between ECT response and brain white matter abnormalities on magnetic resonance images.
Mulsant et al. 1991	42 inpatients (7 men, 35 women) Age 60–89 years (mean ± SD, 73.5 ± 7.3 years) DSM-III major depression	Prospective ECT three times/week; brief pulse; unilateral (*n* = 29, 69%), bilateral (*n* = 3, 7%), or unilateral and then bilateral (*n* = 10, 24%); mean number of ECT treatments, 8.3 (range, 4–13) HRSD, BPRS, and MMSE scores, used for outcome rating, obtained by research nurses	28 patients (67%) had excellent response to ECT (50% decrease in HRSD score). 38 patients had decrease in BPRS score. No significant change in mean MMSE scores for group.
Rubin et al. 1991	101 inpatients (19 men, 82 women) Mean age (± SD), 76.0 ± 6.4 years DSM-III unipolar depression	Retrospective 46 patients (46%) received ECT (technique not described), some in combination with antidepressant drug therapy; 65 (64%) received antidepressant drug therapy only; nonrandomized Nonblinded retrospective outcome rating by unit director	Relative to patients treated with drug therapy, those who received ECT had significantly lower final BDI scores, greater reduction in BDI scores, and higher frequency of ratings of "major improvement" (78% vs. 42% for non-ECT group).
Kellner et al. 1992	15 patients (11 men, 4 women) Age 53–87 (mean, 69.9 years) DSM-III major depression	Prospective Blinded rating of outcome measures including cognitive assessment and antidepressant response Randomized assignment to ECT one time/week or three times/week for 3 weeks; brief pulse; bilateral	All patients improved. Mean HRSD scores decreased from 27 to 12 in three times/week group and from 29 to 20 in one time/week group. No difference in cognitive effects between groups.
Wilkinson et al. 1993	78 patients (23 men, 55 women) Four age groups (18–39, 40–64, 65–74, and 75–88 years) 43 patients > 65 years (mean, 68.96 years in age 65–74 group and 79.50 years in age 75–88 group) DSM-III major depression with melancholia or psychosis	Prospective ECT two times/week; right unilateral in 5 patients (6%), bilateral in remainder; mean number of ECT treatments, 7.9 Nonblinded cognitive and affective ratings Positive response to ECT defined as ≥ 50% reduction in Montgomery Asberg Depression Rating Scale	Positive response to ECT in 73% of patients ≥ 65 years and 54% of patients < 65 years. Age associated with response to ECT, and with more improvement in cognition on MMSE with ECT.
Casey and Davis 1996	19 patients (8 men, 16 women) Mean age 79.5 years DSM-III major depression in 18 patients; bipolar disorder depressed in 1	Retrospective Brief-pulse ECT (22 courses); nonrandomized electrode placement (bilateral, *n* = 13; unilateral, *n* = 1; both, *n* = 8) Nonblinded assessment of "complication," "confusion,"and clinical response (4-point scale)	Clinical response (rating of ≥ 3) achieved in 19 (86.3%) courses. Response associated with younger age, lower ASA rating, and absence of neurological disorder. Complications in 5 patients: dental (1), cardiovascular (2), urinary retention (1), and confusion (1).

(continued)

TABLE 35–1. Studies of electroconvulsive therapy (ECT) as a treatment for geriatric depression *(continued)*

Study	Subjects	Methods	Findings
Tomac et al. 1997	34 patients > 85 years old (79% female) Mean age 81 years (range 85–96) DSM-III-R major depression (85%), bipolar disorder (9%), depressive disorder NOS (3%), delusional disorder (3%), and dementia NOS (59%)	Retrospective Brief-pulse ECT three times/week (mean, 7 ECTs); nonrandomized electrode placement (unilateral, 65%; bilateral, 18%; and both 17%); stimulus dosage at 150%–200% initial seizure threshold Nonblinded assessment of therapeutic response and treatment complications	Significant increase in GAF (mean, 8.2 points, $n = 30$) and significant decrease in HRSD (mean, 5.7 points, $n = 16$) and BPRS (mean, 47.2 points, $n = 18$). Significant increase in MMSE scores (mean, 2.6 points, $n = 20$) Treatment complications in 27 (79%): most common included confusion or delirium (32%), transient hypertension (67%), and arrhythmia (24%)
Gormley et al. 1998	67 patients > 75 years old (73% female) Mean age 79.4 years (range 75–91) ICD-10 recurrent depression (78%), bipolar disorder (15%), or depressive disorder (7%)	Retrospective Brief-pulse ECT twice weekly (mean, 6.7 ECTs); nonrandomized electrode placement (bilateral, 95%; unilateral, 2%; both, 3%) Nonblinded assessment of therapeutic response (4-point scale), "complications," "confusion," and "memory impairment"	Marked improvement in 53% and moderate improvement in 32% Complications in 11% (prolonged confusion, 6.5%; hypomania, 4%; hypertension, 2%; headache, 2%)
Tew et al. 1999	268 women Adults (< age 60 years), 133 patients; young-old (age 60–74 years), 63 patients; old-old (≥ age 75 years), 72 patients DSM-III-R major depression	Prospective Brief-pulse ECT three times/week; nonrandomized electrode placement (bilateral, $n = 22$; unilateral, $n = 136$; both, $n = 87$); stimulus dosage at 2.5 times initial seizure threshold Nonblinded assessment of therapeutic response (HRSD score ≤ 10 at 3 days post last ECT) and of MMSE scores	Adult group had lower response rate (54%) than young-old group (73%), whereas old-old group had an intermediate rate of response (67%); no relation of response to burden of medical illness. Only adult group showed significant decline in MMSE scores at 3 days post ECT.

Note. BDI = Beck Depression Inventory; BPRS = Brief Psychiatric Rating Scale; DSM-III = Diagnostic and Statistical Manual of Mental Disorders, 3rd Edition (American Psychiatric Association 1980); HRSD = Hamilton Rating Scale for Depression; MMSE = Mini-Mental State Exam; WMS = Wechsler Memory Scale.
[a]See Feighner et al. 1972.

Shulman 1984). Previous courses of ECT and increased age at the time of first treatment with ECT have been linked with a slower response rate to ECT, with no effect on eventual positive outcome (Rich et al. 1984b; Salzman 1982; Shapira and Lerer 1999) These limited data should not discourage the clinician from initiating a trial of ECT in patients with any of the aforementioned predictors of nonresponse. Clinical experience suggests that many elderly patients with these putative predictors of nonresponse often will improve with ECT.

Efforts at using biological markers to predict ECT response in elderly patients have met with equivocal success. A variety of probes have been investigated in mixed-age samples, including the dexamethasone suppression test (DST), the thyrotropin-releasing hormone (TRH) test, and other neuroendocrine tests (Decina et al. 1987; Kamil and Joffe 1991; Kirkegaard et al. 1975; Krog-Meyer et al. 1984; Papakostas et al. 1981; Swartz 1993), as well as polysomnographic studies (Coffey et al. 1988; Grunhaus et al. 1996). None of these laboratory studies appear to be strong "state-specific" markers for major depressive illness, and data are conflicting on whether they can be used serially to follow the course of ECT, predict outcome, or predict early relapse. Nevertheless, a report by Devanand et al. (1991) suggests that consideration of complex technical factors in neuroendocrine testing may enhance the clinical utility of such assessments in ECT.

Mania

Although extensive clinical experience indicates that ECT is effective for treating both the manic and depressed phases of bipolar illness in elderly patients, formal data for this population are lacking. A small number of controlled studies involving relatively young mixed-age samples have found ECT to be superior to drug therapy (Mukherjee 1988; Mukherjee et al. 1994; Small et al. 1988, 1991). ECT appeared to be particularly effective in mixed bipolar states and agitated mania, conditions that tend to become more prevalent as the illness becomes more chronic and refractory (Calabrese et al. 1993). Many elderly patients with bipolar disorder have reached this more severe phase of the illness and thus may be expected to have a particularly good response to ECT. Anticonvulsant medications are often effective in mixed bipolar disorder (Calabrese et al. 1993), although we are not aware of efficacy studies testing this use of anticonvulsants in elderly patients. ECT itself also has powerful anticonvulsant properties (Coffey et al. 1995b; Sackeim et al. 1983). Whether bilateral ECT is more effective than nondominant unilateral ECT in the treatment of mania remains controversial (Small et al. 1991).

Schizophrenia and Other Psychotic Disorders

No controlled data exist on the use of ECT in elderly patients with schizophrenia. ECT has been used in relatively younger patients with this illness, and in these patients the presence of affective or catatonic features, an acute onset of illness with relatively brief duration of illness, or a history of response to ECT, correlate with good outcome (American Psychiatric Association 2000). ECT is not very effective for treating the chronic, residual phase of the illness with predominant negative features (Weiner and Coffey 1988). These "deficit" states become more common as the illness progresses (Kaplan and Sadock 1988) and thus should be highly represented in elderly schizophrenic populations, although controlled data on this issue are lacking.

ECT has also been used in elderly patients with other psychotic disorders. Botteron et al. (1991) reported the cases of three elderly patients with late-onset psychosis treated with ECT. None of the patients had major depression or dementia. Two patients with substantial structural brain changes as shown by MR imaging (lateral ventricular enlargement and deep white matter hyperintensities) did not respond to ECT. A third patient with bilateral caudate hyperintensities and normal subcortical white matter did respond to ECT. As will be discussed later, we have noted an excellent response to ECT for major depression in patients with subcortical hyperintensities on magnetic resonance images, including patients with psychotic symptoms and late-age onset (Coffey et al. 1989). To the best of our knowledge, there are no data on the efficacy of ECT in patients with late-onset functional psychoses, such as paraphrenia.

Concomitant Neurological Disease

There is increasing clinical evidence that ECT may be effective for affective disorders in patients with brain disease (Dubovsky 1986; Hsiao et al. 1987; Krystal and Coffey 1997; Weiner et al., in press; Zwil et al. 1992). In some cases, advantage has been taken of the neurobiological effects of ECT in order to treat the neurological disorder. Issues related to modifications of ECT technique in patients with cerebral disease are discussed later in this chapter.

Affective disorder in dementia. Twenty percent to 30% of patients with dementia have marked concomitant depression, and 10%–15% of patients with a diagnosis of dementia actually have the pseudodementia of depression (Price and McAllister 1989; Rummans et al. 1999). Depression may be difficult to diagnose in demented patients. Some dementia patients may be too ill to generate depressive complaints, with affective disorder manifesting itself chiefly as agitated, screaming behavior with neurovegetative signs. Determining whether there is a personal or family history of affective disorder may be helpful in diagnosing depression in these patients (Fogel 1988). Thorough treatment of depression in patients with dementia often does much to enhance quality of life and functional status. (The effectiveness of drug therapy for depression in patients with dementia is discussed in Chapter 34.)

Fisman (1988) reported the case of a man with major depression and profound pseudodementia whose condition was diagnosed incorrectly for 14 years as Alzheimer's disease before his affective disorder was successfully treated with ECT. In a literature review of the cases of 56 patients with dementia and depression treated with ECT, Price and McAllister (1989) found the rate of response of depression to be 73%. ECT effectively treated depression in several subtypes of dementia, including senile dementia of the Alzheimer's type, multi-infarct dementia, and normal-pressure hydrocephalus, as well as the dementias of Parkinson's disease and Huntington's disease (Price and McAllister 1989). Locations of electrodes were not specified in the majority of cases reviewed. Nearly one-third of patients with dementia also had an improvement in cognition after ECT. Delirium was a relatively infrequent complication of ECT in these patients (overall occurrence, 21%), clearing by the time of discharge in all but one patient.

Dementia does not appear to be worsened by ECT. Still, to minimize cognitive side effects of ECT, physicians of patients with dementia may need to pay special attention to issues of concomitant medications, electrode placement, and frequency of treatments (discussed below). Prospective studies are needed to address the efficacy and side effects of ECT in depressed patients with dementia.

Parkinson's disease. As discussed in Chapter 26, depression is common in patients with Parkinson's disease, and treatment of depression with medication may be complicated. Pharmacological treatment of the parkinsonism is also limited. Levodopa therapy for Parkinson's disease often has serious side effects and does little to retard the progression of the illness. Increasing doses of the medication are required to maintain motor function but in turn cause more and more debilitating side effects such as hallucinations, dyskinesias, and the on-off phenomenon. Neuroleptics may improve the psychoses and dyskinesia but increase parkinsonism. This situation has led to recent attempts to graft fetal mesencephalic tissue into the brains of patients with Parkinson's disease (Krauss and Jankovic 1996). Despite some encouraging results, these experi-

ments remain fraught with difficulty at multiple levels (Fahn 1992). Pallidotomy and deep brain stimulation are other neurosurgical procedures that have recently been gaining wider acceptance (Arle and Alterman 1999).

In this setting of limited treatment options, reports of the efficacy of ECT in Parkinson's disease offer the hope of a safe and effective treatment (Table 35–2). Case reports document that ECT is an effective treatment for both the motor manifestations of Parkinson's disease and the commonly associated depression (for a review, see Kellner and Bernstein 1993). Interestingly, some patients experience improvement in motor symptoms but not improvement in mood, or vice versa (Kellner and Bernstein 1993; Young et al. 1985).

A group of Swedish investigators (Andersen et al. 1987) performed the most methodologically rigorous trial of ECT in Parkinson's disease. In this double-blind, controlled, crossover-design comparison of real ECT and sham ECT, 9 (82%) of 11 nondepressed elderly patients with the on-off phenomenon experienced substantial improvement in parkinsonian symptoms with ECT, with the improvement lasting 2–6 weeks. Sham ECT was ineffective. Nine patients received bilateral ECT (8 responded, 1 did not respond) and 2 patients received right unilateral ECT (1 responded, 1 did not respond). A total of five to six treatments was given during the active phase of the trial. The stimulus-dosing strategy was not fully detailed in the report.

In a prospective naturalistic study, Douyon et al. (1989) studied seven patients with both Parkinson's disease and major depression. Major improvement in motor function was noted after only two bilateral treatments. Following an average of seven bilateral ECT treatments with "just above threshold" stimulus dosing, mean New York University Parkinson's Disease Rating Scale scores decreased from 65 to 32 (51% improvement). Patients remained well, without further ECT, for 4 weeks to 6 months. Although initial Hamilton Depression Scale scores were determined for all patients (all scores were greater than 20), follow-up scores were determined for only four. Depression scores decreased by a mean of 50% in these patients. In the report of another prospective naturalistic study, Zervas and Fink (1991) described the successful ECT treatment of four nondepressed elderly patients with severe refractory Parkinson's disease. Three of the four patients received bilateral ECT. Stimulus-dosing strategies were not specified. Improvement in parkinsonism rating scores of 20%–40% was observed. Two patients were successfully treated with ongoing maintenance ECT, but once it was discontinued, both patients relapsed within 4–6 weeks. Finally, ECT has also been found to be effective for neuroleptic-induced

TABLE 35–2. Electroconvulsive therapy (ECT) for the treatment of Parkinson's disease

Study	Number of subjects	Diagnosis	ECT course	Treatment response
Fromm 1959	8	Parkinson's disease	5–6 bilateral ECT treatments	Improvement: 5 patients Mild improvement: 2 patients No improvement: 1 patient
Brown 1973	7	Parkinson's disease and major depression	Average of 8 ECT treatments (electrode placement unknown)	No improvement in Parkinson's symptoms No improvement in depression
Lebensohn and Jenkins 1975	2	Parkinson's disease and depression: 1 patient Parkinson's disease and bipolar disorder, depressed: 1 patient	4–6 ECT treatments (electrode placement unknown)	Improvement in Parkinson's symptoms: 2 patients Improvement in depressive symptoms: 2 patients
Lipper and Bermanzohn 1975	1	Parkinson's disease and psychotic depression	7 ECT treatments (electrode placement unknown)	Marked improvement in depression Improvement in Parkinson's symptoms
Dysken et al. 1976	1	Parkinson's disease and depression	12 bilateral ECT treatments	Improvement in Parkinson's symptoms Improvement in depressive symptoms
Asnis 1977	1	Parkinson's disease and psychotic depression	6 bilateral ECT treatments	Improvement in Parkinson's symptoms Improvement in depressive symptoms
Yudofsky 1979	1	Parkinson's disease and psychotic depression	10 ECT treatments (electrode placement unknown)	Improvement in Parkinson's symptoms Improvement in depressive symptoms
Balldin et al. 1980	5	Parkinson's disease: 5 patients Parkinson's disease and depression: 3 patients	4–8 bilateral ECT treatments	Improvement in Parkinson's symptoms: 5 patients Improvement in depressive symptoms: 3 patients
Balldin et al. 1981	9	Parkinson's disease	3–8 bilateral ECT treatments	Marked improvement: 5 patients Slight improvement: 2 patients No improvement: 2 patients
Ward et al. 1980	5	Parkinson's disease	6 bilateral ECT treatments	No improvement: 5 patients
Holcomb et al. 1983	1	Parkinson's disease and depression	14 ECT treatments (electrode placement unknown)	Improvement in Parkinson's symptoms Improvement in depressed mood
Levy et al. 1983	1	Parkinson's disease and major depression	10 ECT treatments (electrode placement unknown)	Improvement in Parkinson's symptoms Resolution of depressive symptoms
Young et al. 1985	1	Parkinson's disease, major depression, and dementia	7 right unilateral ECT treatments	Improvement in Parkinson's symptoms No improvement in depressed mood or cognitive function
Jaeckle and Dilsaver 1986	1	Parkinson's disease and bipolar disorder, depressed	9 bilateral ECT treatments	Improvement in Parkinson's symptoms Improvement in depressed mood

Study	N	Diagnosis	ECT	Outcome
Andersen et al. 1987	11	Parkinson's disease	Sham control / Bilateral: 9 patients / Right unilateral: 2 patients	Improvement: 9 patients
Burke et al. 1988	3	Parkinson's disease and depression	5–8 right unilateral ECT treatments	Improvement in Parkinson's symptoms: 2 patients / Improvement in depressed mood: 3 patients
Atre-Vaidya and Jampala 1988	1	Parkinson's disease and mania	12 bilateral ECT treatments	Improvement in Parkinson's symptoms / Resolution of manic symptoms
Roth et al. 1988	1	Parkinson's disease and bipolar disorder, manic	10 right unilateral ECT treatments	Improvement in Parkinson's symptoms / Resolution of manic symptoms
Birkett 1988	5	Parkinson's disease and major depression	Right unilateral ECT (number of treatments unknown)	Improvement in Parkinson's symptoms: 4 patients / Improvement in depressive symptoms: 4 patients
Douyon et al. 1989	7	Parkinson's disease and major depression	Average of 7 bilateral ECT treatments	Improvement in depressed mood: 7 patients / Improvement in Parkinson's symptoms: 7 patients
Lauterbach and Moore 1990	1	Parkinson's disease and major depression	9 ECT treatments (electrode placement unknown)	Improvement in Parkinson's symptoms / Improvement in depression
Zervas and Fink 1991	4	Parkinson's disease	8–12 ECT treatments / Bilateral: 3 patients / Right unilateral: 1 patient	Improvement in Parkinson's symptoms: 4 patients
Friedman and Gordon 1992	5	Parkinson's disease and major depression	7–12 ECT treatments / Bilateral: 1 patient / Right unilateral: 3 patients / Electrode placement unknown: 1 patient	Improvement in depressed mood: 4 patients / Improvement in Parkinson's symptoms: 3 patients
Holzer et al. 1992	1	Parkinson's disease and major depression	8 right unilateral ECT treatments	Improvement in Parkinson's symptoms / Improvement in depressed mood
Oh et al. 1992	11	Parkinson's disease and major depression (10 patients) or mania (1 patient)	3–9 ECT treatments / Bilateral: 1 patient / Right unilateral: 9 patients / Unilateral then bilateral: 1 patient	Minor improvement in Parkinson's symptoms: 2 patients / Improvement in psychiatric symptoms: 6 patients / Post-ECT delirium: 7 patients

parkinsonism (Hermesh et al. 1992).

Rasmussen and Abrams (1991) suggested that the primary indication for ECT in Parkinson's disease be refractoriness to, or intolerance of, antiparkinsonian medication in patients with severe disability from the disease. They recommended that ECT for Parkinson's disease be initiated with right unilateral placement at substantially suprathreshold electrical dosage, with a switch to bilateral ECT if no response is seen after three right unilateral treatments. However, some patients with Parkinson's disease may be at increased risk of developing delirium during ECT (Figiel et al. 1991), a complication that could be worsened by use of bilateral electrode placement. For patients who have clearly benefited from ECT, Rasmussen and Abrams (1991) recommended maintenance ECT administered just frequently enough to maintain improvement. Recently, Aarsland et al. (1997) reported on two additional patients whose Parkinson's disease was successfully treated with maintenance ECT.

The mechanism by which ECT benefits patients with Parkinson's disease is unclear. Rudorfer et al. (1988) found significant increases in cerebrospinal fluid homovanillic acid, the primary metabolite of dopamine in the central nervous system, after a course of ECT. In addition to these presumed presynaptic effects, Fochtmann (1988) found increased dopamine, subtype 1 (D_1), receptor binding in the substantia nigra of rats who had electrically induced seizures. She hypothesized that these changes may be associated with other changes in the dopamine system, including upregulation of postsynaptic dopamine, subtype 2 (D_2), receptors in the striatum. Another potential dopamine-enhancing mechanism may be the temporary disruption of the blood-brain barrier seen with ECT (Bolwig et al. 1977), allowing an increase in brain concentrations of levodopa. Whatever the mechanism by which dopamine potentiation may occur, levodopa doses may need to be decreased during a course of ECT to avoid dyskinesia and delirium presumably related to dopamine overactivity.

Poststroke depression. As discussed in Chapter 27, approximately one-third of patients develop marked depression in the 2 years after a stroke (Robinson and Price 1982; Rummans et al. 1999). In a placebo-controlled trial, Lipsey et al. (1984) found a statistically significant improvement in poststroke depression treated with nortriptyline. In other uncontrolled studies, the response rate to psychostimulants in this population was 47%–52% (Finklestein et al. 1987; Lingam et al. 1988). However, patients with stroke are often quite medically ill and debilitated and may be intolerant of pharmacotherapy. In the study by Lipsey et al. (1984), 35% of patients assigned to receive nortriptyline dropped out because of medication intolerance.

Clinical reports suggest that ECT may also be effective for treating poststroke depression. In a retrospective chart review of 14 patients with poststroke depression (mean age, 66 years) treated with ECT at Massachusetts General Hospital, Murray et al. (1986) found that 86% had marked improvement in depression after ECT. Apparently, no patient exhibited any worsening of neurological deficit, and although formal measures of cognitive status were not reported, 5 of the 6 patients with "cognitive impairment" before ECT showed lessening of this deficit after ECT.

Currier et al. (1992) published retrospective data on 20 geriatric patients with poststroke depression treated with ECT at the same hospital, with predominantly nondominant unilateral electrode placement being used. A "marked or moderate response" to ECT was observed in 95% of patients. No patient experienced any exacerbation of preexisting neurological deficits, but 3 patients exhibited "minor encephalopathic complications" (prolonged postictal confusion and amnesia) and two patients developed "severe interictal delirium requiring neuroleptics." Of note, 7 of their patients (37%) relapsed within a mean of 4 months of discontinuation of ECT, despite ongoing maintenance drug therapy.

Elderly psychiatric patients with no clinical history of stroke often have subcortical white matter hyperintensities on magnetic resonance images, which are believed to be evidence of ischemic cerebrovascular disease. Coffey et al. (1989) found a high rate (82%) of response to ECT in depressed patients with these MRI findings, many of whom had been refractory to antidepressant drug therapy. In addition, the majority of the patients tolerated the course of ECT without major systemic or cognitive side effects. This positive outcome with ECT is especially notable given other data that suggest that subcortical ischemic disease may be associated with depressive illness that is resistant to treatment with antidepressant medications (Fujikawa et al. 1996).

In summary, ECT may be effective for poststroke depression, but controlled prospective data are needed to confirm this clinical impression and to identify patients potentially at risk for the adverse cognitive effects of the treatment.

Other neuropsychiatric illnesses. A variety of other mental syndromes secondary to medical conditions in elderly patients may improve with ECT (Hsiao et al. 1987), including catatonia and delirium from many different causes (Fink 1996, 1997; Krystal and Coffey 1997; Strömgren 1997;

Weiner et al. 2000). Indeed, the antidelirium effect of ECT may occur even in the absence of improvement in the conditions that originally caused the delirium. A careful neuropsychiatric evaluation is required in such instances to clarify the etiology, including those conditions that might increase the risk involved in ECT (discussed later in this chapter).

Issues of ECT Technique Relevant to Elderly Patients

Pretreatment Evaluation

When a patient is referred for ECT, a focused evaluation of indications and risk factors for the treatment should ensue (American Psychiatric Press 2000; Coffey 1998). The patient's current mental status, neuropsychiatric history (including recent somatic therapies and history of treatment with ECT), and family psychiatric history should be reviewed. In the evaluation of medical risk factors for the treatment, the focus should be on the brain, the cardiovascular system, the musculoskeletal system, and the upper gastrointestinal tract. Any history of head trauma or surgery, seizures, focal or general neurological complaints, angina, congestive heart failure, bony fractures, osteoporosis, spinal disease or trauma, or esophageal reflux should be elicited. Any personal or family history of problems with anesthesia should be noted.

Handedness should be assessed because of its relevance to nondominant unilateral electrode placement (Kellner et al. 1997). Because the hand used for writing is a fallible indicator, patients should be asked which hand they use to throw a ball, cut with a knife, and so on (American Psychiatric Association 2000). A minority of left-handed patients and patients with mixed dominance may have language localized to the right hemisphere. For this reason, if substantial confusion is observed in a left-handed patient after the first right unilateral ECT treatment, consideration should be given to the use of left unilateral electrode placement at the next session. The time required for the patient to become fully oriented after the treatment can be measured for each type of electrode placement, and the treatment series can then be continued using the placement associated with less confusion (Pratt et al. 1971).

A careful documentation of baseline affective and cognitive status is essential in elderly patients before initiation of ECT. In our clinical experience, the Hamilton or Montgomery Asberg Depression Rating Scales and the Mini-Mental State Exam are often helpful standardized instruments that may be used at intervals throughout the ECT course.

A physical examination and basic laboratory tests (e.g., serum potassium assay) should be performed and an ECG obtained before ECT is initiated in elderly patients. Special care should be given to the neurological examination, including the funduscopic examination to rule out papilledema. Further studies, such as a hemogram, serum chemistries, spine X-rays, EEGs, brain computed tomography (CT) scans or magnetic resonance images, and cardiac functional evaluations (Applegate 1997; Coffey 1998; Rayburn 1997), should be ordered as clinically indicated. Elderly patients have an increased occurrence of clinically important incidental brain findings (e.g., aneurysm, subdural hematoma, undiagnosed primary or metastatic brain tumor, and evidence of increased intracranial pressure), and brain imaging may have predictive value as a tool to detect increased risk for some ECT side effects (discussed in a later section) (Coffey 1996). The EEG can be helpful for differentiating between pseudodementia and dementia in some cases (Leuchter 1991). A baseline EEG to determine background frequency may also be helpful for comparison in cases of prolonged encephalopathy after ECT. Roemer et al. (1990) performed quantitative analyses of pre-ECT EEGs in elderly patients with depression and found that normal anterior interhemispheric coherence in the delta frequency band was associated with more clinical improvement, whereas a poorer clinical response was seen in those patients with lower coherence values.

For patients with serious cardiovascular disease, consultation with a cardiologist is often indicated. Once the decision to proceed with ECT has been made, the cardiologist should be asked how best to maximize the patient's cardiovascular function in preparation for, and during, ECT (McCall 1997).

The patient's medications should be carefully reviewed. Typically, all psychotropics are stopped before ECT, although neuroleptics may be used if necessary (Farah et al. 1995). Lithium taken around the time of ECT has been linked to an increased incidence of delirium and seizures (Weiner et al. 1980). These effects may be related to an increase in brain lithium concentration, due to transient opening of the blood-brain barrier with ECT. Most patients should not receive lithium for several days before or after ECT (Kellner et al. 1991a), although exceptions to this rule should be considered in patients who have demonstrated early relapse when not taking the medication.

Antidepressants are usually stopped to avoid cumulative cardiac and central nervous system side effects (Kellner et al. 1991a), although this practice is now being reconsidered. Studies in the early 1960s found no added benefit with tricyclic antidepressant and ECT combination therapy (Seager and Bird 1962). However, in a retrospective chart review of 84 geriatric patients with depression, Nelson and Benjamin (1989) found improved outcome (i.e., the need for fewer treatments) with tricyclic antidepressant and ECT combination therapy. No increase in side effects occurred in the group receiving combination therapy. The study was severely limited by its retrospective design and by the fact that the ECT-only group presumably included more medically ill patients, in whom antidepressant drug therapy may have been stopped for fear of complication (Nelson and Benjamin 1989). Recently, Lauritzen et al. (1996) demonstrated the safety of ECT combined with paroxetine or imipramine, as well as the ability of both antidepressants to decrease relapse in the 6 months after index treatment (although paroxetine was more effective for relapse prevention than was imipramine).

Benzodiazepines may impair the intensity of the therapeutic seizure, thereby decreasing treatment response (Kellner 1997b; Pettinati et al. 1986). The use of these agents in elderly patients may also theoretically increase their susceptibility to cognitive side effects from ECT. Benzodiazepine use thus should be minimized or stopped before ECT.

In patients with epilepsy, the anticonvulsant effect of ECT itself may allow for a temporary decrease in anticonvulsant dose. There are few reported data about the effects of carbamazepine and valproate on the efficacy of ECT. However, because anticonvulsant medications could interfere with the induction of adequate ECT seizures, anticonvulsants prescribed for psychiatric indications (i.e., not for epilepsy) should usually be tapered and discontinued before ECT (Kellner et al. 1997).

Several other specific pharmacological issues require attention. Theophylline levels should be monitored closely, because high blood levels during ECT have been associated with status epilepticus (Abrams 1997a). Echothiophate, an organophosphate glaucoma medication that irreversibly inhibits cholinesterase and pseudocholinesterase, may cause prolonged apnea when combined with succinylcholine and should not be given (Zorumski et al. 1988). Likewise, donepezil (Aricept) and tacrine (Cognex), reversible cholinesterase inhibitors used as cognition enhancers in patients with Alzheimer's disease, could increase the duration of succinylcholine muscle relaxation (*Physicians' Desk Reference* 1999). Otherwise, patients should take any required cardiac, antireflux, or other medications with a sip of water the morning of the ECT session.

A final and critically important component of the pre-ECT evaluation is the informed consent procedure. According to the 1999 American Psychiatric Association Task Force report on the practice of ECT, adequately informed consent should involve "1) the provision of adequate information, 2) a patient who is capable of under-

standing and acting intelligently upon such information, and 3) the opportunity to provide consent in the absence of coercion" (American Psychiatric Association 2000). Compared with younger patients, those over 65 appear to be less aware that they can refuse ECT (Malcolm 1989). With the increased prevalence of cognitive impairment in elderly patients, competency to consent becomes a major issue, and the education of both patient and family becomes essential. This is also a time in the patient's life cycle when children are becoming increasingly responsible for their parents, and the patient's children should be involved in the consent process whenever possible. Incompetent patients may require the judicial appointment of a legal guardian for consent. (For a pertinent sample of an informed consent document, see American Psychiatric Association 2000).

Recently, there has been a shift to performing ECT on an outpatient basis. Many centers have found this to be a viable and efficient way to offer the treatment, as long as certain precautions are taken (Association for Compulsive Therapy 1996). First, the patient's psychiatric illness must allow for safe management outside the hospital. Clearly, acute suicidality or agitated psychosis will often require inpatient hospitalization. Second, the patient's medical status should be stable enough for safe outpatient management. Additionally, strong social support is required; family members or others must transport the patient to and from the treatment facility, ensure the patient takes nothing by mouth (NPO) for at least 8 hours before a treatment session, and provide supervision between treatments (with particular attention paid to ensuring that the patient refrains from driving and making important financial or personal decisions while experiencing cognitive side effects) (Fink 1994). For some patients, it is helpful to administer the first (or several initial) ECT treatment on an inpatient basis and then switch to outpatient treatments once it has been established that outpatient treatments can be administered safely and comfortably.

ECT Technique

In the United States, ECT is commonly given as a series of single treatments on alternate mornings. Elderly individuals typically receive ECT initially in an inpatient setting. Patients have been previously evaluated for coexisting medical conditions and indications for treatment, and the consent process has been initiated. The treatment team consists of a psychiatrist, an anesthesiologist, and specially trained nursing personnel. ECT is typically given in either a special treatment suite or the recovery area of an operating room suite. Patients should have nothing to eat or drink for at least 8 hours before treatment. Once baseline vital signs and an ECG have been obtained and pulse oximetry has been performed, the short-acting barbiturate methohexital is given at a dosage of approximately 1 mg/kg body weight iv, followed by the depolarizing neuromuscular blocker succinylcholine, given at a dosage of 0.75–1.5 mg/kg body weight iv. Adequacy of neuromuscular blockade is monitored by the use of a peripheral nerve stimulator or by clinical assessment of relaxation, including loss of reflexes and tone.

Throughout the procedure, the patient is ventilated with 100% oxygen and blood oxygen saturation is monitored using a pulse oximeter. Heart rate and blood pressure are also closely monitored. After a specially designed bite block is inserted into the patient's mouth, a predetermined electrical stimulus is delivered across electrodes placed on the patient's properly prepared scalp. Typically, a generalized seizure ensues, lasting from 20 to 90 seconds. The seizure is monitored by electroencephalography and by observation of the motor manifestations of the seizure, a blood pressure cuff having been inflated above systolic pressure on the right ankle to prevent access of the succinylcholine to the right foot. Ventilatory support is continued until the patient emerges from the anesthesia, and further recovery is provided in an environment with as little stimulation as possible. The entire procedure takes about 20 minutes, and patients are often able to have breakfast within an hour of the time of treatment.

A typical course of ECT consists of 6–12 treatments, although occasionally patients may require fewer or more treatments to achieve full response. The treatment schedule is often modified in elderly patients to lessen cognitive side effects, with treatments given once or twice per week rather than three times per week (American Psychiatric Association 2000; Freeman 1995; Lerer et al. 1995; Zervas et al. 1993). ECT is stopped when maximal clinical improvement is thought to have been achieved or when further improvement is not noted between treatments. Special attention is then given to continuation/maintenance treatment with either medication or ECT (discussed in a later section).

Anesthesia Considerations

Brief, light general anesthesia is used during ECT to render the patient unconscious during (and thus amnesic for) the procedure. Methohexital is the agent of choice because it has rapid onset and a brief duration of action and induces minimal postanesthesia confusion. Methohexital also appears to have a lesser anticonvulsant effect than thiopental, propofol, or alfaxalone with alfadolone (Althesin) (Bergsholm and Swartz 1996). Still, because methohexital

is an anticonvulsant, and because the seizure threshold is often increased in elderly patients (see the following section), the lowest effective anesthetic dose is desirable. Because methohexital dosing is based on lean body mass, the required methohexital dosage in many elderly patients may be less than 1 mg/kg total body weight (Fragen and Avram 1990). In some cases, etomidate is a reasonable alternative to methohexital, but it is more expensive and is associated with pain on infusion, longer cognitive recovery time, and short-term adrenocortical suppression.

The preferred neuromuscular blocking agent for ECT is succinylcholine, primarily because it has rapid onset and a brief duration of action. The use of succinylcholine may require special consideration in the elderly patient. Succinylcholine stimulates muscarinic cholinergic receptors in the sinus node and may cause bradycardia, especially if serial doses are required. This effect may be pronounced in patients receiving β-blockers and those with evidence of preexisting conduction delay on ECGs, both frequently the case among elderly patients. Pretreatment with anticholinergics, such as atropine or glycopyrrolate, will block this bradycardiac effect (the use of anticholinergic premedication is discussed in greater detail later in this chapter). Patients with extensive burns or trauma, or with severe spasticity or paralysis, may have an exaggerated extracellular release of potassium in response to succinylcholine (R. D. Miller and Savarese 1990). Use of a nondepolarizing muscle relaxant should be considered in these patients. Myalgia following ECT may be due to either the fasciculation caused by succinylcholine or excessive motor movement during the seizure. Fasciculation may be blocked in subsequent ECT treatments by administering a small pretreatment dose (e.g., 3 mg) of *d*-tubocurarine.

Intragastric pressure also increases with use of succinylcholine, related to abdominal skeletal muscle fasciculation; however, the risk of gastric reflux and aspiration is reduced by a concomitant increase in esophageal pressure above the lower esophageal sphincter (R. D. Miller and Savarese 1990). Certain groups of elderly patients (e.g., those with hiatal hernia, gastroparesis, or morbid obesity) are at risk for substantial gastroesophageal reflux during the procedure, with subsequent risk for aspiration pneumonitis (Zibrak et al. 1988). Smokers are particularly prone to morbidity from aspiration (Lichtor 1990). In these patients, additional strategies beyond requiring NPO status before a session may be considered to decrease gastric volume and acidity during ECT. Premedication with histamine, subtype 2 (H_2), receptor antagonists or sodium citrate decreases gastric acidity, and metoclopramide increases lower esophageal sphincter tone and promotes gastric emptying (Lichtor 1990).

Stimulus Dosing

Seizure threshold (the amount of electricity required to elicit a seizure) increases with age (Coffey et al. 1995a; Sackeim et al. 1991). This effect is believed to be the result of a decrease in the excitability of the brain but may also be partially due to increases in skull thickness (electrical resistance) with aging. Older patients thus require higher ECT stimulus intensities (doses) than do younger patients, but the optimal stimulus dosage for ECT has yet to be determined. Data from mixed-age samples suggest that barely suprathreshold stimulus intensities may be ineffective (especially for unilateral nondominant ECT), whereas excessive stimulus dosing has been linked to more cerebral toxicity (Sackeim et al. 1993; Weiner et al. 1986). Given these data, our clinical practice is to use stimulus dosing in unilateral ECT that is at least 2.5 times the patient's seizure threshold. This method of stimulus dosing requires a determination of the patient's seizure threshold, which may be done routinely at the first ECT session by increasing stimulus intensity in fixed increments over successive stimulations until a seizure results (Coffey et al. 1995a; Kellner et al. 1997; Sackeim et al. 1987). For bilateral ECT, we use a stimulus dose that is 1.5 times the seizure threshold, because the efficacy of this modality appears to be less sensitive to dosing effects than that of unilateral ECT.

Seizure threshold increases during ECT (the well-known anticonvulsant effect), necessitating increases in stimulus dose during the course of therapy (Coffey et al. 1990, 1995b; Kellner et al. 1997; Sackeim 1991; Sackeim et al. 1991). This effect does not appear to be more pronounced in elderly patients, but because this population has a higher initial seizure threshold, some older patients may eventually require stimulus intensities during their course of treatment that exceed the maximal settings of the ECT device. In such instances, we have found administration of caffeine to be an effective and well-tolerated strategy for augmenting ECT seizures in elderly patients (Coffey et al. 1987, 1990; Lurie and Coffey 1990). Higher-powered ECT devices (available in some European countries) are also helpful. The effects of cerebral disease and age-related changes in brain structure on ECT seizure threshold have not been described but are currently under study in our laboratories.

Electrode Placement

The choice of unilateral or bilateral ECT in the elderly patient is often a complex one. Studies in mixed-age samples suggest that right unilateral ECT has fewer cognitive side effects (Weiner et al. 1986). Most research has also found unilateral and bilateral ECT to be equally effective (American Psychiatric Association 2000); however, in those studies in which differences have been noted, bilateral ECT has consistently been found to be more effective (for a review, see Abrams 1997a).

Few studies have addressed the issue of electrode placement specifically in elderly patients. In a meta-analysis of the literature, Pettinati et al. (1986) found a trend for improved efficacy in elderly patients receiving bilateral treatment. In the only reported randomized study, 29 elderly patients with depression were assigned either to unilateral or bilateral ECT two times a week (Fraser and Glass 1980). Stimulus-dosing strategies were unclear. No group differences were observed in terms of therapeutic response or memory performance after ECT, but those subjects randomized to bilateral electrode placement required more time to become reoriented after the fifth ECT treatment (Table 35–1). Whether the effects of cerebral disease or age-related structural brain changes modify the therapeutic or adverse effects of unilateral versus bilateral ECT in elderly patients has not been studied.

Thus, limited data exist to guide the choice of ECT electrode placement in elderly patients with neuropsychiatric illness. Our approach is to begin with right unilateral ECT in elderly patients, switching to bilateral ECT if minimal or no response is seen by the fifth or sixth treatment. Because bilateral ECT may have a more rapid onset of action, it may be considered the treatment of choice in patients in urgent need of care. If intolerable cognitive side effects develop with bilateral ECT, the treatment may be changed to unilateral ECT once the affective disorder has begun to respond. Finally, atypical electrode placements (e.g., left unilateral, right frontotemporal–left frontal, or bifrontal) may be clinically useful in some elderly patients (Kellner 1997a; Letemendia et al. 1993; Manly and Swartz 1994).

Seizure Monitoring

The seizure may be monitored indirectly by observation of the convulsive motor response of a "cuffed" extremity, but more direct monitoring with ictal electroencephalography is preferred. The ECT seizure is monitored to confirm that a seizure has occurred and to determine when it has ended (Kellner et al. 1997; Weiner and Krystal 1993). More recently, the ictal EEG has been studied using sophisticated computer analysis to determine whether various indices such as amplitude, regularity, or coherence may be predictive of treatment efficacy (Krystal et al. 1995, 1996; Weiner and Krystal 1993). These studies suggest that such measures hold promise for indicating seizure adequacy during treatment sessions.

Continuation/Maintenance ECT

Major depression is increasingly recognized as a chronic, relapsing condition. Some studies have found 6-month relapse rates as high as 50% for patients initially responsive to antidepressant medications who are then given no form of continuation/maintenance therapy (Prien and Kupfer 1986). Similarly high rates of relapse have been noted after response to ECT if no form of continuation/maintenance therapy is given (Imlah et al. 1965; Jarvie 1954). Frank et al. (1990) found that relapse rates after response to pharmacotherapy can be substantially reduced by continuation of antidepressant medication at full dose.

ECT is one of the few treatments in modern medicine that is commonly stopped as soon as it has proven effective. Usual clinical practice involves administration of continuation/maintenance pharmacotherapy after successful ECT. Because these patients often failed to respond to medication therapy before ECT, it is not surprising that a 50% relapse rate at 1 year was found for patients receiving maintenance pharmacotherapy after response to ECT (Sackeim et al. 1990). In that study, there was a particular propensity to relapse within 4 months after successful ECT.

Results of a growing number of studies involving mixed-age samples indicate that continuation/maintenance ECT is safe and effective for the prevention of depressive relapse, and there are several promising retrospective studies involving elderly patients (for a review, see Monroe 1991). Thienhaus et al. (1990) described the cases of six elderly patients with major mood disorder treated with maintenance ECT for a period of 1–6 years. While receiving maintenance ECT, patients spent significantly fewer days in the hospital per year on average, compared with the interval prior to beginning maintenance ECT.

Dubin et al. (1992) reported the successful use of maintenance ECT for an average of 22 months in a group of eight patients over age 75. The single patient in the case series who required rehospitalization had been previously withdrawn from maintenance ECT by her attending psychiatrist and placed on fluoxetine. No major adverse events were associated with maintenance ECT in this case series.

Loo et al. (1991) described the use of maintenance ECT in seven elderly patients over an average of 3 years. Mean time in the hospital during this 3-year period decreased to 3 weeks, compared with 27 weeks for patients treated during the 3 years before the introduction of maintenance ECT. Patients had 1.4 recurrences of illness during the maintenance ECT period, compared with 4.7 recurrences for patients during the 3 years preceding maintenance ECT.

In one of the few prospective studies to date, we (Clarke et al. 1989) evaluated 27 patients (mean age, 65 years; range, 26–90 years) not taking psychotropic medications who were assigned to a continuation ECT protocol after initial response to ECT. Only 8% of patients who completed the continuation ECT protocol required rehospitalization, whereas 47% of those who did not complete the protocol relapsed (a statistically significant difference).

Studies comparing continuation/maintenance ECT with continuation/maintenance pharmacotherapy after response to ECT are lacking in the literature. As of this writing, a multisite study comparing treatment with nortriptyline, nortriptyline plus lithium, and placebo after successful ECT is nearing completion (Sackeim 1997) and a second multisite study comparing continuation ECT and treatment with nortriptyline plus lithium has been initiated (C.H. Kellner, A.J. Rush, M. Fink, T. Rummans, unpublished data, 1996). Interim results of the former indicate high relapse rates after ECT for patients (mixed-age group) receiving monotherapy (approximately 75%) compared with patients receiving nortriptyline plus lithium (approximately 40%).

Continuation/maintenance ECT typically involves single treatments given initially at weekly intervals, with the frequency gradually reduced to every 4–8 weeks, as the patient's depressive symptoms allow. The increased interval between maintenance treatments results in fewer cognitive side effects than with an index course of ECT, leading to the suggestion that bilateral treatment may be the modality of choice for continuation/maintenance ECT (Kellner et al. 1991c). Several factors determine whether the treatments can be given on an outpatient basis. Patients must reliably follow NPO orders for 6–8 hours before treatment (patients are permitted only a sip of water to take any required premedications). Patients must also have an adequate support system to assure observation and care for several hours after treatment. If these criteria cannot be met, or if the patient has complex medical or recovery needs, an overnight stay in the hospital may be required.

Adverse Effects of ECT and Their Management

The safety of ECT compares favorably with that of any treatment requiring general anesthesia. The mortality is variously reported as approximating three deaths per 100,000 treatments (the same as for general anesthesia for minor surgery) and may actually be decreasing as medical management of underlying illnesses improves (Abrams 1997a). To put these data into perspective, Abrams (1997b) noted that ECT is 10 times safer than childbirth and that the risk of dying from being struck by lightning is 6 times higher than the risk of dying from ECT.

Kroessler and Fogel (1993) compared the mortality during long-term follow-up of 65 depressed patients age 80 or older who had been treated with ECT with that of patients treated with other modalities. The 2-year survival rate was 54% in the group treated with ECT, versus 90% in the group treated with medications. This group difference was related to more severe depression and physical illness in the patients who had received ECT. The course of ECT itself was remarkably well tolerated by these elderly patients, with a median interval between ECT and time of death of 20 months. The authors called for further attention to medical comorbidity as a prognostic factor in future outcome studies of geriatric depression. Abrams (1997b) noted that the estimated mortality rate among community-dwelling elderly patients (approximately 0.26% per each 3 weeks) was an order of magnitude higher than that observed after a 3-week course of eight ECT treatments in elderly patients (approximately 0.016%).

Cardiovascular Side Effects

A proportion of elderly patients referred for ECT have serious preexisting cardiovascular disease. Common cardiac conditions such as hypertension, angina, previous myocardial infarction, atrial and ventricular arrhythmia, aneurysm, and conduction system disease require evaluation and optimized treatment before ECT, to minimize any adverse effects from the hemodynamic events that occur during ECT.

Uncontrolled retrospective studies comparing the cardiovascular complication rate of ECT in older and younger patients have found an increase in transient and treatable complications in elderly patients. In a non-blinded, retrospective chart review of 293 patients, Alexopoulos et al. (1984) found cardiovascular complications in 9% of the patients age 65 and over, compared with 1% of the patients under 65. Cardiac ischemia, arrhythmia, hypertension, and congestive heart failure were the most common complications, although the vast majority of complications were not clearly temporally related to ECT and did not prevent the completion of treatment. Burke et al. (1987) conducted a similar retrospective chart review of

136 subjects, 30% of whom were age 60 and over. Sine wave bilateral ECT was used in 85% of cases. These investigators found a cardiorespiratory complication rate of 15% in patients age 60 and over, compared with 3% in those under 60. Complications were correlated with the number of cardiovascular medications the patient was receiving, with more medication presumably marking those with more cardiovascular illness. These complications did not affect treatment response. In a chart review of 81 elderly patients, Cattan et al. (1990) found a 36% cardiovascular complication rate with ECT in patients over age 80, compared with 12% in younger geriatric patients. As would be expected, the older patients had notably more medical diagnoses and were receiving more cardiovascular medication than the younger patients.

More recently, two controlled studies of ECT in a total of 66 high-risk patients with cardiovascular disease have demonstrated the safety of ECT in elderly individuals. Zielinski et al. (1993) compared the rate of cardiac complications in a group of 40 depressed patients (mean age, 68.9 years; range, 54–84 years) with serious preexisting cardiac disease (left ventricular impairment, conduction delay, and ventricular arrhythmias) with the rate of such complications in a group of 40 depressed patients (mean age, 68.3 years; range, 55–83 years) without cardiac disease. Not surprisingly, the group with preexisting cardiac disease had more complications. Most of the complications were transient (e.g., brief arrhythmias or increases in ectopy), however, and 38 of the 40 cardiac patients were able to complete their course of ECT. This group of depressed patients with cardiac disease had even more difficulty with adverse cardiac effects from prior trials of tricyclic antidepressants; 11 of 21 patients had been forced to stop tricyclic treatment because of cardiovascular complications. Rice et al. (1994) used a case-control design to compare two groups of patients over age 50 receiving ECT. One group consisted of 26 patients at increased risk for cardiac complications, and 27 patients at standard risk made up the other group. Compared with the patients at standard risk for cardiac complications, patients in the high-risk group were older, had received more pre-ECT medical consultations before ECT, and experienced more minor medical complications from ECT. However, the two groups did not differ in terms of frequency of major medical complications, and no patients died or experienced permanent cardiac morbidity from ECT.

The data just reviewed suggest that ECT is a low-risk procedure, even in elderly patients (Applegate 1997). Still, prospective studies, carefully controlled for severity of cardiovascular and other medical disease, are needed to evaluate the effects of age on cardiovascular complications of ECT.

Increasingly sophisticated medical management during ECT should decrease the cardiovascular risk of treatment in elderly patients (Applegate 1997; Weiner et al., in press). The primary areas of concern are bradycardia, tachycardia, hypertension, and ventricular arrhythmia. Anticholinergic premedications (atropine and glycopyrrolate) may be used to prevent vagally induced bradycardia, but in elderly patients their use may be complicated by confusion, tachycardia, constipation, and urinary retention. We generally reserve the use of anticholinergic premedication for patients who develop unusually prolonged or severe bradyarrhythmias. The method of serial electrical stimulations to determine a patient's seizure threshold (described earlier) may involve administration of subconvulsive stimuli, with a vagal surge unaccompanied by the sympathetic outflow associated with a seizure. The use of this method, as well as the presence of conduction delay on the ECG, may indicate the need for premedication with an anticholinergic, particularly if the patient is also receiving a β-blocker medication.

Hypertension and tachycardia during ECT in elderly patients may be attenuated by short-acting intravenous β-blockers such as labetalol or esmolol (Howie et al. 1990; Stoudemire et al. 1990). It should be kept in mind that β-blockers have anticonvulsant effects, and their use during ECT may limit the intensity of the ECT seizure and, in turn, its therapeutic potency. Kalayam and Alexopoulos (1989) described the safe use of sublingual nifedipine before administration of anesthesia in an elderly patient with a severe hypertensive response to ECT. Hydralazine (an α-adrenergic antagonist), as well as nitroglycerine (sublingual, transdermal, or intravenous), may also be used when clinically indicated. Trimethaphan produces transient sympathetic and parasympathetic ganglionic blockade and has also been used in this setting (Maneksha 1991). Although the hemodynamic responses to ECT are robust, they are well tolerated by most patients, including elderly individuals (Webb et al. 1990). In addition, indiscriminate use of antihypertensive medication may lead to clinically important hypotension in elderly patients. Therefore, we do not routinely blunt the cardiovascular response to ECT in elderly patients unless such changes are extreme or are clearly associated with evidence of cardiovascular compromise. Finally, in patients receiving adrenergic blockers, anticholinergic premedication should be considered so as to prevent a disproportionate decrease of sympathetic tone below parasympathetic tone, with resultant bradycardia (Abrams 1997a).

Marked posttreatment ventricular ectopy (multifocal premature ventricular contractions [PVCs] or several consecutive PVCs) may be treated with lidocaine (1–1.5 mg/kg body weight). Because of its anticonvulsant properties, lidocaine should be given after termination of the seizure (Drop and Welch 1989). Stoudemire et al. (1990) found that ventricular ectopy could also be reduced by pretreatment with labetalol.

Cerebral Side Effects

There is no evidence that ECT causes structural brain damage (Devanand et al. 1994; Weiner 1984). Carefully controlled prospective brain imaging studies in humans reveal no changes in brain structure for up to 6 months after a course of ECT (Coffey 1993; Coffey et al. 1991). Neuropathological studies in animals, including cell counts in regions thought to be at highest risk, reveal no evidence of brain damage when the seizures are induced under conditions that approximate standard clinical practice (i.e., when the seizures are spaced, relatively brief, and modified by oxygenation and muscle relaxation). Furthermore, studies of the pathophysiology of seizure-induced structural brain damage in animals indicate that the conditions necessary for injury do not apply to the modern practice of ECT (Weiner 1984).

The incidence of cerebrovascular complications with ECT is exceedingly rare. ECT has been given successfully to patients with cerebral aneurysms, with close management of blood pressure elevation (Krystal and Coffey 1997). The intracerebral hemorrhage reported in a normotensive patient during ECT was probably related to cerebral amyloid angiopathy (Weisberg et al. 1991). We know of no other reported case of intracerebral hemorrhage with ECT, nor of any documented case of ischemic stroke during the treatment.

The amount of time that must elapse before ECT can be safely administered after an acute cerebral infarction is unclear. Alexopoulos et al. (1984) reported the uneventful delivery of ECT 4 days after a cerebral infarct (whether it was hemorrhagic or ischemic was not specified), and others (Currier et al. 1992; Murray et al. 1986) reported successful ECT 1–2 months after ischemic stroke. Patients with a recent cerebral infarction may have more friable vasculature with a propensity to rebleed. These patients require time for cerebral vessels to heal before ECT, as well as careful management of blood pressure during the procedure. Titratable agents with short half-lives (e.g., esmolol or nitrates) are helpful in this situation. Care must be taken to avoid hypotension in all elderly patients with cerebrovascular disease.

Other intracranial processes are risk factors for ECT. As described earlier, intracranial mass lesions and increased intracranial pressure are among the most serious risk factors for ECT. In a retrospective literature review, Maltbie et al. (1980) examined 28 patients (mean age, 47 years; range, 20–80 years) with brain tumor who were treated with ECT. Only 34% of patients improved, and 74% showed neurological deterioration, with 29% dying from neurological complications within a month of ECT. This study was flawed by a form of recall bias, with cases involving dramatic outcomes more likely to be reported. As well, a previously undiagnosed brain tumor would more likely be diagnosed during a treatment course involving complications than during an uneventful ECT course. Abrams (1997a) and Kellner (1996) reviewed reports of several cases of safe delivery of ECT to patients with brain tumors, mostly meningiomas, and ascribed the lessened risk to the fact that the tumors were small and slow growing and had no associated increased intracranial pressure. There is no report of safely delivered ECT prospectively given to a patient with documented increased intracranial pressure (Abrams 1997a). Subdural hematomas may require evacuation before ECT (Abrams 1997a).

Side Effects in Other Organ Systems

Other organ systems that may be impaired in the elderly patient need to be considered before ECT, including the lungs, bones, eyes, and teeth (Weiner et al. 1999). Pulmonary status should be optimized before ECT. Patients with severe chronic obstructive pulmonary disease and carbon dioxide retention may require special ventilatory strategies during the treatment (Abrams 1997a). Pneumonia secondary to aspiration of gastric contents may occur rarely during ECT (Alexopoulos et al. 1989; Karlinsky and Shulman 1984).

Patients with osteoporosis, spinal disk disease, or spondylosis may require increased muscular relaxation during ECT. Such patients should receive succinylcholine doses of at least 1.0–1.5 mg/kg body weight, and they require careful attention to clinical evidence of adequate relaxation (e.g. loss of reflexes or tone, and disappearance of fasciculation) before delivery of the stimulus. Kellner et al. (1991b) reported the safe treatment of a patient with osteoporosis and cervical spondylosis with multiple subluxations of the cervical spine using succinylcholine doses of 1.3 mg/kg weight.

Because ECT produces a transient increase in intraocular pressure, patients with chronic open-angle glaucoma should receive their eyedrops before ECT. As noted earlier, treatment with echothiophate, an irreversible cholinesterase inhibitor, should be stopped several days before ECT. Patients with acute closed-angle glaucoma or retinal detachment should be stabilized before ECT and watched closely by an ophthalmologist during an ECT course.

When a patient's teeth are loose, decayed, or asymmetrical, the risk of dental injury during ECT may be increased. A major proportion of malpractice litigation with ECT is related to dental issues (Slawson 1985). A specially designed bite block must be inserted before delivery of the ECT stimulus. The tongue, cheeks, and lips must be kept clear of the clenching teeth. The bite block should be used even in edentulous patients. Occasionally, upper or lower dentures may be kept in place during the treatment to facilitate airway management. In patients with only a few remaining, and possibly loose, teeth, dental consultation or alternative bite block strategies (with the aim of shifting bite pressure to the molars) may be helpful (Welch 1993).

Cognitive Side Effects

The cognitive side effects of ECT include acute postictal confusion, impaired retrograde and anterograde memory, and, occasionally, interictal delirium. The severity of these adverse effects is increased with bilateral electrode placement, sine waveform, higher stimulus dose relative to seizure threshold, and more frequent treatments. Conversely, cognitive side effects are reduced with right unilateral electrode placement, brief-pulse waveform, lower stimulus dose relative to seizure threshold, and longer intervals between treatments (American Psychiatric Association 2000). Although it has been suggested that elderly patients may be at greater risk for these cognitive side effects than are younger patients, controlled data on this issue are limited.

Acute postictal disorientation.   In studies involving mixed-age samples of adults, increasing age has been found to be associated with longer or more severe disorientation immediately after ECT (Burke et al. 1987; Calev et al. 1991; Daniel et al. 1987; M.E. Miller et al. 1986; Sackeim et al. 1987). Additional risk factors for post-ECT confusion in elderly patients may include presence of major medical illness or use of psychotropic medications during ECT.

In one of the studies focusing on elderly patients, Fraser and Glass (1978) measured time to recovery of full orientation in nine elderly patients with depression who received ECT in courses in which electrode placement alternated (i.e., unilateral placement in one treatment followed by bilateral placement in the next treatment, and so on). When comparing these reorientation times with those reported in the literature for younger patients, the investigators observed that recovery in elderly patients took five times as long for unilateral treatment and nine times as long for bilateral treatment. Recovery time after bilateral ECT increased cumulatively over the course of ECT, and with closer spacing of treatments. No such relationship was found for unilateral ECT. In a subsequent study of 29 elderly patients with depression randomly assigned to courses of either unilateral (n = 13) or bilateral (n = 16) sine wave ECT, Fraser and Glass (1980) found significantly longer reorientation times after the fifth ECT session among patients receiving bilateral treatments (32.8 minutes) than among those receiving unilateral treatments (9.5 minutes) (Table 35–1). In contrast to the group undergoing bilateral ECT, patients receiving unilateral ECT had a significant reduction in recovery time from the first to the last treatment.

In a study of subjective side effects during ECT, Devenand et al. (1995) found that older patients actually reported fewer severe cognitive symptoms (i.e., confusion/ disorientation and amnesia) than did younger patients.

Agitated delirium on emergence from anesthesia. Approximately 10% of patients receiving ECT experience an acute agitated delirium on emergence from anesthesia, characterized by restlessness, disorientation, combativeness, and poor response to commands. Age does not appear to be a risk factor for this complication (Devanand et al. 1989). The complication is usually effectively treated with intravenous benzodiazepines (e.g., midazolam or diazepam) or other sedatives (e.g., droperidol or methohexital).

Interictal delirium. In a small proportion of patients, ECT is associated with more prolonged disorientation and even frank interictal delirium. Most studies evaluating interictal delirium in elderly patients have used disorientation as a measure, rather than the full DSM-III-R (American Psychiatric Association 1987) or DSM-IV (American Psychiatric Association 1994) criteria for delirium. In a retrospective study involving 136 patients receiving mainly bilateral sine wave ECT, Burke et al. (1987) found disorientation (confusion severe enough to alter the treatment plan) in 18% of patients older than 60 but in 13% of younger patients. This incidence increased to 25% for patients over age 75. In a retrospective study in which mostly bilateral (waveform not specified) ECT was administered, Alexopoulos et al. (1984) found a somewhat greater incidence of confusion (disorientation to time, place, and person) in elderly patients (12.6%) than in younger patients (9.6%). Cattan et al. (1990) conducted a study involving primarily bilateral or combination bilateral-unilateral sine wave ECT and found a nonsignificant trend for more frequent severe disorientation (defined functionally by interference in ward activities) in elderly

patients over 80 (59%, n = 39), compared with those patients 65–80 years old (45%, n = 42).

In the study of Alexopoulos et al. (1984), elderly patients with a history of underlying organic brain disease were found to have higher levels of severe post-ECT confusion than were the younger patients, suggesting that baseline cerebral impairment may increase the risk of adverse cognitive effects of ECT.

In several studies, subcortical structural disease has been implicated in the development of interictal delirium with ECT. We have found subcortical gray and white matter lesions to be more extensive in elderly patients who developed a prolonged interictal delirium during a course of ECT. The majority of these patients were able to continue ECT, with no decline in expected treatment response. All patients were free of delirium 1 week after ECT (Coffey et al. 1989; Figiel et al. 1990). The specificity of subcortical disease in producing delirium after ECT is further suggested by Martin et al. (1992), who found that patients with ischemic lesions of the caudate nucleus had a 92% incidence of delirium during ECT. Patients with a previous stroke in other brain regions had the same incidence of delirium as did a group of elderly depressed control (no stroke) subjects receiving ECT (Martin et al. 1992). In a prospective study of seven consecutive patients with Parkinson's disease, Figiel et al. (1991) found a 100% incidence of interictal delirium during a course of ECT. The delirium lasted 7–21 days, longer than is typical, but 86% of patients recovered from depression. Whether the delirium was due to subcortical disease or to increased intracerebral concentration of levodopa (due to transient breakdown of the blood-brain barrier with ECT) is unknown.

In summary, although the duration and severity of acute post-ECT disorientation may increase with age, the majority of elderly patients appear to recover their orientation within 60–120 minutes of the treatment. In the small percentage of elderly patients who develop more prolonged confusion or frank delirium, underlying cerebral impairment may be contributory, especially dysfunction of the basal ganglia. Clearly, more research is needed in a larger number of elderly patients to characterize post-ECT confusion and to identify its risk factors, including the effects of preexisting cerebral impairment.

Amnesia. A course of ECT is associated with transient disturbances in memory, including both retrograde and anterograde amnesia. Retrograde amnesia (forgetting of material known before the ECT) may extend back to several months before ECT and is more pronounced with bilateral electrode placement, sine waveform, grossly suprathreshold stimulus intensity, and increased treatment frequency (Abrams 1997a). These same factors also increase anterograde amnesia (forgetting of information acquired after the start of ECT). These side effects subside within weeks of completion of ECT, but some patients may have permanent loss of specific memories for some events that occurred before, during, or shortly after the treatment course. Although some patients may report persistent memory difficulties, objective testing has demonstrated that ECT is not likely to produce persistent impairment in the ability to remember past information or acquire new information (American Psychiatric Association 2000).

Given the large body of data on the amnestic effects of ECT, it is surprising that there has been relatively little controlled research on age as a risk factor (Abrams 1997a; Calev et al. 1993; Fink 1979). Some (Fromholt et al. 1973; Heshe et al. 1978) but not all (d'Elia and Raotma 1977; Strömgren et al. 1976) early studies found that ECT-induced amnesia is worse in older patients.

Zervas et al. (1993) examined age effects on memory in a study comparing twice-weekly and three-times-a-week bilateral ECT administered using contemporary techniques (pulse waveform given at "moderately suprathreshold" stimulus intensity). The sample consisted of 42 inpatients with a mean age (± SD) of 53.5 ± 16.1 years; no patient was older than 65 years, however. Correlations were found between age and decrements in retrograde memory 1–3 days after the end of ECT but not 1 month or 6 months posttreatment. Age was also correlated with decrements in verbal anterograde memory acutely and 1 month after ECT (but not 6 months after ECT) and with changes in figural anterograde memory acutely and 6 months after ECT.

McElhiney et al. (1995) examined autobiographical memory in a mixed-age sample (mean age [± SD], 54 ± 13.9 years) of 75 patients with depression randomly assigned with regard to electrode placement and stimulus intensity. Age was found to be a predictor of lower recall of autobiographical memories after ECT. In a follow-up report on this sample, the pre-ECT modified Mini-Mental State Exam score was predictive of the extent of retrograde autobiographical amnesia both 1 week and 2 months after ECT (Sobin et al. 1995). This study provided evidence in support of the conventional clinical wisdom that preexisting cognitive deficit is a risk factor for more severe ECT-induced amnesia. Work is under way by our group to determine whether age-related structural changes on brain images might also be predictive of cognitive impairment after ECT (Coffey 1996).

Memory performance has been reported to improve in elderly patients with the pseudodementia of depression who are treated successfully with ECT (Reynolds et al. 1987; Stoudemire et al. 1995). In the study of Fraser and Glass (1980) described earlier (also see Table 35–1), all elderly patients showed impairment of memory function before ECT, but during treatment, memory improved and was normal in all patients by 3 weeks after completion of the ECT course. No group differences were found on the basis of electrode placement.

There has been relatively little research into the effects of age on subjective memory complaints after ECT. As noted previously, Devanand et al. (1995) found that older patients actually reported fewer severe cognitive symptoms (i.e., confusion/disorientation and amnesia) than did younger patients.

In summary, recent controlled data appear to support the clinical wisdom that elderly patients are at greater risk for the amnestic side effects of ECT. More work is needed in a larger number of elderly patients (especially very old patients) to characterize the extent and severity of ECT-induced amnesia and to identify relevant risk factors, including the effects of preexisting cerebral impairment. Recommendations for lessening ECT amnesia in elderly patients include using unilateral electrode placement and brief pulse stimuli, avoiding maximally suprathreshold stimulus dosing, and lessening the frequency of treatments (e.g., giving ECT on Monday and Friday instead of Monday, Wednesday, and Friday). A variety of pharmacological agents have shown antiamnestic activity in animal models of ECT, but clinical trials in humans have been limited by methodological issues (Prudic et al. 1998).

Psychosocial Issues

In addition to its myriad biological effects, ECT has important intrapsychic and interpersonal effects. A powerful treatment, during which the patient is put to sleep and has an electrical stimulus delivered to the head, may arouse predictable fears and fantasies in the patient. Issues of trust and autonomy over one's body while in a vulnerable position may predominate, especially in patients with a history of trauma. Patient education—in particular, educational videotapes—may be effective and reassuring for these fears. Patients who are vulnerable to idealized fantasies of a nurturant, all-caring, supportive other may overvalue the ECT procedure and practitioner. Conversely, these patients may excessively devalue the treatment when their distorted expectations are not realized. Such patients may be at increased risk for a bad psychological outcome from the treatment. Overidealization of the treatment should be challenged by the ECT practitioner, and the informed consent process should be firmly grounded in factual information.

Patient attitude surveys indicate that those undergoing ECT typically find the experience no more upsetting than a trip to the dentist (Fox 1993; Hughes et al. 1981; Malcolm 1989). In the only study that has systematically examined the effects of age on patients' perception and knowledge of ECT, Malcolm (1989) found that patients over 65 had less knowledge of the procedure before treatment and were also less fearful of it. In addition, fewer elderly patients viewed the treatment as frightening after completing a course of ECT.

Medicolegal issues surrounding the use of ECT in elderly patients include the informed consent process (discussed earlier in this chapter), do-not-resuscitate (DNR) orders, and consideration of driving after ECT. A patient with DNR status may still experience improved quality of life with aggressive treatment of his or her affective disorder and may still be considered for ECT (Sullivan et al. 1992). In such cases, strategies for the management of major complications that could occur during ECT should be discussed with the patient and the family before treatment. Patients should not drive until that point after a course of ECT when cognitive side effects have substantially resolved (Fink 1994). This issue may be an especially sensitive one for elderly patients who consider driving a means of maintaining their mobility and functional independence.

Financial concerns are of increasing importance in today's cost-conscious health care marketplace. A growing literature suggests that ECT has economic advantages over other forms of treatment for severe mood disorders. The cost-effectiveness of ECT has been demonstrated for both inpatient treatment of the index episode as well as for maintenance therapy on an ambulatory basis (Markowitz et al. 1987; McDonald et al. 1998; Olfson et al. 1998; Steffens et al. 1995). Despite these advantages, there remains much variation in ECT reimbursement patterns, and it is not uncommon to encounter payers who will reimburse only for ECT when it is given on an inpatient basis. In addition, reimbursement rates are very low and thus discourage the use of this safe and highly effective treatment.

Transcranial Magnetic Stimulation

Transcranial magnetic stimulation (TMS) is a relatively new technology that uses an electrically induced magnetic field to generate small electrical currents that can depolarize brain neurons. Repeated TMS (rTMS) can cause repeated neuronal firing that (depending on a variety of technical factors related to the TMS, as well as possible host factors) can either augment or suppress neuronal network functioning. Many ECT research groups throughout the world are currently investigating rTMS as a possible anti-depressant treatment. Most studies have been open trials, relatively few elderly patients have been studied, and results indicate that there are minimal side effects but only modest improvements in mood (for a concise review, see George 1998). Although it is unclear what role rTMS will play in the management of elderly patients who are candidates for ECT, rTMS holds great promise as a tool for understanding the neurobiology of mood regulation.

Conclusions

Sixty years after its introduction, ECT remains a cornerstone of the treatment of severe affective disorder and selected other neuropsychiatric illnesses in elderly patients. Recent modifications in ECT technique have reduced the risk of severe side effects in this population. There is, however, a paucity of controlled studies comparing the efficacy and safety of ECT versus pharmacotherapy in elderly patients. ECT also appears to be an effective treatment in patients with preexisting brain disease and in some cases may even have a beneficial effect on the underlying neurological disorder. Further study is needed to determine the impact of age-related changes in brain structure or function and of preexisting cerebral disease on the beneficial and adverse effects of ECT in the elderly.

References

Aarsland D, Larsen JP, Waage O, et al: Maintenance electroconvulsive therapy for Parkinson's disease. Convulsive Therapy 13:274–277, 1997

Abrams R: Electroconvulsive Therapy, 3rd Edition. New York, Oxford University Press, 1997a

Abrams R: The mortality rate with ECT. Convulsive Therapy 13:125–127, 1997b

Alexopoulos GS: Clinical and biological findings in late-onset depression, in American Psychiatric Press Review of Psychiatry, Vol 9. Edited by Tasman A, Goldfinger SM, Kaufman CA. Washington, DC, American Psychiatric Press, 1990, pp 249–262

Alexopoulos GS, Shamoian CJ, Lucas J, et al: Medical problems of geriatric psychiatric patients and younger controls during electroconvulsive therapy. J Am Geriatr Soc 32: 651–654, 1984

Alexopoulos GS, Young RG, Abrams RC: ECT in the high-risk geriatric patient. Convulsive Therapy 5:75–87, 1989

American Psychiatric Association: Diagnostic and Statistical Manual of Mental Disorders, 3rd Edition, Revised. Washington, DC, American Psychiatric Association, 1987

American Psychiatric Association: The Practice of Electroconvulsive Therapy: Recommendations for Treatment, Training and Privileging, 2nd Edition. Washington, DC, American Psychiatric Association, 2000

American Psychiatric Association: Diagnostic and Statistical Manual of Mental Disorders, 4th Edition. Washington, DC, American Psychiatric Association, 1994

Andersen K, Balldin J, Gottfries CG, et al: A double-blind evaluation of electroconvulsive therapy in Parkinson's disease with "on-off" phenomena. Acta Neurol Scand 76:191–199, 1987

Applegate RJ: Diagnosis and management of ischemic heart disease in the patient scheduled to undergo electroconvulsive therapy. Convulsive Therapy 13:128–144, 1997

Arle JE, Alterman RL: Surgical options in Parkinson' disease. Med Clin North Am 83:483–498, 1999

Asnis G: Parkinson's disease, depression, and ECT: a review and case study. Am J Psychiatry 134:191–195, 1977

Atre-Vaidya N, Jampala V: Electroconvulsive therapy in parkinsonism with affective disorder. Br J Psychiatry 152:55–58, 1988

Avery E, Winokur G: Mortality in depressed patients treated with electroconvulsive therapy and antidepressants. Arch Gen Psychiatry 33:1029–1037, 1976

Babigian HM, Guttmacher LB: Epidemiologic considerations in electroconvulsive therapy. Arch Gen Psychiatry 41:246–253, 1984

Balldin J, Eden S, Granerus A-K, et al: Electroconvulsive therapy in Parkinson's syndrome with "on-off" phenomenon. J Neural Transm 47:11–21, 1980

Balldin J, Granerus A-K, Lindstedt G, et al: Predictors for improvement after electroconvulsive therapy in parkinsonian patients with "on-off" symptoms. J Neural Transm 52:199–211, 1981

Benbow SM: The use of electroconvulsive therapy in old age psychiatry. Int J Geriatr Psychiatry 2:25–30, 1987

Benbow SM: The role of electroconvulsive therapy in the treatment of depressive illness in old age. Br J Psychiatry 155:147–152, 1989

Bergman PS, Gabriel AR, Impastato DJ, et al: EEG changes following ECT with the Reiter apparatus. Conferences Neurology 12:347–351, 1953

Bergsholm P, Swartz CM: Anesthesia in electroconvulsive therapy and alternatives to barbiturates. Psychiatric Annals 26:709–712, 1996

Birkett DP: ECT in parkinsonism with affective disorder (letter). Br J Psychiatry 152:712–713, 1988

Black DW, Winokur G, Nasrallah A: A multivariate analysis of the experience of 423 depressed inpatients treated with electroconvulsive therapy. Convulsive Therapy 9:112–120, 1993

Bodley PO, Fenwick PBC: The effects of electroconvulsive therapy on patients with essential hypertension. Br J Psychiatry 112 1241–1249, 1966

Bolwig T, Hertz M, Paulson O, et al: The permeability of the blood-brain barrier during electrically induced seizures in man. J Clin Invest 7:87–93, 1977

Bonne O, Krausz Y, Shapira B, et al: Increased cerebral blood flow in depressed patients responding to electroconvulsive therapy. J Nucl Med 37:1075–1080, 1996

Botteron K, Figiel GS, Zorumski CF: Electroconvulsive therapy in patients with late-onset psychoses and structural brain changes. J Geriatr Psychiatry Neurol 4:44–47, 1991

Braasch ER, Demaso DR: Effect of electroconvulsive therapy on serum isoenzymes. Am J Psychiatry 137:625–626, 1980

Brodersen P, Paulson OB, Bolwig TG, et al: Cerebral hyperemia in electrically induced epileptic seizures. Arch Neurol 28:334–338, 1973

Brown G: Parkinsonism, depression and ECT (letter). Am J Psychiatry 132:1084, 1973

Burke WJ, Rutherford JL, Zorumski CF, et al: Electroconvulsive therapy and the elderly. Compr Psychiatry 26:480–486, 1985

Burke WJ, Rubin EH, Zorumski CF, et al: The safety of ECT in geriatric psychiatry. J Am Geriatr Soc 35:516–521, 1987

Burke W[J], Peterson J, Rubin E: Electroconvulsive therapy in the treatment of combined depression and Parkinson's disease. Psychosomatics 29:341–346, 1988

Calabrese JR, Woyshville MJ, Kimmel SE, et al: Mixed states and bipolar rapid cycling and their treatment with divalproex sodium. Psychiatric Annals 23:70–78, 1993

Calev A, Cohen R, Tubi N, et al: Disorientation and bilateral moderately suprathreshold titrated ECT. Convulsive Therapy 7:99–110, 1991

Calev A, Pass HL, Shapira B, et al: ECT and memory, in The Clinical Science of Electroconvulsive Therapy. Edited by Coffey CE. Washington, DC, American Psychiatric Press, 1993, pp 125–142

Carney MWP, Roth M, Garside RF: The diagnosis of depressive syndromes and the prediction of ECT response. Br J Psychiatry 111:659–674, 1965

Casey DA, Davis MH: Electroconvulsive therapy in the very old. Gen Hosp Psychiatry 18:436–439, 1996

Cattan RA, Barry PP, Mead G, et al: Electroconvulsive therapy in octogenarians. J Am Geriatr Soc 38:753–758, 1990

Clarke TB, Coffey CE, Hoffman GW, et al: Continuation therapy for depression using outpatient electroconvulsive therapy. Convulsive Therapy 5:330–337, 1989

Coffey CE: Structural brain imaging and electroconvulsive therapy, in The Clinical Science of Electroconvulsive Therapy. Edited by Coffey CE. Washington, DC, American Psychiatric Press, 1993, pp 73–92

Coffey CE: Brain morphology in primary mood disorders: implications for ECT. Psychiatric Annals 26:713–716, 1996

Coffey CE: The pre ECT evaluation. Psychiatric Annals 28:506–508, 1998

Coffey CE, Weiner RD, Hinkle PE, et al: Augmentation of ECT seizures with caffeine. Biol Psychiatry 22:637–649, 1987

Coffey CE, Figiel GS, Djang WT, et al: Leukoencephalopathy in elderly depressed patients referred for ECT. Biol Psychiatry 24:143–161, 1988

Coffey CE, Figiel GS, Djang WT, et al: White matter hyperintensity on magnetic resonance imaging: clinical and neuroanatomic correlates in the depressed elderly. J Neuropsychiatry Clin Neurosci 1:135–144, 1989

Coffey CE, Figiel GS, Weiner RD, et al: Caffeine augmentation of ECT. Am J Psychiatry 147:579–585, 1990

Coffey CE, Weiner RD, Djang WT, et al: Brain anatomic effects of ECT: a prospective magnetic resonance imaging study. Arch Gen Psychiatry 48:1013–1021, 1991

Coffey CE, Lucke J, Weiner RD, et al: Seizure threshold in electroconvulsive therapy, I: initial seizure threshold. Biol Psychiatry 37:713–720, 1995a

Coffey CE, Lucke J, Weiner RD, et al: Seizure threshold in electroconvulsive therapy, II: the anticonvulsant effect of ECT. Biol Psychiatry 37:777–788, 1995b

Consensus Conference: electroconvulsive therapy. JAMA 254:2103–2108, 1985

Coryell W, Zimmerman M: Outcome following ECT for primary unipolar depression: a test of newly proposed response predictors. Am J Psychiatry 141:862–867, 1984

Currier MB, Murray GB, Welch CC: Electroconvulsive therapy for post-stroke depressed geriatric patients. J Neuropsychiatry Clin Neurosci 4:140–144, 1992

Daniel WF, Crovitz HF, Weiner RD: Neuropsychological aspects of disorientation. Cortex 23:169–187, 1987

Decina P, Sackeim HA, Kahn DA, et al: Effects of ECT on the TRH stimulation test. Psychoneuroendocrinology 12:29–34, 1987

d'Elia G, Raotma H: Memory impairment after convulsive therapy: influence of age and number of treatments. Acta Psychiat Nervenkr 223:219–226, 1977

Devanand DP, Briscoe KM, Sackeim HA: Clinical features and predictors of postictal excitement. Convulsive Therapy 5:140–146, 1989

Devanand DP, Sackeim HA, Lo ES, et al: Serial dexamethasone suppression tests and plasma dexamethasone levels. Arch Gen Psychiatry 48:525–533, 1991

Devanand DP, Dwork AJ, Hutchinson ER: Does ECT alter brain structure? Am J Psychiatry 151:957–970, 1994

Devanand DP, Fitzsimons L, Prudic J, et al: Subjective side effects during electroconvulsive therapy. Convulsive Therapy 11:232–240, 1995

Douyon R, Serby M, Klutchko B, et al: ECT and Parkinson's disease revisited: a "naturalistic" study. Am J Psychiatry 146:1451–1455, 1989

Drop LJ, Welch CA: Anesthesia for electroconvulsive therapy in patients with major cardiovascular risk factors. Convulsive Therapy 5:88–101, 1989

Dubin WR, Jaffe R, Roemer R, et al: The efficacy and safety of maintenance ECT in geriatric patients. J Am Geriatr Soc 40:706–709, 1992

Dubovsky SL: Using electroconvulsive therapy for patients with neurological disease. Hosp Community Psychiatry 37:819–825, 1986

Dysken M, Evans H, Chan C, et al: Improvement of depression and parkinsonism during ECT: a case study. Neuropsychobiology 2:81–86, 1976

Fahn S: Fetal-tissue transplants in Parkinson's disease. N Engl J Med 327:1589–1590, 1992

Farah A, Beale MD, Kellner CH: Risperidone and ECT combination therapy: a case series. Convulsive Therapy 11:280–282, 1995

Feighner JP, Robins E, Guze SB, et al: Diagnostic criteria for use in psychiatric research. Arch Gen Psychiatry 26:57–63, 1972

Figiel GS, Coffey CE, Djang WT, et al: Brain magnetic resonance imaging findings in ECT-induced delirium. J Neuropsychiatry Clin Neurosci 2:53–58, 1990

Figiel GS, Hassen MA, Zorumski C, et al: ECT-induced delirium in depressed patients with Parkinson's disease. J Neuropsychiatry Clin Neurosci 3:405–411, 1991

Fink M: Convulsive Therapy: Theory and Practice. New York, Raven, 1979

Fink M: Convalescence and ECT. Convulsive Therapy 10:301–303, 1994

Fink M: Neuroleptic malignant syndrome and catatonia: one entity or two? Biol Psychiatry 39:1–4, 1996

Fink M: Catatonia, in Contemporary Behavioural Neurology. Edited by Trimble M, Cummings J. Butterworth/ Heinemann, Oxford, UK, 1997, pp 289–309

Fink M, Abrams R, Bailine S, et al: Ambulatory electroconvulsive therapy: report of a task force of the Association for Convulsive Therapy. Convulsive Therapy 12:42–55, 1996

Finklestein SD, Weintraub RJ, Karmooz N, et al: Antidepressant drug treatment for post-stroke depression: a retrospective study. Arch Phys Med Rehabil 68:772–778, 1987

Fisman M: Intractable depression and pseudodementia: a report of two cases. Can J Psychiatry 33:628–630, 1988

Fochtmann L: A mechanism for the efficacy of ECT in Parkinson's disease. Convulsive Therapy 4:321–327, 1988

Fogel BS: Electroconvulsive therapy in the elderly: a clinical research agenda. Int J Geriatr Psychiatry 3:181–190, 1988

Folstein M[F], Folstein S, McHugh PR: Clinical predictors of improvement after electroconvulsive therapy of patients with schizophrenic, neurotic reactions, and affective disorders. Biol Psychiatry 7:147–152, 1973

Fox HA: Patients' fear of and objection to electroconvulsive therapy. Hosp Community Psychiatry 44:357–360, 1993

Fragen RJ, Avram MJ: Barbiturates, in Anesthesia, 3rd Edition, Vol 1. Edited by Miller RD. New York, Churchill Livingstone, 1990, pp 225–242

Frank E, Kupfer DJ, Perel JM, et al: Three year outcomes for maintenance therapies in recurrent depression. Arch Gen Psychiatry 47:1093–1099, 1990

Fraser RM, Glass IB: Recovery from ECT in elderly patients. Br J Psychiatry 133:524–528, 1978

Fraser RM, Glass IB: Unilateral and bilateral ECT in elderly patients: a comparative study. Acta Psychiatr Scand 62: 13–31, 1980

Freeman CP (ed): The ECT Handbook: The Second Report of the Royal College of Psychiatrists' Special Committee on ECT. London, Royal College of Psychiatrists, 1995

Friedman J, Gordon N: Electroconvulsive therapy in Parkinson's disease: a report on five cases. Convulsive Therapy 8:204–210, 1992

Fromholt P, Christensen AL, Strömgren LS: The effects of unilateral and bilateral electroconvulsive therapy on memory. Acta Psychiatr Scand 49:466–478, 1973

Fromm GH: Observation on the effects of electroshock treatment in patients with parkinsonism. Bulletin of Tulane University 18:71–73, 1959

Fujikawa T, Yokota N, Muraoka M, et al: Response of patients with major depression and silent cerebral infarction to antidepressant drug therapy, with emphasis on central nervous system adverse reactions. Stroke 27:2040–2042, 1996

Gaspar D, Samarasinghe LA: ECT in psychogeriatric practice—a study of risk factors, indications and outcome. Compr Psychiatry 23:170–175, 1982

George MS: Why would you ever want to? Toward understanding the antidepressant effect of prefrontal rTMS. Hum Psychopharmacology 13:307–313, 1998

Gerring JP, Shields HM: The identification and management of patients with high risk for cardiac arrhythmias during modified ECT. J Clin Psychiatry 43:140–143, 1982

Godber C, Rosenvinge H, Wilkinson D, et al: Depression in old age: prognosis after ECT. Int J Geriatr Psychiatry 2:19–24, 1987

Gold L, Chiarella CJ: The prognostic value of clinical findings in cases treated with electric shock. J Nerv Ment Dis 100: 577–583, 1944

Gormley N, Cullen C, Walters L, et al: The safety and efficacy of electroconvulsive therapy in patients over age 75. Int J Geriatr Psychiatry 13:871–874, 1998

Gould L, Gopalaswamy C, Chandy F, et al: Electroconvulsive therapy-induced ECG changes simulating a myocardial infarction. Arch Intern Med 143:1786–1787, 1983

Greenberg L, Fink M: The use of electroconvulsive therapy in geriatric patients. Clin Geriatr Med 8:349–354, 1992

Grunhaus L, Shpley JE, Eiser A, et al: Polysomnographic studies in patients referred for ECT: pre-ECT studies. Convulsive Therapy 12:224–231, 1996

Hermann RC, Dorwart RA, Hoover CW, et al: Variation in the use of ECT in the United States. Am J Psychiatry 152: 869–875, 1995

Hermesh H, Aizenberg D, Friedberg G, et al: Electroconvulsive therapy for persistent neuroleptic-induced akathisia and parkinsonism: a case report. Biol Psychiatry 31:407–411, 1992

Heshe J, Roder E, Theilgaard A: Unilateral and bilateral ECT: a psychiatric and psychological study of therapeutic effect and side effects. Acta Psychiatr Scand Suppl 275:1–180, 1978

Hickie I, Mason C, Gordon P, et al: Prediction of ECT response: validation of a refined sign-based (CORE) system for defining melancholia. Br J Psychiatry 169:68–74, 1996

Holcomb H, Sternberg D, Heninger G: Effects of electroconvulsive therapy on mood, parkinsonism and tardive dyskinesia in a depressed patient: ECT and dopamine systems. Biol Psychiatry 18:865–873, 1983

Holzer JC, Giakas WJ, Mazure CM, et al: Dysarthria during ECT given for Parkinson's disease and depression. Convulsive Therapy 8:201–203, 1992

Howie MB, Black HA, Zvar AD, et al: Esmolol reduces autonomic hypersensitivity and length of seizures induced by electroconvulsive therapy. Anesth Analg 71:384–388, 1990

Hsiao JK, Messenheimer JA, Evans DL: ECT and neurological disorders. Convulsive Therapy 3:121–136, 1987

Huang KC, Lucas LF, Tsueda K, et al: Age-related changes in cardiovascular function associated with electroconvulsive therapy. Convulsive Therapy 5:17–25, 1989

Hughes J, Barraclough BM, Reeve W: Are patients shocked by ECT? J R Soc Med 74:283–285, 1981

Imlah NW, Ryan E, Harrington JA: The influence of antidepressant drugs on the response to electroconvulsive therapy and on subsequent relapse rates. Neuropsychopharmacology 4:438–442, 1965

Jaeckle R, Dilsaver S: Covariation of depressive symptoms, parkinsonism, and post-dexamethasone plasma cortisol levels in a bipolar patient: simultaneous response to ECT and lithium carbonate. Acta Psychiatr Scand 74:68–72, 1986

Jarvie H: Prognosis of depression treated by electric convulsive therapy. BMJ 1:132–134, 1954

Jenike MA: Handbook of Geriatric Psychopharmacology. Littleton, MA, PSG Publishing, 1985

Kahn RL, Pollack M, Fink M: Sociopsychologic aspects of psychiatric treatment in a voluntary mental hospital: duration of hospitalization, discharge ratings and diagnosis. Arch Gen Psychiatry 1:565–574, 1959

Kalayam B, Alexopoulos GS: Nifedipene in the treatment of blood pressure rise after ECT. Convulsive Therapy 5:110–113, 1989

Kamil R, Joffe RT: Neuroendocrine testing in electroconvulsive therapy. Psychiatr Clin North Am 14:961–970, 1991

Kaplan HI, Sadock BJ (eds): Synopsis of Psychiatry, 5th Edition. Baltimore, MD, Williams & Wilkins, 1988, pp 253–269

Karlinsky H, Shulman KI: The clinical use of electroconvulsive therapy in old age. J Am Geriatr Soc 32:183–186, 1984

Kellner CH: The CT scan (or MRI) before ECT: a wonderful test has been overused (editorial). Convulsive Therapy 12:79–80, 1996

Kellner CH: Left unilateral ECT: still a viable option? Convulsive Therapy 13:65–67, 1997a

Kellner CH: Seizure interference by medications: how big a problem (editorial)? Convulsive Therapy 13:1–3, 1997b

Kellner CH, Bernstein HJ: ECT as a treatment for neurologic illness, in The Clinical Science of Electroconvulsive Therapy. Edited by Coffey CE. Washington, DC, American Psychiatric Press, 1993, pp 183–210

Kellner CH, Nixon DW, Bernstein HJ: ECT-drug interactions: a review. Psychopharmacol Bull 27:595–609, 1991a

Kellner CH, Tolhurst JE, Burns CM: ECT in the presence of severe cervical spine disease. Convulsive Therapy 7:52–55, 1991b

Kellner CH, Burns CM, Bernstein HJ, et al: Electrode placement in maintenance electroconvulsive therapy. Convulsive Therapy 7:61–62, 1991c

Kellner CH, Monroe RR, Pritchett J, et al: Weekly ECT in geriatric depression. Convulsive Therapy 8:245–252, 1992

Kellner CH, Coffey CE, Beale MD, et al: Handbook of ECT. Washington, DC, American Psychiatric Press, 1997

Kirkegaard C, Norlem N, Lauridsen UB, et al: Protirelin stimulation test and thyroid function during treatment of depression. Arch Gen Psychiatry 32:1115–1118, 1975

Kramer BA: Use of ECT in California, 1977–1983. Am J Psychiatry 142:1190–1192, 1985

Kramer BA: Electroconvulsive therapy use in geriatric depression. J Nerv Ment Dis 175:233–235, 1987

Kramer BA: Use of ECT in California, revised: 1984–1994. J ECT (in press)

Kroessler D, Fogel B: Electroconvulsive therapy for major depression in the oldest old. Am J Geriatr Psychiatry 1:30–37, 1993

Krog-Meyer I, Kirkegaard C, Kijne B, et al: Prediction of relapse with the TRH test and prophylactic amitriptyline in 39 patients with endogenous depression. Am J Psychiatry 141:945–948, 1984

Krystal AD, Coffey CE: Neuropsychiatric considerations in the use of electroconvulsive therapy. J Neuropsychiatry Clin Neurosci 9:283–292, 1997

Krystal AD, Weiner RD, Coffey CE: The ictal EEG as a marker of adequate stimulus intensity with unilateral ECT. J Neuropsychiatry Clin Neurosci 7:295–303, 1995

Krystal AD, Weiner RD, Gassert D, et al: The relative ability of 3 ictal EEG frequency bands to differentiate ECT seizures on the basis of electrode placement, stimulus intensity, and therapeutic response. Convulsive Therapy 12:13–24, 1996

Krystal AD, Coffey CE, Weiner RD, et al: Changes in seizure threshold over the course of electroconvulsive therapy affect therapeutic response and are detected by ictal EEG ratings. J Neuropsychiatry Clin Neurosci 10:178–186, 1998

Lambourn J, Barrington PC: Electroconvulsive therapy in a sample British population in 1982. Convulsive Therapy 2: 169–177, 1986

Lauritzen L, Odgaard K, Clemmesen L, et al: Relapse prevention by means of paroxetine in ECT-treated patients with major depression: a comparison with imipramine and placebo in medium term continuation therapy. Acta Psychiatr Scand 94:241–251, 1996

Lauterbach E, Moore N: Parkinsonism-dystonia syndrome and ECT. Am J Psychiatry 147:1249–1250, 1990

Lebensohn Z, Jenkins R: Improvement of parkinsonism in depressed patients treated with ECT. Am J Psychiatry 132:283–285, 1975

Lerer B, Shapira B, Calev A, et al: Antidepressant and cognitive effects of twice- versus three-times-weekly ECT. Am J Psychiatry 152:564–570, 1995

Letemendia FJ, Delva NJ, Rodenburg M, et al: Therapeutic advantage of bifrontal electrode placement in ECT. Psychol Med 23:349–360, 1993

Leuchter A: Electroencephalography, in Comprehensive Review of Geriatric Psychiatry. Edited by Sadavoy J, Lazarus LW, Jarvik LF. Washington, DC, American Psychiatric Press, 1991, pp 273–283

Levy L, Savit J, Hodes M: Parkinsonism: improvement by electroconvulsive therapy. Arch Phys Med Rehabil 64: 432–433, 1983

Lichtor JL: Psychological preparation and preoperative medication, in Anesthesia, 3rd Edition, Vol 1. Edited by Miller RD. New York, Churchill Livingstone, 1990, pp 895–928

Lingam VR, Lazarus LW, Groves L, et al: Methylphenidate in treating post-stroke depression. J Clin Psychiatry 49: 151–153, 1988

Lipper S, Bermanzohn P: Electroconvulsive therapy in patients with parkinsonism (letter). Am J Psychiatry 132:457, 1975

Lipsey JR, Robinson RG, Pearlson GD: Nortriptyline treatment of post-stroke depression: a double-blind study. Lancet 1:297–300, 1984

Loo H, Galinowski A, De Carvalho W, et al: Use of maintenance ECT for elderly depressed patients (letter). Am J Psychiatry 148:810, 1991

Lurie SN, Coffey CE: Caffeine-modified ECT in depressed patients with medical illness. J Clin Psychiatry 51:154–157, 1990

Magni G, Fisman M, Helmes E: Clinical correlates of ECT-resistant depression in the elderly. J Clin Psychiatry 49:405–407, 1988

Malcolm K: Patients' perceptions and knowledge of electroconvulsive therapy. Psychiatric Bulletin 13: 161–165, 1989

Malla AK: Characteristics of patients who receive electroconvulsive therapy. Can J Psychiatry 33:696–701, 1988

Maltbie AA, Wingfield MS, Volow MR, et al: Electroconvulsive therapy in the presence of brain tumor. J Nerv Ment Dis 168:400–405, 1980

Mander AJ, Whitfield A, Keen DM, et al: Cerebral and brain stem changes after ECT revealed by nuclear magnetic resonance imaging. Br J Psychiatry 151:69–71, 1987

Maneksha FR: Hypertension and tachycardia during electroconvulsive therapy: to treat or not to treat? Convulsive Therapy 7:28–35, 1991

Manly DT, Swartz CS: Asymmetric bilateral right frontotemporal left frontal stimulus electrode placement: comparisons with bifrontotemporal and unilateral placements. Convulsive Therapy 10:267–270, 1994

Markowitz J, Brown R, Sweeney J, et al: Reduced length and cost of hospital stay for major depression in patients treated with ECT. Am J Psychiatry 144:1025–1029, 1987

Martin M, Figiel G, Mattingly G, et al: ECT-induced interictal delirium in patients with a history of CVA. J Geriatr Psychiatry Neurol 5:149–155, 1992

McCall WV: Cardiovascular risk during ECT: managing the managers (editorial). Convulsive Therapy 13:123–124, 1997

McCall WV, Cohen W, Reboussin B, et al: Pretreatment differences in specific symptoms and quality of life among depressed inpatients who do and do not receive electroconvulsive therapy: a hypothesis regarding why the elderly are more likely to receive ECT. J ECT 15:193–201, 1999

McDonald WM, Phillips VL, Figiel GS, et al: Cost-effective maintenance treatment of resistant geriatric depression. Psychiatric Annals 28:47–52, 1998

McElhiney MC, Moody BJ, Steif BL, et al: Autobiographical memory and mood: effects of electroconvulsive therapy. Neuropsychology 9:501–517, 1995

Mendels J: Electroconvulsive therapy and depression, I: the prognostic significance of clinical factors. Br J Psychiatry 111:675–681, 1965

Messina AG, Paranicas M, Katz B, et al: Effect of electroconvulsive therapy on the electrocardiogram and echocardiogram. Anesth Analg 75:511–514, 1992

Meyers BS, Mei-Tal V: Empirical study on an inpatient psychogeriatric unit: biological treatment in patients with depressive illness. Int J Psychiatry Med 15:111–124, 1985–1986

Miller ME, Siris SG, Gabriel AN: Treatment delays in the course of electroconvulsive therapy. Hosp Community Psychiatry 37:825–827, 1986

Miller RD, Savarese JJ: Pharmacology of muscle relaxants and their antagonists, in Anesthesia, 3rd Edition, Vol 1. Edited by Miller RD. New York, Churchill Livingstone, 1990, pp 389–435

Monroe RR: Maintenance electroconvulsive therapy. Psychiatr Clin North Am 14:947–960, 1991

Mukherjee S: Mechanisms of the antimanic effects of electroconvulsive therapy. Convulsive Therapy 4:74–80, 1988

Mukherjee S, Sackeim HA, Schnur DB: Electroconvulsive therapy of acute manic episodes: a review of 50 years' experience. Am J Psychiatry 151:169–176, 1994

Mulsant BH, Rosen J, Thornton JE, et al: A prospective naturalistic study of electroconvulsive therapy in late-life depression. J Geriatr Psychiatry Neurol 4:3–13, 1991

Murray GB, Shea V, Conn DK: Electroconvulsive therapy for post-stroke depression. J Clin Psychiatry 47:258–260, 1986

Nelson JP, Benjamin L: Efficacy and safety of combined ECT and tricyclic antidepressant drugs in the treatment of depressed geriatric patients. Convulsive Therapy 5:321–329, 1989

Nobler MS, Sackeim HA, Solomou M, et al: EEG manifestations during ECT: effects of electrode placement and stimulus intensity. Biol Psychiatry 34:321–330, 1993

Nobler MS, Sackeim HA, Prohovnik I, et al: Regional cerebral blood flow in mood disorders, III: treatment and clinical response. Arch Gen Psychiatry 51:884–897, 1994

Oh JJ, Rummans TA, O'Conner MK, et al: Cognitive impairment after ECT in patients with Parkinson's disease and psychiatric illness (letter). Am J Psychiatry 149:271, 1992

O'Leary D, Gill D, Gregory S, et al: Which depressed patients respond to ECT? The Nottingham results. J Affect Disord 33:245–250, 1995

Olfson M, Marcus S, Sackeim HA, et al: Use of ECT for the treatment of recurrent major depression. Am J Psychiatry 155:22–29, 1998

Ottosson JO: Experimental studies of the mode of action of electroconvulsive therapy. Acta Psychiatr Scand Suppl 145:1–141, 1960

Oztas B, Kaya M, Camurcu S: Age related changes in the effect of electroconvulsive shock on the blood brain barrier permeability in rats. Mech Ageing Dev 51:149–155, 1990

Pande AC, Grunhaus LJ, Haskett RF, et al: Electroconvulsive therapy in delusional and non-delusional depressive disorder. J Affect Disord 19:215–219, 1990

Papakostas Y, Fink M, Lee J, et al: Neuroendocrine measures in psychiatric patients: course and outcome with ECT. Psychiatry Res 4:55–64, 1981

Pettinati HM, Mathisen KS, Rosenberg J, et al: Meta-analytical approach to reconciling discrepancies in efficacy between bilateral and unilateral electroconvulsive therapy. Convulsive Therapy 2:7–17, 1986

Physicians' Desk Reference, 53rd Edition. Montvale, NJ, Medical Economics, 1999

Post RM: Transduction of psychosocial stress into the neurobiology of recurrent affective disorder. Am J Psychiatry 149:999–1010, 1992

Pratt RTC, Warrington EK, Halliday AM: Unilateral ECT as a test for cerebral dominance, with a strategy for treating left-handers. Br J Psychiatry 119:79–83, 1971

Price TRP, McAllister TW: Safety and efficacy of ECT in depressed patients with dementia: a review of clinical experience. Convulsive Therapy 5:61–74, 1989

Prien R, Kupfer D: Continuation drug therapy for major depressive episodes: how long should it be maintained? Am J Psychiatry 143:18–23, 1986

Prohovnik I, Sackeim HA, Decina P, et al: Acute reductions of regional cerebral blood flow following electroconvulsive therapy: interactions with modality and time. Ann N Y Acad Sci 462:249–262, 1986

Prudic J, Sackeim HA, Decina P, et al: Acute effects of ECT on cardiovascular functioning: relations to patient and treatment variables. Acta Psychiatr Scand 75:344–351, 1987

Prudic J, Sackeim HA, Spicknall K. Potential pharmacologic agents for the cognitive effects of electroconvulsive treatment. Psychiatric Annals 28:40–46, 1998

Rasmussen K, Abrams R: Treatment of Parkinson's disease with electroconvulsive therapy. Psychiatr Clin North Am 14:925–933, 1991

Rayburn BK: Electroconvulsive therapy in patients with heart failure or valvular heart disease. Convulsive Therapy 13:145–156, 1997

Reynolds CF, Perel JM, Kupfer DJ, et al: Open-trial response to antidepressant treatment in elderly patients with mixed depression and cognitive impairment. Psychiatry Res 21:111–122, 1987

Rice EH, Sombrotto LB, Markowitz JC, et al: Cardiovascular morbidity in high-risk patients during ECT. Am J Psychiatry 151:1637–1641, 1994

Rich CL, Spiker DG, Jewell SW, et al: DSM-III, RDC, and ECT: depressive subtypes and immediate response. J Clin Psychiatry 45:14–18, 1984a

Rich CL, Spiker DG, Jewell SW, et al: The efficiency of ECT, I: response rate in depressive episodes. Psychiatry Res 11:167–176, 1984b

Rich CL, Spiker DG, Jewell SW, et al: ECT response in psychotic versus nonpsychotic unipolar depressives. J Clin Psychiatry 47:123–125, 1986

Roberts JM: Prognostic factors in the electroshock treatment of depressive states, I: clinical features from history and examination. Journal of Mental Science 105:693–702, 1959

Robinson RG, Price TR: Post-stroke depressive disorders: a follow-up study of 103 patients. Stroke 13:635–641, 1982

Roemer RA, Shagass C, Dubin W, et al: Relationship between pretreatment electroencephalographic coherence measures and subsequent response to electroconvulsive therapy: a preliminary study. Neuropsychobiology 24:121–124, 1990

Rosenberg R, Vostrup S, Andersen A, et al: Effect of ECT on cerebral blood flow in melancholia assessed with SPECT. Convulsive Therapy 4:62–73, 1988

Roth S, Mukherjee S, Sackeim H: Electroconvulsive therapy in a patient with mania, parkinsonism and tardive dyskinesia. Convulsive Therapy 4:92–97, 1988

Rubin EH, Kinsoherf DA, Wehrman SA: Response to treatment of depression in the old and very old. J Geriatr Psychiatry Neurol 4:65–70, 1991

Rudorfer M, Risby E, Hsaio J, et al: ECT alters human monoamines in a different manner from that of antidepressant drugs. Psychopharmacol Bull 24:396–399, 1988

Rummans TA, Lauterbach EC, Coffey CE, et al: Pharmacologic efficacy in neuropsychiatry: a review of placebo- controlled treatment trials—a report of the ANPA Committee on Research. J Neuropsychiatry Clin Neurosci 11:176–189, 1999

Sackeim HA: Are ECT devices underpowered (editorial)? Convulsive Therapy 7:233–236, 1991

Sackeim HA: What's new with ECT? American Society of Clinical Psychopharmacology Progress Notes 8:27–33, 1997

Sackeim HA, Decina P, Prohovnik I, et al: Anticonvulsant and antidepressant properties of electroconvulsive therapy: a proposed mechanism of action. Biol Psychiatry 18:1301–1310, 1983

Sackeim HA, Decina P, Kanzler M, et al: Effects of electrode placement on the efficacy of titrated, low-dose ECT. Am J Psychiatry 144:1449–1455, 1987

Sackeim HA, Prudic J, Devanand DP, et al: The impact of medication resistance and continuation pharmacotherapy on relapse following response to electroconvulsive therapy in major depression. J Clin Psychopharmacol 10:96–104, 1990

Sackeim HA, Devanand DP, Prudic J: Stimulus intensity, seizure threshold, and seizure duration: impact on the efficacy and safety of electroconvulsive therapy. Psychiatr Clin North Am 14:803–843, 1991

Sackeim HA, Prudic J, Devanand DP, et al: Effects of stimulus intensity and electrode placement on the efficacy and cognitive effects of electroconvulsive therapy. N Engl J Med 328:839–846, 1993

Salzman C: Electroconvulsive therapy in the elderly patient. Psychiatr Clin North Am 5:191–197, 1982

Scott AI, Douglas RH, Whitfield A, et al: Time course of cerebral magnetic resonance changes after electroconvulsive therapy. Br J Psychiatry 156:551–553, 1990

Scott AI, Dougall N, Ross M, et al: Short-term effects of electroconvulsive treatment on the uptake of ^{99m}Tc-exametazime into brain in major depression shown with single photon emission tomography. J Affect Disord 30:27–34, 1994

Seager CP, Bird RL: Imipramine with electrical treatment in depression: a controlled trial. Journal of Mental Science 108:704–707, 1962

Shapira B, Lerer B: Speed of response to bilateral ECT: an examination of possible predictors in two controlled trials. J ECT 15:202–206, 1999

Shettar MS, Grunhaus L, Pande AC, et al: Protective effects of intramuscular glycopyrrolate on cardiac conduction during ECT. Convulsive Therapy 5:349–352, 1989

Slawson P: Psychiatric malpractice: the electroconvulsive therapy experience. Convulsive Therapy 1:195–203, 1985

Small JG, Klapper MH, Kellams JJ, et al: ECT compared with lithium in the management of manic states. Arch Gen Psychiatry 45:727–732, 1988

Small JG, Milstein V, Small IF: Electroconvulsive therapy for mania. Psychiatr Clin North Am 14:887–903, 1991

Sobin C, Prudic J, Devanand DP, et al: Who responds to electroconvulsive therapy? Br J Psychiatry 169:322–328, 1995

Solan WJ, Khan A, Avery DH, et al: Psychotic and nonpsychotic depression: comparison of response to ECT. J Clin Psychiatry 49:97–99, 1988

Staton RD: Electroencephalographic recording during bitemporal and unilateral non-dominant hemisphere (Lancaster position) electroconvulsive therapy. J Clin Psychiatry 42:254–269, 1981

Steffens DC, Krystal AD, Sibert TE, et al: Cost effectiveness of maintenance ECT (letter). Convulsive Therapy 11: 283–284, 1995

Stoudemire A, Knos G, Gladson M, et al: Labetalol in the control of cardiovascular responses to electroconvulsive therapy in high-risk depressed medical patients. J Clin Psychiatry 51:508–512, 1990

Stoudemire A, Hill CD, Morris R, et al: Improvement in depression-related cognitive dysfunction following ECT. J Neuropsychiatry Clin Neurosci 7:31–34, 1995

Strömgren LS: Unilateral versus bilateral electroconvulsive therapy: investigations into the therapeutic effect in endogenous depression. Acta Psychiatr Scand Suppl 240:8–65, 1973

Strömgren LS: ECT in acute delirium and related clinical states. Convulsive Therapy 13:10–17, 1997

Strömgren LS, Juul-Jensen P: EEG in unilateral and bilateral electroconvulsive therapy. Acta Psychiatr Scand 51: 340–360, 1975

Strömgren LS, Christensen AL, Fromholt P: The effects of unilateral brief-interval ECT on memory. Acta Psychiatr Scand 54 336–346, 1976

Sullivan MO, Ward NG, Laxton A: The woman who wanted electroconvulsive therapy and do-not-resuscitate status. Gen Hosp Psychiatry 14:204–209, 1992

Swartz CM: Clinical and laboratory predictors of ECT response, in The Clinical Science of Electroconvulsive Therapy. Edited by Coffey CE. Washington, DC, American Psychiatric Press, 1993, pp 53–71

Tew JD, Mulsant BH, Haskett RF, et al: Acute efficacy of ECT in the treatment of major depression in the old-old. Am J Psychiatry 156:1865–1870, 1999

Thienhaus OJ, Margletta S, Bennett JA: A study of the clinical efficacy of maintenance ECT. J Clin Psychiatry 51: 141–144, 1990

Thompson JW, Weiner RD, Myers CP: Use of ECT in the United States in 1975, 1980, and 1986. Am J Psychiatry 151:1657–1661, 1994

Tomac TA, Rummans TA, Pileggi TS, et al: Safety and efficacy of electroconvulsive therapy in patients over age 85. Am J Geriatr Psychiatry 5:126–130, 1997

Turek IS: EEG correlates of electroconvulsive treatment. Dis Nerv Syst 33:584–589, 1972

Volavka J, Feldstein S, Abrams R, et al: EEG and clinical change after bilateral and unilateral electroconvulsive therapy. Electroencephalogr Clin Neurophysiol 32:631–639, 1972

Volkow ND, Bellar S, Mullani N, et al: Effects of electroconvulsive therapy on brain glucose metabolism: a preliminary study. Convulsive Therapy 4:199–205, 1988

Ward C, Stern GM, Pratt R, et al: Electroconvulsive therapy in parkinsonian patients with the "on-off" syndrome. J Neural Transm 49:133–135, 1980

Webb MC, Coffey CE, Saunders WR, et al: Cardiovascular response to unilateral electroconvulsive therapy. Biol Psychiatry 28:758–766, 1990

Weiner RD: The role of electroconvulsive therapy in the treatment of depression in the elderly. J Am Geriatr Soc 30: 710–712, 1982

Weiner RD: Does ECT cause brain damage? Behav Brain Sci 7:1–53, 1984

Weiner RD, Coffey CE: Indications for use of electroconvulsive therapy, in American Psychiatric Press Review of Psychiatry, Vol 7. Edited by Frances AJ, Hales RE. Washington, DC, American Psychiatric Press, 1988, pp 458–481

Weiner RD, Krystal AD: EEG Monitoring of ECT seizures, in The Clinical Science of Electroconvulsive Therapy. Edited by Coffey CE. Washington, DC, American Psychiatric Press, 1993, pp 93–109

Weiner RD, Whanger AD, Erwin CW, et al: Prolonged confusional state and EEG seizure activity following concurrent ECT and lithium use. Am J Psychiatry 137: 1452–1453, 1980

Weiner RD, Rogers HJ, Davidson JRT, et al: Effects of stimulus parameters on cognitive side effects. Ann N Y Acad Sci 462: 315–325, 1986

Weiner RD, Coffey CE, Krystal AD: Electroconvulsive therapy in the medical and neurological patient, in Psychiatric Care of the Medical Patient, 2nd Edition. Edited by Stoudemire A, Fogel B, Greenberg D. New York, Oxford University Press, 2000

Weisberg LA, Elliott D, Mielke D: Intracerebral hemorrhage following electroconvulsive therapy. Neurology 41:1849, 1991

Welch CA: ECT in medically ill patients, in The Clinical Science of Electroconvulsive Therapy. Edited by Coffey CE. Washington, DC, American Psychiatric Press, 1993, pp 167–182

Welch CA, Drop LJ: Cardiovascular effects of ECT. Convulsive Therapy 5:35–43, 1989

Wesner RB: Prolonged T-wave inversion associated with electroconvulsive therapy. Convulsive Therapy 2:203–206, 1986

Wesner RB, Winokur G: The influence of age on the natural history of unipolar depression when treated with electroconvulsive therapy. Eur Arch Psychiatry Neurol Sci 238:149–154, 1989

Wilkinson AM, Anderson DN, Peters S: Age and the effects of ECT. Int J Geriatr Psychiatry 8:401–406, 1993

Young R, Alexopoulos G, Shamoian A: Dissociation of motor response from mood and cognition in a parkinsonian patient treated with ECT. Biol Psychiatry 20:566–569, 1985

Yudofsky SC: Parkinson's disease, depression and electroconvulsive therapy: a clinical and neurobiologic synthesis. Compr Psychiatry 20:579–581, 1979

Zervas I[M], Fink M: ECT for refractory Parkinson's disease. Convulsive Therapy 7:222–223, 1991

Zervas IM, Calev A, Jandorf L, et al: Age-dependent effects of electroconvulsive therapy on memory. Convulsive Therapy 9:39–42, 1993

Zibrak JD, Jensen WA, Bloomingdale K: Aspiration pneumonitis following electroconvulsive therapy in patients with gastroparesis. Biol Psychiatry 24:812–814, 1988

Zielinski, RJ, Roose SP, Devanand DP, et al: Cardiovascular complications of ECT in depressed patients with cardiac disease. Am J Psychiatry 150:904–909, 1993

Zis AP, Goodwin FK: Major affective disorder as a recurrent illness: a critical review. Arch Gen Psychiatry 36:835–839, 1979

Zorumski CF, Rubin EH, Burke WJ: Electroconvulsive therapy for the elderly. Hosp Community Psychiatry 39:643–647, 1988

Zwil A, McAllister TW, Price TRP: Safety and efficacy of ECT in depressed patients with organic brain disease: review of a clinical experience. Convulsive Therapy 8:103–109, 1992

Zvara DA, Brooker RF, McCall WV, et al: The effects of esmolol on ST-segment depression and arrhythmias after electroconvulsive therapy. Convulsive Therapy 13:165–174, 1997

36

Psychosocial Therapies

Linda Teri, Ph.D.

Susan M. McCurry, Ph.D.

Historically, it was believed that older adults were not good candidates for nonpharmacological, psychotherapeutic interventions. However, in the past several decades, there has been a growing awareness of the psychosocial issues confronting aging adults and of the value of psychotherapy as a tool for managing age-related change and maintaining quality of life. The empirical literature on the treatment of depression in older adults has been summarized in numerous recent reviews (Niederehe 1994, 1996; Scogin and McElreath 1994; Teri et al. 1994). Studies of a number of other treatments related to psychological health in elderly patients have also been reviewed, including behavioral assessment and treatment of anxiety (Hersen and van Hasselt 1992), behavioral management of dementia (C. K. Beck and Shue 1994; Fisher and Carstensen 1990), reminiscence therapy or life review (Haight 1991; Thornton and Brotchie 1987), treatments for sleep and cognitive enhancement (Gatz et al. 1998), and group interventions for family caregivers (Bourgeois et al. 1996; Knight et al. 1993).

In this chapter, we summarize the main psychosocial treatments that have been empirically evaluated in older adults. The focus of the chapter is on psychosocial treatments designed to improve the emotional status of participants. Therefore, the studies reviewed here had as their primary treatment outcomes psychological variables such as depression, anxiety, and other psychiatric symptoms; life satisfaction; interpersonal skills; coping and stress management; and caregiver burden. The emphasis of the chapter is on controlled clinical trials; individual case studies or treatments conducted using single-case design methodologies are not discussed. The majority of the reviewed empirical psychosocial studies involved cognitive-behavioral, brief psychodynamic, or reminiscence-based interventions. Studies of other forms of treatment for geriatric patients, including interventions for alcohol abuse (e.g., Kashner et al. 1992), behavioral treatments for insomnia (e.g., Bliwise et al. 1995; Morin et al. 1999), and cognitive training or memory-enhancement programs (e.g., Quayhagen et al. 1995; Verhaeghen et al. 1992), were excluded unless they included evaluation of mood or psychosocial status as primary outcomes. Also excluded were studies describing treatment of older patients using somatic therapies (e.g., use of light treatment, exercise, massage, or white noise to reduce agitation in patients with dementia [Burgio et al.

1996; Love_l et al. 1995; Snyder et al. 1995]) and studies describing staff training programs in institutional settings (e.g., Baltes et al. 1994; Blair 1995; Heacock et al. 1997; Lantz et al. 1997). In summary, the focus of this chapter is on controlled clinical trials of psychosocial treatments for older adults in which the primary treatment outcomes were psychological.

Psychotherapy for Depression in Older Adults

Much of the psychotherapeutic research involving elderly patients has focused on the treatment of depression. Depression is thought to affect approximately 15% of community-dwelling persons over age 65 and up to 25% of nursing home residents (National Institutes of Health 1991). Depressive symptoms are also prevalent among medically or neurologically ill older adults, including those with dementia and their caregivers (Baker 1996; Gallagher et al. 1989; Teri and Wagner 1992). Nevertheless, epidemiological studies indicate that older adults are underserved by mental health care providers. It has been estimated that only 10% of the older population in need of psychiatric treatment receives this care (National Institutes of Health 1991). Because recurrence of depressive episodes is common throughout the life span, and suicide rates for older adults are greater than for younger adults (Bharucha and Satlin 1997; Reynolds 1997), this lack of psychosocial treatment in geriatric patients is a cause of concern. Fortunately, the literature has generally demonstrated that both acute and continuation therapies can be effective with depressed elderly patients (see Chapter 13). In this section, we review empirical studies of psychosocial interventions that were specifically designed to reduce depression in community-dwelling older adults without dementia.

Cognitive-Behavior Therapy and Psychodynamic Psychotherapy

Cognitive-behavioral approaches have been widely used in the treatment of depression in geriatric outpatients. *Cognitive-behavior therapy* (CBT) refers to an approach that combines the conceptual and applied work of various cognitive and behavioral-social learning theorists such as Beck (see A. T. Beck et al. 1979) and Lewinsohn (see Lewinsohn et al. 1984). In interventions involving CBT, it is generally assumed that psychiatric disturbances are learned and maintained through a combination of cognitive distortions and behavioral or environmental events. Thus, the goal of treatment is to change the cognitive and behavioral context

in which the disturbance occurs, through use of specific techniques such as providing new information, teaching problem-solving strategies, correcting skills deficits, modifying ineffective communication patterns, or changing the physical environment in which problems arise. Homework assignments to supplement in-session interventions are frequently given. Although specific treatment protocols vary, all cognitive-behavioral approaches tend to be active and to be focused on solving specific, current day-to-day problems, rather than on effecting global personality change. In practice, the terms *psychoeducational* and *cognitive-behavioral* are often used interchangeably to refer to similar intervention strategies.

A few controlled studies have compared the use of psychodynamic or insight-oriented approaches with that of either CBT or pharmacotherapy in depressed older subjects. The dynamic approaches used in these studies differ from CBT in their emphasis on the importance of the therapeutic relationship as a mechanism of change and in their focus on historical causes of current patient behavior. Typically, patients are not taught specific skills as a part of therapy, nor is homework outside of session considered an essential aspect of treatment. Rather, greater import is assigned to patients' psychological insight and ongoing emotional experience. Therapeutic techniques such as reflection or interpretation of patient resistance are often used, and the therapist tends to be less directive than in CBT. Brief dynamic or insight-oriented approaches have been developed, however, that emphasize specific problem resolution within a limited number of therapy sessions (Strupp 1982). Among the brief manualized psychodynamic approaches, interpersonal psychotherapy (IPT) (Klerman et al. 1984), has been the most widely used in controlled clinical outcome trials with depressed older patients.

Much of the empirical data on the efficacy of CBT in geriatric subjects have been obtained by L. W. Thompson, Gallagher-Thompson, and their colleagues (Table 36–1). Several of their studies compared cognitive and behavioral treatments with a brief psychodynamic or insight-oriented approach. For example, Gallagher and Thompson (Gallagher and Thompson 1982, 1983; L. W. Thompson and Gallagher 1985) compared the effectiveness of short-term individual cognitive, behavioral, and brief relational-insight therapies in a sample of 30 elderly outpatient volunteers who had no evidence of significant cognitive impairment (Mini-Mental State Exam [MMSE] score of 25 or higher) and in whom a major depressive disorder had been diagnosed. There was a substantial decrease in depressive symptoms in subjects in all three groups by the end of treatment, and this decrease was maintained at 1 year. However, maintenance of treatment gains was not the

TABLE 36–1. Empirical studies of cognitive-behavior or psychodynamic therapy in depressed older adults

Study[a]	Subjects[b]	Subject age (years)	Treatment	Treatment duration
Gallagher and Thompson 1982, 1983; L.W. Thompson and Gallagher 1985	30 outpatients with MDD	Mean, 66–69 (range, 59–80)	Individual CT Individual BT Individual relational-insight therapy	16 sessions in 12 weeks
Jarvik et al. 1982	32 outpatients with MDD (drug trial) 26 outpatients with MDD (group therapy)	Range, 55–81	Imipramine therapy Doxepin therapy Placebo	36 weeks
Steuer et al. 1984	33 outpatient volunteers with MDD	Median, 66 (range, 55–78)	Group CBT Group psychodynamic therapy	46 sessions in 9 months
L.W. Thompson et al. 1983	56 volunteer attendees	Mean, 68 (range, 60–82)	Coping With Depression group course: Professional instructors Nonprofessional instructors	6 weeks
Fry 1984	28 outpatients	Mean, 65 (range, 67–80)	Group CBT Group CBT after wait list	12 sessions in 4 weeks
L.W. Thompson and Gallagher 1984	37 outpatients with MDD	Mean, 67	Individual CT Individual BT Individual dynamic therapy Wait list (control)	16–20 sessions in 3–4 months
Sloane et al. 1985; Schneider et al. 1986	55 outpatients with MDD	Mean, 64 (all subjects > 60)	Individual IPT Nortriptyline therapy Placebo	16 weeks
L.W. Thompson and Gallagher 1986; L.W. Thompson et al. 1987, 1988; Gaston et al. 1988, 1989; Marmar et al. 1989; Gallagher-Thompson et al. 1990; M.G. Thompson et al. 1995	91 outpatients with MDD	Mean, 67	Individual CT Individual BT Individual psychodynamic therapy Wait list (control)	16–20 sessions in 3–4 months
Beutler et al. 1987	56 outpatients with MDD	Mean, 70–71 (all subjects > 65)	Alprazolam therapy Placebo Group CBT and alprazolam therapy Group CBT and placebo	20 sessions

(continued)

TABLE 36–1. Empirical studies of cognitive-behavior or psychodynamic therapy in depressed older adults *(continued)*

Study[a]	Subjects[b]	Subject age (years)	Treatment	Treatment duration
Scogin et al. 1987	29 volunteers with mild depression	Mean, 68–72	Individual cognitive bibliotherapy Individual delayed (cognitive) bibliotherapy Attention-control reading	Self-paced
Scogin et al. 1989, 1990	67 community residents	Mean, 68	Individual cognitive bibliotherapy Individual behavioral bibliotherapy Wait list (control)	4 weeks
L.W. Thompson et al. 1991	67 older adult outpatient volunteers	?	Desipramine therapy Individual CBT Medication and CBT combined	? sessions in 3–4 months
Campbell 1992	103 low-income, community residents with depression	Range, 64–82	Individual CT No treatment (control) Group crafts classes	16 sessions in 8 weeks
Gallagher-Thompson and Steffen 1994	66 family caregivers with depression	Mean, 62	Individual CBT Individual psychodynamic therapy	16–20 sessions in 3–4 months
Reynolds et al. 1992, 1994, 1995, 1996a, 1996b, 1997, 1999a, 1999b; Dew et al. 1997; Opdyke et al. 1996–1997; Miller et al. 1997; Thase et al. 1997; Wolfson et al. 1997	158 consecutively enrolled elderly patients with recurrent MDD	Range, 60–80	After successful open treatment (nortriptyline therapy plus weekly IPT) of index depressive episode, patients are randomly assigned to one of four maintenance therapies: Nortriptyline therapy Nortriptyline therapy and IPT Placebo and IPT Placebo	Monthly for 3 years or until recurrence of major depressive episode
Mossey et al. 1996	76 medical outpatients (recently hospitalized) with subdysthymic depression	Mean, 71 (range, 60–91)	IPT Usual care	10 sessions in 3 months

Note. BT = behavior therapy; CBT = cognitive-behavior therapy; CT = cognitive therapy; IPT = interpersonal psychotherapy; MDD = major depressive disorder.
[a]Studies cited together involved subsamples of the same sample in the larger randomized clinical trial.
[b]A diagnosis of MDD is indicated for subjects in studies in which the diagnosis was specified; other studies may also have included subjects with this diagnosis.

same across the three groups: depressive symptoms increased in subjects in the brief relational-insight therapy group, beginning as early as 6 weeks after treatment, whereas no such relapse was evident in subjects in the other two groups.

Subsequent studies (L. W. Thompson and Gallagher 1984) repeated the comparison of cognitive, behavior, and brief dynamic therapies in elderly patients without dementia and in whom a major depressive disorder had been diagnosed. Significant decreases were noted in depression for all three groups compared to a 6-week, delayed treatment control condition (Gallagher-Thompson et al. 1990; L. W. Thompson and Gallagher 1986; L. W. Thompson et al. 1987). Other research groups have reported similar results. Fry (Fry 1984) found group CBT, both in immediate- and in delayed-treatment form, to be effective in reducing depression in geriatric subjects, although patients were experiencing a wider range of depressive symptoms (including milder symptoms) before treatment than in the studies described previously. Strategies involving CBT have been shown to be effective in treating depression in elderly patients whether such techniques are taught by professional or peer instructors (L. W. Thompson et al. 1983) and through self-paced or time-limited bibliotherapy (Scogin et al. 1987, 1989, 1990).

CBT has also been compared with pharmacotherapy for treating depression in elderly patients. Jarvik, Steuer, and their colleagues (Jarvik et al. 1982; Steuer et al. 1984) conducted two concurrent studies in geriatric outpatients who met DSM-III (American Psychiatric Association 1980) criteria for major depression. In one study (Jarvik et al. 1982), they compared the response of patients who received either imipramine, doxepin, or a placebo. In the other study (Steuer et al. 1984), patients who had no evidence of severe cognitive impairment were assigned to CBT or group psychodynamic therapy. Results indicated that all medication and therapy approaches were better than a placebo in reducing depression, and no significant differences in response between active treatments (imipramine vs. doxepin therapy, CBT vs. dynamic therapy) were observed. Medication therapy initially (at 26 weeks) was associated with a higher full remission rate than was psychotherapy (45% vs. 12%, respectively) (Jarvik et al. 1982). However, in the medication group, the drop-out rate was higher and more subjects showed no improvement by the end of treatment (36 weeks) than in the psychotherapy group. Further, by the end of treatment, 40% of all patients who completed psychotherapy had achieved a full remission in depression, eliminating the early advantage found in medication recipients. Results for the CBT group were slightly better than for the psychodynamic group, but

because subjects were enrolled in an open-trial (nonrandomized) fashion, these conclusions are difficult to interpret (Steuer et al. 1984).

Beutler et al. (1987) compared the relative and combined effectiveness of alprazolam therapy and group cognitive therapy in geriatric patients with major depression. Patients were randomly assigned to a 20-week course of therapy plus medication (alprazolam or placebo) or medication only. Subjects in all treatment groups showed reductions in depressive symptoms (as rated by interviewers using the Hamilton Depression Rating Scale [HDRS]) after 1 month of treatment, and gains were maintained through follow-up sampling (3 months after treatment). However, patient self-reports of depression (as rated using the Beck Depression Inventory [BDI]) and sleep disturbance indicated continued improvement after 1 month and at follow-up only for subjects who received group therapy. Significantly more patients who received cognitive therapy and medication were asymptomatic by the end of follow-up than were those who received medication without psychotherapy. No significant differences were reported for subjects receiving therapy with or without active medication.

More recently, L. W. Thompson and colleagues (1991) compared the efficacy of CBT with that of desipramine therapy, either alone or in combination with CBT, in treating 67 depressed elderly patients. Patients who received combined treatment had significantly greater reductions in depression than did those in the desipramine-only group, but not those who received CBT only. No significant differences in depression measures were observed in subjects who received either desipramine or CBT alone.

IPT has been compared with nortriptyline therapy in some of the most extensive research into psychosocial interventions for treatment of geriatric depression (Table 36–1). Early studies showed that IPT was as effective as nortriptyline therapy at 6 and 16 weeks in the acute treatment of geriatric major depression and that IPT was also associated with lower drop-out rates (Schneider et al. 1986; Sloane et al. 1985). Short-term IPT (six to eight sessions) has also been shown to reduce subdysthymic depression significantly, as evidenced on the Geriatric Depression Scale (GDS), up to 6 months after hospital discharge in elderly outpatients, compared with persons receiving usual medical care (Mossey et al. 1996). In an ongoing double-blind, controlled study, Reynolds and colleagues (1999b) are following a group of cognitively intact elderly individuals who, after successful treatment for recurrent major depression with a combination of IPT and nortriptyline, were randomized to maintenance treatment for 3 years with placebo, nortriptyline, or a combination of

IPT and placebo or IPT and nortriptyline. This study showed that elderly patients are able to benefit from psychological or pharmacological treatment of acute depression, although their rate of response is somewhat slower, and relapse rates appear to be higher, than among younger depressed individuals (Reynolds et al. 1999a).

A variety of factors may influence treatment outcome in studies of CBT and dynamic interventions in older adults. For example, in the Pittsburgh IPT studies, family involvement in educational workshops was linked to improved response to depression treatment and lower drop-out rates (Sherrill et al. 1997). Persons who reported good-quality sleep during the early stages of maintenance therapy have been shown to have significantly lower rates of depression relapse after active antidepressant medication therapy is discontinued and replaced with monthly IPT sessions plus placebo (Reynolds et al. 1997). M.G. Thompson et al. (1995) reported a relationship between major shifts in depressive mood and relapse rate in elderly patients being treated with cognitive, behavioral, or brief psychodynamic therapy. Gallagher-Thompson and Steffen (1994), who treated depressed elderly caregivers with either CBT or brief psychodynamic therapy, reported an interaction between form of treatment and duration of caregiving; individuals who had been caregivers for more than 3.5 years showed greater posttreatment benefit and were less likely to drop out of CBT, whereas those who had been caregivers for a shorter time showed greater improvement with the brief psychodynamic treatment.

Other intra-individual characteristics that have been linked to poor treatment response in elderly patients include endogeneity of depression (Gallagher and Thompson 1983), presence of a personality disorder (L. W. Thompson et al. 1988), and pretreatment defensiveness (Gaston et al. 1988). Commitment to therapy and positive expectations of change have been associated with reductions in depression among elderly patients receiving cognitive therapy but not behavioral or psychodynamic treatment (Gaston et al. 1989; Marmar et al. 1989). Reynolds et al. (1995) outlined many of the logistical challenges of successful depression treatment in this age group, including research recruitment, treatment noncompliance, and selection of appropriate outcome measures. Therapist bias against older adults may be a factor in treatment availability for and outcome with elderly patients (Fry 1986; Lazarus and Weinberg 1982), although few empirical studies have examined the relationship between treatment outcome and therapist variables. Because patients with significant cognitive impairment were generally not enrolled in the existing empirical studies on geriatric depression, there is also little known about the impact of cognitive function (e.g.,

reading ability, conceptualization, or problem-solving skills) on treatment effectiveness or compliance. Future studies are needed to clarify how these or other covariates may influence treatment outcome.

In summary, there is a growing empirical literature showing the effectiveness of CBT and brief psychodynamic therapies in treating depression in physically healthy elderly patients without dementia (studies involving physically frail or cognitively impaired depressed individuals are reviewed later in this chapter). There is evidence that symptom improvements obtained with psychotherapy are equal to those found with pharmacotherapy and that psychotherapy may be associated with lower drop-out rates than pharmacological interventions alone. A wide variety of CBT formats, including individual and group interventions, bibliotherapy, and variants of CBT (cognitive only and behavioral only), have produced reductions in depression. In many studies, treatment gains have been maintained for up to 1 year. The focus of psychotherapy literature has primarily been on community-residing volunteers with a diagnosis of major depression; however, some studies have shown psychotherapy to be effective with milder or chronic depressive symptoms as well. As yet, no empirical studies have examined the efficacy of CBT or psychodynamic treatments in older adults requiring hospitalization for severe depression. However, the research methodologies and standardized assessment instruments that have been used in outpatient studies of CBT and psychodynamic interventions should be applicable in future research with depressed geriatric inpatients as well.

Reminiscence and Life Review Therapies

There is a growing empirical literature on the effectiveness of reminiscence and/or life review therapy in elderly patients. *Reminiscence* is defined as "the act or process of recalling the past . . . a narration of past experiences" (American Heritage Dictionary 1985). In reminiscence therapy, elderly patients are encouraged to remember the past and to share their memories, either with a therapist or with peers, as a way of increasing self-esteem and social intimacy. It is often highly directive and structured, with the therapist choosing each session's reminiscence topic. In life review therapy, not only are past experiences recalled, but an effort is made to help patients reexperience old conflicts and rework them so that there is therapeutic resolution. In other words, life review is one form of reminiscence, designed to produce a better understanding and acceptance of past events (Butler 1963). In the clinical intervention literature, however, *reminiscence* and *life review* are often used interchangeably for any individual or group narrative therapy that encourages patients to remember and describe the past.

Empirical trials have been conducted in which reminiscence and life review were used to reduce depression and anxiety (measured using a variety of self-report measures) and to increase feelings of self-esteem and life satisfaction in older elderly patients (Table 36–2). Although some results have been promising, findings have been inconsistent. For example, Fielden (1990) observed that life satisfaction and socialization increased more among reminiscence group participants than among participants in a "here and now" current events group conducted at a sheltered housing complex. In contrast, Lappe (1987) and Rattenbury and Stones (1989) found that both reminiscence and current events discussion groups were effective in improving elderly patients' ratings of psychological well-being. McMurdo and Rennie (1993) reported reductions in depression among retirement home residents who were enrolled in either reminiscence or exercise groups, although depression decreased more in persons who exercised twice a week. Arean et al. (1993) found that although both reminiscence therapy and problem-solving therapy led to reductions in depression among older adults compared with wait-list control subjects, subjects who underwent reminiscence therapy were significantly more depressed after the conclusion of treatment and at 3-month follow-up than were those who underwent problem-solving therapy. Still other studies have found that reminiscence activities had no significant effects on depression, anxiety, or self-esteem (Hedgepeth and Hale 1983; Perrotta and Meacham 1981).

A number of variables may contribute to the inconsistent impact of reminiscence on psychological well-being, including cognitive function. In most studies conducted so far, persons with obvious cognitive impairment or dementia were excluded from participation, but in almost none of the studies was a formal cognitive screening tool, such as the MMSE or Mental Status Questionnaire, used to assess cognitive function. Other factors that may affect treatment outcome include intervention frequency and duration (Baines et al. 1987; Lappe 1987), patient age (Youssef 1990), whether reminiscence therapy is conducted in a long-term care or community setting (Lieberman and Falk 1971; Molinari and Reichlin 1985) or directed by peer or professional leaders (Fielden 1990; Lieberman and Bliwise 1985), variability in measures of change used to assess treatment outcome (Berghorn and Schafer 1987), and whether environmental stimuli (such as music) are used to enhance the reminiscence process (Bennett and Maas 1988). The amount of structure provided to the reminiscence activity may also affect treatment outcome. For example, systematic life review techniques may be more ther-

apeutic than simple reminiscence, given that life review encourages a reexamination of the emotional outcomes of past events and may enable an individual to put these events in a different, more positive perspective (Parker 1995). Fry (1983) found that "structured" reminiscence was more successful than "unstructured" reminiscence in lowering depression posttest scores and significantly increased the number of reports of self-confidence and adequacy. Haight (1988) compared the effects of structured life review reminiscing in combination with nonstructured "friendly home visits" with the effects of no treatment. Subjects who engaged in life review reported increased amounts of life satisfaction and increased psychological well-being at 8-week posttest, and life satisfaction ratings remained higher for these individuals than for control subjects at 1-year follow-up; however, improvements in other measures of well-being (e.g., affect balance or depression) were no different from those among controls at 1 year (Haight 1992). Structured life review strategies have been found to be as effective as systematic relaxation training (Ingersoll and Silverman 1978) and CBT (Harp-Scates et al. 1986) in reducing anxiety and improving life satisfaction or self-esteem.

The impact of reminiscence techniques may depend on whether they are used in an individual or a group therapy format. For example, some authors have noted that individual reminiscence has produced positive outcomes less consistently than have group interventions (Watt and Wong 1991). However, other authors have reported improvements in mood after individual reminiscence procedures (Fallot 1980; Fry 1983) and have even suggested that individual interventions may be the treatment of choice for life review with geriatric subjects (Haight 1988). There is also some concern that the terms *reminiscence* and *life review* actually describe distinct psychological processes and that these processes may significantly alter the effectiveness of reminiscence as a therapeutic technique (Watt and Wong 1991). Indeed, the conceptual differences between simple reminiscence and active life review have been considered by a number of authors (see Merriam 1980; Molinari and Reichlin 1985; Watt and Wong 1991). However, to date there has been no empirical attempt to define operationally the processes of reminiscence and life review or to test the impact of each on selected clinical populations.

In summary, a number of empirical studies of reminiscence and life review have indicated that both can help reduce negative mood and improve life satisfaction and self-esteem in geriatric outpatients. However, nonsignificant findings have been reported in several studies, which has led to speculation about factors that increase the efficacy of reminiscence strategies. The approach to remi-

TABLE 36–2. Empirical studies of reminiscence therapy in depressed older adults

Study	Subjects	Subject age (years)	Treatment	Treatment duration
Ingersoll and Silverman 1978	17 community residents	Mean, 70	Behavior therapy group	8 sessions
			Reminiscence/life review group	
Fallot 1980	36 female outpatients	Mean, 66 (range, 46–85)	Individual reminiscence	2 sessions
			Individual current or future events	
Perrota and Meacham 1981	21 community residents	Mean, 75–80	Individual reminiscence	5 sessions
			Individual current life events	
			No treatment (control)	
Fry 1983	162 outpatients with depression	Median, 68 (range, 65–82)	Individual structured reminiscence	5 sessions
			Individual unstructured reminiscence	
			Attention only (control)	
Hedgepeth and Hale 1983	60 female outpatients	Mean, 76 (range, 60–98)	Individual reminiscence (past successes)	1 session
			Individual reminiscence (present positive events)	
			No reminiscence (control)	
Harp-Scates et al. 1986	50 outpatients	Mean, 75 (all subjects > 65)	Group cognitive-behavior therapy	6 sessions in 3 weeks
			Reminiscence group	
			Recreational activity	
Lappe 1987	83 NH residents	Mean, 83	Reminiscence group	10 weeks (half met two times/week, half met one time/week)
			Current events group	
Bennett and Maas 1988	26 female NH residents	Mean, 82	Music-based life review group	6 sessions
			Verbal life review group	
Haight 1988, 1992	60 homebound elderly patients	Mean, 76 (range, 61–99)	Individual life review	6 sessions
			"Individual friendly visits" (control)	
			No treatment (control)	
Rattenbury and Stones 1989	24 NH residents	Mean, 83–87	Reminiscence group	8 sessions
			Current topics group	
			No treatment (control)	
Fielden 1990	31 sheltered housing residents	Mean, 74–75	Reminiscence group	9 sessions
			"Here and now" group	
Youssef 1990	66 female NH residents	All subjects > 65	Reminiscence group (65–74 years)	6 sessions in 5 weeks
			Reminiscence group (75+ years)	
			No treatment (control)	

Arean et al. 1993	75 older adults with unipolar, major depressive disorder	Problem-solving therapy
	Mean, 66–68 (range, 55–80)	Reminiscence therapy
		Wait list (control)
		12 sessions
McMurdo and Rennie 1993	49 elderly residents of local-authority residential homes	Exercise to music
	Mean, 81 (range, 64–91)	Reminiscence and music
		2 sessions/week for 7 months

Note. NH = nursing home or long-term residential setting.

niscence or life review used for the treatment of geriatric depression has not been standardized, and many protocol variations exist that could influence treatment outcome. Although the effectiveness of reminiscence remains inconclusive, studies do suggest that structured life review strategies may be more effective than simple narrative reminiscence. However, the lack of objective cognitive screening procedures may have led to a wide variability in subjects' cognitive status across studies and in subsequent ability to remember and to benefit from the reminiscence process. There is also evidence that life review conducted in different formats (individual or group) may produce different effects, but no well-designed comparison studies have been conducted to evaluate this hypothesis. There has also been no attempt to identify which clinical groups are most likely to benefit from reminiscence therapy or under what circumstances alternative treatments should be considered.

Psychotherapy for Depression in Elderly Patients With Dementia

There is growing interest in the psychosocial treatment of depression in patients with dementia because depression is commonly associated with dementia, and treatment of depression can have a positive impact on the functional status of cognitively impaired individuals (Teri and Wagner 1992). In this section, we discuss the empirical studies of treatments specifically geared toward reducing depression in cognitively impaired individuals.

Abraham et al. (1992) randomly assigned 76 nursing home residents with mild to moderate cognitive impairment (based on Modified MMSE scores) and depressive symptoms (GDS scores of at least 11) to CBT, focused visual imagery, or education-discussion groups (Table 36–3). No significant reductions in depression, feelings of hopelessness, or life satisfaction scores were observed for any group after completion of the 24-week intervention, although cognitive test scores did improve slightly over the treatment period. The authors suggested that these negative mood findings may have been due to participants' physical frailty and cognitive impairment and to the limited treatment duration.

A subsequent study involving community-dwelling patients with Alzheimer's disease and their caregivers (Teri et al. 1997) showed that behavior therapy can be effective in the treatment of major or minor depression in outpatients with dementia. Treatment was based on a social-learning model in which depression is viewed as a series of behaviors that are learned and maintained through positive and nega-

TABLE 36–3.   Empirical studies with depressed, cognitively impaired older adults

Study	Subjects	Subject age (years)	Treatment	Treatment duration
Baines et al. 1987	30 NH residents with confusion	Mean, 82 (range, 72–90)	Reality orientation therapy–reminiscence group; No treatment (control)	40 sessions in 16 weeks (treatment group crossover at 8 weeks)
Goldwasser et al. 1987	27 NH residents with dementia	Mean, 82 (range, 70–97)	Reminiscence group; Support (attention/placebo) group; No treatment (control)	10 sessions in 5 weeks
Orten et al. 1989	56 NH residents with dementia	Mean, 83 (range, 58–101)	Reminiscence group; No treatment (control)	16 sessions
Abraham et al. 1992	76 NH residents with depression and mild to moderate cognitive impairment	Mean, 84 (range, 71–97)	Group cognitive-behavior therapy; Visual imagery group; Education–discussion group	24 weeks
Baldelli et al. 1993	23 female NH residents with dementia	Mean, 85 (range, 75–94)	Reality orientation therapy; No treatment (control)	3 sessions/week for 3 months
Teri et al. 1997	72 outpatients with Alzheimer's disease and major or minor depression	Mean, 76	Behavior therapy–pleasant events; Behavior therapy–problem solving; Typical care (control); Wait list (control)	9 sessions

Note.   NH = nursing home or long-term residential setting.

tive reinforcement contingencies (Lewinsohn et al. 1980). Consequently, the central aim of treatment is to reduce or eliminate depressive behaviors by altering the contingencies that maintain them, as well as by introducing new contingencies to stimulate and maintain nondepressive behaviors. In the study by Teri et al. (1997), caregiver-patient pairs were randomly assigned in a double-blind, controlled clinical trial to one of two behavior therapies (behavior therapy–pleasant events or behavior therapy–problem solving) or one of two control protocols (typical care or wait list). Treatment consisted of nine individual, 60-minute sessions, one per week, with patients and caregivers participating in varying degrees. The goals of active treatment were to teach caregivers behavioral strategies for improving patient depression by 1) increasing the number of pleasant events and decreasing the number of unpleasant events and 2) using behavioral problem-solving strategies to alter the contingencies that relate to depression and associated behavior problems.

Significant reductions in depression on standardized measures (including the HDRS, BDI, and Cornell Depression in Dementia Scale) were noted in patients in the behavior therapy groups but not in those in the control groups (Teri et al. 1997). Fifty-two percent of patients assigned to behavior therapy–pleasant events and 68% of those assigned to behavior therapy–problem solving improved over the course of treatment, compared with 20% of subjects in the control groups. Treatment effects were maintained at 6-month follow-up, and baseline severity of depression was the only patient characteristic that predicted treatment response (more depressed subjects were more likely to benefit from treatment). Interestingly, caregivers of patients assigned to behavior therapy showed significant reductions in depression, whereas caregivers of patients on the wait list did not. This latter finding was unexpected, given that patient depression alone was the treatment target. Increased skill in patient management, availability of regular therapeutic support, and reduced depression in the family member with dementia most likely explain these added benefits. Thus, behavioral treatment of patients with dementia may have the additional advantage of improving caregiver affect and caregiving quality, both of which are important and are often not assessed in typical outcome studies (Teri et al. 1992).

Reminiscence and life review techniques have also been used in studies involving confused, depressed elderly patients in long-term care settings (Baines et al. 1987; Goldwasser et al. 1987; Orten et al. 1989). In these studies, reminiscence storytelling was conducted in a group format (Table 36–3). Specific topics or themes were suggested by staff, sometimes with the assistance of personal artifacts, newspapers, music, or other memorabilia used to stimulate residents' memories. All three studies found that simple reminiscing led to reductions in depression and improvements in social functioning for the confused participants. However, changes were not maintained over time in all treatment groups. The inexperience of group facilitators and differing levels of patient impairment may have had a negative impact on long-term treatment effects (Goldwasser et al. 1987; Orten et al. 1989), although it may be that treatment based primarily on cognitive effort (e.g., reminiscence) should not be expected to have long-term effects on mood in persons with a progressive dementing illness. Interestingly, Baines et al. (1987) found that reminiscence groups did improve long-term interactions between nursing home staff and patients, perhaps due to increased staff understanding of patient needs and their caretaking roles.

One final approach to treating depression that has been described for use with dementia patients is reality orientation therapy (Baldelli et al. 1993). This form of therapy was designed to stimulate and consolidate cognitive functions that have not deteriorated. Baldelli et al. (1993) found that subjects who participated in a reality orientation therapy group for 3 months also had significantly lower ratings of depression on the GDS after treatment than did subjects who received no treatment. This study had notable methodological problems, including a lack of random assignment into treatment groups, and the report did not include information about group sample size, describe how the GDS was administered to the cognitively impaired participants, or include follow-up data. The study does, however, provide further indication that depression in patients with dementia may be treatable, and additional research regarding potential forms of treatment is warranted.

In summary, behavior therapy that emphasizes specific skills training and behavior change has been shown to be effective in reducing major and minor depression in outpatients with progressive dementing illnesses such as Alzheimer's disease. There is also evidence that treatment for depression in patients with Alzheimer's disease can improve caregivers' mood, even when treatment does not specifically focus on the caregiver. The empirical literature on the use of CBT in patients with dementia and their caregivers is still in its infancy, and such positive early results support further investigation. In long-term residential settings, reminiscence techniques have been used to improve mood and social functioning in severely impaired patients with dementia. However, changes associated with use of reminiscence are not well sustained once treatment is discontinued; therefore, reminiscence therapy may be most appropriate in settings in which reminiscence groups can be

available as needed for an unrestricted period (e.g., as part of an institutional day activity program). Additional information is also needed regarding the individual patient characteristics (e.g., level of cognitive function) that affect treatment effectiveness in patients with dementia. There are at present too few data to draw conclusions about the usefulness of nonbehavioral treatments (e.g., reality orientation therapy) for reducing depression in this group.

Psychotherapy in Medically Ill Elderly Patients

Elderly patients account for a disproportionally high percentage of the medical illnesses, disabilities, and utilization of health care services in the United States (Keuthen and Wisocki 1991). Because they also represent one of the fastest-growing segments of American society, there is concern that the demand for geriatric medical services will eventually exceed available resources. An increasing number of practitioners have begun exploring the supplemental role of psychosocial interventions in geriatric health care. For example, a number of studies have shown that the use of mental health services leads to a reduction in medical care, particularly in-hospital stays for persons over age 55 (Mumford et al. 1984). Use of behavioral interventions has been shown to improve elderly patients' compliance with difficult medical procedures and their involvement in wellness programs and exercise regimens (Gutman et al. 1977; Kirschenbaum et al. 1987; Matteson 1989). The application and efficacy of psychological interventions in older adults in chronic pain or undergoing medical rehabilitation have been described (Hartke 1991; Saxon 1991).

The majority of controlled experimental studies of psychosocial interventions in medically ill geriatric patients have focused on patients' abilities to cope with chronic or life-threatening illness (Table 36–4). Most of these studies have involved a combination of supportive, educational, and problem-solving strategies drawn from more systematic cognitive-behavioral, insight-oriented, or reminiscence-based approaches. For example, adjustment to declining sensory function has been a focus of some research. Evans et al. (1982) provided problem-solving group therapy by telephone to legally blind elderly patients. Participants showed increases in activity levels and decreases in self-reports of loneliness although no changes in actual social involvement were observed. Andersson and colleagues (1995) taught 12 hearing-impaired elderly patients a combination of relaxation, assertive communication, and problem-solving skills, with the goal of improv-

TABLE 36–4. Empirical studies with medically ill older adults

Study	Subjects	Subject age (years)	Treatment	Treatment duration
Godbole and Verinis 1974	61 rehabilitation inpatients with physical disabilities	Mean, 69 (range, 38–82)	Individual confrontational therapy Individual supportive therapy No treatment (control)	6–12 sessions in 2–4 weeks
Ibrahim et al. 1974	118 patients with cardiac disease	Range, 35–65 (67% of subjects > 50)	Supportive group therapy No treatment (control)	50 weeks
Gruen 1975	70 hospitalized patients with cardiac disease	Range, 40–69	Individual supportive counseling No treatment (control)	5–6 days/week until discharge (mean, 3 weeks)
Kaplan and Kozin 1981	28 female patients with rheumatoid arthritis	Mean, 46–51 (range, 23–63)	Education and supportive counseling group Education group	1 education session and 12 counseling sessions
Spiegel et al. 1981	58 female patients with breast cancer	Mean, 54–55	Support group No treatment (control)	One time/week for 1 year
Evans et al. 1982	84 isolated visually impaired volunteers	Mean, 61–62 (range, 53–78)	Group problem solving by telephone No treatment (control)	8 sessions
Oldenburg et al. 1985	46 patients with cardiac disease	Mean, 56 (range, 29–69)	Individual education/relaxation/ counseling Individual education/relaxation Standard care (control)	10 weeks (counseling); education and relaxation instructions on audiotape
Shearn and Fireman 1985	105 patients with rheumatoid arthritis	Mean, 55–58	Stress management group Support group No treatment (control)	10 sessions
Keefe et al. 1990	99 patients with osteoarthritis	Mean, 64	Pain coping skills (CBT) group Arthritis education group Standard care (control)	10 sessions
Greer et al. 1992	156 patients with cancer	Mean, 51–52 (range, 18–74)	Individual CBT No treatment (control)	0–13 sessions in 4 months (median, 5 sessions)
Rice et al. 1993	229 alcoholic patients	Mean, 39 (range, 18–76; 18% of subjects ≥ 50)	CBT Relationship-enhancement therapy Relationship- and vocational-enhancement therapy	1–2 intake sessions; 1 session/week over 16 weeks; 2 booster sessions (3 months and 1 year after treatment)
Andersson et al. 1995	24 hearing-impaired subjects	Mean, 70 (range, 64–72)	Group CBT No treatment (control)	4 sessions in 5 weeks
Andersson et al. 1997	19 hearing-impaired subjects	Mean, 72 (range, 67–75)	Individual CBT bibliotherapy No treatment (control)	1 in vivo relaxation training session and 4 telephone sessions in 4 weeks

Note.   CBT = cognitive-behavior therapy.

ing patient adjustment to hearing aids and challenging environmental situations (e.g., group conversation where there is background noise). Group participants scored higher on ratings of relaxation and socially appropriate body posture in posttreatment videotaped role plays and, at 1-month follow-up, reported a significantly better ability to handle difficult communication situations than did patients who received no treatment. In a subsequent study (Andersson et al. 1997), hearing-impaired patients who participated in a 4-week bibliotherapy program supplemented with brief weekly telephone contacts had better scores on the Communication Profile for the Hearing Impaired as well as in interpersonal role plays of difficult social situations (e.g., groups) than did control subjects, which suggests that self-help treatment materials may be of value for improving patient adjustment to hearing loss.

Studies have also examined the use of psychotherapy in elderly patients with cancer. Spiegel et al. (1981) found that patients with metastatic breast cancer who participated in a year-long, nondirective support group reported significantly less anxiety, fatigue, and confusion, as well as improved coping strategies, compared with control subjects. Greer et al. (1992) studied patients with newly diagnosed cancer who attended individual CBT sessions to learn a combination of relaxation techniques, cognitive coping strategies, and communication skills for improving interpersonal relationships. These patients reported significantly less anxiety, helplessness, fatalism, and depression and significantly greater adjustment to their disease than did subjects who received no treatment. Statistical improvements were maintained at 4-month follow-up.

Cardiovascular disease (including stroke and heart disease) is another medical problem in geriatric patients that may be amenable to psychotherapeutic intervention (Cohen-Cole 1989; Lipsey and Parikh 1989). Godbole and Verinis (1974) studied 61 older adults with a variety of physical disabilities, including cardiovascular and respiratory disease. Subjects were randomly assigned to "confrontational therapy," supportive therapy, or no treatment. Patients in both active treatment groups showed significant improvements on measures of depression, anxiety, feelings of hopelessness, and somatic complaints compared with control subjects. A number of authors (e.g., Butcher et al. 1984; Imes 1984) have suggested that group psychotherapy can improve social and psychological functioning in patients with stroke. The utility of various depression treatment measures for assessing poststroke depression in geriatric patients has also been described (Agrell and Dehlin 1989). Surprisingly, no empirical studies have demonstrated the efficacy of psychotherapy in this population. Data are available, however, on the use of psychosocial in-

terventions in patients with heart disease.

Ibrahim et al. (1974) compared elderly cardiac patients assigned to a weekly supportive therapy group and control subjects. Therapy group participants had slightly better survival rates and showed a smaller increase in social alienation than did controls during the study period, although no significant differences on psychological, physical, or social measures were obtained. In contrast, Gruen (1975) found that patients who were seen almost daily for supportive counseling and education while in intensive care after a heart attack scored lower on measures of anxiety and depression during hospitalization than did control subjects. Differences in anxiety between groups were maintained at 4-month follow-up, and subjects in the treatment group also tended to be less restricted in activity at follow-up compared with no-treatment control subjects. Oldenburg et al. (1985) found that patients receiving either brief (6–10 sessions) individual counseling and education or education alone after hospitalization for a heart attack reported better psychological and lifestyle functioning at 3-, 6-, and 12-month follow-up than did subjects who received routine care.

There is a growing literature on the impact of psychosocial treatments on disability, pain, and depression in older adults with rheumatoid arthritis or osteoarthritis (Mullen et al. 1987). Keefe et al. (1990) found that patients with osteoarthritic knee pain who received a combination of training in pain coping skills and arthritis education reported significantly lower amounts of pain and psychological disability (anxiety and depression) than did patients who received only arthritis education or standard medical care. However, earlier intervention studies involving patients with rheumatoid arthritis yielded less promising results. For example, Kaplan and Kozin (1981) found no differences between patients with rheumatoid arthritis who only received information about their disease and those who received information and participated in 12 nondirective group counseling sessions. Shearn and Fireman (1985) also found no significant differences in measures of depression, life satisfaction, or functional disability between patients with rheumatoid arthritis who participated in either stress management or mutual support groups for 10 weeks and control subjects. Thus, the effectiveness of interventions designed to treat psychological disability and pain behaviors in medical patients may be different in select populations. Other factors that may have confounding effects on treatment outcome in medically ill elderly patients include patient age and whether the spouse is involved in treatment (Keefe et al. 1990).

In summary, although the number of existing controlled studies is still relatively small and results are mixed, there is evidence that psychosocial interventions are valuable adjunctive treatments for some of the medical conditions that affect older adults. Most studies have included medical outpatients, and all have involved some form of psychoeducational, problem-solving, or supportive intervention strategy. Significant improvements in depression, anxiety, feelings of hopelessness, and coping have been reported in patients with vision and hearing impairment, cancer, heart disease, and arthritis. Slight improvements in survival rate and lower risks for rehospitalization have also been described.

Psychotherapy and Geriatric Caregivers

The American Association of Retired Persons (1986) estimated that more than 5 million community-dwelling elderly people in the United States require some form of assistance to maintain independent living. The vast majority of this assistance comes from family members, usually spouses or grown children who are often themselves elderly or beyond middle age. Caregiving is often a difficult task associated with increased levels of depression, anxiety, insomnia, marital conflict, alcohol and medication use, and medical illness (Cantor 1983; Clipp and George 1990; Coppel et al. 1985; Farkas 1980; Gaynor 1989; Pruchno and Potashnik 1989; Rabins et al. 1982). Research on various psychoeducational, psychotherapeutic, and self-help interventions that have been used with caregivers has been summarized in reviews (Bourgeois et al. 1996; Knight et al. 1993; Toseland and Rossiter 1989; Zarit and Teri 1991). The authors of these reviews noted the lack of methodological rigor in most of these studies and the relatively modest treatment effects reported. They also pointed out the impracticality of expecting short-term supportive or educational interventions to have substantial impact, given the complexity and duration of the caregiving role. Nevertheless, research on the impact of psychosocial interventions with caregivers has rapidly grown over the past decade. This research can be divided into two distinct types: studies of interventions designed to enhance caregiver psychological functioning (here called *caregiver-focused interventions)*, and studies of interventions designed to teach family caregivers to alter patient behavior or psychiatric status (here called *patient-focused interventions)*.

The majority of the empirical treatment studies involving caregivers have been in the caregiver-focused intervention category. A number of these have included heterogeneous groups of caregivers and patient types (Table

36–5). For example, Greene and Monahan (1987, 1989) recruited community-dwelling caregivers whose levels of stress placed their elderly patients at risk for institutionalization. The majority of patients were living with their care providers (77%) and had at least one major medical illness (89%); Alzheimer's disease had been diagnosed in less than one-fifth (14%). Significant reductions in caregiver anxiety, depression, and burden levels were observed after 8 weeks of group counseling that had supportive, educational, and relaxation components. However, improvements were not maintained at 4-month follow-up, and no caregiver or patient characteristics were associated with any outcome. Lovett and Gallagher (1988) studied 107 family caregivers whose patients had a mixture of moderate to severe memory impairment (40% of patients) and a variety of medical conditions and disabilities. Caregivers who participated for 10 weeks in either a behaviorally based group focusing on increasing the number of pleasant events or a cognitive, problem-solving group experienced decreases in depression and increases in morale that were not observed in wait-list control subjects. Perceived self-efficacy was more strongly associated with improvement on outcome measures than was an abundance of pleasant social events in the caregiver's life.

Other investigators have attempted to control for heterogeneity of care providers by focusing on caregivers of patients with specific disabling conditions rather than on caregivers in general. Evans et al. (1988) studied caregivers of stroke patients and found that patients who either 1) participated in educational classes on the physical and psychosocial consequences of stroke or 2) participated in educational classes plus seven CBT sessions scored significantly higher at 6-month and 1-year follow-up on measures of family functioning, communication, and problem solving than did caregivers who did not receive education or CBT. Families receiving CBT had significantly higher levels of patient adjustment than did those receiving education alone or no education or CBT. This finding is particularly important given that 1) anxiety and depression are common after strokes (Gass and Lawhorn 1991); 2) left untreated, depressive symptoms may not spontaneously resolve over time (Egelko et al. 1989); and 3) level of depression and stroke recovery are strongly related to the quality of patients' family relationships and response to stroke-related disability (Evans et al. 1987; S.C. Thompson et al. 1989).

A large number of studies have focused on caregivers of patients with Alzheimer's disease or related dementias. Many of these studies have shown that although caregivers enjoy participation in supportive and psychoeducational groups, these treatments produce limited treatment

TABLE 36–5. Empirical treatment studies with caregiving older adults

Study[a]	Subjects	Subject age (years)	Treatment	Treatment duration
Kahan et al. 1985	40 caregivers of patients with Alzheimer's disease	Range, 16–77 (59% of subjects ≥ 60)	CBT Wait list (control)	8 sessions
Greene and Monahan 1987, 1989	289 caregivers of patients with dementia and medical illnesses (34 groups)	Mean, 58	Group support, education, and relaxation training No treatment (control) (self-selected nonparticipants)	8 sessions
Haley et al. 1987; Haley 1989	54 family caregivers of patients with dementia	Mean, 78	Support group Support and stress management group Wait list (control)	10 sessions in 4 months (7 weekly, 2 every other week, 1 after month delay)
Scharlach 1987	37 daughters (of 24 elderly widowed mothers)	Mean, 50 (range, 38–62)	Group CBT Support/education group Wait list (control)	2 sessions
Zarit et al. 1987	119 family caregivers of patients with dementia	Mean, 62	Support group Individual and family counseling Wait list (control)	8 sessions
Evans et al. 1988	188 caregivers of stroke patients	Mean, 61–63	Education group Education group and individual CBT Standard care (control)	Education group: 2 sessions Education group and CBT: 9 sessions
Lovett and Gallagher 1988	111 caregivers of frail elderly patients	Mean, 59	Behavior therapy group Problem-solving group Wait list (control)	10 sessions
Robinson 1988	20 caregivers of patients with dementia	?	Social skills training group Wait list (control)	8 sessions
Schmidt et al. 1988	20 family caregivers of patients with dementia	Mean, 61–62	Individual problem solving Individual emotional expression and problem solving	4 sessions
Chiverton and Caine 1989	40 spouses of patients with dementia	Mean, 71 (range, 58–87)	Education group No treatment (control)	3 sessions in 4 weeks
Montgomery and Borgatta 1989	541 families caring for 576 elderly persons with physical, functional, or cognitive impairment	?	Full family support services (caregiver seminars, support groups, family consultation services, and respite) Caregiver seminars, support groups, and family consultation only Caregiver seminars and support groups Family consultation services only Respite only No treatment (control)	6 sessions

(continued)

TABLE 36–5. Empirical treatment studies with caregiving older adults *(continued)*

Study[a]	Subjects	Subject age (years)	Treatment	Treatment duration
Toseland et al. 1989	56 daughter/daughter-in-law caretakers of frail elderly patients	Mean, 50–55 (range, 35–66)	Professional-led support and education group Peer-led support group Respite only (control)	8 sessions
Goodman and Pynoos 1990	66 caregivers of patients with dementia	Mean, 63–66	Peer telephone network Telephone mini-lecture series (12 lessons)	2 supportive telephone calls/week for 12 weeks
Mohide et al. 1990	60 caregivers of patients with dementia	Mean, 66–69	Caregiver support program (home visits, respite care, and support group) Conventional care (home nursing) (control)	6 months
Toseland et al. 1990	154 daughter/daughter-in-law caretakers	Mean, 50–52	Individual supportive therapy Support group Respite only (control)	8 sessions
Toseland and Smith 1990	87 daughter/daughter-in-law caretakers	Mean, 50	Individual "action-oriented" therapy with professional counselor Individual "action-oriented" therapy with peer counselor No treatment (control)	8 sessions
Toseland et al. 1992	89 spouses of frail aging veterans	Mean, 64–68	Support groups (support, education, problem solving, stress reduction) No treatment (control)	8 sessions
Mittelman et al. 1993, 1995, 1996	206 spouse caregivers of patients with Alzheimer's disease	87% of subjects ≥65	Individual counseling, family counseling, and support groups Usual care (control)	2 individual and 4 family sessions in 4 months; weekly support group sessions thereafter (groups meet indefinitely)
Robinson and Yates 1994	33 caregivers of family members with dementia	76% of subjects ≥60	Social skills development program (group) Behavioral management skills development program (group) No treatment (control)	6 sessions in 12 weeks
McCurry et al. 1998	36 caregivers of patients with dementia	Mean, 69 (range 50–86)	Group behavioral treatment Individual behavioral treatment Wait list (control)	Group treatment: 6 sessions Individual treatment: 4 sessions

Note. CBT = cognitive-behavior therapy.
[a]Studies cited together involved subsamples of the same sample in the larger randomized clinical trial.

effects. For example, Lawton et al. (1989) found that caregivers (of patients with Alzheimer's disease) who were offered a year of formal respite care, and provided with financial assistance as needed as well as education about the purpose and range of respite services available, were no different afterward, in terms of depression, subjective burden, or ratings of affect, from caregivers who received none of these services. Haley et al. (1987) found no improvements in community-dwelling caregivers' self-reports of psychological or social functioning after participation for 10 weeks in either support-only or support-with-skills-training groups. At 2-year follow-up, although caregivers reported high rates of satisfaction with these groups, there was no evidence of group differences in caregiver outcome, with the exception that group participation may have facilitated placement of patients under skilled nursing care (Haley 1989).

Mohide et al. (1990) compared live-in caregivers who received a combination of education, respite, and group support with caregivers who had standard contact with community home nursing services. Although neither group showed improvements in depression or anxiety after 6 months, caregivers who received the combination treatment did report more increases in perceived quality of life and satisfaction with nursing services and their caregiving role than did the conventional care recipients. Zarit et al. (1987) reported reductions in family caregivers' burden level and psychiatric symptoms after participation in an education and problem-solving support group for 8 weeks or 8 weeks of individual and family counseling, reductions that were maintained at 1-year follow-up. However, these treatment effects were no greater than the changes observed in wait-list control subjects. Finally, as already reviewed, Teri et al. (1997) found caregiver depression decreased with a patient-focused depression treatment program.

There are data showing that caregivers can benefit from brief interventions when the treatment focus is on some specific element of skills training. For example, McCurry et al. (1998) taught caregivers of patients with dementia with sleep disturbance a combination of behavioral strategies to improve sleep (sleep hygiene, stimulus control, and sleep compression) and provided education about caregiving resources and management of patient behavior problems. Caregivers who received individual or group treatment ($n = 21$) had significant improvements in self-reported quality of sleep after treatment discontinuation and at 3-month follow-up compared with wait-list control subjects ($n = 15$), but there were no reported improvements in caregiver depression or burden ratings or in patient behavior as a result of the intervention.

Scharlach (1987) examined whether the relationship between adult daughters and their elderly widowed mothers could be improved while the mothers were still functioning independently. Daughters were assigned to either a cognitive-behavioral intervention, which focused on reducing unrealistic feelings of responsibility, or a supportive-educational intervention, in which daughters were encouraged to become more aware of their mothers' needs. Daughters who attended the cognitive-behavioral seminar had greater reductions in feelings of burden than did control subjects or attendees of the supportive-educational seminar. Further, subjects assigned to a cognitive-behavioral intervention reported subjectively greater improvements in their relationships with their mothers, and the mothers reported significantly less loneliness, after the intervention than did subjects in the other two groups. The results of this study introduce the possibility that psychosocial interventions may serve a preventive function in individuals who are likely to become future caregivers.

A fewer number of controlled trials have been patient-focused interventions that examined the effectiveness of caregiver training programs on the behavior and care outcomes of patients with dementia. In an early study, Schmidt et al. (1988) randomized 20 caregivers to two treatment strategies (problem-solving therapy only and problem-solving therapy plus emotional expression group); there was no control group. After 4 weeks, no significant reductions in caregiver life satisfaction, burden, or psychiatric symptomatology were noted for either treatment. However, caregivers who received the combination treatment reported reduction of conflict with their relatives and greater patient trust and submission to caregiver requests compared with caregivers who underwent problem-solving therapy only. Robinson and Yates (1994) randomized 33 caregivers to one of three treatments: social skills development, behavioral management skills development, or no treatment. Caregivers were offered the option of completing a second (alternative) training after the initial 6-week intervention. At posttest, no significant differences were reported for any groups in caregiver ratings of burden or attitudes toward asking for help (including using senior day programs). Patient behavior problems were rated, although no information about method of assessment or outcome was provided in the report; caregivers who completed a second training ($n = 6$) had significantly lower levels of objective burden compared with control subjects, which suggests that some reduction in patient behavior problems occurred.

Recent studies have suggested that significant treatment effects can be achieved when spousal caregivers are offered more intensive or focused programs of education, individual and family counseling, or ongoing therapeutic support. For example, as reviewed earlier, Teri et al. (1997) found that both outpatients with Alzheimer's disease and their family caregivers experienced significant reductions in depression after completion of a 9-week behavior therapy (focusing on increasing the number of pleasant events or on problem solving) caregiver training program. Mittelman et al. (1993, 1995, 1996) randomly assigned 206 spousal caregivers of patients with Alzheimer's disease to either active treatment or normal care. Caregivers in active treatment received six initial (two individual and four family) psychoeducational sessions over a 4-month period. Caregivers were given information about basic communication, behavior management, and community resources and received a range of emotional and physical support. At the end of the 4 months, caregivers were required to join a support group that met weekly and would continue to meet indefinitely. In addition, caregivers had access to family counselors who were available at any time (including evenings and weekends) for support and assistance. The median time from baseline to nursing home placement was almost 1 year (329 days) longer for spouses of participants in active treatment than for spouses of control subjects, and treatment had the greatest effect when the impaired spouse had mild or moderate dementia.

Regardless of whether the caregiver or the patient is the focus of treatment, a variety of factors may influence treatment effects in caregiver intervention studies. Toseland and colleagues compared the effectiveness of peer-led versus professional-led "action-oriented" support groups for caregivers (Toseland et al. 1989), peer-led versus professional-led individual counseling (Toseland et al. 1990), and group versus individual therapy (regardless of type of leadership) (Toseland and Smith 1990). Significant improvements on measures of well-being and social support and decreases in psychiatric symptoms occurred as a result of both the peer-led and professional-led interventions, regardless of whether caregivers were seen in an individual or group context. However, greater reductions in psychiatric symptoms tended to be associated with individual and professional-led treatment, whereas greater increases in social support were noted with the group and peer-led interventions.

Caregiver relationship to patient may also influence treatment outcome. Montgomery and Borgatta (1989) assigned 541 families caring for impaired elderly individuals to either no treatment or one of five supportive programs with various combinations of education, respite, and family consultation services. After 1 year, they found that adult children caregivers in any of the active treatment groups were less likely than control subjects to have institutionalized their impaired parents, whereas spouses in active treatment groups (except for those with access to a family consultant only) were more likely to have done so.

In summary, the empirical literature on psychosocial interventions with caregivers is growing. There is evidence that brief psychosocial interventions can lead to increased caregiver knowledge, social support, feelings of well-being, patient behavior change, and delays in patient institutionalization. However, treatment effects tend to be modest and inconsistent across studies. There is some evidence that interventions that target specific caregiver problems (e.g., depression or sleep disturbance) may be more likely to have measurable effects, but there have been few studies in which caregiver outcome goals were narrowly defined. Unfortunately, follow-up data are still not always obtained in many caregiver studies, treatment tends to be brief, outcome measures are often poorly tied to intervention hypotheses, and study samples are typically small. Given the design limitations in many caregiver studies, the positive findings that have been reported are impressive and support the need for continued research with caregiver populations.

Psychotherapy and Elderly Patients in Long-Term Care Settings

A move into a long-term care setting can be difficult, or even traumatic, for many older adults. Consequently, there is growing interest in the use of psychosocial interventions to help ease some of the acute adjustment problems associated with long-term residential care. The interventions most commonly used with nursing home residents (Burckhardt 1987; Gugel 1989; Karuza and Katz 1991), the importance of outcome instrument selection in long-term care settings (Rabins et al. 1987), and unique design and administrative issues that affect treatment outcome research (Radebaugh et al. 1996; Rapp et al. 1994; Weiss 1994) have been identified in reviews. As noted at the beginning of this chapter, there are also growing numbers of institutional training programs geared toward teaching staff to manage specific patient behavior problems or improve independence in activities of daily living (Baltes et al. 1994; Blair 1995; Heacock et al. 1997; Lantz et al. 1997). Surprisingly, however, there are few studies that have examined the impact of psychotherapy on patients' psychological well-being and adjustment to nursing home life (Table 36–6).

Dhooper et al. (1993) conducted a pilot project with 16 depressed, cognitively intact nursing home residents. Subjects were randomly assigned to either an active treatment

TABLE 36–6. Empirical studies with older adults in long-term care

Study	Subjects	Subject age (years)	Treatment	Treatment duration
Power and McCarron 1975	30 NH residents with depression	Mean, 84 (range, 70–98)	Individual interactive contact (including physical touching and socialization)	15 sessions
			No treatment (control)	
Langer and Rodin 1976	91 NH residents	Range, 65–90	Resident responsibility-induced group	1 session
			Staff conduct (control)	
Schulz 1976	42 NH residents	Mean, 82 (range, 67–96)	Scheduled visits (visit times chosen by subjects)	2 months
			Scheduled visits (visit times not chosen by subjects)	
			Nonscheduled random visits	
			No visits (control)	
Berger and Rose 1977	25 NH residents	Mean, 77 (range, 48–97)	Individual interpersonal skills training	3 sessions
			Individual discussion (control)	
			Assessment only (control)	
Lindell 1978	39 NH residents	Mean, 81–82 (all subjects > 65)	Supportive group therapy	Therapy: 16 sessions in 8 weeks
			Group discussion (control)	Control: 3 sessions in 8 weeks
Langer et al. 1979	54 NH residents	Mean, 79–80	Individual visit (high self-disclosure)	4 sessions in 6 weeks
			Individual visit (low self-disclosure)	
			No treatment (control)	
			Pretest only (control)	
Dye and Erber 1981	52 new NH residents	Mean, 80	Resident-only group	7 sessions
			Resident-family group	
			No treatment (control)	
Hanley et al. 1981	57 NH residents	Mean, 80	Group reality orientation	4 sessions/week for 12 weeks
			Group reality orientation plus ward orientation	
			No treatment (control)	
Hussian and Lawrence 1981	36 NH residents with depression	Mean, 74 (all subjects > 60)	Social reinforcement for activity	10 sessions in 2 weeks
			Individual problem solving	
			Wait list (control)	
			Social reinforcement and problem solving	
			Problem solving plus social reinforcement	
			Education (control)	

(continued)

TABLE 36–6. Empirical studies with older adults in long-term care *(continued)*

Study	Subjects	Subject age (years)	Treatment	Treatment duration
Moran and Gatz 1987	59 NH residents	Mean, 76	Task-oriented group Insight-oriented group Wait list (control)	12 sessions
Dhooper et al. 1993	16 NH residents with depression	Mean, 78 (range, 64–94)	Cognitive-behavior therapy and reminiscing Unspecified control	9 sessions
Weiss 1994	48 NH residents	? ("young old," 55–74; "old old," 75–100)	Cognitive therapy group Life review group Unspecified ("standard") control	8 sessions
Lantz et al. 1997	14 NH residents	Mean, 81–82	Wellness group No treatment (control)	10 sessions
Rosen et al. 1997	31 NH residents with depression	Mean, 79 (range, 56–96)	Planned leisure activities Wait list (control)	8 weeks

Note.   NHT = nursing home or long-term residential setting.

group (9 weeks of participation in a "Coping Together Group," which included cognitive-behavioral and reminiscence treatment components) or an unspecified control (presumably no treatment) group. Subjects in the active treatment group reported significantly lower post-treatment levels of depression (as rated using the Zung Self-Rating Depression Scale) than did control subjects, although the fact that the study involved small numbers of subjects, no contact control, and apparently nonblinded raters may have influenced treatment outcome. No follow-up data were included in the report.

Dye and Erber (1981) described a program in which 52 new residents participated in support groups (with or without family members) to discuss the events that led to their move, any problems encountered during the admission process, and problem-solving strategies for coping with institutional life. Patients who participated in the resident-only group had lower levels of anxiety and higher internal locus of control scores than did either control subjects or patients who participated in the resident-family group. However, at 6-month follow-up, participants in the resident-only group were significantly more agitated and had lower health self-rating scores than did participants in the family-resident group and control subjects.

In other studies examining residents' adjustment to institutionalization, problems in generalization and long-term maintenance of treatment effects have been reported. Lindell (1978) reported positive changes in self-concept in long-term residential center and nursing home patients who participated in nondirective support groups; however, changes were maintained only in those subjects who continued to meet with their group regularly after the formal research study ended. Hussian and Lawrence (1981) found that depressed nursing home residents initially showed improvements in mood as a result of systematic increases in daily activity or training in problem-solving skills. However, after 2 weeks, only those subjects who both increased their daily activity and learned new problem-solving strategies continued to show improved mood. At 3-month follow-up, no gains were maintained. Thus, although support at the time of transition into a nursing home appears to enhance patients' immediate functioning, this improvement may not be sustained unless other factors are developed to maintain it.

Interpersonal factors have been shown to be particularly influential in patients' psychosocial functioning in long-term settings. For example, Power and McCarron (1975) found that increasing depressed geriatric patients' physical contact with staff, their verbal conversation, and their social interaction with peers led to reductions in self-reported and observed depression in the patients. Similarly, Moran and Gatz (1987) found that nursing home residents who participated in an interpersonal task group (which developed a welcoming project for incoming residents) showed significant improvements in feelings of self-control and increases in scores of life satisfaction. Berger and Rose (1977) found that interpersonal skills could be effectively taught to nursing home residents, although in their study, learned skills were not subsequently used in novel, unpracticed situations. Thus, although increases in quantity and quality of interpersonal contacts may enhance patients' adjustment and functioning in long-term care facilities, it may be necessary for staff to provide ongoing opportunities and assistance if these improvements are to be maintained.

Other studies have suggested that sustained, successful coping in long-term care settings is affected by residents' perception of their autonomy and situational control (Langer and Rodin 1976; Schulz 1976) and that social interaction may be associated with improvements in their immediate memory, alertness, and self-initiation (Langer et al. 1979). Rosen et al. (1997) found that depressed nursing home residents randomly assigned to a control-relevant intervention (in which they were helped to establish an individualized leisure activity program) were more likely to show significant decreases in HDRS scores and to be judged as treatment "responders" by nursing staff than were subjects in a wait-list control group. Responders also showed significant improvements in ratings of community "cohesiveness" or supportiveness after treatment. However, improvements were not maintained once the 8-week intervention was discontinued. Further, the investigators had unexpected problems with recruitment and compliance. Nevertheless, the study provides evidence that interventions designed to empower nursing home residents and to help them reestablish patterns of positive social or recreational activity may be highly effective in ameliorating chronic depression in residential care settings.

In summary, there have been relatively few empirical studies on the use of psychotherapeutic interventions in elderly patients in long-term care settings. A number of those studies are more than 20 years old, and the fact that there are few recent studies is surprising, given the growing number of older adults who are unable to remain independent in their own homes. The existing studies often had small samples and problematic research designs. Nevertheless, the findings do suggest that treatment can improve patient self-concept, reduce depression, and enhance social interaction, although changes may not be well maintained without ongoing therapeutic support. Additional research in this area is clearly needed.

Other Psychotherapeutic Interventions

In the remaining empirical studies of psychotherapy in older adults, a variety of intervention techniques were used to modify depression, anxiety, and other symptoms of emotional distress (Table 36–7). In several studies, meditation-relaxation and cognitive-change techniques were used, and although samples were small, consistent trends were observed. DeBerry (1982) found that 10 weeks of meditation-relaxation training was effective in reducing the number of self-reports of state and trait anxiety, but not depression, in a group of depressed elderly women. Subjects who were assigned continued posttreatment practice with relaxation tapes maintained improvements, whereas state anxiety scores of those who did not practice showed a drift back toward baseline. In a subsequent comparison of meditation-relaxation and cognitive restructuring (DeBerry et al. 1989), the investigators reported significant reductions in state anxiety but not trait anxiety or depression in subjects trained in meditation-relaxation; however, cognitive restructuring produced no significant changes in either depression or anxiety (state or trait). Scogin et al. (1992) offered training in either progressive relaxation or imaginal relaxation techniques to elderly patients with symptoms of tension or anxiety that were at a "subjectively uncomfortable level." Subjects in both treatment groups showed significantly greater improvements in state anxiety and psychiatric symptomatology (as measured by the Symptom Checklist—90) than did delayed-treatment control subjects, although improvements were not maintained at 1-month follow-up. Interestingly, Alexander et al. (1989) found that both meditation and mindfulness (focused attention) training resulted in improvements in cognitive functioning, blood pressure readings, and 3-year survival rates, despite the fact that no changes in anxiety or depression were associated with either intervention.

In some studies, the focus has been on providing skills training to elderly patients with depression. Participation in assertiveness training has been shown to improve effectiveness in interpersonal situations, as well as ratings of self-acceptance (Franzke 1987). Reich and Zautra (1989) found that four sessions of individual therapy, designed to enhance perceived control, significantly increased participation in positive activities by bereaved and disabled elderly subjects and decreased psychological distress as well. However, these improvements were not maintained after the treatment was discontinued.

Other studies have examined the impact of therapy on

TABLE 36–7. Empirical studies (miscellaneous) with older adults

Study	Subjects	Subject age (years)	Treatment	Treatment duration
Nevruz and Hrushka 1969	36 psychiatric inpatients	Mean, 70	Structured therapy group Unstructured therapy group	24 sessions in 12 weeks
Mulligan and Bennett 1977	23 isolated outpatients	Mean, 77 (all subjects > 67)	Social visits (subjects at home) Visit at beginning and end of study (control)	1 hour every 2 weeks for 6 months
Zarit et al. 1981	47 female volunteers	Mean, 64	Memory-training group Personal growth group	7 sessions in 4 weeks
DeBerry 1982	36 women with depression	Mean, 63–79	Relaxation-meditation group Relaxation-meditation group and follow-up tapes Pseudorelaxation group (control)	10 weeks (plus 10 weeks of daily practice for subjects assigned to relaxation-meditation group and follow-up tapes)
Lieberman and Bliwise 1985	108 outpatients	Range, 60–83	Professional-led support group Peer-led support group	36 sessions in 9 months
Franzke 1987	84 community-dwelling subjects	All subjects > 65	Assertiveness training groups No treatment (control)	6 weeks
Ong et al. 1987	20 discharged inpatients (most in day hospital program)	Mean, 74	Support group (psychodynamic and problem solving) No added treatment (control)	Weekly sessions for 9 months
Alexander et al. 1989	73 NH residents	Mean, 81	Transcendental meditation Mindfulness training Mental relaxation No treatment (control)	12 weeks
DeBerry et al. 1989	32 outpatients	Mean, 69 (range, 65–75)	Relaxation-meditation group Cognitive-restructuring group Pseudorelaxation group (control)	20 sessions in 10 weeks
Reich and Zautra 1989	25 bereaved, 25 functionally disabled, and 58 matched control subjects	Mean, 71	Perceived-control intervention Placebo contact No contact (control)	4 sessions in 10 weeks
Viney et al. 1989	30 outpatients with "psychological problems"	Mean, 75	Brief personal construct individual therapy No treatment (control) Criterion group (single contact) (control)	5–13 sessions in 24 weeks

Study	Subjects	Age	Treatment conditions	Duration
Heller et al. 1991	265 women	Median, 74	Time 1 Friendly staff contacts by telephone Assessment only (control) Time 2 (Time 1 staff-contact group only) Staff telephone contact Peer telephone contact (initiators) Peer telephone contact (receivers) Assessment only (control)	Time 1: 10 weeks (two times/week for first 5 weeks, then one time/week) Time 2: 10 weeks
Scogin et al. 1992	71 community residents with anxiety or tension	Mean, 68–69 (all subjects ≥ 60)	Time 1 Progressive relaxation Imaginal relaxation Delayed training (no relaxation training, outcome measures only) Time 2 (delayed-training group only) Delayed progressive training Delayed passive training	4 training sessions

Note. NH = nursing home or long-term residential setting.

subjects' long-term functioning. For example, isolated community-dwelling elderly people who received regular "social visits" in their home for 6 months were more likely to be living independently in the community at 6-month follow-up than were control subjects (Mulligan and Bennett 1977). Geriatric psychiatric patients who participated in weekly psychodynamic problem-solving groups for 9 months had a lower rehospitalization rate, despite the fact that no changes in depressive symptoms were observed in participants (Ong et al. 1987). Therapy has even been shown to influence geriatric psychiatric patients' willingness to leave state hospital wards and try community placement options (Nevruz and Hrushka 1969).

In summary, a variety of nonspecific psychosocial interventions have been used in geriatric subjects. Although a few studies have included psychiatric inpatients, the majority have been conducted with outpatient volunteers. These studies have shown that different combinations of relaxation, cognitive restructuring, emotional support, and skills training can improve self-ratings of depression, anxiety, and self-acceptance. There is also evidence that psychosocial interventions lead to improvements in long-term survival rates and reduced rates of rehospitalization for chronically ill psychiatric patients. However, long-term maintenance of improvements in mood or generalization of newly learned skills has not been consistently reported after therapy discontinuation.

Summary and Future Research Directions

Several conclusions can be drawn from the existing literature on the efficacy of psychosocial interventions in older adults. First, a variety of interventions have been studied in physically healthy, community-dwelling older adults. Cognitive-behavioral strategies have been the subject of most empirical research, although psychodynamic, reminiscence, and various supportive techniques have also been studied in this population. Each treatment has been found effective in decreasing depression, and a few studies have shown this treatment effectiveness to be equal or superior to the effectiveness of pharmacotherapeutic interventions. There is some evidence that improvements resulting from CBT are better maintained at follow-up than those from the other treatment forms, but there are too few long-term outcome comparison studies to evaluate the strength of these findings.

Although research is less plentiful, there is also empirical evidence for the efficacy of CBT and its variants in patients with medical illnesses and dementia, elderly caregivers, and residents of long-term care institutions. A few studies have found that psychodynamic therapy, reminiscence and life review activities, and supportive interventions can also reduce negative mood and improve life satisfaction and self-esteem in disabled or institutionalized older adults and their caregivers. In some cases, long-term improvements (e.g., improved rates of rehospitalization or delayed nursing home placement) were reported even in the absence of reductions in acute depression ratings.

A variety of factors may contribute to differing treatment effects across studies. These factors include patient variables, such as presence or absence of premorbid personality disorders, severity of symptoms at the onset of treatment, cognitive capacity, and patient feelings of commitment to treatment or expectation of change. Specific treatment variables have also been implicated in differing outcomes. For example, structured life review strategies may be more effective than simple reminiscence, participation of family members may enhance treatment impact, and treatment with professional therapists may produce greater reductions in psychiatric symptoms than peer-led interventions. In therapy with patients in long-term settings, and in outpatient therapy with caregivers, maintenance of therapeutic gains appears contingent on ongoing, or at least periodic, therapy. Both group and individual therapies have been successful in older patients.

Although the empirical treatment literature has grown substantially over the past several years, additional research is needed concerning the efficacy of psychosocial interventions in elderly patients. Psychosocial interventions based solely on treatments used in uncontrolled case studies and treatments described in anecdotal reports are still widely used with older adults. The interventions in controlled studies that have been conducted represent a mixture of cognitive-behavioral, psychodynamic, relaxation, supportive counseling, and educational techniques. There are, as yet, no data to indicate which components of particular interventions are efficacious in improving psychological, physical, or social functioning. Although increasing numbers of studies (particularly those focused on depression treatment) now have treatment manuals available, many interventions used with older adults are not manualized or adequately described, making replication or comparison across studies difficult. In these cases, more rigorous treatment definition is needed. There is little empirical research on the impact of therapist or environmental variables on therapy outcome. The cultural, intrapersonal, familial, and health factors that are likely to have an impact on treatment efficacy must be systematically investigated. The intervention literature has tended to focus primarily on the management of pathological cognitive or emotional disorders. The challenges of normal aging deserve attention, as well.

Additional research is needed to determine how long interventions should be continued for maximal treatment impact and to establish strategies for generalization and maintenance once the active treatment phase ends. In the studies reported here, therapy duration ranged from a single session or a few sessions to months or years; in some studies, subjects were exposed to different numbers of sessions over variable lengths of time. Clarifying the significance of this variable may be particularly important for older adults with chronic physical conditions or social circumstances that have precipitated psychosocial intervention. Because therapy outcome is dependent on how psychosocial functioning is defined and measured, research is also needed to identify assessment instruments with good reliability and validity that are sensitive to expected changes and appropriate for use with various elderly populations and in specialized contexts.

Given the growing number of older adults who are medically ill and living in long-term care settings, it is surprising that there are so few controlled studies examining the psychosocial impact of physical disability and institutionalization on geriatric patients. Additional studies of treatment effectiveness in persons with multiple medical, psychiatric, and social disabilities are needed. The use of single-case research design strategies may allow investigators to gather useful information on small numbers of such individuals with little disruption to medical or residential facilities. Validity of results could be maximized by applying such design strategies to multiple settings and using a broad range of reliable assessment instruments. Single-case research design strategies may also permit evaluation of the conjoint impact of pharmacological and psychosocial interventions on functioning in a range of elderly populations.

In summary, although more research is needed, the existing data available on psychosocial interventions in older adults are surprisingly encouraging. A variety of behavioral and supportive interventions have produced improvements in psychological functioning in physically healthy, depressed older subjects, as well as in institutionalized or medically ill geriatric patients and their caregivers. Gains from psychological interventions are often comparable to gains from medical treatments. Efforts now need to be made to clarify which strategies are most efficacious for which patient groups and to develop effective new interventions for elderly patients in both outpatient and inpatient settings.

∎ References

Abraham IL, Neundorfer MM, Currie LJ: Effects of group interventions on cognition and depression in nursing home residents. Nurs Res 41:196–202, 1992

Agrell B, Dehlin O: Comparison of six depression rating scales in geriatric stroke patients. Stroke 20:1190–1194, 1989

Alexander CN, Langer EJ, Newman RI, et al: Transcendental meditation, mindfulness, and longevity: an experimental study with the elderly. J Pers Soc Psychol 57:950–964, 1989

American Association of Retired Persons: A Profile of Older Persons: 1986. Washington, DC, American Association of Retired Persons, 1986

American Heritage Dictionary, 2nd College Edition. Boston, MA, Houghton Mifflin, 1985

American Psychiatric Association: Diagnostic and Statistical Manual of Mental Disorders, 3rd Edition. Washington, DC, American Psychiatric Association, 1980

Andersson G, Melin L, Scott B, et al: An evaluation of a behavioural treatment approach to hearing impairment. Behav Res Ther 33:283–292, 1995

Andersson G, Green M, Melin L: Behavioural hearing tactics: a controlled trial of a short treatment programme. Behav Res Ther 35:523–530, 1997

Arean PA, Perri MG, Nezu AM, et al: Comparative effectiveness of social problem-solving therapy and reminiscence therapy as treatments for depression in older adults. J Consult Clin Psychol 61:1003–1010, 1993

Baines S, Saxby P, Ehlert K: Reality orientation and reminiscence therapy. Br J Psychiatry 151:222–231, 1987

Baker FM: An overview of depression in the elderly: a U.S. perspective. J Natl Med Assoc 88:178–184, 1996

Baldelli MV, Pirani A, Motta M, et al: Effects of reality orientation therapy on elderly patients in the community. Archives of Gerontology and Geriatrics 17:211–218, 1993

Baltes MM, Neumann E-M, Zank S: Maintenance and rehabilitation of independence in old age: an intervention program for staff. Psychol Aging 9:179–188, 1994

Beck AT, Rush AJ, Shaw BF, et al: Cognitive Therapy for Depression. New York, Guilford, 1979

Beck CK, Shue VM: Interventions for treating disruptive behavior in demented elderly people. Nurs Clin North Am 29:143–155, 1994

Bennett SL, Maas F: The effect of music-based life review on the life satisfaction and ego integrity of elderly people. British Journal of Occupational Therapy 51:433–436, 1988

Berger RM, Rose SD: Interpersonal skill training with institutionalized elderly patients. J Gerontol 32:346–353, 1977

Berghorn FJ, Schafer DE: Reminiscence intervention in nursing homes: what and who changes? Int J Aging Hum Dev 24:113–125, 1987

Beutler LE, Scogin F, Kirkish P, et al: Group cognitive therapy and alprazolam in the treatment of depression in older adults. J Consult Clin Psychol 55:550–556, 1987

Bharucha AJ, Satlin A: Late-life suicide: a review. Harv Rev Psychiatry 5:55–65, 1997

Blair CE: Combining behavior management and mutual goal setting to reduce physical dependency in nursing home residents. Nurs Res 44:160–165, 1995

Bliwise D, Friedman L, Nekich JC, et al: Prediction of outcome in behaviorally based insomnia treatments. J Behav Ther Exp Psychiatry 26:17–23, 1995

Bourgeois MS, Schulz R, Burgio L: Interventions for caregivers of patients with Alzheimer's disease: a review and analysis of content, process, and outcomes. Int J Aging Hum Dev 43:35–92, 1996

Burckhardt CS: The effect of therapy on the mental health of the elderly. Res Nurs Health 10:277–285, 1987

Burgio LD, Scilley K, Hardin JM, et al: Environmental "white noise": an intervention for verbally agitated nursing home residents. J Gerontol B Psychol Sci Soc Sci 51:P364–P373, 1996

Butcher J, Smith E, Gillespie C: Short-term group therapy for stroke patients in a rehabilitation centre. Br J Med Psychol 57:283–290, 1984

Butler RN: The life review: an interpretation of reminiscence in the aged. Psychiatry 26:65–76, 1963

Campbell JM: Treating depression in well older adults: use of diaries in cognitive therapy. Issues Ment Health Nurs 13:19–29, 1992

Cantor M: Strain among caregivers: a study of experience in the U.S. Gerontologist 23:597–604, 1983

Chiverton P, Caine ED: Education to assist spouses in coping with Alzheimer's disease: a controlled trial. J Am Geriatr Soc 37:593–598, 1989

Clipp EC, George LK: Psychotropic drug use among caregivers of patients with dementia. J Am Geriatr Soc 38:227–235, 1990

Cohen-Cole SA: Depression and heart disease, in Aging and Clinical Practice: Depression and Coexisting Disease. Edited by Robinson RG, Rabins PV. New York, Igaku-Shoin, 1989, pp 27–39

Coppel DB, Burton C, Becker J, et al: Relationships of cognitions associated with coping reactions to depression in spousal caregivers of Alzheimer's disease patients. Cognitive Therapy and Research 9:253–266, 1985

DeBerry S: The effects of meditation-relaxation on anxiety and depression in a geriatric population. Psychotherapy: Theory, Research and Practice 19:512–521, 1982

DeBerry S, Davis S, Reinhard KE: A comparison of meditation-relaxation and cognitive-behavioral techniques for reducing anxiety and depression in a geriatric population. J Geriatr Psychiatry 22:231–247, 1989

Dew MA, Reynolds CF III, Houck PR, et al: Temporal profiles of the course of depression during treatment. Arch Gen Psychiatry 54:1016–1024, 1997

Dhooper SS, Green SM, Huff MB, et al: Efficacy of a group approach to reducing depression in nursing home elderly residents. Journal of Gerontological Social Work 20:87–100, 1993

Dye CJ, Erber JT: Two group procedures for the treatment of nursing home patients. Gerontologist 21:539–544, 1981

Egelko S, Simon D, Riley E, et al: First year after stroke: tracking cognitive and affective deficits. Arch Phys Med Rehabil 70:297–302, 1989

Evans RL, Werkhoven W, Fox HR: Treatment of social isolation and loneliness in a sample of visually impaired elderly persons. Psychol Rep 51:103–108, 1982

Evans RL, Bishop DS, Matlock A, et al: Prestroke family interaction as a predictor of stroke outcome. Arch Phys Med Rehabil 63:508–512, 1987

Evans RL, Matlock A, Bishop DS, et al: Family intervention after stroke: does counseling or education help? Stroke 19:1243–1249, 1988

Fallot RD: The impact on mood of verbal reminiscing in later adulthood. Int J Aging Hum Dev 10:1979–1980, 1980

Farkas S: Impact of chronic illness on the patient's spouse. Health Soc Work 5:39–46, 1980

Fielden MA: Reminiscence as a therapeutic intervention with sheltered housing residents: a comparative study. British Journal of Social Work 20:21–44, 1990

Fisher JE, Carstensen LL: Behavior management of the dementias. Clin Psychol Rev 10:611–629, 1990

Franzke AW: The effects of assertiveness training on older adults. Gerontologist 27:13–16, 1987

Fry PS: Structured and unstructured reminiscence training and depression among the elderly. Clinical Gerontologist 1:15–37, 1983

Fry PS: Cognitive training and cognitive-behavioral variables in the treatment of depression in the elderly. Clinical Gerontologist 3:25–45, 1984

Fry PS: Depression, Stress, and Adaptations in the Elderly: Psychological Assessment and Intervention. Rockville, MD, Aspen, 1986

Gallagher DE, Thompson LW: Treatment of major depressive disorder in older adult outpatients with brief psychotherapies. Psychotherapy: Theory, Research and Practice 19:482–490, 1982

Gallagher DE, Thompson LW: Effectiveness of psychotherapy for both endogenous and nonendogenous depression in older adult outpatients. J Gerontol 38:707–712, 1983

Gallagher D[E], Rose J, Rivera P, et al: Prevalence of depression in family caregivers. Gerontologist 29:449–456, 1989

Gallagher-Thompson D, Steffen AM: Comparative effects of cognitive-behavioral and brief psychodynamic psychotherapies for depressed family caregivers. J Consult Clin Psycho 62:543–549, 1994

Gallagher-Thompson D, Hanley-Peterson P, Thompson LW: Maintenance of gains versus relapse following brief psychotherapy for depression. J Consult Clin Psychol 58:371–374, 1990

Gass CS, Lawhorn L: Psychological adjustment following stroke: an MMPI study. Psychological Assessment 3:628–633, 1991

Gaston L, Marmar CR, Thompson LW, et al: Relation of patient pretreatment characteristics to the therapeutic alliance in diverse psychotherapies. J Consult Clin Psychol 56:483–489, 1988

Gaston L, Marmar CR, Gallagher D, et al: Impact of confirming patient expectations of change processes in behavioral, cognitive, and brief dynamic psychotherapy. Psychotherapy 26:296–302, 1989

Gatz M, Fiske A, Fox LS, et al: Empirically validated psychological treatments for older adults. Journal of Mental Health and Aging 4:9–46, 1998

Gaynor S: When the caregiver becomes the patient. Geriatric Nursing 10:121–123, 1989

Godbole A, Verinis JS: Brief psychotherapy in the treatment of emotional disorders in physically ill geriatric patients. Gerontologist 14:143–148, 1974

Goldwasser AN, Auerbach SM, Harkins SW: Cognitive, affective, and behavioral effects of reminiscence group therapy on demented elderly. Int J Aging Hum Dev 25:209–222, 1987

Goodman CC, Pynoos J: A model telephone information and support program for caregivers of Alzheimer's patients. Gerontologist 30:399–404, 1990

Greene VL, Monahan DJ: The effect of a professionally guided caregiver support and education group on institutionalization of care receivers. Gerontologist 27:716–721, 1987

Greene VL, Monahan DJ: The effect of a support and education program on stress and burden among family caregivers to frail elderly persons. Gerontologist 29:472–477, 1989

Greer S, Moorey S, Baruch JD, et al: Adjuvant psychological therapy for patients with cancer: a prospective randomised trial. BMJ 304:675–680, 1992

Gruen W: Effects of brief psychotherapy during the hospitalization period on the recovery process in heart attacks. J Consult Clin Psychol 43:223–232, 1975

Gugel R: Psychosocial interventions in the nursing home, in Principles and Practice of Nursing Home Care. Edited by Katz PR, Calkins E. New York, Springer, 1989, pp 212–224

Gutman GM, Herbert CP, Brown SR: Feldenkrais versus conventional exercises for the elderly. J Gerontol 32:562–572, 1977

Haight BK: The therapeutic role of a structured life review process in homebound elderly subjects. J Gerontol 43:P40–P44, 1988

Haight BK: Reminiscing: the state of the art as a basis for practice. Int J Aging Hum Dev 33:1–32, 1991

Haight BK: Long-term effects of a structured life review process. J Gerontol 47:P312–P315, 1992

Haley WE: Group intervention for dementia family caregivers: a longitudinal perspective. Gerontologist 29:478–480, 1989

Haley WE, Brown SL, Levine EG: Experimental evaluation of the effectiveness of group intervention for dementia caregivers. Gerontologist 27:376–382, 1987

Hanley IG, McGuire RJ, Boyd WD: Reality orientation and dementia: a controlled trial of two approaches. Br J Psychiatry 138:10–14, 1981

Harp-Scates SK, Randolph DE, Gutsch KU, et al: Effects of cognitive-behavioral, reminiscence, and activity treatments on life satisfaction and anxiety in the elderly. Int J Aging Hum Dev 22:141–146, 1986

Hartke RJ: Psychological Aspects of Geriatric Rehabilitation. Gaithersburg, MD, Aspen, Inc, 1991

Heacock PR, Beck CM, Souder E, et al: Assessing dressing ability in dementia. Geriatric Nursing 18:107–111, 1997

Hedgepeth BE, Hale WD: Effect of a positive reminiscing intervention on affect, expectancy, and performance. Psychol Rep 53:867–870, 1983

Heller K, Thompson MG, Trueba PE, et al: Peer support telephone dyads for elderly women: was this the wrong intervention? Am J Community Psychol 19:53–74, 1991

Hersen M, van Hasselt VB: Behavioral assessment and treatment of anxiety in the elderly. Clin Psychol Rev 12:619–640, 1992

Hussian RA, Lawrence PS: Social reinforcement of activity and problem-solving training in the treatment of depressed institutionalized elderly patients. Cognitive Therapy Research 5:57–69, 1981

Ibrahim MA, Feldman JG, Sultz HA, et al: Management after myocardial infarction: a controlled trial of the effect of group psychotherapy. Int J Psychiatry Med 5:253–268, 1974

Imes C: Interventions with stroke patients: EMG biofeedback, group activities, cognitive retraining. Cognitive Rehabilitation 2:4–17, 1984

Ingersoll B, Silverman A: Comparative group psychotherapy for the aged. Gerontologist 18:201–206, 1978

Jarvik L, Mintz JM, Steuer J, et al: Treating geriatric depression: a 26-week interim analysis. J Am Geriatr Soc 30:713–717, 1982

Kahan J, Kemp B, Staples FR, et al: Decreasing the burden in families caring for a relative with a dementing illness: A controlled study. J Am Geriatr Soc 33:664–670, 1985

Kaplan S, Kozin F: A controlled study of group counseling in rheumatoid arthritis. J Rheumatol 8:91–99, 1981

Karuza J, Katz PR: Psychosocial interventions in long-term care: a critical overview, in Advances in Long-Term Care, Vol 1. Edited by Katz PR, Kane RL, Mezey MD. New York, Springer, 1991, pp 1–27

Kashner TM, Rodell DE, Ogden SR, et al: Outcomes and costs of two VA inpatient treatment programs for older alcoholic patients. Hosp Community Psychiatry 43:985–989, 1992

Keefe FJ, Caldwell DS, Williams DA, et al: Pain coping skills training in the management of osteoarthritic knee pain: a comparative study. Behavior Therapy 21:49–62, 1990

Keuthen N, Wisocki PA: Behavioral medicine for the health concerns of the elderly, in Handbook of Clinical Behavior Therapy With the Elderly Client. Edited by Wisocki PA. New York, Plenum, 1991, pp 363–381

Kirschenbaum DS, Sherman J, Penrod JD: Promoting self-directed hemodialysis: measurement and cognitive-behavioral intervention. Health Psychol 6:373–385, 1987

Klerman GL, Weissman MM, Rounsaville BJ, et al: Interpersonal Psychotherapy of Depression. New York, Basic Books, 1984

Knight BG, Lutzky SM, Macofsky-Urban F: A meta-analytic review of interventions for caregiver distress: recommendations for future research. Gerontologist 33:240–248, 1993

Langer EJ, Rodin J: The effects of choice and enhanced personal responsibility for the aged: a field experiment in an institutional setting. J Pers Soc Psychol 34:191–198, 1976

Langer EJ, Rodin J, Beck P, et al: Environmental determinants of memory improvement in late adulthood. J Pers Soc Psychol 37:2003–2013, 1979

Lantz MS, Buchalter EN, McBee L: The Wellness Group: a novel intervention for coping with disruptive behavior in elderly nursing home residents. Gerontologist 37:551–556, 1997

Lappe JM: Reminiscing: the life review therapy. J Gerontol Nurs 13:12–16, 1987

Lawton MP, Brody EM, Saperstein AR: A controlled study of respite service for caregivers of Alzheimer's patients. Gerontologist 29:8–16, 1989

Lazarus LW, Weinberg J: Psychosocial intervention with the aged. Psychiatr Clin North Am 5:215–227, 1982

Lewinsohn PM, Sullivan JM, Grosscup SJ: Changing reinforcing events: an approach to the treatment of depression. Psychotherapy: Theory, Research and Practice 17:322–334, 1980

Lewinsohn PM, Antonuccio DO, Steinmetz J, et al: The Coping With Depression Course. Eugene, OR, Castalia, 1984

Lieberman MA, Bliwise NG: Comparisons among peer and professionally directed groups for the elderly: implications for the development of self-help groups. Int J Group Psychother 35:155–175, 1985

Lieberman MA, Falk JM: The remembered past as a source of data for research on the life cycle. Human Development 14:132–141, 1971

Lindell AR: Group therapy for the institutionalized aged. Issues Ment Health Nurs 1:76–86, 1978

Lipsey JR, Parikh RM: Depression and stroke, in Aging and Clinical Practice: Depression and Coexisting Disease. Edited by Robinson RG, Rabins PV. New York, Igaku-Shoin, 1989, pp 186–201

Lovell BB, Ancoli-Israel S, Gevirtz R: Effect of bright light treatment on agitated behavior in institutionalized elderly subjects. Psychiatry Res 57:7–12, 1995

Lovett S, Gallagher D: Psychoeducational interventions for family caregivers: preliminary efficacy data. Behavior Therapy 19:321–330, 1988

Marmar CR, Gaston L, Gallagher D, et al: Alliance and outcome in late-life depression. J Nerv Ment Dis 177: 464–472, 1989

Matteson MA: Effects of a cognitive behavioral approach and positive reinforcement on exercise for older adults. Educational Gerontology 15:497–513, 1989

McCurry SM, Logsdon RG, Vitiello MV, et al: Successful behavioral treatment for reported sleep problems in elderly caregivers of dementia patients: a controlled study. J Gerontol B Psychol Sci Soc Sci 53:P122–P129, 1998

McMurdo MET, Rennie L: A controlled trial of exercise by residents of o d people's homes. Age Ageing 22:11–15, 1993

Merriam S: The concept and function of reminiscence: a review of the research. Gerontologist 20:604–609, 1980

Miller MD, Wolfson L, Frank E, et al: Using interpersonal psychotherapy (IPT) in a combined psychotherapy/medication research protocol with depressed elders: a descriptive report with case vignettes. J Psychother Pract Res 7:47–55, 1997

Mittelman MS, Ferris SH, Steinberg G, et al: An intervention that delays institutionalization of Alzheimer's disease patients: treatment of spouse-caregivers. Gerontologist 33:730–740, 1993

Mittelman MS, Ferris SH, Shulman E, et al: A comprehensive support program: effect on depression in spouse-caregivers of AD patients. Gerontologist 35:792–802, 1995

Mittelman MS, Ferris SH, Shulman E, et al: A family intervention to delay nursing home placement of patients with Alzheimer's disease: a randomized controlled trial. JAMA 276:1725–1731, 1996

Mohide EA, Pringle DM, Streiner DL, et al: A randomized trial of family caregiver support in the home management of dementia. J Am Geriatr Soc 38:446–454, 1990

Molinari V, Reichlin RE: Life review reminiscence in the elderly: a review of the literature. Int J Aging Hum Dev 20:81–92, 1985

Montgomery RJV, Borgatta EF: The effects of alternative support strategies on family caregiving. Gerontologist 29:457–464, 1989

Moran JA, Gatz M: Group therapies for nursing home adults: an evaluation of two treatment approaches. Gerontologist 27:588–591, 1987

Morin CM, Colecchi C, Stone J, et al: Behavioral and pharmacological therapies for late life insomnia: a randomized controlled trial. JAMA 281:991–998

Mossey JM, Knott KA, Higgins M, et al: Effectiveness of a psychosocial intervention, interpersonal counseling, for subdysthymic depression in medically ill elderly. J Gerontol A Biol Sci Med Sci 51:M172–M178, 1996

Mullen PD, Laville EA, Biddle AK, et al: Efficacy of psychoeducational interventions on pain, depression, and disability in people with arthritis: a meta-analysis. J Rheumatol 14:33–39, 1987

Mulligan MA, Bennett R: Assessment of mental health and social problems during multiple friendly visits: the development and evaluation of a friendly visiting program for the isolated elderly. Int J Aging Hum Dev 8:43–65, 1977

Mumford E, Schlesinger HJ, Glass GV, et al: A new look at evidence about reduced cost of medical utilization following mental health treatment. Am J Psychiatry 141:1145–1158, 1984

National Institutes of Health: Diagnosis and Treatment of Depression in Late Life (Consensus Development Conference Statement, vol 9, no 3), November 4–6, 1991

Nevruz N, Hrushka M: The influence of unstructured and structured group psychotherapy with geriatric patients on their decision to leave the hospital. Int J Group Psychother 19:72–78, 1969

Niederehe G: Psychosocial therapies with depressed older adults, in Diagnosis and Treatment of Depression in Late Life: Results of the NIH Consensus Development Conference. Edited by Schneider LS, Reynolds CF, Lebowitz BD, et al. Washington, DC, American Psychiatric Press, 1994, pp 293–315

Niederehe G: Psychosocial treatments with depressed older adults: a research update. American Journal of Geriatric Psychiatry 4:S66–S78, 1996

Oldenburg B, Perkins RJ, Andrews G: Controlled trial of psychological intervention in myocardial infarction. J Consult Clin Psychol 53:852–859, 1985

Ong YL, Martineau F, Lloyd C, et al: A support group for the depressed elderly. Int J Geriatr Psychiatry 2:119–123, 1987

Opdyke KS, Reynolds CF III, Frank E, et al: Effect of continuation treatment on residual symptoms in late-life depression: how well is "well"? Depress Anxiety 4:312–319, 1996–1997

Orten JD, Allen M, Cook J: Reminiscence groups with confused nursing center residents: an experimental study. Soc Work Health Care 14:73–86, 1989

Parker RG: Reminiscence: a continuity theory framework. Gerontologist 35:515–525, 1995

Perrotta P, Meacham JA: Can a reminiscing intervention alter depression and self-esteem? Int J Aging Hum Dev 14:23–30, 1981

Power CA, McCarron LT: Treatment of depression in persons residing in homes for the aged. Gerontologist 27:132–135, 1975

Pruchno R, Potashnik S: Caregiving spouses: physical and mental health in perspective. J Am Geriatr Soc 37:697–705, 1989

Quayhagen MP, Quayhagen M, Corbeil RR, et al: A dyadic remediation program for care recipients with dementia. Nurs Res 44:153–159, 1995

Rabins PV, Mace NL, Lucas MJ: The impact of dementia on the family. JAMA 248:333–335, 1982

Rabins PV, Rovner BW, Larson DB, et al: The use of mental health measures in nursing home research. J Am Geriatr Soc 35:431–434, 1987

Radebaugh TS, Buckholtz N, Khachaturian Z: Behavioral approaches to the treatment of Alzheimer's disease: research strategies. Int Psychogeriatr 8 (suppl 1):7–12, 1996

Rapp CG, Topps-Uriri J, Beck C: Obtaining and maintaining a research sample with cognitively impaired nursing home residents. Geriatric Nursing 15:193–196, 1994

Rattenbury C, Stones MJ: A controlled evaluation of reminiscence and current topics discussion groups in a nursing home context. Gerontologist 29:768–771, 1989

Reich JW, Zautra AJ: A perceived control intervention for at-risk older adults. Psychol Aging 4:415–424, 1989

Reynolds CF III: Treatment of major depression in later life: a life cycle perspective. Psychiatr Q 68:221–246, 1997

Reynolds CF III, Frank E, Perel JM, et al: Combined pharmacotherapy and psychotherapy in the acute and continuation treatment of elderly patients with recurrent major depression: a preliminary report. Am J Psychiatry 149:1687–1692, 1992

Reynolds CF III, Frank E, Perel JM, et al: Treatment of consecutive episodes of major depression in the elderly. Am J Psychiatry 151:1740–1743, 1994

Reynolds CF III, Frank E, Perel JM, et al: Maintenance therapies for late-life recurrent major depression: research and review circa 1995. Int Psychogeriatr 7 (suppl):27–39, 1995

Reynolds CF III, Frank E, Perel JM, et al: High relapse rate after discontinuation of adjunctive medication for elderly patients with recurrent major depression. Am J Psychiatry 153:1418–1422, 1996a

Reynolds CF III, Frank E, Kupfer DJ, et al: Treatment outcome in recurrent major depression: a post hoc comparison of elderly "young old" and midlife patients. Am J Psychiatry 153:1288–1292, 1996b

Reynolds CF III, Frank E, Houck PR, et al: Which elderly patients with remitted depression remain well with continued interpersonal psychotherapy after discontinuation of antidepressant medication? Am J Psychiatry 154:958–962, 1997

Reynolds CF III, Frank E, Perel JM, et al: Nortriptyline and interpersonal psychotherapy as maintenance therapies for recurrent major depression: a randomized controlled trial in patients older than 59 years. JAMA 281:39–45, 1999a

Reynolds CF III, Frank E, Perel JM, et al: Treatment of 70(+)-year-olds with recurrent major depression: excellent short-term but brittle long-term response. Am J Geriatr Psychiatry 7:64–69, 1999b

Rice C, Longabaugh R, Beattie M, et al: Age group differences in response to treatment for problematic alcohol use. Addiction 88:1369–1375, 1993

Robinson KM: A social skills training program for adult caregivers. ANS Adv Nurs Sci 10:59–72, 1988

Robinson K[M], Yates K: Effects of two caregiver-training programs on burden and attitude toward help. Arch Psychiatr Nurs 8:312–319, 1994

Rosen J, Rogers JC, Marin RS, et al: Control-relevant intervention in the treatment of minor and major depression in a long-term care facility. Am J Geriatr Psychiatry 5:247–257, 1997

Saxon SV: Pain Management Techniques for Older Adults. Springfield, IL, Charles C Thomas, 1991

Scharlach AE: Relieving feelings of strain among women with elderly mothers. Psychol Aging 2:9–13, 1987

Schmidt GL, Bonjean MJ, Widem AC, et al: Brief psychotherapy for caregivers of demented relatives: comparison of two therapeutic strategies. Clinical Gerontologist 7:109–125, 1988

Schneider LS, Sloane RB, Staples FR, et al: Pretreatment orthostatic hypotension as a predictor of response to nortriptyline in geriatric depression. J Clin Psychopharmacol 6:172–176, 1986

Schulz R: Effects of control and predictability on the physical and psychological well-being of the institutionalized aged. J Pers Soc Psychol 33:563–573, 1976

Scogin F, McElreath L: Efficacy of psychosocial treatments for geriatric depression: a quantitative review. J Consult Clin Psychol 62:69–74, 1994

Scogin F, Hamblin D, Beutler LE: Bibliotherapy for depressed older adults: a self-help alternative. Gerontologist 27:383–387, 1987

Scogin F, Jamison C, Gochneaur K: Comparative efficacy of cognitive and behavioral bibliotherapy for mildly and moderately depressed older adults. J Consult Clin Psychol 57:403–407, 1989

Scogin F, Jamison C, Davis N: Two-year follow-up of bibliotherapy for depression in older adults. J Consult Clin Psychol 58:665–667, 1990

Scogin F, Rickard HC, Keith S, et al: Progressive and imaginal relaxation training for elderly persons with subjective anxiety. Psychol Aging 7:419–424, 1992

Shearn MA, Fireman BH: Stress management and mutual support groups in rheumatoid arthritis. Am J Med 78:771–775, 1985

Sherrill JT, Frank E, Geary M, et al: Psychoeducational workshops for elderly patients with recurrent major depression and their families. Psychiatr Serv 48:76–81, 1997

Sloane RB, Staples FR, Schneider LS: Interpersonal therapy versus nortriptyline for depression in the elderly, in Clinical and Pharmacological Studies in Psychiatric Disorders. Edited by Burrows GD, Norman TR, Dennerstein L. London, John Libby, 1985, pp 344–346

Snyder M, Egan EC, Burns KR: Interventions for decreasing agitation behaviors in persons with dementia. J Gerontol Nurs 21:34–40, 1995

Spiegel D, Bloom JR, Yalom I: Group support for patients with metastatic cancer. Arch Gen Psychiatry 38:527–533, 1981

Steuer JL, Mintz J, Hammen CL, et al: Cognitive-behavioral and psychodynamic group psychotherapy in treatment of geriatric depression. J Consult Clin Psychol 52:180–189, 1984

Strupp H: Time Limited Dynamic Psychotherapy (TLDP). Nashville, TN, Vanderbilt University, 1982

Teri L ,Wagner A: Alzheimer's disease and depression. J Consult Clin Psychol 3:379–391, 1992

Teri L, Rabins P, Whitehouse P, et al: Management of behavior disturbance in Alzheimer's disease: current knowledge and future directions. Alzheimer Dis Assoc Disord 6:77–88, 1992

Teri L, Curtis J, Gallagher-Thompson D, et al: Cognitive-behavior therapy with depressed older adults, in Diagnosis and Treatment of Depression in Late Life: Results of the NIH Consensus Development Conference. Edited by Schneider LS, Reynolds CF, Lebowitz BD, et al. Washington, DC, American Psychiatric Press, 1994, pp 279–291

Teri L, Logsdon RG, Uomoto J, et al: Behavioral treatment of depression in dementia patients: a controlled clinical trial. J Gerontol B Psychol Sci Soc Sci 52:P159–P166, 1997

Thase ME, Greenhouse JB, Frank E, et al: Treatment of major depression with psychotherapy or psychotherapy-pharmacotherapy combinations. Arch Gen Psychiatry 54:1009–1015, 1997

Thompson LW, Gallagher D: Efficacy of psychotherapy in the treatment of late-life depression. Advances in Behavior Research and Therapy 6:127–139, 1984

Thompson LW, Gallagher D: Depression and its treatment in the elderly. Aging 348:14–18, 1985

Thompson LW, Gallagher D: Psychotherapy for late-life depression. Generations 10:38–41, 1986

Thompson LW, Gallagher D, Nies G, et al: Evaluation of the effectiveness of professionals and nonprofessionals as instructors of "Coping With Depression" classes for elders. Gerontologist 23:390–396, 1983

Thompson LW, Gallagher D, Breckenridge JS: Comparative effectiveness of psychotherapies for depressed elders. J Consult Clin Psychol 55:385–390, 1987

Thompson LW, Gallagher D, Czirr R: Personality disorder and outcome in the treatment of late-life depression. J Geriatr Psychiatry 21:133–153, 1988

Thompson LW Gallagher-Thompson D, Hanser S, et al: Treatment of late-life depression with cognitive/behavioral therapy or desipramine. Poster presented at the annual meeting of the American Psychological Association, San Francisco, CA, August 1991

Thompson MG, Thompson L, Gallagher-Thompson D: Linear and nonlinear changes in mood between psychotherapy sessions: implications for treatment outcome and relapse risk. Psychotherapy Research 5:327–336, 1995

Thompson SC, Sobolew-Shubin A, Graham MA, et al: Psychosocial adjustment following a stroke. Soc Sci Med 28:239–247, 1989

Thornton S, Brotchie J: Reminiscence: a critical review of the empirical literature. Br J Clin Psychol 26:93–111, 1987

Toseland RW, Rossiter CM: Group interventions to support family caregivers: a review and analysis. Gerontologist 29:438–448, 1989

Toseland RW, Smith GC: Effectiveness of individual counseling by professional and peer helpers for family caregivers of the elderly. Psychol Aging 5:256–263, 1990

Toseland RW, Rossiter CM, Labrecque MS: The effectiveness of peer-led and professionally led groups to support family caregivers. Gerontologist 29:465–471, 1989

Toseland RW, Rossiter CM, Peak T, et al: Comparative effectiveness of individual and group interventions to support family caregivers. Soc Work 35:209–217, 1990

Toseland RW, Labrecque MS, Goebel ST, et al: An evaluation of a group program for spouses of frail elderly veterans. Gerontologist 32:382–390, 1992

Verhaeghen P, Marcoen A, Goossens L: Improving memory performance in the aged through mnemonic training: a meta-analytic study. Psychol Aging 7:242–251, 1992

Viney LL, Benjamin YN, Preston CA: An evaluation of personal construct therapy for the elderly. Br J Med Psychol 62 (part 1):35–41, 1989

Watt LM, Wong PT: A taxonomy of reminiscence and therapeutic implications. Journal of Gerontological Social Work 16:37–57, 1991

Weiss JC: Group therapy with older adults in long-term care settings: research and clinical cautions and recommendations. Journal for Specialists in Group Work 19:22–29, 1994

Wolfson L, Miller M, Houck P, et al: Foci of interpersonal psychotherapy (IPT) in depressed elders: clinical and outcome correlates in a combined IPT/nortriptyline protocol. Psychotherapy Research 7:45–56, 1997

Youssef FA: The impact of group reminiscence counseling on a depressed elderly population. Nurse Pract 15:32, 35–38, 1990

Zarit SH, Teri L: Interventions and services for family caregivers. Annual Review of Gerontology and Geriatrics 11:241–265, 1991

Zarit SH, Cole KD, Guider RL: Memory training strategies and subjective complaints of memory in the aged. Gerontologist 21:158–164, 1981

Zarit SH, Anthony CR, Boutselis M: Interventions with caregivers of dementia patients: comparison of two approaches. Psychol Aging 2:225–232, 1987

Neuropsychiatry in Nursing Homes

Barry W. Rovner, M.D.

Ira R. Katz, M.D.

Constantine G. Lyketsos, M.D., M.H.S.

Existing research demonstrates that nursing homes are the modern mental institutions for elderly people in the United States. Unfortunately, training of nursing home staff and physicians, processes of care, and the recognition and treatment of mental disorders do not reflect the current level of scientific knowledge in psychiatry (Rovner and Katz 1992). Consequently, the nursing home represents one of the greatest challenges in clinical geriatric neuroscience. Although it is important to recognize the promise of basic and clinical research for developing treatments that may prevent or cure Alzheimer's disease, it is also necessary to apply scientific knowledge about the relationships between brain disease and behavior to develop strategies for caring for patients with dementia on a day-to-day basis.

Although the prevalence of nursing home residency for those over 65 is approximately 5%, 20%–50% of people over 65 will live in nursing homes at some point before

death (German et al. 1992). The cost of their care is enormous:

> In 1989 the total cost of nursing home care was $47.9 billion, or 8% of all health care expenditures. This was a 12% increase from the year before, and exceeded the 9% average increase observed for the 1980s overall. The bulk (64%) of nursing home expenditures are financed by public programs, either directly through Medicaid (43%) or Medicare (about 3%), or indirectly from transfer payments (i.e., the Medicaid mandated contributions from the resident's social security income; 18%). Given the projected considerable increase in the number and proportion of older Americans, the use of and expense associated with nursing homes has become an issue of considerable national concern. (Wolinsky et al. 1992, p. 173)

The extent of this concern became evident in a study of projected nursing home costs. Kemper et al. (1991) estimated that it will cost $60 billion to pay for future nursing home care for Americans who turned 65 in 1990. This projection is based on data that indicate that 43% of this cohort will enter a nursing home during their lives and will spend an average of 2.8 years there.

Recognizing that the dementia syndrome, so prevalent in this population, is the expression of a brain disease and not the consequence of normal aging has been a major advance, a concept only relatively recently accepted by the nursing home industry and the governmental agencies that regulate it. Gradually, making the diagnosis of dementia (when appropriate) in nursing homes has become an acceptable, indeed a required, practice (e.g., note the PASARR [preadmission screening and annual resident review] regulations of the Omnibus Budget Reconciliation Act of 1987). However, recognizing dementia syndromes as brain diseases has led to a denial, of sorts, of the noncognitive behavioral aspects of these disorders, such as depression, delusions, hallucinations, and states of agitation. Although supervision and provision of assistance in activities of daily living are essential components of care for patients with dementia in nursing homes, these noncognitive psychiatric symptoms frequently accompany the dementia syndrome and determine both the patients' needs for care and the quality of care they receive.

History

The modern nursing home can trace its origins to the almshouses and mental institutions of the nineteenth century, which, transformed incrementally by public policies, have come to resemble hospital facilities. As such, these once-derided places have gained respectability through their identification with more credible medical institutions. Along with that credibility has come the expectation that patients would be cared for using the expertise, knowledge, and technology characteristic of the best hospitals. The policies, procedures, and staffing patterns of most nursing homes are in fact based on this model:

> Indeed, nursing homes appear, at first glance, like a patient-care floor in a general hospital. As in a hospital, the center of activity, and often the physical center of the floor, is a nursing home station. A high-fronted desk, wide enough to permit 2 or 3 people to sit at it, looks out onto the corridor. Behind it and to the sides are books and manuals, miscellaneous supplies, racks filled with patients' charts, lockable medicine cabinets, and perhaps doors to a supply room and a staff bathroom or lounge. Not infrequently, diplomas or state licenses hang on the wall behind the nursing station, along with other official-looking documents, all neatly framed. (Vladeck 1980, p. 7)

Like patients in hospitals, most patients in nursing homes have medical disorders such as high blood pressure, stroke, heart disease, arthritis, or diabetes (Johnson and Grant 1985). They are cared for by nurses and seen by physicians, and they receive medications. The patients are expected more or less to lie in bed passively and receive the care given by the nursing staff.

The reality of the nursing home, however, is not reflected by the sterility of the medical model. Patients have been moved from sickbeds to Gerichairs, and the nursing home now echoes the bedlam of the psychiatric hospital in the era before the development of specific treatments:

> The characteristic picture is that of a dozen residents arrayed in front of a television or sitting in a hall, each staring ahead. If anyone is talking, it is mostly to herself. (Vladeck 1980, p. 26)

Epidemiology

The change in the kinds of patients cared for in nursing homes over the past 20 years is related to the aging of the population and the increasing prevalence of dementing conditions. Patients with these conditions, unlike their primarily medically ill counterparts, are in need of medical attention as a result of their mental, rather than their physical, symptoms. These changes are evident in successive nursing home surveys. The 1977 National Nursing Home Survey indicated that approximately 57% of patients had "chronic brain syndrome" or "senility" (National Center for Health Statistics 1979). By 1985, these conditions were diagnosed in 63% (National Center for Health Statistics 1987).

The Medical Expenditure Panel Survey indicated that, in 1996, 1.6 million persons resided in 16,800 nursing homes and approximately 70%–80% of these residents had dementia (Krauss et al. 1997). However, because only 2,100 nursing homes (12.5%) had dementia special care units, the majority of residents with dementia received general custodial care. In addition, the prevalence of behavior disorders among residents with dementia is high. In the 1987 National Medical Expenditure Survey, the characteristics of a national nursing home sample were examined and 11 behavior problems were grouped into four categories: wandering or safety problems, aggressive behaviors, collecting behaviors, and delusions or hallucinations (Jackson et al. 1997). Predictors of these behaviors included male gender, more severe cognitive impairment, dependence in activities of daily living, incontinence, psychiatric history, receptive communication deficits, and impaired walking and vision. This finding suggests that biological, psychological, and sociocultural factors all contribute to the development of behavior problems. However, nursing homes are ill equipped to treat these problems effectively.

Treatment of mental disorders in nursing homes is impeded by a variety of obstacles, including a shortage of specialized mental health professionals, lack of knowledge and training among nursing staff, lack of adequate payment for mental health care, and difficulty obtaining psychiatric services.

McGrew (1998) noted that although the traditional United States health care system distinguishes between physical and mental health, such a distinction is not made in nursing homes. Further, dementia, for some reason, has been segregated from other mental disorders in nursing homes. Overcoming the barriers that emerge as a consequence will require the cooperation and collaboration of nursing homes, local service providers, states, and the federal government.

Fragmentation of funding also accounts for limitations in mental health care for residents with dementia. Although the nursing home industry is generally a private enterprise, the public sector, largely through Medicare and Medicaid, contributes approximately half of the costs, roughly $40 billion annually. However, both the federal government and the states attempt to shift the cost of mental health care to the other. The best example of this cost shifting is the process known as *transinstitutionalization*, the movement of state-hospitalized psychiatric patients to federally supported nursing homes.

National survey findings indicating an increased prevalence of dementia are based on nonclinician reviews of records and interviews with staff rather than on findings obtained by psychiatrists during direct examination of patients. The former methods cannot reveal whether psychiatric or behavior disorders are the cause or consequence of institutionalization. Thus, until relatively recently, no studies had been carried out on the prevalence of mental disorders among new residents of nursing homes, studies in which psychiatrists examined large, systematically ascertained samples and made diagnoses using modern diagnostic criteria. In 1987–1989, as part of a National Institute of Aging Study, we (Rovner et al. 1990a) evaluated 454 residents newly admitted to a total of eight Baltimore area proprietary nursing homes. The overall objective was to analyze mental morbidity among nursing home residents, establish its magnitude and type, and assess its influence on quality of life.

The following list shows the prevalence of psychiatric disorders divided into four mutually exclusive diagnostic groups on the basis of presence and type of psychopathology:

1. *Dementia complicated:* Patients with dementing disorders complicated by depression, delusions, or delirium (*n* = 123, 27.1% of the entire sample; 40.2% of all patients with dementia)
2. *Dementia only:* Dementia patients without delusions, depression, or delirium (*n* = 183, 40.3% of the entire sample)
3. *Other psychiatric disorders:* Patients without dementia but with affective disorders or schizophrenia (*n* = 58, 12.8% of the entire sample)
4. *No psychiatric disorder:* Residents without any disorder (*n* = 90, 19.8% of the entire sample)

Overall, 364 new residents (80.2%) were considered by the examining research psychiatrists to have psychiatric disorders. The most common diagnosis was dementia (*n* = 306, 67.4%). Primary degenerative dementia of the Alzheimer's type was the most frequent cause of dementia (*n* = 172, 37.9% of the entire sample), followed by multi-infarct dementia (*n* = 81, 17.8% of the entire sample). Other dementia syndromes or causes of dementia included the dementia syndrome of depression, Parkinson's disease, and brain tumor. Of the patients without dementia (*n* = 148, 32.6%), 58 (12.8% of the entire sample) had psychiatric disorders such as affective disorder (*n* = 47, 10.4% of the entire sample; 31.8% of those without dementia) or schizophrenia (*n* = 11, 2.4% of the total; 7.4% of those without dementia).

In 1994–1996, a separate study was conducted to assess the morbidity of nursing home patients with dementia (Tariot et al. 1993). This study involved 187 consecutive patients admitted to Copper Ridge, a model nursing home program for patients with memory disorders and dementia, affiliated with the Johns Hopkins Neuropsychiatry and Memory Group. Sixty percent of the new residents had Alzheimer's disease, 16% had dementia due to cerebrovascular disease, and the remainder had dementia due to other causes, including mixed Alzheimer's and cerebrovascular disease, Parkinson's disease, alcohol-related dementia, and anoxic dementia. The average Mini-Mental State Exam score was 9. Patients also had high rates of noncognitive psychiatric disorders, including delusions (40%), major depression (21%), sleep disorder (36%), and hallucinations (15%). In addition, 40% of patients had been physically aggressive and 49% had wandered in the 2 weeks before admission. Ninety-two percent had at least one of the aforementioned disturbances.

There was also considerable medical comorbidity; patients had a median of five medical disorders. The most common were hypertension, diabetes, heart disease, stroke, eye conditions, and dental problems. Impairment of general health was rated using the Hopkins General Medical Health Rating (Lyketsos et al. 1997). General health was excellent in 12%, good in 42%, fair in 38%, and poor in 8%. It can be concluded, therefore, that on admission to a nursing home, patients with dementia exhibit a substantial degree of medical and psychopathological morbidity in addition to dementia.

These 137 patients were followed for 2 years. There were 47 deaths (mean survival time, 38 months). Cognition steadily declined, with the Mini-Mental State Exam score reaching an average of 5. Rates of behavioral disturbance remained high throughout the 2-year period. Physical aggression was not infrequent: there was a mean of 1.6 incidents per 1,000 resident days. Aggression was most likely to occur on day or evening shifts rather than at night. There was no significant variation in rates of aggression over time, across seasons, or over lunar cycles. Rates of aggression also were not related to resident density nor to the number of recently admitted patients. Therefore, it may be said that dementia patients being admitted to nursing homes exhibit substantially high rates of behavioral disturbance over time, resulting in great demands on staff and other providers of care. These high rates also make necessary an on-site expert psychiatric team to evaluate and treat such disturbances.

We (Katz et al. 1990) reported that the prevalence of major depression in nursing homes was 20% in 1989 and stated that major depression was treatable, even though it was associated with medical disorders that complicated diagnosis and treatment (Parmelee et al. 1989).

In 1991, we (Parmelee et al. 1991) showed that pain was associated with depression in nursing home patients, particularly when a physical problem was present that was a potential source of pain. We hypothesized that either pain causes depression or depression intensifies pain. In 1992, we (Parmelee et al. 1992a) reported an increased mortality rate among nursing home residents with major depression, the increase apparently due to the fact that ill health tends to accompany major depression. In contrast, studying a different sample of nursing home patients and using different methods to control for medical illness, we (Rovner et al. 1991) found that depression was an independent risk factor for mortality over and above severity of medical illness. Depression increased the risk of death in depressed patients by 59%. In 1992, we (Parmelee et al. 1992b) found a 6.6% incidence of major depression over 1 year among nursing home residents and reported that 40% of patients who were depressed at the time of initial evaluation showed

no remission after 1 year.

As high as they are, the rates of diagnosable psychiatric disorders may in fact not reflect the magnitude of the neuropsychiatric problems present in nursing homes. In addition to those patients with major depressive disorder, there are substantial numbers of individuals with less severe but nonetheless clinically significant depressive symptoms, and still others with a persistently flat or blunted affect (Lawton et al. 1996). Moreover, in addition to the large numbers of patients with dementia, there may be others whose more focal deficits in executive functions due to aging (see Chapters 7 and 8 in this volume) or structural brain disease may have contributed to an inability to cope with medical illnesses and function in the community (Royall et al. 1993). Thus, the prevalence and range of nursing home residents with psychiatric disorders requires incorporating basic neuropsychiatric and mental health principles into the design of the care environment.

■ The Nursing Home Environment

In spite of these epidemiological and clinical realities, nursing homes continue to model themselves after general rather than neuropsychiatric hospitals. The medical staffs consist primarily of internists, family practitioners, or general practitioners, and the nursing staff consists primarily of individuals trained in medical-surgical nursing. Because neither the training of the nursing or medical staffs nor their approaches to care have changed to match the changes in the population, the original conceptualization of nursing homes as diminutive hospitals is no longer applicable. Furthermore, the fact that the majority of nursing home patients have conditions known to be associated with states of psychopathology including delirium, depression, delusions, and hallucinations and behavior disorders such as agitation, combativeness, and wandering has added an unanticipated sense of acuity and disturbance to the environment. Overwhelmed, nursing home staff have turned to restraints and psychotropic medications—often in an indiscriminate and uninformed way—to manage these psychiatric syndromes and behavior disorders. Ironically, nursing homes have returned to their origins as mental institutions in that most patients have mental disorders or disruptive behaviors that are difficult to manage and these patients are frequently physically and chemically restrained.

The nursing home environment is also notable for four additional features that have an impact on the treatment of neuropsychiatric disorders: extensive regulatory oversight by federal and state agencies, limited research into treatment, high rates of incapacity to consent to medical care, and special care units. Each feature will be discussed individually here.

Regulatory Oversight

Since the identification of abuses in nursing homes in the 1980s, these facilities have been subject to strict regulations, spelled out in the 1987 Omnibus Budget Reconciliation Act (OBRA; Omnibus Budget Reconciliation Act of 1987). This legislation has improved identification and treatment of mental disorders and has made mandatory the provision of mental health and activity services to residents. OBRA also raised educational standards for staff and initiated the gathering of clinical data on-line. However, some people believe that patient abuse has been defined very broadly in OBRA and that OBRA has created obstacles to the proper use of psychotropic medications and has perpetuated a view of psychotropic drugs as chemical restraints.

Documentation of specific psychiatric diagnoses and behavioral indications is now required when a psychotropic medication is prescribed. Garrard et al. (1991) estimated that had these regulations been in effect from 1976 to 1985, 50% of neuroleptic use in almost 9,000 nursing home residents would have been out of compliance. We (Rovner et al. 1992) found a 36% reduction in the number of prescriptions for neuroleptics from the 3 months before OBRA went into effect until 3 months afterward, but there was no increase in the number of prescriptions for sedative-hypnotics. The same trends existed 1 year later. Although quality assurance data on the prevalence of medical events such as bedsores, weight loss, falls with fractures, adverse incidents, urinary tract infections, and death revealed small but significant changes, the data were difficult to interpret because comparable data from previous years were unavailable.

Along with the pharmacoepidemiological studies demonstrating a nationwide downward trend in the use of psychotropic medications (except for antidepressants), clinical trials have shown that educational efforts may directly facilitate reduction of medication use. Meador et al. (1997) conducted a randomized controlled trial of an educational program to reduce antipsychotic prescribing for patients in nursing homes and found that use of antipsychotics in the six homes offering the educational program decreased from a frequency of 25.3 per 100 days at baseline to 19.7 per 100 days by month 6, a 23% reduction relative to control homes (P = .014). This study showed that focused educational programs may facilitate reduction of antipsychotic prescribing, above and beyond that attributable to regulatory changes. However, the durability of the changed prescribing practices and the degree to which they increase the quality of life for residents remain uncertain. Other studies have also demonstrated the feasibility of reducing use of these medications (Avorn et al. 1992).

Limited Research Into Treatment

Before the implementation of OBRA, depression was often unrecognized and untreated in nursing homes. Heston et al. (1992) found that of 868 persons with depression, only 10% were treated with antidepressants. More patients received neuroleptics and benzodiazepines, but most received no treatment at all. Similar findings were obtained by us (Rovner et al. 1991). Educational efforts to increase recognition of depression (the efforts being fueled by awareness of adverse outcomes of depression, such as mortality and disability) and the availability of newer antidepressants have led to increased antidepressant treatment. Lasser and Sunderland (1998) reported that 69% of nursing home patients referred to a geriatric psychiatry service were taking at least one psychotropic medication. Although many of these patients were taking benzodiazepines (32%) or antipsychotics (42%), antidepressants were most commonly prescribed; 61% of patients prescribed psychotropic medications were taking antidepressants, and 53% of this subgroup were taking serotonin reuptake inhibitors.

Llorente et al. (1998) examined the pharmacy records of 1,573 nursing home residents from the period 1994–1996 and found that 17.7% were receiving antipsychotic medications during that time. Seventy-one percent had appropriate diagnostic indications, 90% were receiving doses within recommended limits, and 90% had documented, appropriate target symptoms. Lower rates of use of anticholinergic agents, low doses of tricyclic antidepressants, and low rates of tricyclic antidepressant use were noted in patients with Alzheimer's disease, findings that reflect the fact that anticholinergic medications should be avoided in such patients, given the cholinergic deficit associated with the disease. In addition, all dosages of psychotropic medications were within the ranges given in the Health Care Financing Administration guidelines. The investigators concluded that newer-generation psychotropics have had a substantial impact on the prescribing practices of primary physicians treating nursing home residents.

Inappropriate medication use by nursing home residents is not limited to psychotropic drugs. Beers et al. (1991) reviewed the literature indicating inappropriate use of antihypertensives, nonsteroidal anti-inflammatory agents, oral hypoglycemics, analgesics, and a variety of other commonly prescribed medications. They proposed explicit criteria for inappropriate use of these medications and also suggested that these criteria might be useful for quality assurance review and clinical practice guidelines.

Borson and Doane (1997) examined psychotropic drug use in 39 skilled nursing facilities during the period 1989–1992 and found that the number of prescriptions for antipsychotics, sedative antihistamines, and sedative-hypnotics decreased significantly and that the prescribing of anxiolytics increased. In addition, they noted that the number of research studies on psychotropic drug use increased after the implementation of OBRA but that few studies focused on the effectiveness of drug treatment. The investigators recommended research into treatment outcomes as the next step to improve the care of this population.

There have been a number of well-designed clinical trials of treatment for agitated nursing home patients with dementia (see also Chapter 22 in this volume). Finkel et al. (1995) found that thiothixene (dose range, 0.25–18 mg) was significantly more effective than placebo in patients who were treated for 11 weeks. There were no notable changes in cognition scores or function. We (Katz et al. 1998) reported the results of a large randomized controlled trial of risperidone in a similar sample. We found that risperidone at 1 mg/day was more effective than placebo in reducing aggression and psychotic symptoms and did not cause significant extrapyramidal symptoms. Treatment at higher doses (2 mg/day) produced marginally better responses but was associated with extrapyramidal symptoms in approximately one-quarter of the patients.

In another study, we (Rovner et al. 1996) evaluated the efficacy of a dementia care program, consisting of activities, guidelines for use of psychotropic medications, and educational rounds. We found that, after 6 months, the program had reduced the number of behavior disorders and the use of antipsychotic medications and restraint, in comparison with the control group. The most important therapeutic element, in our opinion, was the establishment of a safe environment and active routines, to minimize dementia patients' exposure to unstructured situations.

Incapacity to Consent to Medical Care

The Patient Self-Determination Act mandates that federally funded nursing facilities inform patients of their rights under state law 1) to make decisions to accept or refuse medical or surgical treatment and 2) to formulate advance directives (Sabatino 1993). Advance directives allow currently competent patients to record the kind of medical procedures they desire should they become incompetent in

the future. These directives decrease the probability that a guardianship hearing will be necessary. Most states allow two types of advance directives: the living will and the durable power of attorney (see Chapter 41 in this volume).

As previously stated, the prevalence of dementing conditions and other psychiatric disorders in nursing homes is high. This situation suggests that many nursing home patients may not be competent to execute advance directives or to consent to medical procedures. Thus, although the Patient Self-Determination Act may improve autonomy in decision making, its intentions may not be fully realized. We (Janofsky and Rovner 1993) investigated the prevalence of advance directives among 186 nursing home patients. Of 29 residents assessed to be competent, 14 (48%) had a durable power of attorney or a living will. One person (3.5%) had a guardian. The remaining 14 patients (48.5%) had no advance directive. One hundred fifty-seven patients were assessed to be incompetent; 61 (39%) had a durable power of attorney or a living will, 44 (28%) had a guardian, and the remaining 52 (33%) had no form of advance directive. These data showed that substantial numbers of residents lacked either guardians or advance directives.

Special Care Units

Special care units in nursing homes have evolved as potentially innovative approaches to care. The underlying theory of treatment generally is based on the identification and treatment of excess disability, compensation for lost abilities through environmental and social support, and systematic evaluations of residents for potentially reversible medical and neuropsychiatric disorders. These units are usually costly to develop because they require modification of existing designs or creation of new ones, as well as recruitment and training of personnel, to create higher staff-patient ratios. Special care units often charge higher daily rates, and therefore the care may be out of reach for most nursing home patients with dementia.

Ohta and Ohta (1988) were among the first to note the variability among dementia special care units and the heterogeneity of the patients who reside there. Perhaps for these reasons, it has been difficult to assess the effectiveness of special care units. Gold et al. (1991) found that such units appeared to be associated with care of a higher quality than that on traditional units but that the quality of special care units was by no means uniform. Holmes et al. (1990) compared the characteristics of patients with dementia residing on these units with the characteristics of their counterparts on other units within the same facilities and found that the two groups differed in levels of cognitive impairment, behavior, functioning, and physical status. They also found that despite a higher prevalence of behavior disorders among special care patients, staff caring for these patients did not view the disturbances as more severe, and the investigators suggested that the specialized staff were able to adjust to these behaviors. Sloane et al. (1991) conducted a case-control study involving 625 patients with dementia on 31 dementia special care units and 32 traditional units in five states. They found that special care units were associated with reduced use of physical restraints but not of psychotropic drugs and that different variables determined the use of physical restraints and psychotropic medications on the two types of units.

In another study, Sloane et al. (1998) examined the prevalence of agitated behaviors in a representative sample of Alzheimer's disease special care units, to determine the extent to which agitation is associated with aspects of the treatment environment. They found that the proportion of residents exhibiting agitated behavior varied from 0% to 38%. Independent correlates of low agitation levels included favorable scores on measures of the physical environment and of staff treatment activities, low rates of use of physical restraints, small unit size, low levels of resident functional dependency, and fewer comorbid conditions.

Two single-site studies evaluated the outcome of treatment on special care units. Benson et al. (1987) reported increased levels of mental, emotional, and self-care functioning in patients admitted to special care units, and we (Rovner et al. 1990b) found that the functional capacity of patients on special care units remained stable, whereas that of patients on other units declined.

Phillips et al. (1997) examined Minimum Data Set assessments of 77,337 residents in more than 800 facilities, including 1,228 residents in 48 facilities with special care units. They found no statistically significant difference in the rate of decline (nine outcomes were measured) among residents on special care units and residents on traditional units. They concluded that although special care units may have provided unmeasured benefits to families and residents, those benefits did not include slowing rates of functional decline.

Principles of Care

In practice, the perceptions of nursing staff are critical in determining whether or not a behavior disorder is present. Different observers may have differing views about whether a particular behavior is an expected and accepted occurrence or a disturbance that offends or threatens caretakers and the homeostasis of the environment. In this light, the definition of a behavior disorder includes ele-

ments of the dispositions of the patient and of the observer and their interaction within the environment. This point underscores the importance of education of caregivers in nursing homes.

The underlying brain disease exists independent of the environment, but how the disease manifests itself (i.e., whether or not a behavior disorder emerges as a symptom of disease) reflects the interaction of a number of processes. A clarifying distinction in this regard is the recognition of *predisposing features* and *precipitating factors*. Patients with dementia are predisposed to behavioral disturbances on the basis of 1) specific syndromes marked by depression, delusions, and hallucinations; 2) delirium; and 3) poor impulse control, impaired judgment, and poor regulation of mood secondary to the brain damage. Precipitating factors may be environmental events such as recent nursing home placement, a change of rooms, changes of caregivers, uninformed approaches to care, or exposure to threatening activities or circumstances that overwhelm cognitive capacities.

This reasoning leads to parallel but distinctive treatment interventions. From the neuropsychiatric perspective, recognizing that a patient's behavior is the reflection of brain disease, rather than of a willful or manipulative nature, and that depression, delirium, delusions, and hallucinations may represent biological aberrations and symptoms of the underlying disease leads to the directing of treatment toward the somatic therapies found to be beneficial in other patients with these neuropsychiatric symptoms.

Although neurological influences are important in the genesis of behavior disorders, psychosocial influences are important as well. Patients are exposed to environments and persons whom they may not fully comprehend or recognize, predisposing them to a sense of uncertainty, frustration, and lack of direction. Because of these predispositions, the provocations or precipitating factors in the environment may lead to behavioral disturbance. It is thus important to understand the behavior in its social context within the nursing home so that interventions can be designed within that context to prevent the emergence of behavior disorders.

Treatment is optimized when it is possible to evaluate and treat patients on site and transfer patients in need of acute care at a psychiatric hospital. The latter is necessary because some residents require brief psychiatric hospitalization for stabilization. Hospitalizations of agitated patients with dementia are associated with reductions in general psychiatric symptoms and agitation and improvements in depression and global functioning, without adverse effects on cognitive states (Kunik et al. 1996).

◼ Optimizing Care and Related Care Issues

Essential to the success of any psychiatric program in a nursing home is proper education of clinical and administrative staff. This education is an ongoing effort that incorporates use of written material, formal lectures, and hands-on teaching during patient care. Staff should be presented with basic facts and terminology about psychiatric disorders, information about available treatments, and data supporting the efficacy of those treatments. Special attention should be paid to psychopharmacology, electroconvulsive therapy, and the ability to effect change through psychotherapy or environmental and other behavioral interventions.

Staff should learn how to obtain histories from patients and informants, understand the process of neuropsychiatric diagnosis, and develop optimal clinical approaches and environmental modifications. Basic rating scales can be used to facilitate patient evaluation and outcome assessment. We propose the use of the Mini-Mental State Exam (Folstein et al. 1975) or the Severe Impairment Rating Scale (Rabins and Steele 1994) to rate cognition, the Cornell Scale for Depression and Dementia (Alexopoulos et al. 1988) to rate depression and dementia, and the Psychogeriatric Dependency Rating Scale (Wilkinson et al. 1980) or the Neuropsychiatric Inventory (Cummings et al. 1994) to rate behavioral disturbance.

It is also helpful for nursing home staff to develop an accurate understanding of the OBRA regulations. This understanding increases awareness of the restrictions under which nursing homes operate but also clarifies the fact, for example, that any appropriate psychopharmacological treatments are permissible with proper documentation. The intent of the OBRA regulations is not to direct the practice of medicine but rather to ensure the protection of patients. Thus, the practice of neuropsychiatry according to current standards of care is not only possible—it is necessary. Of particular importance in this process is a close alliance with the consulting pharmacists who oversee administration of medications in the nursing home.

Another important aspect of psychiatric practice is patient decision-making capacity. As noted earlier, most patients are not capable of directly providing informed consent and making treatment decisions. It behooves the psychiatrist to involve the patient's family in the clarification of the patient's advance directive soon after the patient has been admitted. The preferred method is to convene a diagnostic conference at which nursing home staff (e.g., a nurse and a social worker) are also present. Such a confer-

ence allows for clear communication between families and staff about treatment preferences, creates rapport between the neuropsychiatrist and the family, and helps the neuropsychiatrist understand how families make health care decisions.

The development of special staff expertise also helps improve care. Given the high volume and complexity of neuropsychiatric disturbances, and the inability of most patients to report response to interventions, the neuropsychiatrist must rely on nursing home staff to appraise a patient's response. This staff can include "psychiatric expert" nurses or aides who understand psychotropic medications and behavioral interventions and who are familiar with standardized rating scales.

The success of a nursing home neuropsychiatric program depends as well on the integration of neuropsychiatric care with all other forms of care, including care by activity therapists, nurses, social workers, occupational and physical therapists, and especially physicians treating the patient's comorbid medical disorders. In addition, the neuropsychiatrist must meet regularly with other health care professionals to evaluate new patients and assess their responses to treatment. At the very minimum, rapid rounds can be conducted each day by nursing staff, with other professionals invited to participate. Such rounds permit identification of patients who are developing new behavioral disturbances or new medical problems. These rounds are best conducted at the change to the evening shift. In addition, a weekly interdisciplinary round is critical, in which all professionals meet to review patient progress and discuss difficult cases. This meeting also serves as a learning opportunity for all professionals in attendance.

Admission evaluations should include a review of the present illness, psychiatric symptoms, family and personal histories, medical history, and current medications. Also at the time of admission, cognitive function, independence in activities of daily living, behavior, and general health should be rated, with input from outside informants taken into account, using standardized scales. An experienced nurse can complete a patient evaluation, rating scales included, in 1–2 hours. The neuropsychiatrist working with the nursing team can review evaluations on rounds, to decide whether further assessment is necessary before treatment is begun. In instances in which patients entering a nursing home are already under psychiatric care by outsider providers, it is important to involve these providers.

In the case of patients who are found not to have neuropsychiatric disorders on admission, reassessment every 6–9 months is useful to detect possible incident changes. Neuropsychiatric reassessment might also be performed in response to a particular change in a patient (e.g., the onset of significant behavioral or mental disturbances) or to a significant change in score on one of the standardized scales (e.g., a decrease in score of more than three points on the Mini-Mental State Exam in a patient without a previous diagnosis of dementia).

The majority of patients admitted to nursing homes have chronic diseases, many of which are progressive or incurable. Most patients are entering the final residence of their lives. The vast majority of nursing home patients will live in the nursing home for an average of approximately 3–4 years before death. For these patients, the goals of care relate to quality of life (being symptom free and comfortable), functioning (maintaining the highest possible levels), longevity, and maintaining of dignity. It is important that staff adopt a can-do philosophy rather than a nihilistic one. Small improvements are almost always possible and can be of tremendous benefit in terms of boosting staff and patient morale.

Knee-jerk responses or prescribing of medications for poorly defined problems should be avoided. The latter often occurs when there is a crisis after hours: a nurse calls a physician to report an "agitated" patient, and the physician prescribes an antipsychotic medication without carefully assessing the patient. Interventions ought to be evidence based as much as possible. Unfortunately, as indicated earlier, scientific evidence regarding outcomes of treatment for neuropsychiatric disorders in nursing homes is sparse. However, an increasing number of studies have been conducted that can inform neuropsychiatric practice. Overall, treatment in the nursing home requires flexibility, optimism, hope, and willingness to work with an interdisciplinary team on all aspects of care.

By the time of admission to the nursing home, most patients have moderate to severe dementia. The underlying disease causing the dementia is typically incurable (see Chapter 24 in this volume). However, for patients with Alzheimer's disease, even at moderate to advanced stages, vitamin E at dosages of 1,000–2,000 IU/day may be prescribed, in an attempt to slow disease progression. For postmenopausal women, estrogen replacement therapy should be considered; this treatment prevents heart attacks and osteoporosis and may slow the progression of dementia. There is also evidence that treatment with nonsteroidal anti-inflammatory agents may slow the progression of disease, although this has not been proven conclusively. In treating vascular dementia, persistent efforts should be made to reduce risk factors for stroke (see Chapter 23 in this volume). Good control of diabetes, hypertension, and heart disease, as well as smoking cessation (required in most nursing homes), is necessary. Treatment with low-dose aspirin or an anticoagulant such as ticlopidine or warfarin may be appropriate.

In addition to treating the disease causing the dementia, the focus of interventions in patients with dementia is on relieving cognitive symptoms and possibly preventing functional decline, using cholinesterase inhibitors.

The use of tacrine and donepezil has been approved for these purposes. The use of other new medications, which are cholinesterase inhibitors as well, appears close to approval. Side effects of treatment with tacrine and donepezil are consistent with those associated with systemic elevations of acetylcholine levels and include increased stomach acid secretion, nausea, vomiting, diarrhea, increased vagal tone with bradycardia and syncope, and muscle cramps. Tacrine also affects the liver; use of the drug requires liver function tests every 2 weeks. The efficacy of treatment with these medications in patients with advanced dementia is not well established. However, because some of these patients may benefit, use of tacrine or donepezil should be considered in all cases.

Perhaps the most important type of care for patients with dementia is supportive care. Stabilization and expert management of comorbid medical conditions are essential. Patients with dementia are vulnerable to delirium, which may manifest itself as uncooperativeness and aggression. Sudden changes in behavior should always be investigated, with the possibility kept in mind that they were caused by a new medical condition (e.g., a urinary tract infection). In addition, patients are vulnerable to the toxic effects of medicines; confirmation, on admission, of medical diagnoses and medications being taken can prevent polypharmacy and the attendant drug interactions.

The three main safety concerns related to patients in nursing homes are falls, wandering, and aggression. Patients should be assessed periodically for gait apraxia and deconditioning, particularly after periods of illness that may have restricted mobility. Physical therapy should be used liberally to improve conditioning. Additionally, in the case of patients who cannot walk, efforts should be made to maintain mobility and independence through the use of devices such as safety chairs that enable walking, wheelchairs, walkers, and canes.

The risk of wandering and leaving the nursing home is high, particularly when a locked unit is not available. Risk factors include sleep disorder, male gender, and advanced dementia. Patients who have a history of wandering benefit from locked units or electronic tags that indicate departure from the nursing home. One of the best ways to prevent wandering is to engage patients in structured activities, so that the boredom and uncertainty that lead to wandering are avoided.

Aggression is a particularly common problem and can

be divided into two types (see Chapter 22 in this volume). The first type of aggression occurs in the context of daily care and is directed at staff attempting to assist the patient. This type of aggression does not respond well to pharmacological therapy and may be best addressed through teaching by staff of practical behavioral management skills. Aggression occurring outside the context of daily care and directed toward other residents or visitors is often unpredictable. Many aggressive patients also have exacerbations of medical problems, delirium, depression, delusions, hallucinations, or very severe dementia. Treatment of other comorbid conditions is important and typically leads to reduced aggression. In rare instances, patients may remain unpredictably aggressive despite environmental and pharmacological interventions. Ongoing trial-and-error approaches, including trials of antipsychotics or benzodiazepines at high doses, may be necessary. Although the use of restraint generally should be avoided, severely aggressive patients require restraint for protection of themselves and others.

Conclusions

Although many of the clinical observations and recommendations in this chapter may seem obvious, and although they are essential elements of care in other medical and neuropsychiatric settings, they are new to the care of patients in nursing homes. One need only recall that recognizing the high prevalence of dementia and the excessive use of restraints and psychotropic medications is a recent advance. Much remains to be accomplished in the area of care for nursing home patients. The lack of knowledge about, lack of interest in, and lack of resources for such care have all contributed to the maintaining of "warehousing" as the standard of care in nursing homes. Because of this approach to care, few administrators or physicians in nursing homes have emphasized the need for psychosocial rehabilitation for dementia patients or organized a system of care to provide it.

Because of the lack of public awareness as well, and the reluctance of federal agencies to provide reimbursement, psychosocial rehabilitation programs are far from being regular and essential aspects of nursing home care. The chief obstacle is cost; lack of mental health professionals trained in geriatrics is another obstacle. With regard to the former, 82% of nursing home administrators and 73.6% of directors of nursing who participated in the 1992 National Telephone Survey of Nursing Homes said that current reimbursement was insufficient for care of residents with dementia and associated behavior disorders (Lombardo 1994). Access to psychiatrists was considered by survey participants to be limited significantly by low Medicaid reimbursement rates. The failure to finance mental health services adequately is the consequence of the division of governmental financing between acute and long-term care and the fragmentation of benefits for medical, social, and income needs.

Fifty percent of participants in a survey of long-term care nursing directors reported that an inadequate number of psychiatrists were available, and 66% reported that psychiatrists, though capably providing diagnostic and medication recommendations, were not offering advice on nonpharmacological management techniques, staff support, and family conflicts (Reichman et al. 1998). These concerns were believed by the nursing directors to be highly important in the day-to-day management and maintenance of mental health in nursing home patients and staff. Reichman et al. (1998) also found that a formal contract for psychiatric services increased the frequency of consultation and satisfaction with the service provided. These data demonstrate the importance of reimbursement mechanisms in terms of determining, at the very least, the frequency and quality of psychiatric care. Reichman and colleagues wrote: "This differential outcome is particularly important with respect to aspects of comprehensive care that are currently non-reimbursable, poorly reimbursed, or burdensome to bill under Medicare-fee-for-service rules. These fall mainly in the domain of liaison function such as psychosocial care planning, staff-support, and help with families" (p. 325)

Unfortunately, the prospect for devoting more resources toward improving psychiatric care in nursing homes is doubtful, given the current national emphasis on cost control. Even if costs could be demonstrated to be offset—by showing, for example, that psychiatric services prevent hip fractures due to mismanagement of psychotropic medications—reimbursement reform would not likely be forthcoming. Until patients and their families demand improvements in mental health care, the situation is not apt to improve. Our hope is that indicators of nursing home quality can be developed, to ensure provision of expert psychiatric care and to establish a rational basis on which care is reimbursed.

Psychosocial rehabilitation programs should become an integral part of reasonable and expected care. Mental health programs should prevent behavior disorders and functional decline due to inactivity and thus enable patients to achieve their highest levels of functioning and well-being. As Bachrach (1992) noted:

[Although] the gains that some can make are so small as to seem out of proportion to the effort it takes on the part of patient and personnel to produce them . . . they are so important that the institution must give each long-term patient encouragement and help to achieve his maximum of restoration. (p. 172)

We are stressing the importance of psychosocial rehabilitation and, even more basically, humanistic treatment of nursing home residents with dementia or other neuropsychiatric disorders. All too often, such appeals set off empty debates about the relative importance of high technology versus highly personal approaches to care. Such debates would be pointless here. There is a need for vigorous approaches to neuropsychiatric diagnosis for all patients with dementia and behavioral disturbances, to identify those with hallucinations, delusions, depression, or delirium. There is also a need for assessment of deficits (e.g., amnesia, aphasia, apraxia, and agnosia) and ensuring that all aspects of nursing home care are carried out with the knowledge of these deficits. Here there must be interactions between clinical neuroscience and front-line staff. If environmental interventions are to prevent or treat behavioral disturbances, they must be more than well-intentioned humanistic endeavors; they must be inferred from what is known about cognitive deficits in dementia, both in general and in the individual patient.

To provide this level of care, a complete revision of the nursing home industry will be required, to meet acceptable standards of neuropsychiatric care for patients in nursing homes. Elon (1993) discussed the disparity between the ideals and the realities of nursing home medical directorship and indicated that to fill the role adequately, greater financial commitment by facilities and reimbursement systems will be necessary. In the absence of such leadership, it will be difficult to implement other promising and innovative efforts, such as enriched educational and practice programs for nursing staff, the use of geriatric nurse practitioners, and collaborative relationships with psychiatrists. Future efforts to improve nursing home care might profitably be modeled on successful approaches already used in modern psychiatric, neuropsychiatric, and rehabilitation hospitals.

Summary

In this chapter, we reviewed the high prevalence of neuropsychiatric conditions and behavioral disturbances in nursing homes. We discussed how nursing homes currently are based on a medical model that may not be appropriate for the problems of their patients. Nursing homes are staffed by personnel who direct their care toward the treatment of medical conditions but not neuropsychiatric ones. This situation may lead to inappropriate use of physical and chemical restraints, an inability to reduce behavior disorders, and failure to improve the psychosocial functioning of patients. Improving the care of nursing home patients with neuropsychiatric disorders requires appreciation of the brain disturbances and how environmental circumstances contribute to both the genesis of problems and the potential for maximizing patients' cognitive, emotional, and physical functioning.

References

Alexopoulos GS, Abrams RC, Young RC, et al: Cornell Scale for Depression in Dementia. Biol Psychiatry 23:271–284, 1988

Avorn J, Soumerai SB, Everitt DE, et al: A randomized trial of a program to reduce the use of psychoactive drugs in nursing homes. N Engl J Med 327:168–173, 1992

Bachrach LL: Psychosocial rehabilitation and psychiatry in the care of long-term patients. Am J Psychiatry 149:1455–1463, 1992

Beers MH, Ouslander JG, Rollingher I, et al: Explicit criteria for determining inappropriate medication use in nursing homes. UCLA Division of Geriatric Medicine. Arch Intern Med 151:1825–1832, 1991

Benson DM, Cameron D, Humbach E, et al: Establishment and impact of a dementia unit within the nursing home. J Am Geriatr Soc 35:319–323, 1987

Borson S, Doane K: The impact of OBRA-87 on psychotropic drug prescribing in skilled nursing facilities. Psychiatr Serv 48:1289–1296, 1997

Cummings JL, Mega M, Gray K, et al: The Neuropsychiatric Inventory: comprehensive assessment of psychopathology in dementia. Neurology 44:2308–2314, 1994

Elon R: The nursing home medical director role in transition. J Am Geriatr Soc 41:131–135, 1993

Finkel SI, Lyons JS, Anderson RL, et al: A randomized, placebo-controlled trial of thiothixene in agitated, demented nursing home patients. Int J Geriatr Psychiatry 10:129–136, 1995

Folstein MF, Folstein SE, McHugh PR: Mini-Mental State: a practical method for grading the cognitive state of patients for the clinician. J Psychiatr Res 12:189–198, 1975

Garrard J, Makriss L, Dunham T, et al: Evaluation of neuroleptic drug use by nursing home elderly under proposed Medicare and Medicaid regulations. JAMA 265:463–467, 1991

German PS, Rovner BW, Burton LC, et al: The role of mental morbidity in the nursing home experience. Gerontologist 32:152–158, 1992

Gold DT, Sloane PD, Mathew LJ, et al: Special care units: a typology of care settings for memory-impaired older adults. Gerontologist 31:467–475, 1991

Heston LL, Garrard J, Makris L, et al: Inadequate treatment of depressed nursing home elderly. J Am Geriatr Soc 40:1117–1122, 1992

Holmes D, Teresi J, Weiner A, et al: Impacts associated with special care units in long-term care facilities. Gerontologist 30:178–183, 1990

Jackson ME, Spector WD, Rabins PV: Risk of behavior problems among nursing home residents in the United States. Journal of Aging and Health 9:451–472, 1997

Janofsky JS, Rovner BW: Prevalence of advance directives and guardianship in nursing home patients. J Geriatr Psychiatry Neurol 6:214–216, 1993

Johnson CL, Grant LA: The Nursing Home in American Society. Baltimore, MD, Johns Hopkins University Press, 1985

Katz IR, Simpson GM, Curlik SM, et al: Pharmacologic treatment of major depression for elderly patients in residential care settings. J Clin Psychiatry 51 (suppl):41–47, 1990

Katz I[R], Jeste DV, Mintzer JE, et al: Risperidone and the treatment of psychosis and aggressive behavior in patients with dementia. Poster presented at the annual meeting of the American Association of Geriatric Psychiatry, San Diego, CA, March 1998

Kemper P, Spillman BC, Murtaugh CM: A lifetime perspective on proposals for financing nursing home care. Inquiry 28:333–344, 1991

Krauss NA, Freiman NP, Rhoades JA, et al: Medical Expenditure Panel Survey, nursing home update, 1996 (AHCPR Publ No 97-0036). Rockville, MD, U.S. Government Printing Office, 1997

Kunik ME, Ponce H, Molinari V, et al: The benefits of psychiatric hospitalization for older nursing home residents. J Am Geriatr Soc 44:1062–1065, 1996

Lasser RA, Sunderland T: Newer psychotropic medication use in nursing home residents. J Am Geriatr Soc 46:202–207, 1998

Lawton MP, Parmelee PA, Katz IR, et al: Affective states in normal and depressed older people. J Gerontol B Psychol Sci Soc Sci 51:P309–P316, 1996

Llorente MD, Olsen EJ, Leyva O, et al: Use of antipsychotic drugs in nursing homes: current compliance with OBRA regulations. J Am Geriatr Soc 46:198–201, 1998

Lombardo NE: Overcoming barriers to mental health services for nursing home residents (AARP Public Policy Institute Publ No 9401). Boston, MA, Hebrew Rehabilitation Center, 1994

Lyketsos CG, Steele CS, Baker L, et al: Major and minor depression in Alzheimer's disease: prevalence and impact. J Neuropsychiatry Clin Neurosci 9:556–561, 1997

McGrew KB: The nursing home as mental health care provider: the mixed message and impact of nursing home reform. The Public Policy and Aging Report 9:1–16, 1998

Meador KG, Taylor JA, Thapa PB, et al: Predictors of antipsychotic withdrawal or dose reduction in a randomized controlled trial of provider education. J Am Geriatr Soc 45:207–210, 1997

National Center for Health Statistics: The 1985 National Nursing Home Survey: 1977 summary for the U.S.: vital and health statistics, series B, no 43 (DHHS Publ No PMS 79-1794). Washington, DC, U.S. Government Printing Office, 1979

National Center for Health Statistics: Preliminary data from the 1985 National Nursing Home Survey: advance data from vital and health statistics, no 142 (DHHS Publ No PMS 87-1250). Hyattsville, MD, Public Health Service, 1987

Ohta RJ, Ohta BM: Special units for Alzheimer's disease patients: a critical look. Gerontologist 28:803–808, 1988

The Omnibus Budget Reconciliation Act of 1987, Nursing Home Reform Amendments, 42 USC 1819

Parmelee P, Katz IR, Lawton MP: Depression among institutionalized aged: assessment and prevalence estimation. Journal of Gerontology 44:M22–M29, 1989

Parmelee P, Katz IR, Lawton MP: The relation of pain to depression among institutionalized aged. Journal of Gerontology 1:P15–P21, 1991

Parmelee P, Katz IR, Lawton MP: Depression and mortality among institutionalized aged. Journal of Gerontology 47:P3–P10, 1992a

Parmelee P, Katz IR, Lawton MP: Incidence of depression and long-term care settings. Journal of Gerontology 47:M189–M196, 1992b

Phillips CD, Sloane PD, Hawes C, et al: Effects of residence and Alzheimer's disease special care units on functional outcomes. JAMA 278:1340–1344, 1997

Rabins PV, Steele CD: A scale to measure impairment in severe dementia and similar conditions. Am J Geriatr Psychiatry 4:247–251, 1996

Reichman WE, Coyne AC, Borson S, et al: Psychiatric consultation in the nursing home: a survey of six states. Am J Geriatr Psychiatry 6:320–327, 1998

Rovner BW, Katz IR: Psychiatric disorders in the nursing home: a selective review of studies related to clinical care. Int J Geriatr Psychiatry 7:75–82, 1992

Rovner BW, German PS, Broadhead J, et al: The prevalence and management of dementia and other psychiatric disorders in nursing homes. Int Psychogeriatr 2:13–24, 1990a

Rovner BW, Lucas-Blaustein J, Folstein MF, et al: Stability over one year in patients admitted to a nursing home dementia unit. Int J Geriatr Psychiatry 5:77–82, 1990b

Rovner BW, German PS, Brandt LJ, et al: Depression and mortality in nursing homes. JAMA 265:993–996, 1991

Rovner BW, Edelman BA, Cox MP, et al: The impact of antipsychotic drug regulations (OBRA 1987) on psychotropic prescribing practices in nursing homes. Am J Psychiatry 149:1390–1392, 1992

Rovner BW, Steele CD, Shmuely Y, et al: A randomized trial of dementia care in nursing homes. J Am Geriatr Soc 44:7–13, 1996

Royall DR, Mahurin RK, True JE, et al: Executive impairment among the functionally dependent: comparisons between schizophrenic and elderly subjects. Am J Psychiatry 150:1813–1819, 1993

Sabatino CP: Surely the wizard will help us, Toto? Implementing the patient self-determination act. hastings Center Report 23:12–16, 1993

Sloane PD, Mathew LJ, Scarborough M, et al: Physical and pharmacologic restraint of nursing home patients with dementia: impact of specialized units. JAMA 265:1278–1282, 1991

Sloane PD, Mitchell SM, Preisser JS, et al: Environmental correlates of resident agitation in Alzheimer's disease special care units. J Am Geriatr Soc 46:862–869, 1998

Tariot PN, Podgorski CA, Blazina L, et al: Mental disorders in the nursing home: another perspective. Am J Psychiatry 150:1063–1069, 1993

Vladeck BC: Unloving Care: The Nursing Home Tragedy. New York, Basic Books, 1980

Wilkinson IM; Graham-White J: Psychogeriatric dependency rating scales (PGDRS): a method of assessment for use by nurses. Br J Psychiatry 137:558–565, 1980

Wolinsky FD, Callahan CM, Fitzgerald JF, et al: The risk of nursing home placement and subsequent death among older adults. Journal of Gerontology 47:S173–S182, 1992

38

Genetic Interventions

Kirk C. Wilhelmsen, M.D., Ph.D.

Genetics, the science that deals with heredity, is having an increasingly pervasive influence on medicine and biological science. This influence is due in large part to the success of genetics in elucidating biological processes in experimental systems and in the identification of genes involved in human disease. Over the last 100 years, investigators have developed the concept of the gene and the chromosomal theory of heredity, which included the elucidation of the structure of DNA (Watson 1987). These developments have resulted in an explosion of information about the organization and structure of genes and their roles in diseases. Genetic analysis is expected to lead to the identification of genes that play key roles in behaviors. The impact of genetics on geriatric neuropsychiatry will be more apparent as DNA analysis is used to predict both favorable and unfavorable responses to medications and establish presymptomatic susceptibility to disease.

Most of the successes of human genetic analysis have been in the identification of rare mutations that produce diseases with simple patterns of inheritance, called *Mendelian traits* (e.g., cystic fibrosis [Kerem et al. 1989a, 1989b; Riordan et al. 1989] and Huntington's disease ("A Novel Gene Containing a Trinucleotide Repeat That Is Expanded and Unstable on Huntington's Disease Chromosomes" 1993). In Mendelian traits, one-fourth or one-half

of the relatives of affected individuals are affected. Non-Mendelian traits do not have predictable modes of inheritance. The causal mutations for most common genetic diseases with Mendelian inheritance have been identified (McKusick and Almon 1998). But it will be many years before mutations are identified for all of the well-described, rare heritable diseases. New mutations are continually being identified, increasing our understanding of gene structure and function.

The work on Mendelian traits has become the foundation for efforts to identify genes that play roles in common diseases produced by the complex interaction between genes and environment, diseases we refer to as *complex traits*. The vast majority of behaviors and diseases of interest to geriatric neuropsychiatry are complex traits.

Because specific genetic findings relevant to geriatric neuropsychiatry are limited, most of this chapter is of a general nature. It will be important for all caregivers and investigators to understand the meaning and context of genetic findings that are made in the next decade.

Genes, Expression, and Diversity

Proteins form the scaffold and machinery in cells and are made of chains of amino acids determined by the structure of DNA. The order of amino acids determines in large part how proteins fold. Some proteins require the assistance of other proteins to adopt the proper three-dimensional structure. The machinery needed to replicate and maintain DNA and to translate its coded information into proteins is made of protein and RNA, a molecule similar in structure to DNA.

DNA is a long macromolecule composed of two paired helical strands of repeating subunits called *nucleotides*. Each nucleotide contains a phosphate group, a five-carbon sugar, and a cyclic nitrogen–containing base. The backbone of each strand is composed of alternating sugars and phosphates with phosphodiester linkages. Cyclic nitrogen bases covalently bond to the sugar group and form hydrogen bonds between the strands, strictly according to base-pairing rules. Thus the bases adenine and thymine are paired, as are guanine and cytosine. RNA differs from DNA in that RNA uses a different sugar and is usually single stranded, and the cyclic nitrogen base uridine replaces thymine.

Cellular machinery replicates DNA by separating its strands and applying hydrogen-bonding rules to reconstruct the paired strands. Similarly, RNA molecules are "transcribed" from one of the temporarily separated DNA strands using base-pairing rules. Elaborate protein- and RNA-containing complexes edit primary RNA transcripts, often "splicing" out internal segments, called *introns*, before making proteins. Proteins are linearly encoded in RNA using a set of three adjacent nucleotides, called a *codon*, to specify the order of polymerization of amino acids in proteins. Additional DNA and RNA nucleotide sequences adjacent to protein coding sequences are used to regulate the timing and level of protein production. The DNA used to encode a protein and its regulatory elements is referred to as a *gene*. Humans have between 50,000 and 100,000 genes encoded in 3.3 billion nucleotide pairs of DNA.

Before cell division, nuclear DNA molecules in cells are replicated. During cell division, nuclear DNA molecules in cells are coiled and condensed into microscopically visible elements called *chromosomes*. One copy of each chromosome ends up in each daughter cell that results from the division of the parental cell. Humans have 22 paired chromosomes and 2 sex chromosomes. One sex chromosome and 1 of each of the 22 paired chromosomes are derived from the chromosomes present in the sperm and oocyte that fuse to form a zygote. Generally speaking, the structure of chromosomes remains intact through the replication of chromosomal DNA, from the time the sperm and oocyte are fused until new sperm and oocytes are produced. During spermatogenesis and oogenesis, the homologous

chromosomes align. They also frequently break and rejoin through a process called *recombination*. Thus a particular maternal chromosome may be derived from both maternal grandparents.

With the exception of genes that are encoded on sex chromosomes, all individuals have two copies of each gene. However, not all genes have identical DNA sequences. Some sequence changes affect how, when, and where genes are expressed, whereas others change the amino acids in the protein product. Common variants in proteins, called *allozymes*, are found throughout the population. However, rare gene variants are frequently referred to as *mutations*, particularly when the DNA changes produce disease or have been the result of recent errors in DNA replication. Sexual reproduction with chromosomal recombination and new mutations creates a limitless variation in genetic constitution. The bulk of human diversity comes from the interaction between common gene variations and environmental factors.

In addition to nuclear DNA, there is also mitochondrial DNA. Mitochondria are intracellular organelles that use oxidation of carbon compounds to produce adenosine triphosphate (ATP), the cellular currency for energy. The mitochondrial genome is a 16,000–base-pair circle of DNA. Each mitochondrion has several genomes that replicate and are divided between daughter organelles as the mitochondrion divides. Most cells have many mitochondria that appear to be divided by chance between daughter cells during division. Rare genetic diseases have been identified with maternal inheritance, a consequence of the fact that all human mitochondria in the zygote come from the oocyte and none come from the sperm. Changes in the sequence of genes also occur during the development and regeneration of tissues in an organism. Some changes stem from errors in DNA replication or repair, called *mutations*, which can cause diseases such as cancer (Hansen and Cavenee 1988; Kinzler and Vogelstein 1996). Other DNA sequence changes in non–germ line cells are the result of cellular processes that affect specific genes. For example, rearrangements in the immunoglobulin gene allow the generation of new types of antibodies (Hayday et al. 1985; Tonegawa 1988).

Processes that do not affect DNA sequence can also affect gene expression. The best studied of these effects are imprinting and X chromosome inactivation. Imprinting is the result of differential expression of maternally and paternally inherited genes (Cassidy and Schwartz 1998; Lewin 1998; Surani 1998). X chromosome inactivation permits balancing of effects of genes on sex chromosomes (Brockdorff and Duthie 1998; Jaenisch et al. 1998). Males have an X chromosome and a Y chromosome, and females have two X chromosomes. This arrangement could result in twice the amount of expression of some X chromosome genes in females. To compensate for this, each female cell has an inactivated X chromosome. This chromosomal inactivation stops genes from being used to make proteins. Thus a female is a mosaic of cells in which the X chromosome from either the mother or the father is inactivated.

In addition to imprinting and inactivation, there are other mechanisms that modulate gene expression, but these mechanisms are less well understood. For example, exposure to certain stimuli can result in long-term changes in gene expression. Technology to measure gene expression for thousands of genes simultaneously has been developed (Lashkari et al. 1997). This technology has allowed investigators to study the correlation of cellular- and tissue-specific patterns of gene expression for large collections of genes after cells or organisms are exposed to drugs, toxins, or other stimuli such as learning.

Effects of Aging of the Genome

Changes in DNA occur as we age. Most changes are non-specific mutations (Osiewacz 1997). Aging is the most important risk factor for cancer that appears to be the direct result of mutations. The extent to which accumulation of mutations affects the process of aging is not certain.

One consistent finding in studies of aging is that mutations can be detected with an increasing frequency in mitochondrial DNA. These studies have focused on the accumulation of specific mutations detected by powerful molecular biology techniques. Most experts would argue that because there are many mitochondria per cell and because mitochondria have more than one copy of DNA, the observed mutations would not have a significant effect on function. On the other hand, all of the deleterious mutations combined could have an effect on function. This view is supported by the observation that certain mitochondrial functions (e.g., cytochrome-c oxidase activity) decline in muscle fibers as we age (Brierley et al. 1997).

It has been widely observed that cells from normal tissue can divide only a limited number of times (Berube et al. 1998; Shore 1998). This finding suggests that there is some cellular mechanism that regulates the number of times a cell divides. One candidate for this mechanism is the shortening of telomere length. Telomeres are the ends of a chromosome's arms. The enzyme that synthesizes a new strand of DNA, DNA polymerase, requires a single strand of DNA with a small bound "primer strand" to add new complementary bases. DNA synthesis with DNA polymerase proceeds in only one direction, and the end of a chromosome is not replicated by DNA synthesis. Thus without another mechanism to regenerate the ends of chromosomes, such chromosomes would become smaller with each round of DNA replication. Some cells have an enzyme, called *telomerase*, that can increase the length of the telomeres. But in most non–germ line cells, telomerase is not made and telomeres become shorter with each cell division.

Whether telomere length plays a physiological role in human aging is not known. Additional work on model systems suggests that there are other mechanisms that regulate cellular life spans. In addition, mutations in genes that can increase the life span of cells and organisms have been identified (Shore 1998). One of the most interesting examples of a mutation that can affect life expectancy in humans was identified by the positional cloning of the gene for Werner's syndrome (Yu et al. 1994, 1997). Patients with Werner's syndrome have a defect in a putative topoisomerase gene, appear to age rapidly, and have an increased risk of developing cancer. A defect in topoisomerase could be predicted to lead to a rapid accumulation of genetic defects.

Molecular Basis of Genetic Analysis

The goal of human genetics is to show that specific gene sequences predispose an individual to specific traits. There are many intermediate observations that can help investigators identify the chromosome location for, and ultimately the genes responsible for, specific traits. This process of using further refinements of the location of a gene to identify a gene is called *positional cloning* (Collins 1995). The positional cloning of the gene for Huntington's disease is an important example.

Linkage Studies

The focus of most previous positional cloning efforts has been on simple Mendelian traits. To find the genes involved in Mendelian disorders, researchers have studied the outcome of chromosomal recombination events in families. Thinking of a chromosome as color coded (see Figure 38–1) allows one to visualize graphically how a simple Mendelian trait would be localized. One would simply look for a correlation between inheriting a specific color-coded chromosome segment and development of a particular disease in a family.

In practice, markers are used to distinguish chromosomes. Markers are tools for monitoring the inheritance of chromosome segments. A marker is any feature that segregates from generation to generation as a simple trait with a

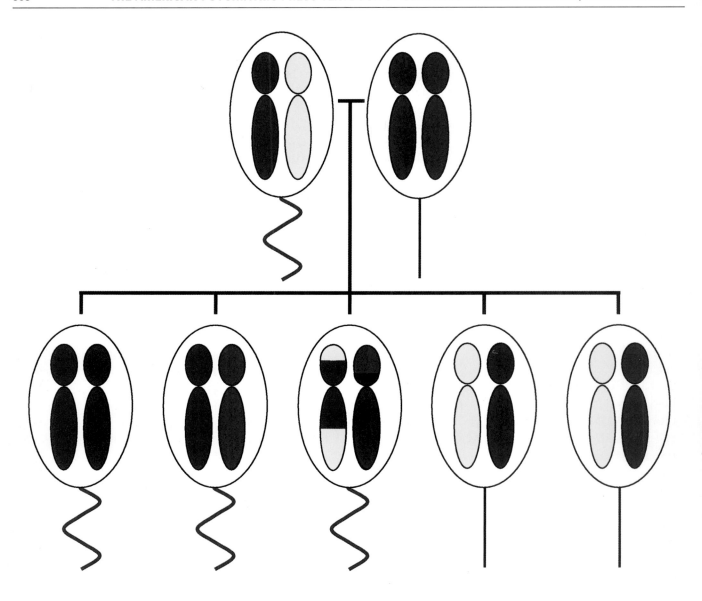

FIGURE 38–1.   Each hypothetical organism represented in this diagram has one shared chromosome and a straight or crooked tail. Each homologous chromosome is a different color in the parental generation *(top)*. During sexual reproduction, one chromosome from each parent is transmitted to the offspring *(bottom)*. In some cases, chromosomes are broken and rejoined, so that an individual receives portions of two grandparental chromosomes. In this example, a red crooked tail is inherited with at least a portion of the red chromosome; individuals with straight tails have inherited the yellow chromosome from their parent with the red tail.

specific chromosome location. The earliest markers were morphological features such as color blindness; these were followed by the more numerous and useful biochemical traits such as ABO blood type. The use of morphological and biochemical markers has largely been supplanted by the study of specific DNA sequence variations (Botstein et al. 1980; Weber and May 1989). Tens of thousands of segments of DNA in which the sequence varies have been identified.

The alternative forms of a marker are called *alleles.* By studying the inheritance of alleles for many different mark-

ers, one can establish the sequence of markers on chromosomes and detect the location of meiotic recombination events. There is usually no direct relationship between the markers used and the trait. In fact, the alleles on the chromosome associated with a disease are often different in different families.

Geneticists have developed mathematical methods to measure the likelihood that a gene for a trait is located at a specific chromosome location given the family structure and the observed marker and clinical data (Ott 1991). Some methods, referred to as *parametric methods*, take into account the effect of allele number (i.e., whether it takes one or two alleles to cause a trait [dominance]), variable age at onset, the possibility that some gene carriers are unaffected (penetrance), and the possibility that multiple genes can produce the same condition (locus heterogeneity). Because parametric methods require estimates of parameters that are difficult to estimate in advance, there has been a trend toward using nonparametric analyses that rely on simple paradigms, particularly for complex traits.

The simplest form of nonparametric analysis is called the *sib-pair method*, in which excess chromosome sharing is looked for (Blackwelder and Elston 1985). When two siblings (a sib pair) are concordant for a trait, it is more likely that they inherited the same chromosome that has the gene for the trait from both parents. In the case of a random chromosome, siblings are expected to have inherited the same chromosome from both parents, the same chromosome from one of their parents, or different chromosomes from both parents (probability of one in four, two in four, and one in four, respectively). In a population of siblings, the average number of chromosomes shared between siblings is one. In a population of siblings concordant for a trait, there is excess chromosome sharing (an average of between one and two) for the chromosomes containing the responsible genes. It is possible to extend this analysis to include large families and information from both affected and unaffected individuals.

The sib-pair method lends itself to simple parameterization including describing the size of particular gene effects and the effects of gene-environment interactions (Hauser et al. 1996; Risch 1990a, 1990b). The most commonly used parameter to describe the size of effects of a particular gene is analogous to the sibling relative risk (λ_s). λ_s is the frequency of a sibling of an affected individual being affected, divided by the population frequency for the trait. λ_s, as it is measured in most conditions, in fact indicates both genetic and environmental effects. Ultimately, it should be possible to break down λ_s to recurrence risk for individual genes and recurrence risk for environmental factors. The interaction between these relative risks, be they additive or multiplicative, will tell us much about the biology of underlying disease. Unfortunately, we cannot yet divide recurrence risk into its primary components in advance. The recurrence risk for common genes will not be greater than the total sibling recurrence risk. Estimating the size of the gene-specific recurrence risk allows one to estimate the sample size needed (Hauser et al. 1996).

With enough relatives of individuals who have specific diseases or traits, it is possible to map susceptibility loci. This approach has been strikingly successful for simple traits. As few as 13 individuals in a nuclear family may be

needed to map a susceptibility locus for an autosomal, dominant, simple Mendelian trait. However, it may take several thousand samples to map a susceptibility locus for complex traits.

The key to all genetic studies is the careful definition of a trait that has a significant heritability, along with the collection of the right family members in order to optimize the efficiency of the analysis. In gene mapping studies, a disease susceptibility locus can usually be localized to a broad chromosomal segment that represents approximately $\frac{1}{100}$–$\frac{1}{600}$ of the entire human genome. Collection of additional samples can often lead to reduction of this segment to less than $\frac{1}{3000}$ of the entire genome, but hundreds to thousands of samples are usually required.

Allelic Association Studies

An approach referred to as *allelic association analysis* has been used to map genes precisely for positional cloning. This approach has been used for many years with the histocompatibility complex, which has as a result been implicated in many diseases, including diabetes, multiple sclerosis, ankylosing spondylitis, and even narcolepsy (Kostyu 1991).

The basis of allelic association studies can be illustrated easily by studying the chromosomes of the descendents of a "founder" with a rare disease (Figure 38–2). The mutation that causes a rare disease in the founder is associated with specific marker alleles along a chromosome. After many generations, all of the individuals who have inherited the founder's mutation have a portion of the founder's chromosome. The likelihood that a specific allele will continue to be associated with a disease after many generations depends on the distance along the chromosome between the sequence and the mutation. As the distance between the mutation and the marker increases, it is increasingly likely that recombination events will break the association on the founder's chromosome.

Allelic association can also be seen with common traits. DNA sequence changes for common traits can either be due to sequence changes that occurred in prehistoric times that have been disseminated throughout the population or be due to the occurrence of many recent mutations. For traits due to ancient mutations, only markers linked extremely closely to the causal sequence variation will show an association because there will have been many opportunities for recombination during the many generations since the founder. Diseases in which there are many new mutations do not show allelic association because there are many founders.

Allelic association studies can be used to localize susceptibility genes precisely. The precision is dependent on

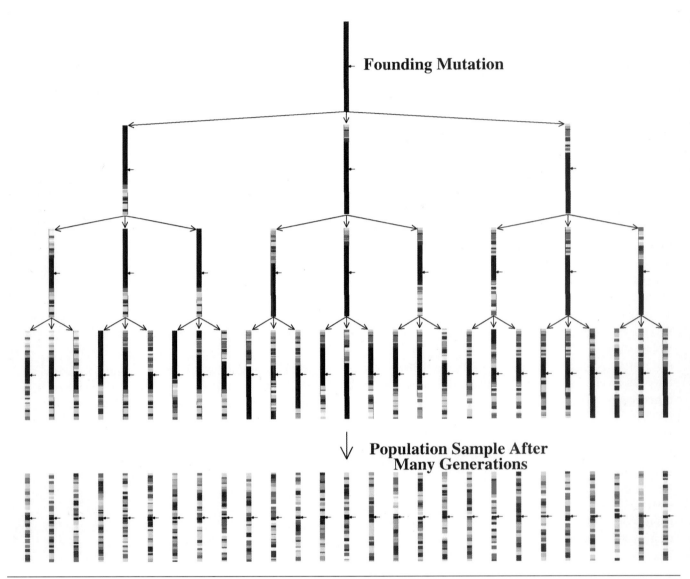

FIGURE 38–2. Chromosomes from a "founder" and his progeny who have inherited a mutation. The location of the mutation on the chromosome is indicated by an arrow. Only chromosomes from affected individuals are shown. The founder's chromosome is in black. Other chromosomes are variegated because there are limitless combinations of possible alleles for each gene and marker. Each meiotic segregation is an opportunity for chromosomes to recombine. With each generation, a smaller portion of the original founder's chromosome is present in the individuals who carry the founder's mutation. After many generations, there is essentially a random distribution of colors at any position on a chromosome, except for segments that contain the mutation.

the number of different mutations, the total number of generations since mutations occurred, and the number of individuals with each mutation. With traits that were established thousands of years ago, it is possible to localize disease susceptibility loci to chromosome segments that represent less than $\frac{1}{3000}$ of a human genome (approximately 1 million base pairs of DNA, or 20–40 genes). Frequently, association studies are used to show that specific DNA sequence variations cause disease. Before strongly associated sequence variations can be considered responsible for a disease, supporting data must usually be obtained.

The most common study design used in allelic association analysis is the case-control design. Use of the case-control design has resulted in the making of spectacular claims that ultimately have not been substantiated. The principal reason for such unsubstantiated conclusions is that there are many reasons an association can be detected, only one of which is significant.

The most common pitfall in case-control designs is population stratification. Case patients and control subjects need to have the same genetic background. The finding that a specific DNA sequence variation is more common among selected short Inuits than among selected tall African tribespeople should not lead one to assume that the DNA sequence variation studied affects stature. It is more likely that the presence of a specific DNA sequence variation is the result of the effects of the separation of the populations for tens of thousands of years. There are apt to be many other sequence changes that also correlate with being part of one of the two populations. Unfortunately, case-control studies are subject to much subtler population-stratification effects. One of the more common errors has been to use laboratory personnel as control subjects in studies of diseases that occur in clinic populations.

Many association studies have been reported in the last decade. The most creditable are extensions of family-based linkage studies in which disease genes are further localized. Frequently, association studies have been conducted to test the hypothesis that a gene plays a role in a disease process. Such hypotheses can be supported but not disproved by association studies. Many reports describing associations between specific DNA sequence variation in the dopamine, subtype 2 (D_2), receptor and the occurrence of alcoholism have been published in recent years (Blum et al. 1990). Since the initial observation by Blum and colleagues, studies that replicated or failed to replicate the original observation have been reported. These discrepant results could mean that alternative D_2 receptor alleles affect susceptibility to alcoholism but that such susceptibility may be detectable only in certain populations with specific genetic backgrounds and environmental influences. An alternative explanation is that subtle effects of population stratification are being detected in some of the case-control studies. In a meta-analysis of all available data, it was concluded that we still do not know whether sequence variation in the D_2 receptor affects susceptibility to alcoholism (Gejman et al. 1994; Gelernter et al. 1993).

Two case-control studies have suggested that the DNA sequence variation of the dopamine, subtype 4 (D_4), receptor leads specifically to novelty-seeking behavior (Benjamin et al. 1996; Ebstein et al. 1996). But one has to question whether these findings were due to a causal relationship between the specific DNA sequences and novelty-seeking behavior or to biases in the collection of samples from individuals who scored similarly on measures of novelty-seeking behavior.

The fundamental problem with the aforementioned studies focusing on alcoholism (Gejman et al. 1994; Gelernter et al. 1993) and novelty seeking (Benjamin et al. 1996; Ebstein et al. 1996) is the case-control design. It is extremely difficult to identify the appropriate control subject for each individual in a population. Recently, two study designs have been introduced in an attempt to overcome the

problems of the case-control design. The first study design, described by Spielman and Ewens (1996), involves the *transmission disequilibrium test* (TDT). In this approach, samples are obtained from a population of affected individuals and from their parents. A comparison is made between the frequency at which alleles are found in affected individuals and the frequency at which nontransmitted parental alleles are found. The nontransmitted parental alleles serve as the control chromosomes for the affected individuals. The rationale for the TDT is that the nontransmitted alleles come from individuals with same genetic background as that of the subjects. The TDT is just now coming into use, but it is recognized as the tool of choice for future association studies.

Unfortunately, particularly in the case of late-onset diseases, it is not always possible to collect DNA samples for genetic analysis from the parents of affected individuals. This limitation can be overcome by performing a family study (i.e., by collecting samples from large numbers of siblings of affected individuals, to reconstruct the genetic constitution of the parents). But more recently, the practical approach of comparing the frequency at which alleles are found in affected individuals with the frequency at which alleles are found in their unaffected siblings has been suggested (Boehnke and Langefeld 1998; Spielman and Ewens 1998). If the siblings have the same genetic background, the disease-associated allele is likely to be underrepresented in the individuals who do not manifest the trait. The likelihood of seeing an association in a discordant–sib-pair study will diminish if there are large numbers of unaffected siblings who have a specific disease susceptibility sequence but, because of other genetic or environmental factors, do not manifest the trait.

Case-control studies can be used with greater confidence when family-based studies demonstrate linkage. Association studies have the power to localize disease genes with extreme precision. It has been suggested that in the future, when it is possible to screen hundreds of thousands of DNA sequence variations, the TDT will be the method of choice for identifying genes for complex traits (Risch and Merikangas 1996).

▌ Dementia

Cognitive decline is a prominent feature associated with aging (see Chapter 8). The general population considers failure to remember recent events and misplacing items not only evidence of aging but a possible harbinger of Alzheimer's disease (AD), the most common form of neurodegenerative cognitive impairment. The importance of cognitive function in the geriatric population is illustrated by the observation that elements of cognitive function can be used to predict life expectancy in normal sexagenarians (Siegler et al. 1982). Although interest in the genetics of normal cognitive function is increasing, most of the effort in human genetics is focused on neurodegenerative diseases that affect cognition. Recent developments in this area have practical import for geriatric neuropsychiatry.

Alzheimer's Disease

The clinical and pathological features of AD have been described in Chapter 24. From a geneticist's point of view, the salient feature of AD is that few patients with AD have positive family histories. The diagnosis of AD is based on the finding of β-amyloid–containing senile plaques and neurofibrillary tangles composed of hyperphosphorylated tau protein. A key to proving that a particular gene plays a role in the pathogenesis of AD is determining how the gene leads to the key pathological findings.

In the rare cases of familial AD, families have mutations in the β-amyloid precursor protein gene, leading to Mendelianly inherited AD (Chartier Harlin et al. 1991). More common mutations in presenilin 1 (Sherrington et al. 1995) and presenilin 2 (Levy-Lahad et al. 1995) also produce Mendelian, inherited AD, with an early age at onset. Presenilin 1 and 2 have no known function, but these mutations affect the biological processing of the amyloid precursor protein, increasing β-amyloid production in experimental models (Scheuner et al. 1996).

More relevant to the current practice of geriatric neuropsychiatry has been the identification of alternative allozymes of apolipoprotein E *(APOE)* as susceptibility loci for AD (Roses 1994). Common variations in the *APOE* gene result in three protein products, referred to as ε2, ε3, and ε4, with allele frequencies of 0.07, 0.77, and 0.16. The risk for developing AD is substantially higher in individuals who have inherited two ε4 alleles (2.5% of the population) than in individuals who have two of the more common ε3 alleles (59% of the population) (Figure 38–3). The average age at onset of AD for individuals with two ε4 alleles is approximately 15 years less than for individuals with two ε3 alleles.

The alternative alleles of the *APOE* gene are appropriately referred to as *allozymes* rather than *mutations*. The sequence variations that result in the three alternative alleles were fixed into the human genome tens, if not hundreds, of thousands of years ago. These alternative alleles have essentially normal function as determined by the final arbiter of genetics, reproductive fitness. They have become widely

distributed throughout the population, which suggests that there is no obvious disadvantage to having the alleles that would predispose a person to AD.

Results of genetic epidemiological analysis suggest that additional genetic susceptibility factors for AD are yet to be identified. Studying families who have late-onset AD has led to the identification of another susceptibility locus, on chromosome 12 (Pericak-Vance et al. 1997). It is uncertain whether this locus plays a major role in the susceptibility to AD in the general population.

Frontotemporal Dementia

In behavioral neurology clinics, frontotemporal dementia (FTD) is the next most common cause of heritable dementia (Brun 1993; "Clinical and Neuropathological Criteria for Frontotemporal Dementia" 1994). Because it may be misdiagnosed as AD, the prevalence of FTD in the population is not clear. In behavioral neurology clinic populations, estimates of the percentage of dementia that results in FTD range from 1% to 15%. Most of the variability in the observed frequency in FTD is probably related to referral biases and different levels of detection sensitivity.

The prototypical forms of FTD characteristically are associated with positive family history in 60% of cases

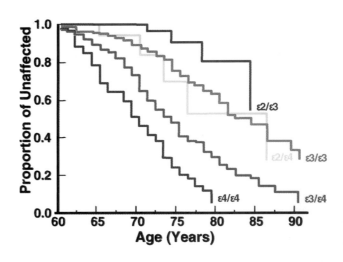

FIGURE 38–3. Onset curves estimated by Kaplan-Meier product limit distributions for apolipoprotein E genotypes. The proportion of individuals without Alzheimer's disease is plotted as a function of time for the five most frequent genotypes.

Source. Reprinted from Roses AD: "Apolipoprotein E Affects the Rate of Alzheimer Disease Expression: Beta-Amyloid Burden Is a Secondary Consequence Dependent on APOE Genotype and Duration of Disease." *Journal of Neuropathology and Experimental Neurology* 53:429–437, 1994. Used with permission.

(Gustafson 1993). Many large families have been identified in which FTD is inherited as a Mendelian trait linked to chromosome 17q21-22 (a region containing the *tau* gene). Mutations in the *tau* gene have been identified in several families with FTD and in individuals with a variety of other clinically and pathologically distinct but overlapping conditions with linkage to 17q21-22. Mutations have also been identified in both coding and presumed regulatory sequences. In the vigorous attempts to find *tau* mutations in other families, the focus has primarily been on the coding sequences. These efforts have failed, but more systematic efforts are under way. It is possible that some cases of FTD are due to mutations in other genes. In one family with FTD, the condition was due to the mutation of another gene on chromosome 3 (Brown et al. 1995).

A characteristic feature in all of the families with *tau* mutations has been the presence of aggregates of hyperphosphorylated tau proteins. Some mutations cause neurofibrillary tangles, as seen in AD. Interestingly, very few amyloid plaques are seen in any individuals with *tau* mutations, and *tau* mutations have not been identified in classic AD. This finding suggests that the neurofibrillary tangles seen in AD are induced by biology of the β-amyloid precursor and that the biochemistry of the *tau* gene may be responsible for neuronal death.

Genetic Testing

When a mutation is identified, it is possible to confirm a diagnosis or make a presymptomatic diagnosis in a relative. As with all genetic diagnostic studies, it is important that testing be performed in the appropriate clinical setting and that genetic counseling occur before and after testing. The clinician should recognize that confirming the diagnosis of a disease by mutation detection can have an effect on family members who may be unwilling participants in the search for knowledge.

DNA from individuals can be sequenced to permit searching for mutations in the amyloid precursor protein, the presenilin genes that are predictors of AD, and the *tau* mutations that cause FTD. These tests are relatively specialized and less widely available than the now routine tests for Huntington's disease. Because mutations in these genes are only rarely responsible for AD and because sequencing is expensive, this type of analysis is usually reserved for subjects with strong family histories. It is uncertain what fraction of FTD cases are due to mutations in *tau*. Because the *tau* gene is large and has complex regulation, it is necessary to screen large segments of DNA sequence for mutations before concluding that a patient has FTD caused by a non-*tau* mutation.

Although it is commercially available, it is inappropriate to use *APOE* genotyping for predictive testing on the general population or on children of patients with AD (Post et al. 1997). The major reason for this is that the available test does not have a high enough predictive value. Many people who have the ε3/ε3 genotype develop AD, and many people who have the ε4/ε4 genotype do not develop AD. Further *APOE* genotyping cannot be used to predict the age at onset of disease, and children of patients with AD may be at risk because of mutations in other genes. In the appropriate setting, *APOE* genotyping can aid in confirming AD diagnosis in populations (Mayeux et al. 1998). Typically, 10% of the patients with a clinical diagnosis of probable AD do not have a pathological diagnosis of AD. A higher concordance rate with pathological diagnosis is observed among patients with a clinical diagnosis who also have at least one ε4 allele. In the near future, *APOE* genotyping may be relevant to clinicians if it can be used to help tailor therapy when multiple therapeutic options are available and their effectiveness is dependent on genotype.

Although medical therapies for most diseases are based on the administration of small molecules, human genetics is spurring the development of alternative strategies. The products of genes identified by human genetic analysis may require delivery to cells in a tissue-specific way. Methods have been developed to insert genes into somatic cells in whole animals. Most approaches rely on the use of modified viruses. The problems of cell targeting, low efficiency, and random DNA insertion are just a few of the obstacles that need to be overcome for this approach to be practical. It is doubtful whether this approach will ever be useful for repairing a mutation that causes a gene to produce a protein with a new toxic function. An approach that has received less attention in the area of genetic disease is the transplantation of tissue to repair an organ (as opposed to organ transplantation). Both fetal neural and autoallogous adrenal tissue have been implanted (Freeman 1997) into the striatum in patients with Parkinson's disease, with mixed results (Kordower et al. 1997; Lieberman et al. 1989) (see Chapter 26). A more practical approach being developed involves transplanting engineered cells grown and selected in vitro.

Summary

Human genetic analysis has already led to the identification of genes that play roles in the most common causes of cognitive decline in the geriatric population. Additional genes will be implicated in these and other traits of interest to geriatricians. In some cases, it is now possible to make presymptomatic diagnoses on the basis of DNA analysis. More important, the identification of genes responsible for human disease offers the opportunity for rational development of drugs to treat and prevent disease. Confirmation of the role of the amyloid precursor protein by the finding of mutations in patients with AD has led to a concerted effort to develop drugs that modify the biochemistry of the gene product. Mice that have pathological features of AD have been genetically engineered to overexpress this gene. These mice are being used as reagents to study the interaction of genes and as systems to test treatment strategies.

Genetic analysis will become an integral part of patient care as treatment is tailored to a patient's genetic constitution. All clinical trials designed to discover agents for the prevention and treatment of AD should now include stratification based on *APOE* genotype. Ideally, therapeutic agents that have general efficacy for the treatment of AD will be developed, but this may not be the case if they have been designed to alter the enzymatic action of APOE.

In the future, analysis of *APOE* through study of a patient's DNA sequence and as-yet unidentified genes will become a routine part of medicine and geriatric neuropsychiatry when genotypes are used to tailor therapy. Despite the promise of genetics to predict our fates, we should recognize that our fate is not entirely determined by our genes. Genetics and epidemiology are becoming increasingly linked, such that it may not be possible to identify genes or environmental factors for some complex traits.

▌ References

Benjamin J, Li L, Patterson C, et al: Population and familial association between the D4 dopamine receptor gene and measures of novelty seeking. Nat Genet 12:81–84, 1996

Berube NG, Smith JR, Pereira-Smith OM: The genetics of cellular senescence. Am J Hum Genet 62:1015–1019, 1998

Blackwelder WC, Elston RC: A comparison of sib-pair linkage tests for disease susceptibility loci. Genet Epidemiol 2:85–97, 1985

Blum K, Noble EP, Sheridan PJ, et al: Allelic association of human dopamine D2 receptor gene in alcoholism. JAMA 263:2055–2060, 1990

Boehnke M, Langefeld CD: Genetic association mapping based on discordant sib pairs: the discordant-alleles test. Am J Hum Genet 62:950–961, 1998

Botstein D, White RL, Skolnick M, et al: Construction of a genetic linkage map in man using restriction fragment length polymorphisms. Am J Hum Genet 32:314–331, 1980

Brierley EJ, Johnson MA, James OF, et al: Mitochondrial involvement in the ageing process: facts and controversies. Mol Cell Biochem 174:325–328, 1997

Brockdorff N, Duthie SM: X chromosome inactivation and the *Xist* gene. Cell Mol Life Sci 54:104–112, 1998

Brown J, Ashworth A, Gydesen S, et al: Familial non-specific dementia maps to chromosome 3. Hum Mol Genet 4:1625–1628, 1995

Brun A: The 2nd International Conference on Frontal Lobe Degeneration of Non-Alzheimer Type, September 11–12, 1992, Lund, Sweden. Dementia 4:(3–4):121–236, 1993

Cassidy SB, Schwartz S: Prader-Willi and Angelman syndromes: disorders of genomic imprinting. Medicine (Baltimore) 77:140–151, 1998

Chartier Harlin MC, Crawford F, Houlden H, et al: Early onset Alzheimer's disease caused by mutations at codon 717 of the beta-amyloid precursor protein gene. Nature 353:844–846, 1991

Clinical and neuropathological criteria for frontotemporal dementia. The Lund and Manchester Groups. J Neurol Neurosurg Psychiatry 57:416–418, 1994

Collins FS: Positional cloning moves from perditional to traditional. Nat Genet 9:347–350, 1995

Ebstein RP, Novick O, Umansky R, et al: Dopamine D4 receptor (D4DR) exon III polymorphism associated with the human personality trait of novelty seeking. Nat Genet 12:78–80, 1996

Freeman TB: From transplants to gene therapy for Parkinson's disease. Exp Neurol 144:47–50, 1997

Gejman PV, Ram A, Gelernter J, et al: No structural mutation in the dopamine D2 receptor gene in alcoholism or schizophrenia: analysis using denaturing gradient gel electrophoresis. JAMA 271:204–208, 1994

Gelernter J, Goldman D, Risch N: The A1 allele at the D2 dopamine receptor gene and alcoholism: a reappraisal. JAMA 269:1673–1677, 1993

Gustafson L: Clinical picture of frontal lobe degeneration of non-Alzheimer type. Dementia 4:143–148, 1993

Hansen MF, Cavenee WK: Tumor suppressors: recessive mutations that lead to cancer. Cell 53:172–173, 1988

Hauser ER, Boehnke M, Guo S-W, et al: Affected-sib-pair interval mapping and exclusion for complex genetic traits: sampling considerations. Genet Epidemiol 13:117–137, 1996

Hayday AC, Saito H, Gillies SD, et al: Structure, organization, and somatic rearrangement of T cell gamma genes. Cell 40:259–269, 1985

Jaenisch R, Beard C, Lee J, et al: Mammalian X chromosome inactivation. Novartis Foundation Symposium 214:200–209, 1998

Kerem BS, Buchanan JA, Durie P, et al: DNA marker haplotype association with pancreatic sufficiency in cystic fibrosis. Am J Hum Genet 44:827–834, 1989a

Kerem B[S], Rommens JM, Buchanan JA, et al: Identification of the cystic fibrosis gene: genetic analysis. Science 245:1073–1080, 1989b

Kinzler KW, Vogelstein B: Lessons from hereditary colorectal cancer. Cell 87:159–170, 1996

Kordower JH, Goetz CG, Freeman TB, et al: Dopaminergic transplants in patients with Parkinson's disease: neuroanatomical correlates of clinical recovery. Exp Neurol 144:41–46, 1997

Kostyu DD: The HLA gene complex and genetic susceptibility to disease. Curr Opin Genet Dev 1:40–47, 1991

Lashkari DA, DeRisi JL, McCusker JH, et al: Yeast microarrays for genome wide parallel genetic and gene expression analysis. Proc Natl Acad Sci U S A 94:13057–13062, 1997

Levy-Lahad E, Wasco W, Poorkaj P, et al: Candidate gene for the chromosome 1 familial Alzheimer's disease locus. Science 269:973–977, 1995

Lewin B: The mystique of epigenetics. Cell 93:301–303, 1998

Lieberman A, Ransohoff J, Berczeller P, et al: Adrenal medullary transplants as a treatment for advanced Parkinson's disease. Acta Neurol Scand Suppl 126:189–196, 1989

Mayeux R, Saunders AM, Shea S, et al: Utility of the apolipoprotein E genotype in the diagnosis of Alzheimer's disease. Alzheimer's Disease Centers Consortium on Apolipoprotein E and Alzheimer's Disease. N Engl J Med 338:506–511, 1998

McKusick VA, Almon V: Mendelian Inheritance in Man: A Catalog of Human Genes and Genetic Disorders. Baltimore, MD, Johns Hopkins University Press, 1998

A novel gene containing a trinucleotide repeat that is expanded and unstable on Huntington's disease chromosomes. The Huntington's Disease Collaborative Research Group. Cell 72:971–983, 1993

Osiewacz HD: Genetic regulation of aging. J Mol Med 75:715–727, 1997

Ott J: Analysis of Human Genetic Linkage. Baltimore, MD, Johns Hopkins University Press, 1991

Pericak-Vance MA, Bass MP, Yamaoka LH, et al: Complete genomic screen in late-onset familial Alzheimer disease: evidence for a new locus on chromosome 12. JAMA 278:1237–1241, 1997

Post SG, Whitehouse PJ, Binstock RH, et al: The clinical introduction of genetic testing for Alzheimer disease: an ethical perspective. JAMA 227:832–836, 1997

Riordan JR, Rommens JM, Kerem B, et al: Identification of the cystic fibrosis gene: cloning and characterization of complementary DNA. Science 245:1066–1073, 1989

Risch N: Linkage strategies for genetically complex traits, I: multilocus models. Am J Hum Genet 46:222–228, 1990a

Risch N: Linkage strategies for genetically complex traits, II: the power of affected relative pairs. Am J Hum Genet 46:229–241, 1990b

Risch N, Merikangas K: The future of genetic studies of complex human diseases. Science 273:1516–1517, 1996

Roses AD: Apolipoprotein E affects the rate of Alzheimer disease expression: beta-amyloid burden is a secondary consequence dependent on APOE genotype and duration of disease. J Neuropathol Exp Neurol 53:429–437, 1994

Scheuner D, Eckman C, Jensen M, et al: Secreted amyloid beta-protein similar to that in the senile plaques of Alzheimer's disease is increased in vivo by the presenilin 1 and 2 and APP mutations linked to familial Alzheimer's disease. Nat Med 2:864–870, 1996

Sherrington R, Rogaev EI, Liang Y, et al: Cloning of a gene bearing missense mutations in early onset familial Alzheimer's disease. Nature 375:754–760, 1995

Shore D: Cellular senescence: lessons from yeast for human aging? Curr Biol 8:R192–R195, 1998

Siegler IC, McCarty SM, Logue PE: Wechsler Memory Scale scores, selective attrition, and distance from death. Journal of Gerontology 37:176–181, 1982

Spielman RS, Ewens WJ: The TDT and other family based tests for linkage disequilibrium and association. Am J Hum Genet 59:983–989, 1996

Spielman RS, Ewens WJ: A sibship test for linkage in the presence of association: the sib transmission/disequilibrium test. Am J Hum Genet 62:450–458, 1998

Surani MA: Imprinting and the initiation of gene silencing in the germ line. Cell 93:309–312, 1998

Tonegawa S: Somatic generation of immune diversity. Biosci Rep 8:3–26, 1988

Watson JD: Molecular Biology of the Gene. Menlo Park, CA, Benjamin Cummings, 1987

Weber JL, May PE: Abundant class of human DNA polymorphisms which can be typed using the polymerase chain reaction. Am J Hum Genet 44:388–396, 1989

Yu CE, Oshima J, Goddard KA, et al: Linkage disequilibrium and haplotype studies of chromosome 8p 11.1-21.1 markers and Werner syndrome. Am J Hum Genet 55:356–364, 1994

Yu CE, Oshima J, Wijsman EM, et al: Mutations in the consensus helicase domains of the Werner syndrome gene. Werner's Syndrome Collaborative Group. Am J Hum Genet 60:330–341, 1997

39

Rehabilitation

Bruce H. Dobkin, M.D.

Goals of rehabilitation programs are to lessen physical and cognitive impairments of patients, increase patients' functional independence, decrease the burden of care provided by significant others, reintegrate patients into their families and communities after illness, and improve the quality of life for patients and their families. Rehabilitation is a problem-solving process with a scope so broad that a specialized team of therapists is needed to make efforts successful.

Physical, cognitive, and behavioral interventions could begin at the first sign of any functional decline in geriatric patients. The causes and natural history of neuropsychiatric disablement in geriatric subjects are not well understood (Wade 1996). More often, efforts are implemented at the time of an accident or of diagnosis of an illness. The most common instigators of a functional evaluation are stroke, traumatic brain injury (TBI), Parkinson's disease, memory loss, dementia from Alzheimer's disease or cerebral ischemia, and injuries secondary to loss of balance, gait dysfunction, and falls. Acute strategies are designed to prevent the medical and psychosocial complications that accompany immobility and new physical and cognitive impairments and disabilities. Evaluation and treatment of impairments and disabilities can take place in an inpatient or outpatient setting. The long-term goal of neuropsychiatric rehabilitation is to lessen disability and handicap.

Assessments, treatments, and outcome measures in rehabilitation are performed by clinicians on at least three levels. *Impairments* include sensorimotor and other neurological, physical, and cognitive deficits, such as a new left hemiparesis and left hemianopsia with hemi-inattention to surroundings. A chronic hip contracture that premorbidly affected walking is a type of impairment that could cause greater disability than one might expect to result from a new stroke. Premorbid impairments in recent memory, word finding, or mood are especially likely to lead to greater-than-expected cognitive dysfunction and disability after a new brain injury. The clinician can use standardized timed tests of physical functioning in elderly patients to obtain a global view of the effects of impairments on important activities. For example, in the Physical Performance Test, a variety of activities are timed, such as walking 50 feet, putting on and removing a jacket, writing a sentence, and climbing a flight of stairs (Reuben and Siu 1990). An obstacle course set up in a hallway was described as a way to assess mobility and balance (Means 1996). Results of tests of postural sway, carried out with or without force plate measures, have been related to the likelihood of falls and disability (Hughes et al. 1996; Wolfson et al. 1992). Significant correlations have been made between speed of walking and levels of independence in activities of daily living (ADLs) in elderly individuals, with speeds of less than 0.3 m/second associated with dependence in one or more activities on the Barthel Index (Potter et al. 1995).

Disabilities are the functional restrictions induced by impairments, such as not being able to walk across a room without assistance because of hemiparesis. The Barthel Index is often used to grade the level of independence in ADLs but does not include a behavioral or cognitive domain. The Functional Independence Measure is another ordinal scale. It includes several broad measures of cognition (Tables 39–1 and 39–2) (Granger et al. 1986; Ottenbacher et al. 1996).

Handicaps arise from impairments and disabilities. Handicaps include the disadvantages that limit or prevent fulfillment of a usual role, such as no longer being able to visit a friend because left hemiparesis prevents stair climbing. In elderly persons, social isolation may follow development of a physical impairment that limits the ability to walk or drive a car. Handicap can be measured in part by the Frenchay Activities Index (Pedersen et al. 1997).

Health-related quality of life is connected to impairment, disability, and handicap. This measure includes a patient's perception of his or her physical functioning, as well as the mental, psychosocial, and emotional state. Health-related quality of life has been measured using the Sickness Index Profile and the Medical Outcomes Study 36-Item Short-Form Health Survey (SF-36) (Garratt et al.

1993). Many other scales have been used in neurorehabilitation and geriatric studies (Dobkin 1996a; Wade 1992).

Disabling neuropsychiatric diseases that are common in the geriatric population cause impairments in sensorimotor skills, cognition, behavior, and emotional control. For example, about half of stroke survivors and persons with chronic multiple sclerosis have cognitive dysfunction, along with about 20% of those with Parkinson's disease (see Chapters 27 and 30). TBI is especially likely to impair attention and executive functions, particularly in older patients after even a mild head injury (see Chapter 28). The combination of physical, cognitive, or behavioral impairments and prescribed and overused centrally acting medications, psychosocial stresses, and other health- and non–health-related issues can lead to profound disability.

TABLE 39–1. **Components of the Functional Independence Measure**

Bladder management
Bowel management
Social interaction
Problem solving
Memory
Comprehension
Bed-to-chair and wheelchair-to-chair transfer
Toilet transfer
Tub and shower transfer
Locomotion (walking or wheelchair)
Climbing stairs
Eating
Grooming
Bathing
Dressing (upper body)
Dressing (lower body)
Toileting

TABLE 39–2. **Scoring for the Functional Independence Measure**

Independence (another person not required for performance of activity; no helper required)

7: Complete independence (all of activity's tasks typically performed safely without modification, use of assistive devices, or use of aids and within reasonable amount of time)

6: Modified independence (performance of activity involves use of assistive device, more than a reasonable amount of time, and/or safety [risk] considerations)

Dependence (another person required for performance of activity, either to supervise or to lend physical assistance, or activity not performed; helper required)

Modified dependence (patient expends ≥ 50% of effort)

5: Supervision or setup required (patient requires no more help than standby assistance, cueing, or coaxing, without physical contact; or helper sets up needed items or applies orthoses)

4: Minimal contact assistance required (with physical contact, patient requires no more help than touching and expends ≥ 75% of effort)

3: Moderate assistance required (patient requires no more help than touching and expends ≥ 50% but < 75% of effort)

Complete dependence (patient expends < 50% of effort; maximal or total assistance required, or activity not performed)

2: Maximal assistance required (patient expends < 50% but ≥ 25% of effort)

1: Total assistance required (patient expends < 25% of effort)

Neuropsychiatric rehabilitation involves not only physicians and nurses but also physical, occupational, recreational, and speech-language therapists; social workers; neuropsychologists; orthotists; dieticians; and sometimes engineers. These professionals work as a team to optimize the physical, cognitive, behavioral, psychosocial, and vocational potential of people who are disabled by their impairments. The primary approach of neuropsychiatric rehabilitation is to lessen disability through training and adaptation. Patients should be able to learn and should be motivated and goal directed. Of course, some geriatric patients may not meet these requirements. An aging brain and body may have confounding effects on rehabilitative therapies; physical, cognitive, and behavioral rehabilitation can be a most difficult challenge for the rehabilitation team.

Rehabilitation services are often organized in relation to the disease being managed. The primary distinction is between acute events such as brain and spinal cord trauma and stroke; the more static conditions in which disability might increase with aging and overuse of muscles and joints, such as cerebral palsy and polio; and the variably progressive disorders such as multiple sclerosis and Parkinson's disease. Services should also be driven by the opportunity to optimize home and community activities and return the patient to the community as soon as possible. A return to the home is often as dependent on the services available in the community as on the severity of the disability and the capacity of the family and caregivers to assist the patient.

▌ Rationale for Gains

Some of the neurobiological mechanisms that might contribute to improvements and, sometimes, increases in impairments and disabilities are outlined in Table 39–3. These mechanisms overlap, and some depend on each other over time. For example, partial recovery of a function because of a partially spared pathway, combined with partial substitution for a function through retraining, may account for gains. Although care must be taken in extrapolating from animal studies of recovery for human interventions (Dobkin 1997), at least a few of these potential mechanisms suggest strategies that can be used by the rehabilitation team to improve outcomes.

Many lines of animal and human research suggest that partial recovery after a stroke can be due to a functional shift to neighboring neurons. Nudo and colleagues (Nudo and Milliken 1996; Nudo et al. 1996) induced an injury of less than 1 mm to the motor cortex of primates in the neu-

rons that represented movement for the arm. The number of perilesional neurons that represented movements of the digits decreased if the monkey did not practice using its hand to scoop pellets out of a narrow well (Nudo and

TABLE 39–3. Neurobiological mechanisms for recovery of function

Network plasticity

1. Recovery of neuronal excitability
   Resolution of cellular toxic-metabolic dysfunction
   Resolution of edema; resorption of blood products
   Resolution of diaschisis
2. Activity in neurons adjacent to injured ones and in partially spared pathways
3. Alternative behavioral strategies
4. Representational adaptations in neuronal assemblies
   Expansion of representational maps
   Recruitment of cells not ordinarily involved in an activity
5. Recruitment of parallel and subcomponent pathways
   Altered activity of distributed functions of cortical and subcortical neural networks
   Activation of pattern generators (e.g., for stepping)
   Recruitment of networks not ordinarily involved in an activity
   Dependence on task-related stimulation

Neuronal plasticity

1. Altered efficacy of synaptic activity
   Activity-dependent unmasking of previously ineffective synapses
   Learning tied to activity-dependent changes (e.g., long-term potentiation, long-term depression) in synaptic strength in peri-injury and remote regions
   Increased neuronal responsiveness from denervation hypersensitivity
   Decrease in number of neurons, as in apoptosis
   Change in number of a variety of receptors
   Change in neurotransmitter release and uptake
2. Regeneration and sprouting of axons and dendrites
   Signaling gene expression for cell viability, growth, and remodeling proteins
   Modulation by neurotrophic factors
   Actions of chemoattractants and inhibitors in milieu
3. Remyelination
4. Transsynaptic degeneration
5. Ion channel changes on fibers for impulse conduction
6. Actions of neurotransmitters and neuromodulators

Source. Adapted from Dobkin 1996a.

Milliken 1996), but the size of neighboring representations for the digits, wrist, and forearm increased with practice (Nudo et al. 1996). Thus, cortical representational changes are especially likely to occur during training that involves learning and the acquisition of specific skills. The neurons of the ischemic penumbra of an acute cerebral infarction may play an important role in functional gains because this region has a large potential for the learning mechanism of long-term potentiation (Dobkin 1998).

Representational plasticity probably arises when previously silent synapses within thalamocortical and intracortical circuits are unmasked (Donoghue 1997). In some instances, this plasticity is accompanied by sprouting of dendritic arbors over short distances (Jones et al. 1996). Indeed, these findings are further evidence for a key principle of behavioral neuroscience, namely, that experience continuously modifies brain structure, especially at the synapse, beyond the period of neurodevelopment and even in the geriatric population. The rules that govern the plasticity of cortical maps appear to parallel those that drive synaptic plasticity (Buonomano and Merzenich 1998). Neocortical modifications in dendritic length, branching, spine density, synapse size and number, glial size and number, and metabolic activity can be produced not only by a stroke or other brain injury but also by aging, sex hormones, neurotrophins, stress, richer environments, and training in specific tasks (Kolb and Whishaw 1998). Although the specific mechanisms that drive these changes are still not certain, they can be related to increases in afferent drives on interneuronal activity, which in turn increase gene expression and protein synthesis. This cascade causes stronger synaptic interactions within neuronal assemblies that participate in a task and leads to behavioral gains.

Substrates for improvements in motor function include the combination of partially spared pathways, flexible neuronal assemblies that represent movements and sensation, and multiple representational maps for movements in a parallel, distributed system. Large anatomical networks also serve cognitive domains, including those for language, spatial awareness, explicit memory and emotional valence, working memory and executive functions, and face and object recognition (Mesulam 1998). The components of each of these networks are interconnected by the convergence of afferent sensory inputs and the divergence of outputs. Thus, afferent drive from practice should modulate neuronal activity, gene expression, learning, and behavioral change. Positron-emission tomography (PET) and functional magnetic resonance imaging (MRI) studies have begun to reveal changes in the organization of these interactions for particular tasks during normal learning and after a cerebral injury (Dettmers et al.

1997; Frackowiak 1994; Karni et al. 1995; Pizzamiglio et al. 1998).

Are the neurobiological mechanisms that have been associated with gains any less likely to evolve when a neuropsychiatric illness affects an aging brain? Few anatomical studies have compared motor recovery in older patients with that in younger patients. Age-related differences in brain regions associated with cognitive processes have been better researched. Greater age has been correlated with a decrease in the number and length of the primary branches of dendrites, the number of dendritic spines, and the density of synapses (Anderson and Rutledge 1996). Because the synapse is the primary site of activity-dependent plasticity, the finding of a decrease in numbers with increasing age beyond 50 years suggests that neuronal adaptations and learning may be limited after a brain injury.

Cognitive rehabilitation strategies have been developed based on the theory that improvements might be mediated by engaging residual links in a distributed cognitive network with therapy (Mountcastle 1997). This strategy is reflected in the primary approaches to cognitive rehabilitation, which include 1) retraining that stresses mental exercises and general cognitive stimulation; 2) training strategies built on theoretical models of specific neuropsychological and neuropsychiatric impairments; 3) techniques drawn from studies in educational, behavioral, and cognitive psychology; and 4) and a psychosocial approach that addresses the cognitive, behavioral, social, and emotional bases and sequelae of any impairment and disability.

A treatment emphasis on behaviorally relevant tasks, with an optimal schedule of practice and feedback, might increase cognitive gains, given that this approach has been found in human and animal studies to enhance upper-extremity and locomotor functions after a brain or spinal cord injury (Dobkin 1996b; Taub and Wolf 1997). This approach may be especially useful for treatment of aphasias, apraxias, and visuospatial, visuoperceptual, attentional, memory, and disruptive behavioral disorders. The optimal duration and intensity of training are uncertain, but more intensive practice seems to enhance subsequent performance (Kwakkel et al. 1997). Unfortunately, most patients receive only a few months of formal inpatient and outpatient retraining, at a modest level of intensity and spread across many tasks.

Physical Approaches

A recent emphasis of geriatric rehabilitation has been on the prevention of falls. Thirty percent of people over age 65 who live in the community fall each year, and this proportion reaches 50% in people over age 80. Falls are a strong predictor of placement in a skilled nursing facility (Tinetti and Williams 1997). A simple test of standing up, walking, and balance can help predict disability in ADLs (Guralnik et al. 1995). Programs of selective muscle strengthening, stretching, and conditioning exercises can improve strength and safety of mobility in frail elderly individuals (Fiatarone et al. 1994). Indeed, frail nonagenarians who participated in an 8-week program of high-intensity resistance training increased their regional muscle mass, gained in strength by an average of 175%, and improved their walking speed by 48% (Fiatarone et al. 1990). Depression may presage a decline in physical performance as well as follow chronic disability in elderly persons (Penninx et al. 1998). Some studies suggest that aerobic exercise improves sleep quality (King et al. 1997) and neuropsychological testing subscores (Dustman et al. 1984).

Exercise programs that bring geriatric patients together in a social setting might lessen the likelihood of physical decline and depressed mood. For many people, a home-based program preceded by instruction is effective. Rehabilitation interventions might have practical goals, such as improving the elderly patient's ability to cross a street within the time limits of a stoplight, climb a flight of stairs, get in and out of a car, or reduce back or leg joint pain that interferes with mobility. A variety of approaches to physical therapy are used.

Exercise and Compensatory Functional Training

Most therapy programs emphasize education about impairments and disabilities, compensatory techniques for ADLs and mobility, and repetitive passive and active exercises to progress from less complex to more functional movements. In the therapeutic-exercise approach, residual motor skills in affected and unaffected extremities are used to compensate for impairments. The acquisition of self-care and mobility skills may take precedence over the quality of movement, as long as patients are safe. Upper-extremity splints, lower-extremity braces such as ankle-foot orthoses, and assistive devices such as walkers and canes tend to be used early in treatment to promote functional compensation. Therapists also make use of general conditioning exercises and energy conservation techniques.

Conditioning and Strengthening

Light resistance exercises are generally safe and effective in improving strength and sometimes function in patients with upper motor neuron (UMN) diseases or diseases of the motor unit, including postpolio syndrome, amyotrophic lateral sclerosis, and myasthenia gravis (Agre et al. 1997; Damiano and Abel 1998; Dobkin 1993; Engardt et al. 1995; Milner-Brown and Miller 1988). Resistance exercises can be carried out without an increase in spasticity in patients with UMN diseases and without muscle injury in patients with neuromuscular diseases. Along with specific retraining programs, medications may be useful, including hormones that limit disuse atrophy, such as androgens and human growth factor (Roy et al. 1991), and drugs that act on the neuromuscular junction, such as pyridostigmine; on muscle, such as β_2-adrenergic agonists (Signorile et al. 1995); or on demyelinated axons, such as the aminopyridines (Bever et al. 1996).

Fitness training is valuable and feasible in patients with UMN, extrapyramidal, or motor unit diseases. For example, treadmill walking has been used with success as an aerobic workout in elderly patients with hemiparetic stroke (Macko et al. 1997).

Neurophysiological Approaches

Approaches have been developed that focus on enhancing the movement of paretic limbs affected by UMN disease (Dickstein 1989). These approaches use sensory stimuli and reflexes to facilitate or inhibit tone, as well as single-muscle and whole limb–muscle movements in and out of mass actions called *synergies*. Some therapists try to administer therapy in a sequence reminiscent of the neurodevelopmental evolution from reflexive to more complex movements. Some techniques permit whereas others inhibit spastic, overflow, or synergistic movements. Mobility activities might be performed in a developmental sequence, with the patient rolling onto the side, with arm and leg flexion on the same side; then extending the neck and legs while prone; lying prone while supporting himself or herself on the elbows; doing static and weight-shifting movements while crawling on all four extremities; sitting; standing; and finally walking.

When these approaches have been compared with other therapies in patients with stroke or cerebral palsy, no real differences in outcomes related to gains in ADLs have been found (Ashburn et al. 1993; Giuliani 1995). However, movement, rather than specific ADLs, is taught in these approaches, so perhaps outcome measures have been inappropriate. More important, the studies in neuroplasticity reviewed earlier suggest that therapy structured around learning new sensorimotor relationships in the wake of altered motor control will be more effective than will methods that aim to foster a developmental sequence.

Motor Learning and Task-Oriented Practice

Another approach involves the use of visual, verbal, and other sensory feedback to achieve task-specific movements, rather than sensory stimuli to facilitate and inhibit movement patterns (Lister 1991). The emphasis is on solving a motor problem rather than on relearning a particular pattern of movement. Studies of motor learning in subjects without brain injuries suggest that practice that is randomly ordered and randomly reinforced produces better posttraining retrieval than do repetitive drills and continuous feedback. Only a few studies have compared these approaches in people with brain injuries, with the same results (Hanlon 1996; Winstein 1999).

Outcomes

Clinical trials that have focused on elderly patients with particular diseases or risk factors for falls have generally shown a significant functional benefit from physical and occupational therapies during inpatient or outpatient rehabilitation. For example, a meta-analysis of the seven randomized trials of interventions to prevent frailty and falls (Frailty and Injuries: Cooperative Studies of Intervention Techniques [FICSIT]) pointed to the benefit of balance, strengthening, and other exercises in terms of reducing falls. Applegate et al. (1990) found that functional assessment and a team approach to medical care, rehabilitation, and psychosocial support were more effective in producing gains in ADLs than was usual community care. Clinical trials of exercise in patients with multiple sclerosis (Di Fabio et al. 1998) or Parkinson's disease (Comella et al. 1994; Patti et al. 1996) pointed to the beneficial effect of an ongoing strengthening and conditioning program on performance of functional activities. Patients with dementia also show physical benefits from an exercise program (Pomeroy 1993).

Rehabilitation outcomes for other common diseases with neuropsychiatric sequelae, such as stroke, TBI, and spinal cord injury, are affected by advanced age. Rehabilitation team efforts, particularly assessments and functionally oriented services performed in an organized way, appear to improve outcomes in elderly stroke patients more than efforts by less organized medical units involving less organized outpatient services (Hui et al. 1995; Indredavik et al. 1997, 1998; Kaste et al. 1995). Functional gains made during stroke rehabilitation were maintained during 2 years of follow-up in patients under age 70 and in patients 70 years and older, although the older group had a greater risk of death and placement in a nursing home (Borucki et al.

1992). After a traumatic head injury necessitating admission for rehabilitation, age greater than 60 years has been associated with longer confusional states, slower recovery, and worse overall outcome, but inpatient and lengthy outpatient programs appear to improve outcomes (D. I. Katz and Alexander 1994). Although the prognosis for functional gains and 2-year survival is worse and the likelihood of nursing home placement is greater after a spinal cord injury in elderly patients than in patients under age 60 (DeVivo et al. 1990; Penrod et al. 1990), gains in ADLs are common with rehabilitation efforts in elderly individuals. Several randomized clinical trials of older persons with an acute stroke demonstrate that both inpatient and outpatient therapy that is task-specific in its treatment strategy will lessen disabilities (Kwakkel 1999; Walker 1999).

■ Cognitive Rehabilitation

Cognitive disturbances are common in patients with recent stroke, TBI, multiple sclerosis, Parkinson's disease, or degenerative brain disease. A prospective study of 227 patients with acute stroke revealed that 35% had measurable cognitive impairments 3 months after onset (Tatemichi et al. 1994) (see Chapter 27). In another study, cognitive decline was observed 3 months after a stroke in 45% of patients ages 55–64 years and in 74% of those ages 75–85 years (Pohjasvaara et al. 1997). Cognitive dysfunction is especially common after TBI (see Chapter 28). Greater severity and longer duration of impairments are associated with lower Glasgow Coma Scale scores on admission for acute care and longer duration of posttraumatic amnesia. Greater severity of cognitive sequelae is strongly associated with age over 60 years (D.I. Katz and Alexander 1994; Levin et al. 1990b). Up to one-half of patients with traumatic spinal cord injury, usually from falls or automobile accidents in geriatric patients, will have cognitive impairments from an associated TBI that may not be obvious early in their care. Of course, any toxic-metabolic or infectious disease will exacerbate cognitive disabilities. A bladder infection or a seizure, for example, often precipitates greater confusion that can last days in a person with dementia or aphasia. Some of the impairments that are often dealt with by the rehabilitation team are listed in Table 39–4. These impairments can also impede gains in mobility, ADLs, and community reintegration.

The amount and rate of recovery of neuropsychological functions vary with the patient's age; the sophistication of the measures used; the type and severity of impairment; the type, severity, and distribution of lesions; and the time since onset. Other more subtle factors, such as the

TABLE 39–4. Cognitive impairments managed during rehabilitation

Language
  Aphasia
  Affective expression
Attention
  Alertness
  Speed of mental processing
  Awareness of disability and impairment
  Focused attention on single stimulus
  Sustained attention to task
  Selective attention during distraction
  Divided or alternating attention among tasks
Memory
  Retrograde and anterograde memory
  Immediate, delayed, cued, and recognition recall
Learning
  Visual learning
  Verbal learning
  Procedural/skills learning
Perception
  Visual perception
  Auditory perception
  Visuospatial perception
Executive functions
  Planning
  Initiation
  Organizational skills
  Maintaining of goals or intentions
  Conceptual reasoning
  Hypothesis testing and ability to shift responses
  Self-appraisal
  Self-monitoring
Intelligence
  Verbal intelligence
  Performance
  Problem solving
  Abstract reasoning

interactions of pathologies, associated sensorimotor and cognitive impairments, and premorbid intellect and education, can affect the efficacy of a particular therapeutic approach, as well as the natural history of gains. Comparisons between interventions are often confounded by differences in intensity and duration of treatment, lack of specification of the methods of treatment, differences in personal interactions between therapist and patient, and the family's level of success in reinforcing desired behaviors.

Overview of Therapy

In addition to cognitive strengths and weaknesses, behaviors of everyday life must be assessed in a cognitive rehabilitation program for a geriatric patient. The assessment should reveal functional capabilities, along with barriers to normal functioning at home and in the community. Functional goals are then set by the team of therapists and physicians with the patient and his or her significant others. Goals must be reasonable for the level of impairment and disability of the individual patient at the time of the evaluation. For a therapeutic approach to be effective outside the hospital or clinic, interventions for neuropsychiatric problems need to be provided under conditions similar to those of the patient's normal environment. Trips to a grocery store, a movie theater, or even the hospital cafeteria provide a chance for the patient and therapist to test the patient's balance, walking ability, selective attention, ability to plan, social communication skills, judgment, and compensatory skills. Goals must be set within the constraints of the amount of therapy available, the safest living arrangement for the patient, the patient's financial state, and the availability of community supportive resources. For example, if a patient with an elderly spouse is able to walk, eat, toilet, and dress with supervision by the end of inpatient rehabilitation for a stroke but acts impulsively and becomes confused or delusional at night, a discharge to the home is suitable only if the patient has a caregiver other than the spouse, who cannot be expected to manage the patient.

General approaches to management include training in particular functional adaptive skills, behavioral modification, and remediation of specific cognitive processes. In the *adaptive approach*, therapy is used in an attempt to circumvent the effects of cognitive impairments on targeted daily activities. Repetition, internally generated and externally generated cues, and cognitive assistive devices are used in training. Learning to perform a particular task usually does not mean that learning to perform other tasks not closely related will follow. *Behavioral modification techniques* are most often used in acute and transitional living settings for patients with TBI. Rewards are given for accomplishing a task or for reducing antisocial actions. In the *cognitive remediation approach*, impairments identified by neuropsychological testing are managed individually through addressing some of the components that make up a particular cognitive skill. The emphasis of the techniques is on interventions that cause the patient to use intact cognitive skills to help compensate for more impaired ones. Techniques usually merge as the team experiments with interventions that address the most difficult problems. Outpatients with TBI are the most likely group to require multimodal programs that stress training in task-specific skills by remediating techniques, awareness about impairments and limitations, and skills needed for independent living and work (Ben-Yishay and Diller 1993).

Aphasia, memory disturbances, and hemi-inattention can cause great disability in older patients. Discussion of these cognitive problems and rehabilitative approaches to them follow.

Aphasia

Incidence. The reported incidence of language disorders in patients with stroke or TBI has varied across studies. In a British health district of 250,000 people, the number of new cases of aphasia in patients with stroke was on average 202 per year (David and Enderby 1990). By 1 month poststroke, 165 of the survivors were potential candidates for speech therapy. In a prospective, community-based Danish study of acute stroke, Pedersen et al. (1995) found that 38% of 881 patients were aphasic on admission, and aphasia was rated as severe on the Scandinavian Stroke Scale in 20% of patients admitted. Nearly one-half of the patients with severe aphasia died shortly after stroke onset, and one-half of the patients with mild aphasia recovered by 1 week. Only 18% of survivors were still aphasic at the time of their acute care and rehabilitation hospital discharge. Patients received speech therapy as needed and were retested at 2-week intervals for 6 months. In 95% of patients with mild aphasia, the highest level of recovery was reached at 2 weeks, whereas best gains were achieved at 6 weeks in those with moderate aphasia and within 10 weeks in those with severe aphasia. Only 8% of patients with severe aphasia fully recovered by 6 months. The best predictor of recovery was a lesser severity of aphasia close to the time of the stroke.

Treatment. Twenty percent to 50% of patients with aphasia have some features of the traditional aphasia subtypes (e.g., nonfluent or Broca's aphasia, fluent or Wernicke's aphasia) (Willmes and Poeck 1993). The traditional classification systems with their lists of broadly defined features often do not take sufficiently into account the underlying disturbances of language, so they may not be optimal for directing rehabilitation treatment. The goal of neurolinguistic assessment of aphasia is to specify problems occurring in the units of language, such as simple words, sentences, and discourse. For each unit, the therapist ascertains how the disturbance affects linguistic forms, such as phonemes, syntax, and meaning.

Speech therapists most often attempt to find ways to help patients compensate for defective language function.

These therapists use a wide variety of stimulation-facilitation techniques, including visual and verbal cueing during picture-matching and sentence-completion tasks, along with frequent repetition and positive reinforcement as the patient approaches the desired responses. Initial treatments also involve tasks that relate to self-care, the immediate environment, and emotionally positive experiences. To prevent patient withdrawal and isolation, it is especially important to quickly find a way to obtain reliable verbal or gestural yes–no responses. Behavioral techniques can be used, particularly for patients with TBI, to help patients improve eye contact skills, initiate and stay on a topic, learn to take turns during conversation, adapt to a listener's needs, and use speech to warn, assert, request, acknowledge, or comment.

In addition to the stimulation-facilitation approach to therapy, a variety of more or less well-defined theoretical models for therapy have been proposed. Therapy techniques have been designed for specific aphasia syndromes and neurolinguistic impairments (Helm-Estabrooks and Albert 1991; LaPointe 1990). Examples of a few of the specific approaches for particular problems follow.

The evidence for the efficacy of melodic intonation therapy (MIT) is especially strong ("Assessment" 1994). In MIT, the therapist and the patient melodically intone multisyllabic words and commonly used short phrases while the therapist taps the patient's left hand to mark each syllable. Gradually, the therapist stops intoning and tapping. MIT works best in patients with Broca's aphasia who have sparse or stereotyped nonsense speech and good auditory comprehension.

Patients in whom a single sound, word, or phrase overwhelms any other attempted output can benefit from a program for Voluntary Control of Involuntary Utterances. In this type of program, pauses and other self-monitoring techniques are used to help the patient gain control over perseverative intrusions.

The agrammatism of Broca's aphasia has been treated using the Helm Elicited Language Program for Syntax Stimulation, in which the goal is for the patient to build increasingly more difficult syntactic constructions. The therapist uses a standard series of drawings of common activities and provides a brief verbal description that ends with a question. The question contains a target phrase. The patient tries to use and build on the words of the target phrase in question. As the patient's responses with target words improve, the patient is asked to complete a story about the drawings without having heard the target sentence.

Some patients with minimal or stereotyped output and impaired comprehension have improved with multiple-input phoneme therapy (Stevens 1989). In this 22-step program, the therapist analyzes phonemes produced spontaneously by the patient and then attempts to elicit first a target phoneme, then blends of consonants, then multisyllabic words, and eventually simple sentences. In another approach, some mute or nonfluent aphasic patients can acquire a limited but useful repertoire of gestures using, for example, American Indian sign language.

Comprehension in patients with global or Wernicke's aphasia has been managed using the sentence-level auditory comprehension program, in which patients are trained to discriminate consonant-vowel-consonant words that are the same or that differ by only one phoneme (e.g., *bill, pill,* and *fill).* Patients then try to associate word sounds with the written form of the word and later try to identify the target word embedded in a sentence. In patients with global aphasia, visual action therapy (in which patients learn to communicate through pantomime) has decreased limb apraxia and improved auditory comprehension. In another technique, the emphasis is on conveying of ideas in face-to-face interactions, rather than on linguistic accuracy. The aim of this technique is to develop any modality that can be used to transmit a message, including hand and facial gestures and drawing.

Acquired dyslexia evolves into one of several varieties that permit specific treatment approaches. In one subject who had phonological dyslexia and read only common whole words, training to go from spelling to sounding out words that were read was associated with a change in brain activation on functional MRI from the left angular gyrus to the left lingual gyrus (Small et al. 1998). Computer software has been designed to aid patients with specific language impairments. For example, the computer provided voiced and printed words along with concept images and storyboards, and improved expressive communication (Steele et al. 1992). Performance of visual-matching and reading comprehension tasks on the computer improved performance of several language tasks not involving a computer (R.C. Katz and Wertz 1997).

Aphasia therapy always includes family training so that those closest to the patient can provide the stimulation and structured environment needed for maximal communication. Frustration and depression in the patient can be managed with behavioral techniques and antidepressant medication (see Chapter 13).

Aging, as well as Alzheimer's and Parkinson's diseases, is often accompanied by impairment in word finding, especially in the finding of proper names. Some of the interventions just described may help, but rehearsal of a person's name before an anticipated meeting or, on making a new acquaintance, repeating the person's name a few times to oneself and linking it to some related image seems to work best. In some instances, a person with high-frequency sensorineural hearing loss who begins wearing hearing aids may realize that he or she may not have clearly heard names of others introduced in the past, which interfered with recall.

Outcome. The wide range of cognitive and linguistic and nonlinguistic communication strengths and weaknesses of people with aphasia has made trials of interventions difficult to perform and the results difficult to interpret. Robey (1998) performed a meta-analysis of 55 trials that met reasonable criteria for inclusion in this analysis of studies of outcomes of speech therapy in patients with aphasia after a stroke. Differences between treated and untreated patients were significant at all stages of recovery. Better outcomes were obtained when therapy was started in the acute stage. Treatments in excess of 2 hours per week produced greater gains than did lesser amounts of therapy. Patients with severe aphasia made large gains when treated by a speech-language pathologist. A language stimulation-facilitation technique was tested in enough cases for the analysis to show its greater-than-average effect. There were not enough studies to permit comparison of effects of treatments across different types of aphasia. Family members, under the direction of a therapist, have been shown to be able to help patients progress.

Memory Disturbances

Memory disturbances can have a profoundly negative influence on compensation and new learning in patients undergoing neurorehabilitation.

Incidence. The incidence of and risk factors for memory loss and dementia caused by one or more strokes have become increasingly appreciated (Desmond et al. 1996; Gorelick 1997; Henon et al. 1997; Kokmen et al. 1996; Moroney et al. 1996; Pohjasvaara et al. 1997; Tatemichi et al. 1992) (also see Chapter 23). The incidence of dementia in population- and community-based studies ranges from nine times greater in the first year after a stroke and two times greater each subsequent year, compared with the expected incidence of dementia in an age-controlled group; to an incidence of about 20% at 3 months after a stroke; to an incidence of 30% among all stroke survivors in a population survey. The frequency of dementia increases with increasing age and varies with the definition used to designate dementia. Even mild aphasia may affect verbal memory and can interfere with verbal learning during rehabilitation (Ween et al. 1996).

Memory impairments after TBI have been related to

the time from injury to assessment as well as to the nature of the memory task and the severity of the injury. A group of 102 patients with TBI, ages 10–60 years, who were hospitalized after any period of unconsciousness or after posttraumatic amnesia of more than 1 hour or with evidence of cerebral trauma were examined at 1 and 12 months postinjury (Dikmen et al. 1987). At 1 month, these patients scored significantly lower on the Wechsler Memory Scale and the Selective Reminding Test than did an age-matched control group. Those who could not follow a command for the longest duration of time beyond 24 hours postinjury scored lower on more subtests of the Wechsler Memory Scale, compared with control subjects. Tests of orientation and short-term memory were not as sensitive to memory deficits as tests that required storage of new information for later use. At 1 year, patients performed better than they had 1 month after onset.

Treatment. Most rehabilitative techniques to improve attention, encoding of new information, recognition, and retrieval have been developed for people with TBI. However, the techniques are applicable to most geriatric patients with neuropsychiatric disturbances. Memory interventions include methods to improve learning ability and assist compensation through the use of memory aids. Rehabilitation of some people with memory impairment may require a different approach than usual. For example, block practice with mass repetition of a drill improves performance during the acquisition of a task or new information in people with normal memory. However, long-term retention is less compared with when random schedules of practice are used. With contextual interference, in which repetition is spaced out or several tasks are intermingled during practice, performance may be worse in the short term. Retention, however, and even generalization of performance under different conditions will greater (Schmidt 1988). Frequency of feedback on performance must also be addressed during training. In normal subjects, constant feedback may improve immediate performance, but an intermittent schedule may improve long-term retention. Much less is known about the optimal way to enhance learning in a patient with an aged brain and with a focal or diffuse brain injury or degenerative disease. Severely amnesic subjects learn poorly with trial-and-error training. More frequent feedback that prevented errors was shown to improve retention (Wilson et al. 1994). On the other hand, a study of people with hemiparesis from a chronic stroke revealed that sensorimotor damage to the brain effects the control and execution of motor skills but not the ability to learn those skills (Winstein 1999).

Because there are differences in how implicit and explicit memories are retained, a variety of approaches to retraining can be used. In priming, amnesic patients are exposed to verbal and especially nonverbal information, and then the patients are aided, through cues and prompts, in recalling that information. Priming does not require semantic processing for encoding. Priming is rather specific to the particular properties of the input and relies on perceptual representations stored by modality-specific memory subsystems, such as those that process word forms and visual objects. Tests of recognition memory are especially sensitive means of detecting residual memory in patients with severe amnesia. This implicit memory can even support the rapid acquisition of novel verbal and nonverbal material. The implicit memory system is independent of the hippocampal and diencephalic structures that are affected in amnesia (Musen and Squire 1992). Priming seems particularly useful during rehabilitation to enhance procedural memory for the acquisition of motor skills.

In cognitive remediation of amnestic disorders, patients are trained in the use of the subcomponent processes that underlie declarative and nondeclarative memory. Therapists can then take a restorative or compensatory approach to affect particular memory skills for functionally important activities. For example, Sohlberg and Mateer (1989) suggested addressing—in order—attentional impairments that could interfere with memory training, through use of strategies to improve focused, sustained, selective, alternating, and then divided attention. Impairments in encoding and recall of information are then addressed by employing associative and external cues meant to prompt an action, with increasingly longer intervals being used.

Many patients with moderate to severe TBI underestimate their memory and emotional impairments, even as they acknowledge physical and other cognitive problems. They may deny having the impairment and withdraw or become angry when attempts at rehabilitation are made. The rehabilitation team must provide the counseling and insight required to overcome this problem. Patients with minor TBI often complain about difficulty in sustained and alternating attention. They struggle to keep information and tasks in mind when forced to deal with more than one item at a time, and they quickly become fatigued when working on a modestly demanding task. The same sort of attentional and executive dysfunction may arise during aging and with neurodegenerative diseases. The most practical rehabilitative interventions for memory, attentional, and executive dysfunction include the patient's limiting subjects to one task at a time, blocking out telephone calls and other interruptions, and writing down the order in which things need to be done.

In patients with moderate to severe TBI, even repetitive drills can have little impact on general recall or on memory outside the training session. Patients can be helped with external aids such as a calendar and appointment diary and internal strategies such as rehearsal and visual imagery. Some memory devices are listed in Table 39–5. Electronic pagers that carry messages (Wilson et al. 1997) or electronic calendars with alarms are especially useful for reminding people to perform daily tasks.

Computers, which might one day serve as neural prostheses, have been tried out extensively in cognitive remediation and skills training. Although software programs abound for working on reaction times, aspects of attention, language, problem solving, and other cognitive tasks, the efficacy of this approach has not been clearly demonstrated. Some amnesic patients have been able to be trained in tasks such as data entry, database management,

TABLE 39–5. Aids and strategies for patients with memory impairment

External aids and strategies

Having others remind

Tape recorder

Writing note on hand

Time reminders

    Alarm clock, telephone call

    Personal organizer, diary

    Calendar, wall planner

    Orientation board

Place reminders

    Labels

    Codes (colors, symbols)

Person reminders

    Name tags

    Clothes that offer a cue

Organizers

    Lists

    Personal organizer, diary

    Posted numbered series of reminders

    Items grouped for use

Electronic pagers

Internal aids and strategies

Mental retracing of events

Visual imagery

Alphabet searching

Making associations to what is already recalled

Rehearsal

First-letter mnemonics

Chunking, grouping items

and word processing because of preserved cognitive abilities, including the ability to respond to partial cues and acquire procedural information (Glisky 1992). This knowledge often will not be carried over when even modest changes are made in the tasks. Through reliance on procedural memory, verbal and visual mnemonic strategies have been used to teach subjects a computer graphics program (Prevey et al. 1991). Cooking and vocational tasks were taught using an interactive software program that cued each subtask in order to build up to the desired task (Kirsch et al. 1992).

Studies involving single subjects and small groups have suggested that some medications may benefit patients with impairments in attention and memory. TBI may lead to damage in a particular neurotransmitter system, such as cholinergic neurons (Schmidt and Grady 1995). Presynaptic cholinergic neurotransmitter concentrations were abnormal in a human postmortem study of TBI (Dewar and Graham 1996). Thus, cognitive rehabilitation trials of cholinergic-enhancing drugs such as donepezil and citicoline (Spiers et al. 1996) seem warranted. Neurotrophic factors have been shown in animal models of trauma to protect cholinergic septal neurons from apoptosis and to improve cognition (Sinson et al. 1997). Replacement therapies for other neurotransmitters, such as dopaminergic (Dobkin and Hanlon 1992; McDowell et al. 1998) and noradrenergic agents (Mattay et al. 1996), have a few human studies to commend them (Plenger et al. 1996; Powell et al. 1996). For example, bromocriptine improved performances on prefrontal tests, such as tests involving carrying out dual tasks, in patients with TBI who had impaired capacities in working memory (McDowell et al. 1998). The ampakines, a new class of drugs that enhance AMPA receptor–mediated currents, show some promise in improving encoding aspects of memory in people with normal memory and may be tried in those who need cognitive rehabilitation (Ingvar et al. 1997).

Outcome. Memory-related processes tend to improve in the first 3 months after a stroke, but the rehabilitation team must be on the watch for any need of compensatory aids or other strategies for patients with memory deficits. After a mild TBI, memory usually recovers by 3 months. The rate and degree of improvement noted varies with the test used to measure severity, the time from injury to testing, and the comparison group (Dikmen et al. 1986). One year after severe closed head injury, patients whose case data were entered in the Traumatic Coma Data Bank had greater impairments in verbal and visual memory, as well as other neurobehaviors such as naming items shown and copying constructions with blocks, compared with healthy individuals (Levin et al. 1990a). Selective rather than global cognitive impairments were likely at 1 year. Memory was disproportionately impaired compared with overall intellectual functioning in 15% of the moderately injured and 30% of the severely injured patients. Subjects in these studies did undergo rehabilitation, but no specific program was provided to all patients.

Hemi-Inattention

Hemiattentional disorders can arise from injury within any node in the cortical-limbic-reticular network that directs attention and integrates the localization and identification of a stimulus, as well its importance to the person (Watson et al. 1994). Unilateral neglect arises from injuries to the posterior parietal cortex, the prefrontal cortex that encompasses the frontal eye fields, and the cingulate gyrus; these regions include representations for sensation, for motor activities such as visual scanning and limb exploration, and for motivational relevance, respectively. Subcortical areas such as the thalamus, striatum, and superior colliculus coordinate the distribution of attention. Atrophy of frontal white matter and the diencephalon contributes to persistent anosognosia (Starkstein et al. 1992). The anterior and posterior extensions of a lesion could also produce impairments in attentional and intentional processes that contribute to neglect (D'Esposito et al. 1993).

Incidence.   In a community-based study involving 281 patients who had had a first acute stroke 3 weeks earlier and who had left or right cerebral lesions, visual neglect was detected in 10% by having subjects copy a Greek Cross and complete the Raven's Colored Progressive Matrices (Sunderland et al. 1987). Only about one-half had hemianopsia or visual extinction. The neglect was modestly associated with poorer ADL scores and slower recovery. Severe neglect was rare beyond 6 months. In another study (Stone et al. 1992), visual neglect, documented by a battery of seven tests by 3 days after a stroke, was greater in right than in left hemisphere cases. In this study and others, however, right-sided inattention was detected in 15%–40% of nonaphasic patients with acute left cerebral infarcts.

Treatment.   The initial choice of intervention depends on the proposed mechanism of unilateral neglect or hemispatial inattention to which the team ascribes (Halligan and Marshall 1994). For example, the patient can be treated for an underaroused injured hemisphere that has difficulty processing sensory inputs. A powerful bias of the intact hemisphere for attention to contralateral space could necessitate finding a way to lessen the imbalance. Some patients have difficulty disengaging from sensory inputs. Other strategies might have to be developed if the mental representation of contralesional space has been degraded or if a unilateral impairment in the activation of motor programs delays or prevents the intention to move to the contralesional side. If the initial theory-based intervention is not successful, others should be tried. Some of the ways that clinicians have tried to manage hemi-inattention are listed in Table 39–6. These approaches have not produced robust or consistent results.

TABLE 39–6.   Interventions for hemi-inattention

Intervention	Study
Multisensory visual and sensory cues, then fading cues	Ben-Yishay and Diller 1993
Verbal elaboration of visual analysis	Hanlon and Dobkin 1992
Visual imagery	Smania et al. 1997
Environmental adaptations	Loverro and Reding 1988
Video feedback	Tham and Tegner 1997
Monocular and binocular patches and prisms	Butter and Kirsch 1992; Dobkin 1996a; Rossi et al. 1990; Serfaty et al. 1995
Warning sound at time of left visual event	Robertson et al. 1999
Left limb movement in left hemispace	Robertson and North 1992
Head and trunk midline adjustments	Karnath et al. 1991; Mennemeier et al. 1994; Simon et al. 1995; Taylor et al. 1994; Wiart et al. 1997
Vestibular stimulation	Rode et al. 1992; Rubens 1985; Vallar et al. 1990
Reduction of hemianoptic defects	Kerkhoff et al. 1994
Pharmacotherapy	Fleet et al. 1987
Computer training	Gray et al. 1992; Robertson et al. 1990

Outcome. In most patients, hemiattentional disorders improve or resolve without specific interventions. Persistence of spatial hemineglect can increase disability. Of 150 consecutive patients with moderate disability after a new stroke, 32% had visual neglect (Kalra et al. 1997). The neglect was modestly associated with poorer ADL scores and slower recovery, though severe neglect was rare beyond 6 months. In another study, only 14 of 84 patients with initial neglect had Barthel Index scores indicating moderate or severe dependence in ADLs in follow-up (Stone et al. 1993). Using data from the National Institute of Neurological Disorders and Stroke (NINDS) Stroke Data Bank, Marshall et al. (1994) examined the effect of hemineglect on the ADL scores at 7–10 days and 1 year after onset of a first stroke. Patients who had anosognosia, visual neglect, tactile extinction, motor impersistence, or auditory neglect had the lowest Barthel Index scores at 1 year, even after adjustment for initial ADL scores and for poststroke rehabilitation.

Recovery from neglect has been reported to be most rapid within the first 2 weeks, regardless of the side of the stroke, and to plateau at 3 months, when most patients have little visual neglect. Severe visual neglect and anosognosia in the first week tend to predict some level of persistent impairment at 6 months. Many patients have more subtle and lingering impairments that are detected only with more sensitive measures. For example, a group of patients with right hemisphere stroke showed a strong, consistent rightward attentional bias soon after stroke onset, as well as an inability to reorient their attention leftward (Mattingley et al. 1994). Twelve months after onset, the attentional bias continued, but they could fully reorient to left hemispace when performing line bisection and cancellation pencil-and-paper tasks.

Behavioral Disorders

Neurobehavioral and affective disorders can be a primary focus of rehabilitation efforts after stroke and TBI and can confound reintegration of a patient into the home or community.

Personality Disorders

Alterations in personality have been reported in up to 75% of patients from 1 to 15 years after TBI and tend not to improve beyond 2 years after onset (Van Zomeran and Saan 1990). In one study (Brooke et al. 1992a), agitated motor and verbal behaviors—which are difficult to define and treat (Fugate et al. 1997)—were found in 11% of patients

with TBI during inpatient rehabilitation, and restlessness was present in 35% of patients. Agitation is an emotional state that may include generalized or more focused fear and anxiety, uncertainty, repetitive behaviors, restlessness, and explosiveness. Agitated patients are not always aggressive. Aggression is common in patients after serious TBI and can be verbal or physical against self, objects, or other people (see Chapter 22). As cognition improves, agitation decreases, but directed and nondirected aggressive, impulsive behavior may evolve. Persistent aggression and emotional dyscontrol suggest premorbid mood and behavioral disorders (Fugate et al. 1997).

Interventions include a medical assessment to determine whether exacerbating problems such as pain and drug-induced confusion exist, behavioral modification with positive and consistently applied reinforcements, a structured milieu, individual and group psychotherapy, and pharmacotherapy. Hypoarousal sometimes improves with administration of stimulants such as methylphenidate and amphetamine or treatment with dopamine agonists. Aggressive or agitated behavior is sometimes decreased by blocking dopaminergic and noradrenergic receptors with haloperidol or risperidone, each of which has a rapid action. Buspirone can be useful for treating aggressive or agitated behavior but may take a week or more to reach a therapeutic level. β-Blockers can also decrease irritability. In a randomized trial of propranolol with a dose escalation to 420 mg/day, there was a reduction in intensity of agitation, but not frequency of episodes, compared with placebo in patients with TBI (Brooke et al. 1992b). Hypomanic behavior may respond to lithium therapy. Anticonvulsants such as carbamazepine sometimes prevent outbursts related to episodic dyscontrol.

Affective Disorders

Depression is very common after stroke (see Chapter 27). In the community-based Framingham Study, depression was diagnosed in 47% of 6-month survivors of stroke and in 25% of age- and sex-matched controls (Wolf et al. 1990). In a population-based cohort of Swedish stroke patients whose mean age was 73 years, the prevalence of major depression was 25% at the time of hospital discharge, 30% at 3 months poststroke, 16% at 1 year, 19% at 2 years, and 29% at 3 years poststroke (Astrom et al. 1993). In this and many other studies, a left anterior infarct, dysphasia, and living alone contributed to depression at time of discharge. At 3 months, greater dependence in ADLs and relative social isolation were associated with depression. Also contributory were few social contacts at 1 and 2 years.

Anxiety is another stroke-related affective disorder

(see Chapters 15 and 27). A generalized anxiety disorder was present in 28% of patients with recent stroke and was associated with greater social isolation and greater dependence in ADLs (Astrom 1996). Apathy was found in about one-quarter of patients within 10 days of a stroke. It was associated with greater cognitive impairment, poorer ADL scores, and some major, but not minor, depression (Starkstein et al. 1993).

Depression is diagnosed in 25%–60% of patients with TBI (see Chapter 28) (Gualtieri and Cox 1991). Late-onset depression has been associated with premorbid psychiatric history and lower psychosocial function (Jorge et al. 1993).

Clinicians should manage mood disorders aggressively, especially when progress in rehabilitation falls short of expectations. Patients with depression may respond to any class of antidepressant medications and require the same care in dosing that is usually taken with any elderly person (Lebowitz et al. 1997). The same medications can help alleviate pseudobulbar emotional incontinence with its involuntary weeping, grimacing, and laughing. Patients must be closely monitored for adverse reactions to the antidepressants, including sedation; insomnia; anticholinergic effects on the bowel, the bladder, and salivation; orthostatic hypotension; cardiac arrhythmias; anxiety; extrapyramidal symptoms; and serotonin syndrome (see Chapter 34).

Treatment of depression after stroke can be quite effective. In natural history studies, 60% of patients who were depressed at less than 3 months after stroke onset were recovered at 1-year follow-up (Astrom et al. 1993). About 20% of patients were found to have a persisting generalized anxiety disorder 3 years after a stroke (Astrom 1996).

Conclusions

A rehabilitation team with experience in the management of physical, behavioral, and cognitive impairments and disabilities can lessen the handicaps and social isolation experienced by some aging patients, especially those with acute or chronic neuropsychiatric disease. Programs of physical exercise and problem solving that promote more independent ADLs and community activities can also lead to a better quality of life.

References

Agre JC, Rodriquez AA, Franke TM, et al: Strength, endurance, and work capacity after muscle strengthening exercise in postpolio subjects. Arch Phys Med Rehabil 78:681–686, 1997

Anderson B, Rutledge V: Age and hemisphere effects on dendritic structure. Brain 119:1983–1990, 1996

Applegate WB, Miller ST, Graney MJ, et al: A randomized, controlled trial of a geriatric assessment unit in a community rehabilitation hospital. N Engl J Med 322:1572–1578, 1990

Arai T, Ohi H, Sasaki H, et al: Hemispatial sunglasses: effect on unilateral spatial neglect. Arch Phys Med Rehabil 78:230–232, 1997

Ashburn A, Partridge C, De Souza L: Physiotherapy in the rehabilitation of stroke: a review. Clinical Rehabilitation 7:337–345, 1993

Assessment: melodic intonation therapy. Report of the Therapeutics and Technology Assessment Subcommittee of the American Academy of Neurology. Neurology 44:566–568, 1994

Astrom M: Generalized anxiety disorder in stroke patients: a 3-year longitudinal study. Stroke 27:270–275, 1996

Astrom M, Adolfsson R, Asplund K, et al: Major depression in stroke patients: a 3-year longitudinal study. Stroke 24:976–982, 1993

Ben-Yishay Y, Diller L: Cognitive remediation in traumatic brain injury: update and issues. Arch Phys Med Rehabil 74:204–213, 1993

Bever CT Jr, Anderson PA, Leslie J, et al: Treatment with oral 3,4 diaminopyridine improves leg strength in multiple sclerosis patients. Neurology 47:1457–1462, 1996

Borucki S, Volpe B, Reding M, et al: The effect of age on maintenance of functional gains following stroke rehabilitation. Journal of Neurological Rehabilitation 6:1–5, 1992

Brooke MM, Questad K, Patterson DR, et al: Agitation and restlessness after closed head injury: a prospective study of 100 consecutive admissions. Arch Phys Med Rehabil 73:320–323, 1992a

Brooke MM, Patterson DR, Questad KA, et al: The treatment of agitation during initial hospitalization after traumatic brain injury. Arch Phys Med Rehabil 73:917–921, 1992b

Buonomano D, Merzenich M: Cortical plasticity: from synapses to maps. Annu Rev Neurosci 21:149–186, 1998

Butter C, Kirsch N: Combined and separate effects of eye patching and visual stimulation on unilateral neglect following stroke. Arch Phys Med Rehabil 73:1133–1139, 1992

Comella CL, Stebbins GT, Brown-Toms N, et al: Physical therapy and Parkinson's disease: a controlled clinical trial. Neurology 44:376–378, 1994

Damiano D, Abel M: Functional outcomes of strength training in spastic cerebral palsy. Arch Phys Med Rehabil 79:119–125, 1998

David R, Enderby P: Speech therapy for aphasia—operating a rationed service. Clin Rehabil 4:245–252, 1990

Desmond DW, Moroney JT, Sano M, et al: Recovery of cognitive function after stroke. Stroke 27:1798–1803, 1996

D'Esposito M, McGlinchey-Berroth R, Alexander MP, et al: Dissociable cognitive and neural mechanisms of unilateral visual neglect. Neurology 43:2636–2644, 1993

Dettmers C, Stephan K, Lemon R, et al: Reorganization of the executive motor system after stroke. Cerebrovascular Disease 7:187–200, 1997

DeVivo MJ, Kartus PL, Rutt RD, et al: The influence of age at time of spinal cord injury on rehabilitation outcome. Arch Neurol 47:687–691, 1990

Dewar D, Graham D: Depletion of choline acetyltransferase activity but preservation of M1 and M2 muscarinic receptor binding sites in temporal cortex following head injury: a preliminary human postmortem study. J Neurotrauma 13:181–187, 1996

Dickstein R: Contemporary exercise therapy approaches in stroke rehabilitation. Critical Reviews in Physical Medicine and Rehabilitation 1:161–181, 1989

Di Fabio RP, Soderberg J, Choi T, et al: Extended outpatient rehabilitation: its influence on symptom frequency, fatigue, and functional status for persons with progressive multiple sclerosis. Arch Phys Med Rehabil 79:141–146, 1998

Dikmen S, McLean A Jr, Temkin NR, et al: Neuropsychologic outcome at one-month postinjury. Arch Phys Med Rehabil 67:507–513, 1986

Dikmen S, Temkin N, McLean A, et al: Memory and head injury severity. J Neurol Neurosurg Psychiatry 50:1613–1618, 1987

Dobkin B: Exercise fitness and sports for individuals with neurologic disability, in Sports and Exercise in Midlife. Edited by Gordon S, Gonzalez-Mestre X, Garrett W. Rosemont, IL, American Academy of Orthopedic Surgeons, 1993, pp 235–252

Dobkin B: Neurologic Rehabilitation. Philadelphia, PA, FA Davis, 1996a

Dobkin B: Recovery of locomotor control. The Neurologist 2:239–249, 1996b

Dobkin B: Experimental brain injury and repair. Curr Opin Neurol 10:493–497, 1997

Dobkin B: Activity-dependent learning contributes to motor recovery. Ann Neurol 44:158–160, 1998

Dobkin B, Hanlon R: Dopamine agonist treatment of antegrade amnesia from a mediobasal forebrain injury. Ann Neurol 33:313–316, 1992

Donoghue J: Limits of reorganization in cortical circuits. Cereb Cortex 7:97–99, 1997

Dustman RE, Ruhling RO, Russell EM, et al: Aerobic exercise training and improved neuropsychological function of older individuals. Neurobiol Aging 5:35–42, 1984

Engardt M, Knutsson E, Jonsson M, et al: Dynamic muscle strength training in stroke patients: effects on knee extension torque, electromyographic activity, and motor function. Arch Phys Med Rehabil 76:419–425, 1995

Fiatarone MA, Marks EC, Ryan ND, et al: High-intensity strength training in nonagenarians: effects on skeletal muscle. JAMA 263:3029–3034, 1990

Fiatarone MA, O'Neill EF, Ryan ND, et al: Exercise training and nutritional supplementation for physical frailty in very elderly people. N Engl J Med 330:1769–1775, 1994

Fleet WS, Valenstein E, Watson RT, et al: Dopamine agonist therapy for neglect in humans. Neurology 37:1765–1770, 1987

Frackowiak R: Functional mapping of verbal memory and language. Trends Neurosci 17:109–115, 1994

Fugate LP, Spacek LA, Kresty LA, et al: Measurement and treatment of agitation following traumatic brain injury, II: a survey of the Brain Injury Special Interest Group of the American Academy of Physical Medicine and Rehabilitation. Arch Phys Med Rehabil 78:924–928, 1997

Garratt AM, Ruta DA, Abdalla MI, et al: The SF36 health survey questionnaire: an outcome measure suitable for routine use within the NHS? BMJ 306:1440–1444, 1993

Giuliani C: Strength training for patients with neurological disorders. Neurology Report 19:29–34, 1995

Glisky E: Computer-assisted instruction for patients with traumatic brain injury: teaching of domain-specific knowledge. Journal of Head Trauma and Rehabilitation 7:1–12, 1992

Gorelick P: Status of risk factors for dementia associated with stroke. Stroke 28:459–463, 1997

Granger C, Hamilton B, Sherwin F: Guide for Use of the Uniform Data Set for Medical Rehabilitation. Buffalo, NY, Buffalo General Hospital, 1986

Gray J, Robertson I, Pentland B, et al: Microcomputer-based attentional retraining after brain damage: a randomised group controlled trial. Neuropsychology and Rehabilitation 2:97–115, 1992

Gualtieri T, Cox D: The delayed neurobehavioral sequelae of traumatic brain injury. Brain Inj 5:219–232, 1991

Guralnik JM, Ferrucci L, Simonsick EM, et al: Lower-extremity function in persons over the age of 70 years as a predictor of subsequent disability. N Engl J Med 332:556–561, 1995

Halligan P, Marshall J: Spatial neglect: position papers on theory and practice. Neuropsychological Rehabilitation 4:103–230, 1994

Hanlon R: Motor learning following unilateral stroke. Arch Phys Med Rehabil 77:811–815, 1996

Hanlon R, Dobkin B: Effects of cognitive rehabilitation following a right thalamic infarct. J Clin Exp Neuropsychol 14:433–447, 1992

Helm-Estabrooks N, Albert M: Manual of Aphasia Therapy. Austin, TX, Pro-Ed, 1991

Henon H, Pasquier F, Durieu I, et al: Preexisting dementia in stroke patients: baseline frequency, associated factors, and outcome. Stroke 28:2429–2436, 1997

Hughes MA, Duncan PW, Rose DK, et al: The relationship of postural sway to sensorimotor function, functional performance, and disability in the elderly. Arch Phys Med Rehabil 77:567–572, 1996

Hui E, Lum CM, Woo J, et al: Outcomes of elderly stroke patients: day hospital versus conventional medical management. Stroke 26:1616–1619, 1995

Indredavik B, Slordahl SA, Bakke F, et al: Stroke unit treatment: long-term effects. Stroke 28:1861–1866, 1997

Indredavik B, Bakke F, Slordahl SA, et al: Stroke unit treatment improves long-term quality of life: a randomized controlled trial. Stroke 29:895–899, 1998

Ingvar M, Ambros-Ingerson J, Davis M, et al: Enhancement by an ampakine of memory encoding in humans. Exp Neurol 146:553–559, 1997

Jones TA, Kleim JA, Greenough WT: Synaptogenesis and dendritic growth in the cortex opposite unilateral sensorimotor cortex damage in adult rats: a quantitative electron microscopic examination. Brain Res 733:142–148, 1996

Jorge RE, Robinson RG, Arndt SV, et al: Comparison between acute- and delayed-onset depression following traumatic brain injury. J Neuropsychiatry Clin Neurosci 5:43–49, 1993

Kalra L, Perez I, Gupta S, et al: The influence of visual neglect on stroke rehabilitation. Stroke 28:1386–1391, 1997

Karnath HO, Schenkel P, Fischer B: Trunk orientation as the determining factor of the "contralateral" deficit in the neglect syndrome and as the physical anchor of the internal representation of body orientation in space. Brain 114:1997–2014, 1991

Karni A, Meyer G, Jezzard P, et al: Functional MRI evidence for adult motor cortex plasticity during motor skill learning. Nature 377:155–158, 1995

Kaste M, Palomaki H, Sarna S: Where and how should elderly stroke patients be treated? A randomized trial. Stroke 26:249–253, 1995

Katz DI, Alexander MP: Traumatic brain injury: predicting course of recovery and outcome for patients admitted to rehabilitation. Arch Neurol 51:661–670, 1994

Katz RC, Wertz RT: The efficacy of computer-provided reading treatment for chronic aphasic adults. J Speech Lang Hear Res 40:493–507, 1997

Kerkhoff G, Munssinger U, Meier EK: Neurovisual rehabilitation in cerebral blindness. Arch Neurol 51:474–481, 1994

King AC, Oman RF, Brassington GS, et al: Moderate-intensity exercise and self-rated quality of sleep in older adults: a randomized controlled trial. JAMA 277:32–37, 1997

Kirsch N, Levine S, Lajiness-O'Neill R, et al: Computer-assisted interactive task guidance: facilitating the performance of a simulated vocational task. Journal of Head Trauma and Rehabilitation 7:13–25, 1992

Kokmen E, Whisnant JP, O'Fallon WM, et al: Dementia after ischemic stroke: a population-based study in Rochester, Minnesota (1960–1984). Neurology 46:154–159, 1996

Kolb B, Whishaw I: Brain plasticity and behavior. Annu Rev Psychol 49:43–64, 1998

Kwakkel G, Wagenaar RC, Koelman TW, et al: Effects of intensity of rehabilitation after stroke: a research synthesis. Stroke 28:1550–1556, 1997

Kwakkel G, Wagenaar RC, Twisk JW, et al: Intensity of leg and arm training after primary middle-cerebral-artery stroke: a randomised trial. Lancet 354(9174):191–196, 1999

LaPointe L: Aphasia and Related Neurogenic Language Disorders. New York, Thieme Medical, 1990

Lebowitz BD, Pearson JL, Schneider LS, et al: Diagnosis and treatment of depression in late life. Consensus statement update. JAMA 278:1186–1190, 1997

Levin HS, Gary HE Jr, Eisenberg HM, et al: Neurobehavioral outcome 1 year after severe head injury: experience of the Traumatic Coma Data Bank. J Neurosurg 73:699–709, 1990a

Levin H[S], Hamilton W, Grossman R, et al: Outcome after head injury, in Handbook of Clinical Neurology, Vol 13: Head Injury. Edited by Braakman R. Amsterdam, Elsevier, 1990b, pp 367–395

Lister M (ed): Contemporary Management of Motor Control Problems: Proceedings of the II Step Conference. Alexandria, VA, Foundation for Physical Therapy, 1991

Loverro J, Reding M: Bed orientation and rehabilitation outcome for patients with stroke and hemianopsia or visual neglect. Journal of Neurological Rehabilitation 2:147–150, 1988

Macko RF, Katzel LI, Yataco A, et al: Low-velocity graded treadmill stress testing in hemiparetic stroke patients. Stroke 28:988–992, 1997

Marshall R, Sacco R, Lee S, et al: Hemineglect predicts functional outcome after stroke (abstract). Ann Neurol 36:298, 1994

Mattay VS, Berman KF, Ostrem JL, et al: Dextroamphetamine enhances "neural network-specific" physiological signals: a positron-emission tomography rCBF study. J Neurosci 16:4816–4822, 1996

Mattingley JB, Bradshaw JL, Bradshaw JA, et al: Residual rightward attentional bias after apparent recovery from right hemisphere damage: implications for a multicomponent model of neglect. J Neurol Neurosurg Psychiatry 57:597–604, 1994

McDowell S, Whyte J, D'Esposito M: Differential effect of a dopaminergic agonist on prefrontal function in traumatic brain injury patients. Brain 121:1155–1164, 1998

Means K: The obstacle course: a tool for the assessment of functional balance and mobility in the elderly. J Rehabil Res Dev 33:413–428, 1996

Mennemeier M, Chatterjee A, Heilman KM: A comparison of the influences of body and environment centred reference frames on neglect. Brain 117:1013–1021, 1994

Mesulam M: From sensation to cognition. Brain 121:1013–1052, 1998

Milner-Brown H, Miller R: Muscle strengthening through high-resistance weight training in patients with neuromuscular disorders. Arch Phys Med Rehabil 69:14–19, 1988

Moroney JT, Bagiella E, Desmond DW, et al: Risk factors for incident dementia after stroke: role of hypoxic and ischemic disorders. Stroke 27:1283–1289, 1996

Mountcastle V: The columnar organization of the neocortex. Brain 120:701–722, 1997

Musen G, Squire L: Nonverbal priming in amnesia. Memory and Cognition 20:441–448, 1992

Nudo RJ, Milliken GW: Reorganization of movement representations in primary motor cortex following focal ischemic infarcts in adult squirrel monkeys. J Neurophysiol 75:2144–2149, 1996

Nudo RJ, Wise BM, SiFuentes F, et al: Neural substrates for the effects of rehabilitative training on motor recovery after ischemic infarct. Science 272:1791–1794, 1996

Ottenbacher KJ, Hsu Y, Granger CV, et al: The reliability of the Functional Independence Measure: a quantitative review. Arch Phys Med Rehabil 77:1226–1232, 1996

Patti F, Reggio A, Nicoletti F, et al: Effects of rehabilitation therapy on Parkinson's disability and functional independence. Journal of Neurological Rehabilitation 10:223–231, 1996

Pedersen PM, Jorgensen HS, Nakayama H, et al: Aphasia in acute stroke: incidence, determinants, and recovery. Ann Neurol 38:659–666, 1995

Pedersen PM, Jorgensen HS, Nakayama H, et al: Comprehensive assessment of activities of daily living in stroke. The Copenhagen Stroke Study. Arch Phys Med Rehabil 78:161–165, 1997

Penninx BW, Guralnik JM, Ferrucci L, et al: Depressive symptoms and physical decline in community-dwelling older persons. JAMA 279:1720–1726, 1998

Penrod LE, Hegde SK, Ditunno JF Jr, et al: Age effect on prognosis for functional recovery in acute, traumatic central cord syndrome. Arch Phys Med Rehabil 71:963–968, 1990

Pizzamiglio L, Perani D, Cappa SF, et al: Recovery of neglect after right hemisphere damage: H2(15)O positron emission tomographic activation study. Arch Neurol 55:561–568, 1998

Plenger PM, Dixon CE, Castillo RM, et al: Subacute methylphenidate treatment for moderate to moderately severe traumatic brain injury: a preliminary double-blind placebo-controlled study. Arch Phys Med Rehabil 77:5 36–540, 1996

Pohjasvaara T, Erkinjuntti T, Vataja R, et al: Dementia three months after stroke: baseline frequency and effect of different definitions of dementia in the Helsinki Stroke Aging Memory Study (SAM) cohort. Stroke 28:785–792, 1997

Pomeroy V: The effect of physiotherapy input on mobility skills of elderly people with severe dementing illness. Clinical Rehabilitation 7:163–170, 1993

Potter JM, Evans AL, Duncan G: Gait speed and activities of daily living function in geriatric patients. Arch Phys Med Rehabil 76:997–999, 1995

Powell JH, al-Adawi S, Morgan J, et al: Motivational deficits after brain injury: effects of bromocriptine in 11 patients. J Neurol Neurosurg Psychiatry 60:416–421, 1996

Prevey ML, Delaney RC, De l'Aune W, et al: A method of assessing the efficacy of memory rehabilitation techniques using a "real-world" memory task: learning a computer language. J Rehabil Res Dev 28:53–60, 1991

Reuben D, Siu A: An objective measure of physical function of elderly outpatients. J Am Geriatr Soc 38:1105–1112, 1990

Robertson IH, Gray JM, Pentland B, et al: Microcomputer-based rehabilitation for unilateral left visual neglect: a randomized controlled trial. Arch Phys Med Rehabil 71:663–668, 1990

Robertson IH, North N: Spatio-motor cueing in unilateral left neglect: the role of hemispace, hand and motor activation. Neuropsychologia 30:553–563, 1992

Robertson IH, Mattingly J, Rorden C, et al: Phasic alerting of neglect patients overcomes their spatial deficits in visual awareness. Nature 395:169–172, 1999

Robey R: A meta-analysis of clinical outcomes in the treatment of aphasia. J Speech Lang Hear Res 41:172–187, 1998

Rode G, Charles N, Perenin MT, et al: Partial remission of hemiplegia and somatoparaphrenia through vestibular stimulation in a case of unilateral neglect. Cortex 28:203–208, 1992

Rossi PW, Kheyfets S, Reding MJ: Fresnel prisms improve visual perception in stroke patients with homonymous hemianopia or unilateral visual neglect. Neurology 40:1597–1599, 1990

Roy R, Baldwin K, Edgerton VR, et al: The plasticity of skeletal muscle: effects of neuromuscular activity, in Exercise and Sports Reviews. Edited by Holloszy J. Baltimore, MD, Williams & Wilkins, 1991, pp 269–312

Rubens A: Caloric stimulation and unilateral visual neglect. Neurology 35:1019–1024, 1985

Schmidt R: Motor Control and Learning. Champaign, IL, Human Kinetics, 1988

Schmidt R, Grady M: Loss of forebrain cholinergic neurons following fluid-percussion injury: implications for cognitive impairment in closed head injury. J Neurosurg 83:496–502, 1995

Serfaty C, Soroker N, Glicksohn J, et al: Does monocular viewing improve target detection in hemispatial neglect? Restorative Neurology and Neuroscience 9:7–13, 1995

Signorile JF, Banovac K, Gomez M, et al: Increased muscle strength in paralyzed patients after spinal cord injury: effect of beta-2 adrenergic agonist. Arch Phys Med Rehabil 76:55–58, 1995

Simon ES, Hegarty AM, Mehler MF: Hemispatial and directional performance biases in motor neglect. Neurology 45:525–531, 1995

Sinson G, Perri BR, Trojanowski JQ, et al: Improvement of cognitive deficits and decreased cholinergic neuronal cell loss and apoptotic cell death following neurotrophin infusion after experimental traumatic brain injury. J Neurosurg 86:511–518, 1997

Small SL, Flores DK, Noll DC: Different neural circuits subserve reading before and after therapy for acquired dyslexia. Brain Lang 62:298–308, 1998

Smania N, Bazoli F, Piva D, et al: Visuomotor imagery and rehabilitation of neglect. Arch Phys Med Rehabil 78:430–436, 1997

Sohlberg M, Mateer C: Introduction to Cognitive Rehabilitation. New York, Guilford, 1989

Spiers PA, Myers D, Hochanadel GS, et al: Citicoline improves verbal memory in aging. Arch Neurol 53:441–448, 1996

Starkstein SE, Fedoroff JP, Price TR, et al: Anosognosia in patients with cerebrovascular lesions: a study of causative factors. Stroke 23:1446–1453, 1992

Starkstein SE, Fedoroff JP, Price TR, et al: Apathy following cerebrovascular lesions. Stroke 24:1625–1630, 1993

Steele R, Kleczewska M, carlson G, et al: Computers in the rehabilitation of chronic, severe aphasia: C-VIC cross modal studies. Aphasiology 6:185–194, 1992

Stevens E: Efficacy of multiple input phoneme therapy in the treatment of severe expressive aphasia and apraxia of speech. Physical Medicine and Rehabilitation: State of the Art Reviews 3:194–199, 1989

Stone SP, Patel P, Greenwood RJ, et al: Measuring visual neglect in acute stroke and predicting its recovery: the Visual Neglect Recovery Index. J Neurol Neurosurg Psychiatry 55:431–436, 1992

Stone SP, Patel P, Greenwood RJ: Selection of acute stroke patients for treatment of visual neglect. J Neurol Neurosurg Psychiatry 56:463–466, 1993

Sunderland A, Wade D, Langton-Hewer R, et al: The natural history of visual neglect after stroke. International Disability Studies 9:55–59, 1987

Tatemichi TK, Desmond DW, Mayeux R, et al: Dementia after stroke: baseline frequency, risks, and clinical features in a hospitalized cohort. Neurology 42:1185–1193, 1992

Tatemichi TK, Desmond DW, Stern Y, et al: Cognitive impairment after stroke: frequency, patterns, and relationship to functional abilities. J Neurol Neurosurg Psychiatry 57:202–207, 1994

Taub E, Wolf S: Constraint induced movement techniques to facilitate upper extremity use in stroke patients. Topics in Stroke Rehabilitation 3:38–61, 1997

Taylor D, Ashburn A, Ward C, et al: Asymmetrical trunk posture, unilateral neglect and motor performance following stroke. Clinical Rehabilitation 8:48–53, 1994

Tham K, Tegner R: Video feedback in the rehabilitation of patients with unilateral neglect. Arch Phys Med Rehabil 78:410–413, 1997

Tinetti M, Williams C: Falls, injuries due to falls, and the risk of admission to a nursing home. N Engl J Med 337:1279–1284, 1997

Vallar G, Sterzi R, Bottini G, et al: Temporary remission of left hemianesthesia after vestibular stimulation: a sensory neglect phenomenon. Cortex 26:123–131, 1990

Wade D: Measurement in Neurological Rehabilitation. New York, Oxford University Press, 1992

Wade D: Epidemiology of disabling neurological disease: how and why does disability occur? J Neurol Neurosurg Psychiatry 61:242–249, 1996

Walker MF, Gladman JR, Lincoln NB, et al: Occupational therapy for stroke patients not admitted to hospital: a randomised controlled trial. Lancet 354(9175):278–280, 1999

Watson RT, Valenstein E, Day A, et al: Posterior neocortical systems subserving awareness and neglect. Neglect associated with superior temporal sulcus but not area 7 lesions. Arch Neurol 51:1014–1021, 1994

Ween JE, Verfaellie M, Alexander MP: Verbal memory function in mild aphasia. Neurology 47:795–801, 1996

Wiart L, Come AB, Debelleix X, et al: Unilateral neglect syndrome rehabilitation by trunk rotation and scanning training. Arch Phys Med Rehabil 78:424–429, 1997

Willmes K, Poeck K: To what extent can aphasic syndromes be localized? Brain 116:1527–1540, 1993

Wilson BA, Baddeley A, Evans J, et al: Errorless learning in the rehabilitation of memory impaired people. Neuropsychology and Rehabilitation 4:307–326, 1994

Wilson BA, Evans JJ, Emslie H, et al: Evaluation of NeuroPage: a new memory aid. J Neurol Neurosurg Psychiatry 63:113–115, 1997

Winstein CJ, Merians AS, Sullivan KJ: Motor learning after unilateral brain damage. Neuropsychologia 37(8):975–987, 1999

Wolf P, Bachman D, Kelly-Hayes M, et al: Stroke and depression in the community: the Framingham Study. Neurology 40 (suppl 1):416, 1990

Wolfson L, Whipple R, Derby CA, et al: A dynamic posturography study of balance in healthy elderly. Neurology 42:2069–2075, 1992

40

Ethical Issues

Peter J. Whitehouse, M.D., Ph.D.

A variety of ethical issues confront geriatric neuropsychiatrists and other health care professionals caring for elderly persons with illnesses that may affect decision-making abilities. Dealing with conflicts of human values and with different views of what it means to be a healthy human being is an important part of the care. Yet it is this art, which is not well understood or well taught, that differentiates the physician from the technologist. Practicing this art in geriatric neuropsychiatry raises special issues of relevance to healer, patient, and society.

The practice of geriatric neuropsychiatry is challenging from an ethical point of view for several specific reasons. First, much of ethics, particularly in the Western world, is based on engaging a rational autonomous self (Engelhardt 1996; Whitehouse and Deal 1995). Neuropsychiatric diseases threaten the rationality and autonomy of our patients. Second, the later stages of life are associated with specific concerns about quality of life and, eventually,

quality of death (Whitehouse and Rabins 1992).

Moral and ethical issues will become more prevalent in the future practice of geriatric neuropsychiatry. One reason stems from the fact that there will be a greater number of older individuals, not only in the Western world but also in countries that are currently less industrialized (see Chapter 2). Thus, the ethical problems surrounding the care of older patients with neurological and psychiatric disease will increase. A second reason that moral and ethical issues will become more prevalent is that the revolution in molecular medicine, particularly genetics, will continue to lead to new technologies, with attendant moral issues (see Chapter 38). Third, revolutions in health care system economics, which are occurring, in part, in response to the graying of our population, will themselves generate new value conflicts for physicians and other providers.

The history of ethics extends back centuries—certainly most notably, in Western traditions, to the Greek philosophers. It is beyond the scope of this chapter to

This work was supported by the National Institute on Aging, Sir John Templeton, and various grants from the pharmaceutical industry. I thank Professor Stephen Post for his contributions to this chapter and dedicate this chapter to Professor Van Rensselaer Potter.

review the world's literature on how human beings have explored their differences concerning fundamental issues about life. However, it is critical—particularly as our clinical practices include patients from more and more ethnic groups—that we respect the vastly different cultural beliefs concerning self, family, community, society, and spirit. At the same time, we need to recognize the universal issues relevant to human beings with neuropsychiatric diseases.

The field of bioethics itself is new; the word *bioethics* was not coined until 1970 (Brody 1992; Chambers 1998; Fox 1990; Potter 1971, 1988; Reich 1995). A consideration of this modern time may be most helpful to the geriatric neuropsychiatrist to understand the current methods of biomedical ethicists. But we must not forget, as physicians and scientists frequently do, that these considerations occur in rich historical and cultural contexts.

Bioethicists are becoming more unified and the field is becoming more professionalized, as illustrated by the merging of several organizations to form the new American Society for Bioethics and Humanities. The field will continue to evolve as members of this organization and others consider the rules for specialization in clinical bioethics consultation and the content of new doctoral programs in bioethics. Defining the knowledge base of this inherently interdisciplinary field is challenging. Tensions exist between those who approach ethics through philosophy and those who approach it through practical clinical issues. There is much discussion within the field about the future of bioethics, the emergence of bioethics as a professional field, and the contribution of bioethics to society (Carter 1998; Pellegrino 1993). Issues associated with geriatrics and neuropsychiatry will play important roles in this evolution of bioethics.

In this chapter, I first discuss the concept of bioethics and consider its methods, particularly in relationship to ethics consultations. I then review issues that arise in the clinical practice of geriatric neuropsychiatry and issues that arise in research. Finally, I discuss issues that will likely be more prominent in geriatric neuropsychiatry and in biomedical ethics in years to come. One theme in this chapter will be constant: an understanding of ethical issues requires a knowledge of the science and practice of medicine, plus a view of the broader social context combined with a passion for human beings as individuals and humanity as a whole.

Some of the ethical problems that I discuss in this chapter are general ones faced by all health care providers. More attention is paid in this chapter to those issues specific to the practice of geriatric neuropsychiatry. It is, of course, the patient populations (and, to a certain extent, the types of research) that define the ethical problems that need to be considered. I consider that the practice of geriat-

ric neuropsychiatry is focused on three broad groups of patients: those patients with mental retardation, those with newly acquired cognitive impairments such as dementia, and those with mental illness. Each of these groups brings special issues to the table for ethical deliberation. Patients with mental retardation have never had entirely normal intellects and may never have been able to understand fully or even appreciate that there are ethical issues involved in their participation in research or their receiving of clinical care. Patients with an acquired dementia may have had the opportunity to write advance directives or at least to converse with others about their health care. Patients with mental illness, such as schizophrenia or depression, often have fluctuating decision-making ability. Combinations of mental retardation, dementia, mental illness, and other conditions such as delirium can occur in individual patients. In the case of all three groups of patients, the caregivers—either substitute decision makers by legal definition or close family members with intimate knowledge of the patient and his or her values—play important roles in the resolving of ethical dilemmas.

Methods in Ethics

As mentioned earlier, an ethical issue involves conflict of human values or differences of opinion about what constitutes good or poor quality of life. An ethicist assists others, be they professionals or patients, in exploring and resolving such conflicts. What are the methods by which an ethicist would accomplish this aim?

The dominant mode of ethical practice for those exposed to contemporary bioethics is based on understanding and application of three principles: autonomy, beneficence, and justice (Beauchamp and Childress 1989). Each ethical situation is analyzed in terms of these three ideas. *Autonomy* refers to the preservation of the right of the individual to make decisions about his or her life course. *Beneficence* relates to the responsibilities of human beings to each other, particularly the principle of nonmaleficence (i.e., doing no harm to others). Finally, *justice* involves extending the scope of ethical analysis to include society, with questions asked about the fairness of health care decisions in terms of their impact not only on the patient and the patient's immediate family but on society at large.

In geriatric neuropsychiatry, these principles can be applied in various ways. In clinical practice and research, we wish to respect the rights of individuals to make their own choices as much as possible. However, in the case of an individual who is decisionally impaired, we need to consider how to provide health care that reflects the values of the patient as expressed through a substitute decision maker or that reflects consideration of the best interests of the patient. In research, the principal issue is how to balance potential risk and benefit to the individual and to society. As the number of elderly individuals with neuropsychiatric conditions increases, the issues of distributive justice (e.g., in discussions of health care rationing) will become more important. The question of how much health care should be provided to individuals with severe dementia, for example, might be considered with the concept of distributive justice in mind.

Although ethical analysis based on these three principles has been helpful, there are other ways of approaching ethical issues. Another important approach is *discourse* or *communicative ethics* (Post et al. 1994). In contrast to principle-based ethics—in which the focus is generally on abstract principles and in which the ethicist may assume a philosopher role rather than a more clinical role—discourse ethics takes its cue from the practical, real-world struggle that individuals face in the care of someone with a neuropsychiatric condition. The focus here is on the quality of communication between the parties involved in the ethical dispute. Ethics consultation frequently involves considerable effort to clarify the positions of the different parties involved in a dispute and to facilitate more effective communication among these parties.

Two other methods in ethics that are relevant to physicians are *casuistry* and *narrative ethics* (Jonsen and Toulmin 1988; Nussbaum 1992). In both these forms of ethical deliberation, the focus is on the life stories of the individuals and groups dealing with value issues. The importance of how a story is told is made clear with these approaches. Much of medicine involves a stylized presentation of people's life histories. What is selected and what is ignored are critical in the definition and resolution of ethical problems. In both casuistry and narrative ethics, the true richness of an individual life is stressed. The value conflicts involved in a particular life situation are exceedingly complex. Any ethics consultation should be undertaken with humility and respect for this complexity.

There is a dynamic tension between ethics and law (see Chapter 41). Practitioners, and especially ethicists, must be aware of the laws of the various jurisdictions in which they practice. Ethical issues are broader in scope and may not be addressed by specific laws. However, it is often difficult to do what is perceived to be right if it is different from what is legal. Every health care organization has a set of ethical guidelines concerning certain common clinical dilemmas such as "Do not resuscitate" orders, medical futility, and physician impairment. Professional organizations frequently develop ethical guidelines for their members as well.

Clinical Ethics

Diagnostic Disclosure

In geriatric neuropsychiatry, labeling an individual as a patient has ethical implications. Labeling an individual as having a disease, such as schizophrenia, can profoundly affect the behavior of other individuals toward this person. What information should be provided to the patient and his or her family concerning the diagnosis and prognosis is often not clear. This is particularly true in the case of a condition such as Alzheimer's disease, with its grave prognosis. Most physicians, at least in this country, support the principle of autonomy and believe individuals should be informed of their diagnosis, but how much information should be provided is often less clear. The clinician should attempt to understand the patient and his or her family's prior understanding of the disease and share new information on the basis of this understanding. The clinician must also remember that what one tells people (or thinks one tells) is often different from what is heard.

Selection of Therapeutic Agents

Geriatric neuropsychiatrists are able to suggest a variety of interventions to patients with neurological and mental disease. Many of these interventions are nonpharmacological, namely individual and group psychosocial therapies (see Chapter 36). In many cases, the efficacy of these interventions is not well understood. Selection of therapy is often based on training biases or personal experiences as much as on scientific findings.

The selection of medication is a similarly complex process, in which trade-offs between different benefits and side effects are made. Particularly in neuropsychiatry, with the strong influence of pharmaceutical companies, physicians must attempt to ensure that the decision to use particular medications is based on the best scientific evidence.

Physician involvement in the business of medicine also raises ethical issues. Geriatric neuropsychiatrists who have a financial interest in health care may have a conflict of interest. Use of equipment or admission of a patient to a particular facility should not be determined by the financial reward to the physician involved in the care of that patient. Establishing appropriate guidelines for pharmaceutical company involvement in the continuing education of physicians is a difficult task. Conflicts or confluences of interest are part of life and are issues of growing importance in clinical and research practice (Kodish et al. 1996).

Managed Care

The business of medicine is rapidly changing. Physicians have experienced a significant loss of control over the individual care for their patients as care pathways, limited drug formularies, and other mechanisms have been introduced that limit physician choice in diagnosis and treatment. The most startling change in the health care system in the United States (similar forces are at work in all industrialized countries) has been the introduction of managed care. In a fee-for-service environment, the ethical dilemma facing physicians is that the more tests and interventions a patient undergoes, the more the patient's physician's income is likely to increase. Thus, incentives exist for ordering more tests and procedures rather than conserving diagnostic and therapeutic resources. In managed care, in which a certain dollar amount is provided to the health organization for a specified set of health care benefits, the incentives are reversed. It may be to the financial advantage of the physician, or at least the health care organization with which he or she is affiliated, if fewer tests and interventions are performed and fewer hospitalizations occur. The ethics of managed care is a growing part of biomedical ethics (Berenson 1998) and is evolving as some of the original excesses of managed care (e.g., the gag rule to prevent physicians from fully discussing treatment options with patients) are being eliminated. The balance of power among the forces at work—consumers, professionals, governments, and the private sector—will continue to shift, to reflect, it is to be hoped, wise social policies.

Driving health care reform in Western Europe, North America, and Japan is the fact that health care costs are becoming an increasing burden on the economy. The growing number of older individuals, combined with lower birth rates, creates dependency ratios with fewer workers in the economy supporting more retirees. As the introduction of expensive technology continues, the dilemma becomes that of providing care in face of escalating costs. Some form of health care rationing already occurs, as in the state of Oregon, and such rationing will likely become more common. Ideally, rationing should be based not only on the cost of the intervention but also on the intervention's efficacy. Even efficacy (i.e., data adequate for regulatory approval) is not enough, as effectiveness (i.e., contribution to a meaningful population impact) is becoming a central issue. Much of the practice of medicine is *not* based on results of well-controlled, randomized, double-blind trials. Medicine is becoming more outcome-research based and evidence based. However, randomized trials of all interventions that geriatric neuropsychiatrists wish to consider offering their patients cannot be performed as they would

be too expensive. Outcome research will be helpful, but improving society's processes for long-term decision making will be more critical. Thus, scientific and political processes for weighing evidence and making decisions about what interventions are effective and congruent with social values will continue to be exceedingly complex (Bulger et al. 1995).

Moreover, even when we have decided whether an intervention is valued appropriately in terms of cost, questions remain: Who shall pay? Who shall be eligible for these services? In the United States, we have been ambivalent about whether a basic minimal package of health care should be available to all, regardless of income, and if such a package were made available, what mental health care should be included.

These decision-making issues about allocation of resources indicate that, in the future, the organizational aspects of health care may be as much a concern in bioethics as bedside dilemmas. In general, ethicists—especially physician and other clinical ethicists—are used to focusing on value conflicts in individual cases. In the future, value conflicts within and among organizations may well become more important in the theories and practice of bioethics. The use and distribution of power among the major players in health care will be topics of particular interest (Brody 1992).

End-of-Life Care

A particularly important subject of ethical discussion for geriatric health care providers is end-of-life care. Too often in American medicine, there has been a preoccupation with the goal of preventing death from illness (i.e., quantity rather than quality of life). Physicians have considered themselves failures when their patients died. However, people do die, and older people are at more risk for death. The fact that the hospice movement has grown is a good sign. Some people believe that hospice care is appropriate for those with conditions besides cancer, conditions including severe Alzheimer's disease (Post and Whitehouse 1998b; Whitehouse et al. 1996).

Major changes have also occurred in our country in attitudes toward physician-assisted suicide and euthanasia. Geriatric neuropsychiatrists may become involved in deciding whether specific treatments (or, for example, provision of food and fluids in the case of patients with severe dementia) should be considered at the end of life. As a rule, all of the current laws and regulations that relate to the issue of euthanasia or assisted suicide require a patient to be competent to participate in the procedure. In the future, we will have to ask whether advance directives concerning euthanasia in later stages of severe neuropsychiatric disease are appropriate means for expressing values of patients. The Royal Dutch Medical Society is preparing a report on this topic as it relates to patients with dementia or other neuropsychiatric conditions. The concept of human dignity figures large in this analysis of physician involvement and social sanctions of assisted death in patients with dementia. Ethical exploration of the concept of dignity in health care will be essential in the future (Moody 1998).

Advance Directives

The use of advance directives has been encouraged, for good reason, by a variety of patient and professional groups (see Chapter 41). It makes sense for individuals to express in writing their wishes concerning care in circumstances in which they may not be able to make their own decisions. The rules regarding how advance directives should be used, particularly in circumstances in which cognitive impairment is involved, vary from state to state. The advance directive can take the form of a *living will*, a document that lists conditions or events that may occur in the future and the patient's desired responses to those situations. Another form of advance directive is a *durable power of attorney*, by which a patient appoints an individual who would make decisions if the patient became incompetent. In my view, advance planning should incorporate both features. In the event that the patient becomes incompetent, the clinician can weigh the evidence from written documents concerning the patient's wishes and the wishes of the identified substitute decision maker. The surrogate decision maker can make the decision on the basis of how he or she believes the patient would have made the decision under the circumstances—a true substituted judgment. Another decision standard is *best interest*, which reflects the surrogate decision maker's views concerning what is judged optimal for the patient at the time of decision making. Both forms of reasoning are appropriate but should be made explicit because substitute decision makers may not entirely follow the wishes of the impaired individual.

Geriatric neuropsychiatrists will have to ensure that advance directives play an appropriate role in their provision of health care. Currently, only a relatively small number of individuals execute advance directives.

Competency Assessment

Geriatric neuropsychiatrists may be called on to attest to the competency of patients (Appelbaum and Grisso 1995). The declaration of competency is made by a judge. Ideally, if the advance directives are used to identify surrogate deci-

sion makers, legal proceedings can be minimized. However, a durable power of attorney must be executed when the patient is competent to designate such decision maker. If the patient is already incompetent, the courts may need to appoint a guardian.

A variety of approaches have been suggested for making a recommendation to the courts about a patient's competency (see Chapter 41). Formal neuropsychological tests can be administered, as can mental status tests with a focus on judgment or problem-solving abilities. The clinician can discuss with the patient circumstances that are similar to the decision facing that individual and can evaluate the patient's ability to make judgments about these practical, real-world problems.

Levels of competency are definable. At the lowest level, the patient recognizes that there is a decision to be made. Competency at higher levels (defined legally in a hierarchical fashion) includes an understanding of the contexts and possible ramifications of decisions beyond the immediate situation.

Also during the assessment for competency, the clinician should assess who would be an appropriate surrogate decision maker, should one need to be appointed by the court. In situations in which the courts are involved, there are frequently conflicts among family members. Assessment of the family structure and process is as important as assessment of the individual patient.

Ethical Issues in Research

Conflict of Interest

A variety of conflicts of interest can occur in research (Levine 1998). When a professional is both a clinician and a researcher, a conflict of interest exists. A clinician must consider currently available therapies for his or her patient first and participation by the patient in research second. Being involved in research gives the professional the incentive to recruit the individual into the protocol. This conflict of interest should be made explicit to potential subjects and the research team. If the conflict is of sufficient magnitude, an independent individual should be assigned the role of obtaining informed consent. Clinicians and researchers alike must recognize that patients and families often find these conceptual differences between the roles of patient and subject difficult to understand.

Financial conflicts of interest may also exist. Increasingly, scientists and clinicians have financial stakes in the performance of products being evaluated in research. These stakes are frequently bigger for basic biological scientists, who may, for example, start biotechnology companies after making basic research discoveries. Clinicians may, for example, consult for or obtain grants from pharmaceutical companies whose products they are testing. Most authors agree that there are different levels of conflict of interest, the levels depending on the nature of the relationship and the amount of potential financial gain. Serving as a one-time speaker for a company is considerably different from being a major stockholder in that same company. Research institutions of various kinds are required by granting agencies such as the National Institutes of Health to have formal policies on this topic.

The procedure most widely used to address the problem of conflict of interest is disclosure. For example, a clinician reporting the results of a study would identify support from the pharmaceutical industry or elsewhere. Disclosure is now required to the appropriate administrative structure within the organization conducting research. The extent of the disclosure (i.e., to whom and in what detail) can vary, however, which is a problem. Writing down one's conflicts of interest on a piece of paper that is subsequently filed and viewed by only a small group of people would hardly meet a requirement for public disclosure.

A fine line will continue to exist between appropriate and inappropriate conflict of interest. If we are to facilitate academic, industry, and governmental collaboration, sharing of resources and expertise is required. Thus, at least a confluence of interest is necessary and desirable for advancement of science and treatment methods. On the other hand, a few absolute proscriptions should probably exist. For example, individuals who have major financial stakes that depend on the profitability of particular products should probably not be involved in testing them.

Research Design

Although not always seen as an ethical issue, the quality of science proposed in a research project is of ethical concern (Kass et al. 1996; Levine 1988). A requirement of research design is that the experimental hypotheses actually be addressed by the study in an appropriate fashion. In other words, the study should actually produce answers to (or at least provide credible evidence relating to) important questions.

Certain specific aspects of the research design may also be ethically problematic. I will use as examples two issues in the field of Alzheimer's disease, with consequences on practice (see also Chapter 24).

One issue concerns the use of placebos. Donepezil, the second drug approved for use as a symptomatic cognitive enhancer in patients with Alzheimer's disease, is viewed by some as the pharmacological standard. Tacrine, the first approved agent, had many side effects, and clinical and market interest in tacrine did not match the interest in donepezil. Given the efficacy of the standard drug (donepezil), should equivalence studies (or studies with similar designs) comparing other drugs with the standard drug be performed instead of placebo-controlled studies? This issue is complex and requires the defining of the clinical standard of practice, as well as a consideration of the scientific, and ultimately social, consequences of using designs that do not incorporate placebos (Karlawish and Whitehouse 1998).

Who should decide whether placebo use is appropriate in trials involving patients with schizophrenia or dementia is another facet of the issue of placebo use. Most ethical formulations have focused on the role of clinicians and professionals in such social judgments. For example, the concept of clinical equipoise asserts that there ought to be a condition of uncertainty about the state of knowledge in the minds of practitioners. Thus, a randomized controlled trial becomes essential for obtaining knowledge needed to advance practice (Karlawish and Whitehouse 1998). Community equipoise is an extension of clinical equipoise to involve more than just clinical. I believe that assessment of the state of the field and decisions concerning research designs such as placebo-controlled trials should incorporate the voices and values of patients and families as well as professionals.

For example, representatives from the Alzheimer's Association in Cleveland (Post and Whitehouse 1995), the Alzheimer's Society of Canada (Cohen et al. 1999), and Alzheimer's Disease International (Brodaty et al. 1999) considered topics such as therapeutic goals, the role of spirituality, and informed consent in research. A variety of approaches can be used to obtain grassroots input. Professional input should be combined with lay input to develop new ways of analyzing issues. Eventually, approaches involving computer networks may improve community discourse.

A second ethical issue that arises in therapeutic trials involving patients with Alzheimer's disease has to do with drug therapies that are presented as more than symptomatic treatments of cognition, that is, as treatments that actually slow progression of disease. Studies have suggested that treatment with estrogens, vitamin E, or anti-inflammatory agents may slow the deterioration (Sano et al. 1997; Whitehouse 1998). Vitamin E is increasingly used in clinical practice today with that therapeutic goal in mind. Consensus has not been achieved, however, regarding how one would design a study so that, after completion of the study, a regulatory claim could be made that treatment with the study drug results not only in prolonged symptomatic improvement but also in alteration of the disease course (Whitehouse et al. 1998). One design involves withdrawal of a medication that has been demonstrated to be more effective in improving the patients' symptoms than placebo. The protocol to demonstrate a modifying effect on disease course thus involves withdrawing the medication and observing what happens to the patients once the medication is withdrawn. If the drug's effects are purely symptomatic, one would expect the conditions of the patients taking the drug to deteriorate to the same level as those of the patients who had been taking the placebo for the entire study. If treatment with the drug has a prolonged or sustained benefit, then the patients' conditions might deteriorate but would never fall to the level of those of the patients taking the placebo. Thus, the ethical issue in this design is that one must give a medicine, demonstrate that it is effective, and then withdraw it to try to differentiate a symptomatic from a sustained effect. Ultimately, a principal issue in research ethics is the balance between opportunity and risk for the individual and the benefits and dangers to society of certain research policies and procedures.

Informed Consent

Clinical research is dependent on the obtaining of voluntary consent from informed patients. Federal guidelines exist for research involving prisoners and children. However, attempts to develop such regulations for those with mental illness, mental retardation, or cognitive impairment have failed because of the political tensions between the clinician-scientists and the patient groups. Scientists have been concerned that regulations would impede scientific progress, whereas the patient groups have been concerned that subjects would not have adequate protection. A variety of national and international groups are now examining the issue of informed consent in those who are cognitively impaired. I and my colleagues have worked with Alzheimer's Disease International and the World Health Organization to develop guidelines to educate ethics review committees globally (Brodaty et al. 1999). In ethical deliberations, the approval and monitoring of protocols should be close to the patient, family, and community (e.g., local ethics review committees) but should be guided by broader global, societal, and cultural input. Most important in the United States are the efforts of the National Bioethics Advisory Committee. The focus of these efforts is on genetics (e.g., cloning) and participation in research (e.g., informed consent and mental illness).

The issue of informed consent is complex because a variety of different regulatory bodies—from national groups such as the Office for Protection and Research and the Federal Drug Administration to state law and local ethical review committees (institutional review boards)—are involved in the area of informed consent. The basic standard of practice is to assess whether a patient is competent to decide on his or her own about participation and, if the patient does not appear to be competent, to inquire of an appropriate family member or other representative whether approval for participation should be granted. In practice, often two signatures are collected and the precise legal standing of the substitute decision maker is not always identified. Efforts to clarify the roles of proxy decision makers are ongoing.

Questions relating to the issue of informed consent include the following: How should competence to make research decisions be established? How should a surrogate decision maker be identified? What are the absolutes (e.g., patients with cognitive incapacity should not participate in risks research that has no possible therapeutic benefit) that can help the surrogate decision maker decide what kinds of research should or should not be permitted? Finally, what kinds of monitoring should be performed to ensure that informed consent is obtained correctly and adequate informed consent is obtained (and the actual study is conducted well)?

Future Ethical Issues

As discussed earlier, ethical issues in geriatric neuropsychiatry are evolving rapidly, for several reasons. First, the science surrounding geriatric neuropsychiatry is exciting and is likely to lead to findings that have important therapeutic and diagnostic implications. Second, the population with geriatric neuropsychiatric conditions is growing. Third, the field of biomedical ethics itself is evolving, and topics that relate directly to geriatric neuropsychiatry, from genetic testing to health care rationing, are being addressed. In this section, I review some of the important issues that are likely to become more prominent in the near future.

It is likely that different genes that either cause or increase susceptibility to a variety of neuropsychiatric conditions will be identified (Gershon et al. 1998) (see Chapter 38). This is particularly the case in neurodegenerative diseases, such as Alzheimer's disease and Huntington's disease (Post and Whitehouse 1998a). In the case of autosomal dominant forms of these diseases, presymptomatic genetic testing is already theoretically feasible in families with specific identified mutations. Guidelines have been created for such testing, which provide family members at risk with information about the presence or absence of the specific mutation. However, although many potential patients initially express interest in this type of testing, relatively little presymptomatic testing has been done, at least for Alzheimer's disease.

Another area of genetics that will be problematic is the identification of further susceptibility loci. For example, one locus in Alzheimer's disease on chromosome 19, the apolipoprotein E *(APOE)* gene, modifies the risk of individuals having Alzheimer's disease (see Chapter 24). Being *APOE4*-positive makes a diagnosis of Alzheimer's disease more likely if cognitive impairment is present. Testing for the autosomal dominant mutations and susceptibility loci is available commercially. Strong statements have been made in support of their current use (often by those who have a financial stake in this use). Yet susceptibility testing is fraught with scientific as well as ethical difficulties. A principal problem relates to the extent to which research samples are representative of patients most likely to be seen by clinicians. For example, there is evidence to suggest that the increased risk associated with being *APOE4*-positive varies with gender and ethnic background. If the ethnic background of the clinician's patient is different from those of research samples, the clinician may find it impossible to assign a specific risk in association with an *APOE4*-positive state. Confidentiality is also an issue. For example, should insurance companies have access to genetic information that might allow them to prevent an individual from obtaining health care insurance or at least to charge higher premiums?

Related to the use of genetic testing in living patients is the use of genetic material from tissue specimens obtained from persons while still alive or at autopsy. There are a number of questions regarding this issue: Should researchers who obtain genetic material be able to use this material for research in areas that are different from the areas specified by the patient? How long should tissues be stored? What rights should patients have to profits from the commercialization of any technology developed in association with the use of the patients' tissue? Genetic issues in geriatric neuropsychiatry will continue to yield questions relating to individuals' rights and social justice.

Another trend is the consideration of broad cultural issues when ethical issues in neuropsychiatric disease are considered. Already, multisite, multinational studies are often conducted in which protocol approval needs to be obtained from ethics review boards representing many different nationalities and cultures. Even within the United States, with its diverse populations, different cultural attitudes toward research and therapeutic goals are evident. The attitudes of African Americans are still affected by the Tuskegee "experiments." In this long-running study, black men with untreated syphilis were observed even after penicillin (an effective agent against syphilis) was discovered. The revelations of the National Radiation Research Review Committee suggest the problems of obtaining adequate informed consent and monitoring studies are still with us (Faden 1996). In the study described, adults and children with or without mental impairment were exposed to radiation in various forms without being told the risks or even that they were being exposed to radioactive substances.

Moreover, because of a variety of factors, principally the financial health of individual nations, the standard of practice may vary in different countries. Here are a few examples: There is considerable controversy concerning AIDS research in African nations that do not have access to the modern medications that are available in the United States. Given that the standard of care is different in Africa, is it acceptable that studies be done in Africa that would be considered unethical in the United States? In the case of Alzheimer's disease, treatment with donepezil may become such a standard of practice in the United States that conducting placebo-controlled studies may be viewed as unethical. Could an American scientist then conduct placebo-controlled research in a country where this use of donepezil had not been approved or where it had been approved but the drug was not affordable for a large segment of the population? A critical issue in this area of international ethics is the relative benefit to various parties, especially the developing country that is the site of the research.

Finally, it is likely that the discipline of bioethics will continue to evolve in ways that will affect geriatric neuropsychiatry practice. Modern medical bioethics evolved from considerations of the impact of medical technologies. For example, the Kennedy Institute, which was founded in 1970, used the word *bioethics* in its title and was principally organized to address ethical issues associated with the care of patients with mental retardation and the use of reproductive technologies. However, the original formulation of bioethics by Van Rensselaer Potter involved a much broader vision of the relationship between science and philosophy and between biology and values. Potter's vision was that bioethics would be a bridge to the future. His bioethics was rooted in land and environmental ethics (McKim 1997). Potter and I developed the idea of creating a bridge between medical and ecological ethics. The survival of human beings and other species, along with environmental stewardship, ought to be the principal focus of a deep bioethics (Potter and Whitehouse 1998; Whitehouse 1998). The word *deep* in *deep bioethics* is borrowed from the phrase *deep ecology*, which is used to describe the approach in which we are to look beyond the numerous individual environmental crises and develop a vision of our individual and species' relationships to nature. Scientific and certain religious beliefs have been interpreted as granting permission to dominate natural processes. Like Potter, deep ecologists ask us to develop individual creeds to guide our own behavior as citizens and professionals. As a species, we should view ourselves as stewards rather than controllers of nature.

In the future, greater concerns will be raised regarding the deterioration of our environment, partly occurring as a result of scientific "progress." The growth of the world's population continues to be a concern. A special part of this growth is the increase in the proportion of elderly individuals. Thus, the ethically appropriate and wise use of our scientific knowledge and technology will be critically important. However, thoughtless application, purely for short-term economic progress and without regard for long-term consequences, will be the death of civilization and perhaps our species.

The next millennium will bring revolution in the biological and informational sciences. Geriatric neuropsychiatry will remain an exciting field but will remain a really important one only if we balance our passions for scientific progress and professional security with sincere and genuine humility regarding our role in the community of human beings and other living creatures.

References

Appelbaum PS, Grisso T: The MacArthur Treatment Competence Study, I: mental illness and competence to consent to treatment. Law Hum Behav 19:105–126, 1995

Beauchamp TL, Childress JF: Principles of Biomedical Ethics, 3rd Edition. New York, Oxford University Press, 1989

Berenson RA: The doctor's dilemma revisited: ethical physician decisions in a managed care environment. Generations, Summer 1998, pp 63–68

Brodaty H, Dresser R, Eisner M, et al: Alzheimer's Disease International and International Working Group for Harmonization of Dementia Drug Guidelines for research involving human subjects with dementia. Alzheimer Dis Assoc Disord 13:71–79, 1999

Brody H: The Healer's Power. New Haven, CT, Yale University Press, 1992

Bulger RE, Bobby EM, Fineberg HV: Society's Choices: Social and Ethical Decision Making in Biomedicine. Washington, DC, National Academy Press, 1995

Carter MA: Assessing the field from within. Medical Humanities Review 12:44–47, 1998

Chambers T: Retrodiction and the histories of bioethics. Medical Humanities Review 12:9–22, 1998

Cohen CA, Whitehouse PJ, Post SG, et al: Ethical issues in Alzheimer disease: the experience of a national Alzheimer society task force. Alzheimer Dis Assoc Disord 13:66–70, 1999

Engelhardt HT Jr: The Foundations of Bioethics, 2nd Edition. New York, Oxford University Press, 1996

Faden R: The Advisory Committee on Human Radiation Experiments: reflections on a presidential commission. Hastings Cent Rep 26:5–10, 1996

Fox RC: The evolution of American bioethics: a sociological perspective, in Social Science Perspectives on Medical Ethics. Edited by Weisz G. Dordrecht, The Netherlands, Kluwer Academic, 1990, pp 201–217

Gershon ES, Badner JA, Goldin LR, et al: Closing in on genes for manic-depressive illness and schizophrenia. Neuropsychopharmacology 18:233–242, 1998

Jonsen AR, Toulmin S: The Abuse of Casuistry. Berkeley, CA, University of California Press, 1988

Karlawish J, Whitehouse PJ: Is the placebo control obsolete in a world after donepezil and vitamin E? Arch Neurol 55:1420–1424, 1998

Kass NE, Sugarman J, Faden R, et al: Trust: The fragile foundation of contemporary biomedical research. Hastings Cent Rep 26:11–24, 1996

Kodish E, Murray T, Whitehouse PJ: Conflict of interest in university-industry research relationships: realities, politics, and values. Acad Med 71:1287–1290, 1996

Levine RJ: The Ethics and Regulation of Clinical Research, 2nd Edition. New Haven, CT, Yale University Press, 1988

McKim R: Environmental ethics: the widening vision. Religious Studies Review 23:245–250, 1997

Moody HR: Why dignity in old age matters, in Dignity and Old Age. Edited by Disch R, Dobrof R, Moody HR. Haworth, 1998, pp 13–38

Nussbaum MC: Love's Knowledge: Essays on Philosophy and Literature. Oxford, UK, Oxford University Press, 1992

Pellegrino ED: The metamorphosis of medical ethics: a 30-year retrospective. JAMA 269:1158–1162, 1993

Post SG, Whitehouse PJ: Fairhill guidelines on ethics of the care of people with Alzheimer's disease: a clinical summary. J Am Geriatr Soc 43:1423–1429, 1995

Post SG, Whitehouse PJ: Genetic Testing for Alzheimer Disease: Ethical and Clinical Issues. Baltimore, MD, Johns Hopkins University Press, 1998a

Post SG, Whitehouse PJ: The moral basis for limiting treatment: hospice and advanced progressive dementia, in Hospice Care for Patients With Advanced Progressive Dementia. Edited by Volicer L, Hurley A. New York, Springer, 1998b, pp 117–131

Post SG, Ripich DN, Whitehouse PJ: Discourse ethics: research, dementia and communication. Alzheimer Dis Assoc Disord 8:58–65, 1994

Potter VR: Bioethics, Bridge to the Future. Englewood Cliffs, NJ, Prentice-Hall, 1971

Potter VR: Global Bioethics Building on the Leopold Legacy. East Lansing, MI, Michigan State University Press, 1988

Potter VR, Whitehouse PJ: Deep and global bioethics for a livable third millennium. The Scientist, January 5, 1998, p 9

Reich WT: The word "bioethics": the struggle over its earliest meanings. Kennedy Institute of Ethics Journal 5:19–34, 1995

Sano M, Ernesto C, Thomas RG, et al: A controlled trial of selegiline and alpha-tocopherol or both as treatment for Alzheimer's disease. N Engl J Med 336:1216–1222, 1997

Whitehouse PJ: Future Drug Development for Alzheimer's Disease (Blue Books of Practical Neurology Series on the Dementias, Vol 19). Woburn, MA, Butterworth Heinemann, 1998, pp 359–372

Whitehouse PJ, Deal WE: Situated beyond modernity: lessons for Alzheimer's disease research (editorial). J Am Geriatr Soc 43:1314–1315, 1995

Whitehouse PJ, Rabins PV: Quality of life and dementia (editorial). Alzheimer Dis Assoc Disord 6:135–138, 1992

Whitehouse PJ, Post SG, Sachs GA: Dementia care at the end of life: empirical research and international collaboration. Alzheimer Dis Assoc Disord 10:3–4, 1996

Whitehouse PJ, Kittner B, Roessner M, et al: Clinical trial designs for demonstrating disease-course-altering effects in dementia. Alzheimer Dis Assoc Disord 12:281–294, 1998

41

Competency and Related Forensic Issues

J. Edward Spar, M.D.

Neuropsychiatric illness in elderly patients commonly leads to abnormalities in mood, memory and other cognitive functions, and the ability to perform activities of daily living. When these deficits become grossly evident, concerns about the mental capacity or competency of the affected individual tend to arise. Health care providers may question the patient's ability to give informed consent for medical treatment or to make end-of-life decisions regarding resuscitation and life support. Attorneys may become concerned about future challenges to the provisions of wills, gifts, and trusts, and concerned friends or relatives may recommend that durable powers of attorney be executed or may contemplate guardianship or conservatorship. If the impaired patient has a driving-related mishap (e.g., gets lost or has an accident), his or her competency to drive may be challenged, and the right to drive may be lost.

In this chapter, I first consider the broad legal construct of *mental capacity* or *competency* (the two terms, as well as the term *competence*, are used interchangeably here) and then discuss the specific social contexts in which the geriatric neuropsychiatrist is likely to perform a contemporaneous or retrospective evaluation of competency. Several re-

lated forensic issues (e.g., limitations on the requirement for informed consent, elder abuse, and undue influence) are addressed in this discussion.

CAVEAT: For purposes of illustration and discussion, I refer in this chapter to *California law*. Because statutory and governing case laws differ considerably from state to state, the reader is strongly urged to check the law applicable to his or her jurisdiction.

What Is Competency?

In the literature on competency, the term *competency* is generally used in reference to decision making and communicating capacity. The President's Commission for the Study of Ethical Problems in Medicine and Biobehavioral Research (President's Commission 1982) defined *competency* as "the ability to make autonomous decisions; to reason and deliberate and to understand and communicate information; and the possession of goals and values" (p. 57). Hoge et al. (1997) defined *decisional competence* as "the capacity to: understand information relevant to the issue at hand; think rationally about alternative courses of action; appreciate one's situation as a person confronted with a specific decision; and express a choice among alternatives" (pp. 146–147).

The presence of terms such as *ability* and *capacity* in statutory definitions of competency has an important practical implication. The court in *Estate of Jenks* made the distinction (as it applies in the testamentary context) thus: "It is the generally recognized rule that testamentary capacity requires only that the testator have *capacity* to know and understand the nature and extent of his bounty, as distinguished from the requirement that he have *actual knowledge* thereof" *(Estate of Jenks* 1971, emphasis added).

It is a presumption in common law that every adult is competent for all legal purposes until proven otherwise, and a formal, legally binding determination of incompetency can be made only by a court. Still, the vast majority of competency determinations are informal and are made by physicians, attorneys, police officers, and other professional and nonprofessional workers in the course of everyday practice. Physicians and other health care professionals make competency judgments when they seek informed consent for risky or invasive medical procedures, lawyers informally assess their clients' competency before taking on estate planning assignments or when designing a criminal defense, and police officers make implicit judgments of competency when deciding whether certain detained individuals should be taken to the police station for booking or to the local emergency room for psychiatric evaluation.

The consequences of a formal determination of incompetency are generally twofold. On the one hand, as an instance of the state acting in *parens patriae* (as a "benevolent parent"), the judgment confers certain protections: appointment of a conservator or guardian protects the individual from the consequences of his or her own poor financial decisions, or inability to secure food, clothing, shelter, or medical care; and a judgment of lack of contractual capacity may excuse an individual from the performance required of an otherwise valid contract. On the other hand, the individual found to be incompetent also pays a price for this protection, namely the loss of certain rights of self-determination, such as the rights to accept or refuse treatment, to enter a plea or to stand trial, to enter into contracts, and to make a will. Some formal judgments of incompetence derive more from the police power of the state and are legitimized by society's concern for the potential victims of the incompetent individual. A finding of incompetence in this context is likely to involve involuntary hospitalization or medical treatment. By contrast, informal judgments of incompetency generally lead to the withholding of certain professional services, at least until further steps are taken.

Formal competency determinations are made in both criminal and civil contexts. Although geriatric neuropsychiatrists are relatively unlikely to become involved in the criminal justice system, this chapter would be incomplete without at least a brief consideration of criminal competency. A more detailed and comprehensive discussion of civil competency follows this section on criminal competency.

Competency in Criminal Law

Mr. J, an 83-year-old retired attorney, had early vascular dementia when the Securities and Exchange Commission initiated an investigation of insider trading. By the time the commission had compiled enough evidence to prosecute him, Mr. J's cognitive function had deteriorated dramatically. He was disoriented to year, month, season, and date; did not know his address or telephone number; and had moderate to severe impairment of new learning, recent recall, and remote memory. He was unable to name any presidents including the current one, even when given clues, and could not recall the names of any of his past employers or the ages of his children, the names of their spouses, or whether they had children. A neuropsychiatrist consulted by the court opined that Mr. J lacked the capacity to stand trial or to plead guilty.

In the criminal context, the two major types of competency have traditionally been *competency to plead guilty* and *competency to stand trial*. In *Dusky v. United States* (1960), the Supreme Court stated that a defendant is competent to stand trial if "[the defendant] has sufficient present ability to consult with his lawyer with a reasonable degree of rational understanding—and . . . a rational as well as factual understanding of the proceedings against him." According to this definition, both decisional competency *and* actual understanding are required. In the case cited above, the neuropsychiatrist opined that Mr. J did not meet either of these criteria. Given that defense attorneys question their clients' ability to meet the Supreme Court's standard in 8%–15% of felony cases, it has been estimated that 25,000 competency evaluations of criminal defendants occur per year (Hoge et al. 1997), making this by far the most common formal determination of competency. In 1993, the Supreme Court held that competency to plead guilty and competency to stand trial are in fact the same *(Godinez v. Moran* 1993). Issues related to this "composite" competency, which has been termed *adjudicative competence* by Hoge et al. (1997), have led to the creation of a substantial literature on the topic (review of which is beyond the scope of this chapter, as are the related issues of diminished capacity and the insanity defense), aimed at the problem of specifying criteria, screening for, and ultimately determining adjudicative competence in criminal defendants. Hoge and colleagues (1997) provided a review of this topic.

Competency in Civil Law

The types of civil competency most likely to concern geriatric neuropsychiatrists are competency 1) to give informed consent for medical care, 2) to execute an advance directive, 3) to give informed consent for enrollment in a study, 4) to enter into (and be held accountable for) a contract (contractual capacity), 5) to execute a will (testamentary capacity) or trust, 6) to provide self-care (provide oneself with food, clothing, shelter, and medical care), and 7) to manage one's finances.

Competency to Give Informed Consent for Medical Care

The capacity to give informed consent for medical care is probably the most studied of all the varieties of civil competency. Four components of decisional competency in the medical setting were distinguished by Appelbaum and Grisso (1988) and have been accepted by most authors: the ability to communicate a choice, to understand relevant information, to appreciate the situation and its consequences, and to manipulate information rationally. Though seemingly straightforward, this definition raises several questions. First, it is not always clear what "rationally manipulating information" means; it has been often noted that the treating physician is most likely to conclude that the manipulation is not rational if the outcome of the manipulation (i.e., the patient's decision to accept or reject the proposed intervention) does not agree with what the physician believes makes the most sense. On this point Appelbaum and Grisso (1988) stated: "Rational manipulation involves the ability to reach conclusions that are logically consistent with the starting premises. This requires both weighing the risks and benefits of a single option and the usually more complex process of weighing multiple options simultaneously . . ." (p. 1636). The notion of appreciation may also be obscure to many clinicians. Schaffner (1991) defined *appreciation* as "not only factual understanding and rational manipulation of the information, but an additional facility for applying general information to particular circumstances and for comprehending the crucial nature of certain data" (p. 255), and Appelbaum and Roth (1982) stated that " 'appreciation' is taken to be an affective, as well as a cognitive, recognition of the nature of the situation" (p. 955).

A thornier problem in the application of the four components of decisional competency is the question of operationalization, that is, what observable criteria would satisfy the definitions of the relevant terms. That is, with the meaning of the terms having been clarified, how does the clinician determine whether understanding and appreciation are present or rational manipulation of information is actually taking place? A potentially important step toward resolution of this problem was taken by Grisso and colleagues (1997), who developed the MacArthur Competence Assessment Tool-Technique, a semistructured interview procedure that guides clinicians and patients through a process of disclosure of information related to informed consent, and an assessment of patients' capacities to make decisions based on the information. Information specific to the patient's situation is used, and only 15–20 minutes are required for the procedure. Preliminary data obtained using this instrument in patients with schizophrenia and schizoaffective disorder suggest that it has acceptable reliability, validity, and clinical feasibility. However, the authors recognized that the elements of decisional competence assessed by this instrument "are not the only factors in ultimate clinical or legal judgments of competence" and anticipated that the main use for the tool would be in "the midrange of ambiguous cases of competence . . . especially when clinicians have reason to believe that their judgments might later be questioned—for example, in legal proceedings about a patient's capacity to decide or about the reasonableness of a clinician's decision to accept a patient's decision or to turn instead to a surrogate" (Grisso et al. 1997, p. 1419)

Capacity is only one of three equally important components of informed consent for medical care. The President's Commission (1982) concluded that the patient must be provided with appropriate information regarding the recommended medical intervention (the categories of information required by California law are listed in Table 41–1) and that the consent must be given voluntarily—that is, it cannot be a result of coercion or threats (discussed in a later section).

Even when a proposed medical intervention is associated with enough risk to warrant seeking informed consent from the patient, there are limits to the kind and amount of information that the clinician must provide, and there are circumstances in which the intervention may proceed without informed consent. In nonemergent situations, courts have ruled that physicians have the responsibility to exercise "therapeutic privilege"—that is, to approach the process of obtaining informed consent in a clinically sensitive and appropriate manner. *Natanson v. Kline* (1960) established that a clinician should provide the information

TABLE 41–1. Requirements of informed consent: what patients must be told about a proposed treatment

The nature and seriousness of the illness, disorder, or defect that the person has

The nature of the medical treatment that is being recommended by the person's health care providers

The probable degree and duration of any benefits and risks of any medical intervention that is being recommended by the person's health care providers, and the consequences of lack of treatment

The nature, risks, and benefits of any reasonable alternatives

Source. Data from California Probate Code § 813.

that the hypothetical "reasonable medical practitioner" would provide to his or her patient. But in *Canterbury v. Spence* (1972) the court turned this reasoning around, concluding that the person receiving the information (the hypothetical "reasonable person") should determine what information is provided. In both of these landmark cases, the notion of reasonability was used in setting lower and upper limits on the information imparted; that is, too much information was considered possibly to be as unreasonable as too little information. In *Natanson v. Kline*, the court noted that full disclosure "could so alarm the patient that it would, in fact, constitute bad medical practice," and in *Canterbury v. Spence* the court recognized that, for some patients, disclosing certain information could "foreclose a rational decision, or complicate or hinder the treatment, or perhaps even pose psychological damage to the patient." In a 1985 Massachusetts case *(Precourt v. Frederick)*, the court was even more explicit, stating: "A physician is not required to inform a patient of remote risks" and "There must be a reasonable accommodation between the patient's right to know, and fairness to physicians and society's interest that medicine be practiced . . . without unrealistic and unnecessary burdens on practitioners."

Informed consent is generally not required in an emergent situation, in which significant harm would come to a patient (or to others, in the case of a violent patient) if the intervention were delayed so that informed consent could be obtained. Under these circumstances, the principle of implied consent applies—that is, the physician may perform the intervention to which a reasonable, self-interested patient would consent, given the opportunity. Similarly, if the patient is unconscious or otherwise incompetent to participate in the consent process, and no substitute decision maker (e.g., guardian or conservator, attorney-in-fact for health care, or, in some jurisdictions, next of kin) or advance directive is available, the physician may ad-

minister appropriate treatment until the patient is able to consent. In California, *emergency medical care* is defined as "those medical services required for the immediate diagnosis and treatment of medical conditions which, if not immediately diagnosed and treated, could lead to serious physical or mental disability or death" (California Health and Safety Code § 1799.110b; see also California Probate Code § 3210). However, the definition of *emergency* may differ in other jurisdictions, and the reader is advised to check applicable local law.

Competency to Execute an Advance Directive

> Mrs. R, an 88-year-old woman with advanced Alzheimer's disease, was admitted to a long-term care facility. As was routine at the facility, on the day of admission Mrs. R was asked to execute a durable power of attorney for health care, appointing her daughter as her attorney-in-fact. She complied, and later that day Mrs. R's daughter was approached for consent to administer neuroleptic medications to her mother. Is anything wrong with this picture?

Advance directives are legal instruments intended to ensure that appropriate decisions regarding medical care are made when a patient becomes incompetent to give informed consent. The Patient Self-Determination Act (Omnibus Budget Reconciliation Act of 1990), which became federal law on December 1, 1991, mandates that hospitals, nursing homes, and other health care organizations provide information to patients concerning availability and use of these instruments.

There are generally two types of advance directives: *proxy directives*, such as the durable power of attorney for health care (DPAHC) or health care proxy, and *instruction directives*, such as the living will. DPAHC allows an individual (the *principal*) to authorize another person, usually a family member or spouse (the *attorney-in-fact*), to give or withhold consent for medical care for the principal if the principal becomes incompetent: "A durable Power of attorney is a power of attorney by which a principal designates another his attorney in fact and the writing contains the words, 'This power of attorney shall not be affected by disability of the principal,' or 'This power of attorney shall become effective upon the disability or incapacity of the principal' or similar words showing the intent of the principal that the authority conferred shall be exercisable notwithstanding the principal's subsequent disability or incapacity" (Uniform Durable Power of Attorney Act). Some states have enacted similar laws creating the health care proxy.

A living will, a document that is created by an individual when he or she is of sound mind, specifies the limits of care to be given by health care providers if the individual "become[s] unable to participate in decisions regarding . . . medical care." One widely circulated version (the source of the previous quotation and available from the Society for the Right to Die, 250 West 57th St., New York, NY 10107) directs the attending physician "to withhold or withdraw treatment that merely prolongs . . . dying" if the individual develops "an incurable or irreversible mental or physical condition with no reasonable expectation of recovery." It also has a section in which the individual can specify particular treatments that he or she does not want, as well as particular preferences regarding treatment and the end of his or her life (e.g., the preference to die at home).

There are clear advantages and disadvantages to both types of directives. A proxy has much more flexibility than an "instructive" has, and a proxy can respond to circumstances that may not have been anticipated by the principal. On the other hand, a proxy can also betray the trust of the principal by making decisions that the principal would not have endorsed. In some states, a living will and DPAHC or health care proxy can be combined, resulting in an instrument that requires the attorney-in-fact or proxy to follow the provisions of the living will and authorizes the exercise of his or her judgment in circumstances not covered by the will.

Obviously, advance directives are intended to be executed when the principal *is* competent to give or withhold consent for medical care, and one might think that the standard for competency to execute an advance directive would be the same as the standard for competency to consent to medical care. Yet California law states: "A natural person having the *capacity to contract* may execute a power of attorney" (California Probate Code § 4120, emphasis added). However, different standards for competency to execute an advance directive may obtain in other states. Therefore, depending on the prevailing definitions of *capacity* to give informed consent to medical treatment and capacity to execute an advance directive, the long-term care facility's handling of Mrs. R (in the previous case example) could be appropriate—that is, she could simultaneously have the capacity to execute a DPAHC and not have the capacity to consent to treatment with a neuroleptic. In a similar vein, the powers of the attorney-in-fact differ from state to state. California law prohibits the attorney-in-fact from consenting to placement in a mental health treatment facility, convulsive treatment, psychosurgery, sterilization, or abortion (California Probate Code § 4722) and also prohibits the attorney-in-fact from consenting to health care

or consenting to the withholding or withdrawal of health care "necessary to keep the principal alive, if the principal objects to the health care or to the withholding or withdrawal of the health care. In such a case, the case is governed by the law that would apply if there were no durable power of attorney for health care" (California Probate Code § 4724). This section appears to reflect the will of the California legislature that individuals retain the authority to make end-of-life decisions, even if they are incompetent to make other medical decisions.

Much has been written about the question of which rules should govern the decisions of substitute decision makers such as attorneys-in-fact. The prevailing view is known as the doctrine of "substituted judgment," according to which the substitute decision maker should act, as much as possible, in accordance with the wishes, values, and goals of the principal. The alternative, "best interests," approach calls upon the substitute decision maker to perform an "objective assessment of the burdens and benefits for this patient" as the basis for his or her decision (Fellows 1998, p. 924). The court in a New Jersey case (*In re Conroy* 1985) spelled out a three-step protocol for analyzing the patient's wishes. First, consider any statements or other directives made by the patient. If these are not conclusive, then attempt to deduce the patient's wishes from his or her more generally held values, religious beliefs, and so on. Finally, if these steps leave the issue in doubt, revert to what a person in the patient's situation might reasonably choose.

Competency to Consent to Enrollment in a Research Study

The considerations just discussed regarding competency to consent to medical care generally apply to competency to consent to enrollment in a study. Before an investigator can claim to have secured informed consent, the subject must have been supplied with appropriate information, *voluntary* consent must have been obtained, and the subject must have been considered competent. In 1982, the President's Commission clearly spelled out the disclosures required under ordinary circumstances (Table 41–2), and in 1996, the Food and Drug Administration published an "exception to informed consent" rule intended to govern research conducted in medically emergent circumstances (Federal Register 1996). To date, however, no comparable guidelines have been articulated for the conduct of research using cognitively impaired (marginally competent or frankly incompetent) subjects in nonemergent situations, although the National Bioethics Advisory Commission (created by President Clinton in 1995) is in the process of drafting a report on this issue (Marwick 1998). Such

TABLE 41–2.   **Disclosures required for research subjects**

The fact that research is being performed and the purposes of the research

Reasonably foreseeable risks

Reasonably expected benefits

Appropriate alternatives

A statement about the maintenance of confidentiality

An explanation about possible compensation if injury occurs, in cases of research involving more than minimal risk

Information about how the subject can have pertinent questions answered

A statement about voluntary participation, indicating that refusal to participate involves no penalties or loss of benefits

guidelines are likely to have important implications for research involving patients with dementia.

Several authors have addressed the problems associated with the use of proxy decision makers for incompetent research subjects. Kapp (1994) identified three "axes" of concern. The first axis is the question of who should act as a proxy decision maker for the impaired research subject, how that person should be selected, and what procedural safeguards should exist to prevent exploitation of the subject by the proxy. In order of decreasing formality, the approaches he discussed included 1) appointment (by a court) of a regular guardian with explicit authority to consent to the principal's participation in research; 2) appointment (by a court) of a guardian *ad litem* (a person appointed to act on behalf of a principal for a specific task) with explicit authority to consent to the principal's participation in a particular research project; 3) execution (when the principal is clearly competent) of a durable power of attorney for research participation, in jurisdictions where such an instrument is available; 4) reliance on the informed consent of family members, in states that have statutes authorizing family members to act as proxies for health care decisions in the absence of an advance directive; and 5) reliance on the informal informed consent of family members, in states that do not have statutes authorizing family members to act as proxies for health care decisions in the absence of an advance directive. Of these, Kapp clearly endorsed the third approach, considering the fourth a backup procedure and the first an approach of last resort. The second axis of concern is the proxy's role and the criteria to be used to make decisions regarding research participation. Kapp agreed with most authorities that the proxy should first protect the subject from harm, but Kapp stated that as long as the wishes of the subject on this point were clear, substituted judgment could permit the proxy to accept whatever de-

gree of risk the subject would have accepted, had he or she been competent. The third axis of concern is the type of research and the kind and quantity of risk to the subject—both considerations, in Kapp's view, being proper foci of the attention of proxy decision makers.

Bonnie (1997) expanded on Kapp's third-axis concerns, recommending that institutional review boards follow the "operative standard of informed consent used in everyday clinical and research practice[, which] varies according to the degree of risk" (p. 110). Bonnie suggested that proxy decision makers be used to provide concurrent authorization for research participation by impaired subjects who are capable only of assenting and, in some cases, even for participation by those fully capable of informed consent (a kind of reverse second opinion). For example, an 85-year-old, mildly cognitively impaired patient agrees to participate in a clinical trial of a cognitive-enhancing medication. The investigator believes that the patient is capable of giving informed consent for study participation and obtains that consent but also obtains written informed consent from the attorney-in-fact for health care. The latter consent serves as a confirmation of the investigator's judgment that the patient's consent is a true expression of the patient's goals and values.). Bonnie also stated that statutory authorization of family members to act as proxies for *health care* decisions in the absence of an advance directive "can reasonably be construed to cover research with potential therapeutic benefit that is properly linked with clinical care, and the statutes can be amended to clarify their application to research settings" (Bonnie 1997, p. 110).

Competency to Enter Into a Contract or Make a Gift

Mr. M, an 86-year-old developer who owned a chain of long-term care facilities, was dying of lung cancer. Shortly before his death, his 51-year-old wife of 10 years convinced him to transfer all of his assets to her in exchange for a very modest monthly stipend. The execution of the transfer took place in Mr. M's hospital room and was attended by several attorneys, who had the foresight to have the proceedings videotaped. After Mr. M died, his daughter challenged the transfer on the basis of the claim that he lacked contractual capacity. A neuropsychiatrist reviewed his medical records, which clearly documented moderately severe delirium on the date of the videotape session, and also reviewed the videotape, which equally clearly demonstrated Mr. M's distractibility, inattention, recent memory impairment, and obvious lack of understanding of the meaning and consequences of the transfer.

Whereas the traditional view of contract versus property law distinguishes between the "future orientation" of contracts and the "present orientation" of a gift, competency to enter into a contract and competency to give a gift during one's lifetime (inter vivos) are treated as essentially the same in contemporary legal literature (Meiklejohn 1988–1989). Geriatric neuropsychiatrists are likely to become involved in legal action related to contractual competency in two situations: 1) when an individual who has entered into a contract or made a gift (the *grantor*) attempts to escape responsibility for the future performance demanded by the contract or to retrieve assets already transferred per the terms of the contract or gift, on the basis of the claim that he or she lacked contractual competency at the time; and 2) when the establishment of a conservatorship of estate (discussed shortly) is under contemplation by a court because a proposed conservatee is thought to be unable, on the basis of mental incapacity, to manage his or her finances or resist fraud or undue influence. Although courts have the authority to grant exceptions in specific cases, the establishment of a conservatorship generally creates an irrebuttable presumption that the conservatee lacks contractual and donative (but not testamentary) capacity.

Definitions of *contractual capacity* vary widely by jurisdiction. The Restatement (Second) of Contracts (1979) provides as follows: "A person incurs only voidable contractual duties by entering into a transaction if by reason of mental illness or defect (a) he is unable to understand in a reasonable manner the nature and consequences of the transaction, or (b) he is unable to act in a reasonable manner in relation to the transaction and the other party has reason to know of his condition." But until 1996, California law stated: "A person entirely without understanding has no power to make a contract of any kind" (California Civil Code § 38) and "A conveyance or other contract made by a person of unsound mind, but not entirely without understanding, made before his incapacity has been judicially determined, is subject to rescission" (California Civil Code § 39a). In part because of the vagueness of this standard, a new section (California Civil Code § 39b) was added to the California code (as part of the Due Process in Competence Determinations Act) in 1996. This section is intended to anchor contractual capacity to the statutory definition of persons who qualify for a conservatorship of estate. It states: "A rebuttable presumption affecting the burden of proof that a person is of unsound mind shall exist if the person is substantially unable to manage his or her own financial resources or resist fraud or undue influence." This statute provides a partial remedy for situations in which an individual, typically elderly and cognitively impaired, who qualifies for but has not (yet) been provided a conservator of estate has entered into an unwise contract (e.g., for unneeded home improvements) because of impaired judg-

ment. If it can be proven that a conservatorship *could* have been established, the usual assumption that every adult is competent for all legal purposes is reversed, and the other party to the contract must prove that the elderly individual possessed contractual capacity (Hankin 1995).

> Mr. K, a 92-year-old man with early Alzheimer's disease, had been a shrewd and successful businessman in his youth. Within the past 2 years, he had invested a large amount of money in an extremely unwise business venture of a distant friend and had loaned large sums of money to several acquaintances without securing collateral and, in one case, with no documentation at all. His oldest son petitioned the probate court to appoint a conservator of estate. After appointing an attorney for Mr. K and obtaining a psychiatric evaluation, the court complied, over Mr. K's objection. The conservator immediately initiated legal proceedings under California Civil Code § 39b to rescind the prior investments and recover some of the assets that had been loaned away.

When a claim of contractual or donative incompetency is adjudicated, courts tend to give substantial weight to facts besides the degree of mental impairment of the grantor, such as the substantive fairness (i.e., the terms of the contract or gift, as opposed to the procedural fairness) of the transaction in question. In other words, the fact that the grantor agreed to an obviously bad deal may be regarded as evidence supporting the claim that the grantor was incompetent.

Competency to Make a Will

> Mr. R, an 84-year-old retired tractor repairman, owned a small house in the countryside, where he had lived alone for almost 50 years. His cousin Lem was his only living relative. Mr. R had moved to a board-and-care facility at the onset of cognitive decline, and after several years he decided to write a will leaving his house to Lem. The attorney called in by the board-and-care facility at Mr. R's request recognized that Mr. R was obviously cognitively impaired and arranged to have Mr. R evaluated by a geriatric neuropsychiatrist. Mr. R was found to be severely impaired in all cognitive spheres, with a Mini-Mental State Exam score of 10 and comparably low scores on several supplementary standardized instruments. But when asked about his will, Mr. R said, "When I die, I'm leaving the house to my cousin Lem. It's all I got, and Lem is my only family. I want it that way in my will. That's all." During an hour-long interview, Mr. R added little to that remark but said nothing suggestive of delusional thought.

Most states define *testamentary capacity* as the capacity to "understand the nature of the testamentary act, understand

and recollect the nature and situation of his or her property, and remember and understand his or her relations to his or her living descendants, spouse, and parents, and those whose interests are affected by the will." Some states require only one or two of these criteria to be met, and many states also require that "the testator [be] also free of . . . delusions or hallucinations [that] result in the person's devising his or her property in a way which, except for the existence of the delusions or hallucinations, he or she would not have done" (California Probate Code § 6100.5). In general, if lack of testamentary capacity is proven, the entire will or codicil (modification to an existing will) is invalid. Testamentary capacity is generally recognized as "only a modest level of competence ('the weakest class of sound minds')" (*Estate of Rosen* 1982), and legal presumptions relating to this competency have traditionally also helped to set the bar fairly low. Accordingly, despite advanced dementia, Mr. R clearly met these criteria for testamentary capacity.

Besides the general presumption that the testator was competent at the time the will was executed, it has also been stated that "when one has a mental disorder in which there are lucid periods, it is presumed that his will has been made during a time of lucidity" (*Estate of Goetz* 1967). The trend of more recent cases, though, has been toward increasing recognition that—at least in the case of progressive illnesses, such as Alzheimer's disease and vascular dementia—once testamentary capacity has been lost, it is unlikely to return, even for brief periods.

Despite the fact that testamentary capacity is a low standard, wills are vulnerable to challenge if an aggrieved party can produce any evidence of mental impairment in the testator, and a medical record containing the mere diagnosis of a neuropsychiatric illness is almost always enough, all things else being equal, to encourage contestants to proceed. Although it is common knowledge among neuropsychiatrists that a diagnosis alone does not imply any particular level of intellectual function or automatically determine the presence or absence of any type of competency, many judges, attorneys, and juries are not in possession of this insight and may need to be educated through expert testimony.

In many will contests, the allegation that the testator lacked testamentary capacity at the time the will was executed is accompanied by the allegation that the will, or parts of it, is the product of undue influence. Because testamentary capacity is such a low standard, and because prospective evaluation of the testator is rarely performed (and if it is, it is almost always at the request of a competent testator or by his or her anticipated beneficiaries), it is usually very difficult to prove that a testator did not possess testa-

mentary capacity at the precise moment that the contested will was signed (executed). Accordingly, an allegation of undue influence often proves to be the stronger case for the contestant. Any part of a will that is proven to be a result of undue influence is overturned, but the remainder remains valid if the will without the influenced provisions still makes sense and the testator otherwise had testamentary capacity. Undue influence is discussed later in this chapter.

Competency to Execute a Trust

Trusts are increasingly popular instruments with which to determine the disposition of one's assets after death, and to that extent a trust serves the same function as a will and the relatively low standard for testamentary capacity should apply. But even if it did, the testamentary standard of understanding the nature of the testamentary act would almost always require more intact intellectual function than that required for a will because trusts are generally more complicated than wills, with more, and more detailed, provisions. Moreover, whereas a will is simply a piece of paper with a set of instructions, a trust is a more abstract entity that requires relatively intact higher intellectual functions to grasp. Some courts have differentiated the standards of competency for trusts and wills on the basis of the fact that establishing a trust entails a step in addition to merely signing a set of instructions: the creator of the trust must also transfer his or her property to the trust. This act would seem to require contractual or donative capacity, which is widely but not universally regarded as a higher level of competency than mere testamentary capacity. (For example, in *Citizen's National Bank v. Pearson* [1978], the court stated: "Greater mental capacity is required to make a deed than is required to execute a will.") Another path to the same conclusion is the argument that because the trustee is endowed with the authority to enter into contracts involving the trust assets, the creator of the trust should possess contractual capacity. The question regarding which standard applies to trusts may admit of different answers, depending on the specific details of the trust and the state in which it is created. An approach under development in California is to require contractual capacity for the creation of a trust and testamentary capacity for execution of amendments to a trust that affect only the after-death disposition of the trust estate.

Undue Influence: The Question of Voluntariness

As mentioned earlier, the question of undue influence is commonly raised in conjunction with a claim of lack of testamentary capacity and in connection with contested trusts, contracts, and gifts. Susceptibility to undue influence is also one of the criteria for establishment of a conservatorship of estate in California and some other states, and the underlying question of voluntariness is also relevant to the issue of informed consent for medical care. Yet, undue influence is a complex and poorly defined legal concept at best. In the legal literature, the question of undue influence tends to be reduced to the "will substitution test"—that is, was the testator's mind so controlled by another person that his or her will is actually the will of another person? Depending on the situation, this "will substitution" may require an element of "coercion, compulsion, or restraint," as in the testamentary context, or merely consist "1) [i]n the use, by one in whom a confidence is reposed by another, or who holds a real or apparent authority over him, of such confidence or authority for the purpose of obtaining an unfair advantage over him; 2) [i]n taking an unfair advantage of another's weakness of mind; or, 3) [i]n taking a grossly oppressive and unfair advantage of another's necessities or distress" (California Civil Code § 1575) with regard to *contracts*. Courts generally approach the issue of undue influence from two closely related legal perspectives, each of which can be thought of as a legal "theory" of undue influence. Although the assumption that undue influence is wielded by a stronger party to the detriment of a weaker party is common to both, the presumption model and the susceptibility model differ in their relative weighting of the evidence (Wrosch 1992). In the presumption model, the evidence focused on is the relationship between the donor and the receiver of the gift or bequest. In some jurisdictions, the mere existence of a confidential and trusting relationship, such as that between an elderly patient with neuropsychiatric illness and his or her primary caregiver, may be enough to shift the burden of proof to the recipient, who then must prove that undue influence did not occur. The presumption of undue influence is strengthened if the donor is mentally weak; a diagnosis of mental illness or retardation is generally adequate to support this claim, and in some cases even recognition that the donor is passive or manipulable will suffice. The presumption of undue influence is also strengthened if the recipient is a clerical, church, or spiritual adviser who fails to ascertain that a donor has received competent and independent advice, or if the recipient actively procures the gift or bequest, or if the recipient unduly benefits from the gift or bequest.

A somewhat weaker set of factors are widely regarded as indicia (that is, they serve to strengthen a claim of undue influence but do not, by themselves, establish a presumption) of undue influence in a testamentary context. These include "unnatural provisions in the will, provisions in the will that are inconsistent with prior or subsequent expressions of the testator's intentions, and a relationship between the testator and the beneficiary that created an opportunity to control the testamentary act" (Spar and Garb 1992).

In the susceptibility model, the focus is more on the relative mental weakness of the donor or testator. But even if it is shown by clear and convincing evidence that the donor or testator was susceptible to undue influence (for example, by expert neuropsychiatric testimony that the donor or testator was mentally impaired), it would still be necessary to show that some kind of improper influence was exerted by the recipient and that the influence sufficed to replace the will of the donor or testator with that of the recipient.

In both the presumption and susceptibility models, a diagnosis of neuropsychiatric illness in the allegedly influenced party will generally support a claim of undue influence, but such a diagnosis is rarely more than just one consideration of many. Singer (1992) identified six additional factors that "are prominent in undue influence situations. They are the production of isolation, the creation of the 'siege mentality,' the fostering of dependence, the creation of powerlessness, the use of fear and deception, and keeping the victim unaware of the manipulative program put into place to influence and control the person and to obtain the signing of documents which benefit the manipulators at the cost of the signer" (p. 8). These factors notwithstanding, it is important to remember that influence, even that which is clearly coercive, is not undue if it does not change the preexisting disposition of the testator. That is, if the bequest or gift would have been made anyway, absent the influence, then no undue influence has occurred. Obviously, knowledge of the testator's long-term wishes and intentions is critical to the establishment of this defense.

Geriatric neuropsychiatrists are likely to become involved in undue-influence evaluations in the clinical context when an individual is believed by friends or family to be vulnerable to exploitation and a conservatorship or guardianship of estate is under consideration. A typical situation involves an elderly divorced or widowed person with vascular or Alzheimer's dementia who has fallen under the sway of a much younger individual who has gradually taken over many caregiving functions and, in some cases, has even become romantically involved with the elderly person. Particularly if there is no close family, or if preexisting family dynamics are distant or conflictful, it may be an easy matter for the younger person to create several of the circumstances listed by Singer (1992). Naive family members may exacerbate the situation by opposing the relationship or by suggesting that mental impairment is present, both of which responses may facilitate the creation of the siege mentality. Inappropriate gifts, excessive payments for services rendered, new trusts and wills, and even late-life marriages are typical results of this situation, especially if there are substantial assets. This scenario presents a major dilemma for lawmakers, adult protective service workers, and the courts. Establishment of a conservatorship may protect whatever assets are left by the time the court has acted, but it is not a particularly effective remedy for already lost assets. Laws against fiduciary abuse may serve the function of intimidating some victimizers, but even this approach is often too little, too late. At the same time, social and legal preventive and remedial maneuvers must also take into consideration the fact that older individuals, even those with neuropsychiatric illness, can make authentic, reasoned changes in their long-held values, and some May-December romances are real.

Competency to Care for Oneself and Manage One's Finances

Laws exist in all 50 states and the District of Columbia providing for the appointment by a court of a guardian or conservator for persons found incompetent to care for themselves or manage their finances. In California, the term *conservator* is used for both the individual appointed to make personal decisions *(conservator of person)* and the individual appointed to make financial decisions *(conservator of estate)*, but in most states the former is called a "guardian." (California reserves the term *guardian* for minors.) Criteria for appointment of a conservator of person or estate (both roles may be assumed by the same person) are as follows: a conservator of person "may be appointed for a person who is unable to provide properly for his or her personal needs for physical health, food, clothing, or shelter" (California Probate Code § 1801[a]), and a conservator of estate "may be appointed for a person who is substantially unable to manage his or her own financial resources or resist fraud or undue influence" (California Probate Code § 1801[b]). These criteria clearly refer to complex social behavior rather than to the cognitive (i.e., decisional) impairments that presumably underlie the functional deficits. In some states, a more cognitively oriented definition is used, following the Uniform Probate Code (§ 5-103), which defines an incapacitated individual as someone who is "impaired by reason of mental illness, mental deficiency, physical illness or disability, advanced age, chronic use of drugs, chronic intoxication, or other cause (except minority) to the extent that he lacks sufficient understanding or capacity to make or communicate responsible decisions concerning his person."

In general, the powers of the conservator of person and the conservator of estate are quite broad: the conservator of person has the power to make decisions regarding place of residence and administration of medical care, and the conservator of estate has the power to manage property, assets, and income (this includes the power to enter into contractual arrangements on behalf of the principal). In California, the conservator of person can consent to medical care, but not over the objection of the conservatee, unless the court has granted general or specific medical power—that is, the power to consent to all medical care (general power) or to consent to a specific treatment (specific power) even over the objection of the conservatee. The establishment of a conservator of estate automatically renders the conservatee incompetent to contract or to transfer property but does not establish lack of testamentary capacity.

Conservatorship and guardianship are clearly radical solutions to the competency problems occasioned by neuropsychiatric and other illnesses. The process of appointment of a guardian or conservator is often demeaning and embarrassing to the conservatee, and disagreement over the need for conservatorship and the motivations of those who support or resist it may lead to long-lasting intrafamilial conflict and resentment. The appointment is also expensive and time-consuming. In response to these shortcomings, most states have provision for limited conservatorship and guardianship, wherein only some of the powers just discussed are granted to the conservator, while the rest remain with the conservatee, as determined by the court on a case-by-case basis. But even this approach is costly and demeaning to the patient and, despite court oversight, sometimes conducive to fiduciary and even physical abuse by guardians. And the process of adjudication of conservatorship and guardianship itself has been criticized. "Guardianship petitions often recite minimal facts in support of the claim of incompetence; often, in fact, they simply restate the circular and conclusory language of the statutory definitions of incompetency. . . . Far too often, [courts] are satisfied with only a perfunctory assessment of the alleged incompetent's mental capacity. . . . Typically, evidence is limited to a brief letter from a physician stating that the patient is incompetent. A complete psychiatric evaluation and formal mental status exam are rarely included" (Rosoff and Gottlieb 1987, pp. 15–16). Clearly, alternatives to conservatorship and guardianship are highly desirable, and fortunately there are several. Wilber and Reynolds (1995) reviewed these alternatives, which are displayed and partly explained in Table 41–3.

TABLE 41–3. Characteristics of financial and health-related services available to older persons

	Capacity		Appropriateness to address risk to the older person			Complexity
Service	Required for execution	Survives incapacity	Personal risk: high, medium, low	Financial risk: high, medium, low	Oversight or recourse	Ability to address complex financial or medical issues
Power of attorney	Yes	No	Low	Medium	By family; legal action	Medium
Bill-paying service	Yes	Not usually	Low	Medium	Agency audit; legal action	Low
Joint accounts/joint tenancy	Yes	Yes	Low	Low	Virtually none; legal action	Low
Durable power of attorney	Yes	Yes	Low	High	By family; legal action	Medium
Durable power of attorney for health care	Yes	Yes	Medium	Low	By family; legal action	Medium
Representative payee	No	Yes	Medium	Medium	Virtually; none by fed govt agency	Low
Personal trusts	Yes	Yes, if drawn properly	Medium	High	Internal audit; banking commissioner, legal action	High
Limited guardianship	No	Yes	High	High	Court; legal action	High
Plenary guardianship	No	Yes	High	High	Court; legal action	High

Source. Reprinted from Wilber KH, Reynolds SL: "Rethinking Alternatives to Guardianship." *The Gerontologist* 35:248–257, 1985. Used with permission.

Elder Abuse

One of the consequences of diminished competency in elderly individuals, and one of the indications for establishment of guardianship and conservatorship, is vulnerability to various forms of abuse. This issue was placed on the national agenda beginning with a report entitled "Elder Abuse: The Hidden Problem" (U.S. House Select Committee on Aging 1980). Estimates of the prevalence of abuse in the 1980s indicated that 10% of Americans over age 65 were victims of some type of abuse (Clark 1984), with 4% subjected to moderate or severe abuse (U.S. House Subcommittee on Health and Long-Term Care of the Select Committee on Aging 1985). More recent studies from England (Ogg and Bennett 1992) and Canada (Podkieks 1992) have supported those estimates. From the beginning, the medical profession assumed a major role in the identification and prevention of this problem. In its Resolution 112, the American Medical Association (AMA) urged the development of diagnostic and treatment guidelines and the proposal of model legislation, and an AMA re-

port in 1992 stated that physicians "are in an ideal position to recognize, manage, and prevent elder mistreatment" (American Medical Association 1992). The legislative program has been quite successful, and there are now elder abuse statutes in every state; all statutes except those in Colorado, New York, and Wisconsin include mandatory reporting laws. Definitions of elder abuse tend to vary from state to state, although most states recognize some combination of physical abuse, neglect, and financial exploitation (known as *fiduciary abuse* in California when perpetrated by caregivers or others), but definitions within those categories also vary greatly, depending on the statutory distinctions between physical and psychological harm, harmful effects and harmful intentions, and acts of omission versus acts of commission (Brewer and Jones 1989).

The success of the medical profession's recognition-and-management agenda has been less impressive. Rosenblatt et al. (1996) looked at elder abuse reports in Michigan between 1989 and 1993 and found that physicians contributed only 2% of the 17,238 reported cases of elder abuse. The study's authors cited inconsistent definitions of abuse, denial (by the patient and by the physician), fear of the consequences of reporting abuse, and ageism and lack of knowledge (on the part of physicians) as reasons for this low rate. They also suggested that physicians may be hesitant to report for fear of making the problem worse, may wish to maintain relationships with the patients and families and avoid court involvement, and may have little faith that state intervention will result in a better outcome. In states in which statutory protection is not provided, physicians may also fail to report suspected abuse for fear of legal liability. The American College of Emergency Physicians (1998) published a policy statement opposing mandatory reporting of abuse to the criminal justice system if the patient is competent, and calling for immunity from liability (in states with mandatory reporting requirements) for persons who do report abuse. They also called for standardized definitions of elder abuse, written protocols on recognition and treatment of elder abuse, and further research in the area.

Lachs et al. (1997) followed 2,812 community-dwelling older adults (median age, 75 years) in Connecticut for 9 years and identified cases of reported and verified elder mistreatment (including abuse, neglect, exploitation, and abandonment) through a state social service agency. They found poverty, nonwhite race, functional disability, and worsening cognitive impairment to be risk factors for reported elder mistreatment and suggested that reporting bias may have led to overestimation of the effects of race and poverty. The total number of cases of corroborated mistreatment was only 47 (30 cases of neglect, 9 of abuse, and 8 of exploitation), resulting in a sampling adjusted 9-year prevalence of 1.6%. Adult children were the most common perpetrators of abuse (45%), followed by spouses (26%), grandchildren, and paid caregivers. A significantly higher prevalence of elder abuse was reported by Comijs and colleagues, who studied a population-based sample of 1797 older people living independently in Amsterdam, The Netherlands. They found a 1.2% 1-year prevalence of physical aggression, 1.4% for financial mistreatment, and 0.2% for neglect. And there is evidence that elder abuse has significant effects on mortality. Lachs and colleagues (1998) followed the community-dwelling cohort described above for an additional 4 years and found that subjects seen for elder mistreatment during the follow-up period had lower rates of survival (95) than the noninvestigated cohort members (40%) ($P < .001$). After statistically correcting for demographic characteristics, chronic diseases, functional status, social networks, cognitive status, and depressive symptomatology, the risk of death remained higher for those subjected to elder treatment (odds ratio, 3.1; 95% confidence interval, 1.4–6.7) when compared with other members of the cohort.

Competency to Drive

The proportion of the American population that drives is rapidly aging, and it is estimated that by the year 2024, one in four drivers in the United States will be over age 65. Declining competency among these drivers is well documented: among older drivers, as a group, the frequency of crashes per mile is approximately twice that among younger drivers, and older drivers incur more fatalities per mile driven than any other age group except males under age 25 (Owsley 1997). Fife et al. (1984) found that vehicle crashes are the second major reason (falls were first) for injury-related emergency room visits among older adults, and Reuben et al. (1988) reported that crashes are the leading cause of injury-related deaths among seniors. Multiple age-related factors are likely to contribute to this phenomenon, including declining visual and auditory acuity, effects of physical and neuropsychiatric illnesses and their treatments, and declining decisional competence due to slowing of cognitive processes and reaction time and deficits in attention, concentration, and visuospatial functions (see Chapter 8).

Although available data are not adequate to determine the precise contribution of each of these factors, some generalizations are possible. McCloskey et al. (1994) found that several ophthalmological problems that affect vision and would seem likely to increase crash risk in fact did not. These included retinal disorders, macular degeneration, myopia and presbyopia, and monocular vision. Glaucoma, however, was associated with an (increased) relative risk (odds ratio) of 1.5. In another study, Foley et al. (1995) found that having cataracts severe enough to preclude reading a newspaper or recognizing a friend across the street was associated with an odds ratio of only 0.9 (the difference was not statistically significant). Similarly, hearing impairment did not increase crash risk, but when a hearing aid was worn while driving, the risk of crashing was increased by an odds ratio of 1.9 (McCloskey et al. 1994).

Koepsell et al. (1994) looked at other medical conditions common among elderly persons, including stroke; coronary disease including heart attack, angina, and coronary disease requiring surgery; chronic obstructive pulmonary disease; cancer; asthma; osteoarthritis and rheumatoid arthritis; and diabetes and found that only coronary disease (odds ratio, 1.4) and diabetes (odds ratio, 2.6) were associated with increased crash risk. Certain medications are also important contributors to crash risk. In a study involving older drivers in Tennessee, Ray et al. (1992) found that current use of benzodiazepines was statistically significantly associated with a relative risk of injurious crashes of 1.5, whereas current use of cyclic antidepressants was associated with a twofold increased risk. Foley et al. (1995) reported that neither the use of opioids nor the use of antihistamines was associated with increased crash risk, but use of nonsteroidal anti-inflammatory agents was found to carry a relative risk of 1.9.

Foley and colleagues (1995) also studied the contribution of physical limitation, reduced ability to perform activities of daily living, various chronic symptoms such as back pain, and depressive symptoms and cognitive deficits to the risk of injurious crash in an undiagnosed population (the geographically defined Established Populations for Epidemiological Study of the Elderly cohort, comprising rural residents of Iowa over age 65). Back pain within the past 12 months and scoring in the highest quintile of depressive symptoms were both associated with an odds ratio of 1.5, whereas scoring poorly on a delayed-recall test (recalling fewer than three words) was associated with an odds ratio of 1.4.

As is suggested by the latter finding, dementia is a well-established risk factor for crashes among elderly patients. Fitten et al. (1995) conducted a prospective study comparing elderly subjects with mild Alzheimer's disease and mild vascular dementia with an age-matched, cognitively intact, healthy control group; an age-matched control group with diabetes; and a young, healthy control group. Subjects completed a standardized driving test, conducted on a course designed to reproduce low-level traffic conditions similar to a suburban drive. Both groups of subjects with dementia performed significantly more poorly on the driving test than any of the control groups. Moreover, subjects with dementia committed more serious driving errors, particularly in the more complex parts of the course. Scores on the Mini-Mental State Exam and on the Sternberg test (another test of short-term memory), along with measures of visual tracking, were the best predictors of driving scores. The healthy elderly control subjects performed as well as the healthy younger control subjects.

In an attempt to characterize more precisely the types of driving errors made by patients with dementia, Dobbs (1997) studied 115 cognitively impaired seniors (average age, 72 years), all of whom were still driving. Each subject drove a road course involving 37 maneuvers and a route requiring approximately 40 minutes of driving time. A driving evaluator in the car (who had control of an auxiliary brake pedal) recorded each driving error. Subjects were also given a battery of cognitive and motor tests considered to be predictive of driving performance. Control groups of cognitively intact elderly individuals (average age, 69 years) and cognitively intact young subjects (average age, 36 years) were studied as well.

Three types of driving errors were observed. The most serious errors were characterized as errors that "could have resulted in a crash had the driving instructor not taken control of the vehicle or the traffic adjusted" (Dobbs 1997, p. 10). These errors were made almost exclusively by subjects with dementia, and three of the four control subjects who made errors of this type were subsequently found, by cognitive testing, to have dementia or be otherwise cognitively impaired. Another, less serious, type of error (e.g., poor positioning on turns or observational errors) was made by drivers in each group but more frequently by the subjects with dementia, and the third type of error, the sort typically made by experienced drivers (e.g., rolling stops), was not committed more often by members of any one study group. Interestingly, Mini-Mental State Exam scores did not identify *individuals* who performed poorly on the driving test, and 25% of the subjects with dementia demonstrated driving competence within the range of that of the control subjects. The latter finding is consistent with previous reports indicating that early-stage Alzheimer's disease is not associated with increased crash risk (Drachman and Swearer 1993).

Dobbs (1997) concluded that diminished driving competence among individuals with dementia is most likely to be picked up by a test protocol (course and scoring procedure) that focuses on very serious errors, but the author also acknowledged that subjecting every cognitively impaired driver to an extensive and detailed road test would be prohibitively costly. Moreover, Dobbs observed that road testing of more impaired drivers is too dangerous to undertake without specially trained evaluators and specially equipped vehicles.

Two alternative approaches for determining competency to drive have been explored and reported in the literature: cognitive assessment and driving simulation. The first involves attempts to determine the specific type and magnitude of sensory and cognitive impairments that lead to serious driving errors, and to develop practical test procedures that could be applied to large numbers of individuals. Several groups have conducted such investigations (Ball et al. 1993; Parasuraman and Nestor 1991), and deficits in attentional processes have emerged as the best predictors of incompetent driving. Most specifically, measuring *useful field of view* (UFOV), the area of the visual field in which information can be rapidly extracted without eye and head movements, appears to be valuable in this context. Three functions contribute to the ability to extract information in this way: the ability to quickly process what is seen, the ability to divide attention, and the ability to distinguish target from background. Impairments in each of these functions can result in diminished UFOV (Ball 1997). Because many neuropsychiatric illnesses common among elderly individuals can lead to deficits in these functions, driving competency evaluations based on UFOV promise to be applicable across the spectrum of diagnoses, not just Alzheimer's or vascular dementia. Early results indicate that subjects with cognitive impairment and intact UFOV do not crash at a higher rate than mentally intact subjects with comparable UFOV. Ball and colleagues (1993) used greater-than-40% reduction in UFOV to distinguish high-risk from low-risk drivers, regardless of diagnosis, and were able to identify a group of high-risk drivers that were 6 times as likely to crash as age-matched low-risk drivers. Further research is expected to clarify the role of UFOV testing in the determination of competency to drive.

Other mediating factors besides UFOV may also be important in patients with Alzheimer's disease. Rizzo and colleagues (1998) examined the perception of movement and shape in 41 subjects with mild to moderate Alzheimer's disease (mean age 72.3 years) compared with 22 subjects without dementia (mean age 71.7 years), and found that the demented subjects had significantly higher thresholds for perceiving shapes defined by motion cues that did nondemented control subjects. They concluded that this deficit could negatively affect the ability to navigate and to recognize objects in relative motion.

The second approach to the assessment of driving competency involves the use of driving simulators, and some preliminary findings suggest that such simulators, designed in light of information regarding crash risk (e.g., the usefulness of measures of UFOV), may represent a practical approach to screening for incompetent drivers. To date, though, prospective studies that would allow meaningful calculation of the diagnostic confidence (i.e., the positive and negative predictive values) of such measures have yet to be published (Bylsma 1997). Lundberg et al. (1997) also suggested that in individuals with dementia, the driving simulator may measure the ability to perform a novel task (i.e., driving a simulator) more than real-life driving ability per se.

Despite the preliminary nature of the research discussed here, the problems posed by drivers with dementia have generated a significant amount of attention in scientific and policy-making circles, and several states have passed legislation requiring physicians to report individuals with dementia or other conditions involving cognitive impairment to the health department. In 1994, the Swedish National Road Administration invited representatives from several research groups in North America and Europe to meet and prepare a consensus statement on dementia and driving based on available scientific data. That group concluded the following: "1) . . . Individuals with moderate and severe dementia should not drive; 2) There is not, at present, sufficient knowledge about the way in which different cognitive impairments influence driving ability. Much research is needed before general conclusions can be drawn concerning if and when persons with mild dementia should stop driving; 3) In the meantime, these cases should be carefully evaluated in an individualized manner" (Johansson and Lundberg 1997, p. 67). The group did not specify criteria for distinguishing moderate from severe dementia, but the article including the conference findings implied that a score of 2–3 on the Washington Clinical Dementia Rating Scale would suffice.

This emerging consensus notwithstanding, the clinician who encounters an elderly patient with cognitive or other impairment that increases the likelihood of driving difficulties, including crashes, may find himself or herself in a position involving conflicts of both obligation and interest. Loss of what many people perceive as the right to drive is experienced by some older patients as an intolerable deprivation of autonomy and freedom (even if the deprivation is of more symbolic than practical significance), and the clinician is clearly obligated to protect his or her patient from the practical inconvenience and psychological pain related to this loss, whenever it is reasonable to do so. At the same time, the clinician has an obligation to try to protect the patient from the possible untoward consequences of his or her impairment, and the clinician also has an obligation to society to protect it from the dangers posed by the significantly impaired driver. The physician's interest may be jeopardized by the legal consequences of failure to report the diagnosis of dementia, but his or her interest may also be jeopardized by reporting such a diagnosis, if the angry patient fires or sues the physician. And none of these conflicts is necessarily resolved by the development of better, more scientifically based criteria to determine high risk, for even when such criteria become available, some patients will not agree with them or will believe that theirs is the exceptional case and will mistrust and be resentful of the physician for offering sincere advice and/or for following a legal mandate. This appears to be one aspect of clinical geriatric practice that is not likely to be ameliorated by scientific or technological progress.

Loss of Competence and Cognitive Impairment: Which Cognitive Functions Are Critical?

Although it is clear that cognitive functions decline with advancing age even in the healthy individual, the rate of this decline and the order in which specific functions are lost vary greatly from person to person, and only broad generalizations are supported by the published data (see Chapter

8). These data suggest that normal aging is typically accompanied by mild generalized slowing of cognitive processes; mild declines in complex attention, executive functions, verbal fluency, and immediate, working, and implicit memory; and moderate declines in recent memory (Spar and La Rue 1997). Wolinsky and colleagues (Wolinsky and Johnson 1991, 1992a, 1992b; Wolinsky et al. 1992a, 1992b), using items from the Activities of Daily Living Scale and the Instrumental Activities of Daily Living Scale, identified three distinct dimensions of everyday function. These dimensions, termed *basic ADLs* (basic activities of daily living) (bathing, dressing, and toileting), *household ADLs* (meal preparation, housework, and shopping), and *advanced ADLs* (e.g., completing a medical history form, ordering merchandise from a catalog, computing taxi rates, or determining the amount due on a telephone bill), were later verified by Fitzgerald et al. (1993), who also showed that ratings for advanced ADLs (but not for the more basic categories) were predictive of scores on the Short Portable Mental Status Questionnaire. It follows that in elderly adults without dementia, the ability to perform these more cognitively complex advanced ADLs is likely to deteriorate before the ability to perform the basic and household ADLs, but data are lacking to link deterioration in these functions with impairments in specific cognitive functions.

Similarly, the specific cognitive changes associated with loss of competency in pathological states such as Alzheimer's disease are only beginning to be understood. Marson et al. (1995) studied 29 patients with probable Alzheimer's disease and 15 cognitively intact elderly control subjects. Using stepwise multiple regression analysis, they found that measures of word fluency best predicted the capacity to "provide rational reasons" for a treatment choice in both groups, although the associations were not strong (R^2: control subjects, .33; patients with Alzheimer's disease, .36). The study also produced a two-variable nonparametric discriminant function that achieved a classification rate for the entire sample of 93%, and the authors concluded that "measures of semantic word fluency/executive function . . . and of simple attention represent cognitive functions that are integrally related to the competency status of both normal control subjects and patients with [Alzheimer's disease] under a rational reasons standard" (Marson et al. 1995, p. 958).

▌ Expert Consultation and Testimony on Competency

In addition to the inevitable competency determinations that arise in their clinical practices, such as those related to

driving, geriatric neuropsychiatrists are also particularly qualified to provide expert forensic consultation and testimony regarding questions of competency and susceptibility to undue influence. Accordingly, neuropsychiatrists need to be familiar with local statutes and case laws defining the various forms of competency. The neuropsychiatric expert may be asked to perform a contemporaneous evaluation of an individual's competency or susceptibility to undue influence or state an opinion on the competency and susceptibility to undue influence of an individual who has since died. Guidelines for such evaluations in the testamentary context have been published previously (Spar and Garb 1992) and are applicable to each of the forms of decisional competency discussed in this chapter but will not be reviewed here. However, I suggest two revisions to those guidelines.

First, it is recommended that the medical expert avoid testifying on the issue of undue influence per se because it is a legal conclusion beyond the expertise of the physician who is not also an attorney. Rather, medical expert testimony should be restricted to the question of the presence and severity of mental impairment and how the patient's *vulnerability* to influence, persuasion, manipulation, being taken advantage of, and so on is affected by that impairment. If circumstances permit, testimony on whether particular decisions made by the impaired individual are the direct result of such manipulation and persuasion may also be justified and may be permitted.

The second revision is based on Rule 703 of the Federal Rules of Evidence, which states: "The facts or data in the particular case upon which an expert bases an opinion or inference may be those perceived by or made known to the expert at or before the hearing. If of a type reasonably relied upon by experts in the particular field in forming opinions or inferences upon the subject, the facts or data need not be admissible in evidence." When the neuropychiatrist's expert opinion is based on retrospective evaluation, direct examination should elicit testimony that clinical assessment and diagnosis of neuropsychiatric illness in the elderly is commonly reliant on information provided by sources (such as spouses, relatives, caregivers, and medical records) other than direct examination of the patient, especially if the patient is severely cognitively impaired, uncooperative, mute, or catatonic. This explanation may be important testimony if the court is inclined to believe, as some clearly are, that retrospective evaluation is not part of reasonable clinical practice and therefore not "protected" by Rule 703 and of highly questionable probative value. Anticipating and correcting this misperception can be of great value in preserving the proper weight of expert testimony.

However it is performed, the expert role is substantially different from the role of clinician, and somewhat different ethical principles obtain. The clinician's obligation to act in the best interests of the patient is replaced by the consultant's mandate to provide an honest and objective opinion and, in the testimonial context, to express that opinion in a convincing manner. Because the two obligations can easily conflict, it is usually not recommended for one individual to assume both roles for the same patient.

Implications for Clinicians

As the population ages and the public becomes increasingly aware of conditions such as Alzheimer's disease, circumstances calling for formal assessment of competency and susceptibility to undue influence are likely to arise more frequently, and neuropsychiatrists who perform these evaluations need to be familiar with applicable statutory and case law. Moreover, because the need for competency assessment is not always anticipated by patients or their attorneys, neuropsychiatrists can also provide a potentially valuable service by performing routine clinical evaluations that include enough content (e.g., comments on how the observed impairments are likely to affect competency and susceptibility to undue influence) to support future retrospective assessments of their patients' competency and susceptibility to influence.

Similarly, even if their patient contact is largely consultative in nature, neuropsychiatrists may find themselves in a position to recognize and report signs of elder abuse, to identify individuals whose deteriorating mental functions warrant consideration of guardianship or conservatorship (or less restrictive forms of assistance), and to diagnose and report conditions that may adversely affect driving safety. Accordingly, they should stay abreast of local laws and regulations that delimit the clinician's responsibilities in these areas as well.

Summary and Recommendations

There are many legal definitions of mental competency, depending on the specific task and the jurisdiction. And, as Marlowe (1994) observed, "legal concepts often do not have immediately discernible scientific counterparts . . . [and] it is therefore necessary for clinicians operationally to define or translate legal concepts into observable, definable, and measurable scientific terms" (p. 12). In a study designed in part to assess how successfully this translation has been effected by psychiatric expert witnesses, colleagues and I (Spar et al. 1995) submitted the following open-ended statement to 300 probate judges around the United States: "Psychiatric expert testimony on matters of mental capacity and susceptibility to undue influence would be most useful to the court if physicians would . . ." (p. 396). The only recurring response (provided by 14 of the 73 who completed the statement) was, in essence, "use lay terms and avoid technical language." A large majority of 119 respondents to other, more structured, survey questions also agreed that psychiatric testimony on impaired mental capacity and susceptibility to undue influence should focus on the specific mental function deficits that underlie the observed impairment (Spar et al. 1995), and a slightly smaller majority agreed that experts should use standardized tests in their evaluations.

Supported by these results, the two senior authors, assisted by a coalition of attorneys and other experts, drafted and helped pass a California law called the Due Process in Competence Determinations Act (DPCDA), which went into effect January 1, 1996. Under the DPCDA (Table 41–4), judges are authorized to require experts testifying on impaired competency to specify at least one mental function deficit that accounts for the alleged incompetency and to explain how that deficit is connected to that impairment. (For example: "Mr. P demonstrated profound deficits in remote memory, as evidenced by an inability to name any presidents, identify the countries that fought in the Gulf War, or recall the names of all of his children or that he had four grandchildren. Because of this deficit, he lacked the capacity to remember and understand his relations to his living descendants and therefore failed to meet one of the criteria for testamentary capacity.") The statute includes a list of mental functions that we believed would be familiar to mental health professionals in many disciplines and comprehensible to attorneys, judges, and jurors and that describes functions that lend themselves to measurement or, at a minimum, description in numbered terms used by widely available assessment instruments. Glass (1997), concluding a review of proposed approaches to competency determination published during the past two decades, stated: "There is still no agreement on either the exact criteria or the methods of assessing mental competency" (p. 32). Although the DPCDA is not offered as a solution to this problem, it is hoped that by facilitating the process of direct and cross-examination, demystifying the process of psychiatric evaluation, and encouraging measurement, more consistent and therefore more just outcomes of formal competency determinations will follow.

TABLE 41–4. Due Process in Competence Determinations Act

810. The Legislature finds and declares the following:

(a) A person who has a mental or physical disorder may still be capable of contracting, conveying, marrying, making medical decisions, executing wills or trusts, and performing other actions.

(b) A judicial determination that a person suffers from one or more mental deficits so substantial that, under the circumstances, the person should be deemed to lack the legal capacity to perform a specific act, should be based on evidence of a deficit in one or more of the person's mental functions rather than on a diagnosis of a person's mental or physical disorder.

811. (a) A determination that a person is of unsound mind or lacks the capacity to make a decision or do a certain act, including, but not limited to, the incapacity to contract, to make a conveyance, to marry, to make medical decisions, to vote, or to execute wills or trusts, shall be supported by evidence of a deficit in at least one of the following mental functions, subject to subdivision (b):

(1) Alertness and attention, including, but not limited to, the following:

(A) Level of arousal or consciousness.

(B) Orientation to time, place, person, and situation.

(C) Ability to attend and concentrate.

(2) Information processing, including, but not limited to, the following:

(A) Short- and long-term memory, including immediate recall.

(B) Ability to understand or communicate with others, either verbally or otherwise.

(C) Recognition of familiar objects and familiar persons.

(D) Ability to understand and appreciate quantities.

(E) Ability to reason using abstract concepts.

(F) Ability to plan, organize, and carry out actions in one's own rational self-interest.

(G) Ability to reason logically.

(3) Thought processes. Deficits in these functions may be demonstrated by the presence of the following:

(A) Severely disorganized thinking.

(B) Hallucinations.

(C) Delusions.

(D) Uncontrollable, repetitive, or intrusive thoughts.

(4) Ability to modulate mood and affect. Deficits in this ability may be demonstrated by the presence of a pervasive and persistent or recurrent state of euphoria, anger, anxiety, fear, panic, depression, hopelessness or despair, helplessness, apathy or indifference, which is inappropriate in degree to the individual's circumstances.

(b) A deficit in the mental functions listed above may be considered only if the deficit, by itself or in combination with one or more other mental function deficits, significantly impairs the person's ability to understand and appreciate the consequences of his or her actions with regard to the type of act or decision in question.

(c) In determining whether a person suffers from a deficit in mental function so substantial that the person lacks the capacity to do a certain act, the court may take into consideration the frequency, severity, and duration of periods of impairment.

(d) The mere diagnosis of a mental or physical disorder shall not be sufficient in and of itself to support a determination that a person is of unsound mind or lacks the capacity to do a certain act.

Source. From California Probate Code §§ 810 and 811.

References

American College of Emergency Physicians: Management of elder abuse and neglect. Ann Emerg Med 31:149–150, 1998

American Medical Association: Diagnostic and Treatment Guidelines on Elder Abuse and Neglect. Chicago, IL, American Medical Association, 1992

Appelbaum PS, Grisso T: Assessing patients' capacities to consent to treatment. N Engl J Med 319:1635–1638, 1988

Appelbaum PS, Roth L: Competency to consent to research: a psychiatric overview. Arch Gen Psychiatry 39:951–958, 1982

Ball K: Attentional problems and older drivers. Alzheimer Dis Assoc Disord 11 (suppl 1):42–47, 1997

Ball K, Owsley C, Sloane M, et al: Visual attention problems as a predictor of vehicle crashes in older drivers. Invest Ophthalmol Vis Sci 34:3110–3123, 1993

Bonnie RJ: Research with cognitively impaired subjects: unfinished business in the regulation of human research. Arch Gen Psychiatry 54:105–111, 1997

Brewer RA, Jones JS: Reporting elder abuse: limitations of statutes. Ann Emerg Med 18:1217–1221, 1989

Bylsma FW: Simulators for assessing driving skills in demented patients. Alzheimer Dis Assoc Disord 11 (suppl 1):17–20, 1997

Cal Civil Code §§ 38, 39, 1575

Cal Health and Safety Code § 1799.110b

Cal Prob Code §§ 810, 811, 813, 1801, 3210, 4120, 4722, 4724, 6100.5

Canterbury v Spence, 464 F2d 772, 787 (DC Cir 1972)

Citizen's National Bank v Pearson, 67 Ill App3d 457, 459, 384 NE2d 548, 550 (1978)

Clark CB: Geriatric abuse—out of the closet. Journal of the Tennessee Medical Association 77:470–471, 1984

Comijs HC, Pot AM, Smit JH, et al: Elder abuse in the community: prevalence and consequences. J Am Geriatr Soc 46(7):885-888, 1998

Dobbs AR: Evaluating the driving competence of dementia patients. Alzheimer Dis Assoc Disord 11 (suppl 1):8–12, 1997

Drachman DA, Swearer J: Driving and Alzheimer's disease: the risk of crashes. Neurology 43:2448–2456, 1993

Due Process in Competence Determinations Act, SB 730 Mello, Chap 842 Stats of 1995

Dusky v United States, 362 US 402;80 S Ct 788 (1960)

Estate of Goetz, 253 Cal App2d 107, 114 (1967)

Estate of Jenks, 189 NW2d 695, 697 (Minn 1971)

Estate of Rosen, 447 A2d 1220, 1222 (Me 1982)

Fed R Evid 703

Federal Register 61 51498 (1996)

Fellows LK: Competency and consent in dementia. J Am Geriatr Soc 46:922–926, 1998

Fife D, Barancik JI, Chatterjee BF: Northeastern Ohio Trauma Study, II: injury rates by age, sex, and cause. Am J Public Health 74:473–478, 1984

Fitten LJ, Perryman KM, Wilkinson CJ, et al: Alzheimer and vascular dementias and driving: a prospective road and laboratory study. JAMA 273:1360–1365, 1995

Fitzgerald JF, Smith DM, Martin DK, et al: Replication of the multidimensionality of activities of daily living. J Gerontol 48:S28–S31, 1993

Foley DJ, Wallace RB, Eberhard J: Risk factors for motor vehicle crashes among older drivers in a rural community. J Am Geriatr Soc 43:776–781, 1995

Glass KC: Refining definitions and devising instruments: two decades of assessing mental competence. Int J Law Psychiatry 20:5–33, 1997

Godinez v Moran, 509 US 389 (1993)

Grisso T, Appelbaum PS, Hill-Fotouhi C: The MacCAT-T: a clinical tool to assess patients' capacities to make treatment decisions. Psychiatr Serv 48:1415–1419, 1997

Hankin MB: A brief introduction to the Due Process in Competence Determinations Act: a statement of legislative intent. California Trusts and Estates Quarterly 1:36–50, 1995

Hoge SK, Bonnie RJ, Poythress N, et al: The MacArthur Adjudicative Competence Study: development and validation of a research instrument. Law Hum Behav 21:141–179, 1997

In re Conroy, 98 NJ 21, 486 A2d 1209 (1985)

Johansson K, Lundberg C: The 1994 International Consensus Conference on Dementia and Driving: a brief report. Alzheimer Dis Assoc Disord 11 (suppl 1): 62–69, 1997

Kapp MB: Proxy decision making in Alzheimer disease research: durable powers of attorney, guardianship, and other alternatives. Alzheimer Dis Assoc Disord 8 (suppl 4):28–37, 1994

Koepsell TD, Wolf ME, McCloskey L, et al: Medical conditions and motor vehicle injuries in older adults. J Am Geriatr Soc 42:695–700, 1994

Lachs MS, Williams C, O'Brien S, et al: Risk factors for reported elder abuse and neglect: a nine-year observational cohort study. Gerontologist 37:469–474, 1997

Lachs MS, Williams CS, O'Brien S, et al: The mortality of elder mistreatment. JAMA 280(5):428–432, 1998

Lundberg C, Johansson K, Ball K, et al: Dementia and driving: an attempt at consensus. Alzheimer Dis Assoc Disord 11:28–37, 1997

Marlowe DB: Psycholegal decision making in clinical practice, in Psychiatric-Legal Decision Making by the Mental Health Practitioner. Edited by Bluestone H, Travin S, Marlowe DB. New York, Wiley, 1994, p 12

Marson DC, Cody HA, Ingram KK, et al: Neuropsychologic predictors of competency in Alzheimer's disease using a rational reasons legal standard. Arch Neurol 52:955–959, 1995

Marwick C: Improved protection for human research subjects. JAMA 279:344–345, 1998

McCloskey LW, Koepsell TD, Wolf ME, et al: Motor vehicle collision injuries and sensory impairments of older drivers. Age Ageing 23:267–273, 1994

Meiklejohn AM: Contractual and donative capacity. Case Western Reserve Law Review 39:307–387, 1988–1989

Natanson v Kline, 300 P2d 1093, 1104, 1106 (1960)

Ogg J, Bennett G: Elder abuse in Britain. BMJ 305:988–989, 1992

Omnibus Budget Reconciliation Act of 1990, PL 101-508, § 4206 and 4751, 104 Stat 1388, 1388-115, and 1388-204 (classified respectively at 42 USC 1395cc(f) (Medicare) and 1396a(w)(Medicaid) (1994))

Owsley C: Clinical and research issues on older drivers: future directions. Alzheimer Dis Assoc Disord 11(suppl 1):3–7, 1997

Parasuraman R, Nestor PG: Attention and driving skills in Alzheimer's disease. Hum Factors 33:539–558, 1991

Podnieks E: National survey on abuse of the elderly in Canada. Journal of Elder Abuse and Neglect 4:5–58, 1992

Precourt v Frederick, 395 Mass 689, 481 NE2d 1144 (1985)

President's Commission for the Study of Ethical Problems in Medicine and Biomedical and Behavioral Research: Making Health Care Decisions, Vol 1: A Report on the Ethical and Legal Implications of Informed Consent in the Patient-Practitioner Relationship. Washington, DC, U.S. Government Printing Office, 1982

Ray WA, Fought RL, Decker MD: Psychoactive drugs and the risk of injurious motor vehicle crashes in elderly drivers. Am J Epidemiol 136:873–883, 1992

Restatement (Second) of Contracts § 15(1) (1979)

Reuben DB, Silliman RA, Traines M: The aging driver: medicine, policy, and ethics. J Am Gerontol Soc 36:35–42, 1988

Rizzo M, Nawrot M: Perception of movement and shape in Alzheimer's disease. Brain 121 (pt 12):2259–2270, 1998

Rosenblatt DE, Cho K-H, Durance PW: Reporting mistreatment of older adults: the role of physicians. J Am Geriatr Soc 44:65–70, 1996

Rosoff AJ, Gottlieb GL: Preserving personal autonomy for the elderly: competency, guardianship, and Alzheimer's disease. J Leg Med 8:1–47, 1987

Schaffner KF: Competency: a triaxial concept, in Competency. Edited by Cutter MAG, Shelp EE. Dordreht, The Netherlands, Kluwer Academic, 1991, pp 253–281

Singer M: Undue influence and written documents: psychological aspects. Journal of Questioned Document Examination 1:4–13, 1992

Spar JE, Garb AS: Assessing competency to make a will. Am J Psychiatry 149:169–174, 1992

Spar JE, La Rue A: Concise Guide to Geriatric Psychiatry, 2nd Edition. Washington, DC, American Psychiatric Press, 1997

Spar JE, Hankin M, Stodden A: Assessing mental capacity and susceptibility to undue influence. Behav Sci Law 13: 391–403, 1995

Uniform Durable Power of Attorney Act. § 1, 8A USA 278 (1983)

Uniform Probate Code (ULA). Vol. 8, § 5-103, pp 327–328

U.S. House Select Committee on Aging: Elder abuse: the hidden problem. Committee publication 96-220, U.S. Congress, 1980

U.S. House Subcommittee on Health and Long-Term Care of the Select Committee on Aging: Elder abuse: a national disgrace. Committee publication 99-502. U.S. Congress, 1985

Wilber KH, Reynolds SL: Rethinking alternatives to guardianship. Gerontologist 35:248–257, 1995

Wolinsky FD, Johnson RJ: The use of health services by older adults. J Gerontol 46:S345–S357, 1991

Wolinsky FD, Johnson RJ: Perceived health status and mortality among older men and women. J Gerontol 47: S304–S312, 1992a

Wolinsky FD, Johnson RJ: Widowhood, health status, and the use of health services by older adults: a cross-sectional and prospective approach. J Gerontol 47:S8–S16, 1992b

Wolinsky FD, Johnson RJ, Fitzgerald JF: Falling, health status, and the use of health services by older adults: a prospective study. Med Care 30:587–597, 1992a

Wolinsky FD, Callahan CM, Fitzgerald JF, et al: The risk of nursing home placement and subsequent death among older adults. J Gerontol 47:S173–S182, 1992b

Wrosch AP: Undue influence, involuntary servitude and brainwashing: a more consistent interests-based approach. Loyola of Los Angeles Law Review 25:499–554, 1992

Index

Page numbers printed in **boldface** *type refer to tables or figures.*